E/S/C/O/P
MONOGRAPHS

The Scientific Foundation for
Herbal Medicinal Products

E/S/C/O/P
MONOGRAPHS

The Scientific Foundation for
Herbal Medicinal Products

Second edition
Completely revised and expanded

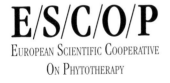

E/S/C/O/P

EUROPEAN SCIENTIFIC COOPERATIVE
ON PHYTOTHERAPY

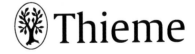

Thieme

Published by ESCOP, the European Scientific Cooperative on Phytotherapy,
Argyle House, Gandy Street, Exeter EX4 3LS, United Kingdom
in collaboration with
Georg Thieme Verlag, Rüdigerstrasse 14, D-70469 Stuttgart, Germany,
and
Thieme New York, 333 Seventh Avenue, New York NY 10001, USA

ISBN 1-901964-07-8 (ESCOP)
ISBN 3-13-129421-3 (GTV)
ISBN 1-58890-233-1 (TNY)

Cover illustration by Trevor Wilson
Cover and text design by Martin Willoughby
Typeset in Optima by Roberta Hutchins
Printed and bound in Great Britain by Biddles Ltd, King's Lynn, Norfolk

CONTENTS

MONOGRAPHS

FOREWORD

This book is an important step in the development of scientific standards for herbal medicinal products in Europe. The eighty revised or completely new monographs represent the state of the art in the phytomedical evidence base. They are compiled by an international team of expert authors: the ESCOP Scientific Committee, supported by a panel of Supervising Editors and numerous invited experts.

ESCOP monographs are formally submitted to the Herbal Medicinal Products Working Party, which is destined to become the Committee for Herbal Medicinal Products, at the European Medicines Evaluation Agency (EMEA) as a basis for establishing core data on the leading herbal medicinal products in Europe. They are therefore a major contribution to the harmonization of standards for herbal medicines across the European Union.

ESCOP is an organization of volunteers. All members of the Scientific Committee, contributing experts, the panel of Supervising Editors and Board of ESCOP give their time freely to their work in pursuit of the highest standards for herbal medicinal products. This book really is a labour of love. We at the Board of ESCOP are very proud of the many who have contributed to these monographs and are most grateful to them.

Professor Dr. med. Dr. h.c. mult. Fritz H. Kemper
Chairman of the Board of ESCOP

PREFACE

This second edition of *ESCOP Monographs* is the culmination of 14 years work by ESCOP Scientific Committee since its first meeting, held in London in August 1989. Overall, it has involved the work of about 50 committee delegates from 15 European countries with contributions from some 30 experts on particular topics and from the ESCOP Board of Supervising Editors, a panel of distinguished academics in the field of herbal medicine.

In the European Union (EU), which will be enlarged to 25 member states in 2004, a key word is "harmonization" - not of our rich tapestry of languages and cultures, but of legislation and systems, to promote a more uniform approach to products, services and the environment. When ESCOP was formed in 1989, as the European umbrella organization of national societies and associations for phytotherapy, it was already evident that the EU Review of Medicines (scheduled for completion by the end of 1990) had not achieved any reasonable degree of harmonization of herbal medicinal products. ESCOP identified a need for scientific monographs on the therapeutic uses of herbal medicines, providing a consensus of viewpoints from European countries (not limited to those within the EU).

The Scientific Committee of ESCOP made rapid progress in this work and 15 of the early monographs were submitted to the EU's Committee for Proprietary Medicinal Products (CPMP) for assessment between 1990 and 1992. On the recommendation of the CPMP, the relatively simple format of initial monographs was replaced by the more demanding and comprehensive format (particularly with respect to pharmacodynamics, pharmacokinetics and safety data) of the Summary of Product Characteristics (SPC). The SPC is an integral part of an application for authorization to market a medicinal product for human use within the European Union; it is "a definitive statement between the competent authority and the marketing authorization holder, and the common basis of communication between the competent authorities of all the member states". Since data sheets for medicinal products are based on them, SPCs ultimately provide information for prescribers and users of medicinal products.

The Scientific Committee was grateful for financial support from the European Commission from 1994 to 1996 while participating in the Biomedical and Health Research Programme (BIOMED 1). This added impetus to the project and, through intensive work, the target of 50 monographs by 1996 was achieved. These 50 and a further 10 monographs were progressively published in loose-leaf form with a ring binder in 1996, 1997 and 1999. Over the past few years all the monographs have been fully revised to a higher standard and expanded with new data, and a further 20 monographs have been prepared. The second edition, as a hard-back book, presents the updated monographs in a more convenient form. An important feature of ESCOP monographs is that they are firmly based on published scientific literature and include journal/book citations in the original language of publication; almost 5000 full citations appear in the text of this book.

The preparation of monographs by delegates and external experts with differing first languages and cultures has been a formidable venture. Happily, it has also proved to be a model of European cooperation - and indeed social as well as scientific harmony. Over the years some 70 weekend meetings of the Scientific Committee have been held in various locations across Europe, from Sweden to the French Riviera and Tuscany, and from Dublin to Vienna, to discuss and refine the draft monographs prior to circulation to the independent Board of Supervising Editors for comment and criticism. When finalized, the texts are now submitted on request, together with all referenced scientific literature, to the Herbal Medicinal Products Working Party (HMPWP) of the European Medicines Evaluation Agency (EMEA). They form the basis for assessment in the preparation of what are called "core data" documents on individual herbal drugs - in effect, official versions of SPCs. Besides making a significant contribution to the regulatory evaluation of herbal medicines, it was always the intention to make the texts available to a wider readership and this book is the outcome.

Clearly, the monograph work of ESCOP is not finished. Research data on herbal medicines continue to be published at a rapid rate. The existing monographs will inevitably need to be updated in due course and additional texts are in preparation.

To all those who have laboured long and burned the midnight oil to prepare and revise monograph drafts, or contributed in other ways to the preparation of this book, ESCOP extends its sincere gratitude. We hope the reader will find the text both informative and stimulating. It is by no means the end of the story.

MEMBERS OF ESCOP

Österreichische Gesellschaft für Phytotherapie	*Austria*
Société Belge de Phytothérapie	*Belgium*
Dansk Selskab for Fytoterapi	*Denmark*
Association Française pour le Médicament de Phytothérapie	*France*
Gesellschaft für Phytotherapie	*Germany*
Irish Association on Phytotherapy	*Ireland*
Società Italiana di Fitochimica	*Italy*
Nederlandse Vereniging voor Fytotherapie	*Netherlands*
Norsk Selskap for Fytoterapi	*Norway*
Sociedad Española de Fitoterapia	*Spain*
Svenska Sällskapet för Fytoterapi	*Sweden*
Schweizerische Medizinische Gesellschaft für Phytotherapie	*Switzerland*
British Herbal Medicine Association	*United Kingdom*

ESCOP SCIENTIFIC COMMITTEE

PRESENT MEMBERS

Anna Rita Bilia	*Italy*
Peter R. Bradley	*United Kingdom*
Jan G. Bruhn	*Sweden*
Desmond Corrigan	*Ireland*
Jozef G. Corthout	*Belgium*
Marijke Frater	*Switzerland*
Lene Gudiksen	*Denmark*
Didier Guédon	*France*
Stephan F.A.J. Horsten	*Netherlands*
Liselotte Krenn	*Austria*
Frédérique Lafforgue	*France*
Norbert Linnenbrink	*Switzerland*
Antonella Riva	*Italy*
Georg Seidel	*Germany*
Barbara Steinhoff	*Germany*
Frans M. van den Dungen	*Netherlands*
Martin J. Willoughby	*United Kingdom*
Jens K. Wold	*Norway*

PAST MEMBERS

M.-L. Abou-Chacra	*France*	S. Palm	*Sweden*
M.-C. Bonjean	*France*	A. Pereira da Silva	*Portugal*
M.R.H. Brautigam	*Netherlands*	S. Philianos	*Greece*
L. Brimer	*Denmark*	C. Röhl	*Switzerland*
K. Brühwiler	*Switzerland*	F. Sandberg	*Sweden*
P. Chaumelle	*France*	G. Schönbeck	*Austria*
F. Chialva	*Italy*	D. Semeelen	*Belgium*
B. Eberwein	*Germany*	E. Sezik	*Turkey*
V. Etges	*Germany*	N.M. Sitaras	*Greece*
M.J.M. Gijbels	*Netherlands*	B. Søholm	*Denmark*
A. Groubert	*France*	W. Spincemaille	*Belgium*
C. Harvala	*Greece*	S. Throm	*Germany*
P. Jean-Jean	*France*	F.F. Vincieri	*Italy*
R. Kalbermatten	*Switzerland*	C. Violon	*Belgium*
B.F. Knudsen	*Denmark*	H.H. Zeylstra	*United Kingdom*
C. Nicolai	*Germany*		

PRESENT CO-CHAIRPERSONS

P.R. Bradley	*United Kingdom*
B. Steinhoff	*Germany*

PRESENT CO-SECRETARIES

M. Frater	*Switzerland*
L. Krenn	*Austria*

CONTRIBUTING EXPERTS

Professor Dr. Rudolf Bauer	*Germany*
Professor Dr. Wolfgang Blaschek	*Germany*
Dr. Cornelia Bellstedt-Suhr	*Germany*
Dr. Normann Boblitz	*Germany*
Dr. Werner Busse	*Germany*
Professor Dr. Reinhold Carle	*Germany*
Dr. Anke Esperester	*Germany*
Dr. Frits Fischer	*Netherlands*
Professor Jacques Fleurentin	*France*
Dr. Jörg Grünwald	*Germany*
Dr. Martina Hecker	*Germany*
Dr. Karl-O. Hiller	*Germany*
Dr. Ingrid Hook	*Ireland*
Dr. Wiltrud Juretzek	*Germany*
Dr. David Knight	*United Kingdom*
Dr. Ulrike Kroll	*Germany*
Dr. Elke Leng-Peschlow	*Germany*
Patricia Lüer	*Germany*
Professor Dr. Beat Meier	*Switzerland*
Dr. Ulrich Mengs	*Germany*
Dr. Paolo Morazzoni	*Italy*
Dr. Orlando Petrini	*Switzerland*
Christine von Platen	*Germany*
Dr. Fabio Soldati	*Switzerland*
Ute Stammwitz	*Germany*
Dr. Christopher Theurer	*Germany*
Tankred Wegener	*Germany*
Dr. Rommert Wijnsma	*Netherlands*
Professor Dr. Hilke Winterhoff	*Germany*

BOARD OF DIRECTORS OF ESCOP

MONOGRAPHS

ABSINTHII HERBA

Wormwood

E/S/C/O/P
MONOGRAPHS
Second Edition

DEFINITION

Wormwood consists of the basal leaves or slightly leafy flowering tops, or of a mixture of these dried, whole or cut organs, of *Artemisia absinthium* L. It contains not less than 2 ml/kg of essential oil, calculated with reference to the dried drug.

The material complies with the monograph of the European Pharmacopoeia [1].

CONSTITUENTS

Sesquiterpene lactones (0.15-0.4%) [2], which give the bitter taste to the drug; principally the guaianolides absinthin and artabsin [3-5] with various others [4,6-9].

Essential oil (0.2-1.5%), varying considerably in composition [2,10]. Depending on the source and chemotype the principal components, any of which may constitute over 40% of the oil, are usually *cis*-epoxyocimene [11,12], β-thujone [12-15], *trans*-sabinyl acetate [12,14,15] and/or chrysanthenyl acetate [12]; lesser amounts of α-thujone (usually less than 3%) may occur [12-15]; many other monoterpenes and various sesquiterpenes are present [11-15].

Other constituents include flavonol glycosides [16], phenolic acids [17], tannins [18], homoditerpene peroxides [19] and 24ζ-ethylcholesta-7,22-dien-3β-ol [20].

CLINICAL PARTICULARS

Therapeutic indications
Anorexia [2,10,21-26], for example after illness [22]; dyspeptic complaints [2,10,21-26].

Posology and method of administration

Dosage

Adult single dose: 1-1.5 g of the drug per 150 ml of water as an infusion or decoction, up to 3 times daily [2,10,22-24,27].
Elderly: dose as for adults.
Children: proportion of adult dose according to body weight.

The dosage may be adjusted according to the bitterness sensitivity of the individual.

Method of administration

For oral administration. In anorexia, administered half to one hour before meals [10,23,24]; for dyspeptic complaints, taken warm after meals [22,24].

Duration of administration

Wormwood should not be taken continuously for periods of more than 3-4 weeks [22].
Prolonged use could induce a distinct aversion to wormwood preparations [21].

Contra-indications

Gastric and duodenal ulcers [24,28].

Special warnings and special precautions for use

None required.

Interaction with other medicaments and other forms of interaction

None reported.

Pregnancy and lactation

Wormwood should not be used during pregnancy and lactation [29].

Effects on ability to drive and use machines

None known.

Undesirable effects

None reported when used as recommended [10,23, 28].

The toxicological risk from use of conventional wormwood preparations is considered to be very low [21,22].

Overdose

Excessive doses of wormwood preparations may cause vomiting, severe diarrhoea, retention of urine or dazed feelings [28].

Overdosage of alcoholic wormwood preparations or the use of the essential oil may cause CNS disturbances, which can lead to convulsions and ultimately to unconsciousness and death [25,28].

PHARMACOLOGICAL PROPERTIES

Pharmacodynamic properties

In vitro experiments

Cholinergic receptor binding activity
Investigations were carried out to evaluate the human CNS cholinergic receptor binding activity of an ethanolic extract of wormwood. In homogenates of human cerebral cortical cell membranes the extract concentration-dependently displaced $[^3H]-(N)$-nicotine and $[^3H]-(N)$-scopolamine from nicotinic and muscarinic receptors respectively with IC_{50} values of < 1 mg/ml. Choline, a weak nicotinic ligand (IC_{50}: 3×10^{-4} M), was found in the extract at concentrations of 10^{-6} to 10^{-5} M, but these concentrations could not account for more than 5% of the displacement activity observed [30].

Antimicrobial activity
Wormwood essential oil diluted 1:1000 exhibited antibacterial and antifungal activity against, for example, *Staphylococcus aureus* and *Candida albicans* [31].

Antimalarial activity
Two homoditerpene peroxides isolated from wormwood exhibited *in vitro* antimalarial activity against *Plasmodium falciparum* with an EC_{50} of 1 μg/ml [19].

In vivo experiments

Effects on the digestive system
A decoction equivalent to 5 g of wormwood had a choleretic effect when administered intravenously to dogs, inducing a 3-fold increase in the secretion of bile [32].

Absinthin given orally to dogs stimulated secretion of gastric juice and increased the acidity of the stomach. This was not observed when absinthin was administered directly into the stomach by gavage, indicating that gastric secretion was reflexively stimulated from the mouth by this bitter principle [32].

Hepatoprotective effects
A dry 80%-methanolic extract from wormwood showed hepatoprotective effects after oral administration to rodents. Whereas acetaminophen (paracetamol) at 1 g/kg body weight caused 100% mortality in mice, pre-treatment of the animals with the extract at 500 mg/kg reduced the death rate to 20%. Pre-treatment of rats with the extract at 2×500 mg/kg for 2 days prevented acetaminophen (640 mg/kg)- and carbon tetrachloride (CCl_4, 1.5 ml/kg)-induced increases in serum levels of glutamate oxaloacetate transaminase and glutamate pyruvate transaminase ($p<0.01$ and $p<0.05$ with respect to acetaminophen and CCl_4). Post-treatment with three successive doses of the extract at 6-hour intervals restricted acetaminophen-induced hepatic damage ($p<0.01$), but CCl_4-induced hepatotoxicity was not significantly altered [33].

Sedative effect
A dry 80%-methanolic wormwood extract, orally administered to mice at 500 mg/kg body weight, prolonged pentobarbital-induced sleeping time from 81 minutes to 117 minutes ($p<0.05$) [33].

Antipyretic activity
A sterol isolated from an ethanolic extract of wormwood alleviated yeast-induced pyrexia in rabbits

[20]. Hexane, chloroform and water-soluble fractions from wormwood had a similar antipyretic effect in rabbits (p<0.05) [34].

Analgesic activity
Subcutaneously administered (–)-3-isothujone (= α-thujone), a constituent of wormwood essential oil, produced antinociceptive effects in mice in the hot plate and Nilsen tests with ED_{50} values of 6.5 and 14.1 mg/kg respectively [35].

Pharmacological studies in humans
A dry alcoholic extract of wormwood (20 mg; suspended in 10 ml of water) was administered by gavage to 15 patients with hepatopathy. Compared to resting activity, a significant increase in gastro-intestinal secretions (p<0.01) was demonstrated by measurement of alpha-amylase, lipase, bilirubin and cholesterol in duodenal fluid [36].

Pharmacokinetic properties
α-Thujone incubated with rabbit liver cytosol in the presence of NADPH gave thujol and neothujol in low yield. On incubation with mouse liver cytosol alone, α-thujone was stable, but in the presence of NADPH it was rapidly metabolized, the major product being 7-hydroxy-α-thujone together with 4-hydroxy-α-thujone, 4-hydroxy-β-thujone and other minor metabolites [37].

In mice treated intraperitoneally with α-thujone, the brain levels of α-thujone and 7-hydroxy-α-thujone were dose- and time-dependent, but α-thujone appeared at much lower levels and was less persistent than 7-hydroxy-α-thujone. The latter compound is less toxic to mice; at 50 mg/kg administered intra-peritoneally, α-thujone was lethal but 7-hydroxy-α-thujone and other metabolites were not lethal [37].

Preclinical safety data

Acute toxicity
Single oral doses of a dry 80%-methanolic wormwood extract at up to 4.0 g/kg body weight caused neither mortality nor behavioural changes in mice [33].

Reproductive toxicity
A significant anti-implantation effect (66% reduction in the number of pregnancies) was detected after oral administration of a dry 50%-ethanolic extract of wormwood to rats at 200 mg/kg body weight for 7 days [38].

Mutagenicity
In the Ames mutagenicity test a tincture and a fluid extract (1:1, 30% ethanol) of wormwood at 200 µl/plate revealed no mutagenic potential in *Salmonella typhimurium* strains TA98 or TA100, with or without S9 metabolic activation [39].

Toxicity of wormwood oil and thujone
The acute oral LD_{50} of wormwood oil (thujone content not stated) in rats was determined as 0.96 g/kg; the acute dermal LD_{50} in rabbits exceeded 5 g/kg. The oil applied topically at 2% in petrolatum produced neither irritation nor sensitization in humans and undiluted oil produced no phototoxic effects in mice or pigs [40].

Subcutaneous LD_{50} values determined in mice were 87.5 mg/kg body weight for α-thujone and 442.4 mg/kg for β-thujone [35]; thus α-thujone is more toxic than β-thujone, which is usually present as a much higher proportion of the oil [12-15,37,41]. α-Thujone is a convulsant, the intraperitoneal LD_{50} in mice being about 45 mg/kg. At 60 mg/kg it is lethal to mice within 1 minute whereas at 30-45 mg/kg the mice either die or recover. The mechanism of α-thujone neurotoxicity has recently been elucidated; it is a reversible modulator of the γ-aminobutyric acid (GABA) type A receptor, but it is rapidly metabolized and detoxified [37].

Intravenous administration of thujone-containing wormwood essential oil to dogs and cats led to convulsions. The minimal convulsive dose in cats was 0.03-0.04 ml of a 1:20 alcoholic dilution of the essential oil [32].

Because of the neurotoxic potential of thujone the use of isolated essential oil of wormwood (in earlier times an ingredient of the liqueur absinthe) and the content of thujone in foods and beverages, is either strictly regulated or prohibited [42]. However, the wormwood oil content of conventional herbal medicines is so low that no injurious effects are to be expected [22]. Wormwood extracts free from thujone can be prepared by using appropriate extraction procedures [43,44].

REFERENCES

1. Wormwood - Absinthii herba. European Pharma-copoeia, Council of Europe.

2. Hose S. Der Wermut - *Artemisia absinthium* L. Arzneipflanze für Kranke und "Kultige". Z Phytotherapie 2002;23:187-94.

3. Schneider G, Mielke B. Zur Analytik der Bitterstoffe Absinthin, Artabsin und Matrizin aus *Artemisia absinthium* L. Teil I: Nachweis in der Droge und Dünnschichtchromatographie. Dtsch Apoth Ztg 1978;118:469-72.

4. Schneider G, Mielke B. Zur Analytik der Bitterstoffe Absinthin, Artabsin und Matrizin aus *Artemisia absinthium* L. Teil II: Isolierung und Gehaltsbest-immungen. Dtsch Apoth Ztg 1979;119:977-82.

5. Beauhaire J, Fourrey J-L, Vuilhorgne M, Lallemand JY.

Dimeric sesquiterpene lactones: structure of absinthin. Tetrahedron Letters 1980;21:3191-4.

6. Beauhaire J, Fourrey J-L, Lallemand JY, Vuilhorgne M. Dimeric sesquiterpene lactone. Structure of isoabsinthin. Acid isomerization of absinthin derivatives. Tetrahedron Letters 1981;22:2269-72.

7. Beauhaire J, Fourrey J-L. Structure of artabsinolides. Photooxygenation studies on artabsin. J Chem Soc Perkin I 1982;1:861-4.

8. Beauhaire J, Fourrey J-L, Guittet E. Structure of absintholide, a new guaianolide dimer of Artemisia absinthium L. Tetrahedron Letters 1984;25:2751-4.

9. Safarova AG, Serkerov SV. Sesquiterpene lactones of Artemisia absinthium. Khim Prir Soedin 1997:834-6. Translated into English as: Chem Nat Compd 1997; 33:653-4.

10. Hänsel R, Keller K, Rimpler H, Schneider G, editors. Artemisia. In: Hagers Handbuch der Pharmazeutischen Praxis, 5th ed. Volume 4: Drogen A-D. Berlin: Springer-Verlag, 1992;357-77.

11. Ariño A, Arberas I, Renobales G, Arriaga S, Domínguez JB. Essential oil of Artemisia absinthium L. from the Spanish Pyrenees. J Essent Oil Res 1999;11:182-4.

12. Chialva F, Liddle PAP, Doglia G. Chemotaxonomy of wormwood (Artemisia absinthium L.). I. Composition of the essential oil of several chemotypes. Z Lebensm Unters Forsch 1983;176:363-6.

13. Nin S, Arfaioli P and Bosetto M. Quantitative determination of some essential oil components of selected Artemisia absinthium plants. J Essent Oil Res 1995;7:271-7.

14. Vostrowsky O, Brosche T, Ihm H, Zintl R, Knobloch K. Über die Komponenten des ätherischen Öls aus Artemisia absinthium L. Z Naturforsch 1981;36c:369-77.

15. Sacco T, Chialva F. Chemical characteristics of the oil from Artemisia absinthium collected in Patagony (Argentina). Planta Med 1988;54:93.

16. Hoffmann B, Herrmann K. Flavonolglykoside des Beifuss (Artemisia vulgaris L.), Estragon (A. dracunculus L.) und Wermut (A. absinthium L.). Z Lebensm Unters Forsch 1982;174:211-5.

17. Swiatek L, Grabias B, Kalemba D. Phenolic acids in certain medicinal plants of the genus Artemisia. Pharm Pharmacol Lett 1998;8:158-60.

18. Shlyapyatis YY. Biology and biochemistry of the common wormwood: 8. Accumulation dynamics of tannic substances, ascorbic acid and carotene. Liet TSR Mokslu Akad Darb Ser C Biol Mokslai 1975;1:43-8, through Biol Abstr 1976;61:28166.

19. Rücker G, Manns D, Wilbert S. Homoditerpene peroxides from Artemisia absinthium. Phytochemistry 1992;31:340-2.

20. Ikram M, Shafi N, Mir I, Do MN, Nguyen P, Le Quesne PW. 24ζ-Ethylcholesta-7,22-dien-3β-ol: A possibly antipyretic constituent of Artemisia absinthium. Planta Med 1987;53:389.

21. Hänsel R, Sticher O, Steinegger E. Wermutkraut. In: Pharmakognosie - Phytopharmazie, 6th ed. Berlin-Heidelberg-New York: Springer-Verlag, 1999:486-8.

22. Weiss RF and Fintelmann V. Artemisia absinthium, Wormwood. In: Herbal Medicine, 2nd ed. (translated from the 9th German edition of Lehrbuch der Phytotherapie). Stuttgart-New York: Thieme, 2000:117-9.

23. Frohne D. Absinthii herba - Wermutkraut. In: Wichtl M, editor. Teedrogen und Phytopharmaka. Ein Handbuch für die Praxis auf wissenschaftlicher Grundlage, 4th ed. Stuttgart: Wissenschaftliche Verlagsgesellschaft, 2002:3-6.

24. Wichtl M, Neubeck M. Wermutkraut - Absinthii herba. In: Hartke K, Hartke H, Mutschler E, Rücker G and Wichtl M, editors. Kommentar zum Europäischen Arzneibuch. Stuttgart: Wissenschaftliche Verlagsgesellschaft, 1999(12. Lfg.):W 16.

25. Gessner O. Gift- und Arzneipflanzen von Mitteleuropa, 3rd ed. Heidelberg: Carl Winter Universitätsverlag 1974:258-60.

26. Paris RR, Moyse H. Absinthe. In: Précis de matière médicale, 2nd ed, Vol. III. Paris: Masson, 1976:418-9.

27. Artemisia absinthium. In: British Herbal Pharmacopoeia 1983. Bournemouth: British Herbal Medicine Association, 1983:32-3.

28. Roth L, Daunderer M, Kormann K. Artemisia absinthium L. In: Giftpflanzen - Pflanzengifte. Vorkommen, Wirkung, Therapie, Allergische und phototoxische Reaktionen, 4th ed. Landsberg: ecomed, 1994:146.

29. McGuffin M, Hobbs C, Upton R, Goldberg A, editors. Artemisia absinthium L. In: American Herbal Products Association's Botanical Safety Handbook. Boca Raton-Boston-London: CRC Press, 1997:15.

30. Wake G, Court J, Pickering A, Lewis R, Wilkins R, Perry E. CNS acetylcholine receptor activity in European medicinal plants traditionally used to improve failing memory. J Ethnopharmacol 2000;69:105-14.

31. Kaul VK, Nigam SS, Dhar KL. Antimicrobial activities of the essential oils of Artemisia absinthium L., Artemisia vestita Wall. and Artemisia vulgaris L. Indian J Pharm 1976;38:21-2.

32. Kreitmair H. Artemisia absinthium L. - der echte Wermut. Pharmazie 1951;6:27-8.

33. Gilani AH, Janbaz KH. Preventive and curative effects of Artemisia absinthium on acetaminophen and CCl$_4$-induced hepatotoxicity. Gen Pharmacol 1995;26:309-15.

34. Khattak SG, Gilani SN, Ikram M. Antipyretic studies on some indigenous Pakistani medicinal plants. J Ethnopharmacol 1985;14:45-51.

35. Rice KC, Wilson RS. (-)-3-Isothujone, a small non-nitrogenous molecule with antinociceptive activity in mice. J Med Chem 1976;19:1054-7.

36. Baumann JC. Über die Wirkung von Chelidonium, Curcuma, Absinth und Carduus marianus auf die Galle- und Pankreassekretion bei Hepatopathien. Med Mschr 1975;29:173-80.

37. Höld KM, Sirisoma NS, Ikeda T, Narahashi T, Casida JE. α-Thujone (the active component of absinthe): γ-aminobutyric acid type A receptor modulation and metabolic detoxification. Proc Natl Acad Sci USA 2000;97:3826-31.

38. Rao VSN, Menezes AMS, Gadelha MGT. Antifertility screening of some indigenous plants of Brasil. Fitoterapia 1988;59:17-20.

39. Schimmer O, Krüger A, Paulini H, Haefele F. An evaluation of 55 commercial plant extracts in the Ames mutagenicity test. Pharmazie 1994;49:448-52.

40. Opdyke DLJ. Monographs on fragrance raw materials: artemisia oil (wormwood). Food Chem Toxicol 1975;13, 721-2.

41. Lawrence BM. Progress in essential oils. Perfumer & Flavorist 1998;23 (Jan/Feb):39-50.

42. Council of Europe. Artemisia absinthium L. In: Natural Sources of Flavourings. Report No. 1. Strasbourg: Council of Europe Publishing, 2000.

43. Tegtmeier M, Harnischfeger G. Methods for the reduction of thujone content in pharmaceutical preparations of Artemisia, Salvia and Thuja. Eur J Pharm Biopharm 1994;40:337-40.

44. Stahl E, Gerard D. Entgiftung von Absinthkraut durch CO_2-Hochdruckextraktion. Planta Med 1982; 45:147.

AGNI CASTI FRUCTUS

Agnus Castus

E/S/C/O/P
MONOGRAPHS
Second Edition

DEFINITION

Agnus castus consists of the whole, ripe, dried fruits of *Vitex agnus castus* L. It contains not less than 0.08 per cent of casticin ($C_{19}H_{18}O_8$; M_r 374.4), calculated with reference to the dried drug.

The material complies with the monograph of the Pharmacopoea Helvetica [1].

CONSTITUENTS

The main characteristic constituents are:

Bicyclic diterpenes of the labdane and clerodane types, particularly rotundifuran (up to 0.3%) [2-7].

Iridoid glycosides such as agnuside (0.02-0.4%) [2,5] and aucubin [2,5,8].

Lipophilic flavonoids such as casticin (3',5-dihydroxy-3,6,7,4'-tetramethoxyflavone, approx. 0.02-0.2%), penduletin and chrysosplenol-D [2,9,10]. Hydrophilic flavones of *O*- or *C*-glycosidic types including orientin, homoorientin, luteolin-7-glucoside, isovitexin and isovitexin xyloside [11].

Triglycerides with α-linolenic, oleic, stearic, palmitic and linoleic acids as the prevalent fatty acid moieties [4,12].

Essential oil, of which the main components are monoterpenes such as α-pinene, sabinene, β-phellandrene and 4-terpineol, and sesquiterpenes such as β-caryophyllene and germacrene B [13,14].

CLINICAL PARTICULARS

Therapeutic indications
Premenstrual syndrome (PMS) including symptoms such as mastodynia or mastalgia [12,15-23].
Menstrual cycle disorders such as polymenorrhoea, oligomenorrhoea or amenorrhoea [16,24-32].

Posology and method of administration

Dosage
Preparations equivalent to 30-40 mg of the drug daily [12,17,23], or up to 240 mg of the drug daily in patients suffering from PMS [21,22].

Mode of administration
For oral administration.

Duration of administration

Treatment for a minimum of 3 months may be appropriate; the advisability of medical advice should be taken into consideration [4,16,24].

Contra-indications

None known.

Special warnings and special precautions for use

None required.

Interaction with other medicaments and other forms of interaction

None known.

Mutual attenuation of effects might occur in patients under concomitant treatment with dopamine receptor antagonists [12].

Pregnancy and lactation

No published data on pregnancy available. Agnus castus should not be taken during pregnancy [12].

Lactation was inhibited in rats after subcutaneous administration of an agnus castus extract twice daily at about 100 times the human daily dose level [33]. An earlier human study showed an increase in lactation [34].

Effects on ability to drive and use machines

None known.

Undesirable effects

Cases of allergic skin reactions have been reported [12].

Overdose

No toxic effects reported.

PHARMACOLOGICAL PROPERTIES

Pharmacodynamic properties

In vitro experiments

An increase in serum levels of prolactin is a frequent cause of menstrual irregularities, pre-menstrual syndrome and mastodynia. In vitro and in vivo experiments have shown that agnus castus extracts have dopaminergic, prolactin-inhibiting activity. Dopamine has been identified as one of the physiological prolactin-inhibiting factors acting on prolactin-producing lactotropic cells of the pituitary and it has been demonstrated that an extract of agnus castus binds to striatal D_2 receptors and directly suppresses the secretion of prolactin from cultures of rat pituitary cells [35-37].

Diterpenes isolated from the lipophilic fraction of an agnus castus extract have been shown to have dopaminergic activity and to inhibit prolactin secretion. In a test using human recombinant D_2 receptor, the contribution to dopaminergic activity of rotundifuran and 6β,7β-diacetoxy-13-hydroxy-labda-8,14-diene (the diterpenes present in the highest concentrations in the extract) was approximately equal to that of three other diterpenes present in lower amounts but having higher dopaminergic activity on a molar basis. Rotundifuran concentration-dependently inhibited prolactin release from cultured rat pituitary cells, its effect at 10^{-4} being equivalent to that of dopamine at 10^{-6} M [6,38-40].

Five ethanolic agnus castus extracts as well as various extract fractions of different polarity were examined in radioligand binding studies and superfusion experiments. Binding inhibition was observed for dopamine D_2 and opioid receptors (μ and κ subtypes) with IC_{50} values of the native extracts between 40 and 70 mg/ml. There was no significant binding to histamine H_1, benzodiazepine or OFQ receptors, nor to the binding site of the serotonin (5-HT) transporter. Lipophilic fractions which contained the diterpenes rotundifuran and 6β,7β-diacetoxy-13-hydroxy-labda-8,14-diene inhibited dopamine D_2 receptor binding. While inhibition of binding to μ- and κ-opioid receptors was most pronounced in lipophilic fractions, binding to δ-opioid receptors was inhibited mainly by an aqueous fraction. In superfusion experiments, the aqueous fraction from a methanolic extract inhibited the release of acetylcholine in a concentration-dependent manner. Furthermore, the potent D_2 receptor antagonist spiperone antagonised the effect of the extract, suggesting a dopaminergic action mediated by D_2 receptor activation [41].

Methanolic extracts from agnus castus of several different origins (Argentina, Turkey and Croatia) and various agnus castus constituents were examined for their binding capacities to μ-opioid and dopamine D_2 receptors. The extracts showed moderate binding affinities for μ-opioid receptors with IC_{50} values between 10 and 40 μg/ml, whereas binding to dopamine D_2 receptors was weak (IC_{50} > 100 μg/ml). Among individual constituents only rotundifuran inhibited μ-opioid binding with an IC_{50} of 4 μM; the others showed no inhibition at concentrations up to 10 μM [42].

A hydroethanolic extract from agnus castus and various isolated constituents were tested for dopaminergic effects in receptor binding experiments using homogenised calf striatum and ^{3}H-spiroperidol as a ligand. The extract showed an affinity for the dopamine D_2 receptor with an IC_{50} of 40-70 μg/ml at concentrations up to 1000 mg/ml. Substantial effects were also observed with the diterpenes rotundifuran (IC_{50}: 45 μg/ml) and 6β,7β-diacetoxy-13-hydroxy-labda-8,14-diene (IC_{50}: 79 μg/ml) [43].

Small cylindrical-shaped portions of striatum were incubated with ^{3}H-acetylcholine. Electrical stimulation released acetylcholine from the tissue which could be detected and quantified as free ^{3}H-choline in the surrounding medium. Agnus castus extract in the perfusion fluid was found to concentration-dependently inhibit acetylcholine release (IC_{50}: approx. 30 µg/ml). The effect of agnus castus could be partly eliminated by the antidopaminergic ligand spiroperidol or by the anticholinergic atropine. From these results it was concluded that agnus castus may have a dual mechanism: it may exert both dopaminergic and cholinergic activity [4,43].

Determination of the binding affinities of a methanolic agnus castus extract for human opioid receptors gave IC_{50} values of 30, 20 and 190 µg/ml for µ-, κ- and δ-opioid receptors respectively [44].

Oestrogenic activity
A methanolic extract from agnus castus exhibited competitive binding affinity with recombinant human oestrogen receptors α (ERα) and β (ERβ), the 50% inhibitory (IC_{50}) values being 46 and 64 µg/ml respectively, compared to values of 5.6 and 2.5 µg/ml for a comparable red clover extract and 30 and 27 µg/ml for a hop strobile extract. With cultured Ishikawa cells (an ER-positive endometrial adenocarcinoma cell line) the extract at 20 µg/ml showed weak oestrogenic activity, as indicated by up-regulation of progesterone receptor mRNA, but did not induce alkaline phosphatase activity. In S30 breast cancer cells, presenelin-2, another oestrogen-inducible gene, was up-regulated in the presence of the extract at 20 µg/ml [45].

In vivo experiments
In rats subjected to stress by exposure to an ether-saturated atmosphere for 30 seconds (which resulted in a dramatic increase in serum prolactin levels within 2 minutes), intravenous pre-treatment with 60 mg of an agnus castus extract in saline markedly reduced the increase in prolactin compared to animals receiving saline only [46].

Bioassay-guided fractionation of an agnus castus extract yielded a group of bicyclic diterpenes which exerted dopaminergic activity *in vivo* [40].

Pharmacological studies in humans
In an open study 34 women (aged 18-43 years) with hyperprolactinaemia were treated with an agnus castus extract corresponding to 40 mg of crude drug daily for one month. In 27 cases (80%) prolactin levels were markedly reduced. Six women did not respond to treatment and in one case the initial prolactin level increased slightly [16].

Clinical studies

Premenstrual syndrome (PMS)
In a randomized, double-blind, comparative study,
women aged 18-45 years suffering from PMS were assigned to treatment over a span of three menstrual cycles with a 60%-ethanolic agnus castus extract (corresponding to 40 mg of crude drug daily) or pyridoxine hydrochloride (2 × 100 mg daily on days 16-35 of the cycle; placebo only on days 1-15). The intention-to-treat analysis included 127 patients, 61 in the agnus castus group and 66 in the pyridoxine group. Therapeutic response was assessed primarily by means of the premenstrual tension scale (PMTS); secondary endpoints were the rating of six typical PMS complaints and the Clinical Global Impression (CGI) scale. Over the course of treatment mean PMTS scores decreased from 15.2 to 5.1 in the agnus castus group and from 11.9 to 5.1 in the pyridoxine group; according to the 95% confidence intervals there was no significant difference between groups. Scores for typical complaints showed greater improvement in the agnus castus group. The CGI results indicated a marked or very marked improvement in 77.1% and 60.6% of patients in the agnus castus and pyridoxine groups respectively. It was concluded that the two types of treatment were equally effective for premenstrual symptoms [17].

In a randomized, double-blind, placebo-controlled study, 178 women suffering from PMS (of whom 170 were evaluated: 86 verum and 84 placebo) and diagnosed in accordance with DSM-III-R, were treated with 20 mg of an agnus castus dry extract (6-12:1; 60% ethanol) or placebo daily over three consecutive menstrual cycles. Improvement in the main efficacy variable (combined score for patients' self assessment of six symptoms: irritability, mood alteration, anger, headache, breast fullness, other menstrual symptoms including bloating) was significantly greater in the verum group than in the placebo group (p<0.001). The physicians' assessment using the CGI scale (three items) showed significant superiority of verum treatment (p<0.001) and responder rates (a responder being defined as a patient showing a reduction of ≥ 50% in self-assessed symptoms) were 52% in the agnus castus group compared to 24% in the placebo group [22].

In a multicentre observational study 1634 patients suffering from PMS received two capsules daily, each containing 1.6-3.0 mg of an extract (6.7-12.5:1) corresponding to 20 mg of agnus castus. After a treatment period of three cycles, 93% reported a decrease or cessation of complaints such as depression, anxiety, craving and hyperhydration. 85% of the physicians rated the global assessment of clinical efficacy as good or very good, and 81% of the patients assessed their status after treatment as very much or much better. Analysis of the frequency and severity of mastodynia revealed that complaints still present after 3 months were mostly less severe [23].

Data from two open studies [15,21] and three post-marketing surveillance studies [18-20] in patients with premenstrual symptoms showed positive effects in this indication from treatment with various agnus castus preparations.

Cycle disorders
In early studies positive results of agnus castus treatment were reported in cases of secondary amenorrhoea and cycle disorders [25-31].

In a randomized, double-blind, placebo-controlled study, 52 women (aged 19-42 years) with luteal phase defects due to latent hyperprolactinaemia were assigned to daily treatment for 3 months with 20 mg of an agnus castus extract (50-70% ethanol) or placebo. Data from 17 verum and 20 placebo patients was available for evaluation. Inadequate (i.e. too short) luteal phases before treatment (mean: 5.5 and 3.4 days in the verum and placebo groups respectively) significantly lengthened to 10.5 days in the agnus castus group (p<0.005) with no effect on overall cycle duration since initially prolonged follicular phases were correspondingly shortened; no change was observed in the placebo group. Mid-luteal progesterone and oestradiol levels increased significantly during treatment with agnus castus (p<0.001 and p<0.05 respectively in comparison with placebo). A significant reduction in releasable pituitary prolactin reserve (p<0.001) during the mid-follicular phase in the agnus castus group was considered sufficient to improve or normalise the disturbed ovarian function, while no change was observed in the placebo group. Furthermore, only 2 out of 9 patients in the verum group initially suffering from PMS reported the complaint after 3 months of treatment, compared to 11 out of 13 in the placebo group (p<0.05). In the verum group 2 women became pregnant [24].

In an open study 45 women with corpus luteum insufficiency were treated over a span of three menstrual cycles with an agnus castus liquid preparation (daily dose equivalent to about 30 mg of crude drug). Only women who had mid-luteal progesterone levels of less than 12 ng/ml and normal prolactin levels were included. By the end of therapy 7 women (15%) had become pregnant and 25 women had progesterone levels greater than 12 ng/ml, while 7 others showed a marked increase, albeit still under 12 ng/ml [32].

Pharmacokinetic properties
No data available.

Preclinical safety data
No published data available.

Clinical safety data
In an open study 20 male volunteers ingested, each

day for 14 days separated by wash-out periods of 7 days, capsules containing a dry extract of agnus castus at dose levels corresponding to 120, 240 and 480 mg of crude drug, and placebo capsules. The subjective tolerability of the extract was considered good; 13 out of the 20 volunteers reported mild to moderate complaints, particularly at the highest dose of extract (e.g headache, fatigue) but these appeared not to be dose-dependent and many could not be clearly attributed to the treatment. No influence was detected on a wide range of clinical laboratory parameters including serum concentrations of gonadotropin and testosterone [47].

In a randomized study, patients with premenstrual tension syndrome received either an agnus castus dry extract (equivalent to 40 mg of crude drug daily; n = 61) or pyridoxine hydrochloride (2 × 100 mg on days 16-35 of the menstrual cycle; n = 66) over a span of three menstrual cycles. Adverse events occurred in 12 patients taking agnus castus and 6 patients taking pyridoxine: mainly gastro-intestinal or lower abdominal complaints and, in the agnus castus group, two case of skin reactions and one of transient headache. No serious adverse events were observed [17].

In a randomized, double-blind study 86 patients received 20 mg of an agnus castus extract (6-12:1; 60% ethanol) daily over a span of three consecutive menstrual cycles, while 84 patients received placebo. 7 patients (4 verum, 3 placebo) reported mild adverse events (once each), all of which resolved without discontinuation of treatment [22].

During an observational study 1634 patients received an extract corresponding to 40 g of agnus castus daily over a treatment period of three menstrual cycles. Minor adverse events, such as skin reactions or gastrointestinal complaints, were observed in 1.2% of cases [23].

No adverse events occurred in a clinical study in which 17 women with latent hyperprolactinaemia were treated daily for 3 months with 20 mg of an agnus castus extract (50-70% ethanol) [24].

REFERENCES

1. Mönchspfefferfrüchte - Agni casti fructus. Pharmacopoea Helvetica.

2. Meier B, Hoberg E. Agni-casti fructus. Neue Erkenntnisse zur Qualität und Wirksamkeit. Z Phytotherapie 1999; 20:140-58.

3. Hoberg E, Meier B, Sticher O. Quantitative high performance liquid chromatographic analysis of diterpenoids in Agni-casti fructus. Planta Med 2000;66:352-5.

4. Berger D. *Vitex agnus castus*: Unbedenklichkeit und

Wirksamkeit beim prämenstruellen Syndrom [Dissertation]. University of Basel, 1998.

5. Hoberg E. Phytochemical and analytical investigations of Vitex agnus-castus L. [Dissertation]. Swiss Federal Institute of Technology (ETH) Zürich, 1999.

6. Christoffel V, Spengler B, Jarry H, Wuttke W. Prolactin inhibiting dopaminergic activity of diterpenes from Vitex agnus castus. In: Loew D, Blume H, Dingermann T, editors. Phytopharmaka V. Darmstadt: Steinkopff, 1999:209-14.

7. Hoberg E, Sticher O, Orjala JE, Meier B. Diterpene aus Agni-casti fructus und ihre Analytik. Z Phytotherapie 1999;20:149-50.

8. Castagnou MR, Larcebau S, Nicou O. Contribution à l'étude des graines de Vitex agnus castus. Deuxième partie. Bull Soc Pharm Bordeaux 1964;103:189-92.

9. Wollenweber E, Mann K. Flavonole aus Früchten von Vitex agnus castus. Planta Med 1983;48:126-7.

10. Belic I, Bergant-Dolar J, Morton RA. Constituents of Vitex agnus castus seeds. Part I. Casticin. J Chem Soc 1961:2523-5.

11. Gomaa CS, El-Moghazy MA, Halim FA, El-Sayyad AE. Flavonoids and iridoids from Vitex agnus castus. Planta Med 1978;33:277.

12. Abel G, Gorkow C, Wolf H. Vitex. In: Hänsel R, Keller K, Rimpler H, Schneider G, editors. Hagers Handbuch der Pharmazeutischen Praxis, Volume 6: Drogen P-Z. Berlin: Springer-Verlag, 1994:1183-96.

13. Zwaving JH, Bos R. Composition of the essential fruit oil of Vitex agnus-castus. Planta Med 1996;62:83-4.

14. Galetti GC, Russo MT, Bocchini P. Essential oil composition of leaves and berries of Vitex agnus-castus L. from Calabria, Southern Italy. Rapid Commun Mass Spectrom 1996;10:1345-50.

15. Coeugniet E, Elek E, Kühnast R. Das prämenstruelle Syndrom (PMS) und seine Behandlung. Ärztezeitschr Naturheilverfahren 1986;27:619-22.

16. Gorkow C. Klinischer Kenntnisstand von Agni-casti fructus. Klinisch-pharmakologische Untersuchungen und Wirksamkeitsbelege. Z Phytotherapie 1999;20:159-68.

17. Lauritzen C, Reuter HD, Repges R, Bohnert K-J, Schmidt U. Treatment of premenstrual tension syndrome with Vitex agnus castus. Controlled, double-blind study versus pyridoxine. Phytomedicine 1997;4:183-9.

18. Feldmann HU, Albrecht M, Lamertz M, Böhnert K-J. Therapie bei Gelbkörperschwäche bzw. prämenstruellem Syndrom mit Vitex-agnus-castus-Tinktur. Gyne 1990;11:421-5.

19. Dittmar FW, Böhnert K-J, Peeters M, Albrecht M, Lamertz M, Schmidt U. Prämenstruelles Syndrom. Behandlung mit einem Phytopharmakon. TW Gynäkologie 1992;5:60-8.

20. Peters-Welte C, Albrecht M. Regeltempostörungen und PMS. Vitex agnus-castus in einer Anwendungsbeobachtung. TW Gynäkologie 1994;7:49-52.

21. Berger D, Schaffner W, Schrader E, Meier B, Brattström A. Efficacy of Vitex agnus castus L. extract Ze 440 in patients with pre-menstrual syndrome (PMS). Arch Gynecol Obstet 2000;264:150-3.

22. Schellenberg R. Treatment for the premenetrual syndrome with agnus castus fruit extract: prospective, randomised, placebo controlled study. BMJ 2001;322:134-7.

23. Loch E-G, Selle H, Boblitz N. Treatment of premenstrual syndrome with a phytopharmaceutical formulation containing Vitex agnus castus. J Women's Health Gender-Based Med 2000;9:315-20.

24. Milewicz A, Gejdel E, Sworen H, Sienkiewicz K, Jedrzejak J, Teucher T, Schmitz H. Vitex agnus castus-Extrakt zur Behandlung von Regeltempoanomalien infolge latenter Hyperprolaktinämie. Ergebnisse einer randomisierter Plazebo-kontrollierten Doppelblindstudie. Arzneim-Forsch/Drug Res 1993:43:752-6.

25. Probst V, Roth OA. Über einen Pflanzenextrakt mit hormonartiger Wirkung. Dtsch Med Wochenschr 1954; 79:1271-4.

26. Roth OA. Zur Therapie der Gelbkörperinsuffizienz in der Praxis. Med Klin 1956;51:1263-5.

27. Halder R. Über die Anwendungsmöglichkeiten der Vitex agnus castus L. in der Frauenheilkunde unter besonderer Berücksichtigung der Blutungsstörungen [Dissertation]. Universität Tübingen, 1957.

28. Amann W. Amenorrhoe - Günstige Wirkung von Agnus castus (Agnolyt®) auf Amenorrhoe. Z Allg Med 1982; 58:228-31.

29. Loch E-G, Kaiser E. Diagnostik und Therapie dyshormonaler Blutungen in der Praxis. Gynäkol Praxis 1990;14:489-95.

30. Bleier W. Therapie von Zyklus- und Blutungsstörungen und weiteren endokrin bedingten Erkrankungen der Frau mit pflanzlichen Wirkstoffen. Zentralblatt Gynäkol 1959;81:701-9.

31. Kayser H-W, Istanbulluoglu S. Eine Behandlung von Menstruationsstörungen ohne Hormone. Hippokrates 1954;25:717-8.

32. Propping D, Katzorke T, Belkien L. Diagnostik und Therapie der Gelbkörperschwäche in der Praxis. Therapiewoche 1988;38:2992-3001.

33. Winterhoff H, Gorkow C, Behr B. Die Hemmung der Laktation bei Ratten als indirekter Beweis für die Senkung von Prolaktin durch Agnus castus. Z Phytotherapie 1991;12:175-9.

34. Mohr H. Klinische Untersuchung zur Steigerung der Laktation. Dtsch Med Wochenschr 1954;79:1513-6.

35. Jarry H, Leonhardt S, Gorkow C, Wuttke W. In vitro prolactin but not LH and FSH release is inhibited by

compounds in extracts of Agnus castus: direct evidence for a dopaminergic principle by the dopamine receptor assay. Exp Clin Endocrinol 1994;102:448-54.

36. Jarry H, Leonhardt S, Wuttke W, Behr B, Gorkow C. Agnus castus als dopaminerges Wirkprinzip in Mastodynon® N. Z Phytotherapie 1991;12:77-82.

37. Sliutz G, Speiser P, Schultz AM, Spona J, Zeilinger R. Agnus castus extracts inhibit prolactin secretion of rat pituitary cells. Hormone Metab Res 1993;25:253-5.

38. Jarry H, Leonhardt S, Wuttke W, Spengler B, Christoffel V. Auf der Suche nach dopaminergen Substanzen in Agni-casti-fructus-Präparaten: Warum eigentlich? Z Phytotherapie 1999;20:150-2.

39. Jarry H, Christoffel V, Spengler B, Popp M, Wuttke W. Diterpenes isolated from *Vitex agnus castus* BNO 1095 inhibit prolactin secretion via specific interaction with dopamine D2 receptors in the pituitary. In: Abstracts of "Phytotherapie an der Schwelle zum neuen Jahrtausend". 10. Jahrestagung der Gesellschaft für Phytotherapie. Münster, 11-13 November 1999.

40. Christoffel V, Spengler B, Abel G, Jarry H, Wuttke W. Diterpenes from BNO 1095 (*Vitex agnus castus*) inhibit prolactin secretion. Focus on Alternative and Complementary Therapies 2000;5:87-8.

41. Meier B, Berger D, Hoberg E, Sticher O, Schaffner W. Pharmacological activities of *Vitex agnus-castus* extracts

in vitro. Phytomedicine 2000;7:373-81.

42. Weisskopf M, Simmen U, Schaffner W. Binding affinities of various *Vitex agnus castus* extracts to µ-opiod and dopamine$_2$ receptor. In: Abstracts of 3rd International Congress on Phytomedicine. Munich, 11-13 October 2000. *Published as*: Phytomedicine 2000;7(Suppl II):110 (Abstract P-117).

43. Berger D, Burkard W, Schaffner W, Meier B. Rezeptorbindungsstudien mit Extrakten und daraus isolierten Substanzen. Z Phytotherapie 1999;20:153-4.

44. Brugisser R, Burkard W, Simmen U, Schaffner W. Untersuchungen an Opioid-Rezeptoren mit *Vitex agnus-castus* L. Z Phytotherapie 1999;20:154.

45. Liu J, Burdette JE, Xu H, Gu C, van Breemen RB, Bhat KPL et al. Evaluation of estrogenic activity of plant extracts for the potential treatment of menopausal symptoms. J Agric Food Chem 2001;49:2472-9.

46. Wuttke W, Gorkow C, Jarry H. Dopaminergic compounds in *Vitex agnus castus*. In: Loew D, Rietbrock N, editors. Phytopharmaka in Forschung und klinischer Anwendung. Darmstadt: Steinkopff, 1995:81-91.

47. Loew D, Gorkow C, Schrödter A, Rietbrock S, Merz P-G, Schnieders M, Sieder C. Zur dosisabhängigen Verträglichkeit eines Agnus-castus-Spezialextraktes. Z Phytotherapie 1996;17:237-43.

ALLII SATIVI BULBUS

Garlic

DEFINITION

Garlic powder is produced from the bulbs, or from the separated cloves, of *Allium sativum* L., cut and dried at a temperature not exceeding 65°C, or freeze-dried, then powdered. It contains not less than 0.45 per cent of allicin ($C_6H_{10}OS_2$; M_r 162.3), calculated with reference to the dried drug.

The material complies with the monograph of the European Pharmacopoeia [1].

CONSTITUENTS

Carefully dried, powdered material contains about 1 per cent of alliin [(+)-S-allyl-L-cysteine sulphoxide] as the main sulphur-containing amino acid [2]. Other characteristic, genuine constituents are (+)-S-methyl-L-cysteine sulphoxide, gamma-L-glutamyl peptides, S-allyl-cysteine, ubiquitous amino acids, steroids and adenosine [3]. In the presence of the enzyme alliinase, alliin will be converted to allicin (1 mg of alliin is considered to be equivalent to 0.45 mg of allicin) [4].

In turn, allicin is the precursor of various transformation products, including ajoenes, vinyldithiines, oligo-sulphides and polysulphides, depending on the conditions applied [4].

Material derived from garlic by steam distillation or extraction in an oily medium contains various allicin transformation products [4-6].

CLINICAL PARTICULARS

Therapeutic indications
Prophylaxis of atherosclerosis [3,7-16].
Treatment of elevated blood lipid levels insufficiently influenced by diet [8,10,14,17-29].
Also used for upper respiratory tract infections and catarrhal conditions [5,30-32], although clinical data to support this indication is not available.

Posology and method of administration

Dosage

Prophylaxis of atherosclerosis or treatment of elevated blood lipid levels
Adults: The equivalent of 6-10 mg of alliin (approx. 3-5 mg of allicin) daily, typically contained in one clove of garlic or in 0.5-1.0 g of dried garlic powder [3,7-29].

E/S/C/O/P
MONOGRAPHS
Second Edition

Upper respiratory tract infections
Adults: 2-4 g of dried bulb or 2-4 ml of tincture (1:5, 45% ethanol), three times daily [30].

Method of administration
For oral administration.

Duration of administration
Long term treatment is generally advised in the prevention of atherosclerosis and prophylaxis or treatment of peripheral arterial vascular diseases [10,12].

Contraindications
None known.

Special warnings and special precautions for use
Caution is advised after surgical operations [33].

Interaction with other medicaments and other forms of interaction
In two cases an increased International Normalized Ratio has been observed in patients on warfarin who had used garlic products (no further data) [34].

Pregnancy and lactation
There are no objections to use during pregnancy and lactation (because neither long term nutritional experience nor any other important circumstances give reason for suspicion). From a controlled trial it is known that major sulphur-containing volatiles from garlic are transmitted to human milk leading to improved drinking habits of the babies [35].

Effects on ability to drive and use machines
Nothing reported.

Undesirable effects
In rare cases gastro-intestinal irritation or allergic reactions [36].

Overdose
No toxic effects reported.

PHARMACOLOGICAL PROPERTIES

Pharmacodynamic properties

Garlic exerts antiatherogenic, lipid-lowering, anti-hypertensive, antiaggregatory, vasodilatory and antioxidant effects. The effects are primarily due to allicin and its transformation products [3].

In vitro experiments

Antiatherogenic and lipid-lowering effects
Inhibitory effects of extracts and isolated fractions from garlic on cholesterol biosynthesis were observed in chicken hepatocytes and monkey livers. At equivalent doses, both the drug and its lipophilic and hydrophilic fractions caused 50-75% inhibition of cholesterol biosynthesis [37].

Inhibition of cholesterol biosynthesis by allicin and ajoene was evaluated in cultivated rat hepatocytes and the human liver cell line HepG2. In rat hepatocytes, ajoene inhibited sterol biosynthesis with an IC_{50} of 15 µM; alliin was almost ineffective. In HepG2 cells both allicin and ajoene inhibited sterol biosynthesis with IC_{50} values of 7 and 9 µM respectively. The inhibition was exerted at the level of HMG-CoA-reductase [38].

Standardized garlic powder (1.3% alliin) inhibited cholesterol biosynthesis in rat hepatocytes with an IC_{50} of 90 µg/ml [39,40]. In HepG2 cells cholesterol biosynthesis was inhibited by the garlic powder with an IC_{50} of 35 µg/ml [40].

The mechanism of action is believed to be an inter-action at the molecular level with the phosphorylation cascade of hydroxymethyl-glutaryl-CoA reductase [38].

Allicin inhibits the incorporation of ^{14}C-acetate into non-saponifiable neutral lipids at concentrations as low as 10 µM and can be regarded as the most active of the sulphur-containing metabolic products of alliin [39].

Inhibition of cholesterol biosynthesis by up to 87% was also observed with petroleum ether, methanol and water extracts of garlic, and a garlic-preparation containing S-allylcysteine [41].

During a 24-hour incubation period garlic powder significantly reduced the level of cholesteryl esters by 26% and free cholesterol by 32% in cells of athero-sclerotic plaques of human aorta (p<0.05) and inhibited their proliferative activity by 55% at 1 mg/ml [15].

Effects on vascular resistance, fibrinolysis and platelet aggregation
In isolated arterial strips from the dog, garlic at 0.2-200 g powder/litre and ajoene at 10^{-6} to 10^{-3} M hyperpolarised membrane potential by 9.3 mV and 4.2 mV, and reduced muscle tone by up to 0.33 g and 0.160 g, respectively [42,43].

Similarly, in human coronary artery smooth muscle garlic at concentrations of 0.0002-0.2 g/litre caused dose-dependent hyperpolarisation (2.7 mV at maximum) and relaxation (20% at maximum); half-maximal effects were obtained at 1.15 mg/litre. Allicin and ajoene produced hyperpolarisation of up to 5.1 mV and 4.4 mV, and diminished vascular tone by 24% and 11%, respectively, with half-maximal effects at 6.2×10^{-9} M and 9.9×10^{-9} M [44].

In isolated rat aorta freeze-dried garlic powder dose-dependently inhibited noradrenaline-induced contractions. The EC_{50} values were 5.28×10^{-3} g/ml in aortas with endothelia and 5.81×10^{-3} g/ml in aortas without endothelia [45].

A two-fold activation of endogenous nitric oxide synthesis was observed in isolated thrombocytes obtained from human volunteers after ingestion of a single dose of 4 g of fresh garlic [46,47].

Garlic preparations and organosulphur compounds from garlic inhibited collagen-stimulated platelet aggregation in platelet-rich plasma with the following IC_{50} values (µg/ml): an aqueous garlic extract 460, total polar constituents 190, alliin 205, allicin 14.0, total thiosulphinates 13.2, adenosine 0.11, guanosine > 20. In whole blood the strongest effects were exhibited by allicin (IC_{50}:14.0 µg/ml) and adenosine (IC_{50}: 0.11 µg/ml) [48].

Diallyldisulphide (40-200 µg/mL) and diallyl-trisulphide (5-100 µg/mL) dose-dependently inhibited platelet aggregation and thromboxane B_2 secretion induced by arachidonic acid, adrenaline, collagen and calcium ionophore A23187 [49].

Antioxidant effects
Allicin inhibited lipid peroxidation induced by an ascorbic acid/Fe^{2+} system at a concentration of 0.18 mM [50].

The antioxidant effect of an aqueous garlic extract obtained from 1 mg of garlic powder was comparable to that of 30 nmol of ascorbic acid or 3.6 nmol of α-tocopherol in a chemiluminescence assay [51,52]. Radical scavenging activity of preparations containing S-allylcysteine has also been demonstrated in both chemiluminescence and 1,1-diphenyl-2-picryl-hydrazyl (DPPH) assays [53].

Garlic powder strongly inhibited superoxide production in phorbol ester-activated granulocytes with an IC_{50} of 390 µg/ml, whereas an alliin-enriched but alliinase-inactivated garlic extract did not inhibit superoxide production at concentrations up to 1 g/ml [54].

An aqueous solution of garlic powder (1.3% alliin) reduced radicals generated by the Fenton reaction and liberated by cigarette smoke [55].

Other effects
An aqueous extract from fresh garlic (100-500 µg/ml) increased the proliferation and improved the morphological characteristics of cultured human fibroblasts (more thin, long and spindly cells instead of large, flat cells) [56].

A similar extract non-competitively and irreversibly inhibited cyclooxygenase activity in rabbit platelets and in lung and vascular aortic tissues with IC_{50} values of 0.35, 1.10 and 0.9 mg respectively; boiled garlic had only modest effects [57].

Anti-aggregatory [48,58], antibacterial [59-61], anti-mycotic [62], antiviral [32] and anti-tumour effects [63,64] of garlic have also been demonstrated.

In vivo experiments

Lipid-lowering and antiatherogenic effects
Earlier studies on lipid-lowering and antiatherogenic effects of garlic have been reviewed [3,13].

Garlic powder (0.6% allicin) fed to rats for 11 days at 0.25, 0.5 or 1 g/kg body weight protected against isoprenaline-induced myocardial damage, as shown by histological examination and biochemical analysis [65].

In the isolated, perfused heart (Langendorff model) from rats which had been given 1% of garlic powder (1.3% alliin) in their diet for 10 weeks, the size of the ischaemic zone (32% vs 41% of total heart tissue; p<0.05), incidence of ventricular tachycardia (0% vs 35%; p<0.05) and incidence of ventricular fibrillation (50% vs 90%; p<0.05) were significantly reduced in comparison with untreated controls [66,67].

A petroleum-ether extract of garlic (corresponding to dried garlic at 1 g/kg body weight), fed to rats for 5 days in combination with an atherogenic diet, significantly prevented elevation of serum cholesterol and triglyceride levels (92.4 and 93 mg/dl respectively, compared to 320 and 370 mg/dl in control animals; p<0.001), and reduced the incidence and grade of atherosclerotic lesions (p = 0.0027) compared to animals fed on the atherogenic diet alone [68].

Rabbits were given cholesterol in their diet at 0.5 g/kg body weight daily for 2 months, then fed for 3 months on a normal diet with or without the addition of fresh garlic at 1 g/kg daily. Compared to rabbits receiving a normal diet over the 3-month period, those given garlic had reduced plaque areas with half as many lesions [69].

After de-endothelialisation of the carotid artery, rats were given a diet containing 2% of cholesterol with or without the addition of 5% of garlic powder (1.3% alliin). After 4 weeks, insertion of a balloon catheter revealed only modest inhibition of the growth of neointima in the rats given garlic compared to those given cholesterol alone. However, the garlic inhibited elevation of serum cholesterol by 42% (p<0.05) and protected enzymes of the glutathione system, which were strongly impaired under hypercholesterolaemia [70].

Antihypertensive effects

Garlic powder given for several weeks at 1 g/kg body weight to spontaneously hypertensive juvenile rats, starting in their fifth week of life, inhibited the development of hypertension and reduced myocardial hypertrophy. In spontaneously hypertensive adult rats (6-7 month of age), garlic lowered blood pressure and myocardial hypertrophy ($p<0.01$) [71].

Garlic powder (1.3% alliin) added at 0.5% to the diet of hypertensive rats significantly prolonged their life span by 22 days ($p<0.02$) compared to 435 days in a control group of hypertensive rats given the normal diet. During the course of the study systolic blood pressure was significantly lower in the garlic group ($p<0.01$) [72].

An aqueous garlic extract administered orally to hypertensive two-kidney-one-clip Goldblatt model rats as a single dose at 50 mg/kg body weight or in repeated daily doses of 50 mg/kg for 2 weeks exerted a significant antihypertensive effect ($p<0.05$) [73].

Other effects

Antiviral [74], antihepatotoxic [75,76] and tumour growth-inhibiting [63,64] effects of garlic have also been demonstrated.

Pharmacological studies in humans

Rheological and antiatherosclerotic effects

In a randomized, double-blind, placebo-controlled, crossover study, the influence on cutaneous microcirculation of a single oral dose of 900 mg of garlic powder (1.3% alliin) was evaluated in 10 healthy volunteers. After 5 hours, a significant increase of 55% was observed in erythrocyte velocity in skin capillaries ($p<0.01$) resulting from vasodilatation of precapillary arterioles, which increased in diameter by 8.6% ($p<0.01$) [77].

In a 2-week, randomized, double-blind, placebo-controlled, crossover study involving 10 healthy volunteers, daily ingestion of 600 mg of a standardized garlic powder preparation (1.3% alliin) lowered susceptibility to lipoprotein oxidation by 34% ($p<0.05$) [78].

In an open study involving 101 healthy volunteers, the effects of taking 300-900 mg of standardized garlic powder (1.3% alliin) daily on elastic properties of the aorta were investigated for at least 2 years. Compared to results from an untreated control group, garlic intake attenuated age-related increases in aortic stiffness: significant differences were observed in pulse wave velocity (8.3 vs. 9.8 m/s, $p<0.0001$) and pressure-standardized elastic vascular resistance (0.63 vs. 0.9 $m^2/s^2 \times$ mm Hg, $p<0.0001$); correlation with age was significantly different ($p<0.0001$) for pulse wave velocity (garlic, $r = 0.44$; control, $r = 0.52$) and

systolic blood pressure (garlic, $r = 0.48$; control, $r = 0.54$) [79].

In an open study 8 healthy volunteers took 1 clove of garlic (about 3 g) daily for 16 weeks. Serum thromboxane B_2 was reduced from 243 to 24 ng/ml ($p<0.001$) [57].

Healthy volunteers (n = 30) took 10 g of fresh garlic daily for 2 months. Clotting time increased from 4.15 to 5.02 min ($p<0.001$) and fibrinolytic actitivity (euglobulin clot lysis time) decreased from 4.17 to 3.26 hour ($p<0.001$). There were no changes in the control group [80].

Lipid-lowering effects

In a randomized, double-blind, placebo-controlled study, significant reductions of up to 30% in fasting and postprandial plasma triglycerides were observed in 24 volunteers after 6 weeks of daily treatment with 900 mg of garlic powder ($p<0.05$ for intergroup differences in fasting plasma triglycerides) [81].

In a randomized, double-blind, placebo-controlled study, the effects of taking 600 mg of standardized garlic powder (1.3% alliin) daily were evaluated in 68 volunteers (initial total cholesterol: verum group 222 mg/dl, placebo group 217 mg/dl). After 15 weeks total cholesterol and triglycerides showed a tendency to decrease in the verum group [82].

In an open study 8 healthy volunteers (initial total cholesterol, 6.1 mmol/litre) took 1 clove of garlic (about 3 g) daily for 16 weeks. Total cholesterol decreased by 21% ($p<0.02$) [57]. In another study, total cholesterol decreased by 15.5% ($p<0.001$) in 30 healthy volunteers who took 10 g of garlic daily for 2 months; no change was observed in an untreated control group [80].

Clinical studies

The effect of garlic on total serum cholesterol has been assessed in four meta-analyses [83-86]. In all of them it was concluded that the available data showed garlic to be superior to placebo in reducing total cholesterol; however, only a modest effect was indicated from one meta-analysis [85]. In another meta-analysis the effect of garlic on blood pressure was evaluated; the results suggested that garlic powder may have some clinical use in mild hypertension [87].

Antihypertensive effects

In a randomized, double-blind, placebo-controlled study, 52 patients with hypercholesterolaemia were treated with 900 mg of standardized garlic powder (1.3% alliin) daily for 6 months. Systolic and diastolic blood pressure (initial values: 145 and 90 mmHg) were reduced by 17% ($p<0.001$) and 10% ($p<0.01$) respectively in the verum group but remained unchanged in the placebo group (p<0.001 for intergroup comparison) [21].

In a randomized study the effects of daily treatment with 600 mg of standardized garlic powder (1.3% alliin, 0.6% allicin release) were compared to those of 1.98 mg of garlic oil in 80 patients with mild hyper-cholesterolaemia. By the end of 4 months of treatment, initial systolic and diastolic blood pressures of 151 and 96 mmHg had decreased by 19 and 17% respectively (both p<0.001) in the garlic powder group whereas no effects were observed in the garlic oil group (p<0.001 for intergroup comparison) [22].

In a randomized, double-blind, placebo-controlled study the effects of 600 mg of standardized garlic powder (1.3% alliin) daily for 12 weeks were evaluated in 47 patients with mild hypertension. In the verum group, initial supine and standing diastolic blood pressures of 102 and 101 mmHg decreased by 13% and 11% respectively (p<0.05), while in the placebo group initial values of 97 and 94 mmHg decreased by 4% and 0.5% respectively (not significant). Initial systolic blood pressures of 171 and 161 mmHg in the verum and placebo groups respectively decreased by 12% (p<0.05) and 6% (not significant). Intergroup comparisons were not reported [18].

In a 12-week randomized, reference-controlled study involving 98 normotensive patients with primary hyperlipoproteinaemia, the effects of daily administration of 900 mg of garlic powder (1.3% alliin) or 600 mg of bezafibrate were compared. Systolic blood pressures of 143.4 mmHg in the garlic group and 140.6 mmHg in the benzafibrate group were reduced by 5.5% and 2% respectively (p<0.05 in favour of garlic). Initial diastolic blood pressures of 82.8 and 82.4 mmHg respectively decreased by 5% in both groups [23].

In a randomized, double-blind, placebo-controlled study 40 patients with moderate hypertension (systolic blood pressure, 178 mmHg; diastolic, 100 mmHg) undergoing concomitant diuretic treatment with triamterene and hydrochlorothiazide received 600 mg of standardized garlic powder (1.3% alliin) or placebo daily. After 12 weeks systolic blood pressure had decreased by 9% in the verum group compared to 3% in the placebo group (p<0.001), while diastolic pressure had decreased by 15% in the verum group compared to 9% in the placebo group (p<0.001) [25].

In a randomized, double-blind study 40 patients with hypercholesterolaemia received 900 mg of standardized garlic powder (1.3% alliin) or placebo daily. After 16 weeks, supine systolic and diastolic blood pressures were significantly lowered in the verum group (p<0.001 and p<0.05 respectively) compared to the placebo group [28].

In a randomized, double-blind study 80 normotensive patients with peripheral arterial occlusive disease received 800 mg of standardized garlic powder (1.3% alliin) or placebo daily. After 12 weeks of therapy the initial diastolic blood pressure of 85 mmHg in the verum group had decreased by 3.5% (p<0.04), while that in the placebo group (initially 83 mmHg) remained unchanged [10].

In a randomized, double-blind study 42 patients with mild hypercholesterolaemia were treated with 900 mg of standardized garlic powder (1.3% alliin) or placebo daily for 12 weeks. At the end of the study systolic and diastolic blood pressures remained unchanged [24].

Rheological and antiatherosclerotic effects

In a randomized, double-blind study, 60 young patients (average age 24 years) with constantly elevated spontaneous platelet aggregation and at increased risk of ischaemic attack were treated with 800 mg of standardized garlic powder (1.3% alliin) or placebo daily for 4 weeks. In the garlic group the ratio of circulating platelet aggregation decreased by 10.3% (p<0.01; placebo group unchanged) and spontaneous platelet aggregation decreased by 56.3% (p<0.01; placebo group unchanged) [9,11].

In a double-blind study 80 patients with peripheral arterial occlusive disease received 800 mg of standardized garlic powder (1.3% alliin) or placebo daily for 12 weeks. In the garlic group plasma viscosity decreased by 3.6% (p<0.0013) and spontaneous platelet aggregation dropped by 59% (p<0.01) while these parameters were unchanged in the placebo group [10].

In a randomized, double-blind study, 23 patients with coronary arterial disease received 900 mg of standardized garlic powder (1.3% alliin) or placebo daily for 3 weeks. The cholesterol content per mg of cell protein decreased from 40 to 28 µg, the LDL oxidation lag-time was prolonged from 133 to 176 min and the LDL-sialic acid content increased from 22 to 33 nmol/mg lipoprotein. In the control group these parameters remained unchanged [14].

In an open study 20 patients with hyper-cholesterolaemia were treated daily for 4 weeks with 600 mg of dried garlic. Fibrinogen decreased by 10% (p<0.01) and fibrinopeptide A by 45% (p<0.01); streptokinase-activated plasminogen increased by 15% (p<0.01) and fibrinopeptide Bβ 15-42 by about 42% (p<0.01) [8].

Incubation of cultured smooth muscle cells for 24 hours with serum from patients with coronary atherosclerosis increased total cell cholesterol by 46.6%. However, incubation with serum taken from the patients 2 hours after ingestion of 300 mg of standardized garlic powder (1.3% alliin) reduced total cell cholesterol to 19.3% [15].

Lipid-lowering effects

Comparative studies
The lipid-lowering effect of 900 mg of garlic powder (standardized to 1.3% alliin) daily (G) was compared to that of 600 mg of bezafibrate daily (B) in 98 patients with hyperlipoproteinaemia. After 12 weeks of treatment, both groups showed significant reductions in total cholesterol (G 25%, B 27%; p<0.001) and LDL-cholesterol (G 32%, B 33%; p<0.001) as well as an increase in HDL-cholesterol (G 51%, B 58%; p<0.001). No significant differences were found between the two groups [23].

In a randomized study the effects of daily treatment with 600 mg of standardized garlic powder (1.3% alliin) or 1.98 mg of garlic oil were compared in 80 patients with mild hypercholesterolaemia. After 4 months of treatment total cholesterol had decreased by 11% in the garlic powder group (p<0.001) and by 3% in the garlic oil group. LDL-cholesterol was reduced by 16% in the garlic powder group (p<0.001) and by 1% in the garlic oil group (intergroup comparison: total cholesterol, not significant; LDL-cholesterol, p<0.001) [22].

Placebo-controlled studies
In a randomized, double-blind, placebo-controlled study the effect of standardized garlic powder tablets (1.3% alliin) was investigated in 261 patients with hyperlipidaemia (initial cholesterol: verum 266, placebo 262 mg/dl). The patients received 800 mg of garlic powder or placebo daily for 16 weeks. In the garlic group mean serum total cholesterol levels dropped by 12% (p<0.001) and triglyceride values by 17% (p<0.001); both results were significant (p<0.001) compared to placebo treatment. A subgroup analysis revealed better results in patients with increased initial lipid levels [26].

In a randomized, double-blind, placebo-controlled study, 42 patients with mild hypercholesterolaemia (serum total cholesterol: verum 262, placebo 276 mg/dl) were treated with 900 mg of standardized garlic powder (1.3% alliin) or placebo daily for 12 weeks. In the garlic group serum total cholesterol decreased by 6% (p<0.01 vs. baseline and placebo) compared to 1% in the placebo group and LDL-cholesterol by 11% (p<0.05 vs. baseline and placebo) compared to 3% in the placebo group [24].

In a randomized, double-blind, placebo-controlled study, 46 patients with mild hypercholesterolaemia (6.5 mmol/dl) were assigned to one of four daily treatments: group I, 900 mg of standardized garlic powder (1.3% alliin); group II, 12 g of fish oil; group III, 12 g of fish oil + 900 mg of standardized garlic powder; group IV, placebo. After 3 weeks of treatment the changes in serum total cholesterol and LDL-cholesterol respectively were: group I, −11.5% and −14.2%; group II, 0% and + 8.8%; group III, −12.2% and −9.5%; group IV, 4.5% and −1.4%. The differences in groups I and III were significant (p<0.01) compared to those in groups II and IV [17].

In a randomized, double-blind study 52 patients with hypercholesterolaemia were treated with 900 mg of standardized garlic powder (1.3% alliin) or placebo daily for 6 months. Baseline serum total cholesterol levels were 6.92 mmol/litre in the garlic group and 7.05 mmol/litre in the placebo group. Serum total cholesterol and LDL-cholesterol respectively decreased by 9% (p<0.01 vs. baseline, p<0.05 vs. placebo) and 10% (p<0.05 vs. baseline) in the verum group and by 4% and 6% in the placebo group [21].

In a randomized, double-blind study 40 patients with moderate hypertension (systolic and diastolic blood pressure 178 and 100 mmHg) and hypercholesterolaemia (280 mg/dl) received 600 mg of standardized garlic powder (1.3% alliin) or placebo daily. After 12 weeks serum total cholesterol had decreased by 10% (p<0.05) and triglycerides by 8% (p<0.05); no changes were observed in the placebo group [25].

In a randomized, double-blind study, 40 patients with hypercholesterolaemia received 900 mg of standardized garlic powder (1.3% alliin) or placebo daily. After 16 weeks of treatment, serum total cholesterol had decreased by 21% in the verum group and 3% in the placebo group (intergroup difference p<0.001). Serum triglycerides decreased by 24% in the verum group and 3% in the placebo group (p<0.05) [28].

In a randomized, double-blind study 23 patients with coronary artery disease (determined by selective coronaroangiography) received 900 mg of standardized garlic powder (1.3% alliin) or placebo daily. Initial serum total cholesterol levels were 218 mg/dl in the verum group and 219 mg/dl in the placebo group. After 3 weeks of treatment HDL-cholesterol had increased by 16% in the verum group (p<0.05); total cholesterol and triglycerides remained unchanged [14].

In a randomized, double-blind study, 80 patients with peripheral arterial occlusive disease (determined by angiography) were assigned to treatment with 800 mg of standardized garlic powder (1.3% alliin) or placebo daily for 12 weeks. Initial serum total cholesterol levels of 266.5 and 264.4 mg/dl in the verum and placebo groups respectively decreased by 12% and 4% (intergroup comparison p<0.011) [10].

In a randomized, double-blind study the effects of 600 mg of standardized garlic powder (1.3% alliin) or placebo daily for 12 weeks were compared in 47 patients with mild hypertension. The baseline serum total cholesterol level of 268 mg/dl decreased by 14% in the garlic group (p<0.05 vs. baseline) and 6% in the placebo group (not significant). Serum triglycerides decreased by 18% in the garlic group (p<0.05) and 6% in the placebo group (not significant) [18].

Placebo-controlled studies with combined diet
After 8 weeks on an NCEP Step I diet (8-10% of calories from saturated fat, not more than 30% of calories from total fat and less than 300 mg of cholesterol per day), the effects of 900 mg of standardized garlic powder (1.3% alliin) or placebo daily for 12 weeks were compared in a randomized, double-blind study in 50 patients with hyperlipidaemia (initial serum total cholesterol: garlic group 274 mg/dl, placebo group 250 mg/dl). The diet was maintained during the course of study. No intergroup differences were observed in serum total cholesterol or LDL-cholesterol [88].

Over 1200 patients with hypercholesterolaemia embarked on an NCEP Step I diet. After 6 weeks, 115 patients who had not responded to the diet (serum total cholesterol 6.0-8.0 mmol/dL) maintained the diet and were enrolled in a randomized, double-blind study, assigned to 900 mg of standardized garlic powder (1.3% alliin) or placebo daily for 6 months. The baseline serum total cholesterol levels were 6.96 and 6.99 mmol/litre in the garlic and placebo groups respectively. At the end of this study there were no intra- nor inter-group differences in lipid parameters [83].

In a randomized, double-blind, crossover study (2 × 12 weeks, with a wash-out period of 4 weeks) 30 patients with hypercholesterolaemia (serum total cholesterol 6.72 mmol/litre) were treated with 900 mg of standardized garlic powder (1.3% alliin) or placebo daily. All patients maintained an NCEP Step I diet during the study. No effects on serum lipids were observed [89].

After following an NCEP Step II diet (not more than 7% of calories from saturated fat, not more than 30% of calories from total fat and less than 200 mg of cholesterol per day) for 6 months, 30 children with primary familial hypercholesterolaemia participated in a randomized, double-blind study and were assigned to 900 mg of standardized garlic powder (1.3% alliin) or placebo daily for 8 weeks. Baseline serum total cholesterol levels were 6.66 and 7.06 mmol/litre in the garlic and placebo groups respectively. No effects on serum lipid levels were observed except for a 10% increase in apolipoprotein A-I in the garlic group (p = 0.03) [90].

In a randomized, double-blind study, 35 renal transplant patients with serum total cholesterol levels

of 290 mg/dl followed an NCEP Step I diet and were also treated with 1.36 g of an undefined garlic preparation (equivalent to 4 mg of allicin daily) or placebo daily for 12 weeks. After 6 and 12 weeks of treatment serum total cholesterol decreased by 5% in the garlic group (p<0.05) while serum levels in the placebo group remained unchanged. Serum triglycerides increased by 7.5% (not significant) and HDL-cholesterol decreased by 5% (not significant) in the garlic group, while in the placebo group these parameters changed by +17.3% (p<0.05) and −6% (p<0.05) respectively [91].

After following an American Heart Association Step I diet for at least 2 weeks (and maintaining it during the course of study), 50 patients with moderate hypercholesterolaemia (LDL subclass pattern A or B; mean serum LDL cholesterol 166 mg/dl) participated in a randomized, double-blind study, taking 900 mg of standardized garlic powder (1.3% alliin) or placebo daily for 3 months. At the end of the study no significant changes were observed in lipid parameters [92].

Open studies
In an open study 917 volunteers with hypercholesterolaemia (serum total cholesterol 262 mg/dl) following a cholesterol and fat-reduced diet were treated with 600 mg of standardized garlic powder (1.3% alliin) daily for 6-8 weeks. Serum total cholesterol decreased by 2.3% (p<0.01) [29].

In an open study 20 patients with hyperlipoproteinaemia type IV (n = 5) and hypercholesterolaemia (n = 15) were treated daily for 4 weeks with 600 mg of garlic powder. The initial average serum total cholesterol of 278 mg/dl decreased by 7.2% (p<0.01) [8].

In an open study 1873 patients with hyperlipidaemia (serum total cholesterol > 200 mg/dl or elevated triglycerides) were treated with 900 mg of standardized garlic powder (1.3% alliin) for 16 weeks. Initial average serum total cholesterol of 290 mg/dl decreased by 16.4% (p<0.0001), LDL-cholesterol by 15.1% (p<0.0001) and triglycerides by 21% (p<0.0001); HDL-cholesterol increased by 9.4% (p<0.0001) [19].

In an open study 1024 patients with hyperlipidaemia (initial serum total cholesterol 297 mg/dl) took 600-900 mg of standardized garlic powder (corresponding to 3-6 mg of allicin) for 16 weeks. Serum total cholesterol decreased by 15.8%, LDL-cholesterol by 13.3% and triglycerides by 13.7%; HDL-cholesterol increased by 14.3% [20].

In an open study 44 patients with hyperlipidaemia (serum total cholesterol 298 mg/dl, triglycerides > 200 mg/dl) were treated with 1.2 g of standardized garlic powder (1.3% alliin) for 18 weeks. Serum total cholesterol decreased by 11.3% (p<0.001), LDL-cholesterol by 15.7% (p = 0.003) and triglycerides by 13%; HDL-cholesterol increased by 19.9% [27].

Prophylaxis of atherosclerosis
Patients homogenous in all demographic data except age (verum > placebo, p<0.001), with advanced atherosclerotic plaques (measured by ultrasound in the carotid bifurcation and/or femoral arteries) and at least one risk factor (high systolic blood pressure, hypercholesterolaemia, diabetus mellitus, smoking), participated in a randomized, double-blind, placebo-controlled study. They were assigned to treatment with 900 mg of standardized garlic powder (1.3% alliin; n = 140) or placebo (n = 140) daily for 48 months; 152 patients (61 in the garlic group and 91 in the placebo group) completed the study; 38% of patients in the verum group discontinued because of annoyance with odour. In the remaining patients plaque volume decreased by 2.6% in the verum group and increased by 15.6% in the placebo group. The strongest effects (in both directions) were observed in women. There was a strong correlation (p<0.0001) of inhibition of the increase in plaque volume with increasing age [12].

In a randomized study over a period of 3 years, 432 patients who had suffered myocardial infarction were assigned to an oily extract of garlic (n = 222) or placebo (n = 210) daily in addition to other necessary medication. Significant reductions in the non-fatal reinfarction rate (44%; p<0.001) and mortality (31%; p<0.01) were observed in patients taking the oily extract of garlic compared to those taking placebo [7].

Pharmacokinetic properties
The absorption and excretion of orally administered radioactively-labelled ^{35}S-alliin, allicin and vinyl-dithiine were studied in rats. Alliin was absorbed and eliminated much faster than the other compounds. After administration of ^{35}S-alliin at 8 mg/kg body weight maximum blood concentration was reached after 10 minutes (allicin 30-60 minutes, vinyldithiine 120 minutes). The excretion of alliin equivalents was mainly renal [93].

The metabolism of allicin was analyzed in perfusion experiments using isolated rat liver. Allicin could be identified after passage through the liver only after administration of high doses (1.2 mg allicin/minute). After administration of 400 µg allicin/minute 95% was metabolized after the first passage through the liver; in this case allicin metabolites such as diallyl disulphide and allyl mercaptan were found in the liver and gall bladder [94].

S-allylcysteine orally administered to rats, mice and dogs was rapidly and easily absorbed, and distributed mainly in plasma, liver and kidney; the bioavailability

was 98.2% in rats, 103.0% in mice and 87.2% in dogs. It was mainly excreted in the urine as the N-acetyl metabolite in rats, while mice excreted both unchanged and N-acetyl forms [95].

Preclinical safety data

Acute toxicity
The intravenous LD_{50} of allicin in mice was determined as 60 mg/kg; when administered subcutaneously the LD_{50} was 120 mg/kg [60].

Other investigators, using various non-standardized garlic extracts, reported the lowest oral LD_{50} value in rats and mice as 30 ml/kg for a 14.5% ethanolic extract from fresh bulbs [96].

Repeated dose toxicity
Fresh garlic juice orally administered to rats at 5 ml/kg body weight daily for 3 weeks resulted in reduced weight gain, gastric mucosal damage and, in some cases, death of the animals [97].

Daily administration of a raw garlic extract to rats at 200 mg/kg body weight for 4 weeks resulted in weight loss and a fall in serum protein levels [98].

Mutagenicity
The genotoxicity of orally administered garlic was assessed using the micronucleus test in mice; compared to controls no significant changes were found in the bone marrow cells [99]. No mutagenicity was evident in the Ames test [100].

Teratogenicity
No data available.

Clinical safety data
In published studies involving consumption of up to 1.2 g of garlic powder daily, garlic odour was the typical and most common side effect of garlic intake. The incidence might be as much as 50%; however, this effect is not considered to be adverse. Common side effects were gastrointestinal discomfort and in rare cases allergic reactions.

In healthy volunteers 10 g of raw garlic consumed daily for 2 months induced no adverse events [80].

Daily administration of high doses of garlic oil (approx. 120 mg, equivalent to 60 g/day fresh garlic) over a period of 3 months did not result in any toxic effects or adverse events [101].

In 3 cases reduced platelet aggregation and prolonged bleeding time have been reported after intake of raw garlic or garlic powder [33,102,103].

REFERENCES

1. Garlic Powder - Allii sativi bulbi pulvis. European Pharmacopoeia. Council of Europe.

2. Sticher O. Beurteilung von Knoblauchpräparaten. Dtsch Apoth Ztg 1991;131:403-13.

3. Koch HP, Lawson LD, editors. Garlic - The science and therapeutic application of *Allium sativum* L. and related species. 2nd ed. Baltimore-Philadelphia-London: Williams & Wilkins, 1996.

4. Block E. The chemistry of garlic and onions. Sci Am 1985;252:114-9.

5. Block E. Die Organoschwefelchemie der Gattung *Allium* und ihre Bedeutung für die organische Chemie des Schwefels. Angew Chem 1992;104:1158-203. *Translated into English as:* The organosulfur chemistry of the genus *Allium*: implications for the organic chemistry of sulfur. Angew Chem Int Ed Engl 1992;31:1135-78.

6. Lawson LD. Bioactive organosulfur compounds of garlic and garlic products: role in reducing blood lipids. In: Kinghorn AD, Balandrin MF, editors. Human Medicinal Agents from Plants. ACS Symp Ser 534. Washington DC: American Chemical Society, 1993: 306-30.

7. Bordia A. Knoblauch und koronare Herzkrankheit. Wirkungen einer dreijährigen Behandlung mit Knoblauchextrakt auf die Reinfarkt- und Mortalitäts-rate. Dtsch Apoth Ztg 1989;129:(Suppl 15):16-7.

8. Harenberg J, Giese C, Zimmermann R. Effect of dried garlic on blood coagulation, fibrinolysis, platelet aggregation and serum cholesterol levels in patients with hyperlipoproteinemia. Atherosclerosis 1988;74:247-9.

9. Kiesewetter H, Jung EM, Mrowietz C, Koscielny J, Wenzel E. Effect of garlic on platelet aggregation in patients with increased risk of juvenile ischaemic attack. Eur J Clin Pharmacol 1993;45:333-6.

10. Kiesewetter H, Jung F, Jung EM, Blume J, Mrowietz C, Birk A et al. Effects of garlic coated tablets in peripheral arterial occlusive disease. Clin Invest 1993;71:383-6.

11. Kiesewetter H, Jung F, Pindur G, Jung EM, Mrowietz C, Wenzel E. Effect of garlic on thrombocyte aggregation, microcirculation and other risk factors. Int J Clin Pharmacol Ther Toxicol 1991;29:151-5.

12. Koscielny J, Klüßendorf D, Latza R, Schmitt R, Radtke H, Siegel G, Kiesewetter H. The antiatherosclerotic effect of *Allium sativum*. Atherosclerosis 1999;144:237-49.

13. Orekhov AN, Grünwald J. Effects of garlic on atherosclerosis. Nutrition 1997;13:656-63.

14. Orekhov AN, Pivovarova EM, Tertov VV. Garlic powder tablets reduce atherogenicity of low density lipoprotein. A placebo-controlled double-blind study. Nutr Metab Cardiovasc Dis 1996;6:21-31.

15. Orekhov AN, Tertov VV, Sobenin IA, Pivovarova EM. Direct anti-atherosclerosis–related effects of garlic. Ann Med 1995;27:63-5.

16. Reuter HD. Spektrum *Allium sativum* L., 2nd ed. Basel: Aesopus Verlag, 1991.

17. Adler AJ, Holub BJ. Effect of garlic and fish-oil supplementation on serum lipid and lipoprotein concentrations in hypercholesterolemic men. Am J Clin Nutr 1997;65:445-50.

18. Auer W, Eiber A, Hertkorn E, Hoehfeld E, Koehrle U, Lorenz A et al. Hypertension and hyperlipidaemia: garlic helps in mild cases. Br J Clin Pract 1990;44(Suppl 69):3-6.

19. Beck E, Grünwald J. Allium sativum in der Stufen-therapie der Hyperlipidämie. Med Welt 1993;44:516-20.

20. Brewitt B, Lehmann B. Lipidregulierung durch standardisierte Naturarzneimittel. Multizentrische Langzeitstudie an 1209 Patienten. Der Kassenarzt 1991;5:47-55.

21. De A Santos OS, Grünwald J. Effect of garlic powder tablets on blood lipids and blood pressure - a six month placebo controlled double blind study. Br J Clin Res 1993;4:37-44.

22. De A Santos OS, Johns RA. Effects of garlic powder and garlic oil preparations on blood lipids, blood pressure and well-being. Br J Clin Res 1995;6:91-100.

23. Holzgartner H, Schmidt U, Kuhn U. Comparison of the efficacy and tolerance of a garlic preparation vs. bezafibrate. Arzneim-Forsch/Drug Res 1992;42:1473-7.

24. Jain AK, Vargas R, Gotzkowsky S, McMahon FG. Can garlic reduce levels of serum lipids? A controlled clinical study. Am J Med 1993;94:632-5.

25. Kandziora J. Blutdruck- und lipidsenkende Wirkung eines Knoblauch-Präparates in Kombination mit einem Diuretikum. Ärztl Forsch 1988;35:1-8.

26. Mader FH. Treatment of hyperlipidaemia with garlic-powder tablets. Evidence from the German Association of General Practitioners' multicentric placebo-controlled double-blind study. Arzneim-Forsch/Drug Res 1990;40:1111-6.

27. Rinneberg AL, Lehmann B. Therapie der Hyperlipo-proteinämie mit einem standardisierten Knoblauch-pulver-Arzneimittel. Der Kassenarzt 1989;45:40-7.

28. Vorberg G, Schneider B. Therapy with garlic: results of a placebo-controlled, double-blind study. Br J Clin Pract 1990;44(Suppl 69):7-11.

29. Walper A, Rassoul F, Purschwitz K, Schulz V. Effizienz einer Diätempfehlung und einer zusätzlichen Phyto-therapie mit *Allium sativum* bei leichter bis mäßiger Hypercholesterinämie. Medwelt 1994;45:327-32.

30. Allium. In: British Herbal Pharmacopoeia 1983.

Bournemouth: British Herbal Medicine Association, 1983:20-1.

31. Bradley PR, editor. Garlic. In: British Herbal Compendium. Volume 1. Bournemouth: British Herbal Medicine Association, 1992:105-8.

32. Tsai Y, Cole LL, Davis LE, Lockwood SJ, Simmons V, Wild GC. Antiviral properties of garlic: *in vitro* effects on influenza B, Herpes simplex and Coxsackie viruses. Planta Med 1985;51:460-1.

33. German K, Kumar U, Blackford HN. Garlic and the risk of TURP bleeding. Br J Urol 1995;76:518.

34. Sunter W. Warfarin and garlic. Pharm J 1991;246:722.

35. Mennella JA, Beauchamp GK. Maternal diet alters the sensory qualities of human milk and the nursling's behavior. Pediatrics 1991;88:737-44.

36. Siegers C-P. Toxicology, side effects and allergenicity. In: Symposium on the chemistry, pharmacology and medical applications of garlic. Lüneburg, Germany, 23-25 February 1989. Cardiology in Practice 1989; September (Suppl):14-5.

37. Quereshi AA, Abiurmeileh N, Din ZZ, Elson CE, Burger WC. Inhibition of cholesterol and fatty acid bio-synthesis in liver enzymes and chicken hepatocytes by polar fractions of garlic. Lipids 1983;18:343-8.

38. Gebhardt R, Beck H, Wagner KG. Inhibition of cholesterol biosynthesis by allicin and ajoene in rat hepatocytes and HepG2 cells. Biochim Biophys Acta 1994;1213:57-62.

39. Gebhardt R. Inhibition of cholesterol biosynthesis by a water-soluble garlic extract in primary cultures of rat hepatocytes. Arzneim-Forsch/Drug Res 1991;41:800-4.

40. Gebhardt R. Multiple inhibitory effects of garlic extracts on cholesterol biosynthesis in hepatocytes. Lipids 1993;28:613-9.

41. Yeh YY, Yeh S-M. Garlic reduces plasma lipids by inhibiting hepatic cholesterol and triacylglycerol synthesis. Lipids 1994;29:189-93.

42. Siegel G, Emden J, Schnalke F, Walter A, Rückborn K, Wagner KG. Wirkungen von Knoblauch auf die Gefäßregulation. Med Welt 1991;42(Suppl 7a):32-4.

43. Siegel G, Walter A, Schnalke F, Rückborn K, Emden J, Wagner KG. Knoblauch und Senkung des Gefäßtonus. Vasomed 1992;4:8-12.

44. Siegel G, Nuck R, Schnalke F, Michel F. Molecular evidence for phytopharmacological K+ channel opening by garlic in human vascular smooth muscle cell membranes. Phytother Res 1998;12:S149-S151.

45. Öztürk Y, Aydin S, Kosar M, Hüsnü Can Baser K. Endothelium-dependent and independent effects of garlic on rat aorta. J Ethnopharmacol 1994;44:109-16.

46. Das I, Khan NS, Sooranna SR. Potent activation of nitric oxide synthase by garlic: a basis for its therapeutic applications. Curr Med Res Opin 1995;13:257-63.

47. Sooranna S, Hirani J, Khan N, Das I. Garlic and nitric oxide metabolism: the implications during pregnancy. Eur J Clin Res 1996;8:22-3.

48. Lawson LD, Ransom DK, Hughes BG. Inhibition of whole blood platelet aggregation by compounds in garlic clove extracts and commercial garlic products. Thromb Res 1992;65:141-56.

49. Bordia A, Verma SK, Srivastava KC. Effect of garlic (*Allium sativum*) on blood lipids, blood sugar, fibrinogen and fibrinolytic activity in patients with coronary artery disease. Prostagland Leukotr Essent Fatty Acids 1998; 58:257-63.

50. Rekka EA, Kourounakis PN. Investigation of the molecular mechanism of the antioxidant activity of some *Allium sativum* ingredients. Pharmazie 1994; 49:539-40.

51. Lewin G, Popov I. Antioxidant effects of aqueous garlic extract. 2nd communication: inhibition of the Cu^{2+}-initiated oxidation of low density lipoproteins. Arzneim-Forsch/Drug Res 1994;44:604-7.

52. Popov I, Blumstein A, Lewin G. Antioxidant effects of aqueous garlic extract. 1st communication: direct detection using the photochemiluminescence. Arzneim-Forsch/Drug Res 1994;44:602-4.

53. Imai J, Ide N, Nagae S, Moriguchi T, Matsuura H, Itakura Y. Antioxidant and radical scavenging effects of aged garlic extract and its constituents. Planta Med 1994;60:417-20.

54. Siegers CP, Röbke A, Pentz R. Effects of garlic preparations on superoxide production by phorbol ester activated granulocytes. Phytomedicine 1999;6: 13-6.

55. Török B, Belagyi J, Rietz B, Jacob R. Effectiveness of garlic on the radical activity in radical generating systems. Arzneim-Forsch/Drug Res 1994;44:608-11.

56. Sevendson L, Rattan SIS, Clark BFC. Testing garlic for possible anti-aging effects on long-term growth characteristics, morphology and macromolecular synthesis of human fibroblasts in culture. J Ethnopharmacol 1994;43:125-33.

57. Ali M, Thomson M. Consumption of a garlic clove a day could be beneficial in preventing thrombosis. Prostagland Leukotr Essent Fatty Acids 1995;53:211-2.

58. Mayeux PR, Agrawal KC, Tou J-SH, King BT, Lippton HL, Hyman AL et al. The pharmacological effects of allicin, a constituent of garlic oil. Agents Actions 1988;25:182-90.

59. Adetumbi MA, Lau BHS. *Allium sativum* (garlic) - a natural antibiotic. Med Hypotheses 1983;12:227-37.

60. Cavallito CJ, Bailey JH. Allicin, the antibacterial principle of *Allium sativum*. I. Isolation, physical properties and antibacterial action. J Am Chem Soc 1944;66:1950-1.

23

61. Sharma VD, Sethi MS, Kumar A, Rarotra JR. Antibacterial property of *Allium sativum* Linn.: *in vivo* & *in vitro* studies. Indian J Exp Biol 1977;15:466-8.

62. Lutomski J, Maleszka R. Mycostatic properties of garlic preparation. II. International Garlic Symposium: Pharmacy, pharmacology and clinical application of *Allium sativum*. Berlin, 7-10 March 1991.

63. Wargovich MJ. Cancer chemoprevention: organo-sulphur components of garlic. In: II. International Garlic Symposium. Pharmacy, pharmacology and clinical application of *Allium sativum*. Berlin, 7-10 March 1991. Cardiology in Practice 1991; June (Suppl):7.

64. Dorant E, van den Brandt PA, Goldbohm RA, Hermus RJJ, Sturmans F. Garlic and its significance for the prevention of cancer in humans: a critical view. Br J Cancer 1993;67:424-9.

65. Ciplea AG, Richter KD. The protective effect of *Allium sativum* and *Crataegus* on isoprenaline-induced tissue necroses in rats. Arzneim-Forsch/Drug Res 1988;38: 1583-92.

66. Isensee H, Rietz B, Jacob R. Cardioprotective actions of garlic (*Allium sativum*). Arzneim-Forsch/Drug Res 1993; 43:94-8.

67. Jacob R, Ehrsam M, Ohkubo T, Rupp H. Antihypertensive und kardioprotektive Effekte von Knoblauchpulver (*Allium sativum*). Med Welt 1991;42(Suppl 7a):39-41.

68. Lata S, Saxena KK, Bhasin V, Saxena RS, Kumar A, Srivastava VK. Beneficial effects of *Allium sativum*, *Allium cepa* and *Commiphora mukul* on experimental hyperlipidemia and atherosclerosis - a comparative evaluation. J Postgrad Med 1991;37:132-5.

69. Mand JK, Gupta PP, Soni GL, Singl R. Effect of garlic on experimental atherosclerosis in rabbits. Indian Heart J 1985;37:183-8.

70. Heinle H, Betz E. Effects of dietary garlic supplement-ation in a rat model of atherosclerosis. Arzneim-Forsch/ Drug Res 1994;44:614-7.

71. Jacob R, Isensee H, Rietz B, Makdessi S, Sweidan H. Cardioprotection by dietary interventions in animal experiments. Pharm Pharmacol Lett 1993;3:131-4.

72. Brändle M, Al Makdessi S, Weber RK, Dietz K, Jacob R. Prolongation of life span in hypertensive rats by dietary interventions. Effects of garlic and linseed oil. Basic Res Cardiol 1997;92:223-32.

73. Al-Qattan KK, Alnaqeeb MA, Ali M. The anti-hypertensive effect of garlic (*Allium sativum*) in the rat two-kidney-one-clip Goldblatt model. J Ethno-pharmacol 1999;66:217-22.

74. Nagai K. Experimental studies on preventive effect of garlic extract against infections with influenza and Japanese encephalitis viruses in mice. J Jap Assoc Infect Dis 1973;47:111-5 [Japanese].

75. Hikino H, Tohkin M, Kiso Y, Namiki T, Nishimura S, Takeyama K. Antihepatotoxic actions of *Allium sativum* bulbs. Planta Med 1986;52:163-8.

76. Nakagawa S, Kasuga S, Matsuura H. Prevention of liver damage by aged garlic extract and its components in mice. Phytotherapy Res 1989;3:50-3.

77. Jung EM, Jung F, Mrowietz C, Kiesewetter H, Pindur G, Wenzel E. Influence of garlic powder on cutaneous microcirculation. A randomized placebo-controlled double-blind cross-over study in apparently healthy subjects. Arzneim-Forsch/Drug Res 1991;41:626-30.

78. Phelps S, Harris WS. Garlic supplementation and lipoprotein oxidation susceptibility. Lipids 1993; 28:475-7.

79. Breithaupt-Grögler K, Ling M, Boudculas H, Belz GG. Protective effect of chronic garlic intake on elastic properties of aorta in the elderly. Circulation 1997; 96:2649-55.

80. Gadkari JV, Joshi VD. Effect of ingestion of raw garlic on serum cholesterol level, clotting time and fibrinolytic activity in normal subjects. J Postgrad Med 1991;37:128-31.

81. Rotzsch W, Richter V, Rassoul F, Walper A. Post-prandiale Lipämie unter Medikation von *Allium sativum*. Arzneim Forsch/Drug Res 1992;42:1223-7.

82. Saradeth T, Seidl S, Resch KL, Ernst E. Does garlic alter the lipid pattern in normal volunteers? Phytomedicine 1994;1:183-5.

83. Neil A, Silagy C, Lancaster 1, Hodgeman J, Moore JW, Jones L, Fowler GH. Garlic powder in the treatment of moderate hyperlipidaemia: a controlled trial and meta-analysis. J Royal Coll Physicians London 1996; 30:329-34.

84. Silagy C, Neil A. Garlic as a lipid lowering agent - a meta-analysis. J Royal Coll Physicians London 1994; 28:39-45.

85. Stevinson C, Pittler MH, Ernst E. Garlic for treating hypercholesterolemia. A meta-analysis of randomized clinical trials. Ann Intern Med 2000;133:420-9.

86. Warshafsky S, Kamer RS, Sivak SL. Effect of garlic on total serum cholesterol. A meta-analysis. Ann Intern Med 1993;119:599-605.

87. Silagy CA, Neil HAW. A meta-analysis of the effect of garlic on blood pressure. J Hypertension 1994; 12:463-8.

88. Isaacsohn JL, Moser M, Stein E, Dudley K, Davey JA, Liskov E, Black HR. Garlic powder and plasma lipids and lipoproteins. Arch Int Med 1998;158:1189-94.

89. Simons LA, Balasubramaniam S, von Konigsmark M, Parfitt A, Simons J, Peters W. On the effect of garlic on plasma lipids and lipoproteins in mild hyper-cholesterolaemia. Atherosclerosis 1995;113:219-25.

90. McCrindle BW, Helden E, Conner WT. Garlic extract therapy in children with hypercholesterolemia. Arch

Pediatr Adolesc Med 1998;152:1089-94.

91. Lash JP, Cardoso LR, Mesler PM, Walczak DA, Pollak R. The effect of garlic on hypercholesterolemia in renal transplant patients. Transplant Proceedings 1998;30: 189-91.

92. Superko HR, Krauss RM. Garlic powder, effect on plasma lipids, postprandial lipemia, low-density lipoprotein particle size, high-density lipoprotein subclass distribution and lipoprotein (a). J Am Coll Cardiol 2000;35:321-6.

93. Lachmann G, Radeck W. Pharmakokinetik von ^{35}S-Alliin bei Ratten. Med Welt 1991;42(Suppl 7a):48.

94. Egen-Schwind C, Eckard R, Kemper FH. Stoffwechsel von Allicin in der isoliert perfundierten Rattenleber. Hoher First-pass-Effekt von Allicin nachgewiesen. Med Welt 1991;42(Suppl 7a):49.

95. Nagae S, Ushijima M, Hatono S, Imai J, Kasuga S, Matsuura H et al. Pharmacokinetics of the garlic compound S-allylcysteine. Planta Med 1994;60:214-7.

96. Nakagawa S, Masamoto K, Sumiyoshi H, Harada H. Acute toxicity test of garlic extract (Japanese). J Toxicol Sci 1984;9:57-60.

97. Nakagawa S, Masamoto K, Sumiyoshi H, Kunihiro K, Fuwa T. Effect of raw and extracted garlic juice on growth of young rats and their organs after peroral administration (Japanese). J Toxicol Sci 1980;5:91-112.

98. Shashikanth KN, Basappa SC, Murthy VS. Effect of feeding raw and boiled garlic extracts on the growth, cecal microflora and serum proteins of albino rats. Nutr Rep Int 1986;33:313-9.

99. Abraham SK, Kesavan PC. Genotoxicity of garlic, turmeric and asafoetida in mice. Mutat Res 1984;136: 85-8.

100. Yoshida S, Hirao Y, Nakagawa S. Mutagenicity and cytotoxicity tests of garlic. J Toxicol Sci 1984;9:77-86.

101. Bordia A, Joshi HK, Sanadhya YK, Bhu N. Effect of essential oil of garlic on serum fibrinolytic activity in patients with coronary artery disease. Atherosclerosis 1978;28:155-9.

102. Burnham BE. Garlic as a possible risk for postoperative bleeding. Plastic Reconstr Surg 1995;95:213.

103. Rose KD, Croissant PD, Parliament CF, Levin MB. Spontaneous spinal epidural hematoma with associated platelet dysfunction from excessive garlic ingestion: a case report. Neurosurgery 1990;26:880-2.

ALOE
CAPENSIS
Cape Aloes

DEFINITION

Cape aloes consists of the concentrated and dried juice of the leaves of various species of *Aloe*, mainly *Aloe ferox* Miller and its hybrids. It contains not less than 18.0 per cent of hydroxyanthracene derivatives, expressed as barbaloin ($C_{21}H_{22}O_9$; M_r 418.4) and calculated with reference to the dried drug.

The material complies with the monograph of the European Pharmacopoeia [1].

CONSTITUENTS

The main active constituents are aloins A and B and 5-hydroxyaloin A, which are aloe-emodin anthrone-C-glycosides. Aloinosides A and B, which are anthrone-C- and O-glycosides, are also considered as active constituents contributing to the sum of hydroxyanthracene glycosides [2,3]. Other constituents include 2-acetonyl-5-methyl-chromones (also known as aloeresins), small quantities of 1,8-dihydroxy-anthraquinones (e.g. aloe-emodin), cinnamic acid and 1-methyl-tetralin derivatives [4-11].

CLINICAL PARTICULARS

Therapeutic indications
For short term use in cases of occasional constipation[12,13].

Posology and method of administration

Dosage
The correct individual dosage is the smallest required to produce a comfortable soft-formed motion.

Adults and children over 10 years: preparations equivalent to 10-30 mg of hydroxyanthracene derivatives, calculated as barbaloin, to be taken once daily at night [12-14].
Elderly: dose as for adults.
Not recommended for use in children under 10 years of age.
The pharmaceutical form must allow lower dosages.

Method of administration
For oral administration.

Duration of administration
Stimulant laxatives should not be used for periods of more than 2 weeks without medical advice.

E/S/C/O/P
MONOGRAPHS
Second Edition

Contra-indications

Intestinal obstruction and stenosis, atony, inflammatory colon diseases (e.g. Crohn's disease, ulcerative colitis), appendicitis; abdominal pain of unknown origin; severe dehydration states with water and electrolyte depletion [15,16].
Children under 10 years.

Special warnings and special precautions for use

As for all laxatives, aloes should not be given when any undiagnosed acute or persistent abdominal symptoms are present.

If laxatives are needed every day the cause of the constipation should be investigated. Long term use of laxatives should be avoided. Use for more than 2 weeks requires medical supervision. Chronic use may cause pigmentation of the colon (pseudo-melanosis coli) which is harmless and reversible after drug discontinuation. Abuse, with diarrhoea and consequent fluid and electrolyte losses, may cause: dependence with possible need for increased dosages; disturbance of the water and electrolyte (mainly hypokalaemia) balance; an atonic colon with impaired function. Intake of anthranoid-containing laxatives for more than a short period of time may result in aggravation of constipation. Hypokalaemia can result in cardiac and neuromuscular dysfunction, especially if cardiac glycosides, diuretics or corticosteroids are taken. Chronic use may result in albuminuria and haematuria.

In chronic constipation, stimulant laxatives are not an acceptable alternative to a change in diet [5,15-17].

Note: A detailed text with advice concerning changes in dietary habits, physical activities and training for normal bowel evacuation should be included on the package leaflet. An example is given in the booklet "Médicaments á base de plantes" published by the French health authority (Paris: Agence du Médicament, 1998).

Interaction with other medicaments and other forms of interaction

Hypokalaemia (resulting from long term laxative abuse) potentiates the action of cardiac glycosides and interacts with antiarrhythmic drugs and with drugs which induce reversion to sinus rhythm (e.g. quinidine). Concomitant use with other drugs inducing hypokalaemia (e.g. thiazide diuretics, adreno-corticosteroids and liquorice root) may aggravate electrolyte imbalance [16].

Pregnancy and lactation

Pregnancy

Experimental studies, as well as many years of experience, do not indicate undesirable or damaging effects during pregnancy or on the foetus when used at the recommended dosage [18-21]. However, in view of experimental data concerning a genotoxic risk from several anthranoids (e.g. aloe-emodin), avoid during the first trimester or take only under medical supervision.

Lactation

Breastfeeding is not recommended as there are insufficient data on the excretion of metabolites in breast milk. Small amounts of active metabolites (rhein) may appear in breast milk. However, a laxative effect in breast-fed babies has not been reported [15,22].

Effects on ability to drive and use machines

None.

Undesirable effects

Abdominal spasms and pain, in particular in patients with irritable colon; yellowish-brown or red (pH dependent) discolouration of urine by metabolites, which is not clinically significant [15,16,23,24].

Overdose

The major symptoms are griping and severe diarrhoea with consequent losses of fluid and electrolytes, which should be replaced [16]. Treatment should be supportive with generous amounts of fluid. Electrolytes, especially potassium, should be monitored; this is particularly important in the elderly and the young.

PHARMACOLOGICAL PROPERTIES

Pharmacodynamic properties

1,8-dihydroxyanthracene derivatives possess a laxative effect [25,26]. Aloins A and B, 5-hydroxyaloin A and the aloinosides A and B are precursors which are not absorbed in the upper gut. Studies in conventional and germ-free animals have established that glycosidases from the intestinal flora are responsible for the breakdown of glycosides. The ability to metabolize various anthranoids varies greatly across species depending upon the composition of intestinal flora [16,27,28]. In male rats which reacted positively to aloin A, the effect of aloins A and B has been determined with an ED_{50} of approximately 20 mg/kg [29]. In humans, anthranoid glycosides ingested orally pass into the colon unmodified. Human intestinal flora are able to break down O-glycosides easily but only to some extent C-glycosides of most anthranoids [30,31]. The main active metabolite is aloe-emodin-9-anthrone, which acts specifically on the colon [32].

There are two different mechanisms of action [33]:

(i) an influence on the motility of the large intestine (inhibition of the Na^+/K^+ pump and of Cl^- channels at the colonic membrane) resulting in accelerated colonic transit [32,34,35], and

(ii) an influence on secretion processes (stimulation of mucus and chloride secretion) resulting in enhanced fluid secretion [32,36,37].

The motility effects are mediated by direct stimulation of colonic neurons [32] and possibly by prostaglandins [38].

Defecation takes place after a delay of 6-12 hours due to the time taken for transport to the colon and metabolization into the active compound.

Pharmacokinetic properties

Aloins A and B, 5-hydroxyaloin A and aloinosides A and B pass directly into the large intestine where they are metabolized by bacterial enzymes into the active anthrone compounds.

In a human pharmacokinetic study with aloes (equivalent to 16.4 mg of hydroxyanthracene derivatives) administered orally for 7 days, aloe-emodin was detected as a metabolite in the plasma only sporadically and with maximum concentrations of less than 2 ng/ml [39]. In the same study rhein was detected in the plasma in concentrations ranging from 6-28 ng/ml (median c_{max} 13.5 ng/ml at median t_{max} 16 h) after single dose administration. In 7-day administration there was no evidence of accumulation of rhein [39].

From another study it was concluded that free anthranoids absorbed systemically in humans are partly excreted in the urine as rhein or as conjugates [40]. It is not known to what extent aloe-emodin anthrone is absorbed. However, in the case of senna, animal experiments with radio-labelled rheinanthrone administered directly into the caecum show that only a very small proportion (less than 10%) of rhein-anthrone is absorbed [41].

It has also been detected that *Eubacterium* sp. strain BAR isolated from human faeces is necessary to observe aloin A-induced diarrhoea in the rat [42]. This bacterial strain is capable of transforming aloin A into the active metabolite aloe-emodin-9-anthrone [30].

Systemic metabolism of free anthranoids depends upon their ring constituents [43,44]. In the case of aloe-emodin, it has been shown in animal experiments that at least 20-25% of an oral dose will be absorbed. The bioavailability of aloe-emodin is much lower than the absorption, because it is quickly oxidized to rhein and an unknown metabolite, or conjugated. Maximum plasma values of aloe-emodin were reached 1.5-3 hours after administration. Maximum concentrations in plasma were about 3 times higher than those in ovaries and 10 times higher than those

in testes [45].

Preclinical safety data

Aloes as crude drug or extract, as well as aloin A, showed low acute and subchronic toxicity in rats and mice after oral treatment with effective laxative dosages [18,20,46].

No specific toxicity was observed when aloes extract (up to 50 mg/kg daily for 12 weeks) and aloin A (up to 60 mg/kg daily for 20 weeks) were administered orally to mice [47,48].

There was no evidence of any embryolethal, teratogenic or foetotoxic effects in rats after oral treatment with aloes extract (up to 1000 mg/kg body weight) or aloin A (up to 200 mg/kg body weight) [18,19].

Results from *in vitro* (gene mutation and chromosome aberration) tests and *in vivo* (micronucleus test in mice bone marrow cells) genotoxicity studies, as well as human and animal pharmacokinetic data, indicate no genotoxic risk from Cape aloes [21,45,49-61].

Data on the carcinogenicity of aloes is not available. However, a standardized senna-glycoside extract which contained the putative mutagen aloe-emodin in quantities similar to the content of aloe-emodin in aloes (0.14%) showed no evidence of induced tumours in any of the tissues examined when it was given orally for 2 years to male and female rats [62]. An ethanolic fraction of Cape aloes was reported to have anti-tumour activity *in vivo* against Sarcoma 180 and Ehrlich ascites cancer cells [63].

In a 2-year study, male and female F344/N rats were exposed to 280, 830 or 2500 ppm of emodin in the diet, corresponding to an average daily dose of emodin of 110, 320 or 1000 mg/kg body weight in male rats and 120, 370 or 1100 mg/kg in female rats. No evidence of carcinogenic activity of emodin was observed in male rats. A marginal increase in the incidence of Zymbal's gland carcinoma occurred in female rats treated with the high dosage but was interpreted as questionable [64].

In a further 2-year study, on B6C3F$_1$ mice, males were exposed to 160, 312 or 625 ppm of emodin (corresponding to an average daily dose of 15, 35 or 70 mg/kg body weight) and females to 312, 625 or 1250 ppm of emodin (corresponding to an average daily dose of 30, 60 or 120 mg/kg). There was no evidence of carcinogenic activity in female mice. A low incidence of renal tubule neoplasms in exposed males was not considered relevant [64].

Clinical safety data

In a case control study with retrospective and

prospective evaluation, no causal relationship between anthranoid laxative use and colorectal cancer could be detected [65,66].

REFERENCES

1. Aloes, Cape - Aloe capensis. European Pharmacopoeia, Council of Europe.

2. Rauwald HW, Beil A. High-performance liquid chromatographic separation and determination of diasteromeric anthrone-C-glucosyls in Cape aloes. J Chromatogr 1993;639:359-62.

3. Rauwald HW, Beil A. 5-Hydroxyaloin A in the genus *Aloe*. Thin-layer chromatographic screening and high performance liquid chromatographic determination. Z Naturforsch 1993;48c:1-4.

4. Hänsel R, Keller K, Rimpler H, Schneider G, editors. Aloe. In: Hagers Handbuch der Pharmazeutischen Praxis, 5th ed. Volume 4: Drogen A-D. Berlin: Springer, 1992:209-32.

5. Steinegger E, Hänsel R. Aloe. In: Pharmakognosie, 5th ed. Berlin: Springer, 1992:428-31.

6. Speranza G, Manitto P, Cassara P, Monti D, de Castri D, Chialva F. Studies on *Aloe*, 12. Furoaloesone, a new 5-methylchromone from Cape aloe. J Nat Prod 1993; 56:1089-94.

7. Speranza G, Manitto P, Monti D, Pezzuto D. Studies on *Aloe*, Part 10. Feroxins A and B, two O-glucosylated 1-methyltetralins from Cape aloe. J Nat Prod 1992;55:723-9.

8. Speranza G, Manitto P, Monti D, Lianza F. Feroxidin, a novel 1-methyltetralin derivative isolated from Cape aloe. Tetrahedron Lett 1990;31:3077-80.

9. Speranza G, Gramatica P, Dada G, Manitto P. Aloeresin C, a bitter C,O-diglucoside from Cape aloe. Phytochemistry 1985;24:1571-3.

10. Gramatica P, Monti D, Speranza G, Manitto P. Aloe revisited. The structure of aloeresin A. Tetrahedron Lett 1982;23:2423-4.

11. Schmidt AH, Hiller KO. HPLC Determination of aloe-emodin in Aloe (article in German). GIT Fachz. Lab. 1996;40:1100-2.

12. Semler P. Über den laxierenden Effekt von Aristochol® Konzentrat Granulat. Med Welt 1975;26:2197-8.

13. USA Department of Health and Human Services: Food and Drug Administration. 21 CFR Part 334. Laxative drug products for over-the-counter human use; Tentative final monograph. Federal Register 1985; 50:2124-58.

14. Gutsche H. Langzeitbehandlung mit einem Phytocholagogum. Ärztliche Praxis 1977;29:3999-4000.

15. Reynolds JEF, editor. Martindale - The Extra Pharmacopoeia. 31st ed. London: Royal Pharmaceutical Society, 1996:1202-3,1240-1.

16. Brunton LL. Agents affecting gastrointestinal water flux and motility, emesis and antiemetics; bile acids and pancreatic enzymes In: Hardman JG, Limbird LE, Molinoff PB, Ruddon RW, Gilman AG, editors. Goodman & Gilman's The Pharmacological Basis of Therapeutics, 9th ed. New York: McGraw-Hill, 1996: 917-36.

17. Müller-Lissner S. Adverse effects of laxatives: fact and fiction. Pharmacology 1993;47(Suppl 1):138-45.

18. Bangel E, Pospisil M, Roetz R, Falk W. Tierexperimentelle pharmakologische Untersuchungen zur Frage der abortiven und teratogenen Wirkung sowie zur Hyperämie von Aloe. Steiner-Informationsdienst 1975;4:1-25.

19. Schmähl D. Henk-Pharma; Internal Report, 1975.

20. Schmidt L. Vergleichende Pharmakologie und Toxikologie der Laxantien. Arch Exper Path Pharmakol 1955;226:207-18.

21. Westendorf J. Anthranoid Derivatives - *Aloe* Species. In: De Smet PAGM, Keller K, Hänsel R, Chandler RF, editors. Adverse Effects of Herbal Drugs, Volume 2. Berlin: Springer, 1993:119-23.

22. Faber P, Strenge-Hesse A. Relevance of rhein excretion into breast milk. Pharmacology 1988;36(Suppl 1):212-20.

23. Tedesco FJ. Laxative use in constipation. Am J Gastroenterol 1985;80:303-9.

24. Ewe K, Karbach U. Factitious diarrhoea. Clin Gastroenterol 1986;15:723-40.

25. Fairbairn JW. Chemical structure, mode of action and therapeutical activity of anthraquinone glycosides. Pharm Weekblad Sci Ed 1965;100:1493-9.

26. Fairbairn JW, Moss MJR. The relative purgative activities of 1,8-dihydroxyanthracene derivatives. J Pharm Pharmacol 1970;22:584-93.

27. Dreessen M, Lemli J. Studies in the field of drugs containing anthraquinone derivatives. XXXVI. The metabolism of cascarosides by intestinal bacteria. Pharm Acta Helv 1988;63:287-9.

28. De Witte P. Metabolism and pharmacokinetics of anthranoids. Pharmacology 1993;47(Suppl 1):86-97.

29. Ishii Y, Tokino Y, Toyo'oka T, Tanizawa H. Studies of Aloe. VI. Cathartic effect of isobarbaloin. Biol Pharm Bull 1998;21:1226-7.

30. Hattori M, Kanda T, Shu YZ, Akao T, Kobashi K, Namba T. Metabolism of barbaloin by intestinal bacteria. Chem Pharm Bull 1988;36:4462-6.

31. Che QM, Akao T, Hattori M, Kobashi K, Namba T. Isolation of a human intestinal bacterium capable of transforming barbaloin to aloe-emodin anthrone. Planta Med 1991;57:15-9.

32. Ishii Y, Tanizawa H, Takino Y. Studies of Aloe. III. Mechanism of cathartic effect. (2). Chem Pharm Bull 1990;38:197-200.

33. Ewe K. Therapie der Obstipation. Dtsch Med Wschr 1989;114:1924-6.

34. Hönig J, Geck P, Rauwald HW. Inhibition of Cl⁻-channels as a possible base of laxative action of certain anthraquinones and anthrones. Planta Med 1992; 58(Suppl 1):586-7.

35. Rauwald HW, Hönig J, Flindt S, Geck P. Different influence of certain anthraquinones/anthrones on energy metabolism: An approach for interpretation of known synergistic effects in laxative action? Planta Med 1992; 58(Suppl 1):587-8.

36. Ishii Y, Tanizawa H, Takino Y. Studies of Aloe. IV. Mechanism of cathartic effect. (3). Biol Pharm Bull 1994;17:495-7.

37. Ishii Y, Tanizawa H, Takino Y. Studies of Aloe. V. Mechanism of cathartic effect. (4). Biol Pharm Bull 1994;17:651-3.

38. Capasso F, Mascolo N, Autore G, Duraccio MR. Effect of indomethacin on aloin and 1,8-dioxianthraquinone-induced production of prostaglandins in rat isolated colon. Prostaglandins 1983;26:557-62.

39. Schulz HU. Investigation into the pharmacokinetics of anthranoids after single and multiple oral administration of Laxatan® Dragees (Study in 6 healthy volunteers). Research Report, LAFAA, March 1993.

40. Vyth A, Kamp PE. Detection of anthraquinone laxatives in the urine. Pharm Weekblad Sci Ed 1979;114:456-9.

41. De Witte P, Lemli J. Excretion and distribution of [¹⁴C]rhein and [¹⁴C]rhein anthrone in rat. J Pharm Pharmacol 1988;40:652-5.

42. Akao T, Che QM, Kobashi K, Hattori M, Namba T. A purgative action of barbaloin is induced by Eubacterium sp. strain BAR, a human intestinal anaerobe, capable of transforming barbaloin to aloe-emodin anthrone. Biol Pharm Bull 1996;19:136-8.

43. De Witte P, Lemli J. Metabolism of ¹⁴C-rhein and ¹⁴C-rhein anthrone in rats. Pharmacology 1988;36(Suppl 1):152-7.

44. Sendelbach LE. A review of the toxicity and carcinogenicity of anthraquinone derivatives. Toxicology 1989;57:227-40.

45. Lang W. Pharmacokinetic-metabolic studies with ¹⁴C-aloe emodin after oral administration to male and female rats. Pharmacology 1993;47(Suppl 1):110-9.

46. Nelemans FA. Clinical and toxicological aspects of anthraquinone laxatives. Pharmacology 1976;14(Suppl 1):73-7.

47. Siegers CP, Younes M, Herbst EW. Toxikologische Bewertung anthrachinonhaltiger Laxantien. Z Phytotherapie 1986;7:157-9.

48. Siegers CP, Siemers J, Baretton G. Sennosides and aloin do not promote dimethylhydrazine-induced colorectal tumors in mice. Pharmacology 1993;47(Suppl 1):205-8.

49. Bootman J, Hodson-Walker G, Dance C. U.-No. 9482: Assessment of clastogenic action on bone marrow erythrocytes in the micronucleus test. Eye, LSR, Internal Report 1987:87/SIR 004/386.

50. Bootman J, Hodson-Walker G, Dance C. Reinsubstanz 104/5 AA (Barbaloin): Assessment of clastogenic action on bone marrow erythrocytes in the micronucleus test. Eye, LSR, Internal Report 1987:87/SIR 006/538.

51. Brown JP, Dietrich PS. Mutagenicity of anthraquinone and benzanthrone derivatives in the Salmonella/microsome test: activation of anthraquinone glycosides by enzymic extracts of rat caecal bacteria. Mutat Res 1979;66:9-24.

52. Brown JP. A review of the genetic effects of naturally occurring flavonoids, anthraquinones and related compounds. Mutat Res 1980;75:243-77.

53. Heidemann A, Miltenburger HG, Mengs U. The genotoxicity status of Senna. Pharmacology 1993; 47(Suppl 1):178-86.

54. CCR, Salmonella typhimurium reverse mutation assay with EX AL 15. Rossdorf 1992: Project No. 280416.

55. CCR, Chromosome aberration assay in Chinese hamster ovary (CHO) cells in vitro with EX AL 15. Rossdorf 1992: Project No. 280438.

56. CCR, Gene mutation assay in Chinese hamster V79 cells in vitro with EX AL 15. Rossdorf 1992: Project No. 280427.

57. Marquardt H, Westendorf J, Piasecki A, Ruge A, Westendorf B. Untersuchungen zur Genotoxizität von Bisacodyl, Sennosid A, Sennosid B, Aloin, Aloe-Extrakt. Steiner Internal Report; Hamburg 1987.

58. Morimoto I, Watanabe F, Osawa T, Okitsu T, Kada T. Mutagenicity screening of crude drugs with Bacillus subtilis rec-assay and Salmonella/microsome reversion assay. Mutat Res 1982;97:81-102.

59. Westendorf J, Poginsky B, Marquardt H, Kraus Lj, Marquardt H. Possible carcinogenicity of anthraquinone-containing medicinal plants. Planta Med 1988;54:562.

60. Westendorf J, Marquardt H, Poginsky B, Dominiak M, Schmidt J, Marquardt H. Genotoxicity of naturally occurring hydroxyanthraquinones. Mutat Res 1990; 240:1-12.

61. Wölfle D, Schmutte C, Westendorf J, Marquardt H. Hydroxyanthraquinones as tumor promoters: enhancement of malignant transformation of C3H mouse fibroblasts and growth stimulation of primary rat hepatocytes. Cancer Res 1990;50:6540-4.

62. Lydén-Sokolowski A, Nilsson A, Sjöberg P. Two-year carcinogenicity study with sennosides in the rat: emphasis on gastrointestinal alterations. Pharmacology

1993;47(Suppl 1):209-15.

63. Soeda M. Studies on the anti-tumor activity of Cape aloe. J Med Soc Toho University 1969;16:365-9.

64. NTP Technical Report 493. Toxicology and carcinogenesis studies of emodin (CAS No. 518-82-1) in F344/N rats and B6C3F$_1$ mice. NIH Publication No.

99-3952, 1999.

65. Loew D, Bergmann U, Schmidt M, Überla KH. Anthranoidlaxantien. Ursache für Kolonkarzinom? Dtsch Apoth Ztg 1994;134:3180-83.

66. Loew D. Pseudomelanosis coli durch Anthranoide. Z Phytotherapie 1994;16:312-8.

ALTHAEAE RADIX

Marshmallow Root

E/S/C/O/P
MONOGRAPHS
Second Edition

DEFINITION

Marshmallow root consists of the peeled or unpeeled, whole or cut, dried roots of *Althaea officinalis* L.

The material complies with the monograph of the European Pharmacopoeia [1].

CONSTITUENTS

Characteristic constituents of the dried root are mucilage polysaccharides (from 5% to 11% or more in biennial roots; highest in late autumn and winter) consisting of a mixture of galacturonorhamnans, arabinans, glucans and arabinogalactans [2-15], but mainly of acidic polysaccharides [13]. The mucilage can withstand temperatures of 40-60°C but not very strong sunlight [16].

Other constituents include flavone glycosides (ca. 0.2% as aglycones) [17], principally isoscutellarein 4'-methyl ether 8-glucoside-2''-sulphate and hypolaetin 8-glucoside, phenolic acids, the coumarin scopoletin [18], starch, pectin [14,15] and tannins [19].

CLINICAL PARTICULARS

Therapeutic indications
Dry cough; irritation of the oral, pharyngeal or gastric mucosa [15,20-28].

Posology and method of administration

Dosage

Adult single dose
For dry cough and oral or pharyngeal irritation, 0.5-3 g of the drug as an aqueous cold macerate [26,28], or 2-8 ml of syrup [25], repeated if required up to a daily dose equivalent to 15 g of the drug. For gastrointestinal irritation, 3-5 g as an aqueous cold macerate [26,28] up to 3 times daily.

Method of administration
For oral administration.

Duration of administration
No restriction.

Contra-indications
None known.

Special warnings and special precautions for use
None required.

Interaction with other medicaments and other forms of interaction
The absorption of other drugs taken simultaneously may be retarded [15].

Pregnancy and lactation
No data available. In accordance with general medical practice, the product should not be used during pregnancy and lactation without medical advice.

Effects on ability to drive and use machines
None known.

Undesirable effects
None reported.

Overdose
No toxic effects reported.

PHARMACOLOGICAL PROPERTIES

Pharmacodynamic properties
The mucilage from marshmallow root covers the mucosa, especially of the mouth and pharynx, protecting them from local irritation [15,20,26,27,29-31].

In vitro experiments
Mucociliary transport in isolated, ciliated epithelium of the frog oesophagus was inhibited by 17% by 200 µl of a cold, 30-minute macerate of marshmallow root (6.4 g/140 ml) [29].

Extracts of marshmallow root stimulated phagocytosis, as well as the release of oxygen radicals and leukotrienes from human neutrophils. Release of cytokines, interleukin-6 and tumour necrosis factor from monocytes was also induced by the extracts, demonstrating their potential anti-inflammatory and immunomodulatory effects [32].

An acidic polysaccharide isolated from marshmallow root, althaea-mucilage O, exhibited weak anti-complement activity (alternative route) on normal human serum at concentrations of 100-1000 µg/ml [33].

In a study of the bioadhesive effects of purified polysaccharides (> 95%) from medicinal plants on porcine buccal membranes, polysaccharides from marshmallow root showed moderate adhesion to epithelial tissue [34].

In vivo experiments

Antitussive effects
Extracts from marshmallow root and isolated mucilage polysaccharides were administered orally to cats at doses of 50 or 100 mg/kg body weight in order to investigate their antitussive effects in comparison with controls. Both the extract and isolated polysaccharides, as well as syrupus Althaeae (1000 mg/kg), significantly diminished the intensity and amount of coughing induced by mechanical irritation [35-37].

Anti-inflammatory effects
An ointment containing an aqueous marshmallow root extract (20%), applied topically to the external ear of rabbits, reduced irritation induced by ultra-violet irradiation or tetrahydrofurfuryl alcohol; the anti-inflammatory effect was less than that of an ointment containing dexamethasone (0.05%). An ointment containing both active ingredients at these levels had an anti-inflammatory effect superior to that of the individual active ingredients [38].

On the other hand, a dry 80%-ethanolic extract from marshmallow root, administered orally at 100 mg/kg body weight, did not inhibit carrageenan-induced rat paw oedema [39].

Hypolaetin 8-glucoside has been shown to possess anti-inflammatory activity [40-42]. When administered intraperitoneally at 90 mg/kg body weight, it dose-dependently inhibited carrageenan-induced rat paw oedema by 74% after 3 hours (p<0.01) compared to 49% inhibition by phenylbutazone at the same dose. The anti-inflammatory effect of hypolaetin 8-glucoside declined more rapidly than that of phenylbutazone, but did not cause gastric erosions whereas phenylbutazone was damaging [42]. Hypolaetin 8-glucoside also showed gastric anti-ulcer activity in rats [43] and was more potent than troxerutin in inhibiting histamine-induced capillary permeability in rats [41].

Hypoglycaemic activity
Mucilage polysaccharides isolated from marshmallow root and administered intraperitoneally to mice at doses of 10, 30 and 100 mg/kg reduced plasma glucose levels to 74%, 81% and 65% respectively of the control level after 7 hours, demonstrating significant hypoglycaemic activity [44].

Phagocytic activity
Isolated mucilage polysaccharides from marshmallow root, administered intraperitoneally to mice at 10 mg/kg, produced a 2.2-fold increase in phagocytic activity of macrophages in the carbon-clearance test [15,45]. This can be interpreted as a non-specific immunomodulatory effect.

Pharmacokinetic properties
No data available.

Preclinical safety data
No data available.

REFERENCES

1. Marshmallow Root - Althaeae radix. European Pharmacopoeia, Council of Europe.

2. Franz G. Die Schleimpolysaccharide von *Althaea officinalis* und *Malva sylvestris*. Planta Med 1966;14:90-110.

3. Karawya MS, Balbaa SI, Afifi MSA. Investigation of the carbohydrate contents of certain mucilaginous plants. Planta Med 1971;20:14-23.

4. Tomoda M, Kaneko S, Ebashi M, Nagakura T. Plant mucilages. XVI. Isolation and characterization of a mucous polysaccharide, "althaea-mucilage O", from the roots of *Althaea officinalis*. Chem Pharm Bull 1977;25:1357-62.

5. Tomoda M, Satoh N, Shimada K. Plant mucilages. XXIV. The structural features of althaea-mucilage O, a representative mucous polysaccharide from the roots of *Althaea officinalis*. Chem Pharm Bull 1980;28:824-30.

6. Capek P, Toman R, Kardosová A, Rosík J. Polysaccharides from the roots of the marsh mallow (*Althaea officinalis* L.): structure of an arabinan. Carbohydr Res 1983;117:133-40.

7. Akhtardzhiev K, Koleva M, Kitanov G, Ninov S. Pharmacognostic study of representatives of *Arum*, *Althaea* and *Hypericum* species. Farmatsiya (Sofia) 1984;34(3):1-6 [Bulgarian]; through Chem Abstr 1985;102:3234.

8. Rosík J, Kardosová A, Toman R, Capek P. Isolation and characterization of mucilages from *Althaea officinalis* L. and *Malva sylvestris* L. *ssp. mauritiana* (L.) Thell. Cesk Farm 1984;33:68-71.

9. Capek P, Toman R, Rosík J, Kardosová A, Janecek F. Polysaccharides from the roots of *Althaea officinalis* L.: structural features of D-glucans. Collect Czech Chem Commun 1984;49:2674-9.

10. Shimizu N, Tomoda M. Carbon-13 nuclear magnetic resonance spectra of alditol-form oligosaccharides having the fundamental structural units of the Malvaceae plant mucilages and a related polysaccharide. Chem Pharm Bull 1985;33:5539-42.

11. Capek P, Rosík J, Kardosová A, Toman R. Polysaccharides from the roots of the marsh mallow (*Althaea officinalis* L. var. Rhobusta): structural features of an acidic polysaccharide. Carbohydr Res 1987;164:443-52.

12. Capek P, Uhrín D, Rosík J, Kardosová A, Toman R, Mihálov V. Polysaccharides from the roots of the marshmallow (*Althaea officinalis* L. var. Rhobusta): dianhydrides of oligosaccharides of the aldose type. Carbohydrate Res 1988;182:160-5.

13. Madaus A, Blaschek W, Franz G. Althaeae radix mucilage polysaccharides, isolation, characterization and stability [Abstract]. Pharm Weekblad Sci Ed 1987;9:239.

14. Evans WC. Marshmallow root. In: Trease and Evans' Pharmacognosy, 14th ed. London-Philadelphia: WB Saunders, 1996:216.

15. Hänsel R, Keller K, Rimpler H, Schneider G. editors. Althaea. In: Hagers Handbuch der Pharmazeutischen Praxis, 5th ed. Volume 4: Drogen A-D. Berlin-Heidelberg: Springer-Verlag, 1992:233-9.

16. Franz G, Madaus A. Stabilität von Polysacchariden. Untersuchungen am Beispiel des Eibischschleims. Dtsch Apoth Ztg 1990;130:2194-9.

17. Gudej J. Oznaczanie flawonoidów w lisciach, kwiatach i korzeniach Althaea officinalis L. [Determination of flavonoids in leaves, flowers and roots of *Althaea officinalis* L.] Farm Polska 1990;46:153-5

18. Gudej J. Flavonoids, phenolic acids and coumarins from the roots of *Althaea officinalis*. Planta Med 1991;57:284-5

19. Bieloszabska FW, Czucha K. Does radix althea contain tannins? Farm Polska 1966;22:173-6 [Polish]; through Chem Abstr 1966;65:8671.

20. Weiss RF. *Althaea officinalis*, Eibisch. In: Lehrbuch der Phytotherapie, 7th ed. Stuttgart: Hippokrates Verlag, 1991;258-9.

21. Bone K. Marshmallow soothes cough. Brit J Phytotherapy 1993/4;3;93.

22. Ninov S, Ionkova I, Kolev D. Constituents of *Althaea officinalis* var. "Russalka" roots. Fitoterapia 1992;63:474.

23. Barnes J, Anderson LA and Phillipson JD. Marshmallow. In: Herbal Medicines - A guide for healthcare professionals, 2nd ed. London-Chicago: Pharmaceutical Press, 2002:331-2.

24. Sweetman SC, editor. Althaea. In: Martindale - The complete drug reference, 33rd ed. London: Pharmaceutical Press, 2002:1577.

25. Pharmaceutical Society of Great Britain. Syrupus Althaeae. In: British Pharmaceutical Codex 1949. London: Pharmaceutical Press, 1949.

26. Wichtl M. Althaeae radix - Eibischwurzel. In: Wichtl M, editor. Teedrogen und Phytopharmaka. Ein Handbuch für die Praxis auf wissenschaftlicher Grundlage. 4th ed. Stuttgart: Wissenschaftliche Verlagsgesellschaft, 2002:32-3.

27. Braun H (revised Frohne D). *Althaea officinalis* L. - Eibisch. In: Heilpflanzen-Lexikon für Ärzte und Apotheker, 5th ed. Stuttgart-New York: Gustav Fischer, 1987:14-5.

28. Marshmallow root. In: Bradley PR, editor. British Herbal Compendium, Volume 1. Bournemouth: British Herbal Medicine Association, 1992:151-3.

29. Müller-Limmroth W, Fröhlich H-H. Wirkungsnachweis einiger phytotherapeutischer Expektorantien auf den mukoziliären Transport. Fortschr Med 1980;98:95-101.

30. Meyer E. Behandlung akuter und chronischer Bronchitiden mit Heilpflanzen. Therapiewoche 1956;6:537-40.

31. Franz G. Polysaccharides in pharmacy: current applications and future concepts. Planta Med 1989; 55:493-7.

32. Scheffer J, König W. Einfluß von Radix althaeae und Flores chamomillae Extrakten auf Entzündungsreaktionen humaner neutrophiler Granulozyten, Monozyten und Rattenmastzellen. In: Abstracts of 3. Phytotherapie-Kongreß, Lübeck-Travemünde, 3-6 October 1991 (Abstract P9).

33. Yamada H, Nagai T, Cyong J-C, Otsuka Y, Tomoda M, Shimizu N, Shimada K. Relationship between chemical structure and anti-complementary activity of plant polysaccharides. Carbohydrate Res 1985;144:101-11.

34. Schmidgall J, Schnetz E, Hensel A. Evidence for bio-adhesive effects of polysaccharides and polysaccharide-containing herbs in an ex vivo bioadhesion assay on buccal membranes. Planta Med 2000;66:48-53.

35. Nosal'ová G, Strapková A, Kardosová A, Capek P, Zathurecky L, Bukovská E. Antitussive Wirkung des Extraktes und der Polysaccharide aus Eibisch (Althaea officinalis L. var. robusta). Pharmazie 1992;47:224-6.

36. Nosál'ová G et al. Antitussive activity of an alpha-D-glucan isolated from the roots of Althaea officinalis L. var. robusta. Pharm. Pharmacol. Lett. 1992;2:195-7.

37. Nosál'ová G, Strapková A, Kardosová A, Capek P. Antitussive activity of a rhamnogalacturonan isolated from the roots of Althaea officinalis L. var. robusta. J Carbohydr Chem 1993;12:589-96.

38. Beaune A, Balea T. Propriétés expérimentales anti-inflammatoires de la guimauve; son action potentialisatrice sur l'activité locale des corticoides. Thérapie 1966;21:341-7.

39. Mascolo N, Autore G, Capasso F, Menghini A, Fasulo MP. Biological screening of Italian medicinal plants for anti-inflammatory activity. Phytotherapy Res 1987;1:28-31.

40. Alcaraz MJ, Moroney M, Hoult JRS. Effects of hypolaetin-8-O-glucoside and its aglycone in in vivo and in vitro tests for anti-inflammatory agents. Planta Med 1989; 55:107-8.

41. Villar A, Gascó MA, Alcaraz MJ. Some aspects of the inhibitory activity of hypolaetin-8-glucoside in acute inflammation. J Pharm Pharmacol 1987;39:502-7.

42. Villar A, Gascó MA, Alcaraz MJ. Anti-inflammatory and anti-ulcer properties of hypolaetin-8-glucoside, a novel plant flavonoid. J Pharm Pharmacol 1984;36:820-3.

43. Alcaraz MJ, Tordera M. Studies on the gastric anti-ulcer activity of hypolaetin-8-glucoside. Phytother Res 1988;2:85-8.

44. Tomoda M, Shimizu N, Oshima Y, Takahashi M, Murakami M, Hikino H. Hypoglycemic activity of twenty plant mucilages and three modified products. Planta Med 1987;53:8-12.

45. Wagner H, Proksch A. Immunostimulatory drugs of fungi and higher plants. In: Wagner H, Hikino H, Farnsworth NR, editors. Economic and Medicinal Plant Research. Volume 1. London: Academic Press, 1985: 113-53.

ANISI FRUCTUS

Aniseed

E/S/C/O/P
MONOGRAPHS
Second Edition

DEFINITION

Aniseed consists of the whole dry cremocarp of *Pimpinella anisum* L. It contains not less than 20 ml/kg of essential oil.

The material complies with the monograph of the European Pharmacopoeia [1].

CONSTITUENTS

The essential oil (2-6%) contains predominantly *trans*-anethole (80-95%) with smaller amounts of estragole, *cis*-anethole, anisaldehyde and pseudoisoeugenyl-2-methylbutyrate [2-5]; sesquiterpene and mono-terpene hydrocarbons are also present [3,5].

Other constituents include flavonol glycosides [6,7], phenolic acids [8-10], a phenolic glucoside [11,12], furocoumarins [13,14], hydroxycoumarins [2] and fixed oil [14].

CLINICAL PARTICULARS

Therapeutic indications
Dyspeptic complaints such as mild spasmodic gastro-intestinal complaints, bloating, flatulence [2,15-20]. Catarrh of the upper respiratory tract [2,15-20].

Posology and method of administration

Dosage

Adult average daily dose: 3 g of crushed fruits as an infusion or similar preparation [15,17].
Children, average daily dose: 0-1 year of age, 0.5 g of crushed fruits as an infusion; *1-4 years of age*, 1 g; *4-10 years of age*, 2 g; *10-16 years of age*, the adult dose [21].

Method of administration
For oral administration.

Duration of administration
No restriction.
If symptoms persist, consult your doctor.

Contra-indications
Persons with known sensitivity to anethole should avoid aniseed.

Special warnings and special precautions for use
Persons with known sensitivity to anethole should

avoid aniseed [22-25]. The sensitizing potential of aniseed is considered low [26].

Interaction with other medicaments and other forms of interaction
None known. Experimental data on weak enzyme induction in rodents cannot be directly extrapolated to man [27].

Pregnancy and lactation
Aniseed may be used during pregnancy and lactation at the recommended dosage, as aqueous infusions only.

Preparations containing the essential oil [28] or alcoholic extracts should not be used during pregnancy and lactation. Mild oestrogenic activity and antifertility effects of anethole (the major constituent of the essential oil) have been demonstrated in rats [29].

Effects on ability to drive and use machines
None known.

Undesirable effects
Rare cases of contact dermatitis caused by anethole-containing toothpastes and cosmetic creams [24,25].

Overdose
No toxic effects reported [22].

PHARMACOLOGICAL PROPERTIES

Note: The European Pharmacopoeia monograph for Anise Oil permits oils obtained by steam distillation from the fruits of *Pimpinella anisum* L. (aniseed) or *Illicium verum* L. (star anise). *Trans*-anethole is the predominant component of both oils, but the other components are not identical. The term 'anise oil' is therefore avoided in the following text and the terms 'essential oil' or 'oil' refer specifically to essential oil from aniseed.

Pharmacodynamic properties
The medicinal use of aniseed is largely based on the secretolytic, antispasmodic and secretomotor effects of its essential oil [2].

In vitro experiments

Antimicrobial effects
An acetone extract of aniseed inhibited the growth of a range of bacteria including *Escherichia coli* and *Staphylococcus aureus,* and also exhibited antifungal activity against *Candida albicans* and other organisms [30].

Essential oil of aniseed inhibited the growth of *Escherichia coli* (MIC: 0.5% V/V), *Staphylococcus aureus* (MIC: 0.25%), *Salmonella typhimurium* (MIC:

2.0%) and *Candida albicans* (MIC: 0.5%) using the agar dilution method [31]. Antimicrobial activity of the oil has also been demonstrated in other studies [32-34].

A methanolic dry extract of aniseed reduced the resistance of *Pseudomonas aeruginosa* to certain antibiotics when used in combination with the individual antibiotic (both the extract and antibiotic being at concentrations which did not inhibit growth when used alone; antibiotic concentrations were half their minimum inhibitory concentrations). The aniseed extract was particularly effective in combination with chloramphenicol, gentamicin, cephalexin, tetracycline or nalidixic acid against the standard strain of *P. aeruginosa*, causing almost complete inhibition of growth; it was less effective against a particularly resistant strain of *P. aeruginosa*, but inhibited growth by 74% in combination with tetracycline [35].

Secretolytic and expectorant effects
A modest increase in mucociliary transport velocity of isolated ciliated epithelium from the frog oesophagus was observed 90 seconds after application of 200 µl of an infusion from aniseed (4.6 g per 100 ml of water) [36].

Spasmolytic effects
The essential oil at 200 mg/litre produced complete relaxation of carbachol-induced contractions of isolated tracheal smooth muscle from the guinea pig. In contrast, the oil increased the contraction force in electrically-stimulated guinea pig ileal smooth muscle with an EC_{50} of 6-7 mg/litre (a positive inotropic effect) [37].

The essential oil (0.02 ml), an aqueous extract (0.6 ml, equivalent to 1.5 g of aniseed) and an ethanolic extract (0.1 ml, equivalent to 0.25 g of aniseed) exhibited relaxant effects on methacholine-induced contractions of guinea pig tracheal chains (prepared from rings of isolated tracheal smooth muscle). The bronchodilatory effects were significant ($p<0.05$, $p<0.005$, $p<0.001$ respectively) compared to those of controls (0.6 ml of saline for the essential oil and aqueous extract; 0.1 ml of ethanol for the ethanolic extract) [38].

Local anaesthetic activity
Trans-anethole concentration-dependently reduced electrically-evoked contractions of rat phrenic nerve-hemidiaphragm, by 10.3% at 10^{-3} µg/ml, by 43.9% at 10^{-2} µg/ml, by 79.7% at 10^{-1} µg/ml and by 100% at 1 µg/ml [39].

Tumour-inhibiting activity of anethole
Anethole at a concentration below 1 mM has been shown to be a potent inhibitor of tumour necrosis factor (TNF)-induced cellular responses, such as activation of nuclear factor-kappa B (NF-κB) and

other transcription factors, and also to block TNF-induced activation of the apoptotic pathway. This might explain the role of anethole in suppression of inflammation and carcinogenesis [40].

In vivo experiments

Secretolytic and expectorant effects
An emulsion of 2 drops of the essential oil, administered intragastrically to cats, caused hypersecretion of mucus in the air passages and stimulated ciliary removal of mucus (which had been inhibited by opium alkaloids) [41].

A solution of the essential oil in 12% ethanol, administered intragastrically to anaesthetised guinea pigs at 50 mg/kg body weight, induced a 3- to 6-fold increase in respiratory tract fluid during the first 2 hours after administration; even 10 mg/kg caused a 2-fold increase [42]. A similar experiment in anaesthetised rats, dosed orally with the oil at 0.0015 ml/kg, resulted in a 28% increase of respiratory tract fluid without influencing chloride concentration or density [43]. Administration of the oil vapour to anaesthetised rabbits by inhalation (in steam) dose-dependently increased the volume of respiratory secretion by 19-82%; doses added to the vaporizer were 0.7-6.5 g/kg body weight (the amount to which the animals were exposed being considerably less). However, at the highest dose level there were signs of tissue damage and a mortality rate of 20% [44].

Sedative effect
The pentobarbital-induced sleeping time of mice was prolonged by 93.5% (p<0.01) after simultaneous intraperitoneal administration of essential oil at 50 mg/kg body weight; trans-anethole gave similar results [27].

Oestrogenic activity of trans-anethole
Trans-anethole administered orally to immature female rats at 80 mg/kg body weight for 3 days significantly increased uterine weight, to 2 g/kg compared to 0.5 g/kg in controls and 3 g/kg in animals given oestradiol valerate subcutaneously at 0.1 µg/rat/day (p<0.001). The results confirmed that trans-anethole has oestrogenic activity; other experiments showed that it has no anti-oestrogenic, progestational, anti-progestational, androgenic or anti-androgenic activity [29].

Local anaesthetic activity of trans-anethole
In the rabbit conjunctival reflex test, solutions of trans-anethole administered into the conjunctival sac concentration-dependently increased the number of stimuli required to evoke the conjunctival reflex (p<0.01): 9.7 stimuli at 10 µg/ml, 31.8 stimuli at 30 µg/ml and 65.2 stimuli at 100 µg/ml, compared to about 3 stimuli for vehicle controls. The effect was comparable to that of procaine [39].

Anti-tumour activity of trans-anethole
In Swiss albino mice with Ehrlich ascites tumour (EAT) in the paw, anethole administered orally at 500 or 1000 mg/kg on alternate days for 60 days significantly and dose-dependently reduced tumour weight (p<0.05 at 500 mg/kg, p<0.01 at 1000 mg/kg), tumour volume (p<0.01 at 500 mg/kg, p<0.001 at 1000 mg/kg) and body weight (p<0.05 to 0.01) compared to EAT-bearing controls. Mean survival time increased from 54.6 days to 62.2 days (500 mg/kg) and 71.2 days (1000 mg/kg). Histopathological changes were comparable to those after treatment with cyclophosphamide (a standard cytotoxic drug). These and other results demonstrated the anticarcinogenic, cytotoxic and non-clastogenic nature of anethole [45].

Anti-genotoxic activity of trans-anethole
In the mouse bone marrow micronucleus test, oral pre-treatment of mice with trans-anethole at 40-400 mg/kg body weight 2 and 20 hours before intraperitoneal injection of genotoxins led to moderate, dose-dependent protective effects against known genotoxins such as cyclophosphamide, procarbazine, N-methyl-N'-nitrosoguanidine, urethane and ethyl methane sulfonate (p<0.05 to p<0.01 at various dose levels). No significant increase in genotoxicity was observed when trans-anethole (40-400 mg/kg body weight) was administered alone [46].

Enzyme induction
Subcutaneous administration of the essential oil to partially (two-thirds) hepatectomized rats at 100 mg/animal/day for 7 days stimulated liver regeneration (p<0.01) [47].

Experiments in which rats were injected intraperitoneally with a mixture of trans-anethole (100 mg/kg bodyweight) and [14C]parathion (1.5 mg/kg) showed no significant effect of trans-anethole on metabolism and excretion of the insecticide. However, when rats were fed a diet containing 1% of trans-anethole for 7 days and subsequently cell fractions from the livers of these rats were incubated for 2 hours with [14C]parathion, significantly less unchanged parathion (1.6%) was recovered compared to controls (12.5%). The data were interpreted as suggesting that feeding trans-anethole to rats for 7 days induced the synthesis of parathion-degrading liver enzymes [27].

Pharmacokinetic properties

Pharmacokinetics in animals
No data available for aniseed.

In mice and rats trans-anethole is reported to be metabolized by O-demethylation and by oxidative transformation of the C3-side chain. After low doses (0.05 and 5 mg/kg body weight) O-demethylation occurs predominantly, whereas higher doses (up to 1500 mg/kg body weight) give rise to higher yields of oxygenated metabolites [48,49].

Pharmacokinetics in humans
No data available for aniseed.

After oral administration of radioactively-labelled trans-anethole (as the methoxy-^{14}C compound) to 5 healthy volunteers at dose levels of 1, 50 and 250 mg on separate occasions, it was rapidly absorbed. 54-69% of the dose (detected as ^{14}C) was eliminated in the urine and 13-17% in exhaled carbon dioxide; none was detected in the faeces. The bulk of elimination occurred within 8 hours and, irrespective of the dose level, the principal metabolite (more than 90% of urinary ^{14}C) was 4-methoxyhippuric acid [50]. An earlier study with 2 healthy subjects taking 1 mg of trans-anethole gave similar results [51].

Preclinical safety data
Most toxicity studies relevant to aniseed have been conducted on trans-anethole, the major constituent of the essential oil.

Acute toxicity
Oral LD_{50} values per kg body weight have been determined for the essential oil as 2.7 g in rats [52] and for trans-anethole as 1.82-5.0 g in mice, 2.1-3.2 g in rats and 2.16 g in guinea pigs [53].

Intraperitoneal LD_{50} values for trans-anethole have been determined as 0.65-1.41 g/kg in mice and 0.9-2.67 g/kg in rats [53].

Repeated-dose toxicity
No data available for aniseed.

In 90-day experiments in rats, 0.1% of trans-anethole in their diet caused no toxic effects. However, dose-related oedema of the liver was reported at higher levels of 0.3%, 1% and 3%, which have no therapeutic value [53]. Male rats receiving 0.25% of anethole in their diet for 1 year showed no toxic effects, while others receiving 1% for 15 weeks had slight oedematous changes in liver cells [54]. Rats given trans-anethole as 0.2, 0.5, 1 or 2% of their diet for 12-22 months showed no effects at any level on clinical chemistry, haematology, histopathology or mortality. Slower weight gain and reduced fat storage were noted at the 1% and 2% levels [53,55].

Reproductive toxicity
Trans-anethole exerted dose-dependent anti-implantation activity after oral administration to adult female rats on days 1-10 of pregnancy. Compared to control animals (all of which delivered normal offspring on completion of term), trans-anethole administered at 50, 70 and 80 mg/kg body weight inhibited implantation by 33%, 66% and 100% respectively. Further experiments at the 80 mg/kg dose level showed that in rats given trans-anethole only on days 1-2 of pregnancy normal implantation and delivery occurred; in those given anethole only on days 3-5 implantation was completely inhibited; and in those given trans-anethole only on days 6-10 three out of five rats failed to deliver at term. No gross malformations of offspring were observed in any of the groups. The results demonstrated that trans-anethole has antifertility activity. From comparison with the days 1-2 group (lack of antizygotic activity), the lower level of delivery in the days 6-10 group was interpreted as a sign of early abortifacient activity [29].

Mutagenicity
A dry ethanolic aniseed extract was mutagenic at high concentrations (5 mg/plate) to streptomycin-dependent strains of Salmonella typhimurium TA 98 [56]. An ethanolic aniseed extract gave negative results at the maximum non-toxic concentration of 0.1 mg/ml in chromosomal aberration tests using a Chinese hamster fibroblast cell line [57].

The essential oil and trans-anethole were mutagenic at 2 mg/plate in the Ames test using Salmonella typhimurium strains TA 98 and TA 100, and mutagenicity was potentiated by S13 activation [27]. In another study, trans-anethole was mutagenic to Salmonella typhimurium TA 100 in the Ames test with S9 activation, doses of 30-120 µg/plate showing a dose-dependent increase in revertants, which did not exceed twice the number of the control [58]. Other investigations with metabolic activation have confirmed that trans-anethole is weakly mutagenic [53].

Estragole, a minor constituent of anise oil, has also shown mutagenic potential in various Ames tests, demonstrating the need for carcinogenicity studies [59,60].

Carcinogenicity
A 1-year experiment in which mice received trans-anethole in their diet gave no evidence of carcinogenic potential: low levels of DNA adducts were observed in liver tissue [53]. In another chronic study of trans-anethole in mice there were no histological differences between treated and control animals [61]. In a study in rats, the highest dose feeding group (1% trans-anethole for 117 weeks) presented with hyperplastic and partially neoplastic changes in the livers of female (but not male) rats; a review of these results confirmed that the observed neoplastic changes in the liver were not due to a direct genotoxic effect induced by trans-anethole [53].

Genotoxicity studies performed with aniseed extracts, the essential oil, trans-anethole and estragole do not provide adequate data to fully evaluate the carcinogenic risk. However, the carcinogenic risk from aniseed in man is assumed to be low [2,22].

REFERENCES

1. Aniseed - Anisi fructus. European Pharmacopoeia, Council of Europe.

2. Hänsel R, Keller K, Rimpler H, Schneider G, editors. Pimpinella. In: Hagers Handbuch der Pharmazeutischen Praxis, 5th ed. Volume 6: Drogen P-Z. Berlin-Heidelberg-New York-London: Springer-Verlag, 1994:135-56.

3. Kubeczka K-H, von Massow F, Formacek V, Smith MAR. A new type of phenylpropane from the essential fruit oil of *Pimpinella anisum* L. Z Naturforsch 1976;31b:283-4.

4. Kubeczka K-H. Grundlagen der Qualitätsbeurteilung arzneilich verwendeter ätherischer Öle. Acta Horticulturae 1978;73:85-93.

5. Schultze W, Lange G, Kubeczka K-H. Direkte massenspektrometrische Analyse von *Pimpinella anisum* L. - Anispulver und Anisöl. Dtsch Apoth Ztg 1987;127:372-8.

6. El-Moghazi AM, Ali AA, Ross SA, Mottaleb MA. Flavonoids of *Pimpinella anisum* L. growing in Egypt. Fitoterapia 1979;50:267-8.

7. Kunzemann J, Herrmann K. Isolierung und Identifizierung der Flavon(ol)-O-glykoside in Kümmel (*Carum carvi* L.), Fenchel (*Foeniculum vulgare* Mill.), Anis (*Pimpinella anisum* L.) und Koriander (*Coriandrum sativum* L.) und von Flavon-C-Glykosiden im Anis. Z Lebensm Unters-Forsch 1977;164:194-200.

8. Schulz JM, Herrmann K. Analysis of hydroxybenzoic and hydroxycinnamic acids in plant material. II. Determination by gas-liquid chromatography. J Chromatogr 1980;195:95-104.

9. Baerheim Svendsen A. Über das Vorkommen der Chlorogen- und Kaffeesäure in der Pflanzenfamilie der Umbelliferen. Pharm Acta Helv 1951;26:253-8

10. El-Wakeil F, Khairy M, Morsi S, Farag RS, Shihata AA, Badel AZMA. Biochemical studies on the essential oils of some fruits of Umbelliferae family. Seifen-Öle-Fette-Wachse 1986;112:77-80.

11. Dirks U, Herrmann K. 4-(β-D-glucopyranosyloxy)-benzoic acid, a characteristic phenolic constituent of the Apiaceae. Phytochemistry 1984;23:1811-2.

12. Dirks U, Herrmann K. Hochleistungsflüssigkeits-chromatographie der Hydroxycinnamoylchinasäuren und der 4-(β-D-glucopyranosyloxy)-benzoesäure in Gewürzen. Z Lebensm Unters Forsch 1984;179:12-6.

13. Ceska O, Chaudhary SK, Warrington PJ, Ashwood-Smith MJ. Photoactive furocoumarins in fruits of some umbellifers. Phytochemistry 1987;26:165-9.

14. Kartnig T, Scholz G. Über einige Lipoid-Inhaltsstoffe aus den Früchten von *Pimpinella anisum* L. und *Carum carvi* L. Fette Seifen Anstrichmittel 1969;71:276-80.

15. Czygan F-C, Hiller K. Anisi fructus - Anis. In: Wichtl M, editor. Teedrogen und Phytopharmaka. Ein Handbuch für die Praxis auf wissenschaftlicher Grundlage, 4th ed. Stuttgart: Wissenschaftliche Verlagsgesellschaft, 2002: 42-4.

16. Weiss RF. In: Lehrbuch der Phytotherapie, 8th ed. Stuttgart: Hippokrates, 1997:83 and 443.

17. Pimpinella. In: British Herbal Pharmacopoeia 1983. Bournemouth: British Herbal Medicine Association, 1983:160-1.

18. Sweetmann SE, editor. Aniseed, Anise oil. In: Martindale - The complete drug reference, 33rd ed. London: Pharmaceutical Press, 2002:1580.

19. Czygan F-C. Anis (Anisi fructus DAB 10) - *Pimpinella anisum* L. Z Phytotherapie 1992;13:101-6.

20. Hänsel R, Sticher O, Steinegger E. Anis und Anisöl. In: Pharmakognosie- Phytopharmazie, 6th ed. Berlin-Heidelberg-New York-London: Springer-Verlag, 1999:692-5.

21. Dorsch W, Loew D, Meyer-Buchtela E, Schilcher H. In: Kooperation Phytopharmaka, editor. Kinderdosierung von Phytopharmaka, 3rd ed. Teil I. Empfehlungen zur Anwendung und Dosierung von Phytopharmaka, monographierte Arzneidrogen und ihren Zubereitungen in der Pädiatrie: Foeniculi fructus (Fenchelfrüchte). Bonn: Kooperation Phytopharmaka, 2002:70-1.

22. De Smet PAGM. Legislatory outlook on the safety of herbal remedies: *Pimpinella anisum*. In: De Smet PAGM, Keller K, Hänsel R, Chandler RF, editors. Adverse effects of herbal drugs, Volume 2. Berlin: Springer, 1993:62.

23. Barnes J, Anderson LA, Phillipson JD. Aniseed. In: Herbal Medicines - A guide for healthcare professionals, 2nd ed. London-Chicago: Pharmaceutical Press, 2002:51-4.

24. Andersen KE. Contact allergy to toothpaste flavours. Contact Dermatitis 1978;4:195-8.

25. Franks A. Contact allergy to anethole in toothpaste associated with loss of taste. Contact Dermatitis 1998; 38:354.

26. Hausen BM. The sensitizing capacity of sulfuretin. In: Allergiepflanzen - Pflanzenallergene. Part 1. Landsberg/ München: ecomed, 1988:300.

27. Marcus C, Lichtenstein EP. Interactions of naturally occurring food plant components with insecticides and pentobarbital in rats and mice. J Agric Food Chem 1982;30:563-8.

28. Tisserand R, Balacs T. Anise. In: Essential Oil Safety - A Guide for Health Care Professionals. Edinburgh: Churchill Livingstone, 1995:117.

29. Dhar SK. Anti-fertility activity and hormonal profile of

trans-anethole in rats. Indian J Physiol Pharmacol 1995;39:63-7.

30. Maruzzella JC, Freundlich M. Antimicrobial substances from seeds. J Am Pharm Assoc 1959;48:356-8.

31. Hammer KA, Carson CF, Riley TV. Antimicrobial activity of essential oils and other plant extracts. J Applied Microbiol 1999;86:985-90.

32. Ramadan FM, El-Zanfaly RT, El-Wakeil FA, Alian AM. On the antibacterial effects of some essential oils. I. Use of agar diffusion method. Chem Mikrobiol Technol Lebensm 1972;2:51-5.

33. Ibrahim YKE, Ogunmodede MS. Growth and survival of *Pseudomonas aeruginosa* in some aromatic waters. Pharm Acta Helv 1991;66:286-8.

34. Shukla HS, Tripathi SC. Antifungal substance in the essential oil of anise (*Pimpinella anisum* L.). Agric Biol Chem 1987;51:1991-3.

35. Aburjai T, Darwish RM, Al-Khalil S, Mahafzah A, Al-Abbadi A. Screening of antibiotic resistant inhibitors from local plant materials against two different strains of *Pseudomonas aeruginosa*. J Ethnopharmacol 2001; 76:39-44.

36. Müller-Limmroth W, Fröhlich H-H. Wirkungsnachweis einiger phytotherapeutischer Expektorantien auf den mukoziliaren Transport. Fortschr Med 1980;98:95-101.

37. Reiter M, Brandt W. Relaxant effects on tracheal and ileal smooth muscles of the guinea pig. Arzneim-Forsch/Drug Res 1985;35:408-14.

38. Boskabady MH, Ramazani-Assari M. Relaxant effect of *Pimpinella anisum* on isolated guinea pig tracheal chains and its possible mechanism(s). J Ethnopharmacol 2001;74:83-8.

39. Ghelardini C, Galeotti N, Mazzanti G. Local anaesthetic activity of monoterpenes and phenylpropanes of essential oils. Planta Med 2001;67:564-6.

40. Chainy GBN, Manna SK, Chaturvedi MM, Aggarwal BB. Anethole blocks both early and late cellular responses transduced by tumor necrosis factor: effect on NF-κB, AP-1, JNK, MAPKK and apoptosis. Oncogene 2000;19:2943-50.

41. Van Dongen K, Leusink H. The action of opium-alkaloids and expectorants on the ciliary movements in the air passages. Arch Int Pharmacodyn 1953;93:261-76.

42. Boyd EM, Pearson GL. On the expectorant action of volatile oils. Am J Med Sci 1946;211:602-10.

43. Boyd EM. Expectorants and respiratory tract fluid. Pharmacol Rev 1954;6:521-42.

44. Boyd EM, Sheppard EP. The effect of steam inhalation of volatile oils on the output and composition of respiratory tract fluid. J Pharmacol Exp Therap 1968;163:250-6.

45. Al-Harbi MM, Qureshi S, Raza M, Ahmed MM, Giangreco AB, Shah AH. Influence of anethole treatment on the tumour induced by Ehrlich ascites carcinoma cells in paw of Swiss albino mice. Eur J Cancer Prev 1995;4:307-18.

46. Abraham SK. Anti-genotoxicity of *trans*-anethole and eugenol in mice. Food Chem Toxicol 2001;39:493-8.

47. Gershbein LL. Regeneration of rat liver in the presence of essential oils and their components. Food Cosmet Toxicol 1977;15:173-81.

48. Sangster SA, Caldwell J, Smith RL. Metabolism of anethole. II. Influence of dose size on the route of metabolism of *trans*-anethole in the rat and mouse. Food Chem Toxicol 1984;22:707-13.

49. Sangster SA, Caldwell J, Smith RL, Farmer PB. Metabolism of anethole. I. Pathways of metabolism in the rat and mouse. Food Chem Toxicol 1984;22:695-706.

50. Caldwell J, Sutton JD. Influence of dose size on the disposition of *trans*-[methoxy-^{14}C]anethole in human volunteers. Food Chem Toxicol 1988;26:87-91.

51. Sangster SA, Caldwell J, Hutt AJ, Anthony A, Smith RL. The metabolic disposition of [methoxy-^{14}C]-labelled *trans*-anethole, estragole and p-propylanisole in human volunteers. Xenobiotica 1987;17:1223-32.

52. von Skramlik E. Über die Giftigkeit und Verträglichkeit von ätherischen Ölen. Pharmazie 1959;14:435-45.

53. Lin FSD. *Trans*-anethole. In: Joint FAO/WHO Expert Committee on Food Additives. Toxicological evaluation of certain food additives and contaminants. WHO Food Additives Series 28. Geneva: World Health Organization 1991:135-52.

54. Hagan EC, Hansen WH, Fitzhugh OG, Jenner PM, Jones WI, Taylor JM et al. Food flavourings and compounds of related structure. II. Subacute and chronic toxicity. Food Cosmet Toxicol 1967;5:141-57.

55. Le Bourhis B. Propriétés biologiques du trans-anéthole. Essai de détermination de la dose journalière acceptable. Parfums Cosmet Sav Fr 1973;3:450-6.

56. Shashikanth KN, Hosono A. *In vitro* mutagenicity of tropical spices to streptomycin-dependent strains of *Salmonella typhimurium* TA 98. Agric Biol Chem 1986;50:2947-8.

57. Ishidate M, Sofuni T, Yoshikawa K, Hayashi M, Nohmi T, Sawada M, Matsuoka A. Primary mutagenicity screening of food additives currently used in Japan. Food Chem Toxicol 1984;22:623-36.

58. Sekizawa J, Shibamoto T. Genotoxicity of safrole-related chemicals in microbial test systems. Mutat Res 1982;101:127-40.

59. De Vincenzi M, Silano M, Maialetti F, Scazzocchio B. Constituents of aromatic plants: II. Estragole. Fitoterapia 2000;71:725-9.

60. European Commission: Scientific Committee on Food. Opinion of the scientific committee on food on estragole (1-allyl-4-methoxybenzene). 26 September 2001.

61. Miller EC, Swanson AB, Phillips DH, Fletcher L, Liem A, Miller JA. Structure-activity studies of the carcinogenicities in the mouse and rat of some naturally occurring and synthetic alkenylbenzene derivatives related to safrole and estragole. Cancer Res 1983;43: 1124-34.

ARNICAE FLOS

Arnica Flower

DEFINITION

Arnica flower consists of the whole or partially broken, dried flower-heads of *Arnica montana* L. It contains not less than 0.4 per cent m/m of total sesquiterpene lactones expressed as helenalin tiglate, calculated with reference to the dried drug.

The material complies with the monograph of the European Pharmacopoeia [1].

Fresh material may also be used, provided that when dried it complies with the monograph of the European Pharmacopoeia.

CONSTITUENTS

Sesquiterpene lactones of the pseudoguaianolide type, 0.2-0.8%; principally helenalin and 11α,13-dihydro-helenalin and their esters with acetic, isobutyric, methacrylic, tiglic and other carboxylic acids [2-5]. Other constituents [6] include diterpenes [7], arnidiol (a triterpene) [8], flavonols [9-11], flavonol glycosides [12-15], flavonol glucuronides [16], pyrrolizidine alkaloids (tussilagine and isotussilagine) [17,18], poly-acetylenes [19], caffeic acid and derivatives [3,20], coumarins [3], fatty acids [21] and essential oil containing fatty acids [22] and carotenoids [23].

CLINICAL PARTICULARS

Therapeutic indications

External use
Treatment of bruises, sprains [3,6,24-27] and inflammation caused by insect bites [6]; gingivitis and aphthous ulcers [3,6]; symptomatic treatment of rheumatic complaints [3,6,24,26,27].

Posology and method of administration

Dosage

External use
Ointments, creams, gels or compresses made with 5-25% V/V tinctures [3,6] or 5-25% V/V fluid extracts [3]; diluted tincture (1:3 to 1:10), diluted fluid extracts or a decoction of 2.0 g of dried arnica flower in 100 ml of water [6].

Method of administration
Topically as diluted tincture [6], ointment, cream, gel or compress.

E/S/C/O/P
MONOGRAPHS
Second Edition

Duration of administration
If symptoms persist or worsen, medical advice should be sought.

Contra-indications
Allergy to *Arnica* or other members of the Compositae [28-31].

Special warnings and special precautions for use
For external use only. Not to be used on open wounds.

Interaction with other medicaments and other forms of interaction
None reported.

Pregnancy and lactation
No restriction for external use; no harmful effects have been reported.

Effects on ability to drive and use machines
None.

Undesirable effects
Skin irritation has been reported [32-35]. Contact dermatitis from arnica may occur in susceptible individuals [28-32,34-39].

Overdose
Not applicable to external use.

PHARMACOLOGICAL PROPERTIES

Pharmacodynamic properties

In vitro experiments

Anti-inflammatory activity
In enzyme assays performed on mouse and rat liver homogenates and human polymorphonuclear neutrophils, helenalin and 2,3-dihydrohelenalin significantly suppressed various parameters of inflammation; at 5 $\times$ 10^{-5} M they inhibited the chemotactic migration of human polymorphonuclear neutrophils by 100% and 20% respectively [40]. From the series of active sesquiterpene lactones tested it was concluded that unsaturated structures such as α-methylene-γ-lactone and/or α,β-unsubstituted cyclopentenone moieties (helenalin has both) must play a role in the anti-inflammatory activity. In these metabolic studies it was furthermore found that sesquiterpene lactones exert their activities at multiple receptor sites, e.g. by suppression of the synthesis of prostaglandins at 10^{-3} M in a prostaglandin synthetase assay and uncoupling of oxidative phosphorylation of human polymorphonuclear neutrophils at 5 $\times$ 10^{-4} M [40,41].

Transcription factor NF-κB is a central mediator of the human immune response, which regulates the transcription of various inflammatory cytokines such as interleukin-1,-2,-6,-8 and TNF-α. It has been shown that the sesquiterpene lactones helenalin and (to a much lesser degree) 11α,13-dihydrohelenalin inhibit NF-κB activation in response to four different stimuli in T-cells, B-cells and epithelial cells. Inhibition was seen at the μM concentration level and was selective, since the activities of four other transcription factors (Oct-1, TBP, Sp1 and STAT5) were not affected [42]. Inhibition of activation of another transcription factor (NF-AT) has also been demonstrated [43].

The most prominent underlying mechanism of action of the sesquiterpene lactones is their interaction with the sulfhydryl (thiol) groups of proteins [44,45]. It is assumed that other constituents, such as flavonoid glycosides, polyacetylenes and caffeic acid derivatives, also contribute to the pharmacological activity of arnica flower [46].

Antimicrobial activity
Using isolated constituents such as helenalin and 11,13-dihydrohelenalin acetate, antimicrobial activity against the Gram-positive bacteria *Arthrobacter citreus, Bacillus brevis, Bacillus subtilis, Corynebacterium insidiosum, Micrococcus roseus, Mycobacterium phlei, Sarcina lutea* and *Staphylococcus aureus,* and Gram-negative *Proteus vulgaris,* has been demonstrated [6,47,48]. Antifungal activity of helenalin and derivatives against *Botrytis cinerea* has also been demonstrated [47].

Cytotoxic effects
The cytotoxic activity of isolated sesquiterpene lactones against cultivated tumour cell lines (GLC$_4$ and COLO 320) has been demonstrated [49]. Isolated flavonoids from arnica flower, applied to human lung carcinoma cell lines, effectively reduced the cytotoxic activity of helenalin [50]. Inhibition of cellular respiration of Ehrlich ascites cells was also reported [51]. Helenalin and 11,13-dihydrohelenalin, as well as an unspecified extract of arnica flower, inhibited platelet activation [52,53].

Other effects
Aqueous arnica flower extracts (2 mg/ml of dried plant extract redissolved after lyophilisation) had an antihistamine effect on smooth muscle preparations [54].

In vivo experiments

Anti-inflammatory effects
The anti-inflammatory activity of helenalin has been demonstrated in several ways. Intraperitoneal pretreatment with helenalin at 2.5 mg/kg body weight inhibited carrageenan-induced rat paw oedema (p<0.001) [41]. In mice, helenalin injected intraperitoneally at 20 mg/kg bodyweight inhibited the acetic acid-induced writhing reflex (an indicator of inflammation pain) by 93% (p<0.001) [41].

Intraperitoneal treatment of rats with chronic adjuvant arthritis with helenalin at 2.5 mg/kg/day for 3 weeks confirmed that sesquiterpene lactones are the constituents mainly responsible for anti-inflammatory activity [40]. $11\alpha,13$-Dihydrohelenalin acetate and methacrylate applied topically at 1 µmol/cm^2 inhibited croton oil-induced mouse ear oedema by 54 and 77% respectively (p<0.001), compared to 44% inhibition by indometacin at 0.2 µmol/cm^2 [43].

Tumour-inhibiting activity
Sesquiterpene lactones from arnica flower inhibited the growth of Ehrlich ascites in mice and Walker 256 carcinosarcoma in rats [51].

Clinical studies
In a randomized, double-blind, placebo-controlled study, patients with chronic venous insufficiency (primary varicosis of the legs) received basic hydrotherapy treatment and also topical application of an arnica flower extract ointment (n = 39) or a placebo ointment (n = 39) to the lower legs and feet. After 3 weeks, from objective plethysmographic measurements and subjective assessments (feelings of tension and swelling in the legs, pain in the legs), improvements were observed in both groups but the degree of improvement was significantly greater after verum treatment. A further study in 100 patients (verum 50, placebo 50), under identical conditions except using an arnica flower extract gel, showed comparable improvements but no difference between groups [55].

In a small study involving 12 male volunteers, external application of an arnica flower gel was found more effective than a placebo gel in relieving muscle ache [56].

Pharmacokinetic properties
No data available.

Preclinical safety data
The safety of arnica flower has been assessed in a recent review. In general, extracts have been found to have low toxicity in acute tests in mice, rats and rabbits. They were not irritating, sensitizing or phototoxic to mouse or guinea pig skin, nor did they produce significant ocular irritation [57].

The safety profile of arnica flower has also been reviewed with respect to sesquiterpene lactones, flavonoids and pyrrolizidine alkaloids [6,38]. The pyrrolizidine alkaloids tussilagine and isotussilagine [17,18] are considered non-toxic because they lack the key structure, a 1,2-unsaturated necine group, considered to be responsible for the toxicity of certain pyrrolizidine alkaloids [6,18].

In vitro experiments
In the Ames mutagenicity test, a hydroethanolic extract of arnica flower showed weakly mutagenic potential in *Salmonella typhimurium* strain TA98 with or without S9 activation and in strain TA100 with activation; the effects were possibly due to the flavonoids present in the extract [58]. Helenalin showed no mutagenic potential in the Ames test using *Salmonella typhimurium* strains TA98, TA100, TA1535 and TA 1537, but was relatively toxic to the test organisms [59].

The sesquiterpene lactones helenalin and $11\alpha,13$-dihydrohelenalin were cytotoxic against GLC$_4$ (a human small cell lung carcinoma cell line) and COLO 320 (a human colorectal cancer line). IC$_{50}$ values for helenalin after 2-hour incubation were 0.44 µM against GLC$_4$ and 1.0 µM against COLO 320; corresponding values for $11\alpha,13$-dihydrohelenalin were 66.1 and 64.7 µM, compared to 4.6 and 8.8 µM for the reference compound cisplatin. Most flavonoids in arnica flower had low cytotoxic activity at 200 µM after 2-hour incubation [49,57].

In vivo experiments
The oral LD$_{50}$ of arnica flower extract in rats has been reported as > 5g/kg. In mice, oral and intraperitoneal values of arnica flower extract have been reported as 123 mg/kg and 31 mg/kg respectively [57].

LD$_{50}$ values of helenalin were determined as 150 mg/kg body weight in mice, 125 mg/kg in rats, 90 mg/kg in rabbits and 85 mg/kg in hamsters, and estimated as 100-125 mg/kg in sheep [60].

REFERENCES

1.   Arnica Flower - Arnicae flos. European Pharmacopoeia, Council of Europe.

2.   Willuhn G, Leven W, Luley C. Arnikablüten DAB 10. Untersuchungen zur qualitativen und quantitativen Variabilität des Sesquiterpenlactongehaltes der offizinellen Arnikadrogen. Dtsch Apoth Ztg l994;134: 4077-85.

3.   Willuhn G. Arnikablüten. In: Wichtl M, editor. Teedrogen. 2nd ed. Stuttgart: Wissenschaftliche Verlagsgesellschaft 1989:65-9.

4.   List PH, Friebel B. Neue Inhaltsstoffe der Blüten von *Arnica montana* L. Arzneim-Forsch/Drug Res 1974;24: 148-51.

5.   Willuhn G, Röttger P-M, Matthiesen U. Helenalin- und 11,13-Dihydrohelenalinester aus Blüten von *Arnica montana*. Planta Med 1983;49:226-31.

6.   Merfort I. Arnica. In: Hänsel R, Keller K, Rimpler H, Schneider G, editors. Hagers Handbuch der Pharmazeutischen Praxis, 5th ed. Volume 4: Drogen A-D. Berlin: Springer-Verlag, 1992:342-57.

7. Schmidt T, Paßreiter CM, Wendisch D, Willuhn G. First diterpenes from *Arnica*. Planta Med 1992;58(Suppl 1): A713.

8. Santer JO, Stevenson R. Arnidiol and faradiol. J Org Chem 1962;27:3204-8.

9. Merfort I. Methylierte Flavonoide aus *Arnica montana* und *Arnica chamissonis*. Planta Med 1984;50:107-8.

10. Merfort I. Flavonoide aus *Arnica montana* und *Arnica chamissonis*. Planta Med 1985;51:136-8.

11. Merfort I, Marcinek C, Eggert A. Flavonoid distribution in *Arnica* subgenus *chamissonis*. Phytochemistry 1986; 25:2901-3.

12. Merfort I, Wendisch D. Flavonoidglycoside aus *Arnica montana* und *Arnica chamissonis*. Planta Med 1987; 53:434-7.

13. Merfort I. Acetylated and other flavonoid glycosides from *Arnica chamissonis*. Phytochemistry 1988;27: 3281-4.

14. Merfort I, Wendisch D. New flavonoid glycosides from Arnicae flos DAB 9. Planta Med 1992;58:355-7.

15. Pietta PG, Mauri PL, Bruno A, Merfort I. MEKC as an improved method to detect falsifications in the flowers of *Arnica montana* and *A. chamissonis*. Planta Med 1994;60:369-72.

16. Merfort I, Wendisch D. Flavonolglucuronide aus den Blüten von *Arnica montana*. Planta Med 1988;54:247-50.

17. Paßreiter CM, Willuhn G, Röder E. Tussilagine and isotussilagine: two pyrrolizidine alkaloids in the genus *Arnica*. Planta Med 1992;58:556-7.

18. Paßreiter CM. Co-occurrence of 2-pyrrolidineacetic acid with the pyrrolizidines tussilaginic acid and isotussilaginic acid and their 1-epimers in *Arnica* species and *Tussilago farfara*. Phytochemistry 1992;31:4135-7.

19. Schulte KE, Rücker G, Reithmayr K. Einige Inhaltsstoffe von *Arnica chamissonis* und anderer *Arnica*-Arten. Lloydia 1969;32:360-8.

20. Merfort I. Caffeoylquinic acids from flowers of *Arnica montana* and *Arnica chamissonis*. Phytochemistry 1992;31:2111-3.

21. Kating H, Rinn W, Willuhn G. Untersuchungen über die Inhaltsstoffe von *Arnica*-Arten. III. Die Fettsäuren in den ätherischen Ölen der Blüten verschiedener *Arnica*-Arten. Planta Med 1970;18:130-46.

22. Güntzel U, Seidel F, Kating H. Untersuchungen über die Inhaltsstoffe von *Arnica*-Arten. I. Der Gehalt an ätherischem Öl in den Blüten verschiedener *Arnica*-Arten. Planta Med 1967;15:205-14.

23. Vanhaelen M. Identification des carotenoides dans *Arnica Montana*. Planta Med 1973;23:308-11.

24. Hänsel R, Haas H. Arnikablüten. In: Therapie mit Phytopharmaka. Berlin: Springer-Verlag,1983:271-2.

25. Arnica. In: British Herbal Pharmacopoeia 1983. Bournemouth: British Herbal Medicine Association, 1983:30-1.

26. Van Hellemont J. Fytotherapeutisch Compendium. Utrecht/Antwerpen: Bohn, Scheltema & Holkema, 1988:71-5.

27. Weiss RF. Lehrbuch der Phytotherapie. 7th ed. Stuttgart: Hippokrates Verlag, 1990:30-1.

28. Eberhartinger C. Beobachtungen zur Häufigkeit von Kontaktallergien. Z Hautkr 1984;59:1283-9.

29. Hausen BM. Kokardenblumen-Allergie. Dermatosen 1985;33:62-5.

30. Machet L, Vaillant L, Callens A, Demasure M, Barruet K, Lorette G. Allergic contact dermatitis from sunflower (*Helianthus annuus*) with cross-sensitivity to arnica. Contact Dermatitis 1993;28:184-200.

31. Hörmann HP, Korting HC. Allergic acute contact dermatitis due to *Arnica* tincture self-medication. Phytomedicine 1995;2:315-7.

32. Hausen BM. Arnikaallergie. Der Hautarzt 1980;31:10-7.

33. Hausen BM. The sensitizing capacity of Compositae plants III. Test results and cross-reactions in Compositae-sensitive patients. Dermatologica 1979;159:1-11.

34. Roth L, Daunderer M, Kormann K. Giftpflanzen - Pflanzengifte, 3rd ed. Landsberg: ecomed Verlag, 1992:122-4.

35. Reynolds JEF, editor. Arnica Flower. In: Martindale - The Extra Pharmacopoeia, 29th ed. London: The Pharmaceutical Press, 1989.

36. Hausen BM, Herrmann HD, Willuhn G. The sensitizing capacity of Compositae plants I. Occupational contact dermatitis from *Arnica longifolia* Eaton. Contact Dermatitis 1978;4:3-10.

37. Herrmann H-D, Willuhn G, Hausen BM. Helenalin-methacrylate, a new pseudoguaianolide from the flowers of *Arnica montana* L. and the sensitizing capacity of their sesquiterpene lactones. Planta Med 1978; 34:299-304.

38. Hausen BM. Sesquiterpene lactones - *Arnica montana*. In: De Smet PAGM, Keller K, Hänsel R, Chandler RF, editors. Adverse Effects of Herbal Drugs, Volume 1. Berlin: Springer-Verlag, 1992:237-42.

39. Spettoli E, Silvani S, Lucente P, Guerra L, Vincenzi C. Contact Dermatitis caused by sesquiterpene lactones. Am J Contact Derm 1998;9:49-50.

40. Hall IH, Starnes CO, Lee KH, Waddell TG. Mode of action of sesquiterpene lactones as anti-inflammatory agents. J Pharm Sci 1980;69:537-43.

41. Hall IH, Lee KH, Starnes CO, Sumida Y, Wu RY,

Waddell TG et al. Anti-inflammatory activity of sesquiterpene lactones and related compounds. J Pharm Sci 1979;68:537-42.

42. Lyss G, Schmidt TJ, Merfort I, Pahl HL. Helenalin, an anti-inflammatory sesquiterpene lactone from *Arnica,* selectively inhibits transcription factor NF-κB. Biol Chem 1997;378:951-61.

43. Klaas CA, Wagner G, Laufer S, Sosa S, Della Loggia R, Bomme U, Pahl HL, Merfort I. Studies on the anti-inflammatory activity of phytopharmaceuticals prepared from *Arnica* flowers. Planta Med 2002;68:385-91.

44. Kolodziej H. Sesquiterpenlactone. Biologische Aktivitäten. Dtsch Apoth Ztg 1993;133:1795-805.

45. Wijnsma R, Woerdenbag HJ, van der Molen J. Het gebruik van Arnica in de fytotherapie. Pharm Weekbl 1994;129:924-30.
Also published in modified form as: Wijnsma R, Woerdenbag HJ, Busse W. Die Bedeutung von Arnika-Arten in der Phytotherapie. Z Phytotherapie 1995; 16:48-62.

46. Willuhn G. *Arnica montana* L. - Porträt einer Arzneipflanze. Pharm Ztg 1991;136:2453-68.

47. Willuhn G, Röttger P-M, Quack W. Untersuchungen zur antimikrobiellen Aktivität der Sesquiterpenlactone der Arnikablüten. Pharm Ztg 1982;127:2183-5.

48. Lee KH, Ibuka T, Wu RY, Geissman TA. Structural-antimicrobial activity relationships among the sesquiterpene lactones and related compounds. Phytochemistry 1977;16:1177-81.

49. Woerdenbag HJ, Merfort I, Paßreiter CM, Schmidt TJ, Willuhn G, van Uden W et al. Cytotoxicity of flavonoids and sesquiterpene lactones from *Arnica* species against the GLC_4 and the COLO 320 cell lines. Planta Med 1994;60:434-7.

50. Woerdenbag HJ, Merfort I, Schmidt TJ, Passreiter CM, Willuhn G, van Uden W et al. Decreased helenalin-induced cytotoxicity by flavonoids from *Arnica* as studied in a human lung carcinoma cell line. Phytomedicine 1995;2:127-32.

51. Hall IH, Lee K-H, Starnes CO, Eigebaly SA, Ibuka T, Wu Y-S et al. Antitumor agents XXX: Evaluation of α-methylene-γ-lactone-containing agents for inhibition of tumor growth, respiration and nucleic acid synthesis. J Pharm Sci 1978;67:1235-9.

52. Weil D, Reuter HD. Einfluß von Arnika-Extrakt und Helenalin auf die Funktion menschlicher Blutplättchen. Z Phytotherapie 1988;9:26-8.

53. Schröder H, Lösche W, Strobach H, Leven W, Willuhn G, Till U, Schrör K. Helenalin and 11α,13-dihydro-helenalin, two constituents from *Arnica montana* L., inhibit human platelet function via thiol-dependent pathways. Thrombosis Res 1990;57:839-45.

54. Brunelin-Geray J, Debelmas AM. Contribution a l'étude de l'*Arnica montana* L. Plantes Méd Phytothér 1969; 3:15-9.

55. Brock FE. Ergebnisse klinischer Studien bei Patienten mit chronisch venöser Insuffizienz. In: von Raison J, Heilmann J, Merfort I, Schmidt TJ, Brock FE, Leven W et al. Arnika - Arzneipflanze mit Tradition und Zukunft. Z Phytotherapie 2000;21:39-54.

56. Moog-Schulze JB. Een medisch experimenteel onderzoek naar de werkzaamheden van een uitwendige toepassing van Arnica-gelei. Tijdschr Integr Geneeskunde 1993;9:105-12.

57. Anon. Final report on the safety assessment of *Arnica montana* extract and *Arnica montana*. Int J Toxicol 2001;20(Suppl 2):1-11.

58. Göggelmann W, Schimmer O. Mutagenic activity of phytotherapeutical drugs. In: Knudsen I, editor: Genetic Toxicology of the Diet. New York: Alan R Liss, 1986: 63-72.

59. MacGregor JT. Mutagenic activity of hymenovin, a sesquiterpene lactone from western bitterweed. Food Cosmet Toxicol 1977;15:225-7.

60. Witzel DA, Ivie GW, Dollahite JW. Mammalian toxicity of helenalin, the toxic principle of *Helenium microcephalum* DC (smallhead sneezeweed). Am J Vet Res 1976;37:859-61.

BETULAE FOLIUM

Birch Leaf

DEFINITION

Birch leaf consists of the whole or fragmented dried leaves of *Betula pendula* Roth and/or *Betula pubescens* Ehrh. as well as hybrids of both species. It contains not less than 1.5 per cent of flavonoids, calculated as hyperoside ($C_{21}H_{20}O_{12}$; M_r 464.4) with reference to the dried drug.

The material complies with the monograph of the European Pharmacopoeia [1].

Fresh material may also be used, provided that when dried it complies with the monograph of the European Pharmacopoeia.

CONSTITUENTS

1-3% of flavonol glycosides, principally hyperoside and other quercetin glycosides together with glycosides of myricetin and kaempferol [2-11]; other phenolic compounds including 3,4'-dihydroxy-propiophenone 3-glucoside (ca. 0.8% in *B. pendula*, 0.08% in *B. pubescens*) and chlorogenic acid (ca. 2% in *B. pubescens*, 0.02-0.1% in *B. pendula*) [2,3]; triterpene alcohols and malonyl esters of the damm-arane type [7,12-19], previously reported as saponins [20-22].

Other constituents include monoterpene glucosides [23], a sesquiterpene oxide [24], roseoside [25], tannins, traces of essential oil [11] and approx. 4% of minerals, particularly potassium [11,26].

Fresh leaves contain up to 0.5% of ascorbic acid [27].

CLINICAL PARTICULARS

Therapeutic indications
Irrigation of the urinary tract, especially in cases of inflammation and renal gravel, and as an adjuvant in the treatment of bacterial infections of the urinary tract [11,28,29].

Posology and method of administration

Dosage
2-3 g of dried leaf as an infusion, two to three times daily; equivalent preparations [28,30].
Tincture (1:10): 2 ml three times daily.
Fresh juice: 15 ml three times daily.

E/S/C/O/P
MONOGRAPHS
Second Edition

Method of administration
For oral administration.

Duration of administration
No restriction.

Contra-indications
None known.

Special warnings and special precautions for use
Oedema due to impaired heart and kidney function [28].

Interaction with other medicaments and other forms of interaction
None reported.

Pregnancy and lactation
No data available. In accordance with general medical practice, the product should not be used during pregnancy and lactation without medical advice.

Effects on ability to drive and use machines
None known.

Undesirable effects
None reported.

Overdose
No toxic effects reported.

PHARMACOLOGICAL PROPERTIES

Pharmacodynamic properties

In vitro experiments

Diuretic activity
Various flavonoids were investigated for their inhibitory activity on specific neuropeptide hydrolases which regulate the formation of urine through excretion of sodium ions [31]. The results led to the conclusion that certain flavonoids, especially quercetin, and other phenolic compounds present in birch may contribute to accelerated formation of urine [32].

In vivo experiments
After oral administration of an infusion of birch leaf to rabbits, urine volume increased by 30% and chloride excretion by 48% [33]; in mice, urine volume increased by 42% and chloride excretion by 128% [33]; in rats, urine volume did not increase but excretion of urea and chloride increased [34]. Young birch leaves administered orally to mice and rats did not produce these effects, in fact an anti-diuretic action was apparent [35].

Oral administration of powdered birch leaf to dogs at 240 mg/kg body weight increased urine volume by 13.8% after 2 hours; a flavonoid fraction at 14 mg/kg increased urine volume by 2.8% [36].

Further studies in rats showed increased excretion of urine after oral administration of aqueous and alcoholic extracts rich in flavonoids (48, 76 and 148 mg/100 ml). The aquaretic effect correlated with the amount of flavonoids, but no saluretic effect could be demonstrated [28,37,38].

However, diuretic effects do not appear to be due entirely to flavonoids since lesser effects were achieved with isolated flavonoid fractions [29,30,36-39].

Various extracts from birch leaf were administered orally to rats: an extract prepared with ethanol 70% (43 mg flavonoids/kg body weight), a fraction obtained from this extract with butanol (192 mg flavonoids/kg body weight), a butanolic fraction low in flavonoids (14 mg flavonoids/kg body weight) and the aqueous residue from the separation process (0.7 mg flavonoids/kg body weight). No increase in diuresis or saluresis could be demonstrated for any of these preparations [17].

It has been suggested that the potassium content of birch leaf may contribute to the diuretic effect [28,30,37,38]. High potassium-sodium ratios were determined in dried leaf (189:1) and in a 1% decoction (168:1) [26].

Clinical studies
Early studies in humans did not show a significant increase in diuresis after administration of an infusion of birch leaf compared to the effect of pure water [40,41].

In a field study, 1066 patients received a dry aqueous extract of birch leaf (4-8:1) at various daily doses (from 180 mg to 1080 mg or more daily) for irrigation of the urinary tract. In most cases (63%) the treatment period was 2-4 weeks. The patients could be classified into four groups: 73.8% suffered from urinary tract infections, cystitis or other inflammatory complaints, 14.2% from irritable bladder, 9.3% from stones and 2.7% from miscellaneous complaints. 56% of patients in the first group also received antibiotic therapy. After treatment the symptoms disappeared in 78% of patients in the first group, 65% in the second group and 65% in the third group. Symptoms disappeared in 80% of patients treated with, and in 75% of those going without, antibiotics. Both physicians and patients considered efficacy to be very good (39% and 48% respectively) or good (52% and 44% respectively) [42].

In a randomized, double-blind, placebo-controlled pilot study, 15 patients with infections of the lower urinary tract were treated with 4 cups of birch leaf tea or placebo tea daily for 20 days. Microbial counts in the urine of the birch leaf tea group decreased by 39% compared to 18% in the control group. At the end of the study, 3 out of 7 patients in the verum group and 1 out of 6 in the placebo group no longer suffered from a urinary tract infection [43].

Pharmacokinetic properties
No data available.

Preclinical safety data
An extract of birch leaf gave a very weak mutagenic response in the Ames test [44]; no other studies have been performed to confirm this.

Clinical safety data
In an open post-marketing study, mild adverse effects were reported in only 8 out of 1066 patients who received a dry aqueous extract of birch leaf (4-8:1) at daily doses of up to 1080 mg for 2-4 weeks [42].

REFERENCES

1. Birch Leaf - Betulae folium. European Pharmacopoeia, Council of Europe.

2. Keinänen M, Julkunen-Tiitto R. Effect of sample preparation method on birch (Betula pendula Roth) leaf phenolics. J Agric Food Chem 1996;44:2724-7.

3. Ossipov V, Nurmi K, Loponen J, Haukioja E, Pihlaja K. High-performance liquid chromatographic separation and identification of phenolic compounds from leaves of Betula pubescens and Betula pendula. J Chromatogr A 1996;721:59-68.

4. Dallenbach-Tölke K, Nyiredy S, Sticher O. Birkenblätter-Qualität. Vergleich der Einzel- und Gesamtbest-immungsmethoden der Flavonoidglykoside von Betulae folium. Dtsch Apoth Ztg 1987;127:1167-71.

5. Dallenbach-Tölke K, Nyiredy S, Meier B, Sticher O. HPLC-Analyse der Flavonoidglykoside aus Betulae folium. Planta Med 1987;53:189-92.

6. Dallenbach-Toelke K, Nyiredy S, Gross GA, Sticher O. Flavonoid glycosides from Betula pubescens and Betula pendula. J Nat Prod 1986;49:1155-6.

7. Pokhilo ND, Denisenko VA, Makhan'kov VV, Uvarova NI. Terpenoids and flavonoids from the leaves of Siberian species of the genus Betula. Chem Nat Compd 1983;19:374-5, translated from Khim Prir Soedin 1983;392-3.

8. Pawlowska L. Flavonoids in the leaves of Polish species of the genus Betula L. IV. Flavonoids of Betula pubescens Ehrh., B. carpatica Waldst., B. tortuosa Ledeb. and B. nana L. leaves. Acta Soc Bot Pol 1982;51:403-11;

through Chem Abstr 1983;99:155204.

9. Tissut M, Egger K. Les glycosides flavoniques foliaires de quelques arbres, au cours du cycle vegetatif. Phytochemistry 1972;11:631-4.

10. Hörhammer L, Wagner H, Luck R. Isolierung eines Myricetin-3-digalaktosides aus Betula verrucosa und Betula pubescens. Arch Pharm 1957;290:338-41.

11. Steinegger E, Hänsel R. Birkenblätter. In: Pharmakognosie, 5th ed. Berlin-Heidelberg-New York: Springer-Verlag, 1992:564-5.

12. Fischer FG, Seiler N. Die Triterpenalkohole der Birkenblätter. Liebigs Ann Chem 1959;626:185-205.

13. Fischer FG, Seiler N. Die Triterpenalkohole der Birkenblätter II. Liebigs Ann Chem 1961;644:146-62.

14. Baranov VI, Malinovskaya GV, Pokhilo ND, Makhan'kov VV, Uvarova NI, Gorovoi PG. Chemo-taxonomic study of Betula species in the Soviet Far East. Rastit Resur 1983;19(2):159-66; through Chem Abstr 1983;99:35948.

15. Pokhilo ND, Makhev AK, Uvarova NI. Triterpenoids of leaves of Betula pendula growing in high mountain regions of the Altai. Chem Nat Compd 1988;24:396-7, translated from Khim Prir Soedin 1988;(3):460-1.

16. Pokhilo ND, Denisenko VA, Makhan'kov VV, Uvarova NI. Triterpenoids of the leaves of Betula pendula from different growth sites. Chem Nat Compd 1986;22:166-71, translated from Khim Prir Soedin 1986;179-85.

17. Rickling B. Identifizierung hämolytisch aktiver Triterpenester aus Betula pendula [Dissertation]. Rheinischen Friedrich-Wilhelms-Universität, Bonn, 1992.

18. Rickling B, Glombitza K-W. Saponins in the leaves of birch? Hemolytic dammarane triterpenoid esters of Betula pendula. Planta Med 1993;59:76-9.

19. Hilpisch U, Hartmann R, Glombitza K-W. New dammaranes, esterified with malonic acid, from leaves of Betula pendula. Planta Med 1997;63:347-51.

20. Kroeber L. Studienergebnisse einer Reihe von Fluidextrakten aus heimischen Arzneipflanzen. Pharm Zentralhalle 1924;400-4.

21. Kofler L, Steidl G. Über das Vorkommen und die Verteilung von Saponinen in pflanzlichen Drogen. II. Blätter, Früchte, Rinden, Hölzer, Wurzeln und Rhizome. Arch Pharm Ber Dtsch Pharm Ges 1934;272:300-12.

22. Tamas M, Hodisan V, Grecu L, Fagarasan E, Baciu M, Muica I. Cercetari asupra saponinelor triterpenice din plante medicinale indigene. Studii Cerc Biochim 1978;21:89-94.

23. Tschesche R, Ciper F, Breitmaier E. Monoterpen-Glucoside aus den Blättern von Betula alba und den Früchten von Chaenomeles japonica. Chem Ber 1977;110:3111-7.

24. Pokhilo ND, Denisenko VA, Novikov VL, Uvarova NI. 14-Hydroxycaryophyllene 4,5-oxide - a new sesquiterpene from *Betula pubescens*. Chem Nat Compd 1984;20:563-7, translated from Khim Prir Soedin 1984;(5):598-603.

25. Tschesche R, Ciper F, Harz A. Roseosid aus *Betula alba* und *Cydonia oblonga*. Phytochemistry 1976;15:1990-1.

26. Szentmihályi K, Kéry Á, Then M, Lakatos B, Sándor Z, Vinkler P. Potassium-sodium ratio for the characterization of medicinal plant extracts with diuretic activity. Phytotherapy Res 1998;12:163-6.

27. Jones E, Hughes RE. A note on the ascorbic acid content of some trees and woody shrubs. Phytochemistry 1984;23:2366-7.

28. Schilcher H. Pflanzliche Diuretika. Urologe B 1987; 27:215-22.

29. Schilcher H. Pflanzliche Urologika. Dtsch Apoth Ztg 1984;124:2429-36.

30. Schilcher H. Birkenblätter. In: Loew D, Heimsoth V, Kuntz E, Schilcher H, editors. Diuretika. Chemie, Pharmakologie und Therapie einschließlich Phytotherapie, 2nd ed. Stuttgart: Georg Thieme Verlag, 1990:268-9.

31. Borman H, Melzig MF. Inhibition of metallopeptidases by flavonoids and related compounds. Pharmazie 2000;55:129-32.

32. Melzig MF, Major H. Neue Aspekte zum Verständnis des Wirkungsmechanismus der aquaretischen Wirkung von Birkenblättern und Goldrutenkraut. Z Phytotherapie 2000;21:193-6.

33. Vollmer H. Untersuchungen über die diuretische Wirkung der Folia betulae an Kaninchen und Mäusen. Vergleich mit anderen Drogen. Naunyn-Schmiedebergs Arch Exp Path Pharmakol 1937;186:584-91.

34. Vollmer H, Hübner K. Untersuchungen über die diuretische Wirkung der Fructus juniperi, Radix levistici, Radix ononidis, Folia betulae, Radix liquiritiae und Herba equiseti an Ratten. Naunyn-Schmiedebergs Arch Exp Path Pharmakol 1937;186:592-605.

35. Elbanowska A, Kaczmarek F. Investigations of the flavonoid compounds content and the diuretic activity of *Betula verrucosa* Ehrh. leaves at different phases of growth. Herba Pol 1966;11:47-56.

36. Borkowski B. Diuretische Wirkung einiger Flavondrogen. Planta Med 1960;8:95-104.

37. Schilcher H, Rau H. Nachweis der aquaretischen Wirkung von Birkenblätter- und Goldrutenkrautauszügen im Tierversuch. Urologe B 1988;28:274-80.

38. Schilcher H, Boesel R, Effenberger S, Segebrecht S. Neuere Untersuchungsergebnisse mit aquaretisch, antibakteriell und prostatotrop wirksamen Arzneipflanzen. Pharmakologische und phytochemische Untersuchungen von Goldrutenkraut, Birkenblättern, Wacholderbeeren, Gewürzsumachwurzelrinde, Liebstöckelwurzel, Queckenwurzel und Medizinal-kürbissamen. Urologe B 1989;29:267-71.

39. Lübben T. Untersuchung von Flavonoiden und Zubereitungen von Folia Betulae und Herba Solidaginis auf die diuretische Wirkung bei der Ratte [Dissertation]. University of Marburg, 1982 (cited in 17).

40. Marx H, Büchmann R. Über harntreibende Heilpflanzen. Dtsch Med Wochenschr 1937;63:384-6.

41. Braun H. Die therapeutische Verwendung wichtiger Drogen der Volksmedizin in der täglichen Praxis. IV. Betula alba (Birke). Fortschr Medizin 1941;59:114-6.

42. Müller B, Schneider B. Anwendungsbereiche eines Trockenextrakts aus Birkenblättern bei Harnwegserkrankungen: Ergebnisse einer Anwendungsbeobachtung. In: Abstracts of Phytotherapie an der Schwelle zum neuen Jahrtausend; 10. Jahrestagung der Gesellschaft für Phytotherapie. Münster, 11-13 November 1999:106-8 (Abstract P16).

43. Engesser A, Bersch U, Berchtold J, Göcking K, Schaffner W. Birkenblättertee (Betulae folium) gegen Infekte der unteren Harnwege - eine Pilotstudie. Arch Pharm Pharm Med Chem 1998;331(Suppl 1):V33.

44. Göggelmann W, Schimmer O. Mutagenic activity of phytotherapeutical drugs. In: Knudsen I, editor. Genetic Toxicology of the Diet. New York: Alan R. Liss, 1986:63-72.

BOLDI FOLIUM

Boldo Leaf

DEFINITION

Boldo leaf consists of the whole or fragmented dried leaves of *Peumus boldus* Molina. The whole drug contains not less than 20.0 ml/kg and not more than 40.0 ml/kg, and the fragmented drug not less than 15.0 ml/kg, of essential oil. It contains not less than 0.1 per cent of total alkaloids, expressed as boldine $(C_{19}H_{21}NO_4; M_r 327.4)$ and calculated with reference to the anhydrous drug.

The material complies with the monograph of the European Pharmacopoeia [1].

CONSTITUENTS

Isoquinoline alkaloids of the aporphine and nor-aporphine types, the major alkaloid being boldine [2-8]; essential oil containing monoterpenic hydro-carbons (mainly limonene, *p*-cymene, β-phellandrene and α-pinene) and oxygenated monoterpenes (mainly ascaridole, 1,8-cineole and linalool) [9-11]. Flavonoids are also present, especially glycosides of rhamnetin, isorhamnetin and kaempferol [12,13].

CLINICAL PARTICULARS

Therapeutic indications
Minor hepatobiliary dysfunction [14-19], symptomatic treatment of mild digestive disturbances [20].

Posology and method of administration

Dosage

Adult daily dose
2-5 g of the drug as a tea infusion [18,20,21].
0.2-0.6 g of the crude drug or equivalent hydro-ethanolic extract [22].
Tincture (1:5, ethanol 80% V/V) [23]: 1-3 ml [18,24].
Fluid extract (1:1, ethanol 80% V/V) [23]: 0.5-1 ml [24].

Method of administration
For oral administration.

Duration of administration
Not more than 4 weeks [20].

Contra-indications
Biliary obstruction [20].

E/S/C/O/P
MONOGRAPHS
Second Edition

Special warnings and special precautions for use

Special warnings
Continuous long-term use not recommended [20].

Precaution for use
None required.

Interaction with other medicaments and other forms of interaction
None reported.

Pregnancy and lactation
In accordance with general medical practice, the product should not be used during pregnancy and lactation without medical advice.

Very high doses of a dry ethanolic boldo leaf extract (800 mg/kg/day) have been reported to cause abortifacient and teratogenic effects in rats [25]; see Reproductive toxicity.

Effects on ability to drive and use machines
None known.

Undesirable effects
No toxic effects reported

Overdose
Emetic effect and spasms with very high doses [26].

PHARMACOLOGICAL PROPERTIES

Pharmacodynamic properties

In vitro experiments

Hepatoprotective effects
Solutions of a hydroethanolic extract of boldo (corresponding to 0.5 and 1 mg of dried leaf per ml) and pure boldine (33 µg/ml) exerted significant hepatoprotection against tert-butyl hydroperoxide-induced hepatotoxicity in isolated rat hepatocytes [27]. Boldine inhibited rat liver microsomal lipid peroxidation by 50% at a concentration of about 0.015 mM [28].

Cytoprotective and antioxidant effects
Boldine inhibited cell damage (trypan blue dye exclusion and lactate dehydrogenase activity) induced by tert-butyl hydroperoxide in a concentration-dependent manner in isolated rat hepatocytes. Preincubation with boldine, or simultaneous addition of boldine (200 µM) and tert-butyl hydroperoxide (0.87 mM), fully protected cell viability [29].

Boldine (12.5-100 µM) protected intact erythrocytes from rats in a time- and concentration-dependent manner against haemolytic damage induced by the free-radical initiator 2,2'-azobis-(2-amidinopropane) (25 and 50 mM) [30].

The lethal effect on Escherichia coli cultures induced by 25 µg/ml stannous chloride (which produces reactive oxygen species through a Fenton-like reaction) was reduced by the presence of 0.50 mM boldine, and the structural conformation of the plasmid pUC 9.1 was not modified by 100 µg/ml stannous chloride in the presence of 1.50 mM boldine. These effects could be explained by the antioxidant activity of boldine [31].

Antioxidant properties of boldine have also been demonstrated by the prevention of rat brain homogenate auto-oxidation and other tests with IC_{50} values of 19.0 to 28.7 µM [32].

In isolated rat hepatocytes boldine (200 µM) completely prevented peroxidative damage (accumulation of thiobarbituric acid reactive substances) induced by tert-butyl hydroperoxide at concentrations equal to or lower than 0.87 mM. However, boldine at the same concentration did not prevent an increase in the level of oxidized glutathione induced by tert-butyl hydroperoxide [29].

Spasmolytic effects
Boldine had a concentration-dependent smooth muscle relaxing effect on acetylcholine-induced contraction of the isolated rat ileum (EC_{50}: 1.7×10^{-4} M) via a competitive antagonist mechanism [33].

Effects on skeletal muscle
The effects of boldine on skeletal muscle were studied using mouse diaphragm and isolated sarcoplasmic reticulum membrane vesicules. At low concentrations (10-200 µM) boldine dose-dependently potentiated ryanodine-induced contraction (2 µM), and at higher concentration (300 µM) induced muscle contraction due to induction of Ca^{2+} release from the sarcoplasmic reticulum and the influx of extracellular Ca^{2+}. Boldine also dose-dependently increased apparent [^{3}H]-ryanodine binding with an EC_{50} of 50 µM [34].

Immunomodulating and cytotoxic effects
The treatment of lymphocytes from healthy donors and from patients with chronic lymphocytic leukaemia or breast cancer with boldine produced, in certain cases, inhibition of lectin-induced blast transformation, enhancement of natural killer cell activity and increased natural and lectin-dependent cell-mediated cytotoxicity. The effects of boldine on cellular immune functions suggested in vitro immunomodulating properties [35].

Antimicrobial activity
The antimicrobial activity of boldo leaf essential oil was assayed against 11 bacteria and one yeast. The more sensitive were Streptococcus pyogenes,

Micrococcus sp. (minimum bactericidal concentration < 0.91 µg/ml) and *Candida* sp. (minimum fungicidal concentration < 0.91 µg/ml) [10].

In vivo experiments

Choleretic effects
Significant choleretic activity, measured by the secretion of bile, was demonstrated in rats after intraduodenal administration of a purified ethanolic extract (250 and 500 mg/kg) [36] or an ethanolic extract (2.5 g/kg) [16] or an infusion of boldo leaf [17]. Most of the actions promoted by crude boldo preparations could be reproduced by the administration of pure boldine [14,15,27,37]. Boldine at 5-20 mg/kg in rats proved effective in increasing the amount of bile [15]. The choleretic activity may imply a synergy between alkaloids and flavonoids [36]. However, subsequent studies have not confirmed the choleretic activity: no significant increases in bile flow were observed after administration of a soft hydroethanolic extract orally to rats at 400 or 800 mg/kg, or intraduodenally to guinea pigs at 200 mg/kg or 800 mg/kg [38], or after intravenous administration of a dry ethanolic extract (4:1) corresponding to boldo leaf at 125-500 mg/kg [27].

Hepatoprotective effects
Significant hepatoprotection against carbon tetra-chloride-induced hepatotoxicity in mice has been demonstrated with a dry hydroethanolic extract containing 0.06-0.115% of boldine at 500 mg/kg (70% protection) and with boldine at 10 mg/kg (49% protection) [27].

Laxative effect
A laxative effect in rats has been described after oral administration of a soft hydroethanolic extract at 400 or 800 mg/kg daily for 8 weeks [38]. This may be due to increased excretion of bile salts modifying colonic motility [39].

Anti-inflammatory effects
Significant and dose-dependent anti-inflammatory effects were observed in the carrageenan-induced rat paw oedema test after intraperitoneal administration of a dry hydroethanolic extract of boldo leaf at 50 and 100 mg/kg; boldine (10 and 20 mg/kg) showed no anti-inflammatory activity in this test [27,40].

Boldine exhibited dose-dependent anti-inflammatory activity in the carrageenan-induced guinea pig paw oedema test with an oral ED_{50} of 34 mg/kg [41].

Boldine administered intrarectally at 100 mg/kg significantly reduced colonic neutrophil infiltration, as measured by myeloperoxidase activity (p = 0.0007), in an experimental model of acute colitis induced in rats by intrarectal administration of 4% acetic acid. Boldine also significantly protected against acid-induced oedema (p<0.05) as shown by decreased total colon weight [42].

Antipyretic effects
Boldine reduced bacterial pyrogen-induced hyperthermia in rabbits during the first 90 minutes of the assay with a mean value of 84% at an oral dose of 60 mg/kg [41].

Cytoprotective effects
Intrarectal administration of boldine at 100 mg/kg to rats with colitis induced by intrarectal administration of 4% acetic acid was found to significantly protect against colonic damage (p<0.05) in terms of major reductions in macroscopic and histologic lesions. Boldine administered intrarectally at 100 mg/kg was also found to maintain colonic fluid transport, a function otherwise markedly affected in the tissue of acid-treated animals [42].

Pharmacological studies in humans
In a double-blind, placebo-controlled, crossover study, 12 healthy volunteers were treated daily with either 2500 mg of a boldo dry extract (ethanol 60% V/V), containing 0.4% of total alkaloids and 0.12% of boldine, or placebo. Each treatment period lasted 4 days with a wash-out interval of 10 days. On the 4th day, 20 g of lactulose was administered and expired hydrogen was collected every 15 minutes. Gastro-intestinal transit time, defined as the time elapsed before expired hydrogen increased by 20 ppm over the fasting level, was significantly prolonged (p<0.05) after administration of the dry boldo extract compared to placebo (112.5 ± 15.4 and 87 ± 11.8 minutes respectively) [43].

Pharmacokinetic properties

In vitro experiments
Addition of boldine at 200 µM to a suspension of isolated rat hepatocytes was followed by an early and rapid accumulation of boldine within the cells, to 1600 µM within 2 minutes. By the end of 60 minutes of incubation the intracellular boldine concentration was 344 µM, still over 50% higher than that initially added to the suspension. When boldine was portally perfused through isolated rat livers, it was concentration-dependently removed from the extra-cellular medium at rates of 6.6, 10.4 and 16.2 nmol/min/0.1 g of liver for 50, 100 and 200 µM boldine respectively [44].

In vivo experiments
Boldine was found in the urine of rats after oral administration of a hydroethanolic boldo leaf extract at 400 and 800 mg/kg [38].

Absorption of boldine was rapid following its oral administration to rats at 25, 50 or 75 mg/kg, maximum plasma concentrations being reached within 15-30 minutes, and the boldine was preferentially concentrated in the liver. Plasma concentrations of boldine declined rapidly with an average half-life of approximately 31 minutes; the elimination appeared to follow a first order type of kinetics [44].

Preclinical safety data

Acute toxicity
Oral administration of a hydroethanolic extract of boldo to rats in single doses as high as 3 g/kg body weight caused no deaths or particularly toxic symptoms [38]. The intraperitoneal LD_{50} in mice of an 80%-ethanolic fluid extract was also low, equivalent to boldo leaf at 6 g/kg [36]. When boldine was administered orally, doses of 500 and 1000 mg/kg were required to cause the death of mice and guinea pigs respectively [14].

Intraperitoneal LD_{50} values in mice of total alkaloids and pure boldine were determined as 420 and 250 mg/kg, corresponding to 75 and 125 g/kg of boldo leaf respectively [36]. In an earlier study, sub-cutaneous injection into dogs of 5 mg/kg of total alkaloids produced vomiting, diarrhoea and, after 40 minutes, epileptic symptoms for about 7 minutes followed by recovery [14].

Subchronic toxicity
Oral administration of a 92.8%-ethanolic dry extract of boldo leaf or boldine to rats daily for 90 days at 200 mg/kg/day caused significant reductions (p<0.05 vs. control) in blood levels of cholesterol, aspartate aminotransferase (AST), total bilirubin, glucose and urea, although cholesterol and AST levels were elevated after 30 and 60 days (p<0.05 vs. control). There were no significant changes in creatinine levels. Doses of 50 mg/kg/day did not produce any significant changes in these parameters over the 90-day period. From histological examination, neither boldo extract nor boldine caused any overt signs of toxicity in the heart or kidneys but alterations of low intensity were observed in liver tissue [25].

Mutagenicity
Boldine showed no genotoxic activity in the SOS chromotest with *Escherichia coli* (up to 10 μg boldine) and no mutagenic potential in the Ames test using *Salmonella typhimurium* strains TA 98, TA 100 and TA 102 (boldine up to 200 μg/plate), with or without metabolic activation. Also, it induced no mutations in haploid *Saccharomyces cerevisiae* cells (boldine up to 200 μg/ml). These results indicate that boldine is not mutagenic in prokaryotic and eukaryotic organisms [45].

Boldine did not induce a statistically significant increase in the frequency of chromosomal aberrations or sister-chromatid exchanges when tested *in vitro* on human peripheral blood lymphocytes (boldine up to 40 μg/ml) or *in vivo* using mouse bone marrow cells (boldine up to 900 mg/kg body weight, administered orally) [46]. A further study has confirmed that boldine, administered intraperitoneally at sublethal doses, induced no signs of genotoxicity in mouse bone marrow as assessed by the micronucleus test [47].

Reproductive toxicity
Groups of 20 pregnant rats were treated orally with a 92.8%-ethanolic dry extract of boldo leaf or boldine at 500 or 800 mg/kg body weight on days 1-5 or days 7-12 of pregnancy (a total of 12 groups including 4 control groups, which were given an equivalent amount of saline 0.9%). Uteri and ovaries were removed for examination on day 19. Daily doses of 500 mg/kg of the extract or boldine did not produce any fetotoxicity but reduced fetal weight by 28-40%. However, daily doses of 800 mg/kg of the extract or boldine produced evidence of abortifacient and teratogenic activity: significant resorption (p<0.5), a low incidence of fetal malformations (1.5% in days 1-5 groups; 3.6% in days 7-12 groups) and also fetal weight decreases of 29-40%. The observations indicated that, at the 800 mg/kg/day level, the boldo leaf extract and boldine had adverse effects at the beginning of egg production and also during implantation [25].

REFERENCES

1. Boldo Leaf - Boldi folium. European Pharmacopoeia, Council of Europe.

2. Schindler H. *Peumus boldus* Mol. Die Stammpflanze der Folia Boldo. Arzneim-Forsch/Drug Res 1957;7:747-53.

3. Rüegger A. Neue Alkaloide aus *Peumus boldus* Molina. Helv Chim Acta 1959;42:754-62.

4. Hughes DW, Genest K, Skakum W. Alkaloids of *Peumus boldus*. Isolation of (+)-reticuline and isoboldine. J Pharm Sci 1968;57:1023-5.

5. Hughes DW, Genest K, Skakum W. Alkaloids of *Peumus boldus*. Isolation of laurotetanine and laurolitsine. J Pharm Sci 1968;57:1619-20.

6. Genest K, Hughes DW. Natural products in Canadian pharmaceuticals. II. *Peumus boldus*. Can J Pharm Sci 1968;3:84-90.

7. Vanhaelen M. Microdosage spectrophotométrique des alcaloïdes dans *Peumus boldus*. J Pharm Belg 1973; 28:291-9.

8. Van Hulle C, Braeckman P, Van Severen R. Influence of the preparation technique on the boldine content of boldo dry extract. J Pharm Belg 1983;38:97-100.

9. Bruns K, Köhler M. Über die Zusammensetzung des Boldoblätteröls. Parfüm und Kosmet 1974;55:225-7.

10. Vila R, Valenzuela L, Bello H, Cañigueral S, Montes M, Adzet T. Composition and antimicrobial activity of the essential oil of *Peumus boldus* leaves. Planta Med 1999;65:178-9.

11. Miraldi E, Ferri S, Franchi GG, Giorgi G. *Peumus boldus* essential oil: new constituents and comparison of oils from leaves of different origin. Fitoterapia 1996;67:227-30.

12. Krug H, Borkowski B. Neue Flavonol-Glykoside aus den Blättern von *Peumus boldus* Molina. Pharmazie 1965;20:692-8.

13. Bombardelli E, Martinelli EM, Mustich G. A new flavonol glycoside from *Peumus boldus*. Fitoterapia 1976;47:3-5.

14. Kreitmair H. Pharmakologische Wirkung des Alkaloids aus *Peumus boldus* Molina. Pharmazie 1952;7:507-11.

15. Borkowski B, Desperak-Naciazek A, Obojska K, Szmal Z. The effect of some aporphine alkaloids on bile secretion in rats. Diss Pharm Pharmacol 1966;18:455-65.

16. Böhm K. Untersuchungen über choleretische Wirkungen einiger Arzneipflanzen. Arzneim-Forsch/Drug Res 1959;9:376-8.

17. Pirtkien R, Surke E, Seybold G. Vergleichende Untersuchungen über die choleretische Wirkung verschiedener Arzneimittel bei der Ratte. Med Welt 1960;33:1417-22.

18. Nussbaumer PA, Buri P, Genequand M. Cholagogues et cholérétiques. Schweiz Apoth Ztg 1968;106:830-4.

19. Nussbaumer PA, Buri P, Genequand M. Cholagogues et cholérétiques. Schweiz Apoth Ztg 1968;106:930-4.

20. Hänsel R. Boldoblätter. In: Phytopharmaka, 2nd ed. Berlin-Heidelberg: Springer-Verlag,1991:189-90.

21. Tisanes. In: Pharmacopée Française, 10th ed. 2000.

22. Peumus. In: British Herbal Pharmacopoeia 1983. Bournemouth: British Herbal Medicine Association, 1983:155-6.

23. Extrait de Boldo (fluide); teinture de Boldo. In: Pharmacopée Française, 8th ed., 1965:458 and 1175.

24. Pharmacopée Française, 9th ed. Fiches de documentation de pratique officinale. Boldo, *Peumus boldus* Mol., 1979.

25. De Almeida ER, Melo AM, Xavier H. Toxicological evaluation of the hydro-alcohol extract of the dry leaves of *Peumus boldus* and boldine in rats. Phytotherapy Res 2000;14:99-102.

26. Braun H. Peumus boldo - Boldo. In: Heilpflanzen Lexikon fur Ärzte und Apotheker Stuttgart: Gustav Fischer, 1981:162.

27. Lanhers MC, Joyeux M, Soulimani R, Fleurentin J, Sayag M, Mortier F et al. Hepatoprotective and anti-inflammatory effects of a traditional medicinal plant of Chile, *Peumus boldus*. Planta Med 1991;57:110-5.

28. Cederbaum AI, Kukielka E, Speisky H. Inhibition of rat liver microsomal lipid peroxidation by boldine. Biochem Pharmacol 1992;44:1765-72.

29. Bannach R, Valenzuela A, Cassels BK, Núnez-Vergara LJ, Speisky H. Cytoprotective and antioxidant effects of boldine on *tert*-butyl hydroperoxide-induced damage to isolated hepatocytes. Cell Biol Toxicol 1996;12:89-100.

30. Jiménez I, Garrido A, Bannach R, Gotteland M, Speisky H. Protective effects of boldine against free radical-induced erythrocyte lysis. Phytotherapy Res 2000;14:339-43.

31. Reiniger IW, da Silva CR, Felzenszwalb I, de Mattos JCP, de Oliveira JF, da Silva Dantas FJ et al. Boldine action against the stannous chloride effect. J Ethnopharmacol 1999;68:345-8.

32. Speisky H, Cassels BK, Lissi EA, Videla LA. Antioxidant properties of the alkaloid boldine in systems undergoing lipid peroxidation and enzyme inactivation. Biochem Pharmacol 1991;41:1575-81.

33. Speisky H, Squella JA, Núñez-Vergara LJ. Activity of boldine on rat ileum. Planta Med 1991;57:519-22.

34. Kang J-J, Cheng Y-W. Effects of boldine on mouse diaphragm and sarcoplasmic reticulum vesicles isolated from skeletal muscle. Planta Med 1998;64:18-21.

35. Gonzáles-Cabello R, Speisky H, Bannach R, Valenzuela A, Fehér J, Gergely P. Effects of boldine on cellular immune functions *in vitro*. J Invest Allergol Clin Immunol 1994;4:139-45.

36. Lévy-Appert-Collin M-C, Lévy J. Sur quelques préparations galéniques de feuilles de Boldo (*Peumus boldus*, Monimiacées). J Pharm Belg 1977;32:13-22.

37. Delso Jimeno JL. Colereticos y colagogos: estudio farmacologico de la hoja del Boldo. Anales Inst Farmacol Esp 1956;5:395-441.

38. Magistretti MJ. Remarks on the pharmacological examination of plant extracts. Fitoterapia 1980;51:67-79.

39. Kirwan WO, Smith AN, Mitchell WD, Falconer JD, Eastwood MA. Bile acids and colonic motility in the rabbit and the human. Part 1. The rabbit. Gut 1975;16:894-902.

40. Lanhers MC, Fleurentin J, Rolland A, Vinche A. Activité anti-inflammatoire d'un extrait de *Peumus boldus* Molina (Monimiaceae). Phytotherapy 1992;38-39:12-3.

41. Backhouse N, Delporte C, Givernau M, Cassels BK, Valenzuela A, Speisky H. Anti-inflammatory and anti-pyretic effects of boldine. Agents Actions 1994;42:114-7.

42. Gotteland M, Jimenez I, Brunser O, Guzman L, Romero S, Cassels BK, Speisky H. Protective effect of boldine in experimental colitis. Planta Med 1997;63:311-5.

43. Gotteland M, Espinoza JM, Cassels BK, Speisky HC. Efecto de un extracto seco de boldo sobre el tránsito intestinal oro-cecal en voluntarios sanos. Rev Méd Chile 1995;123:955-60.

44. Jiménez I, Speisky H. Biological disposition of boldine: *in vitro* and *in vivo* studies. Phytotherapy Res 2000;14:254-60.

45. Moreno PRH, Vargas VMF, Andrade HHR, Henriques AT, Henriques JAP. Genotoxicity of the boldine aporphine alkaloid in prokaryotic and eukaryotic organisms. Mutation Res 1991;260:145-52.

46. Tavares DC, Takahashi CS. Evaluation of the genotoxic potential of the alkaloid boldine in mammalian cell systems in vitro and in vivo. Mutation Res 1994;321:139-45.

47. Speisky H, Cassels BK. Boldo and boldine: an emerging case of natural drug development. Pharmacol Res 1994;29:1-12.

CALENDULAE FLOS

Calendula Flower

E/S/C/O/P
MONOGRAPHS
Second Edition

DEFINITION

Calendula flower consists of the whole or cut, dried, fully opened flowers, which have been detached from the receptacle, of the cultivated, double-flowered varieties of *Calendula officinalis* L. It contains not less than 0.4 per cent of flavonoids, calculated as hyperoside ($C_{21}H_{20}O_{12}$, M_r 464.4) with reference to the dried drug [1].

The material complies with the monograph of the European Pharmacopoeia [1].

Fresh material may also be used, provided that when dried it complies with the monograph of the European Pharmacopoeia.

CONSTITUENTS

Triterpene saponins, mainly oleanolic acid glycosides [2-5]; free and esterified triterpene alcohols, especially faradiol 3-monoesters [2,4-8], carotenoids [2,4,5], flavonoids based on quercetin and isorhamnetin [2,4,5,9,10], polysaccharides [4,5,11], sterols [4,5], sesquiterpenoids [2,4] and essential oil [4,5,12].

CLINICAL PARTICULARS

Therapeutic indications
Symptomatic treatment of minor inflammations of the skin and mucosa; as an aid to the healing of minor wounds [2,5,13-15].

Posology and method of administration

Dosage
External use
Infusion for topical application: 1-2 g of dried flower per 150 ml of water.
Fluid extract 1:1 in 40% ethanol or tincture 1:5 in 90% ethanol [15]. For the treatment of wounds the tincture is applied undiluted; for compresses the tincture is usually diluted at least 1:3 with freshly boiled water [13,16].
Semi-solid preparations containing 2-10% of fluid extract 1:1 [13,15,17].

Method of administration
For topical application.

Duration of administration
No restriction.

Contra-indications
Known sensitivity to members of the Compositae family.

Special warnings and special precautions for use
None required.

Interaction with other medicaments and other forms of interaction
None reported.

Pregnancy and lactation
No data available.
However, there are no objections to external use during pregnancy and lactation.

Effects on ability to drive and use machines
Not relevant.

Undesirable effects
Weak skin sensitisation has been shown experimentally but there are no clearly recorded cases of contact dermatitis [18].

Overdose
Not applicable.

PHARMACOLOGICAL PROPERTIES

Pharmacodynamic properties

In vitro experiments

Immunomodulatory effects
A dry 70% ethanolic extract of calendula flower caused an inhibitory effect in the mitogen-induced lymphocyte proliferation assay. In the mixed lymphocyte reaction the extract showed stimulatory effects at 0.1-10 µg/ml, followed by inhibition at higher concentrations [19].

Isolated polysaccharides from calendula flower were found to stimulate phagocytosis of human granulocytes [11].

Antimicrobial and antiviral effects
Various hydroalcoholic extracts exhibited antibacterial activity [20]. Antifungal activity was observed with a 10% methanol extract [21]. A 70% hydroalcoholic tincture of calendula flower had high virucidal activity against influenza viruses and a marked ability to suppress the growth of herpes simplex virus [22].

A dry extract (dichloromethane-methanol 1:1) exhibited anti-HIV activity in an *in vitro* MTT (dimethylthiazole-diphenyltetrazolium)-based assay. In the presence of 10-30 µg/ml of the extract, 90% inhibition of HIV-1 replication in acutely infected lymphocytic Molt-4 cells was observed. In concentrations of 500 µg/ml the extract suppressed cell fusion and protected uninfected Molt-4 cells against subsequent HIV-induced cytolysis caused by co-cultivation with persistently infected U-937/HIV-1 cells for up to 24 hours. The extract (50, 100 and 200 µg/ml) also caused marked dose- and time-dependent inhibition of HIV-1 reverse transcriptase activity by up to 85% in a cell-free system [23].

Extracts from the flowers have trichomonacidal activity [24,25], which has been attributed to oxygenated terpenes [12].

Antioxidant effects
Extracts of calendula flower of differing polarities exhibited antioxidative effects on liposomal lipid peroxidation induced by Fe^{2+} and ascorbic acid. Marked activity was observed with ether, butanol and aqueous extracts. In combination with pro-oxidants different antioxidative effects were obtained: with pyralene the butanol and aqueous extracts were most effective; with carbon tetrachloride the chloroform and ethyl acetate extracts showed the strongest activity. Combination of the antioxidant fullerenol with each extract resulted in a further decrease in lipid peroxidation [26,27].

Angiogenic effects
The angiogenic activity of a lyophilized aqueous infusion (1:10) of calendula flower was tested in the chick chorioallantoic membrane (CAM) test. The numbers of micro-vessels in tissue sections of treated CAMs were significantly higher (p<0.0001) than in control CAMs. All treated CAMs were positive for hyaluronan, while no hyaluronan was detected in control CAMs [28].

Anti-inflammatory effects
Three isorhamnetin glycosides from calendula flower at concentrations of 1.5×10^{-5} M showed inhibitory effects on arachidonate 12-lipoxygenase from rat lung cytosol [29].

Effects on buccal membranes
In a test system based on porcine buccal membranes, strong concentration-dependent adhesive processes were observed with a low-viscosity, polysaccharide-enriched extract (98% carbohydrates) of calendula flower. These findings suggested that the polysaccharides may contribute to therapeutic effects in the treatment of irritated mucosa [30].

In vivo experiments

Effects on wound healing
Dried alcoholic and aqueous extracts of calendula flower in combination with allantoin, applied topically as a 5% ointment, stimulated epithelization in surgically-inflicted standard wounds in rats [31,32].

In a study in rabbits, the time taken for complete cicatrization of experimental wounds was shortened by approximately 25% after topical treatment with hydrogel or powder preparations containing 10% of an ethanolic dry extract of calendula flower in comparison with vehicle-only controls [33].

Enhanced healing of experimental wounds in buffalo calves was observed after topical treatment with an ointment containing 5% of a dry extract of calendula flower. Epithelization accelerated and histopathological parameters improved in comparison with wounds treated with normal saline only [34].

Experimental incisions in rats were infected with *Staphylococcus epidermidis*. Topical treatment with a calendula cream (not further specified) resulted in accelerated cicatrization compared to controls. The results were confirmed by histological examination [35].

Immunomodulatory effects
Polysaccharide fractions from aqueous extracts of calendula flower appeared to enhance phagocytosis in the carbon clearance test in mice [36]. The unsaponifiable fraction of a hydroalcoholic extract, administered intraperitoneally, protected mice from lethal sepsis due to *Escherichia coli* [37].

Anti-inflammatory effects
A lyophilized extract suppressed inflammatory effects and leukocyte infiltration induced by simultaneous injection of carrageenan and prostaglandin E_1 into rats [38].

A dry 80% ethanolic extract of calendula flower, given orally 1 hour before oedema elicitation, inhibited carrageenan-induced rat paw oedema by 11% at a dose of 100 mg/kg body weight. In the same experiment indometacin at 5 mg/kg resulted in 45% inhibition of oedema [39].

A 70% alcoholic extract and a supercritical CO_2 extract were applied topically in the croton oil ear oedema test in mice. The hydroalcoholic extract had a mild dose-dependent effect, inhibiting oedema by 20% at a dose of 1200 µg/ear, corresponding to 4.16 mg of crude drug. The CO_2 extract produced 30% inhibition at 150 µg/ear, corresponding to 3.6 mg of the crude drug, and 71% inhibition at 1200 µg/ear, corresponding to 28.6 mg of crude drug. The activity at the higher concentration was comparable to that of indometacin at 120 µg/ear [40]. In the same model, triterpenoids were shown to be the most important anti-inflammatory principles in the CO_2 extract [6].

In the same test system in male albino Swiss mice, a faradiol monoester mixture, faradiol-3-myristic acid ester, faradiol 3-palmitic acid ester and ψ-taraxasterol isolated from calendula flower all showed significant (p<0.05) anti-oedematous activity compared to controls at doses of 240 and 480 µg/cm² [8]. Faradiol (which is not present in the free form in calendula flower) proved to be even more active than the esters with an anti-oedematous effect comparable to that of an equimolar dose of indometacin, but 3-esterification reduces the activity by more than 50% [6,8].

Helianol and ψ-taraxasterol from calendula flower inhibited inflammation induced by 12-*O*-tetra-decanoylphorbol-13-acetate (1 µg per ear topically) in female ICR mice. The 50% inhibitory doses were 0.1 mg/ear for helianol and 0.4 mg/ear for ψ-taraxasterol, compared to 0.3 mg/ear for indometacin [7].

Antitumour effects
A triterpene-enriched fraction given orally to mice inoculated with Ehrlich mouse carcinoma prevented the development of ascites and increased survival time compared to controls [41].

Other effects
An isolated saponin fraction administered orally at 50 mg/kg body weight to hyperlipaemic rats reduced the serum lipid level [42-44].

Clinical studies
In a randomized, open, controlled study, the effects of three ointments were compared after topical treatment of patients with 2nd or 3rd degree burns for 17 days: a calendula flower ointment (prepared by digestion in vaseline) (n = 53) or vaseline only (n = 50) or a proteolytic ointment (n = 53). The success rates were considered to be 37/53 for calendula flower ointment, 27/50 for vaseline and 35/53 for the proteolytic ointment. Calendula flower ointment was marginally superior to its base, vaseline (p = 0.05) [45].

In an open, uncontrolled pilot study 30 patients with burns or scalds (degrees 1 and 2a) were treated 3 times per day for up to 14 days with a hydrogel containing 10% of a hydroethanolic extract. The symptoms reddening, swelling, blistering, pain, soreness and heat sensitivity were scored before, during and at the end of treatment. The total score and individual scores for each symptom improved [46].

Pharmacokinetic properties
No data available.

Preclinical safety data

Acute toxicity
For an aqueous extract from calendula flower administered to mice, the intravenous LD_{50} was determined as 375 mg/kg body weight and the

intraperitoneal LD_{100} as 580 mg/kg [47]. For a hydroalcoholic extract (drug to extract ratio 1:1, 30% ethanol) the subcutaneous LD_{50} was 45 mg in mice and the intravenous LD_{50} was 526 mg/100 g in rats [48]. An ethylene glycol extract (drug to extract ratio 2:1) was non-toxic in albino mice after subcutaneous administration of 10 ml/kg [49].

Chronic toxicity
An aqueous extract was reported to be non-toxic in chronic administration to mice [47]. No symptoms of toxicity were observed after oral administration of a calendula flower extract (solvent unspecified) at 0.15 g/kg body weight to hamsters over 18 months and to rats over 21 months [50]. No toxic symptoms appeared in rats after daily oral administration of calenduloside B at 200 mg/kg body weight for 2 months [51].

Mutagenicity
In the Ames test using *Salmonella typhimurium* strains TA 1535, TA 1537, TA 98 and TA 100, a fluid extract (60% ethanol) was non-mutagenic at concentrations of 50-5000 μg/plate. With *Aspergillus nidulans* diploid strain D-30, genotoxic effects with mitotic crossing over and chromosome malsegregation were observed at higher concentrations of 0.1-1.0 mg/ml, at which a concentration-dependent increase of cytotoxicity also occurred. These findings were not confirmed *in vivo* in the mouse bone marrow micronucleus test; after oral administration of the extract at up to 1 g/kg body weight for two days no increase in the number of micronucleated poly-chromated erythrocytes was observed [52].

Six saponins from calendula flower (at 400 μg/plate) were non-mutagenic in the Ames test using *Salmonella typhimurium* TA 98 with and without S9 activation [53].

Carcinogenicity studies with calendula flower extract have been performed in rats over a period of 22 months and in hamsters over a period of 18 months with a daily oral dose of 0.15 g/kg body weight. The extract was not carcinogenic in either species [50].

Sensitizing potential
An oily extract from calendula was tolerable to mucosa in the Draize primary mucosa irritation test using the rabbit eye [4].

Clinical safety data
No side effects or irritations were observed in 30 patients with burns or scalds during treatment with a hydrogel containing 10% of a hydroethanolic extract 3 times daily for up to 14 days [46].

In a randomized study involving 156 patients with 2nd or 3rd degree burns a calendula ointment was significantly better tolerated (p = 0.002) than a proteolytic ointment [45].

REFERENCES

1. Calendula Flower - Calendulae flos. European Pharmacopoeia, Council of Europe.

2. Scheffer JJC. De goudsbloem (*Calendula officinalis* L.) als geneeskruid in verleden en heden. Pharm Weekbl 1979;114:1149-57.

3. Vidal-Ollivier E, Balansard G, Faure R, Babadjamian A. Revised structures of triterpenoid saponins from the flowers of *Calendula officinalis*. J Nat Prod 1989; 52:1156-9.

4. Isaac O. Die Ringelblume. Botanik, Chemie, Pharmakologie, Toxikologie, Pharmazie und therapeutische Verwendung. Stuttgart: Wissenschaftliche Verlagsgesellschaft, 1992:65-6.

5. Willuhn G. Calendulae flos - Ringelblumen. In: Wichtl M, editor. Teedrogen, 3rd ed. Stuttgart: Wissenschaftliche Verlagsgesellschaft, 1997:119-22.

6. Della Loggia R, Tubaro A, Sosa S, Becker H, Saar St, Isaac O. The role of triterpenoids in the topical anti-inflammatory activity of *Calendula officinalis* flowers. Planta Med 1994;60:516-20.

7. Akihisa T, Yasukawa K, Oinuma H, Kasahara Y, Yamanouchi S, Takido M et al. Triterpene alcohols from the flowers of Compositae and their anti-inflammatory effects. Phytochemistry 1996;43:1255-60.

8. Zitterl-Eglseer K, Sosa S, Jurenitsch J, Schubert-Zsilavecz M, Della Loggia R, Tubaro A et al. Anti-oedematous activities of the main triterpendiol esters of marigold (*Calendula officinalis* L.). J Ethnopharmacol 1997; 57:139-44.

9. Komissarenko NF, Chernobai VT, Derkach AI. Flavonoids of inflorescences of *Calendula officinalis*. Khim Prir Soedin 1988;795-801, as English translation in Chem Nat Compd 1988;24:675-80.

10. Vidal-Ollivier E, Elias R, Faure F, Babadjamian A, Crespin F, Balansard G, Boudon G. Flavonol glycosides from *Calendula officinalis* flowers. Planta Med 1989; 55:73-4.

11. Varljen J, Lipták A, Wagner H. Structural analysis of a rhamnoarabinogalactan and arabinogalactans with immuno-stimulating activity from *Calendula officinalis*. Phytochemistry 1989;28:2379-83.

12. Gracza L. Oxygen-containing terpene derivatives from *Calendula officinalis*. Planta Med 1987;53:227.

13. Willuhn G. Pflanzliche Dermatika - Eine kritische Übersicht. Dtsch Apoth Ztg 1992;132:1873-83.

14. Weiss RF and Fintelmann V. *Calendula officinalis*, Marigold. In: Herbal Medicine, 2nd ed. (translated from the 9th German edition of Lehrbuch der Phytotherapie). Stuttgart-New York: Thieme, 2000:312.

15. Isaac O. Calendula. In: Hänsel R, Keller K, Rimpler H, Schneider G, editors. Hagers Handbuch der

Pharmazeutischen Praxis, 5th ed. Volume 4: Drogen A-D. Berlin-Heidelberg: Springer-Verlag, 1992:597-615.

16. Van Hellemont J. Fytotherapeutisch compendium, 2nd ed. Utrecht: Bohn, Scheltema & Holkema, 1988;113-4.

17. Calendula: Crema 10 per cento. In: Farmacopoea Italiana.

18. Hausen BM, Vieluf IK. Allergiepflanzen Pflanzen-allergene: Handbuch und Atlas der allergie-induzierenden Wild- und Kulturpflanzen. 2nd ed. Landsberg, München: Ecomed Verlagsgesellschaft, 1997:85-6.

19. Amirghofran Z, Azadbakht M, Karimi MH. Evaluation of the immunomodulatory effects of five herbal plants. J Ethnopharmacol 2000;72:167-72.

20. Dumenil G, Chemli R, Balansard G, Guiraud H, Lallemand M. Étude des propriétés antibactériennes des fleurs de Souci Calendula officinalis L. et des teintures mères homéopathiques de C. officinalis L. et C. arvensis L. Ann Pharm Fr 1980;38:493-9.

21. Wolters B. Die Verbreitung antibiotischer Eigenschaften bei Saponindrogen. Dtsch Apoth Ztg 1966;106:1729-33.

22. Bogdanova NS, Nikolaeva IS, Scherbakova LI, Tolstova TI, Moskalenko NYu, Pershin GN. A study into antiviral properties of Calendula officinalis. Farmakol Toksikol 1970;33:349-55.

23. Kalvatchev Z, Walder R, Garzaro D. Anti-HIV activity of extracts from Calendula officinalis flowers. Biomed & Pharmacother 1997;51:176-80.

24. Samochowiec E, Urbanska L, Manka W, Stolarska E. Assessment of the action of Calendula officinalis and Echinacea angustifolia extracts on Trichomonas vaginalis in vitro. Wiad Parazytol 1979;25:77-81.

25. Fazakas B, Rácz G. Actiunea unor produse vegetale asupra protozoarului Trichomonas vaginalis. Farmacia (Bucharest) 1965;13:91-3.

26. Popovic M, Kaurinovic B, Mimica-Dukic N, Vojinovic-Miloradov M, Cupic V. Combined effects of plant extracts and xenobiotics on liposomal lipid peroxidation. Part 1. Marigold extract-ciprofloxacin/pyralene. Oxid Commun 1999;22:487-94.

27. Popovic M, Kaurinovic B, Mimica-Dukic N, Vojinovic-Miloradov M, Djordjevic A. Combined effects of plant extracts and xenobiotics on liposomal lipid peroxidation. Part 2. Marigold extract-CCl$_4$/fullerenol. Oxid Commun 2000;23:178-86.

28. Patrick KFM, Kumar S, Edwardson PAD, Hutchinson JJ. Induction of vascularisation by an aqueous extract of the flowers of Calendula officinalis L. the European marigold. Phytomedicine 1996;3:11-8.

29. Bezáková L, Masterová I, Paulíková I, Psenák M.. Inhibitory activity of isorhamnetin glycosides from Calendula officinalis L. on the activity of lipoxygenase.

Pharmazie 1996;51:126-7.

30. Schmidgall J, Schnetz E, Hensel A. Evidence for bio-adhesive effects of polysaccharides and polysaccharide-containing herbs in an ex vivo bioadhesion assay on buccal membranes. Planta Med 2000;66:48-53.

31. Klouchek-Popova E, Popov A, Pavlova N, Krusteva K. Experimental phytochemical, pharmacological and cytomorphological studies of the regenerative action of fractions C1 and C5 isolated from Calendula officinalis. Savremenna Med 1981;32:395-9.

32. Klouchek-Popova E, Popov A, Pavlova N, Krusteva S. Influence of the physiological regeneration and epithelization using fractions isolated from Calendula officinalis. Acta Physiol Pharmacol Bulg 1982;8:63-7.

33. Oana I, Mates N, Ognean L, Muste A, Aldea M, Neculoiu D, Banciu C. Studies concerning the wound healing action of some medicinal herb extracts. Buletinul Universitatii de Stiinte Agricole - Seria Zootehnie si Medicina Veterinara 1995;49:461-5.

34. Ansari MA, Jadon NS, Singh SP, Kumar A, Singh H. Effect of Calendula officinalis ointment, charmil and gelatin granules on wound healing in buffaloes - a histological study. Indian Vet J 1997;74:594-7.

35. Perri de Carvalho PS, Tagliavini DG, Tagliavini RL. Cutaneous cicatrization after topical application of calendula cream and comfrey, propolis and honey association in infected wound of skin. Clinical and histological study in rats. Rev Ciênc Bioméd (São Paulo) 1991;12:39-50.

36. Wagner H, Proksch A, Riess-Maurer I, Vollmar A, Odenthal S, Stuppner H et al. Immunstimulierend wirkende Polysaccharide (Heteroglykane) aus höheren Pflanzen. Arzneim-Forsch/Drug Res 1985;35:1069-75.

37. Delaveau P, Lallouette P, Tessier AM. Drogues végétales stimulant l'activité phagocytaire du système réticulo-endothélial. Planta Med 1980;40:49-54.

38. Shipochliev T, Dimitrov A, Aleksandrova E. Study on the antiinflammatory effect of a group of plant extracts. Vet-Med Nauk (Vet Sci Sofia) 1981;18(6):87-94.

39. Mascolo N, Autore G, Capasso F, Menghini A, Fasulo MP. Biological screening of Italian medicinal plants for anti-inflammatory activity. Phytother Res 1987;1:28-31.

40. Della Loggia R, Becker H, Isaac O, Tubaro A. Topical anti-inflammatory activity of Calendula officinalis extracts. Planta Med 1990;56:658.

41. Boucaud-Maitre Y, Algernon O, Raynaud J. Cytotoxic and antitumoral activity of Calendula officinalis extracts. Pharmazie 1988;43:220-1.

42. Bialaschik FJ. Isolierung und chemische Charakterisierung einiger Oleanolsäurederivate aus Beta vulgaris L. und Calendula officinalis L. sowie pharmakologische Untersuchungen ausgewählter Saponinfraktionen aus beiden Arten [Dissertation]. Berlin: Universities of Berlin and Poznan, 1982.

43. Samochowiec L. Pharmakologische Untersuchungen der Saponosiden von *Aralia mandshurica* Rupr. et Maxim. und *Calendula officinalis* L. Herba Pol 1983;29:151-5.

44. Wojcicki J, Samochowiec L. Comparative evaluation of the effect of *Aralia mandshurica* Rupr. et Maxim. and *Calendula officinalis* L. saponosides on the lipid level in blood serum and liver homogenates. Herba Pol 1980;26:233-7, through Chem Abstr 1981;95:180898s.

45. Lievre M, Marichy J, Baux S, Foyatier JL, Perrot J, Boissel JP. Controlled study of three ointments for the local management of 2nd and 3rd degree burns. Clinical Trials and Meta-Analysis 1992;28:9-12.

46. Baranov AP. Calendula - Wie ist die Wirksamkeit bei Verbrennungen und Verbrühungen? Dtsch Apoth Ztg 1999;139:2135-8.

47. Manolov P, Boyadzhiev Tsv, Nikolov P. Antitumorigenic effect of preparations of *Calendula officinalis* on Crocker sarcoma 180. Eksperim Med Morfol 1964;3:41-5, through Chem Abstr 1965;62:9652d.

48. Boyadzhiev Tsv. Sedative and hypotensive effect of preparations from the plant *Calendula officinalis*. Nauchni Tr Vissh Med Inst Sofia 1964:43:15-20, through Chem Abstr 1965;63:1114a.

49. Russo M. Impiego dell'estratto di Calendula (*Calendula officinalis* L.) in cosmetologia. Rivista Italiana Essenze Profumi Piante Officinali 1972;54:740-3.

50. Avramova S, Portarska F, Apostolova B, Petkova S, Konteva M, Tsekova M et al. Marigold (*Calendula officinalis* L.) - Source of new products for the cosmetic industry. MBI Med Biol Inf 1988;(4):28-32.

51. Yatsyno AI, Belova LF, Lipkina GS, Sokolov SYa, Trutneva EA. Pharmacology of calenduloside B - a new triterpene glycoside obtained from rhizomes of *Calendula officinalis*. Farmakol Toksikol (Moscow) 1978;41:556-60.

52. Ramos A, Edreira A, Vizoso A, Betancourt J, López M, Décalo M. Genotoxicity of an extract of *Calendula officinalis* L. J Ethnopharmacol 1998;61:49-55.

53. Elias R, de Méo M, Vidal-Ollivier E, Laget M, Balansard G, Dumenil G. Antimutagenic activity of some saponins isolated from *Calendula officinalis* L., *C. arvensis* L. and *Hedera helix* L. Mutagenesis 1990;5:327-31.

CARVI FRUCTUS

Caraway Fruit

DEFINITION

Caraway fruit consists of the whole, dry mericarp of *Carum carvi* L. It contains not less than 30 ml/kg of essential oil, calculated with reference to the anhydrous drug.

The material complies with the monograph of the European Pharmacopoeia [1].

CONSTITUENTS

Caraway fruit contains 3-7% V/m of essential oil [2,3], consisting largely of (+)-carvone (50-65%) [4] and (+)-limonene (up to 45%) [5-8] with less than 1.5% of carveol and dihydrocarveol [6,9-11]. It also contains 10-18% of fixed oil, of which the main components are petroselinic (30-43%), linoleic (34-37%), oleic (15-25%) and palmitic (4-5%) acids [3,12-17].

Other constituents include about 20% of protein [2,3], about 15% of carbohydrates [2,18], phenolic acids, mainly caffeic acid [19,20], and traces of flavonoids such as quercetin, kaempferol and their glycosides [21,22].

Carvenone [23], carvacrol [9,24] and perillalcohol [9] are found as distillation and storage artefacts.

CLINICAL PARTICULARS

Therapeutic indications

Internal use
Spasmodic gastro-intestinal complaints, flatulence, bloating [2,3,25-30].
Flatulent colic of infants [2,28,29,31].

External use
Flatulent colic of infants [3,30].

Posology and method of administration

Dosage

DRIED FRUITS
Internal use
Adults and children over 10 years of age: 1.5-6 g of caraway fruit daily [31]. 1-5 g of caraway fruit [2], crushed directly before use, covered with 150 ml of boiling water and allowed to stand for 10-15 minutes.

E/S/C/O/P
MONOGRAPHS
Second Edition

A cup of warm tea is taken 1-3 times daily [2,29]. Other equivalent preparations.

Children from 4 to 10 years: 1-4 g daily [31].
Children from 1 to 4 years: 1-2 g daily [31].
Children up to 1 year: 1 g daily [31].

CARAWAY OIL FOR CHILDREN
Internal use
Children above 4 years: 3-6 drops daily [31].
Children from 1 to 4 years: 2-4 drops daily [31].
Children up to 1 year: 1-2 drops daily [31].
External use
10% in a carrier oil, for example olive oil [3,30].

Method of administration
For oral administration [29] or external application to the abdomen [30]. Combination with other gastrointestinal drugs may be beneficial [26,30].

Duration of administration
If symptoms persist or worsen, use should be discontinued and medical advice sought. Acute abdominal pain requires medical attention.

Contra-indications
Sensitivity to Umbelliferae or Compositae [32-35].

Special warnings and special precautions for use
None required.

Interaction with other medicaments and other forms of interaction
None reported.

Pregnancy and lactation
No data available. In accordance with general medical practice, the product should not be used during pregnancy without medical advice.

Effects on ability to drive and use machines
None known.

Undesirable effects
None reported.

Overdose
No toxic effects reported.

PHARMACOLOGICAL PROPERTIES

Pharmacodynamic properties

Carminative effects
Components of the essential oil cause local stimulation of the gastric mucosa, which activates the vagus nerve, leading to an increase of stomach tonus and rhythmic contraction. The result is an eructation of air from the stomach and an increase in gastric secretion [36,37].

In vitro experiments

Antispasmodic effects
The antispasmodic activity of 2.5 and 10.0 ml/litre of a hydroethanolic extract of caraway fruit (1 part drug to 3.5 parts ethanol 31% m/m) was tested on guinea pig ileum, using acetylcholine and histamine as spasmogens. A dose-dependent decrease of the response to acetylcholine and histamine was observed. The maximum contractility produced by histamine was decreased [25]. In the same test system 2.5 and 10.0 ml/litre of extract decreased the contractility produced by carbachol [26].

The relaxant effects of caraway oil were determined on guinea pig tracheal smooth muscle without addition of spasmogen. A 50% decrease in the force of phasic contractions was achieved with 27 mg/litre caraway oil. No antispasmodic effect was observed on electrically stimulated guinea pig ileum [38].

In an experiment which measured the depolarization-induced uptake of $^{45}Ca^{2+}$ into clonal rat pituitary GH_4C_1 cells, caraway fruit dry extract (80% methanol) at 20 mg/ml promoted Ca^{2+} fluxes into the cells with an increase of 26.8% [39].

Antimicrobial effects
Ethanolic and butanolic extracts of caraway fruit (20 g in 50 ml) exhibited antimicrobial activity against numerous test organisms such as *Escherichia coli*, *Staphylococcus aureus*, *Candida albicans* and *Streptomyces venezuelae* [40].

Methanolic and chloroform extracts of defatted caraway fruit (yield 7.5% and 3.0% respectively) at a dose of 10 µg per disc showed activity against *Shigella dysenteriae* type 1 and *Shigella flexneri* similar to that of ampicillin (10 µg). The active compound was identified as a steroid [41].

A methanolic extract of caraway fruit inhibited *Helicobacter pylori* with an MIC_{50} of 100 µg/ml [42].

The essential oil of caraway fruit showed antimicrobial activity against *Staphylococcus aureus* (MIC 700 ppm), *Escherichia coli* (delayed inhibition), *Salmonella typhi* (MIC 900 ppm), *Shigella dysentery* (MIC 1200 ppm) and *Vibrio cholera* (two-fold inhibition at 800 ppm) [43]. The decrease in antimicrobial activity of caraway fruit essential oil and more lipophilic extracts against *Staphylococcus aureus* depended on the content of lipophilic components [44].

Inhibitory effects were observed with (+)-carvone at concentrations of about 0.15 mg/ml against fungi and vermiforms and 4 mg/ml against bacteria [45].

Caraway fruit led to inhibition of the growth and toxin production of *Aspergillus, Epidermatophyton* and *Trichophyton* species [46-49]. An aqueous extract of caraway fruit (2:1) exhibited significant antifungal activity against *Saccharomyces pastorianus, Candida albicans, Rhizopus nigricans, Aspergillus fumigatus* and *niger, Penicillium digitatum, Botrytis cinerea, Fusarium oxysporum* and *Trichophyton mentagrophytes* [50].

In vivo experiments

Hypoglycaemic and hypocholesterolaemic effects
Treatment of alloxan-induced diabetic rats with 10 mg of caraway oil per kg body weight for 6 weeks significantly reduced (p<0.001) blood glucose by 55% and serum cholesterol by 74% respectively compared to an untreated diabetic control group [51].

Mucotropic effects
The mucotropic effects of carvone given by steam inhalation to urethanized rabbits were investigated at different times of the year. Carvone (2 mg/kg body weight) produced an 89.6% increase in the volume output of respiratory tract fluid during autumn months, while a 17.5% increase was observed during the rest of the year. Carvone at 1-9 mg/kg body weight produced a dose-dependent decrease in the specific gravity of respiratory tract fluid without significant seasonal variation [52].

Pharmacological studies in humans

Antispasmodic effects
Capsules containing 50 mg of caraway oil inhibited contraction of the gallbladder. In 7 volunteers an increase of 90% in gallbladder volume was determined by means of real-time ultrasonographic measurement. The capsules had no inhibitory effect on small intestine motility [53].

Pharmacokinetic properties

Gastrointestinal absorption
The absorption of carvone from a caraway fruit extract (1:3, ethanol 30% V/V) was tested in everted intestinal sacs prepared from male adult rats. After 30 minutes, the uptake from an extract concentration of 117.4 μg/ml was about 3 μg/cm^2 carvone [54].

Percutaneous absorption
No data available for caraway oil, but (+)-carvone was absorbed within 35 minutes after application to the shaved intact abdominal skin of the mouse [55].

Metabolism and excretion
No data available for caraway, but in rabbits (+)-carvone was oxidized to hydroxycarvone and conjugated with glucuronic acid [56].

Preclinical safety data

Acute toxicity
The acute oral LD_{50} of caraway oil in rats has been determined as 3.5 ml/kg [57] and 6.68 g/kg body weight [58]. The acute dermal LD_{50} of caraway oil in rabbits was reported as 1.78 ml/kg [57].

In the brine shrimp lethality bioassay an ethanolic extract of caraway yielded LC_{50} values in the range 85-266 μg/ml [59].

Subchronic and chronic toxicity
A study in rats demonstrated that 1% of (+)-carvone in the diet for 16 weeks caused growth retardation and testicular atrophy, while 0.1% for 28 weeks and 0.25% for one year had no effects [60]. Based on short-term and long-term toxicity studies in rodents, including a no-observed-effect level of 93 mg/kg body weight/day in rats, the World Health Organization has established an ADI (acceptable daily intake) for (+)-carvone of 0-1 mg/kg body weight/day [61].

Mutagenicity and carcinogenicity
Mutagenic screening of chloroform and methanol caraway fruit extracts showed an apparent increase in the number of *Salmonella typhimurium* strain TA 100 revertants, but these observations were accompanied by a reduction in the background lawn of bacterial growth. Therefore the results require further investigation. No mutagenicity was observed with aqueous extracts [62].

The mutagenicity induced by N-methyl-N'-nitro-N-nitrosoguanidine and methylazoxymethanol acetate in the Ames test was inhibited by a hot water extract of caraway fruit, which also prevented the formation of aberrant crypts in the colons of rats after administration of 1,2-dimethylhydrazine [63].

An ethanolic caraway fruit extract at a dose of 10 mg was added to two strains of *Salmonella typhimurium* (TA 98 and TA 102). The extract was non-mutagenic in strain TA 98 and intermediately mutagenic in strain TA 102 [59].

Up to 75 mg of caraway fruit as aqueous, methanolic and hexanic extracts was not mutagenic in *Salmonella typhimurium* strains TA 98 and TA 100 [64].

No data are available on the carcinogenicity of caraway fruit and caraway oil. In a feeding study with mice no carcinogenicity of (+)-carvone could be demonstrated [61]. (+)-Carvone was administered intraperitoneally at 6.0 and 1.20 g/kg to 20 A/He mice 3 times per week for 8 weeks. No significant increase in lung tumours was observed compared to a control group [65].

Powdered caraway fruit fed to rats as 20% of the diet

for 25 weeks significantly decreased (p<0.05) the percentage of rats with 7,12-dimethylbenz(a)-anthracene-induced tumours (42.8% protection) and the mean number of tumours per rat (50.6% protection), and significantly increased (p<0.05) the mean latency period of tumour appearance (17.6 weeks compared to 14.4 weeks in control animals) [66].

Hexane and ethyl acetate extracts of caraway fruit (obtained by successive extraction) showed anti-tumour promoting activity on 12-O-tetradecanoyl-phorbol-13-acetate-enhanced ^{3}H-choline incorporation into phospholipids of C3H10T1/2 cells by 29.3% and 34.3% respectively [67].

Carvone and limonene isolated from caraway oil induced the detoxifying enzyme glutathione S-transferase (GST) in several mouse target tissues. Both compounds increased GST activity in the liver by a factor of 2 compared to the control; carvone exhibited the highest activity in the small intestinal mucosa, while limonene had only a small effect. In the colon, GST activity was significantly increased (p<0.05) by both substances. Carvone also increased glutathione significantly in the lung, colon and small intestinal mucosa (p<0.005, p<0.05 and p<0.05 respectively) [68].

Sensitizing potential
Caraway oil applied to the backs of hairless mice produced no irritating effects. However, oil applied to intact or abraded rabbit skin was irritating. At a concentration of 4% in petrolatum the oil produced no irritation in a 24-hour closed-patch test in humans [57].

Caraway has been characterized as a species with low sensitizing potential [33]. Experimental sensitization (FCA test in guinea pigs) with (+)-carvone (1% in vaseline) yielded a quotient of the sum of reactions and the number of animals of 1.25 [33]. In a maximization test carried out on 25 volunteers, neither (+)-carvone nor caraway oil at concentrations of 2 and 4% in petrolatum produced any sensitization reactions [57,69].

From HPLC analysis caraway fruit contained no detectable sensitizing compounds such as furo-coumarins. However, traces of 5-methoxypsoralen and 8-methoxypsoralen were detected using an ultrasensitive bioassay. Both compounds were at the limit of detection (10^{-9} g) and their levels in the seeds could be estimated only approximately as <0.005 µg/g [70].

Normal mice which had been sensitized 14 days previously by intraperitoneal injection of a caraway fruit extract showed a significant anaphylactic reaction (p<0.001) when challenged on the abdominal wall by the same extract. Their vascular permeability value was 70 compared to 10 in the non-sensitized control group, indicating that caraway fruit had allergenic potential in this system [71].

REFERENCES

1. Caraway Fruit - Carvi fructus. European Pharmacopoeia, Council of Europe.

2. Czygan F-C. Carvi fructus. In: Wichtl M, editor. Teedrogen, 3rd ed. Stuttgart: Wissenschaftliche Verlagsgesellschaft, 1997:134-5.

3. Steinegger E, Hänsel R. Kümmel und Kümmelöl. In: Pharmakognosie, 5th ed. Berlin-Heidelberg: Springer, 1992:313-4.

4. Wagner H. Carvi fructus (Semen) - Kümmel. In: Pharmazeutische Biologie, 5th ed. Volume 2. Drogen und ihre Inhaltsstoffe. Stuttgart-New York: Gustav Fischer, 1993:68.

5. von Schantz M, Ek BS. Über die Bildung von ätherischem Öl in Kümmel, *Carum carvi* L. Sci Pharm 1971;2:82-101.

6. El-Wakeil F, Khairy M, Morsi S, Farag RS, Shihata AA, Badel AZMA. Biochemical studies on the essential oils of some fruits of Umbelliferae family. Seifen Öle Fette Wachse 1986;112:77-80.

7. von Schantz M, Huhtikangas A. Über die Bildung von Limonen und Carvon im Kümmel, *Carum carvi*. Phytochemistry 1971;10:1787-93.

8. Salveson A, Baerheim Svendsen A. Gas liquid chromatographic separation and identification of the constituents of caraway seed oil. I. The monoterpene hydrocarbons. Planta Med 1976;30:93-6.

9. Rothbächer H, Suteu F. Über Hydroxylverbindungen des Kümmelöls. Planta Med 1975;28:112-23.

10. Lawrence BM. New trends in essential oils. Perfum Flavor 1980;5:6-16.

11. Salveson A, Baerheim Svendsen A. Gaschromatographische Trennung und Identifizierung der Bestandteile des Kümmelöles. II. Die sauerstoffhaltigen Monoterpene. Sci Pharm 1978;46:93-100.

12. Seher A, Gundlach U. Isomere Monoensäuren in Pflanzenölen. Fette Seifen Anstrichmittel 1982;84:342-9.

13. Stepanenko GA, Gusakova SD, Umarov AU. Lipids of Carum carvi and Foeniculum vulgare seeds. Khim Prir Soedin 1980;(6):827-8; through Chem Abstr 1981; 94:136161.

14. Kartnig T, Scholz G. Über einige Lipoid-Inhaltsstoffe aus den Früchten von *Pimpinella anisum* (L.) und *Carum carvi* (L.). Fette Seifen Anstrichmittel 1969; 71:276-80.

15. Stahl-Biskup E. Carum. In: Hänsel R, Keller K, Rimpler

H, Schneider G, editors. Hagers Handbuch der pharmazeutischen Praxis, 5th ed. Volume 4: Drogen A-D. Berlin-Heidelberg: Springer-Verlag, 1992:693-700.

16. Salzer U-J. Über die Fettsäurezusammensetzung der Lipoide einiger Gewürze. Fette Seifen Anstrichmittel 1975;77:446-50.

17. Reiter B, Lechner M, Lorbeer E. The fatty acid profiles - including petroselinic and cis-vaccenic acid - of different Umbelliferae seed oils. Fett/Lipid 1998; 100:498-502.

18. Hopf H, Kandler O. Characterization of the 'reserve cellulose' of the endosperm of *Carum carvi* as a β-(1-4)-mannan. Phytochemistry 1977;16:1715-7.

19. Dirks U, Herrmann K. Hochleistungsflüssigkeits-chromatographie der Hydroxycinnamoylchinasäuren und der 4-(β-D-Glucopyranosyloxy)-benzoesäure in Gewürzen. 10. Über Gewürzphenole. Z Lebensm Unters Forsch 1984;179:12-6.

20. Schulz JM, Herrmann K. Über das Vorkommen von Hydroxibenzoesäuren und Hydroxizimtsäuren in Gewürzen. IV. Über Gewürzphenole. Z Lebensm Unters Forsch 1980;171:193-9.

21. Kunzemann J, Herrmann K. Isolierung und Identifizierung der Flavon(ol)-O-glykoside in Kümmel (*Carum carvi* L.), Fenchel (*Foeniculum vulgare* Mill.), Anis (*Pimpinella anisum* L.) und Koriander (*Coriandrum sativum* L.) und von Flavon-C-glykosiden im Anis. I. Gewürzphenole. Z Lebensm Unters Forsch 1977; 164:194-200.

22. Harborne JB, Williams CA. Flavonoid patterns in the fruits of the Umbelliferae. Phytochemistry 1972;11: 1741-50.

23. Rothbächer H, Suteu F. Ursprung und Bildung des Carvenons in Oleum Carvi. Planta Med 1974;26:283-8.

24. Rothbächer H, Suteu F. Zur Entstehung des Carvacrols im Kümmelöl. Chemiker-Ztg 1978;102:260-3.

25. Forster HB, Niklas H, Lutz S. Antispasmodic effects of some medicinal plants. Planta Med 1980;40:309-19.

26. Forster H. Spasmolytische Wirkung pflanzlicher Carminativa. Tierexperimentelle Untersuchungen. Z Allg Med 1983;59:1327-33.

27. Maiwald L. Phytotherapie der Oberbaucherkrankungen. Z Phytotherapie 1984;5:908-18.

28. Reynolds JEF, editor. Caraway. In: Martindale - The Extra Pharmacopoeia, 31st ed. London: Pharmaceutical Press, 1996:1686.

29. Wichtl M and Henke D. Kummel - Carvi fructus. In: Hartke K, Hartke H, Mutschler E, Rücker G and Wichtl M, editors. Arzneibuch-Kommentar. Wissenschaftliche Erläuterungen zum Europäischen Arzneibuch und zum Deutschen Arzneibuch. Stuttgart: Wissenschaftliche Verlagsgesellschaft, 1998 (9. Lfg):K 32.

30. Fintelmann V. Möglichkeiten und Grenzen der Phytotherapie bei Magen-Darm-Krankheiten. Z Phytotherapie 1989;10:29-30.

31. Dorsch W, Loew D, Meyer-Buchtela E, Schilcher H. Carvi fructus (Kümmelfrüchte). In: Kinderdosierungen von Phytopharmaka, 2nd ed. Bonn: Kooperation Phytopharmaka, 1998:47-8.

32. Hausen BM. Zahnpasta-Allergie. Dtsch Med Wschr 1984;109:300-2.

33. Hausen BM, Vieluf IK. In: Allergiepflanzen-Pflanzenallergene. Handbuch und Atlas der allergie-induzierenden Wild- und Kulturpflanzen, 2nd ed. Landsberg/München: Ecomed, 1997:261,304-5 and 506.

34. Wüthrich B, Hofer T. Nahrungsmittelallergie: das "Sellerie-Beifuß-Gewürz-Syndrom". Dtsch Med Wschr 1984;109:981-6.

35. Wüthrich B, Dietschi R. Das "Sellerie-Karotten-Beifuss-Gewürz-Syndrom": Hauttest- und RAST-Ergebnisse. Schweiz Med Wschr 1985;115:358-64.

36. Schilcher H. Pharmakologie und Toxikologie ätherischer Öle. Anwendungshinweise für die ärztliche Praxis. Therapiewoche 1986;36:1100-12.

37. Schilcher H. Ätherische Öle - Wirkungen und Neben-wirkungen. Dtsch Apoth Ztg 1984;124:1433-42.

38. Reiter M, Brandt W. Relaxant effects on tracheal and ileal smooth muscles of the guinea pig. Arzneim-Forsch/Drug Res 1985;35:408-14.

39. Rauha J-P, Tammela P, Summanen J, Vuorela P, Kähkönen M, Heinonen M et al. Actions of some plant extracts containing flavonoids and other phenolic compounds on calcium fluxes in clonal rat pituitary GH_4C_1 cells. Pharm Pharmacol Lett 1999;9:66-9.

40. Maruzzella JC, Freundlich M. Antimicrobial substances from seeds. J Am Pharm Assoc 1959;48:356-8.

41. Ali MA, Kabir MH, Quaiyyum MA, Rahman MM, Uddin A. Antibacterial activity of caraway against *Shigella* spp. Bangladesh J Microbiol 1995;12:81-5.

42. Mahady GB, Pendland SL, Stoia A, Hamill FA. *In vitro* susceptibility of *Helicobacter pylori* to botanicals used traditionally for the treatment of gastrointestinal disorders [Poster]. In: Abstracts of 3rd International Congress on Phytomedicine. Munich, 11-13 October 2000. *Published as:* Phytomedicine 2000;7(Suppl. 2):95 (P-79).

43. Syed M, Khalid MR, Chaudhary FM, Bhatty MK. Antimicrobial activity of the essential oils of the Umbelliferae family. Part V. *Carum carvi, Petroselinum crispum* and *Dorema ammoniacum* oils. Pakistan J Sci Ind Res 1987;30:106-10.

44. Fricke G, Hoyer H, Wermter R, Paulus H. Einfluß lipophiler Stoffe auf die mikrobiologische Hemmwirkung von Aromaextrakten am Beispiel von *Staphylococcus aureus*. Arch Lebensmittelhyg 1998; 49:107-11.

45. Göckeritz D, Weuffen W, Höppe H. Terpene und Terpenderivate vom Carvon- und Camphertyp - ihre antimikrobiellen und verminoxen Eigenschaften. Pharmazie 1974;29:339-44.

46. Kurita N, Miyaji M, Kurane R, Takahara Y. Antifungal activity of components of essential oils. Agric Biol Chem 1981;45:945-52.

47. Farag RS, Daw ZY, Abo-Raya SH. Influence of some spice essential oils on *Aspergillus parasiticus* growth and production of aflatoxins in a synthetic medium. J Food Sci 1989;54:74-6.

48. Hitokoto H, Morozumi S, Wauke T, Sakai S, Kurata H. Inhibitory effects of spices on growth and toxin production of toxigenic fungi. Appl Environ Microbiol 1980;39:818-22.

49. Janssen AM, Scheffer JJC, Parhan-van Atten AW, Baerheim Svendsen A. Screening of some essential oils for their activities on dermatophytes. Pharm Weekbl Sci Ed 1988;10:277-80.

50. Guérin J-C, Réveillère H-P. Activité antifongiques d'extraits végétaux à usage thérapeutique. II. Étude de 40 extraits sur 9 souches fongiques. Ann Pharm Fr 1985;43:77-81.

51. Modu S, Gohla K, Umar IA. The hypoglycaemic and hypocholesterolaemic properties of black caraway (*Carum carvi* L.) oil in alloxan diabetic rats. Biokemistri (Nigeria) 1997;7:91-7.

52. Boyd EM, Sheppard EP. An autumn-enhanced mucotropic action of inhaled terpenes and related volatile agents. Pharmacology 1971;6:65-80.

53. Goerg KJ, Spilker T. Simultane sonographische Messung der Magen- und Gallenblasenentleerung mit gleichzeitiger Bestimmung der orozökalen Transitzeit mittels H$_2$-Atemtest. In: Loew D and Rietbrock N, editors. Phytopharmaka II: Forschung und klinische Anwendung. Darmstadt: Steinkopff, 1996:63-72.

54. Kelber O, Kroll U, Maidonis P, Weiser D, Okpanyi SN. Study of gastrointestinal absorption of plant extracts and their phytomedicinal combination (STW 5) in an ex vivo/in vitro model. In: Abstracts of 3rd International Congress on Phytomedicine. Munich, 11-13 October 2000. *Published as*: Phytomedicine 2000; 7(Suppl. 2): 119 (P-139).

55. Meyer F, Meyer E. Percutane Resorption von ätherischen Ölen und ihren Inhaltsstoffen. Arzneim-Forsch/Drug Res 1959;9:516-9.

56. Hildebrandt H. Über das Verhalten von Carvon und Santalol im Thierkörper. Hoppe-Seyler's Z physiol Chem 1902;36:441-51.

57. Opdyke DLJ. Monographs on fragrance raw materials: Caraway oil. Food Cosmet Toxicol 1973;11:1051.

58. von Skramlik E. Über die Giftigkeit und Verträglichkeit von ätherischen Ölen. Pharmazie 1959;14:435-45.

59. Mahmoud I, Alkofahi A, Abdelaziz A. Mutagenic and toxic activities of several spices and some Jordanian medicinal plants. Int J Pharmacognosy 1992;30:81-5.

60. Hagan EC, Hansen WH, Fitzhugh OG, Jenner PM, Jones WI, Taylor JM et al. Food flavourings and compounds of related structure. II. Subacute and chronic toxicity. Food Cosmet Toxicol 1967;5:141-57.

61. World Health Organization. Toxicological evaluation of certain food additives and contaminants: (+)- and (–)-carvone. WHO Food Additives Series: 28. Geneva: World Health Organization, 1991:155-67.

62. Rockwell P, Raw I. A mutagenic screening of various herbs, spices, and food additives. Nutrition and Cancer 1979;1:10-5.

63. Purintrapiban J, Shaheduzzaman SM, Vinitketkumnuen U, Kinouchi T, Kataoka K, Higashimoto M et al. Inhibitory effect of caraway seeds on mutation by alkylating agents. Environ Mut Res Commun 1995; 17:99-105.

64. Higashimoto M, Purintrapiban J, Kataoka K, Kinouchi T, Vinitketkumnuen U, Akimoto S et al. Mutagenicity and antimutagenicity of extracts of three spices and a medicinal plant in Thailand. Mutation Res 1993; 303:135-42.

65. Stoner GD, Shimkin MB, Kniazeff AJ, Weisburger JH, Weisburger EK, Gori GB. Test for carcinogenicity of food additives and chemotherapeutic agents by the pulmonary tumor response in strain A mice. Cancer Res 1973;33:3069-85.

66. Shwaireb MH, El-Mofty MM, Rizk AM, Abdel-Galil A-MM, Harasani HA. Inhibition of mammary gland tumorigenesis in the rat by caraway seeds and dried leaves of watercress. Oncology Reports 1995;2:689-92.

67. Okuyama T, Matsuda M, Masuda Y, Baba M, Masubuchi H, Adachi M et al. Studies on cancer bio-chemoprevention of natural resources. X. Inhibitory effect of spices on TPA-enhanced ^{3}H-choline incorporation in phospholipids of C3H10T1/2 cells and on TPA-induced mouse ear edema. Chinese Pharmaceut J 1995;47:421-30.

68. Zheng G, Kenney PM, Lam LKT. Anethofuran, carvone, and limonene: potential cancer chemopreventive agents from dill weed oil and caraway oil. Planta Med 1992; 58:338-41.

69. Opdyke DLJ. Monographs on fragrance raw materials: *d*-Carvone. Food Cosmet Toxicol 1978;16:673-4.

70. Ceska O, Chaudhary SK, Warrington PJ, Ashwood-Smith MJ. Photoactive furocoumarins in fruits of some umbellifers. Phytochemistry 1987;26:165-9.

71. Tsuda Y, Kataoka H, Semma M, Ito Y. Studies on substances contained in spices inducing allergic reaction. Shokuhin Eiseigaku Zasshi (J Food Hyg Soc Japan) 2000;41:307-11.

CENTAURII HERBA

Centaury

DEFINITION

Centaury consists of the whole or cut dried flowering aerial parts of *Centaurium erythraea* Rafn [*C. minus* Moench, *C. umbellatum* Gilib., *Erythraea centaurium* (L.) Pers.].

The material complies with the monograph of the European Pharmacopoeia [1].

Fresh material may also be used, provided that when dried it complies with the monograph of the European Pharmacopoeia.

CONSTITUENTS

The characteristic, bitter-tasting constituents are secoiridoid glucosides, principally swertiamarin and smaller amounts of gentiopicroside (gentiopicrin) and sweroside, with bitterness values of about 12,000 [2-6]. Two intensely bitter *m*-hydroxybenzoyl esters of sweroside, centapicrin and deacetylcentapicrin, with bitterness values of about 4,000,000, are also present [4,5,7]. Other iridoids include centauroside (a dimeric secoiridoid), secologanin, 6'-*m*-hydroxy-benzoyl-loganin [8], dihydrocornin (a cyclopentane iridoid), gentioflavoside [9] and the secoiridoid alkaloid gentianine [10,11].

Various methoxylated xanthones are present [2-5,12-16] including eustomin (1-hydroxy-3,5,6,7,8-penta-methoxyxanthone) [17] and 8-demethyl-eustomin [13,17,18].

Other constituents include phenolic acids, such as *p*-coumaric, *o*-hydroxyphenylacetic, ferulic, proto-catechuic, sinapic, vanillic [19,20], hydroxytere-phthalic and 2,5-dihydroxyterephthalic acids [21]; also phytosterols (β-sitosterol, stigmasterol, camp-esterol and others) [22,23], and triterpenoids [24].

CLINICAL PARTICULARS

Therapeutic indications
Dyspeptic complaints; lack of appetite [3,25-28].

Posology and method of administration

Dosage

Adults: 1-4 g of the drug as a maceration, infusion or decoction in 150 ml of water, up to 3 times daily [3,25-28]; 2-4 ml of liquid extract (1:1, ethanol 25%

E/S/C/O/P
MONOGRAPHS
Second Edition

V/V), up to 3 times daily [3,27,28]; tincture (1:5, ethanol 70% V/V), 2-5 g daily [3].

Children: proportion of adult dose according to age or body weight, in ethanol-free dosage forms.

The dosage may be adjusted according to the bitterness sensitivity of the individual.

Method of administration
For oral use in liquid preparations. For lack of appetite, administered half to one hour before meals [3]; for dyspepsia, taken after meals.

Duration of administration
No restriction. If symptoms persist, consult your doctor.

Contra-indications
As with other drugs containing bitter substances, peptic ulcers are a contra-indication for centaury [3].

Special warnings and special precautions for use
None required.

Interaction with other medicaments and other forms of interaction
None reported.

Pregnancy and lactation
No data available. In accordance with general medical practice, the product should not be used during pregnancy or lactation without medical advice.

Effects on ability to drive and use machines
None known.

Undesirable effects
None reported.

Overdose
No toxic effects reported.

PHARMACOLOGICAL PROPERTIES

Pharmacodynamic properties
The bitter principles of centaury reflexively stimulate secretion of gastric juice and bile and thereby enhance appetite and digestion [29,30].

In vitro experiments
A lyophilized hot water extract of centaury (7.5:1) exhibited antioxidant activity as shown by scavenging of superoxide radical in the NADH/PMS system (IC_{50}: 120.2 μg/ml) and also xanthine oxidase inhibitory activity (IC_{50}: 73.2 μg/ml) [31].

In vivo experiments
In the air pouch granuloma test in rats a dry aqueous extract of centaury (3.8:1), applied topically as 5% and 10% creams, exhibited significant transdermal anti-inflammatory activity compared to placebo cream controls (p<0.01) [32]. Anti-inflammatory activity of the same extract was also demonstrated in Freund's adjuvant-induced polyarthritis, in rats treated orally with 10-500 mg per day (p<0.01) [32]. A dry ethanolic extract of centaury, administered orally to rats at 100 mg/kg body weight, inhibited carrageenan-induced paw oedema by 40% compared to controls (p<0.01) [33].

The antipyretic activity of a dry aqueous extract of centaury (3.8:1) was demonstrated in rats after administration of 50-100 mg by gavage in a yeast-induced fever test (p<0.05) [32].

A diuretic effect was shown in rats after oral administration of 8% or 16% aqueous extracts of centaury at 10 ml/kg body weight daily for one week. From the fifth day of treatment urine volume increased significantly (p<0.05) with the lower dose and both doses led to a significant increase of sodium, chloride and potassium excretion (p<0.01 to p<0.001). At the end of treatment a diminution in creatinine clearance was observed (p<0.05 for the lower dose) [34].

Isolated gentiopicroside significantly inhibited the production of tumour necrosis factor in carbon tetrachloride-induced and bacillus Calmette-Guérin/lipopolysaccharide-induced models of hepatic injury in mice after intraperitoneal injection at 30 mg/kg (p<0.05) or 60 mg/kg body weight (p<0.01) daily for 5 days [35].

Isolated protocatechuic acid significantly (p<0.02 to p<0.0009) inhibited azoxymethane-induced colon tumour development after dietary administration to rats at 500 and 1000 ppm [36].

Isolated swertiamarin showed anticholinergic activity, significantly inhibiting carbachol-induced contractions of the proximal colon in rats in a dose-dependent manner (p<0.05) after oral administration at 150 mg/kg and 300 mg/kg body weight [37].

Gentianine administered orally to mice at 30 mg/kg body weight had a depressive effect on the central nervous system, inhibiting spontaneous movement activity (p<0.001) and increasing hexobarbital-induced sleeping time (p<0.05). When administered to rats at 100 mg/kg body weight it showed anti-ulcerogenic activity in the water immersion stress test (p<0.01) and an inhibitory action against gastric secretion (p<0.05) [38].

Clinical studies
No published clinical data are currently available.

Pharmacokinetic properties
By anaerobic incubation with a mixture, and with

individual strains, of human intestinal bacteria, swertiamarin was converted to three metabolites: erythrocentaurin, 5-hydroxymethylisochroman-1-one and gentianine. This demonstrated that orally administered swertiamarin can be transformed into a nitrogen-containing, biologically active substance by flora of the human gastrointestinal tract [39].

Preclinical safety data

Centaury extracts have been evaluated in the Ames mutagenicity test using *Salmonella typhimurium* strains TA98 and IA100 (with and without activation by S9 mix), with rather conflicting results. An inspissated extract showed weak mutagenicity in TA98, but negative results were obtained with a fluid extract and a tincture in strains TA98 and TA100 [40]. In another study, a fluid extract and a tincture showed weak mutagenicity in strain TA100, but not in strain TA98 [41].

In more recent Ames tests, an ethanolic extract of centaury at 200 µl/plate displayed markedly antimutagenic potency in *Salmonella typhimurium* strains TA98 and TA100, inhibiting mutagenicity induced by 2-nitrofluorene (2-NF) and 2-amino-anthracene (2-AA) by over 50%. Furthermore, isolated eustomin at 50 µg/plate showed strong inhibition, 76% against 2-NF and 64% against 2-AA in strain TA100; 8-demethyleustomin was also active, with results of 43% and 39% respectively, but no inhibition was detected from secoiridoid or polar fractions of centaury [17].

REFERENCES

1. Centaury - Centaurii herba. European Pharmacopoeia, Council of Europe.

2. van der Sluis WG. Secoiridoids and xanthones in the genus *Centaurium* Hill (Gentianaceae), a pharmacognostical study [Dissertation]. University of Utrecht, 1985.

3. Hänsel R, Keller K, Rimpler H, Schneider G, editors. Centaurium. In: Hagers Handbuch der Pharmazeutischen Praxis, 5th ed. Volume 4: Drogen A-D. Berlin-Heidelberg: Springer-Verlag, 1992:756-63.

4. van der Sluis WG. Chemotaxonomical investigations of the genera *Blackstonia* and *Centaurium* (Gentianaceae). Plant Syst Evol 1985;149:253-86.

5. Schimmer O, Mauthner H. *Centaurium erythraea* Rafn - Tausendgüldenkraut. Z Phytotherapie 1994;15:299-306.

6. Jankovic T, Krstic D, Savikin-Fodulivic K, Menkovic N, Grubisic D. Comparative investigation of secoiridoid compounds of *Centaurium erythraea* grown in nature and cultured in vitro. Pharm Pharmacol Lett 1998;8:30-2.

7. Sakina K, Aota K. Studies on the constituents of *Erythraea centaurium* (Linné) Persoon. I. The structure of centapicrin, a new bitter secoiridoid glucoside. Yakugaku Zasshi 1976;96:683-8.

8. Takagi S, Yamaki M, Yumioka E, Nishimura T, Sakina K. Studies on the constituents of *Erythraea centaurium* (Linné) Persoon. II. The structure of centauroside, a new bis-secoiridoid glucoside. Yakugaku Zasshi 1982;102:313-7.

9. Do T, Popov S, Marekov N, Trifonov A. Iridoids from Gentianaceae plants growing in Bulgaria. Planta Med 1987;53:580.

10. Rulko F, Witkiewicz K. Gentiana alkaloids. Part VII. Alkaloids of centaury (*Erythrea centaurium* Pers.). Diss Pharm Pharmacol 1972;24:73-7.

11. Bishay DW, Shelver WH, Wahba Khalil SK. Alkaloids of *Erythraea centaurium* Pers. growing in Egypt. Planta Med 1978;33;422-3.

12. Neshta NM, Nikolaeva GG, Sheichenko VI, Patudin AV. A new xanthone compound from *Centaurium erythraea*. Khim Prir Soedin 1982:258 [Russian], translated into English as: Chem Nat Compd 1982:18;240-1.

13. Neshta NM, Glyzin VI, Nikolaeva GG, Sheichenko VI. A new xanthone compound from *Centaurium erythraea*. Khim Prir Soedin 1983:106-7 [Russian], translated into English as: Chem Nat Compd 1983:19;105.

14. Neshta NM, Glyzin VI, Savina AA, Patudin AV. A new xanthone compound from *Centaurium erythraea*. III. Khim Prir Soedin 1983:787 [Russian], translated into English as: Chem Nat Compd 1983:19;750-1.

15. Neshta NM, Glyzin VI, Patudin AV. A new xanthone compound from *Centaurium erythraea*. IV. Khim Prir Soedin 1984:110 [Russian], translated into English as: Chem Nat Compd 1984:20;108.

16. Valentão P, Areias F, Amaral J, Andrade P, Seabra R. Tetraoxygenated xanthones from *Centaurium erythraea*. Nat Prod Lett 2000;14:319-23.

17. Schimmer O, Mauthner H. Polymethoxylated xanthones from the herb of *Centaurium erythraea* with strong antimutagenic properties in *Salmonella typhimurium*. Planta Med 1996;62:561-4.

18. Jankovic T, Krstic D, Savikin-Fodulovic K, Menkovic N, Grubisic D. Xanthone compounds of *Centaurium erythraea* grown in nature and cultured in vitro. Pharm Pharmacol Lett 2000;10:23-5.

19. Hatjimanoli M, Debelmas A-M. Étude de *Centaurium umbellatum* Gil. Identification des acides phénols. Ann Pharm Fr 1977;35:107-11.

20. Dombrowicz E, Swiatek L, Zadernowski R. Phenolic acids in bitter drugs. Part III. Examination of Herba Centaurii. Farm Pol 1988;44:657-60.

21. Hatjimanoli M, Favre-Bonvin J, Kaouadji M, Mariotte A-M. Monohydroxy- and 2,5-dihydroxy terephthalic

acids, two unusual phenolics isolated from *Centaurium erythraea* and identified in other Gentianaceae members. J Nat Prod 1988;51:977-80.

22. Popov S. Sterols of the Gentianaceae family. Compt Rend Acad Bulg Sci 1969;22:293-6.

23. Aquino R, Behar I, Garzarella P, Dini A, Pizza C. Composizione chimica e proprietà biologiche della *Erythraea centaurium* Rafn. Boll Soc Ital Biol Sper 1985;61:165-9.

24. Bellavita V, Schiaffella F, Mezzetti T. Triterpenoids of *Centaurium erythraea*. Phytochemistry 1974;13:289-90.

25. Bisset NG, editor (translated from Wichtl M, editor. Teedrogen). Centaurii herba - Lesser centaury. In: Herbal Drugs and Phytopharmaceuticals. Stuttgart: Medpharm, Boca Raton-London: CRC Press, 1994:134-6.

26. Leung AY, Foster S. Centaury. In: Encyclopedia of Common Natural Ingredients, 2nd ed. New York-Chichester: John Wiley, 1996:143-5.

27. Barnes J, Anderson LA and Phillipson JD. Centaury. In: Herbal Medicines - A guide for healthcare professionals, 2nd ed. London-Chicago: Pharmaceutical Press, 2002:121-2.

28. Centaurium. In: British Herbal Pharmacopoeia 1983. Bournemouth: British Herbal Medicine Association, 1983:55-6.

29. Paris RR, Moyse H. Gentianaceae. In: Précis de Matière Médicale, 2nd ed. Volume 3. Paris: Masson, 1971:100-7.

30. Schmid W. Zur Pharmakologie der Bittermittel. Planta Med 1966;14(Suppl):34-41.

31. Valentão P, Fernandes E, Carvalho F, Andrade PB, Seabra RM, Bastos ML. Antioxidant activity of *Centaurium erythraea* infusion evidenced by its superoxide radical scavenging and xanthine oxidase inhibitory activity. J Agric Food Chem 2001;49:3476-9.

32. Berkan T, Üstünes L, Lermioglu F, Özer A. Antiinflammatory, analgesic and antipyretic effects of an aqueous extract of *Erythraea centaurium*. Planta Med 1991;57:34-7.

33. Capasso F, Mascolo N, Morrica P, Ramundo E. Phytotherapeutic profile of some plants used in folk medicine. Boll Soc Ital Biol Sper 1983;59:1398-404.

34. Haloui M, Louedec L, Michel J-B, Lyoussi B. Experimental diuretic effects of *Rosmarinus officinalis* and *Centaurium erythraea*. J Ethnopharmacol 2000;71:465-72.

35. Kondo Y, Takano F, Hojo H. Suppression of chemically and immunologically induced hepatic injuries by gentiopicroside in mice. Planta Med 1994;60:414-6.

36. Tanaka T, Kojima T, Suzui M, Mori H. Chemoprevention of colon carcinogenesis by the natural product of a simple phenolic compound, protocatechuic acid: suppressing effects on tumor development and biomarkers expression of colon tumorigenesis. Cancer Res 1993;53:3908-13.

37. Yamahara J, Kobayashi M, Matsuda H, Aoki S. Anticholinergic action of *Swertia japonica* and an active constituent. J Ethnopharmacol 1991;33:31-5.

38. Yamahara J, Konoshima T, Sawada T, Fujimura H. Biologically active principles of crude drugs: pharmacological actions of *Swertia japonica* extracts, swertiamarin and gentianine. Yakugaku Zasshi 1978;98:1446-51.

39. El-Sedawy A, Yue-Zhong Shu, Hattori M, Kobashi K, Namba T. Metabolism of swertiamarin from *Swertia japonica* by human intestinal bacteria. Planta Med 1989;55:147-50.

40. Schimmer O, Krüger A, Paulini H, Haefele F. An evaluation of 55 commercial plant extracts in the Ames mutagenicity test. Pharmazie 1994;49:448-51.

41. Göggelmann W, Schimmer O. Mutagenic activity of phytotherapeutical drugs. In: Knudsen I, editor. Genetic toxicology of the diet. New York: Alan R Liss, 1986:63-72.

CHELIDONII HERBA

Greater Celandine

DEFINITION

Greater celandine consists of the dried aerial parts of *Chelidonium majus* L. collected during flowering. It contains not less than 0.6 per cent of total alkaloids, expressed as chelidonine ($C_{20}H_{19}NO_5$; M_r 353.4) and calculated with reference to the dried drug.

The material complies with the monograph of the European Pharmacopoeia [1].

CONSTITUENTS

Benzylisoquinoline alkaloids (0.01-1% by the Ph. Eur. assay method) of the berberine, protoberberine and benzophenanthridine types, the principal alkaloid being coptisine together with chelidonine, protopine, berberine, chelerythrine, sanguinarine, allocryptopine and others; over 20 alkaloids have been identified [2,3]. Several hydroxycinnamic acid derivatives including caffeoylmalic acid (typically around 1.2%) are also present [2,4,5].

CLINICAL PARTICULARS

Therapeutic indications
Symptomatic treatment of mild to moderate spasms of the upper gastrointestinal tract; minor gall bladder disorders; dyspeptic complaints such as bloating and flatulence [6-10].

Posology and method of administration

Dosage
Daily dose for adults and children over 12 years
1.2-3.6 g of the drug as a tea infusion [10].
125-700 mg of standardized hydroalcoholic extracts corresponding to 9-24 mg of total alkaloids, calculated as chelidonine [6-8].
Tincture (1:10): 2-4 ml, 3 times daily [2].
Fluid extract (1:1): 1-2 ml, 3 times daily [2].

Method of administration
For oral administration.

Duration of administration
If symptoms persist for more than two weeks, medical advice should be sought.

Contra-indications
Biliary obstructions; existing or previous liver disease, concomitant use of substances contra-indicated in liver disease [11-13].

E/S/C/O/P
MONOGRAPHS
Second Edition

Special warnings and special precautions for use

Special warnings
In long-term use for more than 4 weeks, checks on liver enzyme activity are recommended [11-13].

Precautions for use
In cases of gallstones, the product should not be used without medical advice.

Interaction with other medicaments and other forms of interaction
None reported [8].

Pregnancy and lactation
No data available. In accordance with general medical practice, the product should not be used during pregnancy and lactation without medical advice.

Effects on ability to drive and use machines
None known.

Undesirable effects
Mild gastrointestinal disturbances, such as stomach upset, nausea or diarrhoea, sometimes occur [6-8]. In rare cases, hepatic inflammation and an increase in liver enzyme activity and serum bilirubin have been reported, reversible on discontinuation of therapy [11-13].

Overdose
Abdominal pain, gastrointestinal cramps, urinary urgency, drowsiness and haematuria may result from an overdose due to the alkaloids [14]. In this case, treatment must be stopped immediately.

PHARMACOLOGICAL PROPERTIES

Pharmacodynamic properties

In vitro experiments

Antispasmodic effects
Hydroethanolic extracts of greater celandine, the alkaloids coptisine, protopine, chelidonine, berberine and allocryptopine, and also caffeoylmalic acid, have shown concentration-dependent antispasmodic activities in the isolated guinea pig and rat ileum and fundus [15-20].

Dry extracts from greater celandine (total alkaloid content 2-3%), with a defined content of the main alkaloids chelidonine (0.4-0.6%), protopine (0.4-0.5%) and coptisine (0.3%), were active in three different models used for testing antispasmodic effects in the guinea pig ileum. Depending on the test, 250 to 500 µg/ml of the extracts resulted in 50% spasmolytic activity. Carbachol-induced spasms were antagonized by coptisine, chelidonine and protopine in a dose-dependent manner. Coptisine was a competitive antagonist (pA$_2$ value of 5.95), whereas chelidonine and protopine were non-competitive antagonists. In the model for inducing contractions through an electrical field, protopine was the most active among the alkaloids, followed by coptisine and then chelidonine. In the barium chloride-stimulated ileum, chelidonine and protopine exhibited papaverine-like musculotropic action, whereas coptisine (up to 3.0×10^{-5} g/ml) was ineffective in this model [15].

In the model of acetylcholine-induced spasm in isolated guinea pig ileum, protopine showed clear anticholinergic activity. Cumulative dose-response curves were parallel-shifted towards the right with increasing protopine concentration and a pA$_2$ value of 5.87 was derived. In the same model, atropine was 660 times more potent than protopine [16].

The antispasmodic activity of pure protopine was examined in isolated rat ileum. Noradrenaline-induced tonic contractions were antagonized in a dose-dependent manner in the range 25-100 µg/ml, whereas phasic contractions were only inhibited at the highest concentration examined (100 µg/ml). Addition of protopine at the plateau of the noradrenaline-induced tonic contraction caused a relaxation which was antagonized neither by indometacin nor by methylene blue [17].

In another study, acetylcholine-induced contractions in isolated guinea pig ileum were antagonized by protopine and allocryptopine with IC$_{50}$ values of 1.3 µM and 2.3 µM respectively, whereas berberine potentiated the contractions. The EC$_{50}$ for the agonistic effect of berberine was 57 µM [18].

The antagonistic activities of coptisine and berberine on carbachol-induced contractions of the smooth muscle of isolated rat fundus were examined. Berberine (0.1 mM) resulted in 60% relaxation, whereas the same concentration of coptisine yielded only 25% reduction. The IC$_{50}$ for berberine was determined as 0.034 mg/ml [19].

The antispasmodic activities of a hydroethanolic greater celandine extract (containing 0.81% total alkaloids, assayed by the Ph. Eur./DAB 10 method), and of coptisine and caffeoylmalic acid, were evaluated in the isolated rat ileum muscle immediately after addition of acetylcholine. The extract (2×10^{-4} g/ml), coptisine (10^{-5} g/ml) and caffeoylmalic acid (2.5×10^{-5} g/ml) showed weak antispasmodic activities (12.7%, 16.5% and 7% respectively) [20].

Choleretic effects
The choleretic activity of a greater celandine hydroethanolic extract was confirmed by experiments with isolated perfused rat liver. The extract (70% ethanol V/V, 5:1, 1.6% total alkaloids and 1.9% of

hydroxycinnamic acid derivatives), and alkaloid and phenolic fractions from it, caused an increase in bile flow. At the same time, bile acid concentrations were reduced, indicating a hydro-choleretic effect. The amount of bile was more than doubled after 40 minutes compared to the pretreatment value at a concentration of 10 mg extract/ml/min. Choleresis induced by the total extract could not be assigned clearly to either the alkaloid or the phenolic fraction [21].

Anti-inflammatory effects
An extract made from a tincture of fresh greater celandine juice, and the alkaloids chelidonine, berberine, chelerythrine and sanguinarine, were tested for anti-inflammatory activity with respect to their ability to inhibit 5- and 12-lipoxygenase (5-LO and 12-LO) in an enzyme assay. The most active inhibitor of both enzymes was sanguinarine (IC_{50}: 0.4 μM for 5-LO and 13 μM for 12-LO) followed by chelerythrine (IC_{50}: 0.8 μM for 5-LO and 33 μM for 12-LO). Chelidonine and berberine were inactive. The greater celandine extract (containing 0.68% of total alkaloids calculated as chelidonine) inhibited 5-LO activity with an IC_{50} of 1.9 μM (calculated on the basis of alkaloid content in terms of chelidonine). The extract showed neither oxidative nor antioxidant properties indicating a specific enzyme interaction rather than a non-specific redox mechanism [22].

In another enzyme assay, the elastase-inhibiting effects of coptisine, berberine and sanguinarine on human sputum elastase (HSE) and porcine pancreatic elastase (PPE) were investigated. All three alkaloids markedly inhibited enzyme activity in both systems. IC_{50} values for the elastase-inhibiting effects were as follows [23]:
coptisine chloride   2.5 μM (HSE);16 μM (PPE)
berberine chloride   3.2 μM (HSE);22 μM (PPE)
sanguinarine chloride 6.2 μM (HSE);16 μM (PPE)

In vivo experiments

Anti-inflammatory effects
No studies are available on greater celandine.

The anti-inflammatory activity of protopine was evaluated in the carrageenan-induced rat paw oedema model. The mean paw volume after an intraperitoneal dose of 50 mg/kg was significantly reduced by 29% compared with the non-treated control (p<0.01). After a dose of 100 mg/kg the reduction was 62% (p<0.001). Reductions caused by the positive control, acetylsalicylic acid at 150 and 300 mg/kg, were 28 and 71% respectively [24].

Hepatoprotective effects
Solutions of a hydroethanolic extract prepared in accordance with the Homeopathic Pharmacopeia of the United States 1978 (HPUS78) by extraction with 41-45% ethanol exerted significant hepato-

protection against carbon tetrachloride toxicity in two studies in rats. In the first study, the extract was administered via a gastric tube twice weekly over 3 weeks as an aqueous suspension of 12.5 mg/ml. This treatment resulted in significant protection against hepatic tissue injury. Increased plasma activities of the enzymes alanine amino-transferase (ALAT), aspartate aminotransferase (ASAT), alkaline phosphatase (AlP) and lactate dehydrogenase (LDH) as well as increased bilirubin, all induced by carbon tetrachloride, were significantly decreased by the extract (p<0.001 for ALAT, ASAT, LDH, p<0.01 for AlP and bilirubin). Cholesterol, which first decreased as a result of carbon tetrachloride injury, significantly increased during the course of treatment with greater celandine extract (p<0.01). On histopathological evaluation of the liver cells, a marked reduction in the number of necrotic cells was observed [25]. In a subsequent study using the same material, it was shown that accumulation of lipids, a reversible toxic response caused by carbon tetrachloride, was considerably less in rats after daily treatment with the extract at 125 mg/kg over 3 weeks compared to controls. Fibrotic changes were prevented with 62.5 and 125 mg/kg [26].

Pharmacological studies in humans
The choleretic effects of greater celandine have been confirmed in patients with liver diseases and in healthy volunteers. A hydroethanolic extract containing 1.5% of total alkaloids calculated as chelidonine in water and administered intragastrically, increased bile flow significantly (p<0.01) as measured by increases in bilirubin, cholesterol, pancreatic lipase and α-amylase compared to basal flow [27,28].

Clinical studies
The efficacy of a greater celandine extract (daily dose: 700 mg of a hydroalcoholic extract 5.3-7.5:1, corresponding to 24 mg of total alkaloids calculated as chelidonine) was confirmed in a double-blind, placebo-controlled study over 6 weeks with 60 patients suffering from epigastric complaints or cramps in the biliary system and/or the upper gastrointestinal tract. The outcome criteria included global assessment by the clinicians and patients using the von Zerssen complaint scale [29]. After 6 weeks of treatment 60% of the verum patients and 27% of the placebo group were considered responders (p = 0.0038). The self-rating score was significantly lower after verum treatment than after placebo (difference after 6 weeks 15%, p = 0.003). Most of the predominant symptoms, i.e. stomach-aches, bile-related complaints, flatulence, nausea and bloating, showed a trend towards full remission in the verum group only [6].

During the course of a retrospective study over 6 months, 206 patients with epigastric complaints related to gall stones or cholecystectomy were treated with a greater celandine preparation in capsules and/or as a liquid. The mean daily dose of the solid preparation was 125 mg of a hydromethanolic extract corresponding to 0.675 mg of chelidonine. The liquid preparation was administered as 3 × 20 drops daily, corresponding to 0.15 mg of chelidonine. Symptoms such as bloating, flatulence, diarrhoea or constipation, lasting abdominal pain, and parameters such as duration of colic-free intervals or food intolerance improved. Previously increased levels of gamma glutamyltransferase and an increased erythrocyte sedimentation rate were normalized [7].

In a multicentre, prospective observational study, 608 patients (403 women and 205 men, mean ages of 59 and 55 years respectively) with dyspeptic complaints or cramp-like pains in the upper gastrointestinal tract, were treated with a hydroethanolic greater celandine extract (5-7:1, mean daily dose 375-500 mg of extract corresponding to 9-12 mg of total alkaloids as determined by HPLC). According to the physicians' global assessment of efficacy (4-point scale), the response after an average of 22 days of treatment was good or very good in 87.4% of the patients. The onset of effect was observed within 30 minutes in 62.3% of patients [8].

In another observational study, 92 patients suffering from biliary disorders were treated with a fluid extract of greater celandine at a dosage of 3 × 20 drops daily, corresponding to 0.15 mg chelidonine. Considerable reductions in pain and other symptoms like bloating and flatulence were observed after 4 weeks of treatment. The mean pain index decreased significantly (p = 0.001) from 3.1 to 1.0 on a 6-point scale [30].

Pharmacokinetic properties
No data available.

Preclinical safety data

Single-dose toxicity
No data on greater celandine available.

Toxicity data for chelidonine indicate low toxicity in mice and rats. The LD_{50} for chelidonine in mice was determined as 1300 mg/kg, while in rats it was higher than 2000 mg/kg. Intraperitoneal administration of chelidonine in sublethal doses caused sedation, ptosis, tremor and decreased body temperature. Chelidonine in doses of one-tenth and one-twentieth of the LD_{50} did not affect motor coordination in mice or rats during a period of 120 minutes after injection [31].

Hepatotoxicity
Certain alkaloids, i.e. chelerythrine and sanguinarine, which in greater celandine are present mainly in the roots and rhizome (0.7-1.1% of chelerythrine and 0.1-0.4% of sanguinarine) and only in minor amounts in aerial parts (about 0.04% of chelerythrine and 0.01% of sanguinarine) [3] can cause significant hepatotoxicity in rats. Intraperitoneal doses of 10 mg/kg caused hepatic cell injury, confirmed histologically, and increases in alanine aminotransferase and aspartate aminotransferase activity of 50% and 100% respectively were also noted [32,33].

Studies on various greater celandine extracts and the alkaloids coptisine, chelidonine, protopine, chelerythrine and sanguinarine in a cytotoxicity test system using primary rat hepatocytes indicated a correlation between alkaloid content of the extracts and the degree of cytotoxicity. EC_{50} values for the alkaloids were determined as follows: sanguinarine 5 µg/ml, chelerythrine 8 µg/ml, coptisine 13 µg/ml, protopine 100 µg/ml, chelidonine > 100 µg/ml. The median EC_{50} value of 34 different extracts and/or products was around 5000 µg/ml [34].

Repeated-dose toxicity
No data available on greater celandine.

Administration of chelerythrine and sanguinarine to rats at 0.2 mg/kg/day for 56 days did not cause signs of hepatic cell injuries [32,33].

Mutagenicity
The micronucleus test with mouse bone marrow (oral doses of greater celandine hydroethanolic extract containing 0.48% of chelidonine up to 2000 mg/kg) gave negative results, indicating no evidence of induced chromosomal or other damage leading to micronucleus formation in polychromatic erythrocytes of treated mice after 24, 48 or 72 hours [35].

REFERENCES

1. Greater Celandine - Chelidonii herba. European Pharmacopoeia, Council of Europe.

2. Hänsel R, Keller K, Rimpler H, Schneider G, editors. Chelidonii herba. In: Hagers Handbuch der Pharmazeutischen Praxis, 5th ed. Volume 4: Drogen A-D. Berlin: Springer-Verlag, 1992:839-48.

3. Fulde G, Wichtl M. Analytik von Schöllkraut. Das Hauptalkaloid ist Coptisin. Dtsch Apoth Ztg 1994; 134:1031-5.

4. Boegge SC, Nahrstedt A, Linscheid M, Nigge W. Distribution and stereochemistry of hydroxy-cinnamoylmalic acids and of free malic acids in Papaveraceae and Fumariaceae. Z Naturforsch 1995; 50c:608-15

5. Schilcher H. Schöllkraut - *Chelidonium majus* L. Portrait einer Arzneipflanze. Z Phytother 1997;18:356-66.

6. Ritter R, Schatton WFH, Gessner B, Willems M. Clinical trial on standardised celandine extract in patients with functional epigastric complaints: results of a placebo-

controlled double-blind trial. Complementary Therapies in Medicine 1993;1:189-93.

7. Ardjah H. Therapeutische Aspekte der funktionellen Oberbauchbeschwerden bei Gallenwegserkrankungen. Fortschr Med 1991;109(Suppl 115):2-8.

8. Kniebel R, Urlacher W. Therapie krampfartiger Abdominalschmerzen. Hochdosierter Schöllkrautextrakt bei krampfartigen Abdominalschmerzen. Z Allg Med 1993;69:680-4.

9. Fintelmann V, Menßen HG, Siegers CP. In: Phytotherapie Manual, 2nd ed. Stuttgart: Hippokrates, 1993: 204-5.

10. Wichtl M, editor. Chelidonii herba. In: Teedrogen und Phytopharmaka, 3rd ed. Stuttgart: Wissenschaftliche Verlagsgesellschaft, 1997:147-9.

11. Greving I, Meister V, Monnerjahn C, Müller KM, May B. Chelidonium majus; rare reason of a severe hepatotoxic reaction? Pharmacoepidemiol Drug Safety 1998;7:S66-69.

12. Benninger J, Schneider HT, Schuppan D, Kirchner T, Hahn EG. Acute hepatitis induced by greater celandine (Chelidonium majus). Z Gastroenterol 1999;117:1234-7.

13. Strahl S, Ehret V, Dahm HH, Maier KP. Nekrotisierende Hepatitis nach Einnahme pflanzlicher Heilmittel. Dtsch med Wschr 1998;123:1410-4.

14. Hänsel R. Schöllkraut. In: Phytopharmaka. Grundlagen und Praxis, 2nd ed. Berlin: Springer, 1991:190-1.

15. Hiller K-O, Ghorbani M, Schilcher H. Antispasmodic and relaxant activity of chelidonine, protopine, coptisine and Chelidonium majus extracts on isolated guinea-pig ileum. Planta Med 1998;64:758-60.

16. Üstünes L, Laekeman GM, Gözler B, Vlietinck AJ, Özer A, Herman AG. In vitro study of the anticholinergic and antihistaminic activities of protopine and some derivatives. J Nat Prod 1988;51:1021-2.

17. Ko FN, Wu TS, Lu ST, Wu YC, Huang TF, Teng CM. Ca^{2+}-channel blockade in rat thoracic aorta by protopine isolated from Corydalis tubers. Jap J Pharmacol 1992; 58:1-9.

18. Piacente S, Capasso A, De Tommasi N, Jativa C, Pizza C, Sorrentino L. Different effects of some isoquinoline alkaloids from Argemone mexicana on electrically induced contractions of isolated guinea-pig ileum. Phytotherapy Res 1997;11:155-7.

19. Lin WC, Chang HL. Relaxant effects of berberine on the rat fundus. Res Commun Molec Pathol Pharmacol 1995;90:333-46.

20. Boegge SC, Kesper S, Verspohl EJ, Nahrstedt A. Reduction of ACh-induced contraction of rat isolated ileum by coptisine, (+)-caffeoylmalic acid, Chelidonium majus, and Corydalis lutea extracts. Planta Med 1996;62:173-4.

21. Vahlensieck U, Hahn R, Winterhoff H, Gumbinger HG, Nahrstedt A, Kemper FH. The effect of Chelidonium majus herb extract on choleresis in the isolated perfused rat liver. Planta Med 1995;61:267-70.

22. Vavrecková C, Gawlik I, Müller K. Benzophenanthridine alkaloids of Chelidonium majus; I. Inhibition of 5- and 12-lipoxygenase by a non-redox mechanism. Planta Med 1996;62:397-401.

23. Tanaka T, Metori K, Mineo S, Hirotani M, Furuya T, Kobayashi S. Inhibitory effects of berberine-type alkaloids on clastase. Planta Med 1993;59:200-2.

24. Saeed SA, Gilani AH, Majoo RU, Shah BH. Anti-thrombotic and anti-inflammatory activities of protopine. Pharmacol Res 1997;36:1-7.

25. Mitra S, Gole M, Samajdar K, Sur RK, Chakraborty BN. Antihepatotoxic activity of Chelidonium majus. Int J Pharmacognosy 1992;30:125-8.

26. Mitra S, Sur RK, Roy A, Mukherjee AS. Effect of Chelidonium majus L. on experimental hepatic tissue injury. Phytotherapy Res 1996;10:354-6.

27. Baumann JC. Über die Wirkung von Chelidonium, Curcuma, Absinth und Carduus marianus auf die Galle- und Pankreassekretion bei Hepatopathien. Medizinische Monatsschrift 1975;29:173-80.

28. Baumann JC, Heintze K, Muth HW. Klinisch-experimentelle Untersuchungen der Gallen-, Pankreas- und Magensaftsekretion unter den phytocholagogen Wirkstoffen einer Carduus marianus-Chelidonium-Curcuma-Suspension. Arzneim-Forsch/Drug Res 1971; 21:98-101.

29. von Zerssen D. Die Beschwerden-Liste. Manual. Weinheim: Beltz Test GmbH, 1976.

30. Knöpfel SA. Auch gegen Gallenleiden ist ein Kraut gewachsen. Therapeutikon 1991;4:205-8.

31. Jagiello-Wojtowicz E, Jusiak L, Szponar J, Kleinrok Z. Preliminary pharmacological evaluation of chelidonine in rodents. Pol J Pharmacol Pharm 1989;41:125-31.

32. Dalvi RR. Sanguinarine: its potential as a liver toxic alkaloid present in the seeds of Argemone mexicana. Experientia 1985;41:77-8.

33. Ulrichova J, Walterova D, Vavreckova C, Kamarad V, Simanek V. Cytotoxicity of benzo[c]phenanthridinium alkaloids in isolated rat hepatocytes. Phytotherapy Res 1996;10:220-3.

34. Gebhardt R, Gaunitz F. Testung Schöllkraut-Alkaloide. Bericht zur Cytotoxizitäts-Untersuchung. Internal Report by Firmenverbund and BAH, Bonn. Leipzig, March 1999.

35. Bootman J. Test substance batch No. 181287: Assessment of clastogenic action on bone marrow erythrocytes in the micronucleus test. Eye, Life Science Research, Internal Report by Steiner Arzneimittel 1988: 88/SIR 013/292.

CIMICIFUGAE RHIZOMA

Black Cohosh

E/S/C/O/P
MONOGRAPHS
Second Edition

DEFINITION

Black cohosh consists of the dried rhizomes and roots of *Cimicifuga racemosa* (L.) Nutt.

A draft monograph on black cohosh, intended for inclusion in the European Pharmacopoeia, has been published [1].

CONSTITUENTS

The characteristic constituents are triterpene glycosides, a complex mixture from which over 30 compounds have been isolated in recent investigations [2-10]. The major triterpene glycosides appear to be cimicifugoside[1] [7,8,11-14], actein [3,4,7-15], a compound formerly known as 27-deoxyactein [6-8,16] but recently re-designated as 23-*epi*-26-deoxyactein [3], and cimiracemosides A [8,9], C and F [8]. All these glycosides are 3-*O*-xylosides or 3-*O*-arabinosides of aglycones of the cycloartane type [2,3,6-10].

Other constituents include fukiic and piscidic acid esters, especially fukinolic (2-*E*-caffeoylfukiic) acid [17,18]; aromatic acids such as caffeic, ferulic and isoferulic acids [12-14,17-19]; and various phenyl-propanoid esters such as methyl caffeate [19], peta-siphenol and cimiciphenol (3,4-dihydroxyphenyl-2-oxopropyl caffeate and isoferulate respectively) [18] and cimiracemates A-D (phenylpropanoid ester dimers) [19].

The isoflavone formononetin was reported to be present in 1985 [20] but has not been detected in sub-sequent investigations [18,21-23], which included an analysis of thirteen different populations of black cohosh in eastern USA [21]. Biochanin A (another isoflavone) has also been reported [22] but not detected in a recent investigation [18].

CLINICAL PARTICULARS

Therapeutic indications
Climacteric symptoms such as hot flushes, profuse sweating, sleep disorders and nervous irritability [24-33].

---

[1] Cimicifugoside (cimigenol 3-*O*-β-D-xyloside) as isolated by He et al. [7], Shao et al. [8] and earlier by Piancatelli and coworkers [11]; in some literature it is called cimigoside or cimifugoside. A different 'cimicifugoside' has been isolated from black cohosh by Kusano et al. [10]; it is the 3-*O*-xyloside of an aglycone with a cyclolanost-7-en structure.

Posology and method of administration

Dosage

Adult daily dose: Isopropanolic (40% V/V) [24-27] or ethanolic (40-60% V/V) [28-34] extracts corresponding to 40-140 mg of the drug; equivalent preparations.

Method of administration
For oral administration.

Duration of administration
No restriction.

Onset of action can be expected within 2-4 weeks [24,25,27,28,35]. For further improvement medication should be taken for at least 6-8 weeks; maximum effects are seen within 3 months [24,27,28].

If symptoms persist, medical advice should be sought.

Contra-indications
None known.

Special warnings and special precautions for use
The use of black cohosh in patients with existing oestrogen-dependent tumours should be approached with caution. The weight of evidence from *in vitro* [36-42] and *in vivo* [43,44] pharmacological studies suggests that black cohosh extracts do not influence the latency or development of mammary tumours, and may have inhibitory effects [36,37,40,41]; however, contradictory results have been obtained in several *in vitro* experiments [45-47]. Clinical experience suggests a lack of risk [48,49], but relevant human toxicological data are unavailable [48].

Interactions with other medicaments and other forms of interaction
None reported.

Pregnancy and lactation
Black cohosh should not be used during pregnancy and lactation [50-52].

Effects on ability to drive and use machines
None known.

Undesirable effects
Occasional gastrointestinal disturbances [29,53-56].

Overdose
Old publications report the occurrence of toxic symptoms after ingestion of 5 g of the unprocessed drug or 12 g of fluid extract [cited in 56]. Since further data are lacking, these reports must be assessed as irrelevant.

Doses of up to 200 mg of the unprocessed drug or equivalent amounts of extracts have been used without apparent adverse effects [27,57].

Earlier texts recommended daily doses of up to 4 g of the unprocessed drug [58].

PHARMACOLOGICAL PROPERTIES

Pharmacodynamic properties

In vitro experiments

Influence on oestrogen receptor-positive breast cancer cells
The majority of studies evaluating the effects of black cohosh extracts on human oestrogen receptor-positive breast cancer cell lines have demonstrated inhibition of proliferation, or at least a lack of proliferative effects:

- A 40%-isopropanolic extract from black cohosh at dilutions corresponding to native dry extract at 1-100 µg/ml significantly and dose-dependently inhibited proliferation of the oestrogen receptor-positive human breast adenocarcinoma cell line MCF-7 under oestrogen-deprived conditions (p<0.05) and also inhibited oestrogen-induced proliferation of the cells (p<0.05 vs. oestradiol 10^{-8} M control). Furthermore, the proliferation-inhibiting effect of tamoxifen at 10^{-6} M was enhanced by the extract. The results suggested a non-oestrogenic or oestrogen-antagonistic effect of the black cohosh extract [36].

- No oestrogenic activities were exhibited by two black cohosh extracts (one ethanolic, the other isopropanolic) in proliferation assays of oestrogen receptor-positive MCF-7 cells; the extracts antagonized oestradiol-induced stimulation of proliferation of the cells at concentrations > 1 µg/ml [37].

- The growth of oestrogen-dependent human breast cancer MCF-7 cells was not stimulated by 48-hour treatment with an alcoholic extract from black cohosh (extraction solvent not further defined) at dilutions from 1:500 to 1:5000. In contrast, in the same test, growth of MCF-7 cells was induced concentration-dependently by dong quai (*Angelica sinensis*; 27-fold at 1:500 dilution, p<0.001) and ginseng (16-fold at 1:500 dilution, p<0.05); however, since these herbal drugs showed no oestrogenic activity as measured in a transient gene expression assay and an *in vivo* bioassay in mice, the authors considered the effect on MCF-7 cells to be independent of oestrogenic activity [38].

- A 50%-ethanolic extract of black cohosh (2 g/

10 ml) at a concentration of 2 µl/ml caused no stimulation of proliferation of oestrogen receptor-positive T47D human breast cancer cells, assessed by measuring the increase/decrease in total protein in cell cultures for 9 days [39].

- A similar extract significantly inhibited the growth of oestrogen receptor-positive T47D human breast cancer cells at concentrations of 0.1 and 1% V/V [40].

- An isopropanolic extract of black cohosh caused significant inhibition of proliferation of oestrogen receptor-positive human mammary carcinoma cell line 435 at concentrations of 2.5-25 µg/ml [41].

- In S30 breast cancer cells the oestrogen-inducible gene presenelin-2 was not up-regulated in the presence of a methanolic extract from black cohosh [42].

In contrast, proliferative effects of black cohosh extracts have been demonstrated in other studies; the reason for these conflicting results is not clear.

- 50%-Ethanolic and 96%-ethanolic extracts of black cohosh at concentrations of 0.1-10 µg/ml and 0.01-1 µg/ml respectively caused proliferation of oestrogen receptor-positive MCF-7 human breast cancer cells; this effect could be antagonized with the specific anti-oestrogen ICI 182,780 [45,59].

- After determination by MTT assay of the optimal concentration of black cohosh for the culture of human breast cancer MCF-7 cells, growth curves of MCF-7 cells in the presence of black cohosh at 4.75 µg/litre or 17β-oestradiol at 0.3 nM were observed for 5 days. The time taken for doubling of cell growth was 32.1 and 31.7 hours in the presence of black cohosh and 17β-oestradiol respectively, compared to 35.3 hours in the blank control. Furthermore, from indirect immunofluorescence assay by flow cytometry, black cohosh at 4.75 µg/litre significantly increased oestrogen receptor levels in the MCF-7 cells ($p<0.01$ compared to control) [46].

- Reporter gene (luciferase) expression was stimulated by more than 200% in oestrogen receptor α- and β-expressing MCF-7 breast cancer cells by treatment with the lipophilic fraction from an ethanolic black cohosh extract (35 µg/ml) or oestradiol (10 nM). This effect was totally blunted by the specific anti-oestrogen ICI 182,780 [47].

One constituent isolated from black cohosh has shown proliferative effects:

- Fukinolic acid isolated from black cohosh increased the proliferation of oestrogen-dependent MCF-7 cells by up to 120% at 5×10^{-7} M ($p<0.05$) and 126% at 5×10^{-8} ($p<0.001$). While these effects were equivalent to the activity of oestradiol at a lower concentration of 10^{-10} M, fukinolic acid showed no significant activity at 5×10^{-9} M [17].

Oestrogen receptor affinity

A chloroform fraction from a methanolic extract of black cohosh exhibited binding to oestrogen receptors of the rat uterus. Formononetin isolated from this fraction showed weak binding to the receptors (1.15% of that of 17β-oestradiol) [20]. However, formononetin has not been detected in black cohosh in more recent studies [18,21-23].

A black cohosh extract (not further defined) at 1:20 dilution to full strength did not inhibit [³H]-oestradiol binding to cytosolic oestrogen receptor from livers of mature ovariectomized rats, whereas extracts from hop strobile or dong quai exerted dose-dependent inhibition [60].

Binding to oestrogen receptors from porcine uteri was demonstrated with an ethanolic extract of black cohosh [47].

In a radioimmunoassay for determination of oestrogenic compounds, increasing sample volumes (5-100 µl) of two different 60%-ethanolic extracts of black cohosh dose-dependently displaced radioactively-labelled oestradiol bound to a specific oestradiol antiserum, paralleling the curve obtained with non-labelled oestradiol. This indicated competition with oestradiol for binding sites on the antibody molecules [61].

A methanolic extract from black cohosh gave negative results in assays for oestrogenic activity: no competitive binding affinity for recombinant human oestrogen receptors α (ERα) and β (ERβ), and no induction of alkaline phosphatase activity or up-regulation of progesterone receptor mRNA in cultured Ishikawa cells (an ER-positive endometrial adenocarcinoma cell line). In contrast, methanolic extracts from red clover (*Trifolium pratense*) and hop strobile gave positive results in these assays [42].

An alcoholic extract from black cohosh (not further defined) at 1:500 dilution did not significantly transactivate human oestrogen receptors ERα or ERβ in a transient gene expression assay using HeLa cells co-transfected with an estrogen-dependent reporter plasmid, whereas 17β-oestradiol at 10^{-9} M increased transcriptional activity through human ERα and ERβ by 20-fold and 10-fold respectively [38].

To determine whether active substances present in a

dry 58%-ethanolic extract of black cohosh bind to either of the two known subtypes of the oestrogen receptor (ERα and ERβ), subtype-specific oestrogen receptor ligand-binding assays were conducted using recombinant human ERα or ERβ. Although the extract displaced radiolabelled oestradiol from binding sites of cytosol preparations from porcine or human endometrium (containing both ERα and ERβ), no such displacement of oestradiol by the extract was achieved when either recombinant human ERα or ERβ was used. Dopaminergic activity of the black cohosh extract was demonstrated in an assay using recombinant human dopamine D_2 receptor protein, and application of countercurrent chromatography to the extract enabled separation of oestrogenic and dopaminergic activities into two distinct fractions. The researchers suggested that substances not yet identified in the extract bind to an as yet unknown oestrogen-binding site (a putative ERγ) in the endometrium, and also that as yet unknown dopaminergic compounds in the extract may contribute to the pharmacological profile of the extract [62].

Inhibition of prolactin secretion
An extract of black cohosh at 100 and 10 µg/ml significantly inhibited both basal and stimulated prolactin secretion in primary cell cultures of the rat pituitary gland. As these effects could be reduced by the dopamine antagonist haloperidol the findings were interpreted as dopaminergic activity [63].

Vasoactive effects
Isolated fukinolic acid and cimicifugic acid D at a concentration of 3×10^{-4} M caused sustained relaxation of rat aortic strips precontracted with norepinephrine; cimicifugic acids A, B and E and fukiic acid showed no vasoactivity at this concentration [64].

Antioxidant activity
A methanolic extract from black cohosh scavenged 1,1-diphenyl-2-picrylhydrazyl (DPPH) free radicals with an IC_{50} of 99 µg/ml, and at concentrations up to 200 µg/ml dose-dependently inhibited DNA single-strand breaks and oxidation of DNA bases induced by the quinone menadione. Of nine compounds (all hydroxycinnamic acid derivatives) identified as antioxidants in the extract, six reduced menadione-induced DNA damage in cultured S30 breast cancer cells, the most potent being methyl caffeate, caffeic acid and ferulic acid. The data suggested that black cohosh can protect against cellular DNA damage caused by reactive oxygen species by acting as an antioxidant [65].

In vivo experiments

Influence on oestrogen receptor-positive mammary tumours
As an oestrogen-receptor positive breast cancer model,

mammary tumours were induced in female rats by intragastric administration of 7,12-dimethyl-benz[a]anthracene (DMBA); the animals were then ovariectomized, allowed to recover, randomized into groups and treated orally for 6 weeks with an isopropanolic extract from black cohosh at daily dose levels of 0.714, 7.14 or 71.4 mg/kg (comparable to 1, 10 or 100 times the human therapeutic dose respectively) or with mestranol (an oestrogenic steroid) at 450 µg/kg/day as a positive control, or vehicle only as a negative control. Six weeks later, whereas tumour growth had been stimulated in the mestranol-treated group (p<0.05), no significant differences could be detected in tumour number or size between the black cohosh groups and the vehicle-only control group. A trend (not statistically significant) towards tumour reduction was observed in the black cohosh groups compared to the control, suggesting a possible inhibitory effect. Serum levels of prolactin, follicle-stimulating hormone (FSH) and luteinizing hormone (LH), organ weights and endometrial proliferation were also unaffected by the black cohosh extract in comparison with the vehicle-only group [43].

In another recent study the animals used were MMTV-neu transgenic female mice, which develop primary and metastatic mammary tumours through spontaneous activation of the proto-oncogene neu (erbB2, HER2), the most common oncogene of breast cancer. Black cohosh (not specified as, but assumed to be, an extract), administered orally to sexually mature female MMTV-neu mice in their diet (40 mg/1800 calories of diet, comparable to women receiving 40 mg/day) from 2 months of age until the maximum age of 16 months, did not alter the latency or incidence of mammary tumours compared to MMTV-neu females maintained on a control diet. However, in females which had developed primary mammary tumours, black cohosh negatively influenced progression to metastatic disease (disease transferred from one part of the body to another); the percentage of detectable lung tumours at necropsy in the black cohosh-treated animals (27.1%, n = 96) was higher than in those on a control diet (10.9%; n = 110). Furthermore, the number of lung tumours per female was higher after long-term exposure to black cohosh. It has not yet been determined whether black cohosh accelerated the development of metastatic disease or increased its incidence. These results suggested that black cohosh does not influence (adversely or beneficially) a woman's risk of developing breast cancer [44]. The observed metastatic effects (in transgenic animals predisposed to the development of tumours) requires further investigation.

Endocrinological activities
A dry 60%-ethanolic black cohosh extract administered intraperitoneally to ovariectomized rats (12 mg of extract twice daily, corresponding to 96 mg/kg body weight/day) caused a clear decrease in serum

concentration of luteinizing hormone (LH) after 3 days. After 1 or 14 days, however, no differences between extract and control solution could be detected. No changes were observed in serum levels of follicle stimulating hormone (FSH) or prolactin. In a similar experiment, a dichloromethane extract (total dose: 27 mg of extract per animal, divided into 9 doses over a period of 4 days, corresponding to 108 mg/kg body weight) also significantly reduced LH levels; serum prolactin and vaginal cytology were unchanged [66].

The dried chloroform-soluble fraction from a methanolic extract of black cohosh (crude drug to chloroform fraction ratio approx. 35:1), administered intraperitoneally to ovariectomized rats as a total dose of 108 mg, corresponding to approx. 568 mg/kg body weight, in divided doses over 4 days, reduced serum levels of LH from 657 ng/ml (injection vehicle as control) to 339 ng/ml [20].

Oral administration of a 50%-ethanolic black cohosh extract at 6, 60 or 600 mg/kg body weight/day to immature mice for 3 days followed by uterus weight tests, and subcutaneously to mature ovariectomized rats followed by vaginal smear tests, did not reveal any oestrogenic effects [67]. In another study, oral administration of a 50%-ethanolic extract of black cohosh to ovariectomized female mice in doses of 50-600 mg daily for 3 days did not produce any oestrogenic effects (cornification) in vaginal smears [68].

Ovarectomized rats showed no effects on uterine weight or oestrogen-regulated genes in the uterus after 7 days or 3 months of daily treatment with 62.5 mg of a black cohosh extract (extraction solvent not specified). However oestrogenic effects, mimicking many of the effects of oestradiol, could be seen in bone, liver and aorta [69,70].

Treatment of ovariectomized mice with 500 μl of an alcoholic black cohosh extract (not further defined) by oral gavage daily for 4 days did not increase uterine weight compared to untreated controls, whereas 17β-oestradiol administered subcutaneously at 100 μg/kg/day caused a 1.7-fold increase [38].

Daily subcutaneous administration of the dichloromethane fraction from an ethanolic black cohosh extract to ovariectomized rats for 7 days at 60 mg/rat had no effect on uterine weight, whereas oestradiol at 8 μg/rat significantly increased uterine weight (p<0.05); both the black cohosh extract and oestradiol significantly reduced serum LH levels (p<0.05) [47].

In contrast, increases in uterine weights after oral administration of black cohosh have been observed in two studies. An unspecified black cohosh extract added to the diet of ovariectomized rats for 3 weeks increased uterine weights and significantly decreased

LH levels (25% reduction, p<0.05); the authors interpreted these findings as oestrogenic activity [71]. In a more recent study, when black cohosh was administered to immature female mice by gavage at 75, 150 or 300 mg/kg body weight daily for 14 days, uterine weights (measured when oestrus was observed) increased with the increasing dosage of black cohosh and the days of oestrus were significantly prolonged in the 300 mg/kg group (p<0.05) [46].

Recent findings suggest that in its mode of action black cohosh may be described as a Selective Oestrogen Receptor Modulator (SERM) [32,47,48,59,69, 70,72,73]. It is now known that there are at least two oestrogen receptors, ERα and ERβ. Many plant compounds show a greater affinity for binding to ERβ than to ERα [74]. Since these receptors are differently expressed in various organs, oestrogenic effects of a substance need to be assessed for each individual tissue, because the same substance can exert oestrogenic and non-/anti-oestrogenic effects depending on the specific tissue. This may explain observations of both oestrogenic and anti-oestrogenic effects of black cohosh [75].

Effects on autonomic nervous system

Hot flush equivalents in oviarectomized rats (rapid and short-term increases of more than 1°C in peripheral body temperature, measured by an implanted sensor and transmitter) were reduced in frequency by oestradiol valerate (2 mg/kg/day; p<0.05) or the anti-dopaminergic drug veralipride (100 mg/kg/day), indicating a response and sensitivity comparable to hot flushes in women. Oral administration of a dry 58%-ethanolic extract of black cohosh to the rats at 100 mg/kg body weight daily for 5 days also significantly reduced the number of hot flush equivalents per day (p<0.05 on days 3-5); the frequency returned to pre-treatment levels after cessation of treatment [76]. In earlier experiments using the same technique, 50%-ethanolic and 40%-isopropanolic black cohosh extracts, orally administered at 100 mg/kg for 4 days, also reduced skin flushes in ovariectomized rats [77].

An extract of black cohosh, orally administered to mice in a range between 25 and 100 mg/kg body weight, caused a distinct and dose-dependent fall in body temperature one hour after gavage, 100 mg/kg having an effect comparable to that of bromocriptine (a dopamine D_2 agonist) given intraperitoneally at 5 mg/kg. The fall in body temperature was inhibited by pretreatment with the dopamine D_2/D_3 receptor antagonist sulpiride at 100 mg/kg, but not by the selective D_1 receptor antagonist SCH 23390. Furthermore the extract prolonged ketamine-induced sleeping time in mice, an effect which also occurred after bromocriptine injection but could be blocked by sulpiride and was unchanged by SCH 23390. These results indicated central activity of the extract mediated by central D_2 receptors [63].

Osteoprotective effects

Treatment of ovariectomized rats with a black cohosh extract at 33 mg/day per animal (added to the diet) for 3 months had osteoprotective effects; compared to ovariectomized but untreated rats, significant reductions in loss of bone mineral density in tibia (p<0.05) and reduced serum levels of osteocalcin (a marker of bone turnover, produced by osteoblasts; p<0.05) were observed. The extract also significantly reduced the sizes of a paratibial (foreleg) fat depot (p<0.05), an abdominal fat depot (p<0.05) and hence body weight (p<0.05), and also serum concentrations of the hormone leptin (an indicator of lipocyte activity; p<0.05). Oral 17β-oestradiol at 0.325-0.35 mg/day per animal had similar and somewhat stronger effects but, in contrast to the black cohosh extract, also significantly reduced serum crosslaps (another marker of bone turnover, produced by osteoclasts; p<0.05), significantly increased uterine weight (p<0.05) and significantly influenced expression of oestrogen-regulated uterine genes, inhibiting ERβ (p<0.05) and stimulating IGF-1 (insulin-like growth factor, which stimulates proliferation of the endometrium; p<0.05). Since the black cohosh extract exerted significant oestrogenic effects in the bone (particularly in osteoblasts, cells which rebuild absorbed bone) and fat tissue of ovariectomized rats, but not in the uterus, it appeared to contain organ-specific selective oestrogen receptor modulators (SERMs), with effects in some, but not all, oestrogen-sensitive organs [73].

From a recent review, it was concluded that in ovariectomized rats a black cohosh extract showed many of the beneficial effects of 17β-oestradiol, including effects in the brain/thalamus to reduce serum LH levels, effects in the bone to prevent osteoporosis and estrogenic effects in the urinary bladder, but had no uterotrophic effect. If clinical studies confirm these results, the extract would appear to be a selective oestrogen receptor modulator (SERM) and may therefore be an alternative to hormone replacement therapy [48].

Other authors concluded, from a recent systematic review of 15 *in vitro* and 15 *in vivo* studies on black cohosh, that the results suggested a central activity rather than a hormonal effect [78].

Other effects

In the tail suspension test in mice (a behavioural test for antidepressant activity) a dry 58%-ethanolic extract of black cohosh, administered by gavage at 50 or 100 mg/kg, reduced the period of immobility (p<0.05), as did imipramine at 30 mg/kg (p<0.05); this effect was observed 60 minutes after a single dose and also after 8 days of treatment [76].

Weak vascular, anti-inflammatory and hypoglycaemic effects of black cohosh have been reported [cited in 56]. However, these old reports provide inadequate information on methods and effects [56] and do not meet modern scientific requirements.

Pharmacological studies in humans

Some studies appear to demonstrate an oestrogen-like mode of action for black cohosh. In a placebo-controlled study in 110 menopausal women of mean age 52 years, daily oral administration of 8 mg of a hydroethanolic extract of black cohosh for 2 months induced a significant (p<0.05) decrease in serum LH levels in the verum group (n = 55) compared to the placebo group (n = 55); FSH levels were similar in both groups [79].

Vaginal cytological parameters also seemed to be influenced in an oestrogenic manner. In a double-blind randomized study, women (aged between 46 and 58 years) with menopausal symptoms received daily for 3 months 8 mg of a black cohosh extract (n = 30) or 0.625 mg of conjugated estrogens (n = 30) or placebo (n = 20). The black cohosh extract increased the degree of proliferation of the vaginal epithelium from 2-3 to 3-4 on the Schmitt scale for vaginal cytology (p<0.01 compared to placebo) [24]. Similar effects were seen in an open controlled study in 60 patients (mean age 54 years), using the karyopyknotic index and eosinophilic index [28]. On the other hand, in a study in 60 women suffering from climacteric complaints following hysterectomy, no significant changes in serum LH and FSH levels were observed during 6 months of treatment with 8 mg/day of a black cohosh extract [25].

However, in a more recent double-blind, randomized study in which women (aged 42-60 years) with climacteric symptoms were assigned to daily treatment for 24 weeks with either 40 mg (n = 76) or 127 mg (n = 76) of a 40%-isopropanolic extract of black cohosh, no significant changes in serum levels of oestradiol, LH, FSH, prolactin or sexual hormone binding globulin could be detected in either group compared to pre-treatment levels. Vaginal cytological parameters also remained unchanged [27].

Investigations on 28 postmenopausal women (mean age 56.4 years), who had taken approx. 136 mg of a 40% isopropanolic extract of black cohosh daily for 3 months, revealed no effect on endometrial thickness (assessed by transvaginal sonography), vaginal cytology or serum levels of LH, FSH, prolactin and oestradiol [72].

In a 12-week randomized, double-blind study in postmenopausal women patients, neither placebo (n = 20) nor a dry 58%-ethanolic extract of black cohosh (daily dose equivalent to 2 × 20 mg of crude drug, n = 20) influenced endometrial thickness, measured by transvaginal ultrasound, whereas conjugated oestrogens (CE, 2 × 0.3 mg daily, n = 22) increased endometrial thickness by more than 1 mm.

The black cohosh extract slightly increased the amount of superficial cells in vaginal smears (10% increase from baseline; p = 0.0542) compared to a significant increase of 38% after CE (p<0.01) and a decrease of 10% after placebo. Analysis of markers of bone metabolism in serum indicated beneficial effects in both the black cohosh and CE groups. Serum levels of "CrossLaps" (metabolic products of bone-specific collagen-1a1, generally accepted as markers of bone degradation) decreased slightly after black cohosh and significantly after CE (p = 0.0181), compared to an increase in the placebo group. On the other hand, serum levels of bone-specific alkaline phosphatase (a metabolic marker for bone formation) increased significantly in the black cohosh group (p = 0.0358 vs. placebo, p = 0.0498 vs. CE) while increasing only slightly in the CE group and remaining almost unchanged in the placebo group. Combined as a Bone Turnover Index, i.e. log (bone-specific alkaline phosphatase/CrossLaps), the beneficial effects on bone metabolism after black cohosh or CE were comparable and significant (p = 0.0138 vs. placebo in both cases). From these results, together with modest improvement in climacteric complaints (summarized under Clinical studies), the authors concluded that the black cohosh extract had selective oestrogen receptor modulator (SERM) activities, i.e. caused desired effects in the hypothalamus, in the mesolimbic brain regions, in bones and on vaginal epithelium, but without oestrogenic effects in the uterus [32].

Clinical studies

Clinical studies performed with a 40%-isopropanolic dry extract of black cohosh (8 mg/day)
The corresponding amounts of unprocessed drug were not stated in the respective papers, but were within the range of 48-140 mg [75]

In a randomized, double-blind, three-armed study, women aged 46-58 years received one of the following treatments daily for 12 weeks: 8 mg of the black cohosh extract (n = 30) or 0.625 mg of conjugated oestrogens (n = 30) or placebo (n = 20). The patients suffered from menopausal complaints such as hot flushes, sweating, palpitations, depressed mood and sleep disorders; they also had vaginal complaints due to oestrogen deficiency. Effects on climacteric symptoms were assessed by the Kupperman Menopause Index and Hamilton Anxiety Scale (HAMA). Compared to placebo the extract produced a significant decrease in the Kupperman Index (mean value from 34 to 14; p<0.001) and the HAMA (p<0.001). Vaginal cytology parameters also improved significantly (p<0.001) [24].

In an open, randomized, comparative study, 60 women under 40 years of age who had undergone hysterectomy but retained at least one intact ovary and complained of climacteric symptoms were treated daily for 24 weeks with 1 mg of oestriol (n = 15) or 1.25 mg of conjugated oestrogens (n = 15) or an oestrogen-progesterone sequence preparation (n = 15) or 8 mg of the black cohosh extract (n = 15). From assessment at 4, 8, 12 and 24 weeks using a modified Kupperman Menopause Index, statistically significant decreases in climacteric symptoms were observed in all treatment groups (p<0.01). Conjugated oestrogens and the oestrogen-progesterone combination appeared to be slightly superior but differences between the groups were not statistically significant [25].

In another open study, 50 women with climacteric symptoms, who had previously been treated every 4-6 weeks with intramuscular injections of a combination of oestradiol valerate 4 mg and prasteronenantate 200 mg, were alternatively treated with the black cohosh extract for 6 months. 28 patients (56%) required no further injections, 21 patients (44%) required one injection during the 6 months and 1 patient required two injections. The Kupperman Menopause Index decreased on average from 17.6 to 9.2 (p<0.001) [26].

Clinical studies performed with a 40%-isopropanolic dry extract of black cohosh (comparison between 40 and 127 mg of unprocessed drug/day)

In a randomized, double-blind study, 152 peri- and postmenopausal women outpatients (aged 42-60 years) with a Kupperman Menopause Index score ≥ 20 (i.e. climacteric symptoms of at least moderate severity) were assigned to daily treatment for 24 weeks with the black cohosh extract at dose levels corresponding to either 39 mg (n = 76) or 127.3 mg (n = 76) of unprocessed drug; the study was not placebo-controlled. Of the initial participants, 123 completed the first 12 weeks and 116 completed 24 weeks. Similar therapeutic effects were evident in both treatment groups after 2 weeks; after 24 weeks the initial median Kupperman scores of 30.5-31.0 had decreased to 7-8 and this was maintained to the end of the 6-month study period in both groups. The number of responders (defined by a Kupperman score < 15) after 3 months was 70% in the 39 mg group and 72% in the 127.3 mg group. No significant difference in results was evident between the two groups either from intention-to-treat or per-protocol analysis, indicating that a daily dose corresponding to 40 mg of unprocessed drug was adequate [27].

Clinical studies performed with a 60% ethanolic extract of black cohosh (80 drops/day)
The corresponding amounts of unprocessed drug were not stated in the respective papers, but were within the range of 48-140 mg [75]

In an open, comparative, three-armed study, 60

women aged 45-60 years with climacteric symptoms received daily for 12 weeks 0.6 mg of conjugated oestrogens (n = 20) or 2 mg of diazepam (n = 20) or the black cohosh extract (n = 20). All three forms of treatment led to reductions in a modified Kupperman Menopause Index (which included hot flushes, nocturnal sweating, nervousness, headache and palpitations), the Hamilton Anxiety Scale and a Self-assessment Depression Scale. Conjugated oestrogens and (in contrast to other studies) the black cohosh extract showed a trend towards oestrogenic stimulation, with increased proliferation of the vaginal epithelium (as shown by increases in karyopyknosis and eosinophil indices) [28].

In an open study in 50 women aged 45-60 years with climacteric complaints (mainly neurovegetative), the black cohosh extract reduced symptoms assessed as moderate by the Kupperman Menopause Index to "requiring no therapy" after 12 weeks (p<0.001) [29].

In another open study, in 36 women aged 45-62 years with climacteric symptoms, treatment with the black cohosh extract for 12 weeks led to a statistically significant average decrease (p<0.001) in the Kupperman Menopause Index compared to the initial value [30].

In a open, multicentre drug-monitoring study of 629 patients, menopausal symptoms such as hot flushes, profuse sweating, headache, vertigo, nervousness and depression improved in over 80% of cases after 6-8 weeks of treatment with the black cohosh extract [31].

Clinical studies performed with a 58%-ethanolic extract of black cohosh (daily dose corresponding to 40 mg of unprocessed drug)

In a randomized, double-blind, placebo-controlled, three-armed multicentre study, postmenopausal women patients (i.e. perimenopausal women, aged 40-60, with well-defined postmenopausal hormone levels and climacteric complaints) were treated daily for 12 weeks with capsules of identical appearance containing a 58%-ethanolic dry extract from black cohosh (daily dose equivalent to 2 × 20 mg of unprocessed drug; n = 20) or 2 × 0.3 mg of conjugated oestrogens (CE, n = 22) or placebo (n = 20). Out of 97 patients initially randomized as intention-to-treat, almost one-third were subsequently found to have hormone levels not in accordance with the protocol and data on only 62 women were considered evaluable. With regard to the primary efficacy criterion, the menopause rating scale (MRS; 10 criteria, rated by the patients), superiority to placebo was evident after both black cohosh extract (p = 0.0506) and CE (p = 0.0513), but did not quite reach statistical significance due to a high placebo effect. When combinations of MRS criteria were evaluated, the results for "atrophy" (4 criteria) were significant in the black cohosh group (p = 0.0218), while the results for "hot flushes" (3 criteria) were significant in the CE group (p = 0.0461). Results from this study with respect to effects on the endometrium and bone metabolism are summarized under Pharmacological studies in humans [32].

A subsequent and longer randomized, open study assessed the effects of a 58%-ethanolic dry extract from black cohosh (daily dose equivalent to 2 × 20 mg of unprocessed drug; n = 90) on hot flushes caused by tamoxifen (20 mg daily) in young premenopausal breast cancer survivors (aged 35-52 years) who had undergone surgery (lumpectomy or mastectomy), irradiation therapy and/or chemotherapy. Patients in the black cohosh group (n = 90) also took tamoxifen, while those in a control group (n = 46) took tamoxifen only over a period of 12 months. Treatment with black cohosh extract significantly reduced the number and severity of hot flushes (p<0.01). Almost half (46.7%) of patients in the black cohosh group were free from hot flushes (none in the tamoxifen-only group). Severe hot flushes were reported by 24.4% of patients in the black cohosh group compared to 73.9% of those in the tamoxifen-only group [33].

Other recent clinical studies

Patients who had previously received chemotherapy and radiation therapy for breast cancer and were experiencing daily hot flushes participated in a randomized, double-blind, placebo-controlled study to assess the effect of black cohosh (2 tablets of a commercial product daily for 2 months; no further details given) on the frequency and intensity of hot flushes on a 1 to 3 scale. Some patients also used tamoxifen concomitantly (for the management of breast cancer). Of the 85 study participants, 42 (of whom 29 used tamoxifen) were assigned to treatment with black cohosh and 43 (of whom 30 used tamoxifen) were assigned to placebo; 69 patients completed the study. Both the black cohosh and placebo groups reported declines in the frequency (about 27% overall) and intensity of hot flushes during the study, but differences between groups were not significant. Both groups reported improvements in seven menopausal symptoms (heart palpitations, excessive sweating, headaches, poor sleep, depression and irritability or nervousness) during the study, but only sweating was significantly reduced in the black cohosh group compared to the placebo group (p = 0.04). Small changes in serum levels of follicle-stimulating hormone and luteinizing hormone also did not differ between groups [80].

In an open study, 50 postmenopausal women patients were treated daily for 6 months with a black cohosh extract (type and amount not stated). An excellent response was reported in subjective complaints assessed by the Kupperman Menopause Index and

Hamilton Anxiety Scale; only 10% of patients had no relevant improvement after 3 months. Endometrial thickness (measured by endovaginal ultrasound) remained unchanged after 6 months [81].

Pre-1970 clinical studies
From 1957 to 1964 a number of case reports and uncontrolled studies were published describing the successful treatment of numerous women with climacteric symptoms or menstrual disorders with black cohosh extracts [53, 82-91].

Clinical reviews
A 1998 review of clinical and human pharmacological studies, assessing the efficacy of black cohosh for menopausal symptoms, concluded that it may be a safe and effective alternative to oestrogen replacement therapy in patients for whom oestrogen replacement therapy is contraindicated or refused [55].

From a more recent systematic review (2002) of four randomized, controlled clinical studies [24,25,28,80] it was concluded that, in spite of plausible mechanisms of action, the clinical efficacy of black cohosh for the treatment of menopausal symptoms has not yet been convincingly demonstrated; further rigorous studies are warranted [92].

Pharmacokinetic properties
No data available.

Preclinical safety data

Chronic toxicity
A 40%-isopropanolic dry extract of black cohosh, administered to rats daily for 6 months at a dose equivalent to 535.5 mg/kg body weight of the unprocessed drug (approximately 700 times the human therapeutic dose), produced no relevant clinical or histopathological changes [75].

Mutagenicity
In the Ames test the same extract revealed no mutagenic potential at up to the equivalent of 30.3 mg of unprocessed drug per plate [75].

Acute toxicity of actein
Minimum lethal single doses of actein were determined [93] as:

Mouse, intraperitoneal:	> 500 mg/kg
Rat, oral:	> 1000 mg/kg
Rabbit, intravenous:	> 70 mg/kg

Subchronic toxicity of actein
Minimal lethal doses of actein administered daily for 30 days were determined [93] as:

Mouse, intraperitoneal:	> 10 mg/kg
Rabbit, oral:	> 6 mg/kg

Clinical safety data
A critical evaluation of the safety of black cohosh concluded that human clinical trials, postmarketing surveillance studies and other reports involving over over 2,800 patients demonstrated a low incidence of adverse events (5.4%). Of the reported adverse events, 97% were minor and did not result in discontinuation of therapy. No severe adverse events were attributed to black cohosh [49].

A recent systematic review of data from clinical studies and also from spontaneous reporting programmes of the World Health Organization and national regulatory bodies suggested that adverse events arising from the use of black cohosh are rare, mild and reversible, the most common being gastrointestinal upsets and rashes. It was concluded that, although definitive evidence is not available, black cohosh seems to be a safe herbal medicine [94].

In another review the author concluded that clinical studies and case reports have demonstrated good tolerance of, and low risk of side effects from, ethanolic and isopropanolic extracts of black cohosh [95].

REFERENCES

1. Black Cohosh - Cimicifugae rhizoma. Pharmeuropa 2002;14:353-5.

2. Chen S-N, Fabricant DS, Lu Z-Z, Fong HHS, Farnsworth NR. Cimiracemosides I-P, new 9,19-cyclolanostane triterpene glycosides from *Cimicifuga racemosa*. J Nat Prod 2002;65:1391-7.

3. Chen S-N, Li W, Fabricant DS, Santsariero BD, Mesecar A, Fitzloff JF, Fong HHS, Farnsworth NR. Isolation, structure elucidation and absolute configuration of 26-deoxyactein from *Cimicifuga racemosa* and clarification of nomenclature associated with 27-deoxyactein. J Nat Prod 2002;65:601-5.

4. Watanabe K, Mimaki Y, Sakagami H, Sashida Y. Cyclo-artane glycosides from the rhizomes of *Cimicifuga racemosa* and their cytotoxic activities. Chem Pharm Bull 2002;50:121-5.

5. Wende K, Mügge C, Thurow K, Schöpke T, Lindequist U. Actaeaepoxide 3-O-β-D-xylopyranoside, a new cycloartane glycoside from the rhizomes of *Actaea racemosa* (*Cimicifuga racemosa*). J Nat Prod 2001; 64:986-9.

6. Bedir E, Khan IA. Cimiracemoside A: a new cyclo-lanostanol xyloside from the rhizome of *Cimicifuga racemosa*. Chem Pharm Bull 2000;48:425-7.

7. He K, Zheng B, Kim CH, Rogers L, Zheng Q. Direct analysis and identification of triterpene glycosides by LC/MS in black cohosh, *Cimicifuga racemosa*, and in several commercially available black cohosh products. Planta Medica 2000;66:635-40.

8. Shao Y, Harris A, Wang M, Zhang H, Cordell GA,

Bowman M, Lemmo E. Triterpene glycosides from *Cimicifuga racemosa*. J Nat Prod 2000;63;905-10.

9. Ganzera M, Bedir E, Khan IA. Separation of *Cimicifuga racemosa* triterpene glycosides by reversed phase high performance liquid chromatography and evaporative light scattering detection. Chromatographia 2000;52: 301-4.

10. Kusano A, Takahira M, Shibano M, In Y, Ishida T, Miyase T and Kusano G. Studies on the constituents of *Cimicifuga* species. XX. Absolute stereostructures of cimicifugoside and actein from *Cimicifuga simplex* Wormsk. Chem Pharm Bull 1998;46:467-72.

11. Piancatelli G. Nuovi triterpeni dall'*Actea racemosa*. Nota IV. Gazz Chim Ital 1971;101:139-48.

12. Beuscher N. *Cimicifuga racemosa* L. Die Traubensilberkerze. Z Phytother 1995;16:301-10.

13. Bradley PR, editor. Black cohosh. In: British Herbal Compendium, Volume 1. Bournemouth: British Herbal Medicine Association, 1992:34-6.

14. Harnischfeger G, Stolze H. Bewährte Wirksubstanzen aus Naturstoffen. Traubensilberkerze. notabene medici 1980;10:446-50.

15. Linde H. Die Inhaltsstoffe von *Cimicifuga racemosa*. 2. Mitt. Zur Struktur des Acteins. Arch Pharm (Weinheim) 1967;300:885-92.

16. Berger S, Junior P, Kopanski L. 27-Deoxyactein: a new polycyclic triterpenoid glycoside from *Actaea racemosa*. Planta Med 1988;54:579-80 (Abstract P1-19).

17. Kruse SO, Löhning A, Pauli GF, Winterhoff H, Nahrstedt A. Fukiic and piscidic acid esters from the rhizome of *Cimicifuga racemosa* and the *in vitro* estrogenic activity of fukinolic acid. Planta Med 1999;65:763-4.

18. Hagels H, Baumert-Krauss J, Freudenstein J. Composition of phenolic constituents in *Cimicifuga racemosa*. In: Abstracts of International Congress and 48th Annual Meeting of the Society for Medicinal Plant Research. Zürich, 3-7 September 2000 (Abstract P1B/03).

19. Chen S-N, Fabricant DS, Lu Z-Z, Zhang H, Fong HHS, Farnsworth NR. Cimiracemates A-D, phenylpropanoid esters from the rhizomes of *Cimicifuga racemosa*. Phytochemistry 2002;61:409-13.

20. Jarry H, Harnischfeger G, Düker E. Untersuchungen zur endokrinen Wirksamkeit von Inhaltsstoffen aus *Cimicifuga racemosa*. 2. *In vitro*-Bindung von Inhaltsstoffen an Östrogenrezeptoren. Planta Med 1985; 51:316-9.

21. Kennelly EJ, Baggett S, Nuntanakorn P, Ososki AL, Mori SA, Duke J et al. Analysis of thirteen populations of black cohosh for formononetin. Phytomedicine 2002; 9:461-7.

22. McCoy J, Kelly W. Survey of *Cimicifuga racemosa* for phytoestrogenic flavonoids. In: Abstracts of 212th American Chemical Society National Meeting, Orlando, Florida, 25-29 August 1996 (Abstract 082).

23. Struck D, Tegtmeier M, Harnischfeger G. Flavones in extracts of *Cimicifuga racemosa*. Planta Med 1997; 63:289.

24. Stoll W. Phytotherapeutikum beeinflusst atrophisches Vaginalepithel: Doppelblindversuch *Cimicifuga* vs. Oestrogenpräparat. Therapeutikon 1987;1:23-31.

25. Lehmann-Willenbrock E, Riedel H-H. Klinische und endokrinologische Untersuchungen zur Therapie ovarieller Ausfallserscheinungen nach Hysterektomie unter Belassung der Adnexe. Zentralbl Gynäkol 1988;110: 611-8.

26. Pethö A. Klimakterische Beschwerden. Umstellung einer Hormonbehandlung auf ein pflanzliches Gynäkologikum möglich? Bei über 50 Prozent der mit Hormonen vorbehandelten Patientinnen wurde unter einer Cimicifuga-Therapie eine weitere Hormongabe überflüssig. Ärztl Praxis 1987;39:1551-3.

27. Liske E, Hänggi W, Henneicke von Zepelin H-H, Boblitz N, Wüstenberg P, Rahlfs VW. Physiological investigation of a unique extract of black cohosh (Cimicifugae racemosae rhizoma): a 6-month clinical study demonstrates no systemic estrogenic effect. J Women's Health Gender-Based Med 2002;11:163-74.
Previously published in German as:
Liske E, Boblitz N, Henneicke-von Zepelin H-H. Therapie klimakterischer Beschwerden mit *Cimicifuga racemosa* - Daten zur Wirkung und Wirksamkeit aus einer randomisierten kontrollierten Doppelblindstudie. In: Rietbrock N, editor. Phytopharmaka VI. Darmstadt: Steinkopff Verlag, 2000:247-57.

28. Warnecke G. Beeinflussung klimakterischer Beschwerden durch ein Phytotherapeutikum. Erfolgreiche Therapie mit Cimicifuga-Monoextrakt. Med Welt 1985;36:871-4.

29. Vorberg G. Therapie klimakterischer Beschwerden. Erfolgreiche hormonfreie Therapie mit Remifemin®. Z Allgemeinmed 1984;60:626-9.

30. Daiber W. Klimakterische Beschwerden: ohne Hormone zum Erfolg! Ein Phytotherapeutikum mindert Hitzewallungen, Schweißausbrüche und Schlafstörungen. Ärztl Praxis 1983;35;65:1946-7.

31. Stolze H. Der andere Weg, klimakterische Beschwerden zu behandeln. Gyne 1982;3:14-6.

32. Wuttke W, Seidlová-Wuttke D, Gorkow C. The *Cimicifuga* preparation BNO 1055 vs. conjugated estrogens in a double-blind placebo-controlled study: effects on menopause symptoms and bone markers. Maturitas 2003;44 (Suppl 1):S67-S77.

33. Hernández Muñoz G, Pluchino S. *Cimicifuga racemosa* for the treatment of hot flushes in women surviving breast cancer. Maturitas 2003;44 (Suppl 1):S59-S65.

34. Rote Liste® Service GmbH, editors. Section 46: Gynäkologika; subsection 7.A.1.1. Pflanzliche Mittel bei klimakterischen Beschwerden; Einzelstoffe;

Cimicifuga racemosa In: Rote Liste 2001. Aulendorf: Editio Cantor Verlag, 2001:46-148 to 46-163.

35. Anon. Chapter 11. Menopause: Complementary approaches. In: The Canadian Consensus Conference on Menopause and Osteoporosis. Reprinted from J SOGC 1998;20 (13 and14). Toronto: Ribosome Communications, 1998:55-62.

36. Bodinet C and Freudenstein J. Influence of *Cimicifuga racemosa* on the proliferation of estrogen receptor-positive human breast cancer cells. Breast Cancer Res Treatment 2002;76:1-10.

37. Zierau O, Bodinet C, Kolba S, Wulf M, Vollmer G. Antiestrogenic activities of *Cimicifuga racemosa* extracts. J Steroid Biochem Molec Biol 2002;80:125-30.

38. Amato P, Christophe S, Mellon PL. Estrogenic activity of herbs commonly used as remedies for menopausal symptoms. Menopause 2002;9:145-50.

39. Zava DT, Dollbaum CM, Blen M. Estrogen and progestin bioactivity of foods, herbs and spices. Proc Soc Exp Biol Med 1998;217:369-78.

40. Dixon-Shanies D, Shaikh N. Growth inhibition of human breast cancer cells by herbs and phytoestrogens. Oncology Reports 1999;6:1383-7.

41. Neßelhut T, Schellhase C, Dietrich R, Kuhn W. Untersuchungen zur proliferativen Potenz von Phytopharmaka mit östrogenähnlicher Wirkung bei Mammakarzinomzellen. Arch Gynecol Obstet 1993; 254:817-8.

42. Liu J, Burdette JE, Xu H, Gu C, van Breemen RB, Bhat KPL et al. Evaluation of estrogenic activity of plant extracts for the potential treatment of menopausal symptoms. J Agric Food Chem 2001;49:2472-9.

43. Freudenstein J, Dasenbrock C, Nißlein T. Lack of promotion of estrogen-dependent mammary gland tumors *in vivo* by an isopropanolic *Cimicifuga racemosa* extract. Cancer Res 2002;62:3448-52.

44. Davis VL, Jayo MJ, Hardy ML, Ho A, Lee H, Shaikh F et al. Effects of black cohosh on mammary tumor development and progression in MMTV-neu transgenic mice. In: Abstracts of 94th Annual Meeting of American Association for Cancer Research. 11-14 July 2003, Washington, D.C. (Abstract R910). *Published as*: Proc Amer Assoc Cancer Res 2003;44(2nd ed.):R910.

45. Löhning A, Verspohl EJ, Winterhoff H. *Cimicifuga racemosa*: in vitro findings using MCF-7 cells. In: Abstracts of Gesellschaft für Phytotherapie Congress: Phytopharmakaforschung 2000. Bonn, 27-28 Nov 1998:72-73 (Abstract P07).
Brief results also given in Ref. 59.

46. Liu ZP, Yu B, Huo JS, Lu CQ, Chen JS. Estrogenic effects of *Cimicifuga racemosa* (black cohosh) in mice and on estrogen receptors in MCF-7 cells. J Med Food 2001;4: 171-8.
Also published in Chinese (with English summary) as: Liu Z, Yang Z, Zhu M, Huo J. Estrogenicity of black

cohosh (*Cimicifuga racemosa*) and its effect on estrogen receptor level in human breast cancer MCF-7 cells. Weisheng Yanjiu (Journal of Hygiene Research) 2001; 30:77-80.

47. Jarry H, Leonhardt S, Düls C, Popp M, Christoffel V, Spengler B et al. Organ-specific effects of *Cimicifuga racemosa* in brain and uterus [Poster]. 23rd International LOF-Symposium on "Phyto-Oestrogens". Gent, 15 January 1999.

48. Wuttke W, Jarry H, Becker T, Schultens A, Christoffel V, Gorkow C, Seidlová-Wuttke D. Phytoestrogens: endocrine disrupters or replacement for hormone replacement therapy? Maturitas 2003;44(Suppl 1):S9-S20.

49. Low Dog T, Powell KL, Weisman SM. Critical evaluation of the safety of *Cimicifuga racemosa* in menopause symptom relief. Menopause 2003;10:299-313.

50. Lepik K. Safety of herbal medications in pregnancy. Can Pharm J 1997;(April):29-33.

51. Barnes J, Anderson LA and Phillipson JD. Cohosh, Black. In: Herbal Medicines - A guide for healthcare professionals, 2nd ed. London-Chicago: Pharmaceutical Press, 2002:141-6.

52. Blumenthal M, Goldberg A, Brinckmann J, Foster S. Black cohosh root. In: Herbal Medicine. Expanded Commission E Monographs. Austin, Texas: American Botanical Council; Newton, Massachusetts: Integrative Medicine Communications, 2000:22-6.

53. Földes J. Die Wirkungen eines Extraktes aus *Cimicifuga racemosa*. Ärztl Forsch 1959;13:623-4.

54. Liske E. Therapeutic efficacy and safety of *Cimicifuga racemosa* for gynecologic disorders. Advances in Therapy 1998;15:45-53.

55. Lieberman S. A review of the effectiveness of *Cimicifuga racemosa* (black cohosh) for the symptoms of menopause. J Women's Health 1998;7:525-9.

56. Beuscher N. Cimicifuga. In: Blaschek W, Hänsel R, Keller K, Reichling J, Rimpler H, Schneider G, editors. Hagers Handbuch der Pharmazeutischen Praxis. Folgeband 2: Drogen A-K. Berlin-Heidelberg-New York: Springer-Verlag, 1998:369-81.

57. Cimicifuga (Black Cohosh). In: Schedule 1, Table A, of United Kingdom Statutory Instrument 1984 No. 769. The Medicines (Products Other Than Veterinary Drugs) (General Sale List) Order 1984, as amended by Statutory Instrument 1990 No. 1129.

58. Madaus G. Cimicifuga. In: Lehrbuch der biologischen Heilmittel. Leipzig: G. Thieme Verlag, 1938:983-7.

59. Winterhoff H, Butterweck V, Jarry H, Wuttke W. Pharmakologische und klinische Untersuchungen zum Einsatz von *Cimicifuga racemosa* bei klimakterischen Beschwerden. Wien Med Wschr 2002;152:360-3.

60. Eagon CL, Elm MS, Eagon PK. Estrogenicity of traditional Chinese and Western herbal remedies. Proc Amer Assoc Cancer Res 1996;37:284 (Abstract #1937).

61. Jarry H, Gorkow C, Wuttke W. Treatment of menopausal symptoms with extracts of Cimicifuga racemosa: *in vivo* and *in vitro* evidence for estrogenic activity. In: Loew D, Rietbrock N, editors. Phytopharmaka in Forschung und klinischer Anwendung. Darmstadt: Steinkopff, 1995:99-112.

62. Jarry H, Metten M, Spengler B, Christoffel V, Wuttke W. In vitro effects of the *Cimicifuga racemosa* extract BNO 1055. Maturitas 2003;44(Suppl 1):S31-S38.

63. Löhning A, Verspohl EJ, Winterhoff H. Pharmacological studies on the dopaminergic activity of *Cimicifuga racemosa* [Poster]. 23rd International LOF-Symposium on "Phyto-Oestrogens". Gent, 15 January 1999.

64. Noguchi M, Nagai M, Koeda M, Nakayama S, Sakurai N, Takahira M, Kusano G. Vasoactive effects of cimicifugic acids C and D, and fukinolic acid in Cimicifuga rhizome. Biol Pharm Bull 1998;21:1163-8.

65. Burdette JE, Chen S-N, Lu Z-Z, Xu H, White BEP, Fabricant DS et al. Black cohosh (*Cimicifuga racemosa* L.) protects against menadione-induced DNA damage through scavenging of reactive oxygen species: bioassay-directed isolation and characterization of active principles. J Agric Food Chem 2002;50:7022-8.

66. Jarry H, Harnischfeger G. Untersuchungen zur endokrinen Wirksamkeit von Inhaltsstoffen aus *Cimicifuga racemosa*. 1. Einfluß auf die Serumspiegel von Hypophysenhormonen ovariektomierter Ratten. Planta Med 1985;51:46-9.

67. Einer-Jensen N, Zhao J, Andersen KP, Kristoffersen K. *Cimicifuga* and *Melbrosia* lack oestrogenic effects in mice and rats. Maturitas 1996;25:149-53.

68. Knüvener E, Korte B, Winterhoff H. Cimicifuga and physiological estrogens. Phytomedicine 2000;7(Suppl 2):12 (Abstract SL-11).

69. Wuttke W, Jarry H, Heiden I, Seidlová-Wuttke D. Effects of *Cimicifuga racemosa* on estrogen-dependent tissues [Abstract]. Maturitas 2000;35(Suppl 1):S34.

70. Wuttke W, Jarry H, Heiden I, Westphalen S, Seidlová-Wuttke D, Christoffel V. Selective estrogen receptor modulator (SERM) activity of the *Cimicifuga racemosa* extract BNO 1055: pharmacology and mechanisms of action. Phytomedicine 2000;7(Suppl 2):12 (Abstract SL-10).

71. Eagon CL, Elm MS, Teepe AG, Eagon PK. Estrogenicity of medicinal botanicals in rat liver and other tissues. Hepatology 1997;26:502A (Abstract 1494).

72. Nesselhut T, Liske E. Pharmacological measures in postmenopausal women with an isopropanolic aqueous extract of Cimicifugae racemosae rhizoma. In: Abstracts of 10th Annual Meeting of the North American Menopause Society (NAMS). New York, 23-25 September 1999 (Abstract No. 99.012).

73. Seidlová-Wuttke D, Jarry H, Becker T, Christoffel V, Wuttke W. Pharmacology of *Cimicifuga racemosa* extract BNO 1055 in rats: bone, fat and uterus. Maturitas 2003;44(Suppl 1):S39-S50.

74. Kuiper GGJM, Lemmen JG, Carlsson B, Corton JC, Safe SH, van der Saag PT et al. Interaction of estrogenic chemicals and phytoestrogens with estrogen receptor β. Endocrinology 1998;139:4252-63.

75. Boblitz N, Liske E, Wüstenberg P. Traubensilberkerze - Wirksamkeit, Wirkung und Sicherheit von *Cimicifuga racemosa* in der Gynäkologie. Dtsch Apoth Ztg 2000; 140:2833-8.

76. Winterhoff H, Spengler B, Christoffel V, Butterweck V, Löhning A. *Cimicifuga* extract BNO 1055: reduction of hot flushes and hints of antidepressant activity. Maturitas 2003;44(Suppl 1):S51-S58.

77. Löhning A, Verspohl EJ, Winterhoff H. *Cimicifuga racemosa* extracts reduce the frequency of skin flushing episodes in ovariectomized rats. In: Abstracts of Joint Meeting of the ASP, AFERP, GA and PSE; 2000 Years of Natural Products Research - Past, Present and Future. Amsterdam, 26-30 July 1999 (Abstract 327).

78. Borrelli F, Izzo AA, Ernst E. Pharmacological effects of *Cimicifuga racemosa*. Life Sci 2003;73:1215-29.

79. Düker E-M, Kopanski L, Jarry H, Wuttke W. Effects of extracts from *Cimicifuga racemosa* on gonadotropin release in menopausal women and ovariectomized rats. Planta Med 1991;57:420-4.

80. Jacobson JS, Troxel AB, Evans J, Klaus L, Vahdat L, Kinne D et al. Randomized trial of black cohosh for the treatment of hot flashes among women with a history of breast cancer. J Clin Oncol 2001;19:2739.

81. Georgiev DB, Iordanova E. Phytoestrogens - the alternative approach. Maturitas 1997;27(Suppl 1):213 (Abstract P309).

82. Schotten EW. Erfahrungen mit dem Cimicifuga-Präparat Remifemin. Landarzt 1958;34:353-4.

83. Stefan H. Ein Beitrag zu den Erscheinungsformen und zur Therapie hormonal bedingter Biopathiesyndrome der Frau. Ringelheimer Biol Umschau 1959;14(10):149-52 and 1959;14(11):157-62.

84. Stiehler K. Über die Anwendung eines standardisierten Cimicifuga-Auszuges in der Gynäkologie. Ärztl Praxis 1959;11:916-7.

85. Brücker A. Beitrag zur Phytotherapie hormonaler Störungen der Frau. Med Welt 1960;44:2331-3.

86. Heizer H. Kritisches zur Cimicifuga-Therapie bei hormonalen Störungen der Frau. Med Klin 1960;55:232-3.

87. Görlich N. Behandlung ovarieller Störungen in der Allgemeinpraxis. Ärztl Praxis 1962;14:1742-3.

88. Schildge E. Beitrag zur Behandlung von prämenstruellen und klimakterischen Verstimmungs- und Depressions-Zuständen. Ringelheimer Biol Umschau 1964;19(2):18-22.

89. Starfinger W. Therapie mit östrogen-wirksamen Pflanzenextrakten. Med Heute 1960;9(4):173-4.

90. Langfritz W. Beitrag zur Therapie von Regeltempo-anomalien und deren Begleiterscheinungen bei jungen Mädchen und jungen Frauen. Med Klin 1962;57:1497-9.

91. Kesselkaul O. Über die Behandlung klimakterischer Beschwerden mit Remifemin. Med Monatsschr 1957; 11(2):87-8.

92. Borrelli F, Ernst E. *Cimicifuga racemosa*: a systematic review of its clinical efficacy. Eur J Clin Pharmacol 2002;58:235-41.

93. Genazzani E, Sorrentino L. Vascular action of acteina: active constituent of *Actaea racemosa* L. Nature 1962; 194:544-5.

94. Huntley A, Ernst E. A systematic review of the safety of black cohosh. Menopause 2003;10:58-64.

95. Foster S. Black cohosh: *Cimicifuga racemosa*. A literature review. HerbalGram 1999;(45):35-49.

CINNAMOMI CORTEX

Cinnamon

DEFINITION

Cinnamon consists of the dried bark, freed from the outer cork and the underlying parenchyma, of the shoots grown on cut stock of *Cinnamomum zeylanicum* Nees. It contains not less than 12 ml/kg of essential oil.

The material complies with the monograph of the European Pharmacopoeia [1].

Where used below, the term 'cinnamon bark oil', refers to essential oil obtained from the bark of *Cinnamomum zeylanicum* Nees.

CONSTITUENTS

Cinnamon contains up to 4% of essential oil consisting principally of cinnamaldehyde (60-75%) together with cinnamyl acetate and eugenol (both about 1-5%), β-caryophyllene (1-4%), linalool (1-3%) and 1,8-cineole (1-2%) [2-12].

Other constituents include oligomeric procyanidins [13], mucilage polysaccharides [14,15], cinnamic acid and phenolic acids [16], and the pentacyclic diterpenes cinnzeylanol and its acetyl derivative cinnzeylanine [17].

CLINICAL PARTICULARS

Therapeutic indications
Dyspeptic complaints such as gastrointestinal spasms, bloating and flatulence [2,18-25]; loss of appetite [2,18-25]; diarrhoea [19-21].

Posology and method of administration

Dosage

Adult daily dose: 1.5-4 g of dried bark or as an infusion [2,18-22]; 0.5-1.0 ml of fluid extract (1:1, 70% ethanol) [19,20]; 2-4 ml of tincture [2,19,20].
Elderly: dose as for adults.
Children: for infantile diarrhoea [19], proportion of adult dose according to age and body weight in alcohol-free preparations.

Method of administration
For oral administration.

Duration of administration
No restriction.

E/S/C/O/P
MONOGRAPHS
Second Edition

Contra-indications

Patients with known allergy to cinnamon, cinnamon bark oil or cinnamaldehyde [26-31].

Special warnings and special precautions for use

None required.

Interaction with other medicaments and other forms of interaction

None reported.

Pregnancy and lactation

Only limited data available [19,22]. In accordance with general medical practice, the product should not be used during pregnancy and lactation without medical advice.

Effects on ability to drive and use machines

None known.

Undesirable effects

None reported.

Overdose

Not applicable to cinnamon. Cinnamon bark oil and cinnamaldehyde in doses over 0.2 g/day (equivalent to 15-20 g of crude drug) have irritant properties [2,18,22].

PHARMACOLOGICAL PROPERTIES

Pharmacodynamic properties

In vitro experiments

Flatulence

Anti-foaming activity of cinnamon bark oil has been demonstrated in a foam generator as a model for flatulence, using artificial gastric and intestinal fluids, by breaking foam with a corresponding release of gas [32].

Spasmolytic activity

Papaverine-like spasmolytic effects of cinnamon bark oil (EC_{50} 41 mg/litre) and cinnamaldehyde were observed in tests on guinea pig tracheal and ileal smooth muscle. Smooth muscle contractions in dog ileum, colon and stomach were inhibited by cinnamon bark oil and cinnamaldehyde [22,33,34].

Antifungal properties

Powdered cinnamon, dry extracts of cinnamon (acetone, alcohol, chloroform, ether), cinnamon bark oil (in concentrations ranging from 1% to 0.0025%) and cinnamaldehyde inhibited growth of the following fungi and yeasts including their mycotoxin production: *Aspergillus flavus, A. niger, A. parasiticus* (cinnamon bark oil at 200 ppm and cinnamaldehyde at 150 ppm), *Candida albicans, C. lipolytica, C. parakrusei,*

Debaryomyces hansenii, Fusarinum oxysporum, Hansenula anomala, Kloeckera apiculata, Lodderomyces elongisporus, Penicillium italicum, P. viridicatum, P. cladosporioides, Rhodotolrula rubra, Saccharomyces cerevisiae, Torulopis glabrata. Cinnamon bark oil inhibited the growth of the following dermatophytes: *Epidermophyton floccosum, Microsporum canis, Trichophyton mentagrophytes and T. rubrum* [35-42]. The inhibitory zone induced by cinnamon bark oil in solid media was 28 mm in diameter [35-42], comparable to the 20-25 mm zone induced by ketoconazole at 100 µg/ml [39]. Aflatoxin production of *A. parasiticus* was completely inhibited by a cinnamon extract (10:1) [35].

Antibacterial properties

Cinnamon bark oil in concentrations from 0.1% to 0.0025% [42], the vapour of the oil and supercritical CO_2 extracts of cinnamon inhibited the growth of Gram-positive and Gram-negative bacteria: *Bacillus anthracis, B. brevi, B. mycoides, B. subtilis, B. pumilus, Bordetella bronchiseptica, Escherichia coli, Lactobacillus plantarum, Micrococcus citreus, M. pyogenes var. albus, Mycobacterium avium, Proteus morganii, Pseudomonas aeruginosa, P. mangiferae indicae, Salmonella typhi, Sarcina lutea, Staphylococcus albus, S. aureus, S. epidermidis, Streptococcus faecium, Xanthomonus campestris* [37,41-45]. Minimum inhibitory concentrations varied from 0.050 to 0.250 mg/ml [41]. The inhibitory zone of cinnamon bark oil (0.2 ml/20 ml agar plate) was up to 23 mm in diameter, comparable to the 17 mm zone of streptomycin sulfate (1 mg/ml) for *B. mycoides* [43]. Powdered cinnamon and certain isolated constituents of cinnamon also exhibited antibacterial effects in 24 foodborne bacteria [46].

Anti-inflammatory activity

Cinnamon bark oil inhibited cyclooxygenase activity and prostaglandin formation [47].

Effects on human spermatozoa

Cinnamon bark oil had a spermicidal effect on human spermatozoa *in vitro* with a minimum effective concentration of 1:400 V/V [48].

Cytotoxicity

Petroleum ether (25:1) and chloroform (68:1) extracts of cinnamon exhibited cytotoxic effects with respective ED_{50} values of 60 and 58 µg/ml in human cancer (KB) cells and 24 and 20 µg/ml in mouse leukaemia L1210 cells [49]. Cinnamaldehyde was also cytotoxic to rat hepatocyte suspensions after 2 hours at a threshhold concentration of 10^{-3} M, measured by lactate dehydrogenase leakage. Intracellular glutathione was progressively depleted by cinnamaldehyde in a concentration-dependent manner from 10^{-4} to 10^{-3} M [49-51]. Cinnamaldehyde exhibited cytotoxic effects with ED_{50} values of 4.8 µg/ml in mouse L1210 cell cultures [51].

In vivo experiments
In rats and dogs cinnamon bark oil inhibited stomach motility; in mice it inhibited intestinal motility and stress- or serotonin-induced ulcers [22,34]. Cinnamaldehyde administered intravenously to rats at 5 and 10 mg/kg body weight had a stimulating effect on the cardiovascular system and inhibited gastric contraction. When administered intravenously to dogs at 5 and10 mg/kg body weight cinnamaldehyde had a dose-dependent hypotensive effect [34].

Anti-inflammatory activity
In the cotton pellet granuloma test, dry ethanolic extracts of cinnamon administered orally to rats at 400 mg/kg body weight showed anti-inflammatory activity [52].

Antinociceptive activity
Dry ethanolic extracts of cinnamon administered orally to mice at 200 and 400 mg/kg body weight exhibited analgesic effects in the hot-plate and acetic acid-induced writhing tests [52].

Clinical studies
In a randomized, placebo-controlled study, 23 patients with *Helicobacter pylori* infections were assigned to treatment daily for 4 weeks with 2 × 40 mg of a 95% ethanolic extract of cinnamon (n = 15) or placebo (ethanol 95%, n = 8). The amount of *H. pylori* colonization was measured by the ^{13}C urea breath test (UBT) before and after therapy. Over the treatment period mean UBT counts increased from 22.1 to 24.4 in the cinnamon group and from 23.9 to 25.9 in the placebo group. From these results it was concluded that at the dosage used the treatment was ineffective in eradicating *H. pylori* [53].

Pharmacokinetic properties
A benzene-methanol (9:1) extract of cinnamon (80 µl of 180 mg/ml extract) induced "substrate binding" spectral interactions *in vitro* with rat hepatic microsomal cytochrome P-450 [54].

Preclinical safety data

Acute toxicity
The oral LD_{50} of cinnamon bark oil in rats has been determined as 4.16 g/kg [55] and 3.4 ml/kg [27] body weight. The dermal LD_{50} of cinnamon bark oil in rabbits has been reported as 0.69 ml/kg. Undiluted oil was severely irritating to the intact skin of rabbits and mildly irritating when applied to the backs of hairless mice; however, when tested at 8% in petrolatum it produced no irritation in 25 human subjects [27].

Subacute and chronic toxicity
Cinnamaldehyde added to the diet of rats for 16 weeks at 1% resulted in slight swelling of hepatic cells and slight hyperkeratosis of the squamous portion of the stomach; the no-effect level was 0.25% [22,56].

Mutagenicity, genotoxicity and carcinogenicity
Although cinnamon extracts, cinnamon bark oil and cinnamaldehyde showed no mutagenic potential in several studies using the Ames test [57-59], more recent studies, also using the Ames test, have revealed mutagenic activity of these substances [60-62].

Cinnamon bark oil was mutagenic in the *Bacillus subtilis* DNA repair test (rec assay) [63-65]. Cinnamon bark oil and cinnamaldehyde gave positive results in chromosomal aberration tests using Chinese hamster cell cultures as substrate [60,66].

Cinnamaldehyde showed genotoxic effects in *Drosophila* test systems [67,68]. An aqueous extract of cinnamon gave a negative result in a similar *Drosophila* test system [69].

The available data on mutagenicity of cinnamon are rather contradictory. In part the discrepancies have been explained by the fact that cinnamon bark oil and cinnamaldehyde exhibit antimicrobial as well as cytotoxic effects, which could account for observed "antimutagenic" effects when concentrations of the oil are in the range which could cause growth retardation of *Salmonella* strains or borderline toxicity in cell cultures [49-51,70-75]. This explanation is supported by the fact that cinnamon extracts and cinnamaldehyde were cytotoxic in KB human carcinoma and L1210 mouse leukaemia cell lines. ED_{50} levels were 50-60 µg/ml and 20-24 µg/ml for petroleum ether and chloroform extracts respectively [49] and 4.8 µg/ml for cinnamaldehyde [50] in these cell lines.

Overall, the data on mutagenicity and genotoxicity are considered insufficient to fully evaluate the carcinogenic risk of cinnamon [21,22].

Teratogenicity
Cinnamaldehyde was reported to exhibit teratogenic effects in chick embryos [76]. The teratogenic dose was closely related to the toxic dose of cinnamaldehyde (0.5 mmol/embryo) with 58.2% malformations and 49% lethality. However, a methanol extract of cinnamon given by gastric intubation was not teratogenic in rats [77]. These data are considered to be of limited value in risk assessment for humans [21,22].

REFERENCES

1. Cinnamon - Cinnamomi cortex. European Pharmacopoeia, Council of Europe.

2. Hänsel R, Keller K, Rimpler H, Schneider G, editors. Cinnamomum. In: Hagers Handbuch der Pharma-

zeutischen Praxis, 5th ed. Volume 4: Drogen A-D. Berlin-Heidelberg-New York-London: Springer-Verlag, 1993:884-911.

3. Wichtl M, Schäfer-Korting M. Zimtrinde. In: Hartke K, Hartke H, Mutschler E, Rücker G, Wichtl M, editors. Kommentar zum Europäischen Arzneibuch. Stuttgart: Wissenschaftliche Verlagsgesellschaft, 1999(11.Lfg.): Z 1.

4. Evans WC. Cinnamon and cinnamon oil. In: Trease and Evans' Pharmacognosy, 14th ed. London-Philadelphia-Toronto: WB Saunders, 1996:275-8.

5. Wijesekera ROB. The chemistry and technology of cinnamon. Crit Rev Food Sci Nutr 1978;10:1-30.

6. Wijesekera ROB, Jayewardene AL, Rajapakse LS. Volatile constituents of leaf, stem and root oils of cinnamon (Cinnamomum zeylanicum). J Sci Food Agric 1974;25:1211-20.

7. Ross MSF. Analysis of cinnamon oils by high-pressure liquid chromatography. J Chromatogr 1976;118:273-5.

8. Senanayake UM, Lee TH, Wills RBH. Volatile constituents of cinnamon (Cinnamomum zeylanicum) oils. J Agric Food Chem 1978;26:822-4.

9. Formácek V, Kubeczka K-H. Cinnamon oil. In: Essential oils analysis by capillary gas chromatography and carbon-13 NMR spectroscopy. Chichester-New York: John Wiley, 1982:43-9.

10. Lawrence BM. Progress in essential oils. Perfumer & Flavorist 1998;23:39-50.

11. Tateo F, Chizzini F. The composition and quality of supercritical CO_2 extracted cinnamon. J Ess Oil Res 1989;1:165-8.

12. De Medici D, Pieretti S, Salvatore G, Nicoletti M, Rasoanaivo P. Chemical analysis of essential oils of Malagasy medicinal plants by gas chromatography and NMR spectroscopy. Flavour Fragrance J 1992;7:275-81.

13. Nonaka G, Morimoto S, Nishioka I. Tannins and related compounds. Part 13. Isolation and structures of trimeric, tetrameric and pentameric proanthocyanidins from cinnamon. J Chem Soc Perkin Trans I 1983:2139-45.

14. Gowda DC, Sarathy C. Structure of an L-arabino-D-xylan from the bark of Cinnamomum zeylanicum. Carbohydrate Res 1987;166:263-9.

15. Sarathy C, Gowda DC. Structural features of a D-glucan from the stem bark of Cinnamomum zeylanicum. Indian J Chem 1988;27B:694-5.

16. Schulz JM, Herrmann K. Über das Vorkommen von Hydroxibenzoesäuren und Hydroxizimtsäuren in Gewürzen. IV. Über Gewürzphenole. Z Lebensm Unters Forsch 1980;171:193-9.

17. Isogai A, Suzuki A, Tamura S, Murakoshi S, Ohashi Y, Sasada Y. Structures of cinnzeylanine and cinnzeylanol,

polyhydroxylated pentacyclic diterpenes from Cinnamomum zeylanicum Nees. Agric Biol Chem 1976;40:2305-6.

18. Czygan F-C. Zimtrinde. In: Bisset NG, editor (translated from Wichtl M, editor. Teedrogen, 2nd. ed.). Herbal Drugs and Phytopharmaceuticals. A handbook for practice on a scientific basis. Stuttgart: Medpharm, Boca Raton: CRC Press, 1994:148-50.

19. Barnes J, Anderson LA and Phillipson JD. Cinnamon. In: Herbal Medicines - A guide for healthcare professionals, 2nd ed. London-Chicago: Pharmaceutical Press, 2002:135-6.

20. Cinnamomum. In: British Herbal Pharmacopoeia 1983. Bournemouth: British Herbal Medicine Association, 1983:68.

21. Cortex Cinnamomi. In: WHO Monographs on Selected Medicinal Plants, Volume 1. Geneva: World Health Organization, 1999:95-104.

22. Keller K. Cinnamomum Species. In: De Smet PAGM, Keller K, Hänsel R, Chandler RF, editors. Adverse Effects of Herbal Drugs, Volume 1. Berlin-Heidelberg-New York: Springer-Verlag 1992:105-14.

23. Leung AY, Foster S, editors. Cinnamon (and Cassia). In: Encyclopedia of common natural ingredients used in food, drugs and cosmetics, 2nd ed. New York-Chichester: John Wiley, 1996:167-70.

24. Reynolds JEF, editor. Cinnamon. In: Martindale - The Extra Pharmacopoeia, 31st ed. London: Royal Pharmaceutical Society, 1996.

25. Schneider E. Cinnamomum verum - Der Zimt. Z Phytotherapie 1988;9:193-6.

26. Hausen BM, Nothdurft H. Cinnamomum zeylanicum Blume. In: Allergiepflanzen-Pflanzenallergene. Teil 1. Kontaktallergene. Landsberg/München: Ecomed Verlagsgesellschaft, 1988:95-7.

27. Opdyke DLJ. Monographs on fragrance raw materials: cinnamon bark oil, Ceylon. Food Cosmet Toxicol 1975;13 (Suppl):111.

28. Calnan CD. Cinnamon dermatitis from an ointment. Contact Dermatitis 1976;2:167-70.

29. Nater JP, De Jong MCJM, Baar AJM, Bleumink E. Contact urticarial skin responses to cinnamaldehyde. Contact Dermatitis 1977;3:151-4.

30. Mathias CGT, Chappler RR, Maibach HI. Contact urticaria from cinnamic aldehyde. Arch Dermatol 1980;116:74-6.

31. Nixon R. Cinnamon allergy in a baker. Australasian J Dermatol 1995;36:41.

32. Harries N, James KC, Pugh WK. Antifoaming and carminative actions of volatile oils. J. Clin. Pharmacy 1978;2:171-7.

33. Reiter M, Brandt W. Relaxant effects on tracheal and

ileal smooth muscles of the guinea pig. Arzneim-Forsch/Drug Res 1985;35:408-14.

34. Harada M, Yano S. Pharmacological studies on Chinese Cinnamon. II. Effects of cinnamaldehyde on the cardiovascular and digestive systems. Chem Pharm Bull 1975;23:941-7.

35. Sharma A, Ghanekar AS, Padwal-Desai SR, Nadkarni GB. Microbiological status and antifungal properties of irradiated spices. J Agric Food Chem 1984;32:1061-3.

36. Conner DE, Beuchat LR. Effects of essential oils from plants on growth of food spoilage yeasts. J Food Sci 1984;49:429-34.

37. Janssen AM, Chin NLJ, Scheffer JJC, Baerheim Svendsen A. Screening for antimicrobial activity of some essential oils by the agar overlay technique. Statistics and correlations. Pharm Weekbl Sci Ed 1986;8:289-92.

38. Saito M, Kawasumi T, Kusumoto K-i. Antifungal effects of herbs, spices, vegetables, fruit and volatile compounds. Rep Natl Food Res Inst 1991;55:15-8.

39. Lima EO, Gompertz OF, Giesbrecht AM, Paulo MQ. In-vitro antifungal activity of essential oils obtained from officinal plants against dermatophytes. Mycoses 1993;36:333-6.

40. Bullerman LB. Inhibition of aflatoxin production by cinnamon. J Food Sci 1974;39:1163-5.

41. Raharivelomanana PJ, Terrom GP, Bianchini JP, Coulanges P. Contribution à l'étude de l'action antimicrobienne de quelques huiles essentielles extraites de plantes Malgaches. II. Les Lauracées. Arch Inst Pasteur Madagascar 1989;56:261-71.

42. Ehrich J, Bauermann U, Thomann R. Antimikrobielle Wirkung von CO_2-Gewürzextrakten von Bohnenkraut bis Ceylon-Zimt. Lebensmitteltechnik 1995;(11):51-3.

43. Chaurasia SC, Jain PC. Antibacterial activity of essential oils of four medicinal plants. Indian J Hosp Pharm 1978;15:166-8.

44. Maruzzella JC, Henry PA. The in vitro antibacterial activity of essential oils and oil combinations. J Am Pharm Assoc 1958;47:294-6.

45. Maruzzella JC, Sicurella NA. Antibacterial activity of essential oil vapors. J Am Pharm Assoc 1960;49:692-4.

46. Billing J, Sherman PW. Antimicrobial functions of spices: why some like it hot. Quart Rev Biol 1998; 73:3-49.

47. Wagner H, Wierer M, Bauer R. In vitro-Hemmung der Prostaglandin-Biosynthese durch etherische Öle und phenolische Verbindungen. Planta Med 1986;52:184-7.

48. Buch JG, Dikshit RK, Mansuri SM. Effect of certain volatile oils on ejaculated human spermatozoa. Indian J Med Res 1988;87:361-3.

49. Chulasiri MU, Picha P, Rienkijkan M, Preechanukool

K. Cytotoxic effect of petroleum ether and chlorofrom extracts from Ceylon cinnamon (Cinnamomum zeylanicum Nees) barks on tumor cells in vitro. Int J Crude Drug Res 1984;22:177-80.

50. Moon KH, Pack MY. Cytotoxicity of cinnamic aldehyde on leukemia L1210 cells. Drug Chem Toxicol 1983; 6:521-35.

51. Swales NJ, Caldwell J. Studies on trans-cinnamaldehyde II: mechanisms of cytotoxicity in rat isolated hepatocytes. Toxicol in Vitro 1996;10:37-42.

52. Atta AH, Alkofahi A. Anti-nociceptive and anti-inflammatory effects of some Jordanian medicinal plant extracts. J Ethnopharmacol 1998;60:117-24.

53. Nir Y, Potasman I, Stermer E, Tabak M and Neeman I. Controlled trial of the effect of cinnamon extract on Helicobacter pylori. Helicobacter 2000;5:94-7.

54. Wickramasinghe RH, Müller G, Norpoth K. Spectral evidence of interaction of spice constituents with hepatic microsomal cytochrome P-450. Cytobios 1980;29:25-7.

55. von Skramlik E. Über die Giftigkeit und Verträglichkeit von ätherischen Ölen. Pharmazie 1959;14:435-45.

56. Hagan EC, Hansen WH, Fitzhugh OG, Jenner PM, Jones WI, Taylor JM et al. Food flavourings and compounds of related structure. II. Subacute and chronic toxicity. Food Cosmet Toxicol 1967;5:141-57.

57. Sekizawa J, Shibamoto T. Genotoxicity of safrole-related chemicals in microbial test systems. Mutat Res. 1982;101:127-40.

58. Lijinsky W, Andrews AW. Mutagenicity of vinyl compounds in Salmonella typhimurium. Teratog Carcinog Mutagen 1980;1:259-67.

59. Prival MJ, Sheldon AT, Popkin D. Evaluation, using Salmonella typhimurium, of the mutagenicity of seven chemicals found in cosmetics. Food Chem Toxicol 1982;20:427-32.

60. Ishidate M, Sofuni T, Yoshikawa K, Hayashi M, Nohmi T, Sawada M, Matsuoka A. Primary mutagenicity screening of food additives currently used in Japan. Food Chem Toxicol 1984;22:623-36.

61. Mahmoud I, Alkofahi A, Abdelaziz A. Mutagenic and toxic activities of several spices and some Jordanian medicinal plants. Int J Pharmacognosy 1992;30:81-5.

62. Sivaswamy SN, Balachandran B, Balanehru S, Sivaramakrishnan VM. Mutagenic activity of South Indian food items. Indian J Exp Biol 1991;29:730-7.

63. Ungsurungsie M, Paovalo C, Noonai A. Mutagenicity of extracts from Ceylon cinnamon in the rec assay. Food Chem Toxicol 1984;22:109-12.

64. Paovalo C, Chulasiri MU. Bacterial mutagenicity of fractions from chloroform extracts of Ceylon cinnamon. J Food Protect 1986;49:12-3.

65. Ungsurungsie M, Suthienkul O, Paovalo C. Mutagenicity

screening of popular Thai spices. Food Chem Toxicol 1982;20:527-30.

66. Kasamaki A, Takahashi H, Tsumura N, Niwa J, Fujita T, Urasawa S. Genotoxicity of flavouring agents. Mutat Res 1982;105:387-92.

67. Venkatasetty R. Genetic variation induced by radiation and chemical agents in *Drosophila melanogaster*. Diss Abstr Int B 1972;32:5047-8.

68. Woodruff RC, Mason JM, Valencia R, Zimmering S. Chemical mutagenesis testing in *Drosophila*. V. Results of 53 coded compounds tested for the National Toxicology Program. Environ Mutagenesis 1985;7:677-702.

69. Abraham SK, Kesavan PC. A preliminary analysis of the genotoxicity of a few spices in *Drosophila*. Mutat Res 1985;143:219-23.

70. Rutten B, Gocke E. The "antimutagenic" effect of cinnamaldehyde is due to a transient growth inhibition. Mutat Res 1988;201:97-105.

71. Hayashi M, Sofuni T, Ishidate M Jr. A pilot experiment for the micronucleus test. The multi-sampling at multi-dose levels method. Mutat Res 1984;141:165-9.

72. Marnett LJ, Hurd HK, Hollstein MC, Levin DE, Estebauer H. Naturally occurring carbonyl compounds are mutagens in Salmonella tester strain TA104. Mutat Res 1985;148:25-34.

73. Mortelmans K, Haworth S, Lawlor T, Speck W, Tainer B. Salmonella mutagenicity tests II. Results from the testing of 270 chemicals. Environ Mutagenesis 1986;8 (Suppl):1.

74. Ohta T, Watanabe K, Moriya M, Shirasu Y, Kada T. Antimutagenic effects of cinnamaldehyde on chemical mutagenesis in *Escherichia coli*. Mutat Res 1983;107: 219-27.

75. De Silva HV, Shankel DM. Effects of the antimutagen cinnamaldehyde on reversion and survival of selected Salmonella tester strains. Mutat Res 1987;187:11-9.

76. Abramovici A, Rachmuth-Roizman P. Molecular structure-teratogenicity relationships of some fragrance additives. Toxicology 1983;29:143-56.

77. Lee E-B. Teratogenicity of the extracts of crude drugs. Korean J Pharmacog 1982;13:116-21.

CRATAEGI FOLIUM CUM FLORE

Hawthorn Leaf and Flower

E/S/C/O/P
MONOGRAPHS
Second Edition

DEFINITION

Hawthorn leaf and flower consists of the whole or cut, dried flower bearing branches of *Crataegus monogyna* Jacq. emend. Lindm., *C. laevigata* (Poiret) D.C. (*C. oxyacanthoides* Thuill.) or their hybrids or, more rarely, other European *Crataegus* species including *C. pentagyna* Waldst. et Kit. ex Willd., *C. nigra* Waldst. et Kit. and *C. azarolus* L. It contains not less than 1.5 per cent of flavonoids, expressed as hyperoside ($C_{21}H_{20}O_{12}$; M_r 464.4) and calculated with reference to the dried drug.

The material complies with the monograph of the European Pharmacopoeia [1].

CONSTITUENTS

The major constituents are:

Flavonoids (up to 2%) such as vitexin-2″-rhamnoside, acetylvitexin-2″-rhamnoside, hyperoside, vitexin and rutin [2-7].

Procyanidins based on the condensation of catechin and/or epicatechin with varying degrees of polymerisation [2,4,5,8]. The most important are oligomeric procyanidins [2,4-6,9] containing from 2 to 8 monomeric units [2,4]. The content of oligomeric procyanidins is approx. 3% [4,5,10].

Other constituents include triterpenes such as ursolic acid, oleanolic acid and crataegolic acid; phenolic acids such as chlorogenic acid and caffeic acid; amines such as choline; xanthines; and minerals (mainly potassium salts) [4,8].

CLINICAL PARTICULARS

Therapeutic indications

Preparations based on hydroalcoholic extracts
Declining cardiac performance corresponding to Functional Capacity Class II [11] as defined by the New York Heart Association (NYHA)[12-21].

Herbal teas and other preparations different from the above
Nervous heart complaints. Support of cardiac and circulatory functions [22-24].

Classification of Functional Capacity by the New York Heart Association [11]

Class I. Patients with cardiac disease but without resulting limitation of physical activity. Ordinary physical activity does not cause undue fatigue, palpitation, dyspnea, or anginal pain.

Class II. Patients with cardiac disease resulting in slight limitation of physical activity. They are comfortable at rest. Ordinary physical activity results in fatigue, palpitation, dyspnea, or anginal pain.

Class III. Patients with cardiac disease resulting in marked limitation of physical activity. They are comfortable at rest. Less than ordinary activity causes fatigue, palpitation, dyspnea, or anginal pain.

Class IV. Patients with cardiac disease resulting in inability to carry on any physical activity without discomfort. Symptoms of heart failure or the anginal syndrome may be present even at rest. If any physical activity is undertaken, discomfort is increased.

Posology and method of administration

Dosage

Preparations based on hydroalcoholic extracts
Hydroalcoholic extracts (drug to extract ratio 4-7:1) with defined content of oligomeric procyanidins or flavonoids, 160-900 mg daily [12-21].

Herbal teas and other preparations
1-1.5 g of comminuted drug as an infusion, 3-4 times daily [22,23].
Powdered drug, 2-5 g daily; tincture (Codex Fr. IX), 20 drops 2-3 times daily; fluid extract (Codex Fr. IX), 0.5-2.0 g daily, 60-120 drops 3 times daily; dry extract (Belg Farm V), 50-300 mg 3 times daily; glycerol macerate, 50 drops 3 times daily [23].

Method of administration
For oral administration.

Duration of administration
No restriction.

Contra-indications
None known.

Special warnings and special precautions for use
A physician must be consulted in cases where symptoms continue unchanged for longer than 6 weeks, or when fluid accumulates in the legs. Medical intervention is absolutely necessary when pains occur in the region of the heart, spreading out to the arms, upper abdomen or the area around the neck, or in cases of respiratory distress (dyspnoea).

Interaction with other medicaments and other forms of interaction
None reported.

Pregnancy and lactation
No *human* data available. In accordance with general medical practice, the product should not be used during pregnancy or lactation without medical advice.

Effects on ability to drive and use machines
None known.

Undesirable effects
None reported.

Overdose
No toxic effects reported.

PHARMACOLOGICAL PROPERTIES

Pharmacodynamic properties
A review of the pharmacology of *Crataegus* [2], including extracts from leaves, flowers and fruits, confirmed that both *in vitro* and *in vivo* an increase in myocardial contractility (positive inotropic effect) has been observed with *Crataegus* extracts, flavonoids and procyanidins. This effect is probably for the main part due to procyanidins. In several *in vitro* and *in vivo* models an increase in coronary blood flow has been demonstrated after administration of *Crataegus* extracts, flavonoids and procyanidins. This effect is also demonstrable after oral administration. Oligomeric procyanidins seem to have the most marked effect. Some types of *Crataegus* extracts, flavonoids and procyanidins exert various effects on heart frequency in *in vitro* and *in vivo* models. An antiarrhythmic effect has also been observed in the animal model. Aqueous and alcoholic *Crataegus* extracts have a small hypotensive effect after intravenous or oral administration. More recent experiments make it evident that procyanidins are considerably involved.

Increase in cardiac contractility (positive inotropic action)

In vitro experiments
Using Langendorff heart preparations, isolated papillary muscles or isolated myocardial cells, a positive inotropic effect has been demonstrated with extracts [9,25-30], macerates [27], flavonoid fractions [9], procyanidin fractions [9,27] and single constituents: vitexin-2″-rhamnoside [27], vitexin [31], monoacetyl-vitexin-rhamnoside [31,32], luteolin-7-glucoside [32], epicatechin [27], crataegolic acid [27], hyperoside [27,32], rutin [31,32] and biogenetic

amines [27,33]. In the Langendorff heart perfused at constant pressure, 3 µg/ml of an extract standardized on flavonoid content increased contractility by 9.5% [28]. In the Langendorff heart perfused at constant volume, 50-500 µg/ml of a non-standardized extract increased contractility in a dose-dependent manner by 38.3-142.4%. A flavonoid fraction (50-500 µg/ml) produced a dose-dependent increase in contractility of 73.4-259.2% and an oligomeric procyanidin fraction (500 ng/ml to 50 µg/ml) produced a dose-dependent increase in contractility of 35.8-231.7% [9]. Within the range of 30-129 µg/ml, an extract standardized on flavonoid content increased the contraction of isolated myocardial cells, the contraction amplitude reaching a plateau from 120 µg/ml onwards and amounting to 153% of the control value [26].

In isolated, electrically-stimulated muscle strips of left ventricular myocardium from transplant patients with heart failure of NYHA class IV, an extract standardized on oligomeric procyanidin content increased the force of contraction at concentrations higher than 10 µg/ml, improved the force-frequency relationship at 100 µg/ml and exerted competitive inhibition of specific binding of ^{3}H-ouabain to the Na$^+$-K$^+$-ATPase (EC$_{50}$: 95 µg/ml) [25,30]. In isolated electrically-stimulated atrial myocytes from patients who had undergone an aorto-coronary bypass operation and left ventricular myocytes from patients with terminal heart failure, an extract standardized on oligomeric procyanidin content increased the force of contraction at a concentration of 0.1 ng/ml from 4.4% to 10.2% (atrial myocytes; $p<0.05$ from 0.001 ng/ml) and 3.7% to 7.7% (ventricular myocytes; $p<0.05$ from 0.01 ng/ml) [29].

In vivo experiments
In the anaesthetized dog, an extract standardized on oligomeric procyanidin content (7.5-30.0 mg/kg, administered intravenously) increased the maximum left ventricular contraction velocity (dp/dt max.) by 16.8-31.1% [34].

Increase in coronary blood flow and myocardial circulation

In vitro experiments
In Langendorff heart models, coronary blood flow was increased by extracts [9,28,35], macerates [27], flavonoid fractions [9], procyanidin fractions [9,27] and single constituents: hyperoside [31,32,36], vitexin [31,32], monoacetyl-vitexin-rhamnoside [31,32], vitexin-2"-rhamnoside [27,31,32], rutin [32,36,37], luteolin-7-glucoside [32,36,37], crataegolic acid [27], ursolic acid [27] and biogenetic amines [27]. In the Langendorff heart perfused at constant pressure: 3 µg/ml of an extract standardized on flavonoid content produced an increase in coronary perfusion of 64.3% [28]; an extract standardized on oligomeric procyanidin content (1-10 µg/ml) caused a dose-

dependent increase in coronary flow up to about 2-fold, with peak flow rates after about 2 minutes and flow rates remaining enhanced for more than 60 minutes [35]; a non-standardized extract (100 µg/ml) produced an increase in coronary perfusion of 32.1% [9]. A flavonoid fraction (100 µg/ml) increased coronary flow by 63.5% and a fraction of oligomeric procyanidins (10 µg/ml) increased the same parameter by 59.0% [9].

In vivo experiments
In the anaesthetized dog, an extract standardized on oligomeric procyanidin content (7.5-30 mg/kg administered intravenously) produced a dose-dependent increase in coronary blood flow of 46.7-89.4% [34]. In the non-anaesthetized dog, a dose-dependent increase in local myocardial perfusion in the left ventricle of up to 70% of the perfusion at rest was observed over a period of several hours when an oligomeric procyanidin fraction (35-70 mg/kg, three times daily) was administered orally [38].

Negative bathmotropic action

In vitro experiments
In the Langendorff heart, macerates, especially a glycerol/ethanol macerate, exerted protective effects on arrhythmia induced by aconitine, calcium chloride or chloroform/adrenaline and by ischaemic reperfusion [39]. 0.5 µg/ml of an extract standardized on flavonoid content extended the effective refractory time of the ventricular myocardium by 3.8%, which increased in a dose-dependent manner to 9.9% at 10 µg/ml; the extract showed a clear difference from other substances with a positive inotropic effect, i.e. adrenaline, amrinone, milrinone and digoxin, which shortened the effective refractory time [28]. In isolated myocardial cells, at concentrations of 90 µg/ml and higher, the extract also extended the refractory time in a dose-dependent manner from 144 msec under controlled conditions to 420 msec and above; at the maximum concentration of 180 µg/ml, the refractory time was either 1000 msec or no longer measurable [26]. In isolated guinea pig ventricular myocytes an extract standardized on flavonoid content blocked both the delayed and the inward rectifier potassium current, by 25% and 15% respectively at a concentration of 0.01 mg/ml [40].

In isolated guinea-pig cardiac papillary muscles, 0.01 mg/ml of an extract standardized on flavonoid content increased action potential duration by about 10 msec at 20% repolarisation and by 12 msec at 50% and 90% repolarisation. Furthermore, the time constant of recovery of the maximum upstroke velocity of the action potential was prolonged from 8.80 to 22.6 msec [41].

In vivo experiments
Following oral administration in the normotensive

rat, macerates and a fluid extract produced a decrease in heart rate; a glycerol/ethanol macerate (12.5 mg/kg of dried drug) reduced the heart rate from 504 strokes/min to 450 strokes/min (2 hours after application). At oral doses of 25 mg/kg, the preparations had a protective effect on arrhythmia induced by aconitine, calcium chloride and chloroform/adrenaline [42]. An extract standardized on oligomeric procyanidin content and an extract standardized on flavonoid content protected rats from ischaemia- and reperfusion-induced ventricular fibrillation and tachycardia [43-45].

Protection from ischaemia-reperfusion induced damage

In vitro experiments
In the isolated, ischaemic and reperfused working heart, a water-soluble extract (0.05% solution) improved mechanical cardiac function during reperfusion, accelerated the recovery of energy metabolism and reduced the lactate level during ischaemia [46]. In the ischaemic and reperfused Langendorff heart, the increase in lactate dehydrogenase levels was significantly lower (1777.3 mU/min vs. control 3795.3 mU/min; p = 0.01) after pre-treatment of rats with extract standardized on flavonoid content [47]. A glycerol/ethanol macerate and crataegolic and ursolic acids had protective effects against reperfusion-dependent tachycardia [39]. Both luteolin-7-glycoside and acetylvitexin rhamnoside (5×10^{-5} M) reduced the ischaemic area [48].

In vivo experiments
An extract standardized on oligomeric procyanidin content (5 mg/kg, administered intravenously 5 minutes prior to occlusion) reduced the occurrence and duration of reperfusion-induced ventricular fibrillations and tachycardia in rats [44]. Oral pretreatment with this extract (100 mg/kg) for 6 days protected rats completely from lethal ventricular fibrillations (0% vs. control 100%) and hypotensive crises, and reduced the incidence (62% vs. control 100%) and duration (20.0 sec vs. control 47.1 sec) of ventricular tachycardia [43]. Oral administration of 20 mg/kg/day of an oligomeric procyanidin-rich fraction of this extract to rats provided similar protection against ischaemia-reperfusion induced damage [49]. Oral pre-treatment of rats for 3 months with an extract standardized on flavonoid content (2% of extract mixed with the standard diet) reduced the average prevalence of malignant arrhythmias (perfusion stop for 20 min, 51% vs. control 89%; perfusion stop for 18 min, 8% vs. control 48%) [45].

Vasorelaxation, decrease of peripheral vascular resistance

In vitro experiments
In the Langendorff heart an extract standardized on oligomeric procyanidin content (1-10 µg/ml) caused a relaxation of coronary vessels that was completely reversed by a nitric oxide (NO) synthase inhibitor, and enhanced the relaxant effect of the NO donor nitroprusside [35]. In isolated aortic strips six hydroalcoholic extracts reduced the contraction induced by norepinephrine with EC_{50} values from 4.16 mg/litre to 9.80 mg/litre. An aqueous extract was less effective with an EC_{50} of 22.39 mg/litre [50].

In vivo experiments
Following single and chronic oral administration of a fluid extract and macerates of hawthorn leaf and flower, arterial blood pressure was reduced in normotensive and deoxycorticosterone acetate (DOCA)-hypertensive rats. In the normotensive rat, a glycerol/ethanol macerate (single dose of 12.5 mg/kg dried vegetable tissue) reduced blood pressure from 144 mm Hg to 125 mm Hg, and in the DOCA-hypertensive rat from 176 mm Hg to 154 mm Hg [42].

After an oral administration period lasting 30 days, an extract standardized on flavonoid content (300 mg/kg/day) produced a decrease in blood pressure from 132 mm Hg to 123 mm Hg [51]. In anaesthetized rats (30 mg/kg, administered intravenously) and dogs (15 mg/kg, administered intravenously), an extract standardized on oligomeric procyanidin content produced a decrease in total peripheral resistance in both species, in addition to a decrease in arterial blood pressure in the dogs [34]. In anaesthetized dogs, hyperoside (1 mg/kg administered intravenously, followed by an infusion of 0.1 mg/kg/min for 30 minutes) initially produced a drop in blood pressure of 72 mm Hg, and subsequently of 25 mm Hg up to the 30th minute, with a parallel decrease in systemic arterial resistance [52]. In anaesthetized cats, oligomeric procyanidins (3 mg/kg, administered intravenously) lowered the blood pressure from 145.2 mm Hg to 118 mm Hg within 90-120 min after administration [53].

Mechanisms of action
Various *in vitro* studies have indicated possible mechanisms of action: inhibition of cAMP-phosphodiesterase activity [31,48,54-57], inhibition of Na^+-K^+-ATP-ase activity [9,25,30], inhibition of thromboxane (TXA_2) synthesis and stimulation of prostacyclin (PGI_2) synthesis [58-60], antioxidative activities [49,61,62] and inhibition of human neutrophil elastase [49].

Clinical studies

Clinical studies performed with a hydroalcoholic extract of hawthorn leaf and flower standardized to contain 18.75% of oligomeric procyanidins
In 20 patients with NYHA class II cardiac insufficiency and left ventricular ejection fraction < 55%, the extract (oral daily dose: 480 mg, for 4 weeks) increased

the ejection fraction from 40.18% to 43.5% at rest and from 41.51% to 46.56% during exercise (investigation method: radionuclide angiocardiography). Blood pressure decreased slightly at rest and during exercise, and exercise tolerance increased from 703.75 watt (W) × minute to 772.11 W × minute [13]. In 7 patients with NYHA class II-III cardiac insufficiency and left ventricular ejection fraction < 55%, the extract (oral daily dose: 240 mg, for 4 weeks) increased the ejection fraction from 29.8% to 40.45% (investigation method: nuclear resonance scanning) [14].

In two placebo-controlled, double-blind studies, 136 patients [15] and 30 patients [16] with NYHA class II cardiac insufficiency received orally either 160 mg of extract per day or placebo for 8 weeks. The main target parameter was the change in pressure-rate product (systolic blood pressure × heart rate/100) difference, comparing the difference between a 50 W loading and the resting value, from beginning to end of treatment. The verum groups showed statistically significant improvements in exercise tolerance, as indicated by decreases in the difference between pressure rate products: verum – 6.2, placebo + 0.1, p = 0.018 [15]; verum – 11.6, placebo – 4.9, p<0.05 [16]. Decreases in subjective complaints (p<0.05) [15] or in complaints score (verum – 16.5, placebo – 4, p<0.05) [16] were also noted.

In a surveillance study 1011 patients with NYHA class II cardiac insufficiency were treated with 900 mg of extract daily for 24 weeks. During and at the end of the treatment period marked improvements in clinical symptoms (better performance in the exercise tolerance test and reductions in fatigue, palpitations and exercise dyspnoea) were observed. Ankle oedema disappeared in 83% and nocturia in 50% of the patients. The ejection fraction was improved by 6.7%, blood pressure was reduced from 142.9/84.5 mm Hg to 137.0/82.3 mm Hg, and maximal exercise tolerance increased from 88.75 W to 102.5 W [21].

The effects of treatment with a hawthorn leaf and flower extract have also been investigated in patients with a more advanced stage of the disease, chronic congestive heart failure of NYHA class III (necessitating basic diuretic therapy), in a randomized, double-blind, placebo-controlled multicentric study. After a 4-week run-in phase on placebo plus diuretics (50 mg of triamterene and 25 mg of hydrochlorothiazide once daily), the patients received 900 mg (n = 70) or 1800 mg (n = 69) of the extract or placebo (n = 70) daily, with continued diuretic therapy in every case. After 16 weeks of treatment with 1600 mg of extract, maximum tolerated workloads during bicycle exercise showed a significant increase in comparison with both placebo (p = 0.013) and 900 mg of extract (p = 0.01). The patients rated both dose levels of the extract as significantly better than placebo in reducing

typical symptoms of heart failure (p = 0.004 for 1800 mg of extract; p = 0.04 for 900 mg of extract). Both physicians and patients rated efficacy as very good more often in the group treated with 1800 mg of extract than in either of the other two groups. The incidence of adverse events in the 1800 mg of extract group (none serious) was lower than in the other groups, particularly with respect to dizziness and vertigo [63].

Clinical studies performed with a hydroalcoholic extract of hawthorn leaf and flower standardized to contain 2.2% of flavonoids
In a placebo-controlled, double-blind study (oral daily dose: 600 mg of extract, for 8 weeks) involving 78 patients with NYHA class II cardiac insufficiency, exercise tolerance in the verum group increased by 28 W compared to 5 W in the placebo group (p<0.001). Compared to placebo the pressure-rate product was significantly lower (p<0.05) and the subjective symptoms score improved significantly (p<0.001) [17].

In another placebo-controlled, double-blind study (oral daily dose: 900 mg of extract, for 8 weeks) involving 72 patients with NYHA class II cardiac insufficiency, it was possible to demonstrate by ergospirometry that oxygen uptake increased under verum treatment but not with placebo (p<0.05). In the verum group the time taken to reach the anaerobic threshold during exercise increased by 30 seconds; in the placebo group by only 2 seconds. Patients in the verum group also showed significant improvement (p<0.01) in terms of their subjective assessment of symptoms [18].

In a double-blind comparative study, 132 patients with NYHA class II cardiac insufficiency were treated orally with 900 mg of extract or 37.5 mg of captopril daily for 8 weeks. During the course of treatment both groups showed a statistically significant increase (p<0.001) in exercise tolerance, from 83 to 97 W in the verum group and from 83 to 99 W in the captopril group. In both groups the pressure-rate product was reduced and the incidence and severity of symptoms decreased by around 50%. No significant difference was observed between the two treatments [19].

In a placebo-controlled, double-blind study, 85 patients with NYHA class II cardiac insufficiency were treated orally with 300 mg of extract daily for 4 weeks. Compared to placebo the treatment gave a non-significant improvement in exercise tolerance and clinical symptoms [64].

In a surveillance study, the efficacy of treatment with 900 mg of extract daily was assessed in 1476 patients with heart failure of NYHA classes I and II. Evaluation was performed after 4 and 8 weeks by observing changes in well-being relating to nine typical symptoms of heart failure and by measuring blood pressure and heart rate during each consultation. At the end of the surveillance period the symptom score had dropped by a mean of 66.6%; NYHA class I patients were almost free of symptoms. In a subgroup of patients with a stimulated sympathoadrenergic system, reductions were observed in systolic and diastolic blood pressure (160 to 150 mm Hg and 89 to 85 mm Hg respectively), heart rate (89 to 79 per minute) and incidence of arrhythmias [20].

Pharmacokinetic properties

[14]C-labelled procyanidins orally administered to mice, as 0.87 mg of a total oligomeric procyanidins (OPC) fraction, 1.08 mg of trimeric procyanidins or 1.03 mg of higher procyanidins per mouse, showed within 1-7 hours an absorption rate of about 20-30% for the total OPC fraction, 40-81% for trimeric procyanidins and 16-42% for higher oligomeric procyanidins. Elimination of absorbed radioactivity by expiration and in the urine respectively after 7 hours was 0.6% and 6.4% for the total OPC fraction, 47.5% and 1.8% for trimeric procyanidins, and 12.9% and 1.8% for higher oligomeric procyanidins. Daily oral administration of 0.12 mg (= 145 nCi) of the total OPC fraction for 7 days produced an accumulation of radioactivity in the organs on average 2-3 times higher than after a single dose; thus, for example, taking the daily dose administered per animal as 100%, the relative concentration of the total OPC fraction in the myocardium was 9% after 15 hours and 28% after 7 days [65].

Preclinical safety data

Acute toxicity
The oral LD_{50} of a hydroethanolic extract of hawthorn leaf and flower standardized to contain 18.75% of oligomeric procyanidins could not be determined; 3000 mg/kg could be given to rats and mice without causing toxic signs or death. An intraperitoneal LD_{50} of 1170 mg/kg was calculated in the mouse and 750 mg/kg in the rat; toxic signs included sedation, piloerection, dyspnoea and tremor [66].

Repeated dose toxicity
No toxic effects were observed in rats and dogs after oral administration of the same extract at 30, 90 and 300 mg/kg/day over a period of 26 weeks. 300 mg/kg/day could be considered a 'no effect' level for the extract in the rat and dog [66].

Reproduction toxicity
Oral doses of the same extract at up to 1.6 g/kg in rats and rabbits revealed no teratogenic effects. In rats, the extract showed no peri- or postnatal toxicity and no effects on the F1 generation or on their fertility [67].

Mutagenicity
The same extract was neither mutagenic nor clastogenic in a standard battery of mutation and cytogenic tests (Ames test, mouse lymphoma test, cytogenetic analysis in cultured human lymphocytes, mouse micronucleus test) [66].

It has been assumed that mutagenic activity in *Salmonella typhimurium* exhibited by a *Crataegus* fluid extract (1:1) is based on the quercetin content and that induction of sister chromatid exchange is based on the presence of flavone-C-glycosides as well as flavone aglycones. However, in comparison with the amount of quercetin ingested in the diet, the content of of quercetin in the drug is so low that a risk to humans may be practically excluded [68-71].

Carcinogenicity
No data are available on carcinogenicity. Data relating to genotoxicity and mutagenicity suggest that there is little carcinogenic risk relevant to humans.

REFERENCES

1. Hawthorn leaf and flower - Crataegi folium cum flore. European Pharmacopoeia, Council of Europe.

2. Ammon HPT, Kaul R. *Crataegus*. Herz-Kreislauf-Wirkungen von Crataegusextrakten, Flavonoiden und Procyanidinen. Teil 1: Historisches und Wirkstoffe. Dtsch Apoth Ztg 1994;134:2433-6. Teil 2: Wirkungen auf das Herz. *ibid* 1994;134:2521-35. Teil 3: Wirkungen auf den Kreislauf. *ibid* 1994;134:2631-6.

3. Lamaison JL, Carnat A. Teneur en principaux flavonoïdes des fleurs et des feuilles de *Crataegus monogyna* Jacq. et de *Crataegus laevigata* (Poiret) DC. (Rosaceae). Pharm Acta Helv 1990;65:315-20.

4. Bauer I. Crataegus. In: Hänsel R, Keller R, Rimpler R, Schneider G, editors. Hagers Handbuch der Pharmazeutischen Praxis, 5th ed. Volume 4: Drogen A-D. Berlin: Springer-Verlag 1992:1040-62.

5. Kartnig Th, Hiermann A, Azzam S. Untersuchungen über die Procyanidin- und Flavonoidgehalte von *Crataegus monogyna*-Drogen. Sci Pharm 1987;55:95-100.

6. Rehwald A, Meier B, Sticher O. Qualitative and quantitative reversed-phase high-performance liquid chromatography of flavonoids in Crataegus leaves and flowers. J Chromatogr A 1994;677:25-33.

7. Wagner H, Tittel G. HPLC als Analysen- und Standardisierungsmethode von herzwirksamen Drogen. In: Rietbrock N, Schnieders B, Schuster J, editors. Wandlungen in der Therapie der Herzinsuffizienz. Braunschweig: Friedr. Vieweg & Sohn, 1983:33-41.

8. Steinegger E, Hänsel R. Proanthocyanidine; Weißdornpräparate. In: Pharmakognosie, 5th ed. Berlin: Springer-Verlag, 1992:404-7,580-4.

9. Leukel-Lenz A. Untersuchungen zur pharmakologischen Wirkung von Crataegusfraktionen und deren analytische Charakterisierung [Dissertation]. University of Marburg, 1988.

10. Hölzl J, Strauch A. Untersuchungen zur Biogenese der oligomeren Procyanidine von Crataegus. Planta Med 1977;32:141-53.

11. AHA Medical/Scientific Statement. 1994 Revisions to classification of functional capacity and objective assessment of patients with diseases of the heart. Circulation 1994;90:644-5.

12. Loew D. Crataegus-Spezialextrakte bei Herzinsuffizienz. Gesicherte pharmakologische und klinische Ergebnisse. Kassenarzt 1994;15:43-52.

13. Eichstädt H, Bäder M, Danne O, Kaiser W, Stein U, Felix R. Crataegus-Extrakt hilft dem Patienten mit NYHA II-Herzinsuffizienz. Untersuchung der myokardialen und hämodynamischen Wirkung eines standardisierten Crataegus-Präparates mit Hilfe computergestützter Radionuklidventrikulographie. Therapiewoche 1989; 39:3288-96.

14. Weikl A, Noh H-S. Der Einfluß von Crataegus bei globaler Herzinsuffizienz. Herz und Gefäße 1992;516-24.

15. Weikl A, Assmus K-D, Neukum-Schmidt A, Schmitz J, Zapfe G, Noh H-S, Siegrist J. Crataegus-Spezialextrakt WS 1442. Objektiver Wirksamkeitsnachweis bei Patienten mit Herzinsuffizienz (NYHA II). Fortschr Med 1996;114:291-6.

16. Leuchtgens H. Crataegus-Spezialextrakt WS 1442 bei Herzinsuffizienz NYHA II. Eine plazebo-kontrollierte randomisierte Doppleblindstudie. Fortschr Med 1993;111:352-4.

17. Schmidt U, Kuhn U, Ploch M, Hübner W-D. Efficacy of the Hawthorn (Crataegus) Preparation LI 132 in 78 patients with chronic congestive heart failure defined as NYHA functional class II. Phytomedicine 1994;1:17-24.

18. Förster A, Förster K, Bühring M, Wolfstädter HD. Crataegus bei mäßig reduzierter linksventrikulärer Auswurffraktion. Ergospirometrische Verlaufsuntersuchung bei 72 Patienten in doppelblindem Vergleich mit Plazebo. Münch Med Wschr 1994; 136(Suppl 1):S21-6.

19. Tauchert M, Ploch M, Hübner W-D. Wirksamkeit des Weißdorn-Extraktes LI 132 im Vergleich mit Captopril. Multizentrische Doppelblindstudie bei 132 Patienten mit Herzinsuffizienz im Stadium II nach NYHA. Münch Med Wschr 1994;136(Suppl 1):S27-33.

20. Schmidt U, Albrecht M, Podzuweit H, Ploch M, Maisenbacher J. Hochdosierte Crataegus-Therapie bei herzinsuffizienten Patienten NYHA-Stadium I und II. Z Phytotherapie 1998;19:22-30.

21. Tauchert M, Gildor A, Lipinski J. Einsatz des hochdosierten Crataegusextraktes WS 1442 in der Therapie der Herzinsuffizienz Stadium NYHA II. Herz 1999;24:465-74.

22. Wichtl M. Crataegi folium cum flore. In: Wichtl M, editor. Teedrogen und Phytopharmaka. 3rd ed. Stuttgart: Wissenschaftliche Verlagsgesellschaft, 1997:168-72.

23. van Hellemont J. In: Fytotherapeutisch compendium. Utrecht: Bohn, Scheltema & Holkema, 1988:179-80.

24. Pfister-Hotz G. Phytotherapie in der Geriatrie. Schweiz Apoth-Ztg 1997;135:118-21.

25. Brixius K, Frank K, Münch G, Müller-Ehmsen J, Schwinger RHG. WS 1442 (Crataegus-Spezialextrakt) wirkt am insuffizienten menschlichen Myokard Kontraktionskraftsteigernd. Herz Kreislauf 1998;30:28-33.

26. Pöpping S, Fischer Y, Kammermeier H. Crataegus-Wirkung auf Kontraktion und O_2-Verbrauch isolierter Herzzellen. Münch Med Wschr 1994;136(Suppl 1):S39-46.

27. Occhiuto F, Circosta C, Costa R, Briguglio F, Tommasini A. Étude comparée de l'activité cardiovasculaire des pousses, des feuilles et des fleurs de Crataegus oxyacantha L. II. Action de préparations extractives et de principes actifs purs isolés sur le coeur isolé de lapin. Plantes Méd Phytothér 1986;20:52-63.

28. Joseph G, Zhao Y, Klaus W. Pharmakologisches Wirkprofil von Crataegus-Extrakt im Vergleich zu Epinephrin, Amrinon, Milrinon und Digoxin am isoliert perfundierten Meerschweinchenherzen. Arzneim-Forsch/Drug Res 1995;45:1261-5.

29. Schmidt-Schweda S, v Burstin J, Möllmann H, Wollner S, Holubarsch C. Der positiv inotrope Effekt des Crataegus Spezialextraktes WS 1442 in isolierten Myozyten aus menschlichem Vorhof- und Ventrikelmyokard wird vorwiegend durch oligomere Procyanidine vermittelt. Z Kardiol 2000;89(Suppl 5):164 (Abstract 797).

30. Schwinger RHG, Pietsch M, Frank K, Brixius K. Crataegus special extract WS 1442 increases force of contraction in human myocardium cAMP-independently. J Cardiovasc Pharmacol 2000;35:700-7.

31. Schuessler M, Fricke U, Hölzl J, Nikolov N. Effects of flavonoids from Crataegus species in Langendorff perfused isolated guinea pig hearts. Planta Med 1992;58(Suppl 1): A 646-7.

32. Schüssler M, Hölzl J, Fricke U. Myocardial effects of flavonoids from Crataegus species. Arzneim-Forsch/Drug Res 1995;45:842-5.

33. Wagner H, Grevel J. Herzwirksame Drogen IV: Kardiotone Amine aus Crataegus oxyacantha. Planta Med 1982;45:98-101.

34. Gabard B, Trunzler G. Zur Pharmakologie von Crataegus. In: Rietbrock N, Schnieders B, Schuster J, editors. Wandlungen in der Therapie der Herzinsuffizienz. Braunschweig: Friedr. Vieweg & Sohn, 1983:43-53.

35. Koch E, Chatterjee SS. Crataegus extract WS-1442 enhances coronary flow in the isolated rat heart by endothelial release of nitric oxide. Naunyn-Schmiedeberg's Arch Pharmacol 2000;361(Suppl):R48 (Abstr 180).

36. Schuessler M, Hölzl J, Nikolov N, Fricke U. Einfluß verschiedener Flavonoide aus Crataegus species auf den Koronarfluss und die Kontraktilität isoliert perfundierter Meerschweinchenherzen. Pharmazie unserer Zeit 1993;22:154-5.

37. Schüssler M, Gronwald B, Hölzl J, Fricke U. Cardiac effects of flavonoids from Crataegus species. Planta Med 1993;59(Suppl.):A 688.

38. Roddewig C, Hensel H. Reaktion der lokalen Myokarddurchblutung von wachen Hunden und narkotisierten Katzen auf orale und parenterale Applikation einer Crataegusfraktion (oligomere Procyanidine). Arzneim-Forsch/Drug Res 1977; 27:1407-10.

39. Costa R, Occhiuto F, Circosta C, Ragusa S, Busa G, Briguglio F, Trovato A. Étude comparée de l'activité cardiovasculaire des jeunes pousses, des feuilles et des fleurs de Crataegus oxyacantha L. III. Action protectrice sur le coeur isolé de rat vis-a-vis des agents arythmogènes et dans les arythmies par reperfusions. Plantes Méd Phytothér 1986;20:115-28.

40. Müller A, Linke W, Klaus W. Crataegus extract blocks potassium currents in guinea pig ventricular cardiac myocytes. Planta Med 1999;65:335-9.

41. Müller A, Linke W, Zhao Y, Klaus W. Crataegus extract prolongs action potential duration in guinea-pig papillary muscle. Phytomedicine 1996;3:257-61.

42. Occhiuto F, Circosta C, Briguglio F, Tommasini A, De Pasquale A. Étude comparée de l'activité cardio-vasculaire des jeunes pousses, des feuilles et des fleurs de Crataegus oxyacantha L. I. Activité électrique et tension artérielle chez le rat. Plantes Méd Phytothér 1986;20:37-51.

43. Krzeminski T, Chatterjee SS. Ischemia and early reperfusion induced arrhythmias: beneficial effects of an extract of Crataegus oxyacantha L. Pharm Pharmacol Lett 1993;3:45-8.

44. Kurcok A. Ischemia- and reperfusion-induced cardiac injury: effects of two flavonoid containing plant extracts possessing radical scavenging properties. Naunyn-Schmiedeberg's Arch Pharmacol 1992; 345(Suppl):R81 (Abstr 322).

45. Al Makdessi S, Sweidan H, Dietz K, Jacob R. Protective effect of Crataegus oxyacantha against reperfusion arrhythmias after global no-flow ischemia in the rat heart. Basic Res Cardiol 1999;94:71-7.

46. Nasa Y, Hashizume H, Ehsanul Hoque AN, Abiko Y. Protective effect of Crataegus extract on the cardiac mechanical dysfunction in isolated perfused working rat heart. Arzneim-Forsch/Drug Res 1993;43:945-9.

47. Al Makdessi S, Sweidan H, Müllner S, Jacob R.

Myocardial protection by pretreatment with Crataegus oxyacantha. An assessment by means of the release of lactate dehydrogenase by the ischemic and reperfused Langendorff heart. Arzneim-Forsch/Drug Res 1996; 46:25-7.

48. Schüssler M, Acar D, Cordes A, Hölzl J, Rump AFE, Fricke U. Antiischämische Wirkung von Flavonoiden aus Crataegus. Arch Pharm 1993;326:708 (P 77).

49. Chatterjee SS, Koch E, Jaggy H, Krzeminski T. In-vitro- und In-vivo-Untersuchungen zur kardioprotektiven Wirkung von oligomeren Procyanidinen in einem Crataegus-Extrakt aus Blättern mit Blüten. Arzneim Forsch/Drug Res 1997;47:821-5.

50. Vierling W, Brand N, Gaedcke F, Sensch KH, Schneider E, Scholz M. Crataegus-Extrakte - Untersuchungen zur pharmazeutischen und pharmakologischen Äquivalenz. Dtsch Apoth Ztg. 2000;140:5301-6.

51. Fehri B, Aiache JM, Boukef K, Memmi A, Hizaoui B. Valeriana officinalis et Crataegus oxyacantha: Toxicité par administrations réitérées et investigations pharmacologiques. J Pharm Belg 1991;46:165-76.

52. Lièvre M, Andrieu J-L, Baconin A. Etude des effets cardiovasculaires de l'hypéroside extrait de l'aubépine chez le chien anesthésié. Ann Pharm Fr 1985;43:471-7.

53. Rewerski W, Piechocki T, Rylski M, Lewak S. Einige pharmakologische Eigenschaften der aus Weißdorn (Crataegus oxyacantha) isolierten oligomeren Procyanidine. Arzneim-Forsch/Drug Res 1971;21:886-8.

54. Beretz A. Etude de quelques propriétés pharma-cologiques du Crataegus sp. (Rosacées). Effets de polyphenols sur l'AMP 3',5'-cyclique phospho-diesterase [Dissertation]. Université Louis Pasteur de Strasbourg, 1979:49-54.

55. Schüssler M, Fricke U, Nikolov N, Hölzl J. Comparison of the flavonoids occurring in Crataegus species and inhibition of 3',5'-cyclic adenosine monophosphate phosphodiesterase. Planta Med 1991;57(Suppl. 2): A133.

56. Petkov E, Nikolov N, Uzunov P. Inhibitory effect of some flavonoids and flavonoid mixtures on cyclic AMP phosphodiesterase activity of rat heart. Planta Med 1981;43:183-6.

57. Kukovetz WR. Erkenntnisstand von Crataegus (Diskussionsbeitrag). Pharm Ztg 1976;121:1432.

58. Vibes J, Lasserre B, Declume C. Effects of a total extract from Crataegus oxyacantha blossoms on TXA_2 and PGI_2 biosynthesis in vitro and on TXA_2- and PGI_2-synthesising activities of cardiac tissue. Med Sci Res 1991;19:143-5.

59. Vibes J, Lasserre B, Gleye J. Effects of a methanolic extract from Crataegus oxyacantha blossoms on TXA_2 and PGI_2 synthesising activities of cardiac tissue. Med Sci Res 1993;21:435-6.

60. Vibes J, Lasserre B, Gleye J, Declume C. Inhibition of

thromboxane A$_2$ biosynthesis in vitro by the main components of *Crataegus oxyacantha* (Hawthorn) flower heads. Prostagland Leukotr Essent Fatty Acids 1994;50:173-5.

61. Bahorun T, Trotin F, Pommery J, Vasseur J, Pinkas M. Antioxidant activities of *Crataegus monogyna* extracts. Planta Med 1994;60:323-8.

62. Bahorun T, Gressier B, Trotin F, Brunet C, Dine T, Luyckx M et al. Oxygen species scavenging activity of phenolic extracts from hawthorn fresh plant organs and pharmaceutical preparations. Arzneim-Forsch/Drug Res 1996;46:1086-9.

63. Tauchert M. Efficacy and safety of crataegus extract WS 1442 in comparison with placebo in patients with chronic stable New York Heart Association class-III heart failure. Am Heart J 2002;143:910-5.

64. Bödigheimer K, Chase D. Wirksamkeit von Weißdorn-Extrakt in der Dosierung 3mal 100 mg täglich. Multizentrische Doppelblindstudie mit 85 herzinsuffizienten Patienten im Stadium NYHA II. Münch Med Wochenschr 1994;136(Suppl 1):S7-11.

65. Hecker-Niediek AE. Untersuchungen zur Biogenese, Markierung und Pharmakokinetik der Procyanidine

aus Crataegus-Species [Dissertation]. University of Marburg, 1983.

66. Schlegelmilch R, Heywood R. Toxicity of *Crataegus* (Hawthorn) Extract (WS 1442). J Am Coll Toxicol 1994;13:103-11.

67. Albrecht A, Juretzek W. Weißdorn (*Crataegus laevigata, Crataegus monogyna*), Weißdornblätter mit Blüten (Crataegi folium cum flore). Springer: LoseblattSystem Naturheilverfahren 1995.

68. Schimmer O, Haefele F, Krüger A. The mutagenic potencies of plant extracts containing quercetin in *Salmonella typhimurium* TA98 and TA100. Mutat Res 1988;206:201-8.

69. Fintelmann V, Siegers C-P. Johanniskraut weiterhin unbedenklich. Dtsch Apoth Ztg 1988;128:1499-500.

70. Bertram B. Flavonoide. Eine Klasse von Pflanzeninhaltsstoffen mit vielfältigen biologischen Wirkungen, auch mit karzinogener Wirkung? Dtsch Apoth Ztg 1989;129:2561-71.

71. Schimmer O, Krüger A, Paulini H, Haefele F. An evaluation of 55 commercial plant extracts in the Ames mutagenicity test. Pharmazie 1994;49:448-51.

CURCUMAE LONGAE RHIZOMA

Turmeric

DEFINITION

Turmeric consists of the scalded and dried rhizomes of *Curcuma longa* L. (*C. domestica* Valeton). It contains not less than 2.5% of dicinnamoylmethane derivatives, calculated as curcumin ($C_{21}H_{20}O_6$; M_r 368.4), and not less than 25 ml/kg (or not less than 20 ml/kg for the cut drug) of essential oil, both calculated with reference to the dried drug.

The material complies with the monograph of the Deutscher Arzneimittel-Codex [1].

CONSTITUENTS

The major constituents are 3-5% of curcuminoids - a mixture of dicinnamoylmethane derivatives such as curcumin (diferuloylmethane), monodemethoxy-curcumin (*p*-coumaroylferuloylmethane) and bisdemethoxycurcumin (di-*p*-coumaroylmethane) - and 3-5% of volatile oil composed principally of sesquiterpenes, e.g. zingiberene, curcumol, and α- and β-turmerone. The curcuminoid bisdemethoxy-curcumin is characteristic for turmeric [2]. Minor constituents include the acidic arabinogalactans ukonanes A-D [3].

CLINICAL PARTICULARS

Therapeutic indications
Symptomatic treatment of mild digestive disturbances and minor biliary dysfunction [1,2,4,5].

Posology and method of administration

Dosage

Adult average daily dose: 1.5-3 g of the drug or corresponding extracts [1,2,5].
Elderly: dose as for adults.

Method of administration
For oral administration.

Duration of administration
No restriction. If symptoms persist, seek medical advice.

Contra-indications
Biliary obstruction.

E/S/C/O/P
MONOGRAPHS
Second Edition

Special warnings and special precautions for use

Special warnings
Patients with cholelithiasis should take turmeric only after consultation with a physician.

Precautions for use
None required.

Interaction with other medicaments and other forms of interaction
None reported.

Pregnancy and lactation
No human data available. In accordance with general medical practice, the product should not be used during pregnancy and lactation without medical advice.

Effects on ability to drive and use machines
None known.

Undesirable effects
None known.

Overdose
No toxic effects reported.

PHARMACOLOGICAL PROPERTIES

Pharmacodynamic properties
Turmeric exerts choleretic, anti-inflammatory, antioxidative, hepatoprotective, hypolipaemic and antitumour effects. The pharmacologically active constituents are considered to be curcuminoids and the essential oil [2,6,7].

In vitro experiments

Hepatobiliary effects
In the model of the isolated and perfused rat liver a lipophilic fraction from an ethanolic extract of turmeric caused an increase in bile flow (3.7 µl/liver: 25%, AUC p<0.05, 6.4 µl/liver: 46%, AUC p<0.001) and stimulated bile acid production at two lower doses (1.2 µl and 1.8 µl/liver: 12% each). In the same model the residual dried ethanolic extract (15 and 45 mg/liver) increased bile flow (50 and 80%) but did not change bile acid production. The effect of the highest dose was still evident 90 minutes after the final addition of extract to the medium [8,9].

Antioxidative and cell protective effects
An aqueous turmeric extract and isolated curcumin inhibited liposomal lipid peroxidation (70% at 300 ng/µl) and peroxide-induced DNA damage (80% at 100 ng/ml) [10].

Curcumin, demethoxycurcumin and bisdemethoxy-

curcumin exerted strong scavenging effects on superoxide radicals generated by xanthine-xanthine oxidase (IC_{50}: 33, 63 and 198 µM respectively) and interacted with 1,1-diphenyl-2-picrylhydrazyl (DPPH) stable free radicals (IC_{50}: 22, 63 and 98 µM respectively) [11]. Curcumin was found to scavenge superoxide radicals (alkaline DMSO method; 39% at 54 µM), act as a hydroxyl radical scavenger at higher concentrations (5.4 µM: 4.6%, 54 µM: 33.3%) and activate the Fenton reaction at lower concentrations (5.4 µM: 52.7%) [12]. In a cell-free peroxidation system (peroxidation of arachidonic acid by iron/ascorbate), curcumin at 1 µM exerted strongly antioxidative activity of about 50% [13,14]. Curcumin reacted with galvinoxyl and DPPH, and suppressed free radical-induced oxidation of methyl linoleate in homogenous organic solution and in aqueous emulsions, soybean phosphatidylcholine liposomal membranes and rat liver homogenates [15].

Curcumin at lower concentrations (5×10^{-5} to 10^{-3} M) was found to protect rat hepatocytes against paracetamol-induced lipid peroxidation, without protection against paracetamol-induced lactate dehydrogenase leakage and glutathione depletion [16]. Curcumin (4-100 µM) protected human red blood cells and their membranes (red blood cell ghosts) against peroxide-induced lysis and lipid peroxidation [17]. Lipid peroxidation was inhibited dose-dependently by curcumin in rat liver microsomes (IC_{50}: 25 µM) [18]. Similar results were obtained in mouse erythrocytes (IC_{50} 10 µM, compared to 1 µM for dl-α-tocopherol) [19]. Curcumin, mono-demethoxycurcumin and bisdemethoxycurcumin (0.01 to 1.0 mg/ml) exerted a dose-dependent and significant hepatoprotective effect in carbon tetrachloride-induced (p<0.001 for 0.1 and 1.0 mg/ml) and galactosamine-induced (p<0.1 for 0.1 mg/ml and p<0.001 for 1.0 mg/ml) cytotoxicity in primary cultured rat hepatocytes, as measured by decreases in ASAT and ALAT concentrations in the medium [20].

A protein isolated from an aqueous extract of turmeric concentration-dependently inhibited iron/ascorbate-induced lipid peroxidation in rat brain tissue and cod liver oil (50% inhibition at 50 µg/ml) and provided 50% protection of Ca^{2+}-ATPase activity [21].

In a porcine renal tubular cell line (LLC-PK_1), powdered turmeric (100 µg/ml) and curcumin (10 and 100 µg/ml) significantly inhibited (p<0.05) hydrogen peroxide-induced lipid degradation, cytolysis and lipid peroxidation [22].

Anti-inflammatory effects
Curcumin inhibited sheep seminal cyclooxygenase with an IC_{50} of 8.8 µM compared to 1.2 µM for indometacin [23]. In other experiments, curcumin inhibited 5-lipoxygenase in rat peritoneal neutrophils (IC_{50} of 30 µM compared to 0.5 µM for nor-

dihydroguaiaretic acid) and cyclooxygenase in human platelets (IC$_{50}$: 2 µM). It also inhibited platelet aggregation induced by arachidonate, adrenaline and collagen (IC$_{50}$: 32, 100 and 344 µM respectively) and thromboxane B$_2$ production from endogenous [^{14}C]arachidonate in washed platelets (IC$_{50}$: 63 µM) with a concomitant increase in the formation of 12-lipoxygenase-catalysed metabolites such as 12-hydroxyeicosatetraenoic acid. Furthermore, it inhibited incorporation of [^{14}C]arachidonate into platelet phospholipids (32% at 250 µM) and deacylation of arachidonate-labelled phospholipids after stimulation with calcium ionophore A23187 [24]. Similar results have been found in other studies [25,26].

Addition of curcumin at 3, 10, 30 or 100 µM to cytosol from homogenates of mouse epidermis inhibited the metabolic conversion of arachidonic acid to 5-hydroxyeicosatetraenoic acid (5-HETE) by 40, 60, 66 and 83% respectively, and the conversion of arachidonic acid to 8-HETE by 40, 51, 77 and 85% respectively (IC$_{50}$: 5-10 µM). The metabolic conversion of arachidonic acid to prostaglandin E$_2$, prostaglandin F$_2\alpha$ and prostaglandin D$_2$ by epidermal microsomes was inhibited by approximately 50% after the addition of curcumin at 5-10 µM [27].

Antimutagenic effects
In the Ames test an aqueous extract of turmeric, a curcumin-free aqueous extract and isolated curcumin all exhibited antimutagenic effects against various direct-acting mutagens such as 1-methyl-3-nitro-1-nitrosoguanidine, benzo[a]pyrene, dimethyl benzo[a]anthracene and cigarette smoke condensates [28-30]. Curcumin at 5µM inhibited lipopoly-saccharide-induced production of TNF and IL-1 in a human macrophage cell line [31]; it was also shown to inhibit protein kinase activity in mouse fibroblast cells [32] and was cytotoxic to lymphocytes and Dalton's lymphoma cells [33].

Other effects
Curcumin (10^{-3} to 10^{-5} M) inhibited thromboxane B$_2$ production, platelet malondialdehyde synthesis, and adenosine diphosphate- and collagen-induced platelet aggregation in rhesus monkey blood in a con-centration-dependent manner [34,35].

In monkey polymorphonuclear leukocytes curcumin (1 × 10^{-6} to 10^{-3} M) inhibited aggregation induced by a chemotactic peptide and zymosan-activated plasma, but not aggregation induced by arachidonic acid and zymosan. The release of myeloperoxidase by various stimuli was inhibited by curcumin at 1 mM. Curcumin caused dose-dependent inhibition of O^{2-} radicals in neutrophils induced by arachidonic acid, the chemotactic peptide and zymosan [36].

Curcumin was found to be a potent inhibitor of the rat liver enzyme CYP 1A1/1A2 measured as ethoxy-resorufin de-ethylating (EROD) activity in β-naphthoflavone (βNF)-induced microsomes. It was a less potent inhibitor of the enzyme CYP 2B1/2B2, measured as pentoxyresorufin depentylation (PROD) activity in phenobarbital-induced microsomes and a weak inhibitor of the enzyme CYP 2E1, measured as p-nitrophenol (PNP) hydroxylation activity in pyrazole-induced microsomes. K$_i$ values were 0.14 and 76.02 µM for EROD- and PROD-activities; PNP hydroxyl-ation activity was inhibited only by 9% at 30 µM. In EROD and PROD experiments, a competitive type of inhibition was exhibited. Curcumin was also a potent inhibitor of glutathione S-transferase (GST) activity in cytosol from the liver of rats treated with phenobarbital, β-naphthoflavone (βNF) and pyrazole. In liver cytosol from rats treated with phenobarbital, curcumin inhibited GST activity in a mixed-type manner with a K$_i$ of 5.75 µM. In liver cytosol from rats treated with pyrazole or βNF, curcumin exhibited a competitive type of inhibition with K$_i$ values of 1.79 µM and 2.29 µM respectively [37].

In vivo experiments

Biliary effects
In a bile duct fistula model in rats under urethane anaesthesia, orally administered essential oil of turmeric (300 mg/kg body weight) caused an increase of about 17% in bile flow in the first hour after administration, whereas curcumin (300 mg/kg) and 2% carboxymethylcellulose (the vehicle as a control) caused decreases of 2% and 22% respectively [38]. In the same model curcumin, bisdemethoxycurcumin and a mixture of the three main curcuminoids (25 mg/kg intravenously in each case) increased biliary flow over a 2-hour period compared to the control (0.1 N NaOH) by about 80%, 120% and 70% respectively. All the tested curcuminoids caused the same slight and constant decrease in bile acid excretion as the control groups [39,40]. Bisdemethoxycurcumin administered intravenously at 25 mg/kg reduced cyclosporin-induced cholestasis by increasing bile flow and bile acid secretion, whereas curcumin only increased bile flow [39].

In another bile duct fistula study in rats, intravenous administration of curcumin (25 and 50 mg/kg body weight) dose-dependently increased basal bile flow by 100%, biliary bilirubin excretion by 50%, and biliary cholesterol excretion by 13%. Cyclosporin (30 mg/kg, intravenous) reduced bile flow by 34% and biliary excretion of bilirubin and of cholesterol by 67%. Intravenous administration of curcumin at 25 and 50 mg/kg body weight 30 minutes after cyclosporin increased bile flow in a dose-dependent manner to 130% of the basal value for 1 hr and increased biliary excretion of cholesterol and of bilirubin to 100% of basal values for 30 and 150 minutes respectively. When injected 15 minutes before the cyclosporin, curcumin prevented the drop in bile flow at 50 mg/kg and the reduction in biliary bilirubin excretion at 25 mg/kg until the end of the experiment (180 minutes). However, cyclosporin-induced reduction of biliary cholesterol excretion was not prevented by curcumin. Biliary excretion of cyclosporin (1.2 µg/kg/min) and its metabolites (1.2 µg/kg/min) were slightly reduced, to 83% of initial values, by curcumin at 50 mg/kg [41].

Intravenous administration of aqueous and alcoholic turmeric extracts (up to 5 g/kg body weight), sodium curcuminate (up to 25 mg/kg) or essential oil (5 mg/kg) stimulated bile acid secretion in anaesthetized, bile duct-cannulated dogs. The effects on choleresis were measurable for up to 120 minutes after administration and were strongest for sodium curcuminate and the alcoholic turmeric extract [42,43]. Sodium curcuminate increased total excretion of bile acids, bilirubin and cholesterol in these studies [42].

Cytoprotective effects
Curcumin administered orally to mice at 250 mg/kg body weight for 14 days inhibited lipid peroxidation stimulated in various organs by chemical agents such as carbon tetrachloride, paraquat and cyclophosphamide [44]. Curcumin supplementation at 1% in the diet of rats for 10 weeks significantly decreased lipid peroxidation (p<0.01) by 29% in rat liver homogenates and by 35% in rat liver microsomes, and significantly increased (p<0.001) superoxide dismutase by 19%, catalase by 19% and glutathione peroxidase by 20% compared to rats fed on a control diet [45]. When administered orally to mice at 250 mg/kg for 15 days curcumin stimulated glutathione S-transferase (GST) activity in the liver 1.8 fold compared to initial values (p<0.05); doses of 50, 100 and 500 mg/kg were slightly less active [46]. Curcumin administered orally to rats at 30 mg/kg for 10 days lowered liver and serum lipid peroxide levels, serum ALAT, ASAT and lactate dehydrogenase induced by intraperitoneal injection of Fe^{2+} at 30 mg/kg [47]. Curcumin administered orally to rats at 80 mg/kg significantly lowered (p<0.001) ethanol-induced increases in levels of ASAT, ALAT, serum cholesterol, phospholipids and free fatty acids [48].

Hypolipidaemic effects
Significant lowering (p<0.001) of serum total cholesterol by 81% and serum triglycerides by 85% compared to controls was observed 12 hours after a single oral administration of an ethanolic (50% v/v) extract of turmeric at 300 mg/kg body weight to Triton-induced hyperlipidaemic rats [49]. Curcumin added at 0.1, 0.25 and 0.5% to a diet enriched with 1% of cholesterol, fed to rats for 7 weeks, reduced levels of total cholesterol in serum to 125, 122 and 128 mg/100 ml, and in the liver to 720, 957 and 596 mg/100 g fresh weight respectively, compared to 377 mg/100 ml and 1900 mg/100 g fresh weight

respectively in rats fed a diet supplemented with cholesterol alone [50].

Anti-inflammatory effects
Various extracts of turmeric as well as curcumin, administered intraperitoneally, exerted an anti-inflammatory effect in carrageenan-induced rat paw oedema; the ED_{50} (mg/kg body weight) 4 hours after oedema provocation was about 4.7 for an aqueous extract, 8.7 for curcumin, 40.7 for a petroleum ether extract and 309 for an alcoholic extract. The aqueous extract at 40 mg/kg was as effective as indometacin at 5 mg/kg [51]. Carrageenan-induced paw oedema was inhibited by curcumin in mice with an ED_{50} of 100.2 mg/kg compared to 78.0 mg/kg for cortisone, and in rats with an ED_{50} of 48.0 mg/kg compared to 45.0 mg/kg for cortisone and 48.0 mg/kg for phenylbutazone [52]. In another study, curcumin administered by intraplanar injection at 50 mg/kg inhibited carrageenan-induced rat paw oedema by 48% compared to 60% inhibition by phenylbutazone at 100 mg/kg) [53].

In the granuloma pouch test, a petroleum ether extract of turmeric (25 mg/kg body weight), an aqueous extract (20 mg/kg), an alcoholic extract (100 mg/kg) and indometacin (4 mg/kg), administered intraperitoneally for 6 days, significantly decreased granuloma pouch weights (p<0.001), whereas with curcumin (20 mg/kg) the decrease was not significant. The strongest effects were obtained with the aqueous and petroleum ether extracts. Using the same concentrations in the cotton pellet test, the extracts as well as curcumin significantly reduced pellet weights (p<0.001) [51]. Anti-inflammatory and anti-arthritic effects of turmeric essential oil, administered orally at 0.01 ml/kg for 13 days, were demonstrated in Freund's adjuvant arthritis in rats; the effect was significant compared to the control (milk; p<0.01) or cortisone acetate (p<0.05) [54].

Curcumin administered orally at 80 and 160 mg/kg inhibited granuloma formation in the granuloma pouch test by 14.3 and 29.5% respectively, compared to 21.6% by phenylbutazone at 40 mg/kg. In the cotton pellet test curcumin at 80 and 160 mg/kg reduced the formation of granulation tissue by 21.5 and 22.0% respectively, compared to 19.0% by phenylbutazone at 80 mg/kg [52]. In another study using the granuloma pouch test, oral administration of curcumin at 100 and 200 mg/kg body weight inhibited granuloma formation by 21.7 and 30.8% respectively, compared to 26.6 and 32.3% by ibuprofen at 15 and 20 mg/kg respectively. Both compounds significantly prevented increases in liver and granuloma tissue lysosomal enzymes compared to control: acid phosphatase (p<0.01) and cathepsin-D (p<0.05) [55].

In the mouse ear oedema test, topically applied curcumin markedly inhibited epidermal inflammation induced by TPA (32% inhibition by curcumin at 0.2 µM, 99% inhibition at 1.0 µM) or arachidonic acid (60% inhibition by curcumin at 5 µM) [27].

Antitumour and ulcerogenic/ulceroprotective effects
An aqueous extract of turmeric, a curcumin-free aqueous extract and curcumin, each administered intraperitoneally at 3 mg/animal 18 hours before injection of benzo[a]pyrene at 250 mg/kg body weight, significantly inhibited bone marrow micronuclei formation in mice by 43, 76 and 65% respectively (p<0.001). Furthermore, the incidence and multiplicity of forestomach tumours induced by benzo[a]pyrene, administered orally to mice at 1 mg/animal twice weekly for 4 weeks, were significantly inhibited (p<0.001) by the aqueous extract at 3 mg/day, the curcumin-free aqueous extract at 1 mg/day and curcumin at 1 mg/day, administered intragastrically for 2 weeks before, during and for 2 weeks after benzo[a]pyrene treatment [28].

Turmeric administered as 5% of the diet for 4 weeks significantly reduced tumour incidence (p<0.001), by 40% in the model of forestomach tumours in mice and by 80% with respect to oral mucosal tumours in hamsters [56,57]. Dietary turmeric at 0.1, 0.5 and 3% for 4 weeks reduced benzo[a]pyrene-induced DNA adducts in the liver of rats by 61, 76 and 71% [58].

Turmeric fed to rats for 3 months as from 1 to 10% of their diet before a single intraperitoneal injection of benzo[a]pyrene- or 3-methylcholanthrene inhibited the mutagenicity of urine (collected for 24 hours after injection) in the Ames test [59].

Curcuminoids have been shown to reduce solid tumour volume and increase the life span of mice bearing Ehrlich ascites tumour cells [60]. Curcumin given to mice as 2% of their diet for 6 weeks inhibited azoxymethanol-induced hyperproliferation of colonic epithelial cells and the incidence of focal areas of dysplasia [61]. Commercial grade curcumin (containing 77% of curcumin, 17% of demethoxycurcumin and 3% of bisdemethoxycurcumin), given to mice as 0.5-2% of their diet for about 3 weeks, reduced the incidence and size of tumours induced in the forestomach, duodenum and colon by various carcinogens such as benzo[a]pyrene and N-ethyl-N'-nitro-N-nitrosoguanidine by 47-77% [62].

Topical application of curcumin at 1, 3 or 10 µM together with 12-O-tetradecanoylphorbol-13-acetate (TPA) twice weekly for 20 weeks to mice with tumours previously initiated with 7,12-dimethylbenzo[a]-anthracene inhibited the number of TPA-induced tumours per mouse by 39, 77 and 98% respectively [63]. Using the same methodology, similar results have been observed in other studies in mice [64,65]. Topical application of curcumin at 1, 3, and 10 µmol together with 5 nmol of TPA to the shaved backs of

mice inhibited TPA-induced increases in epidermal ornithine decarboxylase mRNA by 66, 81 and 91% respectively [66].

A single oral dose of an ethanolic extract of turmeric at 500 mg/kg body weight was significantly anti-ulcerogenic in rat models of ulceration such as hypothermic restraint stress (35% inhibition, p<0.05), pyloric ligation (66% inhibition, p<0.01) and indometacin (34% inhibition, p<0.001) [67]. Curcumin administered orally to rats at 100 mg/kg for 6 days produced gastric ulceration (not significant), whereas 50 mg/kg had no effect; a marked reduction in the mucin content of gastric juice (p<0.001) was observed after 100 mg/kg [68].

Aqueous and methanolic extracts of turmeric administered intragastrically to rabbits at 132 and 155 mg/kg body weight decreased gastric secretion by 44.4 and 47.9%, acid output by 66.5 and 55.3% and pepsin output by 50.4 and 68.6% respectively [69].

Other effects
A single dose of curcumin administered intra-peritoneally to mice at 25-200 mg/kg body weight inhibited platelet thromboxane production and exhibited anti-thrombotic effects as measured by protection against death or paralysis induced by intravenously administered collagen (15 µg) and adrenaline (30 µM); these effects were dose-dependent [34]. Curcumin administered orally to rats as a single dose of 100-300 mg/kg inhibited collagen-induced platelet aggregation [35].

Pharmacological studies in humans
An infusion of turmeric (200 ml, prepared from 3.2-4 g of drug), administered orally to 19 patients with complaints such as duodenal ulcer or cholecystitis, increased bile secretion approximately two-fold on average [4].

A dry hydroethanolic extract of turmeric, administered to 18 healthy volunteers for 45 days at a daily dose equivalent to 20 mg of curcumin, significantly decreased serum lipid peroxide levels (p<0.05) [70].

Daily administration of 1.5 g of turmeric to 16 chronic smokers for 30 days significantly reduced urinary excretion of mutagens (p<0.001) as measured by the Ames test [71].

Clinical studies

Gastrointestinal effects
In a randomized, double-blind, placebo-controlled, multicentre study, 106 patients with dyspeptic complaints such as abdominal pain, epigastric discomfort, flatulence or belching) were treated daily for 7 days with 2 g of turmeric (n = 38), a herbal

combination including cascara and nux vomica extracts and ginger (n = 30) or placebo (n = 38). At the end of the study 27 patients in the turmeric group, 17 in the herbal extract mixture group and 16 in the placebo group reported a notable improvement. The difference between turmeric and placebo was significant (p = 0.003) [5].

In a randomized study 50 patients with benign gastric ulcers were treated daily over 12 weeks with either 750 mg of turmeric (n = 27) or an antacid preparation containing aluminium and magnesium hydroxides (n = 23). After 6 weeks of treatment, 9 patients in the turmeric group (33.3%) and 15 in the antacid group (65.2%) were completely healed; 14 in the turmeric group (51.9%) and 8 in the antacid group (34.8%) were improved (p<0.05). After a further 6 weeks 70.6% of the patients in the turmeric and 94.1% in the antacid group were completely healed as verified by endoscopy [72].

In contrast, in a double-blind, placebo-controlled study involving 130 patients with duodenal ulcer, treatment with 6 g of turmeric daily for 8 weeks did not prove superior to placebo in the ulcer healing rate: 27% in the turmeric group, 29% in the placebo group [73].

On average, 440 patients with dyspeptic complaints participating in an open surveillance study were treated with 2 × 81 mg of a turmeric extract (13-25:1, 96% ethanol) daily for 4 weeks. Compared to initial values, subjective symptom scores declined by approx. 84% for vomiting, 71% for nausea, 66% for upper abdominal pain, 66% for lower abdominal pain, 61% for feeling of fullness, 58% for flatulence and 58% for constipation; the overall dyspeptic symptom score declined by 66%. From evaluation by the physicians, global efficacy was excellent in 27% of cases and good in 60% [74].

Anti-inflammatory effects
In a randomized, double-blind, cross-over study 18 patients with rheumatoid arthritis treated daily for 2 weeks with 1200 mg of curcumin or 300 mg of phenylbutazone showed significant improvement (p<0.05) in morning stiffness, walking time and joint swelling in both phases compared with baseline values [75].

In another randomized study, following surgery for inguinal hernia or hydrocele, 45 patients were treated daily for 5 days, beginning from the post-operative day, with 1200 mg of curcumin or 300 mg of phenylbutazone or placebo. Improvements in typical post-operative symptoms (spermatic cord oedema, tenderness, pain) was observed in 84% of patients in the curcumin group, 86% in the phenylbutazone group and 62% in the placebo group [76].

Pharmacokinetic properties
Kinetic data are available only for curcumin.

A single dose of 2 g of curcumin administered orally to 8 human volunteers led to undetectable or very low serum concentrations: C_{max} 0.006 ± 0.005 µg/ml, T_{max} 1 hour, AUC_{0-tn} 0.004 µg/hour/ml. Concomitant administration of piperine (an inhibitor of hepatic and intestinal glucuronidation, to enhance the serum concentration, extent of absorption and bioavailability of curcumin) as a single 20 mg dose significantly increased serum concentrations at 0.25 and 0.5 hour (p<0.01) and at 0.75 hour (p<0.001), C_{max} to 0.18 ± 0.03 µg/ml and AUC_{0-tn} to 0.08 µg/hour/ml, while T_{max} decreased to 0.69 hour [77].

Curcumin given orally to rats as a single dose at 2 g/kg body weight resulted in C_{max} of 1.35 ± 0.23 µg/ml, T_{max} of 0.83 ± 0.05 hour, $t_{1/2}$ of 1.70 ± 0.58 hour and AUC_{0-tn} of 2.36 ± 0.28 µg/hour/ml. Concomitant administration of piperine at 20 mg/kg increased C_{max} to 1.80 ± 0.16 µg/ml and AUC_{0-tn} to 3.64 ± 0.31 µg/hour/ml, significantly prolonged T_{max} to 1.29 ± 0.23 hour (p<0.02) and diminished $t_{1/2}$ to 1.05 ± 0.18 hour (p<0.02). Total clearance significantly decreased from 713.00 ± 12.00 to 495.90 ± 37.08 litre/hour (p<0.02) [77].

After oral administration of curcumin to rats at 1 g/kg body weight about 75% was excreted in the faeces and only traces in the urine; plasma and bile concentrations of curcumin were negligible. Following intravenous application, curcumin was excreted via bile [78]. [³H]-labelled curcumin administered orally to rats at 0.6 mg/kg body weight led to faecal excretion of radioactivity of about 89% in 72 hrs and excretion of about 6% via bile. After intraperitoneal administration, about 73% of the radioactivity was excreted in the faeces and about 11% in bile [79]. When a single 400 mg dose of curcumin was administered orally to rats, about 60% was absorbed and 40% excreted unchanged in the faeces over a period of 5 days. No curcumin could be detected in urine and only traces were found in the portal blood, liver and kidney [80].

Studies with isolated perfused rat liver [78] and isolated rat intestine [81] suggested initial metabolism of curcumin in the intestine, producing easily absorbable metabolites, and intensive second metabolism in the liver. Major metabolites were glucuronides of tetrahydrocurcumin and hexahydrocurcumin, with dihydroferulic acid and traces of ferulic acid as further metabolites, all of which were excreted in the bile.

Oral administration of radio-labelled curcumin to rats resulted in radioactivity being found only in liver and kidneys [80,82].

Preclinical safety data

Acute toxicity
No visible signs of toxicity were observed following oral administration of a single dose of an ethanolic extract of turmeric at 0.5, 1 or 3 g/kg body weight to mice [83], or powdered turmeric at 2.5 g/kg or an ethanolic extract at 300 mg/kg to rats, guinea pigs and monkeys [84]. Single oral doses of curcumin at 1-5 g/kg body weight induced no toxic effects in rats [78].

No mortality was observed after administration of curcumin to mice as a single oral or intraperitoneal dose at 2.0 g/kg body weight [52].

Acute intraperitoneal LD_{50} values in mice for petroleum ether, alcoholic and aqueous fractions from turmeric (obtained by successive extraction of the same material) and for curcumin were determined as 0.525, 3.980, 0.430 and 1.5 g/kg body weight respectively [51].

Repeated dose toxicity
Turmeric oleoresin (containing volatile oil and 15-40% of curcuminoids) fed to pigs at dietary levels of 60, 296 and 1551 mg/kg body weight/day for 102-109 days led to a reduction in weight gain at the highest dose (males: $p<0.01$, females: $p<0.001$). Dose-related increases in liver and thyroid weights were observed at all dose levels. Pericholangitis, hyperplasia of the thyroid and epithelial changes in the kidney and urinary bladder occurred after dosage at 296 and 1551 mg/kg [85].

Following 90-day oral administration to mice of an ethanolic extract of turmeric at 100 mg/kg/day, considerable increases in heart and lung weights ($p<0.05$) and decreases in white and red blood cell counts ($p<0.01$) were observed compared to controls [83].

There are conflicting reports on the ulcerogenic potential of curcumin [68]. An ulcerogenic tendency was observed after oral administration of curcumin to rats at 100 mg/kg body weight for 6 days [68]. However, in another study, a single oral dose of an ethanolic extract of turmeric was found to be anti-ulcerogenic (see In vivo experiments: antitumour and ulcerogenic/ulceroprotective effects) [67].

Mutagenicity
Aqueous and alcoholic extracts of turmeric, and also the essential oil and curcumin, have shown no mutagenic potential in the Ames test, with or without metabolic activation [28,86].

No genotoxicity was observed in mouse bone-marrow cells (micronucleus test) after single oral doses of turmeric at up to 5 g/kg body weight [87]. Turmeric

and curcumin given to mice as 0.5% and 0.015% of their diet respectively for 12 weeks, and turmeric given to rats in their diet at 0.5% and 0.05% for 12 weeks, induced no genotoxic effects as measured by the incidence of micronucleated polychromatic erythrocytes and chromosomal aberrations in bone-marrow cells [88]. In contrast to the earlier findings, a single oral dose of a methanolic extract of turmeric at 100, 250 and 500 mg/kg body weight was found to induce an increase in chromosomal aberrations in bone marrow cells of mice [89].

A single intraperitoneal dose of curcumin administered to mice at 5-200 mg/kg body weight induced a dose-dependent increase in sister chromatid exchanges ($p<0.05$) starting at 25 mg/kg [90].

Rats fed for 9 months with curcumin at 0.1, 0.2, 0.5 and 1 mg/kg body weight showed significant increases in chromosomal aberrations in bone marrow cells at the two highest doses ($p<0.05$) [90].

Reproduction toxicity
Turmeric at 0.5% and curcumin at 0.015% of the diet of mice for 12 weeks produced no teratogenic effects, as measured by pregnancy rate, number of live and dead embryos, and total implants [88].

Turmeric at 4 g/kg or curcumin at 0.4 g/kg body weight, administered orally for 14 or 21 days to lactating mice, significantly increased hepatic levels of glutathione S-transferase ($p<0.01$), acid-soluble sulphydryl groups ($p<0.01$) and cytochrome b_5 and P_{450} ($p<0.05$) in both lactating mice and their suckling neonates [91].

Clinical safety data
Over 600 individuals have participated in open and controlled studies with turmeric (up to 6 g daily) or curcumin (up to 1.5 g daily) for several weeks of treatment. No serious or major adverse events have been reported. In a few cases minor adverse events have occurred, mainly involving gastrointestinal discomfort, which may have been due to underlying symptoms [5,73].

A single case of local allergic reaction after topical application of turmeric and curcumin has been reported [92].

REFERENCES

1.   Curcumawurzelstock - Curcumae longae rhizoma. Deutscher Arzneimittel-Codex.

2.   Staesche K, Schleinitz H. *Curcuma*. In: Hänsel R, Keller K, Rimpler H, Schneider G, editors. Hagers Handbuch der Pharmazeutischen Praxis, 5th ed. Volume 4: Drogen A-D. Berlin-Heidelberg-New York-London: Springer-

Verlag, 1992:1084-102.

3. Gonda R, Takeda K, Shimizu N, Tomoda M. Characterization of a neutral polysaccharide having activity on the reticuloendothelial system from the rhizome of *Curcuma longa*. Chem Pharm Bull 1992; 40:185-8.

4. Kalk H, Nissen K. Untersuchungen über die Wirkung der Curcuma (Temoelavac) auf die Funktion der Leber und Gallenwege. Dtsch Med Wschr 1931;57:1613-5.

5. Thamlikitkul V, Dechatiwongse T, Chantrakul C, Nimitnon S, Ayurd CHVE, Punktrut W et al. Randomized double blind study of *Curcuma domestica* Val. for dyspepsia. J Med Assoc Thai 1989;72:613-20.

6. Ammon HPT, Wahl MA. Pharmacology of *Curcuma longa*. Planta Med 1991;57:1-7.

7. Srimal RC. Turmeric: a brief review of medicinal properties. Fitoterapia 1997;68:483-93.

8. Schlepper O, Nahrstedt A, Winterhoff H. Choleretische Eigenschaften des Öles von *Curcuma domestica* Val. in der isoliert perfundierten Rattenleber (IPRL) [Poster]. 10. Jahrestagung der Gesellschaft für Phytotherapie. Münster, Germany, 11-13 November 1999 (Poster P15).

9. Schlepper O, Flume M, Nahrstedt A, Winterhoff H. Pharmacological and analytical investigations on the choleretic properties of *Curcuma domestica* Val. [Poster]. Joint meeting of the ASP, AFERP, GA and PSE. Amsterdam, 26-30 July 1999 (Poster 329).

10. Shalini VK, Srinivas L. Lipid peroxide induced DNA damage: protection by turmeric (*Curcuma longa*). Molec Cell Biochem 1987;77:3-10.

11. Sreejayan N, Rao MNA. Free radical scavenging activity of curcuminoids. Arzneim-Forsch/Drug Res 1996; 46:169-71.

12. Kunchandy E, Rao MNA. Oxygen radical scavenging activity of curcumin. Internat J Pharmaceutics 1990; 58:237-40.

13. Ammon HPT, Anazodo MI, Safayhi H, Dhawan BN, Srimal RC. Curcumin: A potent inhibitor of leukotriene B_4 formation in rat peritoneal polymorphonuclear neutrophils (PMNL). Planta Med 1992;58:226.

14. Ammon HPT, Safayhi H, Mack T, Sabieraj J. Mechanism of antiinflammatory actions of curcumine and boswellic acids. J Ethnopharmacol 1993;38:113-9.

15. Noguchi N, Komuro E, Niki E, Willson R. Action of curcumin as an antioxidant against lipid peroxidation. J Japan Oil Chem Soc (Yukagaku) 1994;43:1045-51.

16. Donatus IA, Sardjoko, Vermeulen NPE. Cytotoxic and cytoprotective activities of curcumin. Effects on paracetamol-induced cytotoxicity, lipid peroxidation and glutathione depletion in rat hepatocytes. Biochem Pharmacol 1990;39:1869-75.

17. Grinberg LN, Shalev O, Tønnesen HH, Rachmilewitz EA. Studies on curcumin and curcuminoids: XXVI. Antioxidant effects of curcumin on the red blood cell membrane. Internat J Pharmaceutics 1996;132:251-7.

18. Pulla Reddy AC, Lokesh BR. Studies on spice principles as antioxidants in the inhibition of lipid peroxidation of rat liver microsomes. Molec Cell Biochem 1992;111: 117-24.

19. Toda S, Ohnishi M, Kimura M, Nakashima K. Action of curcuminoids on the hemolysis and lipid peroxidation of mouse erythrocytes induced by hydrogen peroxide. J Ethnopharmacol 1988;23:105-8.

20. Kiso Y, Suzuki Y, Watanabe N, Oshima Y, Hikino H. Antihepatotoxic principles of *Curcuma longa* rhizomes. Planta Med 1983;49:185-7.

21. Selvam R, Subramanian L, Gayathri R, Angayarkanni N. The anti-oxidant activity of turmeric (*Curcuma longa*). J Ethnopharmacol 1995;47:59-67.

22. Cohly HHP, Taylor A, Angel MF, Salahudeen AK. Effect of turmeric, turmerin and curcumin on H_2O_2-induced renal epithelial (LLC-PK_1) cell injury. Free Rad Biol Med 1998;24:49-54.

23. Wagner H, Wierer M, Bauer R. *In vitro*-Hemmung der Prostaglandin-Biosynthese durch etherische Öle und phenolische Verbindungen. Planta Med 1986;52:184-7.

24. Srivastava KC, Bordia A, Verma SK. Curcumin, a major component of food spice turmeric (*Curcuma longa*) inhibits aggregation and alters eicosanoid metabolism in human blood platelets. Prostaglandins Leukotr Essent Fatty Acids 1995;52:223-7.

25. Flynn DL, Rafferty MF, Boctor AM. Inhibition of 5-hydroxy-eicosatetraenoic acid (5-HETE) formation in intact human neutrophils by naturally-occurring diarylheptanoids: Inhibitory activities of curcuminoids and yakuchinones. Prostaglandins Leukotr Med 1986; 22:357-60.

26. Srivastava, KC. Extracts of two frequently consumed spices - cumin (*Cuminum cyminum*) and turmeric (*Curcuma longa*) - inhibit platelet aggregation and alter eicosanoid biosynthesis in human blood platelets. Prostaglandins Leukotr Essent Fatty Acids 1989;37:57-64.

27. Huang MT, Lysz T, Ferraro T, Abidi TF, Laskin JD, Conney AH. Inhibitory effects of curcumin on in vitro lipoxygenase and cyclooxygenase activities in mouse epidermis. Cancer Res 1991;51:813-9.

28. Azuine MA, Kayal JJ, Bhide SV. Protective role of aqueous turmeric extract against mutagenicity of direct-acting carcinogens as well as benzo[a]pyrene-induced genotoxicity and carcinogenicity. J Cancer Res Clin Oncol 1992;118:447-52.

29. Nagabhushan M, Amonkar AJ, Bhide SV. *In vitro* antimutagenicity of curcumin against environmental mutagens. Food Chem Toxicol 1987;25:545-7.

30. Nagabhushan M, Nair UJ, Amonkar AJ, D'Souza AV,

Bhide SV. Curcumins as inhibitors of nitrosation in vitro. Mutation Res 1988;202:163-9.

31. Chan MM. Inhibition of tumor necrosis factor by curcumin, a phytochemical. Biochem Pharmacol 1995;49:1551-6.

32. Liu J-Y, Lin S-J, Lin J-K. Inhibitory effects of curcumin on protein kinase C activity induced by 12-O-tetradecanoyl-phorbol-13-acetate in NIH 3T3 cells. Carcinogenesis 1993;14:857-61.

33. Kuttan R, Bhanumathy P, Nirmala K and George MC. Potential anticancer activity of turmeric (*Curcuma longa*). Cancer Lett 1985;29:197-202.

34. Srivastava R, Dikshit M, Srimal RC, Dhawan BN. Anti-thrombotic effect of curcumin. Thromb Res 1985; 40:413-7.

35. Srivastava R, Puri V, Srimal RC, Dhawan BN. Effect of curcumin on platelet aggregation and vascular prostacyclin synthesis. Arzneim-Forsch/Drug Res 1986;36:715-7.

36. Srivastava R. Inhibition of neutrophil response by curcumin. Agents Actions 1989;28:298-303.

37. Oetari S, Sudibyo M, Commandeur JNM, Samhoedi R, Vermeulen NPE. Effects of curcumin on cytochrome P450 and glutathione activities in rat liver. Biochem Pharmacol 1996;51:39-45.

38. Ozaki Y, Liang OB. Cholagogic action of the essential oil obtained from *Curcuma xanthorrhiza* Roxb. Shoyakugaku Zasshi 1988;42:257-63.

39. Deters M, Siegers C, Muhl P, Hänsel W. Choleretic effects of curcuminoids on an acute cyclosporin-induced cholestastis in the rat. Planta Med 1999;65:610–3.

40. Siegers C-P, Deters M, Strubelt O, Hänsel W. Choleretic properties of different curcuminoids in the rat bile-fistula model. Pharm Pharmacol Letters 1997;7:87-9.

41. Deters M, Siegers C, Hänsel W, Schneider KP, Hennighausen G. Influence of curcumin on cyclosporin-induced reduction of biliary bilirubin and cholesterol excretion and on biliary excretion of cyclosporin and its metabolites. Planta Med 2000;66:429-34.

42. Ramprasad C, Sirsi M. Curcuma longa and bile secretion – Quantitative changes in the bile constituents induced by sodium curcuminate. J Sci Industr Res 1957;16C:108-10.

43. Ramprasad C, Sirsi M. Studies on Indian medicinal plants: *Curcuma longa* Linn. - Effect of curcumin and the essential oils of *C. longa* on bile secretion. J Sci Industr Res 1956;15C:262-5.

44. Soudamini KK, Unnikrishnan MC, Soni KB, Kuttan R. Inhibition of lipid peroxidation and cholesterol levels in mice by curcumin. Indian J Physiol Pharmacol 1992;36:239-43.

45. Pulla Reddy AC, Lokesh BR. Effect of dietary turmeric (*Curcuma longa*) on iron-induced lipid peroxidation in the rat liver. Food Chem Toxicol 1994;32:279-83.

46. Susan M, Rao MNA. Induction of glutathione S-transferase activity by curcumin in mice. Arzneim-Forsch/Drug Res 1992;42:962-4.

47. Pulla Reddy AC, Lokesh BR. Effect of curcumin and eugenol on iron-induced hepatic toxicity in rats. Toxicology 1996;107:39-45.

48. Rajakrishnan V, Menon VP, Rajashekaran KN. Protective role of curcumin in ethanol toxicity. Phytother Res 1998;12:55-6.

49. Dixit VP, Jain P, Joshi SC. Hypolipidaemic effects of *Curcuma longa* L and *Nardostachys jatamansi* DC in triton-induced hyperlipidaemic rats. Indian J Physiol Pharmacol 1988;32:299-304.

50. Subba Rao D, Chandra Sekhara N, Satyanarayana MN, Srinivasan M. Effect of curcumin on serum and liver cholesterol levels in the rat. J Nutr 1970;100:1307-16.

51. Yegnanarayan R, Saraf AP, Balwani JH. Comparison of anti-inflammatory activity of various extracts of Curcuma longa (Linn). Indian J Med Res 1976;64:601-8.

52. Srimal RC, Dhawan BN. Pharmacology of diferuloyl methane (curcumin), a non-steroidal anti-inflammatory agent. J Pharm Pharmacol 1973;25:447-52.

53. Ali M, Bagati A, Gupta J. Comparison of anti-inflammatory activity of curcumin analogues. Indian Drugs 1995;32:502-5.

54. Chandra D, Gupta SS. Anti-inflammatory and anti-arthritic activity of volatile oil of Curcuma longa (Haldi). Indian J Med Res 1972;60:138-42.

55. Srivastava R, Srimal RC. Modification of certain inflammation-induced biochemical changes by curcumin. Indian J Med Res 1985;81:215-23.

56. Azuine MA, Bhide SV. Chemopreventive effect of turmeric against stomach and skin tumors induced by chemical carcinogens in Swiss mice. Nutr Cancer 1992;17:77-83.

57. Azuine MA, Bhide SV. Adjuvant chemoprevention of experimental cancer: catechin and dietary turmeric in forestomach and oral cancer models. J Ethnopharmacol 1994;44:211-7.

58. Mukundan MA, Chacko MC, Annapurna VV, Krishnaswamy K. Effect of turmeric and curcumin on BP-DNA adducts. Carcinogenesis 1993;14:493-6.

59. Polasa K, Sesikaran B, Krishna TP, Krishnaswamy K. Turmeric (*Curcuma longa*)-induced reduction in urinary mutagens. Food Chem Toxicol 1991;29:699-706.

60. Ruby AJ, Kuttan G, Babu KD, Rajasekharan KN, Kuttan R. Anti-tumour and antioxidant activity of natural curcuminoids. Cancer Lett 1995;94:79-83.

61. Huang M-T, Deschner EE, Newmark HL, Wang Z-Y, Ferraro TA, Conney AH. Effect of dietary curcumin and ascorbyl palmitate on azoxymethanol-induced colonic

epithelial cell proliferation and focal areas of dysplasia. Cancer Lett 1992;64:117-21.

62. Huang M-T, Lou Y-R, Ma W, Newmark HL, Reuhl KR, Conney AH. Inhibitory effects of dietary curcumin on forestomach, duodenal and colon carcinogenesis in mice. Cancer Res 1994;54:5841-7.

63. Huang M-T, Smart RC, Wong C-Q, Conney AH. Inhibitory effect of curcumin, chlorogenic acid, caffeic acid and ferulic acid on tumor promotion in mouse skin by 12-O-tetradecanoylphorbol-13-acetate. Cancer Res 1988;48:5941-6.

64. Huang M-T, Wang ZY, Georgiadis CA, Laskin JD, Conney AH. Inhibitory effects of curcumin on tumor initiation by benzo[a]pyrene and 7,12-dimethyl-benz[a]anthracene. Carcinogenesis 1992;13:2183-6.

65. Nagabhushan M, Bhide SV. Curcumin as an inhibitor of cancer. J Am Coll Nutr 1992;11:192-8.

66. Lu Y-P, Chang RL, Huang M-T, Conney AH. Inhibitory effect of curcumin on 12-O-tetradecanoylphorbol-13-acetate-induced increase in ornithine decarboxylase mRNA in mouse epidermis. Carcinogenesis 1993; 14:293-7.

67. Rafatullah S, Tariq M, Al-Yahya MA, Mossa JS, Ageel AM. Evaluation of turmeric (Curcuma longa) for gastric and duodenal antiulcer activity in rats. J Ethnopharmacol 1990;29:25-34.

68. Gupta B, Kulshrestha VK, Srivastava RK, Prasad DN. Mechanism of curcumin induced gastric ulcer in rats. Indian J Med Res 1980;71:806-14.

69. Sakai K, Miyazaki Y, Yamane T, Saitoh Y, Ikawa C, Nishihata T. Effect of extracts of Zingiberaceae herbs on gastric secretion in rabbits. Chem Pharm Bull 1989; 37:215-7.

70. Ramirez-Boscá A, Soler A, Gutierrez MAC, Alvarez JL, Almagro EQ. Antioxidant Curcuma extracts decrease the blood lipid peroxide levels of human subjects. Age 1995;18:167-9.

71. Polasa K, Raghuram TC, Krishna TP, Krishnaswamy K. Effect of turmeric on urinary mutagens in smokers. Mutagenesis 1992;7:107-9.

72. Kositchaiwat C, Kositchaiwat S, Havanondha J. Curcuma longa Linn. in the treatment of gastric ulcer. Comparison to liquid antacid: a controlled clinical trial. J Med Assoc Thailand 1993;76:601-5.

73. Van Dau N, Ngoc Ham N, Huy Khac D, Thi Lam N, Tong Son P, Thi Tan N et al. The effects of a traditional drug, turmeric (Curcuma longa), and placebo on the healing of duodenal ulcer. Phytomedicine 1998;5:29-34.

74. Deitelhoff P, Petrowicz O, Müller B. Antidyspeptic properties of turmeric root extract. In: Abstracts of 3rd International Congress on Phytomedicine. Munich, 11-13 October 2000. Published as: Phytomedicine 2000;7(Suppl. 2):92 (Poster P-71).

75. Deodhar SD, Sethi R, Srimal RC. Preliminary study on antirheumatic activity of curcumin (diferuloyl methane). Indian J Med Res 1980;71:632-4.

76. Satoskar RR, Shah SJ, Shenoy SG. Evaluation of anti-inflammatory property of curcumin (diferuloyl methane) in patients with postoperative inflammation. Internat J Clin Pharmacol Ther Toxicol 1986;24:651-4.

77. Shoba G, Joy D, Joseph T, Majeed M, Rajendran R, Srinivas PSSR. Influence of piperine on the pharmacokinetics of curcumin in animals and human volunteers. Planta Med 1998;64:353-6.

78. Wahlström B, Blennow G. A study on the fate of curcumin in the rat. Acta Pharmacol Toxicol 1978; 43:86-92.

79. Holder GM, Plummer JL, Ryan AJ. The metabolism and excretion of curcumin (1,7-bis-(4-hydroxy-3-methoxyphenyl)-1,6-heptadiene-3,5-dione) in the rat. Xenobiotica 1978;8:761-8.

80. Ravindranath V, Chandrasekhara N. Absorption and tissue distribution of curcumin in rats. Toxicology 1980;16:259-65.

81. Ravindranath V, Chandrasekhara N. In vitro studies on the intestinal absorption of curcumin in rats. Toxicology 1981;20:251-7.

82. Ravindranath V, Chandrasekhara N. Metabolism of curcumin - studies with [^{3}H]curcumin. Toxicology 1982;22:337-44.

83. Qureshi S, Shah AH, Agee AM. Toxicity studies on Alpinia galanga and Curcuma longa. Planta Med 1992;58:124-7.

84. Bhavani Shankar TN, Shantha NV, Ramesh HP, Murthy IAS, Murthy VS. Toxicity studies on turmeric (Curcuma longa): Acute toxicity studies in rats, guinea pigs and monkeys. Indian J Exp Biol 1980;18:73-5.

85. Bille N, Larsen JC, Hansen EV, and Würtzen G. Subchronic oral toxicity of turmeric oleoresin in pigs. Food Chem Toxicol 1985;23:967-73.

86. Jensen NJ. Lack of mutagenic effect of turmeric oleoresin and curcumin in the Salmonella/mammalian microsome test. Mutation Res 1982;105:393-6.

87. Abraham SK, Kesavan PC. Genotoxicity of garlic, turmeric and asafoetida in mice. Mutation Res 1984; 136:85-8.

88. Vijayalaxmi. Genetic effects of turmeric and curcumin in mice and rats. Mutation Res 1980;79:125-32.

89. Jain AK, Tezuka H, Kada T, Tomita I. Evaluation of genotoxic effects of turmeric in mice. Current Sci 1987; 56:1005-6.

90. Giri AK, Das SK, Talukder G, Sharma A. Sister chromatid exchange and chromosome aberrations induced by curcumin and tartrazine on mammalian cells in vivo. Cytobios 1990;62:111-7.

91. Singh A, Singh SP, Bamezai R. Postnatal modulation of

hepatic biotransformation system enzymes via translactational exposure of F_1 mouse pups to turmeric and curcumin. Cancer Lett 1995;96:87-93.

92. Hata M, Sasaki E, Ota M, Fujimoto K, Yajima J, Shichida T, Honda M. Allergic contact dermatitis from curcumin (turmeric). Contact Dermatitis 1997;36:107-8.

CYNARAE FOLIUM

Artichoke Leaf

DEFINITION

Artichoke leaf consists of the dried basal leaves of *Cynara scolymus* L.

The material complies with the monograph of the Pharmacopée Française [1]. Fresh material [2] may also be used, provided that when dried it complies with the monograph of the Pharmacopée Française.

CONSTITUENTS

The characteristic constituents are caffeoylquinic acids, e.g. chlorogenic acid and 1,5-dicaffeoylquinic acid, flavonoids, e.g. luteolin 7-glucoside (cynaroside) and 7-rutinoside (scolymoside) with a smaller amount of free luteolin, and bitter-tasting sesquiterpene lactones, e.g. cynaropicrin [3-7]. Various aliphatic acids, especially hydroxy acids (e.g. lactic, glycolic, malic and hydroxymethylacrylic acids) [8,9], and caffeic acid [4], are also present.
   Cynarin (1,3-dicaffeoylquinic acid), found only in traces in the fresh or dried leaf, is generated from 1,5-dicaffeoylquinic acid during processing with hot water and is therefore usually present in aqueous extracts [3-7].

Note: The above numbering of 1,3-dicaffeoylquinic acid (cynarin) and 1,5-dicaffeoylquinic acid is in accordance with IUPAC recommendations [10]. Many papers on artichoke still number these compounds as 1,5-dicaffeoylquinic acid (cynarin) and 1,3-dicaffeoyl-quinic acid respectively.

CLINICAL PARTICULARS

Therapeutic indications
Digestive complaints (e.g. stomach ache, nausea, vomiting, feeling of fullness, flatulence) and hepato-biliary disturbances [11-17].
Adjuvant to a low fat diet in the treatment of mild to moderate hyperlipidaemia [12-15,18-22].

Posology and method of administration

Dosage
Adult daily dose: 5-10 g of dried leaf as an aqueous dry extract [11-15,19] or infusion [23]; other equivalent preparations.
Elderly: dose as for adults.
Children over 4 years: proportion of adult dose according to age or body weight.

E/S/C/O/P
MONOGRAPHS
Second Edition

Method of administration
For oral administration.

Duration of administration
No restriction. If symptoms persist, consult your doctor.

Contra-indications
Obstruction of the bile duct; known allergy to artichoke or other species of the Compositae [11].

Special warnings and special precautions for use
Patients with cholelithiasis should take artichoke leaf only after consulting a physician.

Interaction with other medicaments and other forms of interaction
None reported.

Pregnancy and lactation
No data available. In accordance with general medical practice, the product should not be used during pregnancy and lactation without medical advice.

Effects on ability to drive and use machines
None known.

Undesirable effects
Mild gastro-intestinal disturbances may occur in rare cases; allergic reactions might occur in sensitized patients [12,14,16].

Overdose
No toxic effects reported.

PHARMACOLOGICAL PROPERTIES

Pharmacodynamic properties
The pharmacologically active constituents of artichoke leaf are considered to be caffeoylquinic acids and flavonoids, which exert choleretic, hepatoprotective, antioxidant, cholesterol-lowering and lipid-lowering effects.

In vitro experiments

Antioxidant and hepatoprotective effects
Antioxidant and cytoprotective effects of an artichoke leaf aqueous dry extract (4.5:1) were demonstrated in primary cultures of rat hepatocytes exposed to *t*-butyl hydroperoxide (*t*-BHP). When added simultaneously or prior to *t*-BHP, the extract inhibited lipid peroxidation in a concentration-dependent manner down to 0.001 mg/ml [24].

Several characteristic polyphenolic constituents of artichoke leaf were effective in reducing *t*-BHP-induced malondialdehyde production; EC_{50} values were 7, 8.1, 12.5, 15.2 and 28 µg/ml for luteolin, caffeic acid, chlorogenic acid, cynarin and luteolin-

7-glucoside respectively. The extract also prevented loss of intracellular glutathione caused by *t*-BHP [24-28].

The effect of an artichoke leaf aqueous dry extract (4.5:1) on free radical production in human polymorphonuclear cells was tested by flow cytometry using phorbol 12-myristate-13-acetate as the stimulant. The extract strongly inhibited the generation of reactive oxygen species with an EC_{50} of 0.23 µg/ml [29].

Cynarin and caffeic acid showed significant cytoprotective activity (p<0.01 at 1 mg/ml) against carbon tetrachloride in isolated rat hepatocytes, reducing leakage of the liver enzymes glutamic oxaloacetic transaminase and glutamic pyruvic transaminase [30].

Artichoke leaf aqueous dry extract at 1-20 µg/ml retarded Cu^{2+}-mediated oxidation of human low density lipoprotein (LDL) in a dose-dependent manner; the effect was attributed in part to luteolin 7-glucoside (as well as to caffeoylquinic acids) [31].

Inhibitory effects on cholesterol biosynthesis
Artichoke leaf aqueous dry extract (4.5:1) inhibited the biosynthesis of cholesterol from ^{14}C-acetate in primary cultured rat hepatocytes in a concentration-dependent biphasic manner. Extract concentrations of 0.007-0.1 mg/ml produced moderate inhibition of about 20%; at 1 mg/ml the inhibition was about 80% [32,33]. At 50-100 µg/ml, caffeic acid and cynarin produced negligible inhibition, chlorogenic acid 10-15% and cynaroside (luteolin 7-glucoside) 19-22%, but luteolin 51-63% [33]. When cynaroside was incubated with β-glucosidase, maximum inhibition of 50-60% was observed, with an EC_{50} of approx. 30 µM. In human hepatic (HepG2) cells the maximum response of luteolin was more than 80% and the EC_{50} value was slightly higher. It was concluded that luteolin (a minor constituent) and indirectly its glucoside, cynaroside, seem to be mainly responsible for the inhibition of hepatic biosynthesis of cholesterol by artichoke leaf extracts [33,34].

Subsequently it was demonstrated that, while artichoke extracts inhibit cholesterol biosynthesis from ^{14}C-acetate in primary cultured rat hepatocytes, inhibition in human hepatic (HepG2) cells is weak unless they have been pre-treated with β-glucosidase. This was explained by the fact that rat hepatocytes contain more endogenous β-glucosidase, enabling release of luteolin from its glucoside, cynaroside. Since β-glucosidase is present in the intestinal tract and in the liver, release of luteolin from cynaroside may occur in the human body [35].

Hepatobiliary effects
An artichoke leaf aqueous dry extract enhanced the secretion of biliary substances in bile canaliculi

reformed in primary cultures of hepatocytes. A cholestatic effect induced in the cultures by lithocholate was inhibited by the extract [36].

The effect of pressed juice (sap) from fresh artichoke on choleretic activity was investigated in isolated perfused rat liver. Pressed juice, undiluted and diluted 1:3 and 1:5, produced dose-dependent increases in bile flow of up to 150%, 125% and 112% respectively, detectable 20 minutes after addition and reaching maximum values 10 minutes later. Bile acid production remained almost unchanged [37]. By testing fractions of the pressed juice, it was shown that phenolic constituents were mainly responsible for the choleretic action, the strongest effects on both choleresis and bile acid production being exerted by mono- and dicaffeoylquinic acids [38].

In further experiments with isolated perfused rat liver, a different pressed juice (from fresh artichoke flower buds) produced a comparable increase in bile flow and increased bile acid excretion by up to 128%. In contrast, dried pressed juice (16:1, from flower buds) and dry aqueous extract (4:1) from artichoke leaf increased bile flow without significantly increasing bile acid secretion and no correlation with the content of caffeoylquinic acids was evident [39].

In vivo experiments

Hepatobiliary and hepatoprotective effects
A deproteinized aqueous extract of artichoke leaf, administered orally to partially hepatectomized rats at 0.5 ml/animal daily for 21 days, significantly increased liver tissue regeneration as measured by residual liver weight, mitotic index and percentage of binucleated liver cells [40]. In further experiments using the same methodology, the deproteinized extract accelerated the increase in liver weight, induced pronounced hyperaemia, and increased the percentage of binuclear hepatocytes and the content of ribonucleic acid in liver cells [41].

Two hydroethanolic extracts of fresh artichoke [42] were administered intraperitoneally to groups of rats: a total extract (19% caffeoylquinic acids; 200 mg/kg body weight) and a purified extract enriched in phenolic compounds (46% caffeoylquinic acids; 25 mg/kg body weight). Through bile duct cannulation it was shown that both extracts stimulated choleresis, significantly increasing the bile dry residue and total cholate secretion ($p<0.05$) [43]. The same extracts administered orally (400 mg/kg body weight of total extract or 200 mg/kg of purified extract) increased gastrointestinal propulsion in rats by 11% and 14% respectively ($p<0.05$) [43].

An aqueous extract of artichoke leaf (2.2% caffeoylquinic acids, 0.9% luteolin 7-glucoside), administered orally to rats at 500 mg/kg body weight

48 hours, 24 hours and 1 hour before inducing liver intoxication with carbon tetrachloride, improved liver function as measured by decreased levels of bilirubin, glutathione and liver enzymes [44].

In bile duct cannulated rats, an undefined artichoke leaf fluid extract (0.45 mg/kg body weight), administered intraperitoneally, produced increases of 32% in bile flow and 49% in bile acid concentration respectively [45].

Chlorogenic acid administered orally to rats at 5-40 mg/kg body weight significantly stimulated choleresis (70%) and peristaltic activity (40%) in a concentration-dependent manner [46]. A dose-dependent increase in bile flow of up to 95% and an increase in biliary-excreted cholesterol was observed following a single intravenous administration of cynarin (7-166 mg/kg body weight) in the bile fistula rat model. Choleresis was still observed 4 hours after administration of 100 or 166 mg/kg body weight [47-50].

Intraperitoneal administration of a purified, acid-rich, butanolic extract of artichoke leaf at 10 mg/kg protected mice against toxicity induced by ethanol; the LD_{50} for treated mice was 6.8 g ethanol/kg compared to 5.6 g ethanol/kg for the control group. The effect of the artichoke extract could be reproduced by administration of a mixture of citric, malic, succinic and hydroxymethylacrylic acids (2.5 mg/kg; LD_{50} of 7.1 g ethanol/kg) [51].

Lipid-lowering and anti-atherogenic effects
Powdered artichoke aerial parts, administered orally at 110 mg/kg body weight for 120 days to rats fed on an atherogenic diet, lowered increases in serum and liver cholesterol and prevented the formation of atherosclerotic plaques [52-54]. After 60 days on an atherogenic diet, 110 mg/kg body weight of powdered artichoke aerial parts, administered orally to rats daily for 10 weeks, lowered serum cholesterol by 36% compared to 25% in the control group [55].

Two hydroethanolic extracts of fresh artichoke, a total extract (19% caffeoylquinic acids; 100 mg/kg body weight) and a purified extract (46% caffeoylquinic acids; 25 mg/kg body weight), administered intraperitoneally to rats four times over a 28-hour period after inducing hyperlipidaemia with Triton WR 1339, decreased total cholesterol by 14% and 45%, and triglycerides by 18% and 33%, respectively [43].

Cynarin (100 and 200 mg/kg body weight), administered intravenously to rabbits, lowered serum cholesterol by about 20%. Triton WR 1339-induced hypercholesterolaemia in rats was significantly lowered ($p=0.05-0.02$) by cynarin after intraperitoneal administration (2 × 200 mg/kg body weight) [47]. Cynarin injected at 30 mg/kg/day significantly lowered the increases in total serum lipids ($p<0.05$) and esterified serum fatty acids (p<0.001) induced in rats by giving them 15% ethanol instead of drinking water for 70 days [56].

Pharmacological studies in humans

Choleretic effect
In a double-blind, placebo-controlled, cross-over study, the choleretic effect of a single dose of dry aqueous extract (4.5-5:1) of artichoke leaf was investigated in 20 male volunteers with acute or chronic metabolic disorders. To subjects in two randomized groups of 10, either 1.92 g of the extract (the contents of 6 proprietary capsules, each containing 320 mg of extract plus excipients) in 50 ml water or a placebo of similar appearance was administered via an intraduodenal probe, the subjects having empty stomachs on test days. Crossover to the alternative medication followed an 8-day washout phase. Monitoring of bile secretion was accomplished using multichannel probes. Compared to initial values, mean bile secretion was significantly higher (p<0.01) in the verum group: 127% higher 30 minutes after administration, 151% after 60 minutes (the maximum effect) and 94% after 90 minutes; results after 120 minutes and 150 minutes were also significantly higher (p<0.05). Placebo treatment stimulated bile secretion to a lesser extent, with a maximum increase of 39% after 30 minutes. No adverse effects or relevant changes in laboratory safety parameters were observed [17].

Lipid-lowering effects
In a randomized, double-blind, placebo-controlled study, the lipid-lowering effects of an artichoke leaf aqueous dry extract were investigated in 44 healthy volunteers over 12 weeks. The mean initial concentrations of total cholesterol were very low in both the verum (204.2 mg/dl, n_v = 22) and placebo (203.0 mg/dl, n_p = 22) groups. In volunteers with initial cholesterol > 230 mg/dl (n_v = n_p = 3), 640 mg of extract three times daily significantly decreased concentrations of total cholesterol (p = 0.015) and triglycerides (p = 0.01) compared to placebo. In volunteers with initial cholesterol > 220 mg/dl (n_v = n_p = 5), serum cholesterol was not significantly different (p = 0.14) after treatment with the extract compared to placebo; however, a significant difference (p = 0.012) could be detected for triglycerides. In volunteers with initial cholesterol > 210 mg/dl (n_v = 10, n_p = 7), treatment with the extract led to a significant difference (p = 0.022) for triglycerides compared to placebo [19].

Decreases in cholesterol, triglycerides, free fatty acids, phospholipids and β-lipoproteins were observed in 30 healthy elderly subjects after daily administration for 6 weeks of 0.45 or 0.9 g of an undefined artichoke extract containing 0.09% of polyphenols [21].

Daily administration of 900 mg of an artichoke extract with a minimum polyphenolic acids content of 5.5% to 10 industrial workers with long term occupational exposure to carbon disulfide for 30 days significantly lowered blood levels of cholesterol (p<0.02), free fatty acids, phospholipids and total lipids (p<0.05) [20].

Other effects
Two further studies involved workers with long term occupational exposure to carbon disulfide. 43 men were treated daily with an artichoke syrup (40 ml, corresponding to 0.9 g of artichoke extract, containing a minimum of 0.09% polyphenolic acids); after 1 year of treatment pathological electroretinograms became normal in about 28% of subjects [57]. Daily administration of 40 ml of the same syrup to 62 men significantly lowered spontaneous platelet aggregation by the end of 1 year (p<0.01) and 2 years (p<0.001) [58].

Thermometric (energy expenditure, respiratory quotient) and cardiovascular (heart rate, systolic and diastolic blood pressure) monitoring of healthy young volunteers after administration of a single large dose (1.92 g) of dry aqueous extract of artichoke leaf showed no increases in these parameters which would indicate any potential for artichoke leaf as a thermogenic agent in the treatment of human obesity [59].

Clinical studies

Antidyspeptic and lipid-lowering effects
In a multicentre, randomized, placebo-controlled, double-blind study, the effect of a fresh artichoke leaf aqueous dry extract (25-35:1) was investigated in 143 patients with hyperlipoproteinaemia (cholesterol > 280 mg/dl). Patients received either 1800 mg of artichoke extract (n = 71) or placebo (n = 72) daily as coated tablets for 6 weeks. In the verum group, reductions of total cholesterol (18.5%) and LDL-cholesterol (22.9%) from baseline to end of treatment were significantly superior (p= 0.0001) to those in the placebo group (8.6% and 6.3% respectively). The LDL/HDL ratio decreased by 20.2% in the artichoke extract group and 7.2% in the placebo group [18].

A multicentre open study with an average treatment duration of 43.5 days was conducted in 553 patients with dyspeptic complaints. The daily dose was generally 3-6 capsules of artichoke leaf aqueous dry extract (3.8-5.5:1, 320 mg per capsule). Digestive complaints declined in a clinically relevant and statistically significant manner within 6 weeks of treatment, the overall symptoms improving by about 71%. Compared to initial values, the subjective score reduction was approx. 66% for meteorism, 76% for abdominal pain, 82% for nausea and 88% for emesis. In a subgroup of 302 patients, total cholesterol decreased by 11.5% and triglycerides by 12.5%, while HDL-cholesterol showed a minimal rise of

2.3%. Global efficacy assessed by the physicians was excellent or good in 87% of cases [12].

The same extract at a daily dosage of 3-6 capsules (320 mg per capsule) was evaluated in a 6-month open study of 203 patients with dyspeptic complaints. After 21 weeks of treatment, the overall improvement in symptoms was 66% compared to initial values, e.g. vomiting by 84%, abdominal pain by 78%, nausea by 76%, flatulence by 70% and meteorism by 69%. Concentrations of total blood cholesterol and triglycerides, determined in 171 and 170 patients, decreased by 10.9% and 11.0% respectively. From determinations in 159 patients, LDL-cholesterol decreased by 15.8% and HDL-cholesterol increased by 6.3%. Global efficacy assessed by the physicians was excellent or good in 85.7% of cases. No adverse reactions were reported [13].

In a comparative study, 73 patients with primary hypertriglyceridaemia resistant to treatment with clofibrate were treated daily for 1 month with an undefined artichoke extract (9 tablets, each containing 5 mg of polyphenolic acids, n = 25) or with cynarin (0.75 g, n = 28 or 1.5 g, n = 20). The artichoke extract exerted significant total lipid-, triglyceride- and phospholipid-lowering effects in about 56% of the patients, whereas 0.75 g or 1.5 g of cynarin improved lipid parameters in 61% or 40% of the patients respectively [22].

In an open study, 403 patients with functional gall bladder disorders were treated with an undefined artichoke extract (2 tablets twice daily, each containing 375 mg of extract standardized to 1% caffeoylquinic acids). After 4 weeks of treatment, complaints such as nausea, stomach pains or loss of appetite had disappeared in more than 52% of patients and symptoms had improved in more than 80% of patients [16].

Other effects
In a placebo-controlled, double-blind study in malaria patients, a purified aqueous dry extract from fresh artichoke leaf juice administered intramuscularly (100 mg/day) and orally (1600 mg/day) for 3 days, continuing the oral treatment on days 4 to 7 (n = 46), or placebo (n = 46), was given as treatment additional to standard quinine therapy. More rapid improvements in clinical symptoms of malaria observed in patients given artichoke therapy in addition to quinine were attributed to hepatoprotective effects of the artichoke extract [60].

Pharmacokinetic properties
No data available.

Preclinical safety data

Acute toxicity
The oral LD_{50} and intraperitoneal LD_{10} in male rats of a hydroalcoholic total extract of artichoke leaf (19% caffeoylquinic acids) were determined as > 2000 mg/kg and > 1000 mg/kg body weight respectively; with a purified extract (46% caffeoylquinic acids) the oral LD_{40} and intraperitoneal LD_{50} were 2000 mg/kg and 265 mg/kg respectively [42].

The LD_{50} of cynarin in mice was determined as 1900 mg/kg body weight. When administered intraperitoneally to rats at 800 mg/kg or intravenously to rabbits at 1000 mg/kg/hour, cynarin produced no apparent side effects or signs of toxicity [47].

Subacute toxicity
Cynarin administered intraperitoneally to adult rats for 15 days at doses of 50-400 mg/kg/day produced no macroscopic or histological abnormalities or changes in blood parameters [47].

Chronic toxicity
Cynarin administered intraperitoneally to rats daily for 40 days at 50-400 mg/kg/day caused no changes in overall condition or blood parameters. Increased body weight and significantly increased kidney weight (p<0.01) were observed only in animals treated with 400 mg/kg and significantly increased liver weight (p<0.01) in animals treated with 100-400 mg/kg. Some rats treated with cynarin at 100, 200 and 400 mg/kg showed irritative-degenerative changes in liver and kidneys, most evident in rats receiving 400 mg [46]. Young rabbits treated intravenously with cynarin at 50 mg/kg/day for 30 days remained in good condition with no evidence of toxicity from extensive haematological and histological investigation [47].

In primary cultures of rat hepatocytes no cytotoxic effects from an artichoke leaf aqueous dry extract (4.5:1) were observed at concentrations of up to 1 mg per ml of culture medium [24,26,27,61].

Clinical safety data
No major adverse events have been reported from clinical or human pharmacological studies with preparations containing extracts of artichoke leaf involving over 1600 subjects and study durations of up to 2 years. In all, 19 minor adverse events were reported, mainly gastrointestinal complaints [12,13,16-22,57,58,60,62]. A systematic review of published human studies concluded that safety data for artichoke leaf extracts indicate only mild and infrequent adverse effects [63].

REFERENCES

1. Artichaut - Cynara scolymus. Pharmacopée Française.

2. Brand N. Die Artischocke - eine Dekade interdisziplinärer Forschung. Z Phytother 1999;20:292-302.

3. Brand N, Weschta H. Die analytische Bewertung der Artischocke und ihrer Präparate. Z Phytother 1991; 12:15-21.

4. Schilcher H. Pharmazeutische Aspekte pflanzlicher Gallentherapeutika. Z Phytother 1995;16:211-22.

5. Brand N. Cynara scolymus L. - Die Artischocke. Z Phytother 1990;11:169-75.

6. Brand N. Der Extrakt in Artischockenpräparaten. Pharmazeutische Aspekte eines pflanzlichen Wirkstoffes. Dtsch Apoth Ztg 1997;137:3564-78.

7. Wagenbreth D, Grün M, Wagenbreth A-N, Wegener T. Artischocke - Qualitätsdroge aus Arzneipflanzenanbau. Dtsch Apoth Ztg 1996;136:3818-26.

8. Bogaert J-P, Mortier F, Jouany J-M, Pelt J-M, Delaveau P. Acides organiques, en particulier acides-alcools du Cynara scolymus L. (Composées). Ann Pharm Fr 1972; 30:401-8.

9. Bogaert J-P, Mortier F, Jouany J-M, Delaveau P, Pelt J-M. Caractérisation et dosage de l'acide hydroxyméthylacrylique dans les feuilles de Cynara scolymus L. (Compositae). Plantes Méd Phytothér 1974;8:199-203.

10. IUPAC Commission on the Nomenclature of Organic Chemistry (CNOC) and IUPAC-IUB Commission on Biochemical Nomenclature (CBN). Nomenclature of Cyclitols: Recommendations, 1973. Biochem J 1976; 153:23-31.

11. Hänsel R, Keller K, Rimpler H, Schneider G, editors. Cynara. In: Hagers Handbuch der Pharmazeutischen Praxis, 5th ed. Volume 4: Drogen A-D. Berlin: Springer-Verlag, 1992:1117-22.

12. Fintelmann V. Antidyspeptische und lipidsenkende Wirkungen von Artischockenblätterextrakt. Ergebnisse klinischer Untersuchungen zur Wirksamkeit und Verträglichkeit von Hepar-SL® forte an 553 Patienten. Z Allg Med 1996;72 (Suppl 2):3-19.
Clinical data also reported in:
Fintelmann V, Menßen HG. Artischockenblätterextrakt. Dtsch Apoth Ztg 1996;136:1405-14.

13. Fintelmann V, Petrowicz O. Langzeitanwendung eines Artischocken-Extraktes bei dyspeptischem Symptomkomplex. Ergebnisse einer Beobachtungsstudie. Naturamed 1998;13:17-26.

14. Kraft K. Artichoke leaf extract - Recent findings reflecting effects on lipid metabolism, liver and gastrointestinal tracts. Phytomedicine 1997;4:369-78.

15. Barnes J, Anderson LA and Phillipson JD. Artichoke. In: Herbal Medicines - A guide for healthcare professionals, 2nd ed. London-Chicago: Pharmaceutical Press,

2002:61-6.

16. Held C. Tagungsbericht von der 1. Deutsch-Ungarischen Phytopharmakon-Konferenz. Budapest, 20 November 1991. Z Klin Med 1992;47:92-3.

17. Kirchhoff R, Beckers C, Kirchhoff GM, Trinczek-Gärtner H, Petrowicz O, Reimann HJ. Increase in choleresis by means of artichoke extract. Phytomedicine 1994;1:107-15.
Also published in German as:
Kirchhoff R, Beckers C, Kirchhoff G, Trinczek-Gärtner H, Petrowicz O, Reimann H-J. Steigerung der Cholerese durch Artischockenextrakt. Ergebnisse einer plazebokontrollierten Doppelblindstudie. Ärztl Forsch 1993;40(6):1-12.

18. Englisch W, Beckers C, Unkauf M, Ruepp M, Zinserling V. Efficacy of artichoke dry extract in patients with hyperlipoproteinemia. Arzneim-Forsch/Drug Res 2000; 50:260-5.

19. Petrowicz O, Gebhardt R, Donner M, Schwandt P, Kraft K. Effects of artichoke leaf extract (ALE) on lipoprotein metabolism in vitro and in vivo [Abstract]. Atherosclerosis 1997;129:147.

20. Wójcicki J, Winter S. Effect of preparation Cynarex on the blood serum lipids level of the workers exposed to the chronic action of carbon disulphide. Medycyna Pracy 1975;26:213-7 [POLISH/English summary].

21. Wójcicki J, Samochowiec L, Kosmider K. Influence of an extract from artichoke (Cynara scolymus L.) on the level of lipids in serum of aged men. Herba Pol 1981;27:265-8 [POLISH/English summary].

22. Wójcicki J, Olejak B, Pieczul-Mróz J, Torbus-Lisiecka B, Bukowska H, Gregorczyk J. The use of 1,5-dicaffeoylquinic acid in the treatment of hypertriglyceridemia. Przeglad Lek 1982;39:601-6 [POLISH/English summary].

23. Tisanes. In : Pharmacopée Française, Xᵉ ed. 1989.

24. Gebhardt R. Antioxidative and protective properties of extracts from leaves of the artichoke (Cynara scolymus L.) against hydroperoxide-induced oxidative stress in cultured rat hepatocytes. Toxicol Appl Pharmacol 1997; 144:279-86.

25. Gebhardt R, Fausel M. Antioxidant and hepatoprotective effects of artichoke extracts and constituents in cultured rat hepatocytes. Toxicol in Vitro 1997; 11:669-72.

26. Gebhardt R. Protektive antioxidative Wirkungen von Artischockenextrakt an der Leberzelle. Med Welt 1995; 46:393-5.

27. Gebhardt R. Neue experimentelle Erkenntnisse zur Wirkung von Artischockenblätterextrakt. Z Allg Med 1996;72 (Suppl 2):20-3.

28. Gebhardt R, Rexhepaj R, Fausel M. Antioxidative und hepatoprotektive Wirkung von Flavonoiden aus Blattextrakten der Artischocke. Ein Vergleich an Hepatozytenkulturen unter Einwirkung toxischer

Hydroperoxide. Z Phytotherapie 1999;20:97-8.

29. Pérez-García F, Adzet T, Canigueral S. Effect of an artichoke leaf extract on free radical production in human leukocytes. In: Franz G, Vieweger U, editors. Proceedings of 45th Annual Congress of Society for Medicinal Plant Research, Regensburg, 7-12 September 1997 (Abstract H 09).

30. Adzet T, Camarasa J, Laguna JC. Hepatoprotective activity of polyphenolic compounds from Cynara scolymus against CCl_4 toxicity in isolated rat hepatocytes. J Nat Prod 1987;50:612-7.

31. Brown JE, Rice-Evans CA. Luteolin-rich artichoke extract protects low density lipoprotein from oxidation in vitro. Free Radical Res 1998;29:247-55.

32. Gebhardt R. Artischockenextrakt - In-vitro-Nachweis einer Hemmwirkung auf die Cholesterinbiosynthese. Med Welt 1995;46:348-50.

33. Gebhardt R. Inhibition of cholesterol biosynthesis in primary cultured rat hepatocytes by artichoke (Cynara scolymus L.) extracts. J Pharmacol Exp Ther 1998; 286:1122-8.

34. Gebhardt R. Inhibition of hepatic cholesterol biosynthesis by artichoke leaf extracts is mainly due to luteolin [Poster]. Cell Biol Toxicol 1997;13:58.

35. Gebhardt R, Hanika A. Hemmung der Cholesterin-Biosynthese durch Blätterextrakte der Artischocke in HepG2-Zellen. Verstärkung durch Vorinkubation mit β-Glukosidase intensiviert. Z Phytotherapie 1999;20:95-6.

36. Gebhardt R. Hepatocellular actions of artichoke extracts: stimulation of biliary secretion, inhibition of cholesterol biosynthesis and antioxidant properties. In: Abstracts of 2nd International Congress on Phytomedicine, Munich, 11-14 September 1996 (Abstract SL-35). Published as: Phytomedicine 1996;3 (Suppl. 1):51.

37. Matuschowski P, Gumbinger HG, Nahrstedt A, Winterhoff H. Testing of Cynara scolymus L. in the isolated perfused rat liver. In: Abstracts of 44th Annual Congress of Medicinal Plant Research, Prague. 3-7 September 1997. Published as: Planta Med 1997;63 (Suppl.):55 (Abstract P 44).

38. Matuschowski P. Beitrag zur Pharmakologie und Wirkstoff-Findung von Cynara scolymus L. [Dissertation]. University of Münster, Germany, 1998.

39. Flume M, Nahrstedt A, Winterhoff H. Einfluß verschiedener Zubereitungen aus Cynara scolymus L. auf Gallenfluß und Gallensäureausscheidung [Poster]. In: Abstracts of 10. Jahrestagung der Gesellschaft für Phytotherapie, Münster, 11-13 November 1999: Phytotherapie an der Schwelle zum neuen Jahrtausend, 1999:100-1 (Poster P13).

40. Maros T, Rácz G, Katonai B, Kovács VV. Wirkungen der Cynara scolymus-Extrakte auf die Regeneration der Rattenleber, 1. Mitteilung. Arzneim-Forsch/Drug Res 1966;16:127-9.

41. Maros T, Seres-Sturm L, Rácz G, Rettegi C, Kovács VV,

Hints M. Wirkungen der Cynara scolymus-Extrakte auf die Regeneration der Rattenleber, 2. Mitteilung. Arzneim-Forsch/Drug Res 1968;18:884-6.

42. Bombardelli E, Gabetta B, Martinelli EM. Gas-liquid chromatographic and mass spectrometric investigation on Cynara scolymus extracts. Fitoterapia 1977;48:143-52.

43. Lietti A. Choleretic and cholesterol lowering properties of two artichoke extracts. Fitoterapia 1977;48:153-8.

44. Adzet T, Camarasa J, Hernandez JS, Laguna JC. Action of an artichoke extract against CCl_4-induced hepatotoxicity in rats. Acta Pharm Jugosl 1987;37:183-7.

45. García-Giménez MD, de la Puerta Vázquez R, Sáenz-Rodríguez MT. Actividad colerética de distintas especies del género Helichrysum Miller. Rev Farmacol Clin Exp 1990;7:79-83.

46. Czok G, Lang K. Chlorogensäure-Wirkungen am Magen-Darmkanal. Arzneim Forsch 1961;11:545-9.

47. Preziosi P, Loscalzo B. Pharmacological properties of 1,4-dicaffeylquinic acid, the active principle of Cynara scolymus. Arch Int Pharmacodyn 1958;117:63-80.

48. Preziosi P, Loscalzo B, Marmo E. Comparison of choleretic effects of CYN and Na-dehydrocholate. Experientia 1959;15:135-8.

49. Preziosi P, Loscalzo B. L'azione sulla coleresi, sul colesterolo ematico e sulla lipoidosi colesterolica del principio attivo del carciofo e di sostanze ad esso correlate. Fitoterapia 1956;27:666-72.

50. Preziosi P. Loscalzo B, Marmo E, Miele E. Effects of single or repeated treatment with several anti-cholesterolemic compounds on biliary excretion of cholesterol. Biochem Pharmacol 1960;5:251-62.

51. Mortier F, Bogaert J-P, Jouany J-M, Dixneuf P, Delaveau P. Action d'un extrait purifié de Cynara scolymus L. (Composées) sur l'intoxication aiguë par l'éthanol. Plantes Méd Phytothér 1976;10:36-43

52. Samochowiec L. Investigations on experimental atherosclerosis. Part XV. The effect of Cynara scolymus L. and Cynara cardunculus L. on the development of experimental atherosclerosis in white rats. Diss Pharm 1959;11:99-113 [POLISH/English summary].

53. Samochowiec L. The action of herbs and roots of artichokes (Cynara scolymus L.) and cardoons (Cynara cardunculus L.) on the development of experimental atherosclerosis in white rats. Diss Pharm 1962;14:115-22 [POLISH/English summary].

54. Samochowiec L, Habczynska D, Wazna-Bogunska C. The influence of atherogenic diet and artichokes (Cynara scolymus L) and cardoons (Cynara cardunculus L.) on the histopathology of coronary arteries and myocardium in white rats. Patologia Polska 1962;13:337-48 [POLISH/English summary].

55. Samochowiec L. The effect of artichokes (Cynara scolymus L.) and cardoons (Cynara cardunculus L.) on developed atherosclerotic changes in white rats. Folia

Biol 1962;10:75-83.

56. Samochowiec L, Wojcicki J, Kadykow M. The influence of 1,5-dicaffeoylquinic acid on serum lipids in the experimentally alcoholised rat. Panminerva Med 1971; 13:87-8.

57. Palacz O, Czepita D, Wójcicki J. Electroretinographic investigations in subjects in chronic exposure to carbon disulphide. III. Cynarex effect on ERG related to blood lipid pattern. Klin Oczna 1981;83:223-5 [POLISH/English summary].

58. Woyke M, Cwajda H, Wójcicki J, Kosmider K. Platelets aggregation in workers chronically exposed to carbon disulphide and subjected to prophylactic effects of Cynarex preparation. Med Pracy 1981;32:261-4 [POLISH/English summary].

59. Martinet A, Hostettmann K, Schutz Y. Thermogenic effects of commercially available plant preparations aimed at treating human obesity. Phytomedicine 1999; 6:231-8.

60. Wone E, Barondra-Haaby E, de Lauture H. Intérêt de l´intégration systématique du chophytol dans le traitement ambulatoire du paludisme. Afrique Médicale 1986;25:233-40.

61. Gebhardt R. Hepatoprotektion durch Extrakt aus Artischocken. Pharm Ztg 1995;140:34-7.

62. Siedek H, Hammerl H, Pichler O. Cholerese und Cholesterinstoffwechsel. Wiener Klin Wschr 1963; 75:460-3.

63. Pittler MH, Ernst E. Artichoke leaf extract for serum cholesterol reduction. Perfusion 1998;11:338-340.

ECHINACEAE PALLIDAE RADIX

Pale Coneflower Root

DEFINITION

Pale coneflower root consists of the fresh or dried underground parts of *Echinacea pallida* (Nutt.) Nutt., harvested at the end of the vegetation period [1].

A draft monograph on pale coneflower root, intended for inclusion in the European Pharmacopoeia, has been published [2].

CONSTITUENTS

The characteristic constituents are caffeoyl derivatives, especially echinacoside (0.5-1.0%) [1,3-9], essential oil (0.2-2.0%) [1,3-5,10] containing alkenes such as pentadeca-1,8Z-diene [1,10,11], and a range of ketoalkenes and ketoalkenynes [1,3-7,10], principally pentadeca-8Z-ene-2-one [5,10] together with pentadeca-8Z,11Z-diene-2-one, pentadeca-8Z,13Z-diene-11-yne-2-one, tetradeca-8Z-ene-11,13-diyne-2-one and others [1,3-6,10].

8-hydroxyketoalkenynes are produced by oxidation on storage of the dried drug. They include 8-hydroxy-tetradeca-9E-ene-11,13-diyne-2-one, 8-hydroxy-pentadeca-9E-ene-11,13-diyne-2-one and 8-hydroxy-pentadeca-9E,13Z-diene-11-yne-2-one [1,3-6].

Other constituents include glycoproteins and polysaccharides [12].

CLINICAL PARTICULARS

Therapeutic indications
Adjuvant therapy and prophylaxis of recurrent infections of the upper respiratory tract (common cold) [13,14].

Posology and method of administration

Dosage

Adult daily dose: Hydroethanolic extracts corresponding to 900 mg of crude drug [13,14]; other equivalent preparations.
Children: proportion of adult dose according to age or body weight.

Method of administration
For oral administration.

Duration of administration
The duration of treatment should not exceed 8 weeks.

Contra-indications
Known hypersensitivity to plants of the Compositae.

As with all immunostimulants, not recommended in progressive systemic disorders or autoimmune diseases such as tuberculosis, leucoses, collagenoses, multiple sclerosis, AIDS, HIV infections [1].

Special warnings and special precautions for use
None required.

Interaction with other medicaments and other forms of interaction
None reported.

Pregnancy and lactation
In accordance with general medical practice, the product should not be used during pregnancy or lactation without medical advice.

No statistical difference from the control group was seen in terms of pregnancy outcome, delivery method, maternal weight gain, gestational age, birth weight or fetal distress following gestational exposure to oral preparations containing echinacea in a prospective controlled study involving 412 women. The preparations contained extracts mainly from *Echinacea angustifolia* and *E. purpurea*; only one was an *E. pallida* preparation [15].

Effects on ability to drive and use machines
None known.

Undesirable effects
In rare cases hypersensitivity reactions, e.g. skin reactions, may occur [1].

Overdose
No toxic effects reported.

PHARMACOLOGICAL PROPERTIES

Pharmacodynamic properties

In vitro experiments

Influence on immune function
A 90% ethanolic extract (1:10) of pale coneflower root at a concentration of 10^{-2} mg/ml enhanced the phagocytosis index of human granulocytes by 23%; no effect was observed at concentrations of 10^{-6} mg/ml or lower. The chloroform-soluble fraction from the ethanolic extract increased phagocytosis by 39% at 10^{-4} mg/ml, while the water-soluble fraction stimulated phagocytosis by a maximum of only 14% at 10^{-3} mg/ml [16].

A high molecular weight fraction ($M_r > 10,000$ D) containing polysaccharides and glycoproteins from

pale coneflower root enhanced the proliferation of mouse spleen cells, and stimulated the production of interferon (IFNα/β) and immunoglobulin M as well as the number of antibody-producing cells in spleen cell cultures. It also increased the production of cytokines (such as interleukin-1, interleukin-6 and tumour necrosis factor α) and nitric oxide in mouse macrophage cultures [12,17]. Incubation of this fraction with human monocytes enhanced the production of interleukin-1, interleukin-6 and tumour necrosis factor α [17].

Antioxidant activity
Methanolic extracts from pale coneflower root exhibited antioxidant activity, the mechanisms of which include free radical scavenging and transition metal chelating [18,19].

Caffeoyl derivatives (such as echinacoside) protected collagen from free radical-induced degradation in a dose-dependent manner [20].

Antimicrobial activity
The antibacterial activity of echinacoside (8×10^{-3} M) against *Staphylococcus aureus* corresponds to approx. 10 Oxford units of penicillin [21].

Extracts of pale coneflower root exhibited near UV-mediated phototoxic and antifungal activity, measured by inhibition of the growth of *Candida shehata*: the activity was attributed primarily to ketoalkenes and ketoalkynes [22].

A high molecular weight fraction ($M_r > 10,000$ D) containing polysaccharides and glycoproteins from pale coneflower root exhibited antiviral activity against *Herpes simplex* virus type 1 in a plaque-reduction assay [12]. Antiviral activity of echinacoside against vesicular stomatitis virus in L-929 mouse cells was demonstrated in a plaque reduction assay [9].

In vivo experiments

Phagocytosis-stimulating effects
In the carbon clearance test in mice, oral administration of a 90%-ethanolic extract (1:10) of pale coneflower root daily for 2 days at 0.5 ml/kg body weight increased phagocytosis 2.2-fold. When chloroform- and water-soluble fractions of the ethanol extract were administered separately at concentrations corresponding to their content in the original extract, the lipophilic fraction (2.6-fold increase) proved more active than the hydrophilic (1.3-fold increase) [16].

Intravenous injection of 50, 100 or 500 µl of a high molecular weight fraction ($M_r > 10,000$ D) containing polysaccharides and glycoproteins from pale coneflower root significantly increased the concentration of the cytokine interleukin-1 in the serum of mice ($p < 0.05$) [12]. A single oral administration of this

127

fraction to mice at 3.7 mg per animal significantly enhanced antibody production in Peyer's plaque cells [17].

Clinical studies

In a randomized, double-blind study, 160 patients with influenza-like infections of the upper respiratory tract were treated for 8-10 days with either a hydroalcoholic liquid extract of pale coneflower root at a daily dose corresponding to 900 mg of dried root (n = 80) or placebo (n = 80). Significant improvements in four major symptoms, common cold, weakness, pain in arms and legs, and headache (p<0.0001), and in the overall symptom score (p<0.0004), were observed in the verum group compared to the placebo group. Also, the duration of illness was significantly shorter in verum patients (p<0.0001): in those with putative bacterial infections, 9.8 days compared to 13.0 with placebo; in those with putative viral infections, 9.1 days compared to 12.9 with placebo [13].

REFERENCES

1. Liersch R, Bauer R. *Echinacea*. In: Hänsel R, Keller K, Rimpler H, Schneider G, editors. Hagers Handbuch der Pharmazeutischen Praxis, 5th ed. Volume 5: Drogen E-O. Berlin: Springer-Verlag, 1993:1-34.

2. Pale Coneflower Root - Echinaceae pallidae radix. Pharmeuropa 2002;14:137-8.

3. Bauer R. Echinacea - Eine Arzneidroge auf dem Weg zum rationalen Phytotherapeutikum. Dtsch Apoth Ztg 1994;134:94-103.

4. Bauer R, Wagner H. Chapter 4: Chemie der Inhaltsstoffe. In: Echinacea - Handbuch für Ärzte, Apotheker und andere Naturwissenschaftler. Stuttgart: Wissenschaftliche Verlagsgesellschaft, 1990:67-91.

5. Bauer R, Khan IA, Wagner H. TLC and HPLC analysis of *Echinacea pallida* and *E. angustifolia* roots. Planta Med 1988;54:426-30.

6. Bauer R, Wray V, Wagner H. The chemical discrimination of *Echinacea angustifolia* and *E. pallida*. Pharm Weekbl Sci Ed 1987;9:220.

7. Bauer R, Remiger P. Der Einsatz der HPLC bei der Standardisierung von Echinacea-Drogen. Arch Pharm (Weinheim) 1989;322:324.

8. Bauer R, Wagner H. Neue Ergebnisse zur Analytik von *Echinacea*-Wurzeln. Sci Pharm 1987;55:159-61.

9. Cheminat A, Zawatzky R, Becker H, Brouillard R. Caffeoyl conjugates from *Echinacea* species: structures and biological activity. Phytochemistry 1988;27:2787-94.

10. Heinzer F, Chavanne M, Meusy J-P, Maltre H-P, Giger E, Baumann TW. Ein Beitrag zur Klassifizierung der therapeutisch verwendeten Arten der Gattung Echinacea. Pharm Acta Helv 1988;63:132-6.

11. Voaden DJ, Jacobson M. Tumor inhibitors. 3. Identification and synthesis of an oncolytic hydrocarbon from American coneflower roots. J Med Chem 1972; 15:619-23.

12. Beuscher N, Bodinet C, Willigmann I, Egert D. Immunmodulierende Eigenschaften von Wurzelextrakten verschiedener *Echinacea*-Arten. Z Phytother 1995;16:157-66.

13. Bräunig B, Knick E. Therapeutische Erfahrungen mit Echinacea pallida bei grippalen Infekten. Naturheilpraxis 1993;46:72-5.
    Also published, in modified form, as:
    Dorn M, Knick E, Lewith G. Placebo-controlled, double-blind study of Echinaceae pallidae radix in upper respiratory tract infections. Compl Ther Med 1997;5:40-2.

14. Willuhn G. Echinaceae pallidae radix. In: Wichtl M, editor. Teedrogen und Phytopharmaka, 4th ed. Stuttgart: Wissenschaftliche Verlagsgesellschaft, 2002:183-6.

15. Gallo M, Sarkar M, Au W, Pietrzak K, Comas B, Smith M et al. Pregnancy outcome following gestational exposure to echinacea: a prospective controlled study. Arch Intern Med 2000;160:3141-3

16. Bauer R, Jurcic K, Puhlmann J, Wagner H. Immunologische In-vivo- und In-vitro-Untersuchungen mit *Echinacea*-Extrakten. Arzneim-Forsch/Drug Res 1988; 38:276-81.

17. Bodinet K. Immunpharmakologische Untersuchungen an einem pflanzlichen Immunmodulator [Dissertation]. Greifswald, Germany: Ernst-Moritz-Arndt-Universität, 1999.

18. Hu C, Kitts DD. Studies on the antioxidant activity of *Echinacea* root extract. J Agric Food Chem 2000;48: 1466-72.

19. Sloley BD, Urichuk LJ, Tywin C, Coutts RT, Pang PKT, Shan JJ. Comparison of chemical components and antioxidant capacity of different *Echinacea* species. J Pharm Pharmacol 2001;53:849-57.

20. Maffei Facino R, Carini M, Aldini G, Saibene L, Pietta P, Mauri P. Echinacoside and caffeoyl conjugates protect collagen from free radical-induced degradation: a potential use of *Echinacea* extracts in the prevention of skin photodamage. Planta Med 1995;61:510-4.

21. Stoll A, Renz J, Brack A. Isolierung und Konstitution des Echinacosids, eines Glykosids aus den Wurzeln von *Echinacea angustifolia* D.C. Helv Chim Acta 1950; 33:1877-93.

22. Binns SE, Purgina B, Bergeron C, Smith ML, Ball L, Baum BR, Arnason JT. Light-mediated antifungal activity of *Echinacea* extracts. Planta Med 2000;66:241-4.

ECHINACEAE PURPUREAE HERBA

Purple Coneflower Herb

DEFINITION

Purple coneflower herb consists of the fresh or dried, flowering aerial parts of *Echinacea purpurea* (L.) Moench [1].

A draft monograph on purple coneflower herb, intended for inclusion in the European Pharmacopoeia, has been published [2].

CONSTITUENTS

Characteristic constituents are a series of alkamides with the isomeric dodeca-2E,4E,8Z,10E/Z-tetraenoic acid isobutylamides as main compounds [3,4].

Further characteristic constituents are caffeic acid derivatives, predominantly cichoric acid (2,3-*O*-dicaffeoyl-tartaric acid) (1.2-3.1%) [4-6], 2-*O*-feruloyl-tartaric acid and 2-*O*-caffeoyl-3-*O*-coumaroyl-tartaric acid [7].

Polysaccharides (PS) such as PS I (a 4-*O*-methyl-glucuronoarabinoxylan with an average MW of 35,000 D), PS II (an acidic arabinorhamnogalactan of MW 450,000 D) [6,8-11] and a xyloglucan (MW 79,500 D) [6,12] have been isolated from purple coneflower herb. A highly-branched acidic arabino-galactan-protein (average MW of 1.2×10^6 D, with a protein content of less than 10%) [13], inulin-type fructans (average MW 6,000 D) [13] and a pectin-like polysaccharide [6,12] have been isolated from the pressed juice from fresh purple coneflower herb.

Flavonoids (0.48%) such as quercetin, kaempferol and isorhamnetin and their glycosides have been found in the leaves [14].

The essential oil (0.08-0.32%) [15-17] contains borneol, bornyl acetate, pentadeca-8-ene-2-one, germacrene D, caryophyllene and caryophyllene epoxide [18] and a germacrene alcohol, germacra-4(15),5E,10(14)-triene-1β-ol [19].

Minor constituents include 13-hydroxy-octadeca-9Z,11E,15Z-trienoic acid, methyl-*p*-hydroxy-cinnamate, a labdane derivative and polyacetylenes [20,21].

E/S/C/O/P
MONOGRAPHS
Second Edition

CLINICAL PARTICULARS

Therapeutic indications

Internal use
Adjuvant therapy and prophylaxis of recurrent infections of the upper respiratory tract (common colds) and also of the urogenital tract [1,22-27].

External use
As an adjuvant for the treatment of superficial wounds [1,28].

Posology and method of administration

Dosage

Internal use
Adult daily dose: 6-9 ml of pressed juice; other equivalent preparations at comparable dosage [1,22-27]. *Children:* Proportion of adult dose according to age or body weight.

External use
Semi-solid preparations with a minimum of 15% of pressed juice [1,28].

Method of administration
For oral administration and topical application.

Duration of administration
The duration of continuous treatment should not exceed 8 weeks [1]. No adverse reactions have been reported after long term oral administration [29].

Contra-indications

Internal use
Hypersensitivity to plants of the Compositae.

As with all immunostimulants, not recommended in cases of progressive systemic disorders and auto-immune diseases such as tuberculosis, leucoses, collagenoses, multiple sclerosis, AIDS or HIV infections [1,29].

External use
Hypersensitivity to plants of the Compositae.

Special warnings and special precautions for use
None required.

Interaction with other medicaments and other forms of interaction
None reported.

Pregnancy and lactation
In accordance with general medical practice, the product should not be used during pregnancy or lactation without medical advice.

No statistical difference from the control group was seen in terms of pregnancy outcome, delivery method, maternal weight gain, gestational age, birth weight or fetal distress following gestational exposure to oral preparations containing *Echinacea* (including *E. purpurea*) in a prospective controlled study involving 412 women [30] (see Clinical safety data below).

Effects on ability to drive and use machines
None known.

Undesirable effects
In rare cases hypersensitivity reactions, e.g. skin reactions, can occur [29].

Overdose
No toxic effects reported.

PHARMACOLOGICAL PROPERTIES

Pharmacodynamic properties

In vitro experiments

Stimulation of phagocytosis and cell count
A lyophilisate of the pressed juice from purple coneflower herb at a concentration of 5.0 mg/ml increased the ratio of phagocytosing human granulocytes significantly from 79% to 95% and also stimulated phagocytosis of yeast particles significantly by more than 50%. At the highest tested dose of 12.5 mg/ml the number of phagocytosing granulocytes and the phagocytosis index decreased [31].

In vitro stimulation of phagocytosis has been verified in further assays [32-34]. Similar results were reported with the alkamide fraction, polysaccharides and cichoric acid [7,35,36].

Cultures of cytologically unchanged human bone marrow cells showed a significantly enhanced mitotic index of granulo- and monopoesis after incubation for up to 72 hours with 0.2 or 2.0 mg/ml lyophilized pressed juice from purple coneflower herb. In blood cultures of patients suffering from chronic myeloic leukaemia or osteomyelosclerosis, the number of mature granulocytes was mostly unchanged. In blood cultures of patients suffering from acute non-lymphatic leukaemia the total count of functionally mature granulocytes increased. More importantly, there was a highly significant reduction of granuloblasts due to a changed pattern of differentiation [37].

Stimulation of T-lymphocyte populations has been observed in the T-lymphocyte transformation test. Lyophilized pressed juice from purple coneflower herb stimulated incorporation of ^{3}H-thymidine at medium concentrations (50-500 µg/ml), while high concentrations (≥ 2500 µg/ml) showed a suppressive or cytotoxic effect [38].

Stimulation of the cell-defence mechanism
In macrophage cultures from mice, lyophilized pressed juice from purple coneflower herb immediately induced a sharp increase in chemiluminescence [38]. Similar findings were seen in granulocyte cultures from healthy human donors. A 24% increase in the formation of oxygen radicals has been demonstrated after 60 minutes of pre-incubation with 50 µg/ml lyophilized pressed juice and suboptimal stimulation with zymosan, suggesting a significant increase in previously depressed granulocyte activity in accordance with the results of the chemiluminescence method [39].

Cytotoxicity
High concentrations ($\geq$ 2500 µg/ml) of lyophilized pressed juice from purple coneflower herb were cytotoxic in the T-lymphocyte transformation test [38]. Furthermore, 100 µg of a polysaccharide fraction from purple coneflower herb stimulated peritoneal macrophages and bone marrow macrophages to cytotoxicity against P-815 cells in the same manner as 10 units of macrophage activating factor (MAF). It also stimulated phagocytosis and interleukin formation [8,35].

Antiviral and viral resistant activity
Incubation of mouse L-929 cells or HeLa cells with 20 µg/ml of a purple coneflower herb pressed juice preparation for 4-6 hours before viral challenge increased their resistance to influenza, herpes and vesicular stomatitis viruses by 50-80% for at least 24 hours. The presence of hyaluronidase eliminated this effect [40].

In the presence of DEAE dextran a lyophilisate of pressed juice from purple coneflower herb at concentrations of 25-200 µg/ml exhibited antiviral activity against encephalomyocarditis and vesicular stomatitis viruses. No antiviral activity was observed with DEAE dextran or the lyophilisate alone [41].

A decoction and a 30% ethanolic extract from purple coneflower herb inhibited the intracellular propagation of ECHO$_9$ Hill virus in a monkey kidney cell culture [42].

Wound healing activity
Fibroblast populated collagen lattice was used to study the influence of purple coneflower extracts on the collagen contracting ability of C3H10T1/2 mouse fibroblasts. An ethanolic extract prepared from fresh herb (final ethanol concentration 65%) significantly inhibited collagen contraction (p<0.05) when added, at 10 µl or 30 µl per 2 ml of collagen gel, during preparation of the lattice. A corresponding amount of ethanol had no inhibitory effect. With increasing elapsed time between preparation of the gel and addition of the extract there was less inhibition of elongation of fibroblasts and of the process leading to collagen linking. No effect was observed when the extract was added one hour after gel formation [43].

Hyaluronidase inhibiting activity
Hyaluronidase inhibiting activity has been demonstrated in a *Streptococcus mucosus* culture. Hyaluronidase-dependent decapsulation of the bacteria (through depolymerization of hyaluronic acid) was diminished by the addition of 0.1 ml of purple coneflower herb pressed juice to 0.3 ml of the test solution [44].

The hyaluronidase inhibiting activity of cichoric acid has been shown to be greater than that of chlorogenic acid [45].

Free radical scavenging properties
Caffeic acid derivatives characteristic of *Echinacea* species protected collagen from free radical-induced degradation in a dose-dependent manner; the IC$_{50}$ for cichoric acid was 16.5 µM [46].

In vivo experiments
The properdin (β-globulin) level in rabbits was enhanced following intravenous injection of purple coneflower herb pressed juice at 0.6 ml/kg body weight. This appears to be an alternative way of stimulating the release of properdin [47].

Intravenous injection of rabbits with 0.5 ml of purple coneflower herb pressed juice, followed by a second injection 24 hours later, initiated leucocytosis after transient leucopenia [48]. As well as blood leucocytosis, a migration of bone marrow granulocytes into peripheral blood was demonstrated in rabbits following a single injection of 1.5 ml of purple coneflower herb pressed juice. Within 6 hours the number of ^{3}H-labelled lymphocytes had increased from 7% to 40% and granulocytes from 34% to 89% [49].

In the carbon clearance test in mice, an ethanolic extract from purple coneflower herb was used as a solution of 5 mg of extract per 30 ml of normal saline. After oral administration of this solution at 10 ml/kg body weight, three times daily for 2 days, carbon clearance was increased by a factor of 1.5 compared to the control. A chloroform-soluble fraction was even more active (factor 1.6), while the water-soluble fraction was less active (factor 1.3) [36].

Similarly, an ethanolic tincture from fresh purple coneflower herb, administered orally to mice at 0.17 ml/kg three times daily for 2 days, stimulated carbon clearance by a factor of 2.1 [36].

Hyaluronidase inhibiting activity
In a modified spreading test in rats, hyaluronidase-stimulated spreading of dye was inhibited by sub-

cutaneous injection of 0.04 ml of concentrated (7:1) pressed juice from purple coneflower herb. The effect was comparable to that of 1 mg of cortisone [50].

Subcutaneous pretreatment of guinea pigs with a preparation of pressed juice from purple coneflower herb, 0.3 ml administered 48 hours before and a second time 24 hours before infection, reduced the dissemination and intensity of a *Streptococcus* infection. No lethality was observed in the treated group (10 animals) in contrast to the control group, in which some deaths occurred within one week [51].

Wound healing activity
After making a double-circle incision in the left flank of anaesthetized guinea pigs, the wounds were treated daily with 0.15 ml of an ointment containing pressed juice from purple coneflower herb and covered with surgical gauze. By the 6th and 9th days following surgery the wound areas were significantly smaller (p<0.05) in comparison with untreated controls [52].

Clinical studies
In a randomized, double-blind, placebo-controlled study, 120 patients with initial symptoms of acute, uncomplicated upper airways infections were treated orally for up to 10 days with either a preparation containing 80 g of pressed juice from purple cone-flower herb per 100 g, at a dosage of 20 drops every 2 hours for the first day and thereafter three times daily (n = 60) or placebo (n = 60). The time taken to improvement was significantly shorter (p<0.0001) in the verum group. In the subgroup of patients in whom common colds developed, the average time to improvement was 4 days with the expressed juice preparation (n = 24) compared to 8 days with placebo (n = 36) [23].

In a similar randomized, double-blind, placebo-controlled study, 80 patients with common cold were treated orally with 2 × 5 ml of pressed juice from purple coneflower herb or placebo daily over a period of 10 days. The patients documented their symptoms, and the intensity of symptoms, in a daily questionnaire and the effect of treatment was assessed by the modified Jackson score. From intention-to-treat analysis the pressed juice reduced the median number of days of illness to 6, compared to a median of 9 days in the placebo group. Per-protocol analysis confirmed this result. The results were clinically relevant and statistically significant (p = 0.0112 and 0.0180 for intention-to-treat and per-protocol analysis respect-ively) [24].

In a further randomized, double-blind prospective study, 108 patients with a history of more than 3 colds or respiratory infections in the preceding year were treated daily for 8 weeks with 2 × 4 ml of either a preparation containing pressed juice from purple coneflower herb (n = 54) or placebo (n = 54). During

the treatment period 65% of patients in the verum group and 74% in the placebo group had at least one cold or respiratory infection. The average number of colds or respiratory infections per patient and the median duration of these ailments were 0.78 and 4.5 days respectively in the verum group compared to 0.93 and 6.5 days in the placebo group. Within a subgroup of 66 patients (29 verum, 37 placebo) who were especially susceptible to infections (T4/T8 cell ratio < 1.5) verum treatment reduced the average duration of infections by 29% to 5.34 days, compared to 7.54 days in patients given placebo. Although the incidence, duration and severity of colds and respiratory infections tended to be lower in the ver-um group, none of the results reached statistical significance [25].

559 adult volunteers, prone to common cold but otherwise healthy, participating in a randomized, double-blind study were provided with placebos or one of three different preparations of *Echinacea purpurea*, all of identical appearance: (A) 6.78 mg per tablet of a crude extract based on 95% fresh herb and 5% fresh root; (B) 48.27 mg per tablet of the same extract, ie. a 7-fold higher dosage; or (C) 29.60 mg per tablet of a crude extract from fresh root only. The volunteers were instructed to take 2 tablets of the assigned preparation three times daily immediately from onset of the first symptoms of common cold until they felt healthy again, but for no longer than 7 days. 246 volunteers caught a cold during the 6-month study period, of whom 180 fully conformed with the study protocol and were assessed by doctors for relative reduction of a complaint index, based on the severity of 12 symptoms, from day 1/2 to day 5/7. Preparations A (n = 41; p = 0.020) and B (n = 49; p = 0.003), but not C (n = 44; p = 0.060), were significantly more effective than placebo (n = 46). The 7-fold higher dosage of B was only slightly more effective than the dosage of A [27].

In a retrospective open study of 170 patients, intramuscular injection of 1-2 ml of diluted pressed juice from purple coneflower herb (equivalent to 100-200 mg of pressed juice) on three successive days for the treatment of pertussis was comparable to antibiotics alone or in combination therapy. In a group of 63 patients treated only with the pressed juice 35% improved within 5 days of treatment and 81% within 10 days, whereas only 10% in a group of 30 patients treated with antibiotics alone improved within 5 days and 46% within 10 days. Out of a group of 77 patients treated with antibiotics plus intra-muscular pressed juice, 9% improved within 5 days of treatment and 53% within 10 days [53].

Similar results were obtained in a comparative retrospective open study of 1280 patients suffering from bronchitis. Results in a group treated only with pressed juice from purple coneflower herb (intramuscularly, with the same dosage as in the previous study [51]) were better than those in groups treated with antibiotics alone or with antibiotics plus intramuscular pressed juice [54].

In a randomized, double-blind, prospective study, 42 healthy male athletes were treated orally with a preparation containing 80 g of pressed juice from purple coneflower herb per 100 g (8 ml) or a magnesium hydrogen phosphate + magnesium hydrogen citrate preparation (providing 43 mg of Mg++) or placebo daily for 28 days preceding a triathlon competition to investigate the effects on exercise-induced whole body reactions. Compared to placebo, the pressed juice markedly decreased sIL-2R in urine before the competition and enhanced the exercise-induced decrease in serum sIL-2R; it also enhanced exercise-induced increases in urinary IL-6 and serum cortisol. There was no incidence of respiratory infection in the pressed juice group compared to 3 out 13 and 4 out of 13 in the magnesium and placebo groups respectively [55].

In an open comparative study involving 203 patients suffering from recurrent vaginal candidiasis, all patients were treated for 6 days with locally-applied antifungal cream containing econazole nitrate. In addition, groups of patients received pressed juice from purple coneflower herb for 10 weeks: 2 ml subcutaneously twice weekly (n = 20); 2 ml intramuscularly twice weekly (n = 60); 0.5-2 ml intravenously twice weekly (n = 20); or 30 drops orally three times daily (n = 60). Cell-mediated immunity was measured by an intracutaneous test (Multitest Merrieux) with recall antigens, before and 10 weeks after the start of treatment, and showed significant improvement over this period in patients receiving the pressed juice. In the control group (n = 43) patients treated only with econazole nitrate had a very high relapse rate of 60.5% within 6 months, while adjuvant immunostimulation with the pressed juice significantly reduced relapse rates to 5-17% depending on the mode of administration [26].

Positive results have been reported from clinical evaluation of 4598 patients with skin disorders, such as wounds, eczema, herpes simplex and burns, after topical application several times daily of an ointment containing pressed juice from purple coneflower herb. Healing was achieved in 85% of cases [28].

The conclusion from a systematic review of controlled clinical studies with extracts from different species of *Echinacea* was that such preparations can be efficacious immunomodulators. However, further methodologically sound, randomized clinical trials should be conducted [22].

Pharmacokinetic properties
No data available.

Preclinical safety data

Single dose toxicity
Single oral or intravenous doses of pressed juice from purple coneflower herb caused no toxicity in rats or mice at the maximum administrable dose. The LD_{50} in rats is therefore over 15,000 mg/kg orally and over 5,000 mg/kg intravenously; in mice, over 30,000 mg/kg orally and over 10,000 mg/kg intravenously [56].

Repeated dose toxicity
After oral administration of 0, 800, 2400 or 8000 mg/kg of pressed juice from purple coneflower herb daily for 4 weeks to male and female rats, no relevant differences between the groups were evident from laboratory or necropsy results [56].

Mutagenic potential

In vitro experiments
No significant increase in revertant numbers was observed when preparations containing pressed juice from purple coneflower herb at concentrations of up to 5000 µg expressed juice per plate were tested in *Salmonella typhimurium* strains TA 98, TA 100, TA 1535, TA 1537 and TA 1538, with or without S-9 metabolic activation [56].

The same preparations gave no statistically significant increase in the frequency of mutations in the mouse lymphoma assay at concentrations up to 5000 µg/ml, with or without S-9 metabolic activation [56].

There was no evidence of a clastogenic effect in human lymphocyte cultures with the lyophilised product at concentrations of up to 5000 µg/ml, with or without S-9 metabolic activation [56].

There were no significant differences in the frequency of morphologically transformed colonies between controls and groups of Syrian hamster embryo (SHE) cells treated with a preparation of lyophilized pressed juice from purple coneflower herb (5-55 µg/ml) equivalent to 80-880 µg of pressed juice per ml of test medium. Benzo[a]pyrene positive controls showed significant increases in malignant transformed cells [56]. This SHE assay generally correlates well with the findings of long-term carcinogenicity studies, which are not available for pressed juice from purple coneflower herb.

In vivo experiments
A single oral dose of 25 g/kg of a preparation containing 80 g of pressed juice from purple coneflower herb per 100 g and ethanol (22 %) administered to mice did not increase the number of micronucleated polychromatic erythrocytes (PCE) compared to negative controls. Positive controls treated with cyclophosphamide did show a significant increase in micronucleated PCEs [56].

Clinical safety data

In controlled clinical studies involving oral treatment with purple coneflower herb preparations, adverse event rates were comparable to placebo (<15%) and the preparations were very well tolerated [24,27]. In two studies, no adverse events were observed in the purple coneflower herb group [23,55]. Only one study reported a higher rate, with adverse events occurring in 20.4% of patients [25]. After topical treatment, adverse events were observed in 2.3% of 4598 patients in an uncontrolled study [28]. None of the reported adverse events was of a serious nature, the symptoms being mainly gastrointestinal disorders (oral treatment) or burning and itching (topical treatment).

In a prospective controlled study involving 412 women, the pregnancy outcome was investigated following gestational exposure to (undefined) solid or liquid preparations of Echinacea (angustifolia, purpurea and in one case pallida). Of 206 women who used echinacea products during pregnancy, 112 used them in the first trimester. In the echinacea group 13 spontaneous abortions as well as 6 major malformations (4 of these occurring after exposure to echinacea in the first trimester) were reported compared to 7 spontaneous abortions and 7 major malformations in the control group. No statistical difference was seen in terms of pregnancy outcome, delivery method, maternal weight gain, gestational age, birth weight or fetal distress [30].

REFERENCES

1. Liersch R, Bauer R. Echinacea. In: Hänsel R, Keller K, Rimpler H, Schneider G, editors. Hagers Handbuch der Pharmazeutischen Praxis, 5th ed. Volume 5: Drogen E-O. Berlin-Heidelberg: Springer-Verlag, 1993:1-34.

2. Purple Coneflower Herb - Echinaceae purpureae herba. Pharmeuropa 2002;14:138-40.

3. Bohlmann F, Hoffmann H. Further amides from Echinacea purpurea. Phytochemistry 1983;22:1173-5.

4. Bauer R, Remiger P, Wagner H. Echinacea. Vergleichende DC- und HPLC-Analyse der Herba-Drogen von Echinacea purpurea, E. pallida und E. angustifolia (3. Mitt.). Dtsch Apoth Ztg 1988;128:174-80.

5. Alhorn R. Phytochemische und vegetationsperiodische Untersuchungen von Echinacea purpurea (L.) Moench unter Berücksichtigung der Kaffeesäurederivate [Dissertation]. University of Marburg/Lahn, 1992.

6. Bauer R. Echinacea: Biological effects and active principles. Chapter 12 in: Lawson LD, Bauer R, editors. Phytomedicines of Europe. Chemistry and Biological Activity. ACS Symposium Series 691. Washington DC: American Chemical Society, 1998:140-57.

7. Soicke H, Al-Hassan G, Görler K. Weitere Kaffeesäure-Derivate aus Echinacea purpurea. Planta Med 1988; 54:175-6.

8. Wagner H, Proksch A, Riess-Maurer I, Vollmar A, Odenthal S, Stuppner H et al. Immunstimulierend wirkende Polysaccharide (Heteroglykane) aus höheren Pflanzen. Arzneim-Forsch/Drug Res 1985;35:1069-75.

9. Wagner H, Proksch A. Über ein immunstimulierendes Wirkprinzip aus Echinacea purpurea Moench. Z angew Phytother 1981;2:166-71.

10. Wagner H, Proksch A, Riess-Maurer I, VollmarA, Odenthal S, Stuppner H et al. Immunstimulierend wirkende Polysaccharide (Heteroglykane) aus höheren Pflanzen. Arzneim-Forsch/Drug Res 1984;34:659-61.

11. Proksch A, Wagner H. Structural analysis of a 4-O-methylglucuronoarabinoxylan with immuno-stimulating activity from Echinacea purpurea. Phytochemistry 1987;26:1989-93.

12. Stuppner H. Chemische und immunologische Untersuchungen von Polysacchariden aus der Gewebekultur von Echinacea purpurea (L.) Moench [Dissertation]. Ludwig-Maximilians-Universität, Munich, 1985.

13. Classen B, Witthohn K, Blaschek W. Characterization of an arabinogalactan-protein isolated from pressed juice of Echinacea purpurea by precipitation with the β-glucosyl Yariv reagent. Carbohydrate Res 2000; 327:497-504.

14. Malonga-Makosi J-P. Untersuchung der Flavonoide von Echinacea angustifolia DC und Echinacea purpurea Moench [Dissertation]. Heidelberg: Ruprecht-Karls-Universität, 1983.

15. Kuhn A. Zur Chemie der Echinacea. In: Madaus G, editor. Echinacea purpurea Moench. Med-Biol Schriftenreihe. Radebeul/Dresden: Verlag Rohrmoser, 1939;(13):6-8.

16. Neugebauer H. Zur Kenntnis der Inhaltsstoffe von Echinacea. Pharmazie 1949;4:137-40.

17. Bomme U, Hölzl J, Heßler C, Stahn T. Wie beeinflußt die Sorte Wirkstoffgehalt und Ertrag von Echinacea purpurea (L.) Moench im Hinblick auf die pharmazeutische Nutzung? 1. Mitt. Ergebnisse des einjährigen Anbaues. Landwirtschaftliches Jahrbuch 1992;69:149-64.

18. Bos R, Heinzer F, Bauer R. Volatile constituents of the leaves of Echinacea purpurea, E. pallida and E. angustifolia. 19th International Symposium on Essential Oils and Other Natural Substrates, Zurich, 1988.

19. Bauer R, Remiger P, Wray V, Wagner H. A germacrene alcohol from fresh aerial parts of Echinacea purpurea. Planta Med 1988;54:478-9.

20. Becker H, Hsieh WC. Chicoree-Säure und deren Derivate aus Echinacea-Arten. Z Naturforsch 1985; 40c:585-7.

21. Schulte KE, Rücker G, Perlick J. Das Vorkommen von Polyacetylen-Verbindungen in *Echinacea purpurea* Mnch. und *Echinacea angustifolia* DC. Arzneim-Forsch/Drug Res 1967;17:825-9.

22. Melchart D, Linde K, Worku F, Bauer R, Wagner H. Immunomodulation with *Echinacea* - a systematic review of controlled clinical trials. Phytomedicine 1994;1:245-54.

23. Hoheisel O, Sandberg M, Bertram S, Bulitta M, Schäfer M. Echinagard treatment shortens the course of the common cold: a double-blind, placebo-controlled clinical trial. Eur J Clin Res 1997;9:261-8.

24. Schulten B, Bulitta M, Ballering-Brühl B, Köster U, Schäfer M. Efficacy of Echinacea purpurea in patients with a common cold. A placebo-controlled, randomised, double-blind clinical trial. Arzneim-Forsch/Drug Res 2001;51:563-8.

25. Schöneberger D. Einfluß der immunstimulierenden Wirkung von Preßsaft aus Herba Echinaceae purpureae auf Verlauf und Schweregrad von Erkältungs-krankheiten. Forum Immunologie 1992;2:18-22.
The same clinical study has also been published as: Grimm W, Müller H-H. A randomized controlled trial of the effect of fluid extract of *Echinacea purpurea* on the incidence and severity of colds and respiratory infections. Am J Med 1999;106:138-43.

26. Coeugniet E, Kühnast R. Rezidivierende Candidiasis - Adjuvante Immuntherapie mit verschiedenen Echinacin®-Darreichungsformen. Therapiewoche 1986;36:3352-8.

27. Brinkeborn RM, Shah DV, Degenring FH. Echinaforce® and other *Echinacea* fresh plant preparations in the treatment of common cold. A randomized, placebo-controlled, double-blind clinical trial. Phytomedicine 1999;6:1-6.

28. Viehmann P. Erfahrungen mit einer Echinacea-haltigen Hautsalbe. Erfahrungsheilkunde 1978;27:353-8.

29. Parnham MJ. Benefit-risk assessment of the squeezed sap of the purple coneflower (*Echinacea purpurea*) for long-term oral immunostimulation. Phytomedicine 1996;3:95-102.

30. Gallo M, Sarkar M, Au W, Pietrzak K, Comas B, Smith M et al. Pregnancy outcome following gestational exposure to echinacea. A prospective controlled study. Arch Intern Med 2000;160:3141-3.

31. Stotzem CD, Hungerland U, Mengs U. Influence of *Echinacea purpurea* on the phagocytosis of human granulocytes. Med Sci Res 1992;20:719-20.

32. Tympner K-D. Der immunbiologische Wirkungs-nachweis von Pflanzenextrakten. Z angew Phytother 1981;2:181-4.

33. Fanselow G. Der Einfluß von Pflanzenextrakten (*Echinacea purpurea, Aristolochia clematitis*) und homöopathischer Medikamente (Acidum formicicum, Sulfur) auf die Phagozytoseleistung humaner Granulozyten in vitro [Dissertation]. Munich: Ludwig-Maximilians-Universität, 1984.

34. Bittner E. Die Wirkung von Echinacin auf die Funktionen des Retikuloendothelialen Systems [Dissertation]. Freiburg: Albert-Ludwigs-Universität, 1969.

35. Stimpel M, Proksch A, Wagner H, Lohmann-Matthes M-L. Macrophage activation and induction of macrophage cytotoxicity by purified polysaccharide fractions from the plant *Echinacea purpurea*. Infect Immun 1984;46:845-9.

36. Bauer R, Remiger P, Jurcic K, Wagner H. Beeinflussung der Phagozytose-Aktivität durch *Echinacea*-Extrakte. Z Phytother 1989;10:43-8.

37. Krause M. Die Wirkungen von Echinacin auf Knochenmarkkulturen bei zytologisch unverändertem Knochenmark sowie auf Blutkulturen bei chronisch-myeloischer Leukämie, Osteomyelosklerose und akuter nichtlymphatischer Leukämie [Dissertation]. Freie Universität Berlin, 1984.

38. Hoh K. Untersuchungen über immunmodulierende Wirkungen von *Echinacea purpurea* Preßsaft und dafür verantwortliche Inhaltsstoffe [Dissertation]. Freiburg: Albert-Ludwigs-Universität, 1990.

39. Krause W. Untersuchungen zur Wirkung von Ascorbinsäure und Echinacin® auf die Funktion neutrophiler Granulozyten [Dissertation]. Tübingen: Eberhard-Karls-Universität, 1986.

40. Wacker A, Hilbig W. Virushemmung mit Echinacea purpurea. Planta Med 1978;33:89-102.

41. Orinda D, Diederich J, Wacker A. Antivirale Aktivität von Inhaltsstoffen der Composite *Echinacea purpurea*. Arzneim-Forsch/Drug Res 1973;23:1119-20.

42. Skwarek T, Tynecka Z, Glowniak K, Lutostanska E. *Echinacea* L. - Inducer of interferons. Herba Polonica 1996;42:110-7.

43. Zoutewelle G, van Wijk R. Effects of *Echinacea purpurea* extracts on fibroblast populated collagen lattice contraction. Phytotherapy Res 1990;4:77-81.

44. Büsing KH. Hyaluronidasehemmung als Wirkungs-mechanismus einiger therapeutisch nutzbarer Naturstoffe. Arzneim-Forsch/Drug Res 1955;5:320-2.

45. Maffei Facino R, Carini M, Aldini G, Marinello C, Arlandini E, Franzoi L et al. Direct characterization of caffeoyl esters with antihyaluronidase activity in crude extracts from *Echinacea angustifolia* roots by fast atom bombardment tandem mass spectrometry. Il Farmaco 1993;48:1447-61.

46. Maffei Facino R, Carini M, Aldini G, Saibene L, Pietta P, Mauri P. Echinacoside and caffeoyl conjugates protect collagen from free radical-induced degradation: A potential use of *Echinacea* extracts in the prevention of skin photodamage. Planta Med 1995;61:510-4.

47. Büsing KH, Thürigen G. Über die Wirkung von Pflanzeninhaltsstoffen auf das Komplement- und Properdinsystem. Allergie und Asthma 1958;4:29-32.

48. Heuschneider J. Das Verhalten der Leukozyten und der alkalischen Neutrophilenphosphatase nach zweifacher Applikation eines Endotoxins und eines aus Polysacchariden bestehenden Pflanzenextraktes bei Kaninchen [Dissertation]. Universität Gießen, 1970.

49. Choné B. Gezielte Steuerung der Leukozyten-Kinetik durch Echinacin. Ärztl Forsch 1965;19:611-2.

50. Koch FE, Haase H. Eine Modifikation des Spreading-Testes im Tierversuch, gleichzeitig ein Beitrag zum Wirkungsmechanismus von Echinacin. Arzneim-Forsch/Drug Res 1952;2:464-7.

51. Koch FE, Uebel H. Experimentelle Untersuchungen über die lokale Beeinflussung der Gewebsresistenz gegen Streptokokkeninfektion durch Cortison und Echinacin. Arzneim-Forsch/Drug Res 1954;4:551-60.

52. Kinkel HJ, Plate M, Tüllner H-U. Objektivierbare Wirkung von Echinacin®-Salbe auf die Wundheilung. Med Klin 1984;79:580-3.

53. Baetgen D. Erfolge in der Keuchhusten-Behandlung mit Echinacin®. Therapiewoche 1984;34:5115-9.

54. Baetgen D. Behandlung der akuten Bronchitis im Kindesalter. Praxisstudie mit einem Immunstimulans aus Echinacea purpurea. TW Pädiatrie 1988;1:66-70.

55. Berg A, Northoff H, König D, Weinstock C, Grathwohl D, Parnham MJ et al. Influence of Echinacin (EC31) treatment on the exercise-induced immune response in athletes. J Clin Res 1998;1:367-80.

56. Mengs U, Clare CB, Poiley JA. Toxicity of Echinacea purpurea - Acute, subacute and genotoxicity studies. Arzneim-Forsch/Drug Res 1991;41:1076-81.

ECHINACEAE PURPUREAE RADIX

Purple Coneflower Root

DEFINITION

Purple coneflower root consists of the fresh or dried underground parts of *Echinacea purpurea* (L.) Moench, harvested at the end of the vegetation period [1].

A draft monograph on purple coneflower root, intended for inclusion in the European Pharmacopoeia, has been published [2].

CONSTITUENTS

The main constituents are cichoric acid (2,3-*O*-dicaffeoyltartaric acid) (0.6-2.3%) [1,3-5], alkamides (0.01-0.04%) [1,6,7], polyacetylene derivatives [8], polysaccharides and glycoproteins [9-11]. A small amount of essential oil (up to 0.1% V/m) is also present [12].

CLINICAL PARTICULARS

Therapeutic indications

Internal use
Adjuvant therapy and prophylaxis of recurrent infections of the upper respiratory tract (common cold) [1,13,14].

Posology and method of administration

Dosage

Adult daily dose: 3 × 60 drops of a tincture (1:5, ethanol 55% V/V), corresponding to 3 × 300 mg of dried root [1,13]; other equivalent preparations at comparable dosage.
Children: Proportion of adult daily dose according to age or body weight.

Method of administration
For oral administration.

Duration of administration
The duration of treatment should not exceed 8 weeks.

Contra-indications
Known hypersensitivity to plants of the Compositae.

As with all immunostimulants, not recommended in cases of progressive systemic disorders and auto-immune diseases such as tuberculosis, leucoses, collagenoses, multiple sclerosis, AIDS or HIV infections [1].

E/S/C/O/P
MONOGRAPHS
Second Edition

Special warnings and special precautions for use
None required.

Interaction with other medicaments and other forms of interaction
None reported.

Pregnancy and lactation
In accordance with general medical practice, the product should not be used during pregnancy or lactation without medical advice.

No statistical difference from the control group was seen in terms of pregnancy outcome, delivery method, maternal weight gain, gestational age, birth weight or fetal distress following gestational exposure to oral preparations containing *Echinacea* (including *E. purpurea*) in a prospective controlled study involving 412 women [15] (see Clinical safety data below).

Effects on ability to drive and use machines
None known.

Undesirable effects
In rare cases hypersensitivity reactions, e.g. skin reactions, may occur.

Overdose
No toxic effects reported.

PHARMACOLOGICAL PROPERTIES

Pharmacodynamic properties

In vitro experiments

Influence on immune functions
An ethanolic extract of purple coneflower root enhanced phagocytosis by 33% in the granulocyte smear test at a concentration of 10^{-4} mg/ml. Aqueous and lipophilic fractions from the ethanolic extract showed immunostimulatory activity [16].

A purified glycoprotein fraction and polysaccharide fractions from purple coneflower root stimulated the activity of mouse macrophages in the carbon clearance test; this activation included enhanced secretion of interleukin-1 (IL-1) [10,11].

A high molecular weight fraction (MW > 10,000 D) containing polysaccharides and glycoproteins from purple coneflower root enhanced the proliferation of mouse spleen cells; stimulated the production of cytokines such as interferon (IFNα/β) in spleen cell cultures, and interleukin-1 (IL-1), interleukin-6 (IL-6) and tumour necrosis factor-α (TNF-α) in mouse macrophage cultures; increased immunoglobulin M production and the number of antibody-producing cells, and increased NO production of macrophages

[9,17]. Incubation of this fraction with human monocytes also enhanced the production of IL-1, IL-6 and TNF-α [17]. Pre-treatment of mouse macrophages with a polysaccharide fraction from purple coneflower root increased the production of IL-1 [10].

Purple coneflower root powders and various extracts showed a macrophage activating capacity. Extracts standardized to 4% of phenolic compounds (such as chlorogenic and cichoric acid) or to alkylamides were inactive with respect to induction of macrophage cytokine production [18].

Methanolic extracts from purple coneflower root exhibited antioxidant activity, the mechanisms of which include free radical scavenging and transition metal chelating [19,20].

Polyunsaturated isobutylamides have been shown to exert anti-inflammatory activity in the 5-lipoxygenase assay [21,22]. A fraction from purple coneflower root consisting of 10 polyunsaturated isobutylamides had an inhibitory effect on 5-lipoxygenase of 92.5% at 50 µM (calculated for a mean relative molecular mass of 220) [21].

Caffeoyl derivatives such as echinacoside and cichoric acid protected collagen from free radical-induced degradation in a dose-dependent manner [23].

Wound healing activity
Fibroblast-populated collagen lattice was used to study the influence of purple coneflower extracts on the collagen contracting ability of C3H10T1/2 mouse fibroblasts. An ethanolic extract (65% V/V) of purple coneflower root showed a dose-dependent inhibition of collagen gel contraction when added at the time of preparation of the gel. A corresponding amount of ethanol showed no influence. With increase of elapsed time between gel preparation and addition of extract, there was less inhibition of elongation of fibroblasts and of the processes leading to collagen linking. No effect was observed when the extract was added one hour after gel preparation [24].

Antimicrobial activity
Antibacterial activity of polyacetylenic compounds against *Escherichia coli* and *Pseudomonas aeruginosa* has been demonstrated [25].

Extracts of purple coneflower root exhibited near UV-mediated phototoxic and antifungal activity, measured by inhibition of the growth of *Candida* spp. and *Saccharomyces cerevisiae*; the activity was attributed primarily to ketoalkenes and ketoalkynes [26].

A decoction and a 30% ethanolic extract of purple coneflower root inhibited the propagation of ECHO$_9$ Hill virus in monkey kidney cell cultures [27].

A high molecular weight fraction (MW > 10,000 D) containing polysaccharides and glycoproteins from purple coneflower root exhibited antiviral activity against herpes simplex virus and influenza virus [9].

The antiviral activity of cichoric acid and purified fractions from purple coneflower root has been demonstrated [28,29]. Incubation with cichoric acid (125 µg/ml) for 4 hours reduced the infectivity of vesicular stomatitis virus in mouse L-929 cells by more than 50% [29].

In vivo experiments

A 3-fold increase in phagocytosis was demonstrated in the carbon clearance test in mice after oral administration of 10 ml/kg of a solution containing ca. 5 mg of an ethanolic extract of purple coneflower root in 30 ml of physiological saline, three times daily for 2 days. When chloroform and aqueous fractions of this extract were administered separately, the lipophilic fraction proved more active than the hydrophilic. However, the hydrophilic fraction showed considerably more activity than a hydrophilic fraction from *Echinacea pallida* root [16,30].

Oral administration of purple coneflower root extract (0.45 mg/day) to 7-week-old mice for 2 weeks resulted in a doubling of the number of natural killer (NK) cells and monocytes in the bone marrow (site of new cell generation for these lines), and in the spleen (principal site of functional activity of NK cells) [31]. Oral administration of the same amount of root extract to ageing mice (15-16 months old, with an average life-span of 21 months) stimulated the production of new NK cells, leading to a 30% increase in the absolute number of NK cells and a 20% increase in the total functional activity of NK cells in the spleen as measured by the lysis of lymphoma cells *in vitro* [32]. Moreover, oral administration of the powdered root to mice injected with leukaemia cells increased their survival time compared to controls [33]. Powdered root also exhibited a strong adjuvant effect on vaccination with inactivated leukaemia cells [34].

Stimulation of the cell defence mechanism

Production of the cytokines interleukin-1 and interleukin-6 in mice was enhanced by intravenous doses (50, 100 and 500 µg/animal) of a purified high molecular weight fraction containing glycoproteins and polysaccharides from purple coneflower root [9]. Oral administration of this fraction to mice significantly enhanced antibody production in Peyer's plaque cells [17].

Pharmacological studies in humans

In a double-blind study, 24 healthy male volunteers took 3 × 30 drops of an ethanolic extract of purple coneflower root or placebo daily for 5 days. By day 5 a significant increase in phagocytosis of 120% was observed in the verum group, compared to 20% in the placebo group. The effect was transient and phagocytotic activity returned to normal within 6 days [35].

Clinical studies

In a double-blind, placebo-controlled study, 180 patients with influenza, randomized into three groups of 60, were given a tincture of purple coneflower root (1:5, ethanol 55%) at daily dosages corresponding to 450 mg or 900 mg of dried root, or placebo. After 3-4 days and 8-10 days there was no statistical difference in symptoms between the group taking the 450 mg dose and the placebo group. In contrast, the group taking the 900 mg dose showed a highly significant reduction in symptom score at both time points (p<0.0001) [13].

289 volunteers from four military establishments and one industrial plant participated in a double-blind, placebo-controlled study to investigate the efficacy of *Echinacea* extracts in the prevention of upper respiratory tract infections. Randomized groups were instructed to take, twice daily for 12 weeks, 50 drops (ca. 1 ml) of one of three trial preparations: ethanolic extract (plant to extract ratio 1:11 in 30% ethanol) of purple coneflower root (Group A, n = 99) or *Echinacea angustifolia* root (Group B, n = 100), or an ethanolic placebo solution (Group C, n = 90). 244 participants fully conformed with the protocol: 85, 84 and 75 in Groups A, B and C respectively. The average time until first occurrence of first upper respiratory tract infections was 69, 66 and 65 days, and 29%, 32% and 37% of participants had at least one upper respiratory tract infection, in Groups A, B and C respectively. Although perhaps suggesting a relative reduction in risk of infection of 20% for purple coneflower root and 13% for *Echinacea angustifolia* root compared to placebo, the results were not statistically significant [36].

Pharmacokinetic properties

No data available.

Preclinical safety data

No data available on purple coneflower root.

Clinical safety data

No adverse events were reported in a clinical study in which groups of 60 patients with influenza received oral treatment daily for 10 days with a tincture of purple coneflower root, equivalent to 450 mg or 900 mg of dried root; the preparation was well tolerated [13].

In another clinical study, 10 out of 99 subjects who took 2 × 50 drops (2 × 1 ml) of a hydroethanolic extract of purple coneflower root daily for 12 weeks reported

adverse effects, compared to 11 out of 90 subjects in the placebo group; none of the adverse effects were serious or required therapeutic action [36].
.
In a prospective controlled study involving 412 women, the pregnancy outcome was investigated following gestational exposure to (undefined) solid or liquid preparations of Echinacea (angustifolia, purpurea and in one case pallida). Of 206 women who used echinacea products during pregnancy, 112 used them in the first trimester. In the echinacea group 13 spontaneous abortions as well as 6 major malformations (4 of these occurring after exposure to echinacea in the first trimester) were reported compared to 7 spontaneous abortions and 7 major malformations in the control group. No statistical difference was seen in terms of pregnancy outcome, delivery method, maternal weight gain, gestational age, birth weight or fetal distress [15].

REFERENCES

1. Liersch R, Bauer R. Echinacea. In: Hänsel R, Keller K, Rimpler H, Schneider G, editors. Hagers Handbuch der pharmazeutischen Praxis, 5th ed. Volume 5: Drogen E-O. Berlin: Springer-Verlag, 1993:1-34.

2. Purple Coneflower Root - Echinaceae purpureae radix. Pharmeuropa 2002;14:140-1.

3. Becker H, Hsieh WC. Chicoree-Säure und deren Derivate aus Echinacea-Arten. Z Naturforsch 1985; 40c:585-7.

4. Hsieh WC. Isolierung und Charakterisierung von Kaffeesäurederivaten aus Echinacea-Arten [Dissertation]. University of Heidelberg, 1984.

5. Perry NB, Burgess EJ, Glennie VL. Echinacea standardization: analytical methods for phenolic compounds and typical levels in medicinal species. J Agric Food Chem 2001;49:1702-6.

6. Bauer R, Remiger P. TLC and HPLC analysis of alkamides in Echinacea drugs. Planta Med 1989;55: 367-71.

7. Bauer R, Remiger P, Wagner H. Alkamides from the roots of Echinacea purpurea. Phytochemistry 1988;27: 2339-42.

8. Schulte KE, Rücker G, Perlick J. Das Vorkommen von Polyacetylen-Verbindungen in Echinacea purpurea Mnch. und Echinacea angustifolia DC. Arzneim-Forsch/ Drug Res 1967;17:825-9.

9. Beuscher N, Bodinet C, Willigmann I, Egert D. Immunmodulierende Eigenschaften von Wurzel-extrakten verschiedener Echinacea-Arten. Z Phyto-therapie 1995;16:157-66.

10. Beuscher N, Scheit K-H, Bodinet C, Egert D. Modulation of host resistance by polymeric substances from Baptisia tinctoria and Echinacea purpurea. In: Masihi KN, Lange W, editors. Immunotherapeutic prospects of infectious diseases. Berlin-Heidelberg: Springer-Verlag, 1990:59-63.

11. Wagner H, Proksch A, Riess-Maurer I, Vollmar A, Odenthal S, Stuppner H et al. Immunstimulierend wirkende Polysaccharide (Heteroglykane) aus höheren Pflanzen. Arzneim-Forsch/Drug Res 1985;35:1069-75.

12. Heinzer F, Chavanne M, Meusy J-P, Maltre H-P, Giger E, Baumann TW. Ein Beitrag zur Klassifizierung der therapeutisch verwendeten Arten der Gattung Echinacea. Pharm Acta Helv 1988;63:132-6.

13. Bräunig B, Dorn M, Knick E. Echinaceae purpureae radix: zur Stärkung der körpereigenen Abwehr bei grippalen Infekten. Z Phytotherapie 1992;13:7-13.

14. van Hellemont J. Echinacea purpurea. In: Fytothera-peutisch compendium, 2nd ed. Utrecht: Bohn, Scheltema & Holkema, 1994;209-10.

15. Gallo M, Sarkar M, Au W, Peitrzak K, Comas B, Smith M et al. Pregnancy outcome following gestational exposure to echinacea: A prospective controlled study. Arch Intern Med 2000;160:3141-3.

16. Bauer R, Remiger P, Jurcic K, Wagner H. Beeinflussung der Phagozytose-Aktivität durch Echinacea-Extrakte. Z Phythotherapie 1989;10:43-8.

17. Bodinet K. Immunpharmakologische Untersuchungen an einem pflanzlichen Immunmodulator [Dissertation]. Greifswald, Germany: Ernst-Moritz-Arndt-Universität, 1999.

18. Rininger JA, Kickner S, Chigurupati P, McLean A, Franck Z. Immunopharmacological activity of Echinacea preparations following simulated digestion on murine macrophages and human peripheral blood mononuclear cells. J Leukocyte Biol 2000;68:503-10.

19. Hu C, Kitts DD. Studies on the antioxidant activity of Echinacea root extract. J Agric Food Chem 2000;48: 1466-72.

20. Sloley BD, Urichuk LJ, Tywin C, Coutts RT, Pang PKT, Shan JJ. Comparison of chemical components and antioxidant capacity of different Echinacea species. J Pharm Pharmacol 2001;53:849-57.

21. Wagner H, Breu W, Willer F, Wierer M, Remiger P, Schwenker G. In vitro inhibition of arachidonate metabolism by some alkamides and prenylated phenols. Planta Med 1989;55:566-7.

22. Müller-Jakic B, Breu W, Pröbstle A, Redl K, Greger H, Bauer R. In vitro inhibition of cyclooxygenase and 5-lipoxygenase by alkamides from Echinacea and Achillea species. Planta Med 1994;60:37-40.

23. Maffei Facino R, Carini M, Aldini G, Saibene L, Pietta P, Mauri P. Echinacoside and caffeoyl conjugates protect collagen from free radical-induced degradation: a potential use of Echinacea extracts in the prevention of skin photodamage. Planta Med 1995;61:510-4.

24. Zoutewelle G, van Wijk R. Effects of Echinacea purpurea

extracts on fibroblast populated collagen lattice contraction. Phytother Res 1990;4:77-81.

25. Schulte KE, Rücker G, Boehme R. Polyacetylene als Inhaltstoffe der Klettenwurzeln. Arzneim-Forsch/Drug Res 1967;17:829-33.

26. Binns SE, Purgina B, Smith ML, Ball L, Baum BR, Arnason JT. Light-mediated antifungal activity of *Echinacea* extracts. Planta Med 2000;66:241-4.

27. Skwarek T, Tynecka Z, Glowniak K, Lutostanska E. *Echinacea* L. - Inducer of interferons. Herba Polonica 1996;42:110-7.

28. May G, Willuhn G. Antivirale Wirkung wäßriger Pflanzenextrakte in Gewebekulturen. Arzneim-Forsch/Drug Res 1978;28:1-7.

29. Cheminat A, Zawatzky R, Becker H, Brouillard R. Caffeoyl conjugates from *Echinacea* species: structures and biological activity. Phytochemistry 1988;27:2787-94.

30. Bauer R, Jurcic K, Puhlmann J, Wagner H. Immuno-logische in-vivo- und in-vitro-Untersuchungen mit *Echinacea*-Extrakten. Arzneim-Forsch/Drug Res 1988; 38:276-81.

31. Sun LZ-Y, Currier NL, Miller SC. The American coneflower: A prophylactic role involving non-specific immunity. J Altern Complement Med 1999;5:437-46.

32. Currier NL, Miller SC. Natural killer cells from aging mice treated with extracts from *Echinacea purpurea* are quantitatively and functionally rejuvenated. Experim Gerontol 2000;35:627-39.

33. Currier NL, Miller SC. *Echinacea* and melatonin augment natural-killer cells in leukemic mice and prolong life span. J Altern Complement Med 2001;7: 241-51.

34. Currier NL, Miller SC. The effect of immunization with killer tumor cells, with/without feeding of *Echinacea purpurea* in an erythroleukemic mouse model. J Altern Complement Med 2002;8:49-58.

35. Jurcic K, Melchart D, Holzmann M, Martin P, Bauer R, Doenecke A, Wagner H. Zwei Probandenstudien zur Stimulierung der Granulozytenphagozytose durch *Echinacea*-Extrakt-haltige Präparate. Z Phytotherapie 1989;10:67-70.

36. Melchart D, Walther E, Linde K, Brandmaier R, Lersch C. Echinacea root extracts for the prevention of upper respiratory tract infections. A double-blind, placebo-controlled randomized trial. Arch Fam Med 1998;7:541-5.

ELEUTHEROCOCCI RADIX

Eleutherococcus

E/S/C/O/P
MONOGRAPHS
Second Edition

DEFINITION

Eleutherococcus consists of the whole or cut, dried, underground organs of *Eleutherococcus senticosus* (Rupr. et Maxim.) Maxim.

The material complies with the monograph of the European Pharmacopoeia [1].

CONSTITUENTS

Lignans such as eleutheroside E (syringaresinol diglucoside, 0.1%) and eleutheroside B_4 (sesamin, 0.023%), and other phenylpropanoids including eleutheroside B (syringin, 0.5%), sinapyl alcohol and chlorogenic acid; also coumarins, saponins and polysaccharides [2-4].

CLINICAL PARTICULARS

Therapeutic indications
Decreased mental and physical capacities such as weakness, exhaustion, tiredness and loss of concentration, as well as during convalescence [2,3,5-21].

Posology and method of administration

Dosage

Adults: 1-2 ml of fluid extract (1:1, ethanol 40% V/V), 1-3 times daily [2,3,17].
65-195 mg of dry extract (14-25:1, ethanol 40% V/V) daily [21]. Other preparations corresponding to 2-3 g of dried root and rhizome daily [2,3].

Method of administration
For oral administration.

Duration of administration
If symptoms persist or worsen after one month, medical advice should be sought.

Contra-indications
None known.

Special warnings and special precautions for use
Some reports of blood pressure increase have been documented in hypertensive patients. A causal relationship to the use of eleutherococcus could not be established [2,3].

Interaction with other medicaments and other forms of interaction
None reported.

Pregnancy and lactation
No teratogenic or other effects have been observed in studies on pregnant animals [22]. However, in accordance with general medical practice, eleutherococcus should not be used during pregnancy and lactation without medical advice.

Effects on ability to drive and use machines
None known.

Undesirable effects
None confirmed.

Overdose
No toxic effects reported.

PHARMACOLOGICAL PROPERTIES

Pharmacodynamic properties

In vitro experiments

Immunomodulating effects
A solution containing 0.98 g of a hydroethanolic fluid extract of eleutherococcus per 5 ml enhanced phagocytosis by human leucocytes at concentrations between 0.0078 mg/ml and 3.14 mg/ml by 18% [23]. Proliferation of lymphocytes remained unaffected [23,24]. An ethanolic dry extract (15:1) at concentrations between 0.1 and 1 mg/ml increased phagocytosis in human granulocytes by 60 to 240% [24]. The effects were attributed to polysaccharides contained in the drug [25,26]. An ethanolic fluid extract was shown to induce the production of interleukin-1 (IL-1) and interleukin-6 (IL-6). The effective concentration ranged from 0.1 to 1.0 mg/ml for enhancement of IL-1 and from 0.03 to 1.0 mg/ml for IL-6. Interleukin-2 (IL-2) production by human mononuclear cells was not affected. Isolated eleutherosides B and E had no effect in the same model. There was no indication that eleutherococcus extract exerts a direct effect on the proliferation of T and B cells as part of the antigen-specific immunity, where IL-2 is involved [27]. These findings are in line with results from earlier studies [24].

Antiviral activity
An ethanolic fluid extract inhibited the replication of human rhinovirus, respiratory syncytial virus and influenza A virus in cell cultures [28,29]. The ED_{50} of the extract was a 1/120 dilution in the case of rhinovirus and influenza A virus and 1/2240 in the case of respiratory syncytial virus. The effect of the fluid extract was affected neither by heat stress nor by conversion to a dry extract preparation [29].

Antiproliferative effects
A freeze-dried hot water extract exerted a cytotoxic effect on L1210 murine leukaemia cells. The extract inhibited cellular proliferation in a dose-dependent manner starting at 25 µg/ml and reaching a plateau between 200 and 400 µg/ml [30].

Antioxidant effects
A freeze-dried hot water extract was tested for free radical scavenging activity and inhibition of lipid peroxidation by means of 5 different biochemical test methods. The extract showed antioxidant activity *in vitro* with IC_{50} values of 3.9 to 7.9 mg/ml [31].

Endocrine effects
An ethanolic fluid extract (7.7% w/v solids), dried and reconstituted to 10% of its original volume in buffer solution, was found to interact competitively with mineralocorticoid and glucocorticoid receptors [32].

A freeze-dried hot water extract induced an increase in ACTH and luteinizing hormone secretion in primary cultures of rat pituitary cells at concentrations of 0.1 µg/ml and 0.01 or 0.1 µg/ml respectively. Addition of syringin and syringaresinol diglucoside induced a further increase in luteinizing hormone secretion. The release of follicle-stimulating hormone was inhibited. Although an influence of eleutherococcus on the pituitary adrenal system could be verified *in vivo*, there was no evidence of any relevant influence on the pituitary gonadal system [33].

In vivo experiments

Immunostimulating effects
Polysaccharides isolated from eleutherococcus, given intraperitoneally to mice at 10 mg/kg, exerted an immunostimulating effect as demonstrated in the carbon clearance test [34].

Antiviral activity
The antiviral activity of an eleutherococcus ethanolic fluid extract was evaluated in experimental influenza infection. The virus and the extract were simultaneously administered intranasally to mice. The titre of influenza virus in the lungs of the animals was recorded over 6 days. On days 5 and 6 after infection marked virus titres were measured in the lungs of control animals, whereas no virus titre was found in the animals treated with eleutherococcus extract [35].

An ethanolic fluid extract of eleutherococcus, dried and reconstituted in water, was given intraperitoneally to mice in amounts of 2.5 mg, 25 mg or 100 mg. Blood was drawn at regular intervals and tested *in vitro* for inhibition of vesicular stomatitis virus. Maximum inhibition of virus replication was reached 18 hours after administration of the extract and found to be 40%. The effect was attributed to the formation of γ-interferon [36].

Resistance to stress

The protective effects of eleutherococcus against mental and physical stress have been investigated in numerous studies.

Mice were treated daily with subcutaneous doses of 0.1 ml of a 1:10 dilution of an ethanolic fluid extract conforming to the former USSR Pharmacopoeia for 14 days before irradiation with 3 Gy gamma rays. During the 30 days following irradiation, leucocyte counts and nucleic acid levels in the white blood cells of animals pre-treated with the extract were recorded in comparison with a control group. Animals pre-treated with eleutherococcus extract showed markedly higher nucleic acid levels than the controls from day 10 to day 30 of the recovery time [37].

Larvae of the pond snail *Lymnaea stagnalis* (3 days old) were pre-treated for 20 hours with an aqueous extract containing 1% of eleutheroside E and 0.34% of eleutheroside B at concentrations ranging from 0.68 mg/ml to 68 µg/ml. When exposed to heat shock (4 minutes at 43°C), 84% of the larvae in the highest dose group survived compared to 9% in a non-treated control population. Pre-treatment with eleutherococcus extract at 0.34 mg/ml and 0.68 mg/ml protected the larvae against menadione-induced oxidative stress (600 µM for 2 hours) and against toxic exposure to copper (150 µM for 1 hour) [38].

Hepatoprotective effects

A freeze-dried hot water extract of eleutherococcus was administered intragastrically to rats at 100, 300, 500 or 1000 mg/kg body weight, 2 hours before and 2 and 6 hours after administration of a single hepato-toxic dose of paracetamol (acetaminophen), or 2 hours before and 24 and 48 hours after administration of a single hepatotoxic dose of carbon tetrachloride. Control groups received a saline solution or the toxic substance alone. The rats were killed (24 hours after paracetamol administration, 72 hours after carbon tetrachloride) and blood samples were analysed for aspartate aminotransferase (ASAT) and alanine aminotransferase (ALAT) activity as indicators of liver function. Serum ASAT and ALAT activity was significantly lower ($p < 0.005$) in the groups that received 300 or 500 mg of eleutherococcus extract in comparison with the control groups. Liver tissue was less damaged in the eleutherococcus (100, 300 and 500 mg/kg) groups. However, liver damage was greater in animals that had received eleutherococcus extract at 1000 mg/kg [31].

Endocrine effects

A freeze-dried hot water extract of eleutherococcus was administered intraperitoneally to rats as a single dose of 3 mg/kg body weight. As a result, serum levels of corticosteroids increased markedly within 30 minutes compared to a control group that received physiological saline (314 ± 32 ng/ml vs 239 ± 41ng/ml). After 23 hours serum corticosteroids in the treatment group had dropped to control levels [33].

In a stress experiment using the same extract, rats received daily single doses of 100 mg/kg or 500 mg/kg body weight orally or 3.0 mg/kg intraperitoneally for 7 weeks. Controls received water orally or physiological saline intraperitoneally. After 7 weeks each group was divided into 3 subgroups. One group was not submitted to any stress, a second group received a single intravenous injection with physiological saline as an acute form of stress and the third group was treated with corticotrophin-releasing hormone (CRH). Serum ACTH and corticosterone levels were investigated in all groups. In rats not submitted to stress, ACTH was at the control level. In stressed animals that received eleutherococcus extract intraperitoneally or 500 mg/kg orally, ACTH was completely suppressed. Corticosterone increased in the unstressed animals treated intraperitoneally. However, corticosterone release was significantly decreased ($p < 0.05$) following acute stress. The effects were not transmitted through stimulated CRH release [33].

Pharmacological studies in humans

Immunomodulating effects

In vitro and *ex vivo* studies suggest an increase in leukocyte, cytotoxic T-cell, T-helper cell, and B- and T-lymphocyte counts in peripheral blood; in phagocytosis; in natural killer cell and T-cell activity; in stimulation of lymphocyte proliferation and activity; in interferon production; and in chemotactic migration and inhibition of Migration Inhibition Factor [39-44].

The influence on immunological parameters was investigated in 36 healthy volunteers in a double-blind, placebo-controlled study following oral administration of a preparation containing about 6 g of an ethanolic eleutherococcus fluid extract (1:1) or placebo daily for 28 days. The number and state of activation of T-cell sub-populations were determined by quantitative flow cytometry. A significant increase in the number of lymphocytes ($p < 0.0001$), such as T-lymphocytes ($p < 0.0001$), activated T-cells ($p < 0.01$), T-helper cells ($p < 0.00001$), cytotoxic cells ($p < 0.0001$), natural killer cells ($p < 0.1$) and B-lymphocytes ($p < 0.05$), by 30-85% was observed in the active treatment group. These T-cell sub-populations remained almost unchanged in the placebo group [40].

Stimulation of phagocytosis was investigated in 14 healthy volunteers who received orally 2 ml of a fluid extract of eleutherococcus daily for 7 days, while 10 other volunteers received placebo. Blood samples for lymphocyte determination were taken before administration of the extract, after completion of administration on day 7 and in follow-up on day 28. The percentage of active lymphocytes was determined *ex vivo* by the nitroblue-tetrazolium phagocytosis test. A statistically significant (p<0.05) increase in the number of active lymphocytes was observed on days 7 and 28 [41].

The influence of an eleutherococcus fluid extract on immunological parameters was investigated in 35 healthy volunteers following daily oral administration of 75 drops for 30 days. The study was randomized and active-controlled; 15 other volunteers received echinacea pressed juice over the same period. The percentage of lymphocytes with spontaneous blastic transformation and phytohaemagglutinin (LF-7)-induced blastic transformation as an indicator of phagocytic activity increased significantly (p<0.05) in the eleutherococcus group (by 65% and 49% respectively) but remained unchanged in the echinacea group [5].

Resistance to stress; adaptogenic potential
Increases in resistance to various physical stressors (adaptogenic potential) have been investigated in several studies involving healthy volunteers. These include improved tolerance to high altitudes and the extreme temperatures of heat chambers [6-8].

In a placebo-controlled study, 220 healthy men were exposed to high temperature (118-120°C) and low relative humidity (15%) in a sauna for 25 minutes. The subjects had been pre-treated orally with an eleutherococcus fluid extract at 1.0 ml/day for 10 days; a control group received placebo. The primary evaluation criteria were sensomotor reactions to optical and acoustic stimuli, and manual, physical and mental performance parameters (3 tests) before and after the stress situation. The eleutherococcus group showed a decrease in latency periods immediately after exposure compared to the placebo group. The verum group also gave better performances in mental tests, with significant differences compared to placebo in picture-letter combination, figure finding, colour recognition and figure placing tests [6].

In a placebo-controlled study, 117 volunteers were treated orally with an eleutherococcus fluid extract at 1 ml/day for 30 days; 108 volunteers in a control group received a placebo solution. Defined abdominal skin areas were irradiated with UV light for periods of up to 2.5 minutes and erythema formation induced by the UV light was measured. In the eleutherococcus group the time before occurrence of skin irritation (erythema) was prolonged by a factor of 6 compared to placebo (p<0.05) [8].

Capillary resistance, measured by the development of petechiae following the application of low pressure under cupping glasses fixed to the lower arm, was evaluated in a placebo-controlled study involving 212 healthy volunteers; 130 received an eleutherococcus fluid extract orally at 1 ml/day for 30 days while 82 in a control group received placebo. A

significant improvement in capillary resistance (p<0.0001) was observed after eleutherococcus treatment [8].

Effects on psychomotor performance, cognitive function and physical performance
Effects on psychomotor performance and cognitive function were investigated in a placebo-controlled study involving 190 healthy pilots, co-pilots and flight engineers of helicopter crews. The subjects received an eleutherococcus fluid extract or a placebo solution orally at 2 ml/day for 10 days. A battery of psycho-physical tests was applied on day 10 and after a subsequent helicopter flight (15, 60, and 180 minutes after landing): dynamic tremometry test, sensomotor reaction rate/reflexometer, digit-letter recognition test, mental arithmetic test, compass selection test and number arranging/memorizing tests. Subjects in the verum group consistently demonstrated better test outcomes at the different time points compared to those in the placebo group. In several tests these effects persisted for 3 hours following the helicopter flight [10].

The influence of an eleutherococcus fluid extract on physical performance was investigated in 35 healthy volunteers following daily oral administration of 75 drops for 30 days. The study was randomized and active-controlled; 15 other volunteers received echinacea pressed juice over the same period. An ergospirometric test revealed a significantly higher oxygen plateau in the eleutherococcus group compared to the echinacea group: oxygen consumption (litres/kg/min) during maximal effort was 39.24 before and 42.65 after 30 days, compared to 35.03 before and 36.91 after 30 days in the echinacea group (p<0.01) [5].

In a single-blind, placebo-controlled, cross-over study in healthy volunteers, improvement in physical performance was investigated using a bicycle ergometer test. The subjects were treated orally for 8 days with 4 ml/day of an ethanolic fluid extract of eleutherococcus conforming to the former USSR Pharmacopoeia, or with placebo, or remained untreated as controls (n = 6 in each group). Eleutherococcus treatment was superior to the controls for all parameters assessed (significant differences between p<0.005 and p<0.01 compared to controls for maximum oxygen assimilation, oxygen pulse, total ergometer performance and time to exhaustion) [9].

Visual performance was investigated in a placebo-controlled study involving 234 healthy volunteers (train engineers) aged between 24 and 45 years. Those in the eleutherococcus group were treated orally with a fluid extract at 2 ml/day for 40 days. Spectral sensitivity, colour contrast sensitivity and stability of colour perception were determined. Assessments were conducted at baseline and on days

1, 5, 20 and 40, with a follow-up after approximately 2 months, all tests being conducted before and after the work shift of the train engineers. Verum treatment improved the time threshold for red, green and blue light, improved colour perception, contrast sensitivity, visual perception ability for red and green light, and the time threshold for contrast sensitivity. After the 40-day treatment with eleutherococcus visual perception ability had increased by 2.5 to 4.5 times the initial value and this improvement was maintained for 2 to 2.5 months. The placebo group showed no improvement in any of the tests [11].

In a placebo-controlled study 50 volunteers (men and women aged 30 to 50 years) received a single 2 ml dose of an eleutherococcus fluid extract or placebo. Spectral and contrast sensitivity of the eye as well as stability in colour differentiation were evaluated. Improved spectral sensitivity was found in subjects with normal trichromatic vision after administration of eleutherococcus; in the spectral ranges assessed, spectral sensitivity compared to initial values improved by 47% to 82%. No improvements were observed in the placebo group [12].

The effect of eleutherococcus on experimentally-induced vestibular dizziness was investigated in a controlled study involving 40 male healthy volunteers aged between 24 and 38 years, 25 of whom had good vestibular stability and 15 decreased vestibular stability. The volunteers were treated with 4 ml of a fluid extract 40-60 min before beginning the test (swivel chair for coriolis stimulation). Swivel chair training was carried out up to the first signs of malaise, such as hot feeling, salivation or retching. Each volunteer participated in up to 30 training sessions within a period of 2-3 weeks. In the group with low vestibular stability 10 volunteers were treated with eleutherococcus extract and 5 received placebo. Volunteers with good vestibular stability received no treatment and served as an additional control group. Subjects in the placebo group showed severe nausea after 7-12 minutes, but all those in the eleutherococcus group were able to support 15 minutes of swivel chair training without such reactions [13].

The effect of eleutherococcus on cognitive functions (concentration test, selective memory test) was investigated in 24 healthy, middle-aged volunteers (36-58 years) in a randomized, placebo-controlled, double-blind, crossover study. The subjects were treated orally with 1.25 g of eleutherococcus, ginkgo leaf (28.2 mg of flavone glycosides, 7.2 mg of terpene lactones), vitamins or placebo daily for 3 months. No changes were observed in the concentration (D-2) test. The results in a selective memory test significantly improved after eleutherococcus treatment compared to placebo (p<0.02). Participants felt that they were more active while being treated with eleutherococcus (p<0.02) versus ginkgo leaf and vitamins. They rated

25 different visual analogue scales in favour of eleutherococcus (p<0.05) compared to placebo [14].

The adaptogenic effects of eleutherococcus fluid extracts for the organism under stress have been investigated in 30 other studies involving a total of 2100 persons aged between 19 and 72 years, exposed to various stressors (e.g. heat, noise, increased performance or training requirements). The extracts were given orally 1-3 times daily in doses of 2-6 ml/day for up to 60 days [3]. These studies provide supportive evidence for the putative adaptogenic effect of eleutherococcus.

Clinical studies

Prophylaxis against viral infections
The prophylactic effect of an eleutherococcus fluid extract against influenza virus infections and other acute respiratory diseases was investigated in a double-blind, controlled study involving 1376 persons. From the beginning and throughout an influenza virus epidemic the subjects received either 4 ml of fluid extract or placebo daily. Typical symptoms of an influenza infection were recorded. Morbidity rates were determined during the treatment period and in a 3-month follow-up period. Morbidity rates were consistently lower in the eleutherococcus group than in the placebo group, but the differences were not statistically significant. However, administration of eleutherococcus led to a significantly lower frequency of complications (pneumonia, bronchitis, maxillary sinusitis, otitis) arising from infections (p<0.05), indicating milder development of the infections [16].

In another study the prophylactic effect of eleutherococcus against viral infections was investigated in children under school age with signs of suppression of the T-cell system, disorders in the B-cell system and/or an increased number of lymphocytes with low functional activity. The children received an ethanolic eleutherococcus fluid extract or placebo (2 drops per year of age) daily for 2 months prior to the seasons with highest infection risk in October-November and March-April. T- and B-lymphocytes and morbidity rates for acute viral respiratory infections or pneumonia were determined before and after the treatment phase. Total numbers of T- and B-lymphocytes increased and the number of lymphocytes with low functional activity decreased. Morbidity rates for acute viral respiratory infections and influenza decreased by 9.8% and the morbidity rate for pneumonia by 40% in the eleutherococcus group compared to placebo [17].

Administration of eleutherococcus fluid extract (5 days per week, 1 drop per year of age) to 130 infants attending a creche-kindergarten led to an almost 3.6-fold decrease in the incidence of influenza, anginal, acute respiratory and adenoviral infections compared to the incidence in 117 infants of the same age attending a similar establishment nearby. Broadly similar results were obtained in a subsequent and larger study involving 517 children (265 verum, 252 control) aged 1-7 years given the same dosage for one month; the incidence of respiratory-viral infections fell approximately 3-fold [15].

Effects on psychomotor performance and cognitive function

In a double-blind, placebo-controlled study, 40 hospitalized patients (28 women and 12 men aged from 23 to 55 years) with impaired performance due to neurasthenic syndrome for 1-5 years received 120 mg of eleutherococcus dry extract (equivalent to 2.0 ml of fluid extract) or placebo daily for 3 weeks. Mental performance differences between the treatment groups were determined quantitatively and qualitatively by a letter-correction test. Performance improved in the eleutherococcus group compared to the control group after 3 weeks and even after a single administration (stimulating effect, p<0.001) [21].

Other clinical studies

An open study demonstrated lower rates of various post-operative complications in abdominal and pelvic tumour patients given an eleutherococcus extract as part of a multi-faceted regimen prior to and during surgery [18].

The adjuvant use of an eleutherococcus liquid extract, 0.3-0.5 ml/kg body weight daily with penicillin, in 195 children suffering from meningococcal infections was reported to decrease the frequency of acoustic organ complications. Complications were reduced by a factor of 3 and the duration of hospital stays by 5-6 days [19].

In a double-blind, placebo-controlled study, 93 patients were treated orally with 400 mg of an eleutherococcus dry extract or placebo daily for 6 months as a prophylactic approach to recurrent episodes of *Herpes simplex* type II infections. Based on questionnaires (covering the 6 months before treatment commenced and the 6 months of treatment), 75% of patients in the eleutherococcus group reported an improvement in the frequency, severity and duration of outbreaks compared to 34% in the placebo group; the results were significant in favour of the verum group (p = 0.0002 to 0.0007) [20].

Pharmacokinetic properties

The absorption and elimination of ³H-labelled eleutheroside B was studied in rats after intra-peritoneal administration. The highest concentration of eleutheroside in the blood was observed after 15 minutes; it then dropped sharply in the period from 30 minutes to 4 hours after administration. Amounts of radioactivity in the urine and faeces indicated that elimination of eleutheroside B or its metabolites is mainly urinary (90% within 48 hours, compared to not more than 3% in the faeces) [45].

A subsequent study investigated the distribution of ³H-labelled eleutheroside B in major organs after intraperitoneal administration to rats. The liver and kidneys showed maximum incorporation within 75 minutes. High levels of labelled eleutheroside B were also found in the pancreas and medium levels in the hypophysis, adrenals and spleen. Whereas elimination from the spleen was rapid, a more complex relationship was observed in the hypophysis and adrenals. In the hypophysis, the level of radioactivity after 30 minutes fell by 50% within 2 hours but then increased, reaching the initial level again within 4 hours. Adrenal glands also showed a tendency towards accumulation between hours 2 and 4 [46].

Preclinical safety data

Acute toxicity

The acute oral LD_{50} of powdered eleutherococcus was 31.0 g/kg body weight. For a fluid extract of eleutherococcus (1:1, 33% ethanol) the oral LD_{50} in rats was greater than 20 ml/kg body weight and the intraperitoneal LD_{50} in mice was 14.5 ml/kg [22].

The oral LD_{50} of an aqueous extract of eleutherococcus in mice was greater than 3g/kg body weight. LD_{50} values for an ethanolic extract were determined as 23 ml/kg body weight after oral administration and 8 ml/kg body weight after intravenous administration. Deaths observed with the latter were attributed to the alcohol in the drug preparation [47].

Repeated dose toxicity

Eleutherococcus extracts prepared by repeated extraction at 80°C with either ethanol or water were administered to rats in doses of up to 400 mg/kg body weight/day for 33-47 days. There were no appreciable differences in comparison with controls [48]. Rats receiving 5.0 ml/kg/day of an ethanolic extract for 320 days did not show any toxic effects [22].

Reproductive toxicity

Teratogenicity studies in rats, mink, rabbits and lambs using an ethanolic fluid extract of eleutherococcus revealed no abnormalities in the offspring and no adverse effects in the parent animals [22].

Mutagenicity

Mutagenicity testing of aqueous and ethanolic eleutherococcus extracts showed that the extracts were not mutagenic to *Salmonella typhimurium* strains TA 100 and TA 98. The micronucleus test in mice was negative up to doses of 1 g/kg body weight of an ethanolic extract and 0.5 g/kg body weight of an aqueous extract [48].

REFERENCES

1. Eleutherococcus - Eleutherococci radix. European Pharmacopoeia, Council of Europe.

2. Aicher B, Wozniewski T. Eleutherococcus. In: Blaschek W, Hänsel R, Keller K, Reichling J, Rimpler H, Schneider G, editors. Hagers Handbuch der Pharmazeutischen Praxis, 5th ed. Folgeband 2: Drogen A-K. Berlin-Heidelberg-New York: Springer, 1998:556-597.

3. Farnsworth NR, Kinghorn AD, Soejarto DD, Waller DP. Siberian Ginseng (*Eleutherococcus senticosus*): current status as an adaptogen. In: Wagner H, Hikino H, Farnsworth NR, editors. Economic and Medicinal Plant Research, Volume 1. London: Academic Press, 1985:155-215.

4. Hänsel R, Sticher O, Steinegger E. Eleutherococcuswurzel. In: Pharmakognosie - Phytopharmazie. Berlin-Heidelberg-New York: Springer, 1999:811-3.

5. Szolomicki S, Samochowiec L, Wójcicki J, Drozdzik M. The influence of active components of *Eleutherococcus senticosus* on cellular defence and physical fitness in man. Phytother Res 2000;14:30-5.

6. Gubchenko PP. Influence of some plant adaptogens on efficiency rehabilitation after forced weight reduction. In: New Data on Eleutherococcus: Proceedings of the Second International Symposium on Eleutherococcus, Moscow 1984. Part II. Vladivostok: Academy of Sciences of the USSR, Far East Science Center, 1986:252-7.

7. Novozhilov GN, Silchenko KI. The mechanism of adaptogenic action of *Eleutherococcus senticosus* extract on the human body under thermal stress. Fisiol Cheloveka 1985;11:303-6.

8. Dardymov IV, Berdyshev VV, Golikov PP, Fedorets BA. The effect of prolonged administration of eleutherococcus and ascorbic acid on the healthy human body. Institute of biological active societies [Russian]. Lek Sredestva Dalnego Vostoka 1966;7:133-40.

9. Asano K, Takahashi T, Miyashita M, Matsuzaka A, Muramatsu S, Kuboyama M et al. Effect of *Eleutherococcus senticosus* extract on human physical working capacity. Planta Med 1986;52:175-7.

10. Gubchenko PP, Fruentov NK. A comparative study of effectiveness of eleutherococcus and other plant adaptogens as agents for enhancing the working capacity of the flying personnel. In: New Data on Eleutherococcus: Proceedings of the Second International Symposium on Eleutherococcus, Moscow 1984. Part II. Vladivostok: Academy of Sciences of the USSR, Far East Science Center, 1986:240-51.

11. Sosnova TL. Eleutherococcus as a means to raise colour perception of locomotive engineers. In: New Data on Eleutherococcus: Proceedings of the Second International Symposium on Eleutherococcus, Moscow 1984. Part II. Vladivostok: Academy of Sciences of the USSR, Far East Science Center, 1986:258-64.

12. Sosnova TL. Wirkung des Stachel-Eleutherokokk auf die farbunterscheidende Funktion des Sicht-analysators bei Personen mit normal-trichomatischem Sehvermögen. Vestnik Oftalmol 1969;5:59-61.

13. Baburin EF, Tarassow IK, Alexejew WN. The issue of prophylaxis in vertigo. In: Prozesse der Adaption und biologischen Aktivität von Stoffen, 1976.

14. Winther K, Ranløv C, Rein E, Mehlsen J. Russian root (Siberian ginseng) improves cognitive functions in middle-aged people, whereas Ginkgo biloba seems effective only in the elderly [Abstract]. J Neurol Sci 1997;150:S90.

15. Barkan AN, Gaiduchenya LI, Makarenko YA. [Effect of eleutherococcus on the morbidity of viral respiratory infections among children in organized collectives]. Pediatriia (Moscow) 1980;4:65-6.

16. Shadrin AS, Kustikova YG, Belogolovkina NA, Baranov NI, Oleinikova EV, Sigaeva VP et al. Estimation of prophylactic and immunostimulating effects of Eleutherococcus and *Schizandra chinensis* preparations. In: New Data on Eleutherococcus: Proceedings of the Second International Symposium on Eleutherococcus, Moscow 1984. Part II. Vladivostok: Academy of Sciences of the USSR, Far East Science Center, 1986:289-93.

17. Kozlov VK. Motivation of metabolic therapy using "energy complexes" and eleutherococcus preparations for improving adaptation disorders in children. In: New Data on Eleutherococcus: Proceedings of the Second International Symposium on Eleutherococcus, Moscow 1984. Part II. Vladivostok: Academy of Sciences of the USSR, Far East Science Center, 1986:277-81.

18. Staroselsky IV, Lisetsky VA, Kaban AP, Ganul VL, Cherny VA, Kikot VA. Prevention of postoperative complications following surgery for cancer of the lung, esophagus, stomach and colorectal cancer in patients aged over 60 years. Vopr Onkol 1991;37:873-7.

19. Kovalenko TI, Vereshchagin IA. Treating meningococcal infection in children - oral injection of eleutherococcus liquid extract from day 4 in addition to usual therapy. Don Med Inst, 1994.

20. Williams M. Immuno-protection against herpes simplex type II infection by eleutherococcus root extract. Int J Alternat Complement Med 1995;13 (July):9-12.

21. Strokina TI. The changes in higher nervous activity in neurotic patients under treatment with eleutherococcus. Lek Sredestva Dalnego Vostoka 1967;7:201-11.

22. Brekhman II. On antitoxic action of eleutherococcus. Moscow: Verlag der Akademie der Wissenschaften, 1982.

23. Wildfeuer A, Mayerhofer D. Untersuchung des Einflusses von Phytopräparaten auf zelluläre Funktionen der körpereigenen Abwehr. Arzneim-Forsch/Drug Res 1994;44:361-6.

24. Wagner H, Jurcic K. Immunologische Untersuchungen eines Eleutherococcus Trockenextraktes. Internal report. Dr. K. Thomae GmbH, 1993.

25. Wagner H, Proksch A, Riess-Maurer I, Vollmar A,

Odenthal S, Stuppner H et al. Immunstimulierend wirkende Polysaccharide (Heteroglykane) aus höheren Pflanzen (Vorläufige Mitteilung). Arzneim-Forsch/Drug Res 1984;34:659-61.

26. Fang J-N, Proksch A, Wagner H. Immunologically active polysaccharides of *Acanthopanax senticosus*. Phytochemistry 1985;11:2619-22.

27. Steinmann GG, Esperester A, Joller P. Immuno-pharmacological in vitro effects of *Eleutherococcus senticosus* extracts. Arzneim-Forsch/Drug Res 2001;51: 76-83.

28. Wacker A, Eilmes H-G. Virushemmung mit Eleutherokokk Fluid-Extrakt. Erfahrungsheilkunde 1978;27:346-51.

29. Glatthaar-Saalmüller B, Sacher F, Esperester A. Antiviral activity of an extract derived from roots of *Eleutherococcus senticosus*. Antiviral Res 2001;50: 223-8.

30. Hacker B, Medon PJ. Cytotoxic effects of *Eleutherococcus senticosus* aqueous extracts in combination with N^6-(Δ^2-isopentenyl)-adenosine and 1-β-D-arabinofuranosylcytosine against L1210 leukemia cells. J Pharm Sci 1984;73:270-2.

31. Lin C-C, Huang P-C. Antioxidant and hepatoprotective effects of *Acanthopanax senticosus*. Phytother Res 2000;14:489-94.

32. Pearce PT, Zois I, Wynne KN, Funder JW. *Panax ginseng* and *Eleutherococcus senticosus* extracts - *in vitro* studies on binding to steroid receptors. Endocrinol Japon 1982;29:567-73.

33. Nörr H. Phytochemische und pharmakologische Unter-suchungen der Adaptogendrogen *Eleutherococcus senticosus, Ocimum sanctum, Codonopsis pilosula, Rhodiola rosea* und *Rhodiola crenulata* [Dissertation]. Ludwig-Maximilians-Universität München, 1993.

34. Wagner H, Proksch A, Riess-Maurer I, Vollmar A, Odenthal S, Stuppner H et al. Immunstimulierend wirkende Polysaccharide (Heteroglykane) aus höheren Pflanzen. Arzneim-Forsch/Drug Res 1985; 35:1069-75.

35. Protasova SF, Zykov MP. Antiviral effect of eleuthero-coccus in experimental influenza infection. In: New Data on Eleutherococcus: Proceedings of the Second International Symposium on Eleutherococcus, Moscow 1984. Part I. Vladivostok: Academy of Sciences of the USSR, Far East Science Center, 1986: 170-3.

36. Wacker A. Über die Interferon induzierende und immunstimulierende Wirkung von Eleutherococcus. Erfahrungsheilkunde 1983;6:339-43.

37. Minkova M, Pantev T, Topalova S, Tenchova V. Peri-pheral blood changes in Eleutherococcus-pretreated mice exposed to acute gamma radiation. Radiobiol-Radiother 1982;23:675-8.

38. Boon-Niermeijer EK, van den Berg A, Wikman G,

Wiegant FAC. Phyto-adaptogens protect against environmental stress-induced death of embryos from the freshwater snail *Lymnaea stagnalis*. Phytomedicine 2000;7:389-99.

39. Bohn B, Nebe CT, Birr C. Flow-cytometric studies with *Eleutherococcus senticosus* extract as an immuno-modulatory agent. Arzneim-Forsch/Drug Res 1987;37: 1193-6.

40. Bohn B, Nebe CT, Birr C. Immunopharmacological effects of *Eleutherococcus senticosus* extract as determined by quantitative flow cytometry. Int J Immunopharmacol 1988;10(Suppl 1):67.

41. Elkin VM, Zakharova NG, Kingo ZN, Leonov VM, Dyubina TA. Effect of eleutherococcus on factors of the organism's resistance. In: New Data on Eleuthero-coccus: Proceedings of the Second International Symposium on Eleutherococcus, Moscow 1984. Part I. Vladivostok: Academy of Sciences of the USSR, Far East Science Center, 1986:159-63.

42. Kupin VI, Polevaya ES, Sorokin AM, Gamaleya NF. Increased immunologic reactivity of lymphocytes in oncologic patients treated with eleutherococcus extract. In: New Data on Eleutherococcus: Proceedings of the Second International Symposium on Eleutherococcus, Moscow 1984. Part II. Vladivostok: Academy of Sciences of the USSR, Far East Science Center, 1986:294-300.

43. Schmolz MW, Sacher F, Aicher B. The synthesis of Rantes, G-CSF, IL-4, IL-5, IL-6, IL-12 and IL-13 in human whole-blood cultures is modulated by an extract from *Eleutherococcus senticosus* L. roots. Phytotherapy Res 2001;15:268-70.

44. Borchers AT, van de Water J, Kenny TP, Keen CL, Stern JS, Hackman RM, Gershwin ME. Comparative effects of three species of ginseng on human peripheral blood lymphocyte proliferative responses. Int J Immunother 1998;14:143-52.

45. Bezdetko GN, German AB, Shevchenko VP, Mitrokhin YI, Myasoedov NF, Dardymov IV et al. A study of the pharmacokinetics and the mode of action of eleutherococcus glycosides. I. Tritiation of eleutheroside B. Kinetics of its accumulation and excretion from the animal organism. Khim Farm Zh 1981;15:9-13.

46. German AV, Bezdetko GN, Mitrokhin YI, Chirkov GN, Shevchenko VP, Barenboim GM et al. A study of the pharmacokinetics and the mode of action of eleutherococcus glycosides. II. Eleutheroside distribution about organs and subcellular fractions. Khim Farm Zh 1982;16:26-32.

47. Medon PJ, Thompson EB, Farnsworth NR. Hypoglycemic effect and toxicity of *Eleutherococcus senticosus* following acute and chronic administration in mice. Acta Pharmacologica Sinica 1981;2:281-5.

48. Hirosue T, Matsuzawa M, Kawai H, Hosogai Y, Yoshimura H, Takemoto K. Mutagenicity and subacute toxicity of *Acanthopanax senticosus* extracts in rats. J Food Hyg Soc Jpn 1986;27:380-6.

EUCALYPTI AETHEROLEUM

Eucalyptus Oil

DEFINITION

Eucalyptus oil is obtained by steam distillation and rectification from the fresh leaves or the fresh terminal branchlets of various species of *Eucalyptus* rich in 1,8-cineole. The species mainly used are *Eucalyptus globulus* Labill., *Eucalyptus fruticetorum* F. von Mueller (*Eucalyptus polybractea* R.T.Baker) and *Eucalyptus smithii* R.T.Baker.

The material complies with the monograph of the European Pharmacopoeia [1].

CONSTITUENTS

The European Pharmacopoeia monograph for eucalyptus oil specifies a chromatographic profile: 1,8-cineole (= eucalyptol; not less than 70%), limonene (4-12%), α-pinene (2-8%), α-phellandrene (less than 1.5%), β-pinene (less than 0.5%), camphor (less than 0.1%) [1]. To achieve these parameters and to minimise less desirable substances such as aldehydes, the oil obtained from initial steam distillation is rectified by alkaline treatment and fractional distillation [2]. The rectified oil contains 70-90% of 1,8-cineole [2-4].

In addition to constituents specified by the European Pharmacopoeia, a sample of rectified oil was found to contain γ-terpinene (2.2%), *p*-cymene (2.2%), terpinene-4-ol (1.2%), α-terpineol (0.8%), myrcene (0.5%) and terpinolene (0.3%) [3]; sesquiterpenes such as globulol and aromadendrene, which are usually present in unrectified, steam-distilled oil [5], were not detected.

CLINICAL PARTICULARS

Therapeutic indications

Internal use
Adjuvant treatment of chronic obstructive respiratory complaints [6,7] including bronchitis [8] and bronchial asthma [8,9].

Symptomatic relief of colds and catarrh of the upper respiratory tract [2,10].

External use
Symptomatic treatment of colds and rheumatic complaints [2,10].

E/S/C/O/P
MONOGRAPHS
Second Edition

Posology and method of administration

Dosage

Internal use
0.05-0.2 ml per dose [10]; 0.3-0.6 ml daily [2].
In capsules: 100-200 mg, 2-5 times daily [6-9,11].

External use
By inhalation: 12 drops per 150 ml of boiling water [11], or a 1.5% V/V solution prepared from 1 tablespoon (15 ml) per litre of warm water; treatment may be repeated up to three times daily [12].
As a liniment containing 25% V/V of oil [10].
As an ointment containing 1.3% V/m, for adults and children over 12 years: to be applied as a thick layer, up to three times daily [12,13].
As a lozenge: 0.2-15.0 mg dissolved slowly in the mouth, repeated every 0.5-1 hour [12].
As a mouthwash containing 0.91 mg/ml: 20 ml as a gargle twice daily [12].

Method of administration
For oral administration, inhalation or topical application.

Duration of administration
If symptoms persist or worsen, medical advice should be sought.

Contra-indications
Not to be used internally in cases of inflammation of the gastro-intestinal tract or gall bladder, or when liver function is impaired [2].

Special warnings and special precautions for use
Eucalyptus oil and its preparations should not be applied to the face, especially the nose, of babies and very young children [13,14].

Interaction with other medicaments and other forms of interaction
Eucalyptus oil induced hepatic microsomal enzyme activity in both in vitro and in vivo tests. The effects of other drugs may be reduced [15,16].

Pregnancy and lactation
Experiments in mice did not show any embryotoxic or fetotoxic effects after subcutaneous administration of the oil at 135 mg/kg body weight [17]. Since human data is not available, eucalyptus oil should not be used during pregnancy and lactation without medical advice.

Effects on ability to drive and use machines
None known.

Undesirable effects
In rare cases, nausea, vomiting or diarrhoea may occur [2].

Overdose
30 ml of eucalyptus oil is considered lethal [2], but ingestion of as little as 4-5 ml of oil by adults [18] and 1.9 g by a 10-year-old boy [19] has resulted in fatalities. Numerous cases of eucalyptus oil poisoning, particularly in children, have been documented [20-22], but little correlation has been observed between the reported amount of oil ingested and the severity of symptoms [22]; 2.5 ml of eucalyptus oil has caused moderate poisoning in some children [20], while others have apparently ingested larger amounts and remained asymptomatic [22].

Toxic symptoms are rapid in onset and present as epigastric burning, abdominal pain, spontaneous vomiting, respiratory problems, bronchospasm and tachypnoea followed by respiratory depression. Loss of consciousness may progress to coma and convulsions may occur, especially in children. Pinpoint pupils may lead to confusion with opiate poisoning [18], but the odour of eucalyptus on the patient's breath should assist in diagnosis.

Appropriate treatment includes gastrointestinal decontamination with activated charcoal and sorbitol [22]. If gastric lavage is required in children after recent large volume ingestion, it should be performed after general anaesthesia with endotracheal intubation [20].

In cases of minor depression of consciousness, the recommended treatment is frequent observation and intensive nursing. In unconscious states endotracheal intubation, gastric lavage, whole bowel irrigation, activated charcoal and mechanical ventilation are recommended [20].

Excessive topical use of eucalyptus oil can also lead to systemic poisoning. A 6-year-old girl who was treated topically for pruritic urticaria on the limbs and trunk with a home-made remedy, applied with bandages, containing approx. 25 ml (and on the final occasion approx. 50 ml) of eucalyptus oil per application, progressed from slurred speech, ataxia and muscle weakness to complete unconsciousness; after hospital treatment the patient recovered within 24 hours [23].

PHARMACOLOGICAL PROPERTIES

Pharmacodynamic properties

In vitro experiments

Antimicrobial activity
Eucalyptus oil showed inhibitory or bactericidal activity against a range of bacteria. Minimum inhibitory concentrations (MICs, in % V/V) for Gram-positive bacteria included: Listeria monocytogenes 0.25,

Bacillus subtilis 1.0, *Staphylococcus aureus* 2.0 and *Enterococcus* spp. 2.0. MICs for Gram-negative bacteria included: *Shigella flexneri* 0.25, *Klebsiella pneumoniae* 0.50, *Salmonella choleraesuis*, *Proteus mirabilis* and *Enterobacter aerogenes* 2.0. The oil was not effective against *Escherichia coli* or *Pseudomonas aeruginosa* (> 4.0) and in most cases it was less effective than tea tree oil [3].

In another study, eucalyptus oil was particularly effective against a *Streptococcus* isolated from bronchial aspirates, but also showed activity against pathogenic strains of *Staphylococcus aureus*, *Klebsiella*, *Salmonella typhi*, *Proteus* spp. and, in contrast to the above, *Escherichia coli* [24].

Eucalyptus oil showed inhibitory activity against *Herpes simplex* virus (HSV) types 1 and 2 in RC-37 cell cultures using a plaque reduction assay with IC_{50} values of 0.009% and 0.008% respectively, and in viral suspension tests reduced virus titres by 57.9% and 75.4% respectively. The results indicated that the oil was capable of exerting a direct virucidal effect on HSV, affecting the virus before and during absorption, but not after penetration into the host cell [25].

Antioxidant properties
Eucalyptus oil inhibited the liberation of ethene from α-keto-γ-methiol-butyric acid by the Fenton oxidant in a concentration-dependent manner starting with significant inhibition at 0.1% of oil. In another test, which allowed quantification of the degranulation of activated neutrophilic granulocytes in whole blood from human volunteers (using a system which led to the production of hypochlorous acid, HOCl), eucalyptus oil strongly inhibited the liberation by HOCl of ethene from 1-aminocyclopropane-1-carboxylic acid at concentrations above 0.1%, with almost complete inhibition at 0.25% [26].

Anti-inflammatory effects of 1,8-cineole
The inhibitory effect of 1,8-cineole on lipopolysaccharide (LPS)- and interleukin-1β (IL-1β)-stimulated inflammation mediator production was evaluated in human monocytes isolated from the blood of healthy volunteers. With 1,8-cineole at a concentration of 10^{-6} g/ml, significant inhibition of LPS-stimulated production of arachidonic acid metabolites was observed, leukotriene B4 (LTB_4) by 47%, IL-1β by 74% and thromboxane B2 by 91% (all p<0.005); the production of tumour necrosis factor-α was even more strongly inhibited, by 98.8% with LPS stimulation (p = 0.0001) and by 97.8% with IL-1β-stimulation (p = 0.0012) [27].

The effects of 1,8-cineole on inflammation mediator production by monocytes from the blood of healthy volunteers has been compared to the effects of the glucocorticoid budesonide. The monocytes were stimulated with LPS (10 µg/ml) in the presence of 1,8-cineole or budenoside (10^{-10} to 10^{-4} M) for 20 hours, then LTB_4, IL-1β and prostaglandin E2 (PGE_2) were determined by enzyme immunoassay in the culture supernatants. 1,8-Cineole at a therapeutically relevant concentration of 1.5 µg/ml (10^{-5} M) inhibited the production of LTB_4 by 27.9% (p = 0.17), IL-1β by 84.2% (p<0.001) and PGE_2 by 75.5% (p<0.003). In a comparable manner, a therapeutically relevant concentration of budenoside (10^{-8} M) inhibited the production of LTB_4 by 23% (p<0.004), IL-1β by 52% (p<0.002) and PGE_2 by 44% (p<0.02) [28].

Ex vivo experiments

Anti-inflammatory effects of 1,8-cineole
Patients with bronchial asthma (n = 10) and healthy volunteers (n = 12) participated in a study to investigate the effect of 1,8-cineole on production of the representative arachidonic acid metabolites leukotriene B4 (LTB_4) and prostaglandin E2 (PGE_2) by isolated monocytes stimulated with the calcium ionophore A23187. The subjects were treated orally with 3 × 200 mg of 1,8-cineole daily for 3 days and testing of monocytes from their blood samples took place before therapy, after 3 days of treatment (day 4) and 4 days after its discontinuation (day 8). Production of the arachidonic acid metabolites was significantly inhibited on day 4, in monocytes both from patients with bronchial asthma (LTB_4 by 40.3%, p = 0.005, n = 10; PGE_2 by 31.4%, p = 0.1, n = 3) and from healthy volunteers (LTB_4 by 57.9%, p = 0.028, n = 12; PGE_2 by 42.7%, p = 0.012, n = 8) [29].

In vivo experiments
Eucalyptus oil in doses of 10, 50 and 100 mg/kg body weight was administered to guinea pigs by stomach tube. Respiratory tract fluid (RTF) was collected from a tracheal cannula under urethane anaesthesia. Compared to controls treated with 12% ethanol at a dose of 5 ml/kg, eucalyptus oil (50 mg/kg) gave a 172% increase in RTF output after 2 hours. Smaller increases were seen with similar dose levels in rats, rabbits, cats and dogs. No effects were observed on either the specific gravity or chloride content of the RTF [30].

Administration of eucalyptus oil by steam inhalation to urethane-treated rabbits in doses of up to 20 g/kg body weight had no significant effect on RTF output except at the highest dose, which caused deaths in the animals [31].

Eucalyptus oil emulsified in physiological saline was administered to guinea pigs, then cough was generated by mechanical stimulation and the antitussive effect relative to codeine (15 mg/kg) evaluated. Eucalyptus oil (5%) administered by inhalation had an antitussive effect relative to codeine of 0.68 (p<0.05). When administered intraperitoneally in a concentration of 50 mg/kg, the effect relative to codeine was 0.56 (p<0.001) [32].

Pharmacological studies in humans

Eucalyptus oil (10 ml) was administered to 26 male and 5 female volunteers over a period of 5 minutes by means of a face mask. Total nasal resistance to airflow was measured by means of a nasal resistance meter. The results showed that eucalyptus oil had no effect on nasal resistance to airflow, but the majority of subjects reported a cold sensation in the nose with the sensation of improved airflow [33].

During a clinical study [6, summarized under Clinical studies] a test performed on the patients demonstrated that cineole improved ciliary performance. Compared to initial data, after 4 days of oral treatment with 3×200 mg of cineole daily the ciliary frequency of cilia brushed from the inside of the nose (2-3 cm from the orifice), placed in a nutrient solution and observed under a microscope fitted with a photomultiplier increased by 8.2% (p<0.001), whereas corresponding increases after ambroxol and placebo treatment were insignificant (1.1% and 1.7% respectively) [6].

Clinical studies

In a single-blind parallel study 234 subjects with acute respiratory tract infections were divided into 4 treatment groups (vaporised eucalyptus oil, camphor, menthol, or steam control). Nasal airway resistance was measured using a rhinomanometer. Eucalyptus oil was significantly more effective in reducing nasal congestion only over the first hour (p<0.02) [34]. In a number of studies in patients with acute coryzal rhinitis (common cold) no significant differences in nasal decongestant activity between eucalyptus oil (1.3%) in petrolatum and petrolatum placebo were reported [34].

Although few clinical studies have been carried out with eucalyptus oil, several studies involving the oral use of its major component, 1,8-cineole (70-90% of the oil), have been published, as summarized below.

In a randomized, double-blind, placebo-controlled study, 32 patients suffering from steroid-dependent bronchial asthma and being treated orally with 5-24 mg of the glucocorticosteroid prednisolone daily (as the lowest maintenance dose) as well as inhaled steroids and other asthma medications were additionally assigned to receive orally 3×200 mg of cineole or placebo daily for 12 weeks. Oral prednisolone dose levels were reduced by 2.5 mg increments every 3 weeks. A decrease of 36% in daily prednisolone dosage was tolerated in the verum group (mean reduction, 3.75 mg) compared to only 7% (mean reduction, 0.91 mg) in the placebo group (p = 0.006). In the verum group 12 out of 16 patients achieved a reduction in oral glucocorticosteroid dose level compared to 4 out of 16 in the placebo group (p = 0.012) [9].

To compare the effects of secretolytics on lung function, a double-blind, placebo-controlled, three-way cross-over study was carried out in 30 patients with chronic obstructive respiratory complaints. They were treated for periods of 4 days, separated by washout periods of 2-3 days, with 2 capsules (verum or placebo) and 1 tablet (verum or placebo) three times daily providing, in a randomized order, the following *daily* doses: 3×200 mg of cineole (in capsules); 3×30 mg of ambroxol hydrochloride (in tablets); placebo capsules and tablets only. No concomitant medications (theophylline, β-2 adrenergics, mucolytics or antitussives) were permitted during the study. 20 patients completed the full course of treatment. Significant improvements from treatment with cineole and ambroxol were observed with respect to forced vital capacity (FVC), forced expiratory volume in one second (FEV$_1$) and peak expiratory flow (PEV). Compared to initial values before cineole, ambroxol and placebo respectively, FVC values 2.5 hours after completion of treatment on day 4 had increased by 5.3%, 5.5% and 2.2% (p<0.01 in favour of cineole or ambroxol); the changes in FEV$_1$ were + 4.2%, + 4.8% and – 0.3% (p<0.05 in favour of cineole or ambroxol) while PEV values had changed by + 9.1%, + 7.2% and – 0.4% (p<0.05 in favour of cineole or ambroxol). Changes in cough scores were not significant [6].

In a randomized, double-blind, cross-over study, 29 patients suffering from chronic obstructive respiratory complaints were assigned to treatment with 3×200 mg of cineole (in 6 capsules, taken with 3 placebo tablets) or 3×30 mg of ambroxol (in 3 tablets, taken with 6 placebo capsules) daily for 7 days and vice versa after a wash-out period of 3-5 days. Concomitant medication with inhaled steroids and/or oral theophylline was permitted throughout the study. Data from the 24 patients who complied with the protocol was included in the analysis. In lung function tests by body plethysmography, airway resistance (RAW) and specific conductance (sGAW) significantly improved (p<0.01) after treatment with both cineole and ambroxol, while intrathoracic gas volume (ITGV) and residual volume (RV) improved significantly only after cineole (p<0.05). No significant changes were observed in the spirometric lung function parameters FEV$_1$ or FVC; vital capacity (VC) significantly increased with cineole (p<0.05) but not with ambroxol. Scores for dyspnoea, coughing and amount of secretion showed some improvement after both treatments but failed to reach statistical significance. Based on the plethysmographic results, the authors concluded that cineole appears to have a bronchodilator (as well as expectorant) effect [7].

In an open study 100 patients, of whom 81 were suffering from chronic bronchitis and 19 from bronchial asthma and/or emphysema, received orally, after acute deterioration of their condition and in addition to their basic medication (mainly β-2 mimetics and theophylline), 4×200 mg or 3×200 mg of cineole daily for 7 days,. Measurement of clinical parameters of lung function at the end of treatment showed, in comparison with initial values, average increases of 11% in forced vital capacity (FVC), 12% in forced expiratory volume in one second (FEV$_1$) and 19% in peak expiratory flow (PEV), while residual volume after maximum exhalation (RV) decreased by 18%. The physicians and patients assessed the therapeutic effects of cineole treatment as good in 70% and 75% of cases, and satisfactory in 23% and 14%, respectively [8].

Pharmacokinetic properties

Inhalation by mice of 1,8-cineole from 0.5 ml of rosemary oil released into the breathing air resulted in detectable levels of 1,8-cineole in the blood. Elimination of 1,8-cineole from blood was biphasic with a short half-life of 6 minutes during the first phase and a half-life of about 45 minutes during a second phase, indicating elimination in accordance with a two-compartment model [35].

Topical application to rats of an ointment containing *inter alia* 66.5 mg of 1,8-cineole resulted in levels of 10.5 mg of cineole in muscle tissue after 3 hours [36].

Following intravenous administration of a solution of cineole in ethanol to rats, 1% of the administered cineole was found in lung tissue and 4% in liver tissue after 1 hour [37].

Oral administration of 1,8-cineole to brushtail possums (*Trichosorus vulpecula*) gave rise to *p*-cresol, 9-hydroxycineole and cineol-9-oic acid as major urinary metabolites [38].

In humans (n = 10) a plasma half-life of 35.8 minutes was established after a 10-minute inhalation of cineole [39].

Preclinical safety data

Acute toxicity
The oral LD$_{50}$ of eucalyptus oil has been determined as 4.44 g/kg body weight in rats [40] and 3.32 g/kg in mice [41].

The oral LD$_{50}$ of 1,8-cineole was 2.48 g/kg body weight in the rat while the acute dermal LD$_{50}$ exceeded 5 g/kg in rabbits [42].

Subacute toxicity
Groups of male and female rats received eucalyptol (1,8-cineole) for 28 days, either by stomach tube on 5 days/week at 150-1200 mg/kg body weight or in encapsulated form with the diet at 3750-30000 mg, equivalent to 381-3342 mg/kg bw/day for male rats

and 353-3516 mg/kg bw/day for female rats. At dose levels of 600 mg/kg and higher, dose-related decrease in body weight gain and absence of a normal degree of hepatic centrilobar cytoplasmic vacuolization was observed in male rats. In addition, other dose-related lesions in the liver, kidneys and parotid salivary glands were found at all dose levels in male rats fed encapsulated eucalyptol [19].

Chronic toxicity
In a long-term oral study, groups of 52 male, pathogen-free, CFLP mice were given 1,8-cineole at 0, 8 or 32 mg/kg body weight/day by gavage (in a toothpaste base) on 6 days per week for 80 weeks followed by an observation period of 16-24 weeks according to the number of survivors. No treatment-related effects on body weight, food consumption, survival, weight of adrenals, kidneys, liver, lungs or spleen, or on the microscopic appearance of brain, lungs, liver and kidneys, or on tumour incidence, were observed [43].

Reproductive toxicity
Studies in rats showed that 1,8-cineole penetrated placental tissue to give a foetal blood level sufficient to stimulate hepatic enzyme activity after a dose of 500 mg/kg given subcutaneously [16]. Mice treated subcutaneously with eucalyptus oil at a dose of 135 mg/kg body weight during the period of organo-genesis (days 6-15 of gestation) showed no evidence of embryotoxicity or fetotoxicity [17].

Studies in rats have shown that 1,8-cineole probably cannot cross the blood-milk barrier in amounts sufficient to affect hepatic microsomal enzymes in the offspring [44].

Mutagenicity and carcinogenicity
1,8-cineole did not show mutagenic effects in *Salmonella typhimurium* strains TA97a, TA98, TA100 and TA102, with or without metabolic activation [45] nor, in earlier tests, in strains TA98, TA100, TA1535 and TA1537 [19].

In Chinese hamster ovary (CHO) cells, 1,8-cineole did not induce chromosome aberrations with or without metabolic activation. Sister chromatid exchanges were induced in CHO cells only in the absence of metabolic activation at doses that induced cell cycle delay [19]. Sister chromatid exchanges induced by mitomycin C in cultured CHO K-1 cells were not increased by post-treatment with 1,8-cineole [46].

The rec-assay in *Bacillus subtilis* showed no evidence of DNA damage [19].

Eucalyptus oil appeared to be a weak promoter of papilloma formation in mice treated with 9,10-dimethyl-benzanthracene [47].

REFERENCES

1. Eucalyptus oil - Eucalypti aetheroleum. European Pharmacopoeia, Council of Europe.

2. Brand N. Eucalyptus. In: Hagers Handbuch der Pharmazeutischen Praxis, 5th ed. Volume 5: Drogen E-O. Berlin: Springer-Verlag, 1993:115-30.

3. Harkenthal M, Reichling J, Geiss H-K, Saller R. Comparative study on the *in vitro* antibacterial activity of Australian tea tree oil, cajuput oil, niaouli oil, manuka oil, kanuka oil and eucalyptus oil. Pharmazie 1999; 54:460-3.

4. Wilson ND, Watt RA, Moffat AC. A near-infrared method for the assay of cineole in eucalyptus oil as an alternative to the official BP method. J Pharm Pharmacol 2001;53:95-102.

5. Renedo J, Otero JA, Mira JR. Huile essentielle d'*Eucalyptus globulus* L. de Cantabrie (Espagne). Variation au cours de la distillation. Plantes Méd Phytothér 1990;24:31-5.

6. Kaspar P, Repges R, Dethlefsen U, Petro W. Sekretolytika im Vergleich. Änderung der Ziliarfrequenz und Lungen-funktion nach Therapie mit Cineol und Ambroxol. Atemw-Lungenkrkh 1994;20:605-14.

7. Wittman M, Petro W, Kaspar P, Repges R, Dethlefsen U. Zur Therapie chronisch obstruktiver Atemwegser-krankungen mit Sekretolytika. Doppelblinder, randomisierter Cross-over-Vergleich zwischen Cineol und Ambroxol. Atemw Lungenkrkh 1998;24:67-74.

8. Mahlo D-H. Obstruktive Atemwegserkrankungen. Mit Cineol die Lungenfunktionsparameter verbessern. Therapiewoche 1990;40:3157-62.

9. Juergens UR, Dethlefsen U, Steinkamp G, Gillissen A, Repges R, Vetter H. Anti-inflammatory activity of 1,8-cineole (eucalyptol) in bronchial asthma: a double-blind placebo-controlled trial. Respiratory Med 2003;97:250-6.

10. Reynolds JEF, Prasad AB, editors. Martindale - The Extra Pharmacopoeia. 28th ed. London: Pharmaceutical Press, 1982:1017-8.

11. Van Hellemont J. In: Fytotherapeutisch compendium, 2nd ed. Utrecht: Bohn, Scheltema & Holkema, 1988:232.

12. Food and Drug Administration. Over-The-Counter Drugs. Establishment of a monograph for OTC cold, cough, allergy, bronchodilator and antiasthmatic products. Federal Register 1976;41:38408-9.

13. Schilcher H. External applications for respiratory tract diseases. In: Phytotherapy in Paediatrics. Stuttgart: Medpharm, 1997:30.

14. Corrigan D. *Eucalyptus* species. In: De Smet PAGM, Keller K, Hänsel R, Chandler RF, editors. Adverse effects of herbal drugs, Volume 1. Berlin: Springer-Verlag, 1992:125-33.

15. Jori A, Bianchetti A, Prestini PE. Effects of essential oils on drug metabolism. Biochem Pharmacol 1969;18:2081-5.

16. Jori A, Briatico G. Effect of eucalyptol on microsomal enzyme activity of foetal and newborn rats. Biochem Pharmacol 1973;22:543-4.

17. Pages N, Fournier G, Le Luyer F, Marques M-C. Les huiles essentielles et leur propriétés tératogènes potentielles: example de l'huile essentielle d'Eucalyptus globulus, Étude préliminaire chez la souris. Plantes Méd Phytothér 1990;24:21-6.

18. McPherson J. The toxicology of eucalyptus oil. Med J Austral 1925;2:108-10.

19. Scientific Committee on Food. Opinion of the Scientific Committee on Food on eucalyptol. SCF/CS/FLAV/FLAVOUR/20 ADD2 Final. European Commission, Health & Consumer Protection Directorate-General. 17 April 2002. http://europa.eu.int/comm/food/fs/sc/scf/index_en.html

20. Tibballs J. Clinical effects and management of eucalyptus oil ingestion in infants and young children. Med J Austral 1995;163:177-80.

21. Tibballs J, James A. Eucalyptus oil - medicinal therapy or folk remedy? Aust J Hosp Pharm 1995;25:516-9.

22. Webb NJA, Pitt WR. Eucalyptus oil poisoning in childhood: 41 cases in south-east Queensland. J Paediatr Child Health 1993;29:368-71.

23. Darben T, Cominos B, Lee CT. Topical eucalyptus oil poisoning. Australasian J Dermatol 1998;39:265-7.

24. Benouda A, Hassar M, Benjilali B. Les propriétés antiséptiques des huiles essentielles *in vitro* testées contre des germes pathogènes hospitaliers. Fitoterapia 1988;59:115-9.

25. Schnitzler P, Schon K, Reichling J. Antiviral activity of Australian tea tree oil and eucalyptus oil against herpes simplex virus in cell culture. Pharmazie 2001;56:343-7.

26. Graßmann J, Hippeli S, Dornisch K, Rohnert U, Beuscher N and Elstner EF. Antioxidant properties of essential oils. Possible explanations for their anti-inflammatory effects. Arzneim-Forsch/Drug Res 2000;50:135-9.

27. Juergens UR, Stöber M, Vetter H. Inhibition of cytokine production and arachidonic acid metabolism by eucalyptol (1,8-cineole) in human blood monocytes in vitro. Eur J Med Res 1998;3:508-10.

28. Juergens UR, Stöber M, Vetter H. Steroidartige Hemmung des monozytären Arachidonsäure-metabolismus und der IL-1β-Produktion durch 1.8-Cineol. Atemw-Lungenkrkh 1998;24:3-11.

29. Juergens UR, Stöber M, Schmidt-Schilling L, Kleuver T, Vetter H. Antiinflammatory effects of eucalyptol (1,8-cineole) in bronchial asthma: inhibition of arachidonic acid metabolism in human blood monocytes ex vivo. Eur J Med Res 1998;3:407-12.

30. Boyd EM, Pearson GL. On the expectorant action of volatile oils. Am J Med Sci 1946;211:602-10.

31. Boyd EM, Sheppard EP. The effect of steam inhalation of volatile oils on the output and composition of respiratory tract fluid. J Pharmacol Exp Ther 1968; 163:250-6.

32. Misawa M, Kizawa M. Antitussive effects of several volatile oils especially of cedar leaf oil in guinea pigs. Pharmacometrics 1990;39:81-7.

33. Burrow A, Eccles R, Jones AS. The effect of camphor, eucalyptus and menthol vapour on nasal resistance to airflow and nasal sensation. Acta Otolaryngol 1983; 96:157-61.

34. Food and Drug Administration. Final monograph for OTC nasal decongestant drug products. Federal Register 1994;59:43389-91.

35. Kovar KA, Gropper B, Friess D, Ammon HPT. Blood levels of 1,8-cineole and locomotor activity of mice after inhalation and oral administration of rosemary oil. Planta Med 1987;53:315-8.

36. Weyers W, Brodbeck R. Hautdurchdringung ätherischer Öle. Pharm unserer Zeit 1989;18:82-6.

37. Grisk A, Fischer W. Zur pulmonalen Ausscheidung von Cineol, Menthol und Thymol bei Ratten nach rektaler Applikation. Zschr Ärztl Fortbild 1969;63:233-6.

38. Southwell JA, Flynn TM, Degabriele R. Metabolism of α- and β-pinene, p-cymene and 1,8-cineole in the brushtail possum Trichosurus vulpecula. Xenobiotica 1980;10:17-23.

39. Römmelt H, Schnizer W, Swoboda M, Senn E. Pharmakokinetik ätherischer Öle nach Inhalation mit einer terpenhaltigen Salbe. Z Phytotherapie 1988;9:14-6.

40. von Skramlik E. Über die Giftigkeit und Verträglichkeit von ätherischen Ölen. Pharmazie 1959;14:435-45.

41. Ohsumi T, Kuroki K, Kimura T, Murakami Y. Study on acute toxicities of essential oils used in endodontic treatment. Kyushu Shika Gakkai Zasshi 1984;38:1064-71 through Chem Abstr 1985;102:179007.

42. Opdyke DLJ. Eucalyptus oil. Food Cosmet Toxicol 1975;13:107-8.

43. Roe FJC, Palmer AK, Worden AN, Van Abbe NJ. Safety evaluation of toothpaste containing chloroform. I. Long term studies in mice. J Envir Path and Toxicol 1979;2: 799-819.

44. De Vincenzi M, Silano M, De Vincenzi A, Maialetti F, Scazzocchio B. Safety data review. Constituents of aromatic plants: eucalyptol. Fitoterapia 2002;73:269-75.

45. Gomes-Carneiro MR, Felzenszwalb I, Paumgartten FJR. Mutagenicity testing of (±)-camphor, 1,8-cineole, citral, citronellal, (–)-menthol and terpineol with the Salmonella/microsome assay. Mutation Res 1998; 416:129-36.

46. Sasaki YF, Imanishi H, Ohta T, Shirasu Y. Modifying effects of components of plant essence on the induction of sister-chromatid exchanges in cultured Chinese hamster ovary cells. Mutation Res 1989;226:103-10.

47. Roe FJC, Field WEH. Chronic toxicity of essential oils and certain products of natural origin. Food Cosmet Toxicol 1965;3:311-24.

FILIPENDULAE ULMARIAE HERBA

Meadowsweet

DEFINITION

Meadowsweet consists of the whole or cut, dried flowering tops of *Filipendula ulmaria* (L.) Maxim. (= *Spiraea ulmaria* L.). It contains not less than 1 ml/kg of steam-volatile substances, calculated with reference to the dried drug.

The material complies with the monograph of the European Pharmacopoeia [1].

CONSTITUENTS

Flavonoids, up to 6% in the flowers, particularly spiraeoside (quercetin-4'-glucoside), and approx. 3-4% in the flowering herb, including hyperoside, other quercetin derivatives and kaempferol-4'-glucoside [2-8].

Glycosides of salicylaldehyde (monotropitin = gaultherin), of methyl salicylate (spiraein) and of salicyl alcohol (isosalicin) (up to 0.5% in total) [9-13].

Steam distillation of the dried flowers yields a small amount (0.2%) of volatile oil (arising from the phenolic glycosides during drying and storage), of which about 75% is salicylaldehyde [12,14,15]. Previous findings, however, stated that such compounds are only present in fresh flowers [16]; after steam distillation of fresh flowering tops, the proportion of salicylaldehyde in the oil was 36% [17].

Ellagitannins (10-15%) derived from galloyl-4,6-hexahydroxydiphenoyl-β-D-glucose units, the major one being the dimeric compound rugosin D [9,18-23].

The flowers also contain a heparin-like substance, which is bound to plant proteins in the form of a complex [24,25].

CLINICAL PARTICULARS

Therapeutic indications
As supportive therapy for the common cold [9,18, 19,26-28].
Meadowsweet is also used to enhance the renal elimination of water [9,18,19,28-31], although published scientific evidence does not adequately support this indication.

Posology and method of administration

Dosage
Unless otherwise prescribed, the daily dose as a tea

E/S/C/O/P
MONOGRAPHS
Second Edition

157

infusion is:
Adults: 2-6 g of the drug daily [18,32].
Children 1-4 years of age: 1-2 g daily [33].
Children 4-10 years of age: 2-3 g daily [33].
Children 10-16 years of age: adult dose [33].

Liquid extract (1:2), 3-6 ml daily; tincture (1:5), 7.5-15 ml daily [32].

Method of administration
For oral administration.

Duration of administration
No restriction.

Contra-indications
Due to the presence of salicylates, the drug should not be used in cases of hypersensitivity to salicylates [9,18].

Special warnings and special precautions for use
None required.

Interaction with other medicaments and other forms of interaction
None reported. The level of salicylate derivatives makes interaction with anticoagulant agents unlikely.

Pregnancy and lactation
No data available. In accordance with general medical practice, the products should not be used during pregnancy and lactation without medical advice.

Effects on ability to drive and use machines
None known.

Undesirable effects
None reported.

Overdose
No toxic effects reported.

PHARMACOLOGICAL PROPERTIES

Pharmacodynamic properties

Antimicrobial activity

In vitro experiments
Combined 70%-ethanolic and aqueous extracts (1 ml corresponding to 1 g of herb), tested at 5% in the culture medium, inhibited the growth of *Staphylococcus aureus haemolyticus*, *Streptococcus pyogenes haemolyticus*, *Escherichia coli*, *Shigella flexneri*, *Klebsiella pneumoniae* and *Bacillus subtilis* [34].

A tincture from the flowers (70% ethanol, diluted 1:10 and 1:25) inhibited the growth of *Staphylococcus aureus* and *S. epidermis* at both concentrations, and

of *Proteus vulgaris* and *Pseudomonas aeruginosa* at the higher concentration only. No effect was seen with *E. coli* or *Klebsiella* [35].

Anti-inflammatory activity

In vitro experiments
An aqueous, lyophilized extract of meadowsweet leaves inhibited prostaglandin biosynthesis from ^{14}C-arachidonic acid (i.e. inhibited cyclooxygenase) in bovine seminal vesicle microsomes by 36% at 0.2 mg/ml, a relatively low level of activity compared to 88% inhibition by indometacin at 2.8 μM. The same extract strongly inhibited platelet activating factor (PAF)-induced exocytosis (and hence release of the enzyme elastase) in neutrophils from human peripheral blood by 93% at 0.25 mg/ml [36].

Immunomodulatory activity

In vitro experiments
Dry extracts from meadowsweet flowers and herb exhibited strong inhibitory activity towards the classical pathway of the complement system, ethyl acetate (IC_{50}: 5.4 μg/ml) and methanolic (IC_{50}: 14.6 μg/ml) extracts of the flowers, and the methanolic extract (IC_{50}: 14.5 μg/ml) of the herb, being the most effective. As the ethyl acetate extract of the flowers retained its activity after treatment with skin powder, it was concluded that complement inhibitory activity of this fraction is not attributable to tannins [37].

In the same series of experiments, meadowsweet dry extracts from flowers and herb prepared with ether, ethyl acetate, methanol or water inhibited luminol-dependent chemiluminescence (an indicator of the production of reactive oxygen species) generated by zymosan-stimulated human polymorphonuclear leukocytes (PMNs) with IC_{50} values of 66.3 μg/ml, 42.3 μg/ml and 37.4 μg/ml respectively for the flower extracts and 81.9 μg/ml, 44.5 μg/ml, 59.5 μg/ml and 60.8 μg/ml respectively for the herb extracts. The extracts also inhibited T-cell proliferation, with IC_{50} values of 100.4 μg/ml, 173.9 μg/ml and 210.5 μg/ml respectively for ethyl acetate, methanol and aqueous extracts of the flowers, and 195.1 μg/ml, 150.0 μg/ml and 195.2 μg/ml respectively for ether, ethyl acetate and methanolic extracts of the herb [37].

Various extracts of meadowsweet flowers were investigated for *in vitro* modulatory activity towards the classical pathway of complement activation. The highest inhibitory activity was found in the ethyl acetate extract (IC_{50}: 2.9 μg/ml), followed by the ether (IC_{50}: 9.8 μg/ml), light petroleum (IC_{50}: 12.0 μg/ml), methanol (IC_{50}: 12.8 μg/ml) and aqueous (IC_{50}: 53.5 μg/ml) extracts. A purified fraction from the ethyl acetate extract (constituents not identified) also showed strong inhibitory activity (IC_{50}: 0.46 μg/ml), even stronger than that of isolated flavonoids (of which quercetin was the most potent with an IC_{50} of 16.7 µg/ml) [38].

A decoction of the flowers enhanced the growth-stimulating activity of mice peritoneal macrophages *in vitro* and *in vivo* [39].

Elastase-inhibiting activity

In vitro experiments
Extracts (50% ethanolic) of meadowsweet flowers and leaves inhibited the activity of the proteolytic enzyme elastase by 100% and 92% respectively, measured by spectrophotometry using an amino acid-nitroanilide substrate and attributed to the tannin content of the materials [40].

Anticoagulant and fibrinolytic effects

In vivo experiments
A heparin-like complex found in meadowsweet flowers showed some anticoagulant and fibrinolytic properties after intramuscular and intravenous administration to animals, the effect being neutralized by protamine sulphate [24,25].

Intestinal effects/effects on gastric ulcers

In vivo experiments
Orally administered decoctions of meadowsweet flowers (1:10 and 1:20) at doses of 0.5 or 2.5 ml/100 g respectively reduced the formation of stomach lesions induced by fixation, immobilisation or subcutaneous injection of reserpine to rats and mice. The decoctions also prevented acetylsalicylic acid-induced lesions of the stomach and promoted healing of ethanol-induced stomach lesions in rats [41].

An ethanolic spissum extract from meadowsweet, administered to mice (50-1000 mg intraperitoneally), rats (2500 mg/kg orally) and rabbits (15-30 mg/kg intravenously) as a 5% aqueous solution and a decoction (1:20), showed a positive effect on the permeability of vessels provoked by histamine in the trypan blue test system [42].

Quercetin-3'-glucoside from meadowsweet, orally administered as a dose of 0.5 ml of a 5% solution per 10 g body weight, reduced by 50% the occurrence of serious lesions of the rat stomach provoked by immobilisation and intraperitoneal injection of reserpine (2.5 mg/kg) [43].

CNS effects

In vivo experiments
In various animals, a 5% aqueous solution of an ethanolic spissum extract and a decoction (1:20) from meadowsweet showed suppressive effects on the central nervous sytem, such as reduction of motor activity and rectal temperature, myorelaxation and potentiation of the activity of narcotic agents, and prolongation of the life time of mice in closed cages [42].

Anticarcinogenic effects

In vivo experiments
Long-term oral administration of a decoction of meadowsweet flowers inhibited the growth of brain and spinal cord tumours induced by transplacental administration of N-ethyl-N-nitroso-urea in rats. It did not affect the development of cervical and vaginal tumours induced by intravaginal application of 7,12-dimethylbenz[a]anthracene in mice but, when applied intravaginally, the decoction inhibited cervical and vaginal carcinogenesis induced by this compound. Tubal oral administration of the decoction suppressed the growth of transplanted sarcoma-180 as well as the growth and metastasis of transplanted Lewis' carcinoma in mice [39].

Local administration of a decoction of meadowsweet flowers resulted in a 39% decrease in the frequency of squamous-cell carcinoma of the cervix and vagina induced in mice by 7,12-dimethylbenz[a]anthracene treatment [44].

Isolated rugosin D was administered intraperitoneally as a single dose of 10 mg/kg body weight to 6 female mice; 4 days later and at weekly intervals thereafter for 60 days the mice were injected intraperitoneally with 10^5 sarcoma-180 tumour cells. Antitumour activity was calculated as the percentage increase in life-span, %ILS = 100 × (mean survival days of the treated group - mean survival days of the vehicle control group/mean survival days of the vehicle control group). The vehicle control group had a mean survival period of 12.9 days. After 10 mg of rugosin D, the %ILS value was 171.5 and one animal showed no tumours on day 60. The authors suggested that the antitumour activity was likely to be through potentiation of the immunity of host animals rather than direct activity on the tumour cells [45].

Affinity for proteins

In vitro experiments
Isolated rugosin D (a dimer of penta-O-galloyl-β-D-glucose) showed a high capacity for binding to bovine serum albumin (BSA), even higher than penta-O-galloyl-β-D-glucose, the tannin having the highest protein binding capacity in the simple galloyl-D-glucose series [46], whereas 1,2,3-tri-O-galloyl-4,6-hexahydroxydiphenoyl-β-D-glucose had a weaker effect and 2,3-di-O-galloyl-4,6-hexahydroxy-diphenoyl-β-D-glucose a low effect [47].

Effects on cervical mucosa

Clinical study

After local application of an ointment containing a decoction of meadowsweet flowers to 48 patients with cervical dysplasia, a positive response was recorded in 32 patients (67%), including 25 cases (52%) of complete regression of dysplasia. No recurrence was observed within 12 months in 10 completely cured patients [44].

Pharmacokinetic properties

No data available.

Preclinical safety data

For an ethanolic spissum extract of meadowsweet as a 5% aqueous solution, the intraperitoneal LD_{50} in mice and intravenous LD_{50} in rabbits were determined as 1770 mg/kg and 75.7 mg/kg respectively. For a decoction (1:20), the intraperitoneal LD_{50} in male and female mice, and the intravenous LD_{50} in rabbits, were found to be 535 mg/kg, 1050 mg/kg and 141.5 mg/kg respectively [42].

Pharmacological studies of meadowsweet flowers and their extracts in rats and rabbits did not show any influence on liver function [48].

REFERENCES

1. Meadowsweet - Filipendulae ulmariae herba. European Pharmacopoeia, Council of Europe.

2. Lamaison JL, Carnat A, Petitjean-Freytet C. Teneurs en principaux flavonoides de lots commerciaux de *Filipendula ulmaria* (L.) Maxim. Plantes Méd Phytothér 1991;25:1-5.

3. Lamaison JL, Petitjean-Freytet C, Carnat A. Teneurs en principaux flavonoïdes de parties aériennes *Filipendula ulmaria* (L.) Maxim. subsp. *ulmaria* et subsp. *denudata* (J. & C: Presl) Hayek. Pharm Acta Helv 1992;67:218-22.

4. Hörhammer L, Hänsel R, Endres W. Über die Flavonglykoside der Gattungen Filipendula und Spiraea. Arch Pharmaz 1956;289/61:133-40.

5. Scheer T, Wichtl M. Zum Vorkommen von Kämpferol-4'-O-β-D-glucopyranosid in *Filipendula ulmaria* und *Allium cepa*. Planta Med 1987;53:573-4.

6. Hörhammer L, Hänsel R, Kriesmair G, Endres W. Zur Kenntnis der Polygonaceenflavone. I. Über ein mittels α-Glykosidasen spaltbares Querzetinarabinosid aus *Polygonum polystachum*. Arch Pharmaz Ber deutsch pharmaz Ges 1955;288/60:419-25.

7. Shelyuto VL, Glyzin VI, Filipchik VN, Smirnova LP, Ban'kovskii AI. Structure of a flavonoid glycoside from

Filipendula ulmaria. Khim Prir Soedin 1977;(1):113, through Chem Abstr 1977;87:50194.

8. Poukens-Renwart P, Tits M, Wauters J-N, Angenot L. Densitometric evaluation of spiraeoside after derivatization in flowers of *Filipendula ulmaria* (L.) Maxim. J Pharmaceut Biomed Analysis 1992;10:1085-8.

9. Meier B, Meier-Liebi M. Filipendula. In: Hänsel R, Keller K, Rimpler H, Schneider G, editors. Hagers Handbuch der pharmazeutischen Praxis, 5th ed. Volume 5: Drogen E-O. Berlin: Springer-Verlag, 1993: 147-56.

10. Thieme H. Isolierung und Strukturaufklärung des Spiraeins, eines Phenolglykosids aus den Blüten von *Filipendula ulmaria* (L.) Maxim. Pharmazie 1965; 20:113-4.

11. Meier B, Lehmann L, Sticher O, Bettschart A. Salicylate in Arzneipflanzen. Screening-Methoden (HPLC, DC) zum Nachweis. Dtsch Apoth Ztg 1987;127:2401-7.

12. Meier B. Analytik, chromatographisches Verhalten und potentielle Wirksamkeit der Inhaltsstoffe salicylat-haltiger Arzneipflanzen Mitteleuropas [Habilitations-schrift]. Eidg Techn Hochschule (ETH) Zürich, 1987: 161-9.

13. Thieme H. Isolierung eines neuen phenolischen Glykosids aus den Blüten von *Filipendula ulmaria* (L.) Maxim. Pharmazie 1966;21:123.

14. Lindeman A, Jounela-Eriksson P, Lounasmaa M. The aroma composition of the flower of meadowsweet (*Filipendula ulmaria* (L.) Maxim.). Lebensm Wiss Technol 1982;15:286-9.

15. Kozhin SA, Sulina YG. Composition of essential oil from *Filipendula ulmaria* inflorescences. Rastit Resur 1971;567-71; through Chem Abstr 1972;76:297.

16. Piette JL, Lecomte J. Salicyles de la spirée ulmaire et composition du sol. Bull Soc Roy Sci Liège 1981;50:178-84.

17. Valle MG, Nano GM, Tira S. Das ätherische Öl aus *Filipendula ulmaria*. Planta Med 1988;54:181-2.

18. Wichtl M. Spiraeae flos - Mädesüßblüten. In: Wichtl M, editor. Teedrogen und Phytopharmaka, 4th ed. Stuttgart: Wissenschaftliche Verlagsgesellschaft, 2002:587-9.

19. Wichtl M. Monographien-Kommentar: Mädesüßblüten. In: Standardzulassungen für Fertigarzneimittel. Stuttgart: Deutscher Apotheker Verlag, Frankfurt: Govi-Verlag, 1997.

20. Okuda T, Yoshida T, Hatano T. Classification of oligomeric hydrolysable tannins and specificity of their occurrence in plants. Phytochemistry 1993;32: 507-21.

21. Haslam E, Lilley TH, Cai Y, Martin R, Magnolato D. Traditional herbal medicines - the role of polyphenols. Planta Med 1989;55:1-8.

22. Haslam E. Natural polyphenols (vegetable tannins) as

drugs: possible modes of action. J Nat Prod 1996;59:205-15.

23. Gupta RK, Al-Shafi SMK, Layden K, Haslam E. The metabolism of gallic acid and hexahydroxydiphenic acids in plants. Part 2. Esters of (S)-hexahydroxydiphenic acid with D-glucopyranose ($^4C_1$). J Chem Soc Perkin Trans I 1982:2525-34.

24. Kudrjashov BA, Lyapina LA and Aziyeva LD. Heparin-like anticoagulant content in Filipendula ulmaria flowers. Farmakol Toksikol 1990;53(4):39-41.

25. Kudrjashov BA, Amosova YM, Lyapina LA, Osipova NN, Azieva LD, Lyapin GY, Basanova AV. Heparin from Filipendula ulmaria and its properties. Izvest Akad Nauk SSSR, Ser Biol 1991:939-43, through Chem Abstr 1992;116:165953.

26. Schilcher H. Fiebersenkende Phytopharmaka. In: Phytotherapie in der Kinderheilkunde, 2nd ed. Stuttgart: Wissenschaftliche Verlagsgesellschaft, 1992:40-1.

27. Schulz V, Hänsel R, Tyler VE. Meadowsweet flowers. In: Rational Phytotherapy - a physicians' guide to herbal medicine, 4th ed. Berlin-Heidelberg-New York: Springer-Verlag, 2001:173-4.

28. Zeylstra H. Filipendula ulmaria. Br J Phytotherapy 5:8-12.

29. Decaux F. Les propriétés thérapeutiques de la reine de prés (Spiraea ulmaria L.). Rev Phytothérapie 1941;25:13-7.

30. Valnet J. Reine-des-prés. In: Phytothérapie - Traitement des maladies par les plantes. Paris: Editions Maloine, 1976:671-2.

31. Leclerc H. Ulmaire. In: Précis de Phytothérapie, 5th ed. Paris: Masson, 1976:55-6.

32. Mills S, Bone K. Meadowsweet (Filipendula ulmaria L.). In: Principles and Practice of Phytotherapy. Edinburgh-London-New York: Churchill Livingstone, 2000:479-82.

33. Dorsch W, Loew D, Meyer E, Schilcher H. Filipendulae ulmariae flos (Mädesüß). In: Kinderdosierungen von Phytopharmaka, 2nd ed. Bonn: Kooperation Phytopharmaka 1998:62-3.

34. Csedö K, Monea M, Sabau M, Esianu S. The antibiotic activity of Filipendula ulmaria. Planta Med 1993;59 (Suppl):A675.

35. Hintz IC, Hodisan V, Tamas M. Clujul Medical 1983; 56:381-4 (cited in [9]).

36. Tunón H, Olavsdotter C, Bohlin L. Evaluation of anti-inflammatory activity of some Swedish medicinal plants. Inhibition of prostaglandin biosynthesis and PAF-induced exocytosis. J Ethnopharmacol 1995; 48:61-76.

37. Halkes SBA, Beukelman CJ, Kroes BH, van den Berg AJJ, Labadie RP, van Dijk H. In vitro immunomodulatory activity of Filipendula ulmaria. Phytotherapy Res 1997;11:518-20.

38. Halkes SBA, Beukelman CJ, Kroes BH, van den Berg AJJ, van Dijk H, Labadie RP. A strong complement inhibitor from the flowers of Filipendula ulmaria (L.) Maxim. Pharm Pharmacol Lett 1997;7:79-82.

39. Bespalov VG, Limarenko AY, Voitenkov BL. Anticarcinogenic, antitumour and immunomodulating activities of dropwort Filipendula ulmaria flower decoction. Khim Farm Zh 1992;26:59-61, through Chem Abstr 1992;116:227822.

40. Lamaison JL, Carnat A, Petitjean-Freytet C. Teneur en tanins et activité inhibitrice de l'élastase chez les Rosaceae. Ann Pharm Fr 1990;48:335-40.

41. Barnaulov OD, Denisenko PP. Antiulcerogenic action of the decoction from flowers of Filipendula ulmaria (L.) Maxim. Farmakol Toksikol 1980;43:700-5.

42. Barnaulov OD, Kumkov AV, Khalikova NA, Kozhina IS, Shukhobodskij BA. Chemical composition and primary assessment of the pharmacological properties of preparations from Filipendula ulmaria (L.) Maxim. Rastit Resur 1977;13:661-9 [RUSSIAN].

43. Barnaulov OD, Manicheva OA, Shelyuto VL, Konopleva MM, Glyzin VI. Effects of flavonoids on the development of experimental gastric dystrophies in mice. Khim Farm Zh 1984;18:935-41 [RUSSIAN].

44. Peresun'ko AP, Bespalov VG, Limarenko AI, Aleksandrov VA. Clinico-experimental study of using plant preparations from the flowers of Filipendula ulmaria (L.) Maxim for the treatment of precancerous changes and prevention of uterine cervical cancer. Vopr Onkol 1993;39:291-5 [RUSSIAN].

45. Miyamoto K, Kishi N, Koshiura R, Yoshida T, Hatano T, Okuda T. Relationship between the structures and the antitumor activities of tannins. Chem Pharm Bull 1987; 35:814-22.

46. McManus JP, Davis KG, Beart JE, Gaffney SH, Lilley TH, Haslam E. Polyphenol interactions. Part 1. Introduction: Some observations on the reversible complexation of polyphenols with proteins and polysaccharides. J Chem Soc Perkin Trans II 1985:1429-38.

47. Beart JE, Lilley TH, Haslam E. Plant polyphenols - secondary metabolism and chemical defence: some observations. Phytochemistry 1985;24:33-8.

48. Barnaulov OD, Boldina I, Galushko VV, Karamysina GK, Komkov AV, Limarenka AY et al. Pharmacological properties of galenic preparations from the flowers of Filipendula ulmaria (L.) Maxim. Rastit Resur 1979; 15:399-407.

FOENICULI FRUCTUS

Fennel

DEFINITIONS

Bitter fennel consists of the dry, whole cremocarps and mericarps of *Foeniculum vulgare* Miller subsp. *vulgare* var. *vulgare*. It contains not less than 40 ml/kg of essential oil, calculated with reference to the anhydrous drug. The oil contains not less than 60.0 per cent of anethole and not less than 15.0 per cent of fenchone [1].

Sweet fennel consists of the dry, whole cremocarps and mericarps of *Foeniculum vulgare* Miller subsp. *vulgare* var. *dulce* (Miller) Thellung. It contains not less than 20 ml/kg of essential oil, calculated with reference to the anhydrous drug. The oil contains not less than 80.0 per cent of anethole [2].

The materials comply with the monographs of the European Pharmacopoeia [1,2].

CONSTITUENTS

The essential oil of bitter fennel contains predominantly anethole and fenchone with not more than 5% of estragole [1,2]. It also contains α-pinene, limonene, camphene, *p*-cymene, β-pinene, β-myrcene, α-phellandrene, sabinene, γ-terpinene and terpinolene [3-5].

The essential oil of sweet fennel contains predominantly anethole with not more than 10% of estragole and not more than 7.5% of fenchone [2]. Other components include α-pinene and limonene [3] as well as β-pinene, β-myrcene and *p*-cymene [4,5].

The fruits also contain water-soluble glycosides of monoterpenoid, alkyl and aromatic compounds [6-12].

CLINICAL PARTICULARS

Therapeutic indications
Dyspeptic complaints such as mild, spasmodic gastro-intestinal ailments, bloating and flatulence [3,13,14]. Catarrh of the upper respiratory tract [3,13-18].

Posology and method of administration

Dosage

Adult daily dose: 5-7 g of crushed fruits as an infusion or similar preparation [3,13].

Children, average daily dose: 0-1 year of age, 1-2 g of crushed fruits as an infusion; *1-4 years of age*, 1.5-3 g; *4-10 years of age*, 3-5 g; *10-16 years of age*, the adult dose [19].

Method of administration
For oral administration.

Duration of administration
Infusions or similar preparations: no restriction. If symptoms persist, consult your doctor.

Contra-indications
Persons with known sensitivity to anethole should avoid the use of fennel [20,21].

Special warnings and special precautions for use
Persons with known sensitivity to anethole should avoid the use of fennel [20,21].

Interaction with other medicaments and other forms of interaction
None reported for humans.

Pregnancy and lactation
Fennel may be used during pregnancy and lactation [22] at the recommended dosage, as aqueous infusions only.

Preparations containing the essential oil [23] or alcoholic extracts should not be used during pregnancy and lactation. Mild oestrogenic activity and antifertility effects of anethole (the major constituent of the essential oil) have been demonstrated in rats [24].

Effects on ability to drive and use machines
None known.

Undesirable effects
A single case of allergic reaction to fennel has been reported [25].
Rare cases of contact dermatitis caused by anethole-containing preparations [20,21].

Overdose
No toxic effects reported [22].

PHARMACOLOGICAL PROPERTIES

Pharmacodynamic properties

In vitro experiments

Antimicrobial effects
Acetone, *n*-butanol, ethanol and ether extracts of fennel inhibited the growth of a range of bacteria including *Escherichia coli* and *Staphylococcus aureus*, and also exhibited antifungal activity against *Candida albicans* and other organisms [26].

Fennel oil inhibited the growth of *Escherichia coli* (MIC: 0.5% V/V), *Staphylococcus aureus* (MIC: 0.25%), *Salmonella typhimurium* (MIC: 1.0%) and *Candida albicans* (MIC: 0.5%) using the agar dilution method [27]. Significant antibacterial activity of the oil (10µl of undiluted oil added to wells in the agar plates) has been demonstrated against *Brevibacterium linens, Clostridium perfringens, Leuconostoc cremoris* and *Staphylococcus aureus* [28]. Earlier studies also demonstrated antibacterial activity of the oil [29,30].

Antioxidant activity
Antioxidant activity of fennel oil against lipid peroxidation was demonstrated in the thiobarbituric acid reactive species assay and in a micellar model system [28]

Secretolytic and expectorant effects
An increase of about 12% in mucociliary transport velocity was observed in isolated ciliated epithelium from the frog oesophagus 90 seconds after application of 200 µl of an infusion from bitter fennel (4.6 g per 100 ml of water) [18].

Effects on musculature
The essential oil had a spasmogenic effect on smooth muscle of isolated guinea-pig ileum at a concentration of 8×10^{-5} g/ml. On a skeletal muscle preparation of isolated rat phrenic nerve diaphragm it caused contracture and inhibition of the twitch response to nerve stimulation at a concentration of 2×10^{-4} g/ml [31].

A 30%-ethanolic extract from bitter fennel produced a concentration-dependent decrease in acetylcholine- and histamine-induced contractility of isolated guinea pig ileum at concentrations of 2.5-10.0 ml/litre; however, taking into account the effect of ethanol, only the results with histamine were significant (p<0.005 at 10 ml/litre) [32]. In the same test system, the extract at 2.5 and 10.0 ml/litre also concentration-dependently reduced carbachol-induced contractility [33].

Fennel oil significantly and dose-dependently reduced the intensity of oxytocin-induced contractions (p<0.01 at 50 µg/ml) and PGE_2-induced contractions (p<0.01 at 10 and 20 µg/ml) of the isolated rat uterus. The oil also reduced the frequency of contractions induced by PGE_2 (but not by oxytocin) [34].

Local anaesthetic activity
Trans-anethole concentration-dependently reduced electrically-evoked contractions of rat phrenic nerve-hemidiaphragm, by 10.3% at 10^{-3} µg/ml, by 43.9% at 10^{-2} µg/ml, by 79.7% at 10^{-1} µg/ml and by 100% at 1 µg/ml [35].

Tumour-inhibiting activity of anethole
Anethole at a concentration below 1 mM has been

shown to be a potent inhibitor of tumour necrosis factor (TNF)-induced cellular responses, such as activation of nuclear factor-kappa B (NF-κB) and other transcription factors, and also to block TNF-induced activation of the apoptotic pathway. This might explain the role of anethole in suppression of inflammation and carcinogenesis [36].

In vivo experiments

Secretolytic and expectorant effects
Anethole and fenchone vapour were given by inhalation to urethanized rabbits as doses of 1 to 243 mg/kg body weight added to the steam vaporizer (the amount actually absorbed by the animals being considerably less, estimated as not more than 1% of that added to the vaporizer). Inhalation of anethole did not affect the volume but produced a dose-dependent (1-9 mg/kg) decrease in the specific gravity of respiratory tract fluid. Inhalation of fenchone produced a dose-dependent (1-9 mg/kg) augmentation of the volume output of respiratory tract fluid and a dose-dependent (1-27 mg/kg) decline in its specific gravity [37].

Effects on the digestive tract
Fennel administered orally at 24 mg/kg body weight increased spontaneous movement of the stomach in unanaesthetized rabbits and reduced the inhibition of stomach movement induced by sodium pentobarbitone [38].

An aqueous extract of fennel (10% w/v), perfused through the stomach of anaesthetized rats at 0.15 ml/minute and collected over periods of 20 minutes, significantly increased gastric acid secretion (p<0.02) to more than 3-fold compared to the basal secretion determined from perfusion of saline solution [39].

Addition of 0.5% of fennel to the diet of rats for 6 weeks shortened food transit time by 12% (p<0.05) [40].

Anti-inflammatory effects
Oral pre-treatment of rats with a dry 80%-ethanolic extract from sweet fennel at 100 mg/kg body weight inhibited carrageenan-induced paw oedema by 36% (p<0.01) compared to 45% inhibition by indometacin at 5 mg/kg [41].

Oestrogenic effects
Oral administration of an acetone extract from fennel to adult female ovarectomized rats at 0.5-2.5 mg/kg body weight caused dose-dependent oestrogenic effects: induction of the oestrus phase (after 10 days, in 40% of rats at 0.5 mg/kg, in 100% at 2.5 mg/kg), increase in mammary gland weight (p<0.05 at 0.5 mg/kg, p<0.01 at 2.5 mg/kg) and increase in weights of endometrium, cervix and vagina (p<0.01 to p<0.001 at 2.5 mg/kg). Oestrogenic effects were also evident in mature male rats after treatment with the extract at 1.5 or 2.5 mg/kg/day for 15 days: no significant change in body or organ weights but, particularly at the higher dose, significant changes in protein and acid and alkaline phosphatase in the testes, vas deferens, seminal vesicles and prostate [42].

Trans-anethole administered orally to immature female rats at 80 mg/kg body weight for 3 days significantly increased uterine weight, to 2 g/kg compared to 0.5 g/kg in controls and 3 g/kg in animals given oestradiol valerate subcutaneously at 0.1 µg/rat/day (p<0.001). The results confirmed that trans anethole has oestrogenic activity; other experiments showed that it has no anti-oestrogenic, progestational, anti-progestational, androgenic or anti-androgenic activity [24].

Hypotensive effect
A lyophilized aqueous extract of fennel administered orally at 190 mg/kg body weight (equivalent to crude drug at 1000 mg/kg) for 5 days significantly lowered the systolic blood pressure of spontaneously hypertensive (SH) rats (p<0.05), but had no effect on normotensive rats. The extract also significantly increased the urine output of SH rats, by 80% at day 3 (p<0.05), and increased renal excretion of sodium and potassium (p<0.05), suggesting that fennel acted mainly as a diuretic and natriuretic in the SH rats [43].

Anti-tumour activity
In Swiss albino mice with Ehrlich ascites tumour (EAT) in the paw, anethole administered orally at 500 or 1000 mg/kg on alternate days for 60 days significantly and dose-dependently reduced tumour weight (p<0.05 at 500 mg/kg, p<0.01 at 1000 mg/kg), tumour volume (p<0.01 at 500 mg/kg, p<0.001 at 1000 mg/kg) and body weight (p<0.05 to 0.01) compared to EAT-bearing controls. Mean survival time increased from 54.6 days to 62.2 days (500 mg/kg) and 71.2 days (1000 mg/kg). Histopathological changes were comparable to those after treatment with cyclophosphamide (a standard cytotoxic drug). These and other results demonstrated the anti-carcinogenic, cytotoxic and non-clastogenic nature of anethole [44].

Anti-genotoxic activity of anethole
In the mouse bone marrow micronucleus test, oral pre-treatment of mice with trans-anethole at 40-400 mg/kg body weight 2 and 20 hours before intra-peritoneal injection of genotoxins led to moderate, dose-dependent protective effects against known genotoxins such as cyclophosphamide, pro-carbazine, N-methyl-N'-nitrosoguanidine, urethane and ethyl methane sulfonate (p<0.05 to p<0.01 at various dose levels). No significant increase in genotoxicity was observed when trans-anethole (40-400 mg/kg body weight) was administered alone [45].

Enzyme induction

Experiments in which rats were injected intraperitoneally with a mixture of trans-anethole (100 mg/kg bodyweight) and [14C]parathion (1.5 mg/kg) showed no significant effect of trans-anethole on metabolism and excretion of the insecticide. However, when rats were fed a diet containing 1% of trans-anethole for 7 days and subsequently cell fractions from the livers of these rats were incubated for 2 hours with [14C]parathion, significantly less unchanged parathion (1.6%) was recovered compared to controls (12.5%). The data were interpreted as suggesting that feeding trans-anethole to rats for 7 days induced the synthesis of parathion-degrading liver enzymes [46].

Pharmacokinetic properties

Pharmacokinetics in animals
No data available for fennel.

In mice and rats trans-anethole is reported to be metabolized by O-demethylation and by oxidative transformation of the C3-side chain. After low doses (0.05 and 5 mg/kg body weight) O-demethylation occurs predominantly, whereas higher doses (up to 1500 mg/kg body weight) give rise to higher yields of oxygenated metabolites [47,48].

Pharmacokinetics in humans
No data available for fennel.

After oral administration of radioactively-labelled trans-anethole (as the methoxy-14C compound) to 5 healthy volunteers at dose levels of 1, 50 and 250 mg on separate occasions, it was rapidly absorbed. 54-69% of the dose (detected as 14C) was eliminated in the urine and 13-17% in exhaled carbon dioxide; none was detected in the faeces. The bulk of elimination occurred within 8 hours and, irrespective of the dose level, the principal metabolite (more than 90% of urinary 14C) was 4-methoxyhippuric acid [49,50]. An earlier study with 2 healthy subjects taking 1 mg of trans-anethole gave similar results [51].

Preclinical safety data

Acute toxicity
Oral administration of an ethanolic extract of fennel to mice at 0.5, 1 and 3 g/kg body weight caused no mortality and no significant difference in body and vital organ weights or in external morphological, haematological or spermatogenic parameters in comparison with the control group over a period of 24 hours [52].

The oral LD_{50} of bitter fennel oil in rats was determined as 4.52 ml/kg [53]. Values of 3.8 g/kg [54] and 3.12 g/kg [55] have also been reported for fennel oil in rats,

but in a more recent study the oral LD_{50} was estimated to be 1.326 g/kg [34].

Intraperitoneal LD_{50} values for trans-anethole have been determined as 0.65-1.41 g/kg in mice and 0.9-2.67 g/kg in rats [50].

Subchronic toxicity
Oral administration of an ethanolic extract of fennel to mice at 100 mg/kg for 3 months caused no significant differences in mortality or in haematological and spermatogenic parameters in comparison with the control group [52].

Reproductive toxicity
Trans-anethole exerted dose-dependent anti-implantation activity after oral administration to adult female rats on days 1-10 of pregnancy. Compared to control animals (all of which delivered normal offspring on completion of term), trans-anethole administered at 50, 70 and 80 mg/kg body weight inhibited implantation by 33%, 66% and 100% respectively. Further experiments at the 80 mg/kg dose level showed that in rats given trans-anethole only on days 1-2 of pregnancy normal implantation and delivery occurred; in those given anethole only on days 3-5 implantation was completely inhibited; and in those given trans-anethole only on days 6-10 three out of five rats failed to deliver at term. No gross malformations of offspring were observed in any of the groups. The results demonstrated that trans-anethole has antifertility activity. From comparison with the days 1-2 group (lack of antizygotic activity), the lower level of delivery in the days 6-10 group was interpreted as a sign of early abortifacient activity [24].

Mutagenicity and carcinogenicity
Aqueous and methanolic extracts of fennel gave negative results in the Ames test using Salmonella typhimurium strains TA 98 and TA 100, with or without metabolic activation [56,57]. These extracts also gave negative results in the Bacillus subtilis rec-assay [56].

Fennel oil (2.5 mg/plate) and trans-anethole (2 mg/plate) were mutagenic in the Ames test using Salmonella typhimurium strains TA 98 and TA 100, and mutagenicity was potentiated by S13 activation [46]. In another study, trans-anethole was mutagenic to Salmonella typhimurium TA 100 in the Ames test with S9 activation, doses of 30-120 µg/plate showing a dose-dependent increase in revertants which did not exceed twice the number of the control [58]. Other investigations with metabolic activation have confirmed that trans-anethole is weakly mutagenic [50].

Sweet fennel oil gave positive results in the Bacillus subtilis DNA-repair test [58], but fennel oil gave a negative result in the chromosomal aberration test using a Chinese hamster fibroblast cell line [59].

Estragole, a minor constituent of fennel oil, has shown mutagenic potential in a number of Ames tests and proved carcinogenic in animal models [60,61]

Available data is insufficient to evaluate the carcinogenic risk for fennel infusion, but it appears to be relatively low [22].

REFERENCES

1. Fennel, Bitter - Foeniculi amari fructus. European Pharmacopoeia, Council of Europe.

2. Fennel, Sweet - Foeniculi dulcis fructus. European Pharmacopoeia, Council of Europe.

3. Brand N. Foeniculum. In: Hänsel R, Keller K, Rimpler H, Schneider G, editors. Hagers Handbuch der Pharmazeutischen Praxis, 5th ed. Volume 5: Drogen E-O. Berlin-Heidelberg-New York-London: Springer-Verlag, 1993:156-81.

4. Tóth L. Untersuchungen über das ätherische Öl von *Foeniculum vulgare*. Planta Med 1967;15:157-72.

5. Trenkle K. Neuere Untersuchungen an Fenchel (*Foeniculum vulgare* M.). 2. Mitteilung: Das ätherische Öl von Frucht, Kraut und Wurzel fruktifizierender Pflanzen. Pharmazie 1972;27:319-24.

6. Kitajima J, Ishikawa T, Tanaka Y. Water-soluble constituents of fennel. I. Alkyl glycosides. Chem Pharm Bull 1998;46:1643-6.

7. Kitajima J, Ishikawa T, Tanaka Y. Water-soluble constituents of fennel. II. Four *erythro*-anethole glycol glycosides. Chem Pharm Bull 1998;46:1591-4.

8. Ishikawa T, Kitajima J, Tanaka Y. Water-soluble constituents of fennel. III. Fenchane-type mono-terpenoid glycosides. Chem Pharm Bull 1998;46:1599-602.

9. Ishikawa T, Kitajima J, Tanaka Y. Water-soluble constituents of fennel. IV. Menthane-type mono-terpenoids and their glycosides. Chem Pharm Bull 1998;46:1603-6.

10. Kitajima J, Ishikawa T, Tanaka Y, Ono M, Ito Y, Nohara T. Water-soluble constituents of fennel. V. Glycosides of aromatic compounds. Chem Pharm Bull 1998;46:1587-90.

11. Ishikawa T, Kitajima J, Tanaka Y, Ono M, Ito Y, Nohara T. Water-soluble constituents of fennel. VI. 1,8-Cineole type glycosides. Chem Pharm Bull 1998; 46:1738-42.

12. Ishikawa T, Tanaka Y, Kitajima J. Water-soluble constituents of fennel. VII. Acyclic monoterpenoid glycosides. Chem Pharm Bull 1998;46:1748-51.

13. Czygan F-C, Hiller K. Foeniculi amari fructus - Bitterer Fenchel, Foeniculi dulcis fructus - Süßer Fenchel. In: Teedrogen und Phytopharmaka. Ein Handbuch für die Praxis auf wissenschaftlicher Grundlage, 4th ed. Stuttgart: Wissenschaftliche Verlagsgesellschaft, 2002:212-5.

14. Madaus G. Foeniculum. In: Lehrbuch der biologischen Heilmittel. Volume II. Hildesheim-New York: Georg Olms 1976:1354-61.

15. Sweetman SE, editor. Fennel, Fennel oil. In: Martindale - The complete drug reference. 33rd ed. London: Pharmaceutical Press, 2002:1610.

16. Merkes K. Drogen mit ätherischem Öl (XVI): *Foeniculum vulgare* Miller - Fenchel. pta-repetitorium 1980;(12):45-8.

17. Weiss RF. In: Lehrbuch der Phytotherapie, 8th ed. Stuttgart: Hippokrates, 1997:82-83, 443 and 463.

18. Müller-Limmroth W, Fröhlich H-H. Wirkungsnachweis einiger phytotherapeutischer Expektorantien auf den mukoziliaren Transport. Fortschr Med 1980;98:95-101.

19. Dorsch W, Loew D, Meyer-Buchtela E, Schilcher H. In: Kooperation Phytopharmaka, editor. Kinderdosierung von Phytopharmaka, 3rd ed. Teil I. Empfehlungen zur Anwendung und Dosierung von Phytopharmaka, monographierte Arzneidrogen und ihren Zubereitungen in der Pädiatrie: Foeniculi fructus (Fenchelfrüchte). Bonn: Kooperation Phytopharmaka, 2002:70-1.

20. Andersen KE. Contact allergy to toothpaste flavours. Contact Dermatitis 1978;4:195-8.

21. Franks A. Contact allergy to anethole in toothpaste associated with loss of taste. Contact Dermatitis 1998;38:354.

22. Keller K. *Foeniculum vulgare*. In: De Smet PAGM, Keller K, Hänsel R, Chandler RF, editors. Adverse effects of herbal drugs, Volume 1. Berlin-Heidelberg-New York: Springer-Verlag, 1992:135-42.

23. Tisserand R, Balacs T. Fennel (sweet and bitter). In: Essential Oil Safety - A guide for health care professionals. Edinburgh: Churchill Livingstone, 1995:136.

24. Dhar SK. Anti-fertility activity and hormonal profile of *trans*-anethole in rats. Indian J Physiol Pharmacol 1995;39:63-7.

25. Schwartz HJ, Jones RT, Rojas AR, Squillace DL, Yunginger JW. Occupational allergic rhino-conjunctivitis and asthma due to fennel seed. Ann Allergy Asthma Immunol. 1997;78:37-40.

26. Maruzzella JC, Freundlich M. Antimicrobial substances from seeds. J Am Pharm Assoc 1959;48:356-8.

27. Hammer KA, Carson CF, Riley TV. Antimicrobial activity of essential oils and other plant extracts. J Applied Microbiol 1999;86:985-90.

28. Ruberto G, Baratta MT, Deans SG, Dorman HJD. Antioxidant and antimicrobial activity of *Foeniculum vulgare* and *Crithmum maritimum* essential oils. Planta Med 2000;66:687-93.

29. Afzal H, Akhtar MS. Preliminary studies on the antibacterial properties of essential oil extracts from five folk medicines. J Pak Med Assoc 1981;31:230-2.

30. Ramadan FM, El-Zanfaly RT, El-Wakeil FA, Alian AM. On the antibacterial effects of some essential oils. I. Use of agar diffusion method. Chem Mikrobiol Technol Lebensm 1972;2:51-5.

31. Lis-Balchin M, Hart S. A preliminary study of the effect of essential oils on skeletal and smooth muscle in vitro. J Ethnopharmacol 1997;58:183-7

32. Forster HB, Niklas H, Lutz S. Antispasmodic effects of some medicinal plants. Planta Med 1980;40:309-19.

33. Forster HB. Spasmolytische Wirkung pflanzlicher Carminativa. Tierexperimentelle Untersuchungen. Z Allg Med 1983;59:1327-33.

34. Ostad SN, Soodi M, Shariffzadeh M, Khorshidi N, Marzban H. The effect of fennel essential oil on uterine contraction as a model for dysmenorrhea; pharmacology and toxicology study. J Ethnopharmacol 2001;76:299-304.

35. Ghelardini C, Galeotti N, Mazzanti G. Local anaesthetic activity of monoterpenes and phenylpropanes of essential oils. Planta Med 2001;67:564-6.

36. Chainy GBN, Manna SK, Chaturvedi MM Aggarwal BB. Anethole blocks both early and late cellular responses transduced by tumor necrosis factor: effect on NF-κB, AP-1, JNK, MAPKK and apoptosis. Oncogene 2000; 19:2943-50.

37. Boyd EM, Sheppard EP. An autumn-enhanced mucotropic action of inhaled terpenes and related volatile agents. Pharmacology 1971;6:65-80.

38. Niiho Y, Takayanagi I, Takagi K. Effects of a combined stomachic and its ingredients on rabbit stomach motility in situ. Japan J Pharmacol 1977;27:177-9.

39. Vasudevan K, Vembar S, Veeraraghavan K, Haranath PSRK. Influence of intragastric perfusion of aqueous spice extracts on acid secretion in anesthetized albino rats. Indian J Gastroenterol 2000;19:53-6.

40. Platel K, Srinivasan K. Studies on the influence of dietary spices on food transit time in experimental rats. Nutr Res 2001;21:1309-14.

41. Mascolo N, Autore G, Capasso F, Menghini A, Fasulo MP. Biological screening of Italian medicinal plants for anti-inflammatory activity. Phytother Res 1987;1:28-31.

42. Malini T, Vanithakumari G, Megala N, Anusya S, Devi K, Elango V. Effect of Foeniculum vulgare Mill. seed on the genital organs of male and female rats. Indian J Physiol Pharmacol 1985;29:21-6.

43. El Bardai S, Lyoussi B, Wibo M, Morel N. Pharmacological evidence of hypotensive activity of Marrubium vulgare and Foeniculum vulgare in spontaneously hypertensive rats. Clin Exper Hypertension 2001;23:329-43.

44. Al-Harbi MM, Qureshi S, Raza M, Ahmed MM, Giangreco AB, Shah AH. Influence of anethole treatment on the tumour induced by Ehrlich ascites carcinoma cells in paw of Swiss albino mice. Eur J Cancer Prev 1995;4:307-18.

45. Abraham SK. Anti-genotoxicity of trans-anethole and eugenol in mice. Food Chem Toxicol 2001;39:493-8.

46. Marcus C, Lichtenstein EP. Interactions of naturally occuring food plant components with insecticides and pentobarbital in rats and mice. J Agric Food Chem 1982;30:563-8.

47. Sangster SA, Caldwell J, Smith RL. Metabolism of anethole. II. Influence of dose size on the route of metabolism of trans-anethole in the rat and mouse. Food Chem Toxicol 1984;22:707-13.

48. Sangster SA, Caldwell J, Smith RL, Farmer PB. Metabolism of anethole. I. Pathways of metabolism in the rat and mouse. Food Chem Toxicol 1984;22:695-706.

49. Caldwell J, Sutton JD. Influence of dose size on the disposition of trans-[methoxy-^{14}C]anethole in human volunteers. Food Chem Toxicol 1988;26:87-91.

50. Lin FSD. Trans-anethole. In: Joint FAO/WHO Expert Committee on Food Additives. Toxicological evaluation of certain food additives and contaminants. WHO Food Additives Series 28. Geneva: World Health Organization 1991:135-52.

51. Sangster SA, Caldwell J, Hutt AJ, Anthony A, Smith RL. The metabolic disposition of [methoxy-^{14}C]-labelled trans-anethole, estragole and p-propylanisole in human volunteers. Xenobiotica 1987;17:1223-32.

52. Shah AH, Qureshi S, Ageel AM. Toxicity studies in mice of ethanol extracts of Foeniculum vulgare fruit and Ruta chalepensis aerial parts. J Ethnopharmacol 1991;34:167-72.

53. Opdyke DLJ. Monographs on fragrance raw materials: fennel oil, bitter. Food Cosmet Toxicol 1976;14:309.

54. Opdyke DLJ. Monographs on fragrance raw materials: fennel oil. Food Cosmet Toxicol 1974;12:879-80.

55. von Skramlik E. Über die Giftigkeit und Verträglichkeit von ätherischen Ölen. Pharmazie 1959;14:435-45.

56. Morimoto I, Watanabe F, Osawa T, Okitsu T. Mutagenicity screening of crude drugs with Bacillus subtilis rec-assay and Salmonella/microsome reversion assay. Mutat Res 1982;97:81-102.

57. Yamamoto H, Mizutani T, Nomura H. Studies on the mutagenicity of crude drug extracts. I. Yakugaku Zasshi 1982;102:596-601.

58. Sekizawa J, Shibamoto T. Genotoxicity of safrole-related chemicals in microbial test systems. Mutat Res 1982;101:127-40.

59. Ishidate M, Sofuni T, Yoshikawa K, Hayashi M, Nohmi T, Sawada M, Matsuoka A. Primary mutagenicity

screening of food additives currently used in Japan. Food Chem Toxicol 1984;22:623-36.

60. De Vincenzi M, Silano M, Maialetti F, Scazzocchio B. Constituents of aromatic plants: II. Estragole. Fitoterapia 2000;71:725-9.

61. European Commission: Scientific Committee on Food. Opinion of the scientific committee on food on estragole (1-allyl-4-methoxybenzene). 26 September 2001.

FRANGULAE CORTEX

Frangula Bark

DEFINITION

Frangula bark consists of the dried, whole or fragmented bark of the stems and branches of *Rhamnus frangula* L. (*Frangula alnus* Miller). It contains not less than 7.0 per cent of glucofrangulins, expressed as glucofrangulin A ($C_{27}H_{30}O_{14}$; M_r 578.5) and calculated with reference to the dried drug.

The material complies with the monograph of the European Pharmacopoeia [1].

CONSTITUENTS

The main active constituents of the dried bark are glucofrangulins A and B (emodin-6-O-α-L-rhamnosyl-8-O-β-D-glucoside and emodin-6-O-β-D-apiosyl-8-O-β-D-glucoside respectively), frangulins A, B and C (emodin-6-O-α-L-rhamnoside, emodin-6-O-β-D-apioside and emodin-6-O-β-D-xyloside), and emodin-8-O-β-D-glucoside, together with small amounts of other anthraquinone glycosides, dianthrones and aglycones [2-8].

CLINICAL PARTICULARS

Therapeutic indications
For short term treatment of occasional constipation [9-10].

Posology and method of administration

Dosage
The correct individual dose is the smallest required to produce a comfortable soft-formed motion.

Adults and children over 10 years: preparations equivalent to 20-30 mg of glucofrangulins daily, calculated as glucofrangulin A [7].
Elderly: dose as for adults.

Not recommended for use in children under 10 years of age.
The pharmaceutical form must allow lower dosages.

Method of administration
For oral administration.

Contra-indications
Not to be used in cases of: intestinal obstruction and stenosis, atony, inflammatory colon diseases (e.g. Crohn's disease, ulcerative colitis), appendicitis; abdominal pain of unknown origin; severe dehydration

E/S/C/O/P
MONOGRAPHS
Second Edition

states with water and electrolyte depletion.
Not to be used in pregnancy or in children under 10 years of age [7,11].

Special warnings and special precautions for use
As for all laxatives, frangula bark should not be given when any undiagnosed acute or persistent abdominal symptoms are present.

If laxatives are needed every day the cause of the constipation should be investigated. Long term use of laxatives should be avoided. Use for more than 2 weeks requires medical supervision. Chronic use may cause pigmentation of the colon (pseudomelanosis coli) which is harmless and reversible after drug discontinuation. Abuse with diarrhoea and consequent fluid and electrolyte losses may cause: dependence with possible need for increased dosages; disturbance of the water and electrolyte (mainly hypokalaemia) balance; an atonic colon with impaired function. Intake of anthranoid-containing laxatives for more than a short period of time may result in aggravation of constipation. Hypokalaemia can result in cardiac and neuromuscular dysfunction, especially if cardiac glycosides, diuretics or corticosteroids are taken. Chronic use may result in albuminuria and haematuria.

In chronic constipation stimulant laxatives are not an acceptable alternative to a changed diet [7,9-18].

Note: A detailed text with advice concerning changes in dietary habits, physical activities and training for normal bowel evacuation should be included on the package leaflet. An example is given in the booklet "Médicaments á base de plantes" published by the French health authority (Paris: Agence du Médicament).

Interaction with other medicaments and other forms of interaction
Hypokalaemia (resulting from long term laxative abuse) potentiates the action of cardiac glycosides and interacts with antiarrhythmic drugs or with drugs which induce reversion to sinus rhythm (e.g. quinidine). Concomitant use with other drugs inducing hypokalaemia (e.g. thiazide diuretics, adrenocorticosteroids and liquorice root) may aggravate electrolyte imbalance [7].

Pregnancy and lactation

Pregnancy
Not recommended during pregnancy.

There are no reports of undesirable or damaging effects during pregnancy or on the foetus when used in accordance with the recommended dosage schedule. However, experimental data concerning a genotoxic risk from several anthranoids (e.g. emodin and physcion) and frangula bark extract are not

counterbalanced by sufficient studies to eliminate a possible risk [19-27].

Lactation
Breastfeeding is not recommended as there are insufficient data on the excretion of metabolites in breast milk.

Excretion of active principles in breast milk has not been investigated. However, small amounts of active metabolites (e.g. rhein) from other anthranoids are known to be excreted in breast milk. A laxative effect in breast-fed babies has not been reported [11,28].

Effects on ability to drive and use machines
None.

Undesirable effects
Abdominal spasms and pain, in particular in patients with irritable colon; yellow or red-brown (pH dependent) discolouration of urine by metabolites, which is not clinically significant [7,11,29-31].

Overdose
The major symptoms are griping and severe diarrhoea with consequent losses of fluid and electrolyte, which should be replaced.

Treatment should be supportive with generous amounts of fluid. Electrolytes, particularly potassium, should be monitored; this is especially important in the elderly and the young [7].

PHARMACOLOGICAL PROPERTIES

Pharmacodynamic properties
1,8-dihydroxyanthracene derivatives possess a laxative effect. For the greater part the glycosides (frangulins and glucofrangulins) are not absorbed in the upper gut; they are converted by the bacteria of the large intestine into the active metabolite (emodinanthrone). There are two different mechanisms of action:

(i) an influence on the motility of the large intestine (stimulation of peristaltic contractions and inhibition of local contractions) resulting in accelerated colonic transit, thus reducing fluid absorption,

(ii) an influence on secretion processes (stimulation of mucus and active chloride secretion) resulting in enhanced fluid secretion [32-41].

Defecation takes place after a delay of 8-12 hours due to the time taken for transport to the colon and metabolization into the active compound.

In vitro experiments
Emodin inhibited the aggregation of rabbit platelets

induced by arachidonic acid and collagen, without affecting that induced by ADP or PAF. Frangulin B selectively and dose-dependently inhibited collagen-induced aggregation and ATP release in rabbit platelets, without affecting those induced by arachidonic acid, ADP, PAF and thrombin. Frangulin B also inhibited the platelet aggregation induced by trimucytin, a collagen receptor agonist [42].

Frangulin B showed potent inhibitory activity against tumour necrosis factor-α (TNF-α) formation in lipopolysaccharide/γ-interferon-stimulated murine microglial cell line N9 (IC$_{50}$: 42.6 μM, p<0.01) [43].

Pharmacokinetic properties
It is generally assumed (by analogy with sennosides from senna) that the glycosides (frangulins and glucofrangulins) are largely not split by human digestive enzymes in the upper gut and therefore not absorbed to a large extent. They are converted by the bacteria of the large intestine into the active metabolite (emodin-anthrone). Mainly anthraquinone aglycones are absorbed and transformed into their corresponding glucuronide and sulphate derivatives. After oral administration of frangula bark extract, rhein, emodin and traces of chrysophanol are found in human urine [33,41].

Oral administration of emodin to rabbits at 10 mg/kg body weight resulted in a very low serum concentration (approximately 2.5 μg/ml). Emodin was found to be highly bound (99.6%) to serum protein [44].

Preclinical safety data
No studies are available on single dose toxicity, repeated dose toxicity, reproductive toxicity or on *in vivo* carcinogenicity of frangula bark or frangula bark preparations.

Various frangula bark extracts have been shown to be genotoxic in several *in vitro* systems (bacterial mutation, chromosomal aberration and DNA repair in mammalian cells). No increase in mutations was observed in a gene mutation assay with mammalian cells. Emodin, the main laxative principle of frangula bark, was mutagenic in the Ames test but gave inconsistent results in gene mutation assays (V79 HGPRT), positive results in the UDS test with primary rat hepatocytes but negative results in the SCE assay. Other anthraquinone constituents also gave positive results in limited experiments [21-27,45].

In a 2-year study, male and female F344/N rats were exposed to 280, 830 or 2500 ppm of emodin in the diet, corresponding to an average daily dose of emodin of 110, 320 or 1000 mg/kg body weight in male rats and 120, 370 or 1100 mg/kg body weight in female rats. No evidence of carcinogenic activity of emodin

was observed in male rats. A marginal increase in the incidence of Zymbal's gland carcinoma occurred in female rats treated with the high dosage but was interpreted as questionable.

In a further 2-year study, on B6C3F$_1$ mice, males were exposed to 160, 312 or 625 ppm of emodin (corresponding to an average daily dose of 15, 35 or 70 mg/kg body weight) and females to 312, 625 or 1250 ppm of emodin (corresponding to an average daily dose of 30, 60 or 120 mg/kg body weight). There was no evidence of carcinogenic activity in female mice. A low incidence of renal tubule neoplasms in exposed males was not considered relevant [46].

Clinical safety data
Despite a lack of formal preclinical data on frangula bark, epidemiological studies suggest that there is no carcinogenic risk in humans from the use of anthranoid laxatives [47-49].

REFERENCES

1. Frangula Bark - Frangulae cortex. European Pharmacopoeia, Council of Europe.

2. Wagner H, Hörhammer HP. Synthese und endgültiger Strukturbeweis von Glucofrangulin A aus *Rhamnus frangula* L. Z Naturforsch 1969;24b:1408-13.

3. Hörhammer HP, Wagner H. Endgültiger Strukturbeweis und Synthese von Frangulin A. Z Naturforsch 1972; 27b:959-61.

4. Wagner H, Demuth G. 6-O-(D-Apiofuranosyl)-1,6,8-trihydroxy-3-methyl-anthrachinon, ein neues Glykosid (Frangulin B) aus der Rinde von *Rhamnus frangula* L. Z Naturforsch 1974;29c:204-8.

5. Labadie RP. The anthracene derivatives in *Rhamnus frangula* L. I. The aglycones. Pharm Weekbl 1970;105: 189-95.

6. Lemli J, Cuveele J. Les transformations des hétérosides anthroniques pendant le séchage des feuilles de *Cassia senna* et de *Rhamnus frangula*. Planta Med 1978;34:311-8.

7. Hänsel R, Keller K, Rimpler H, Schneider G, editors. Rhamnus. In: Hagers Handbuch der Pharmazeutischen Praxis, 5th ed. Volume 6: Drogen P-Z. Berlin: Springer-Verlag, 1994:392-410.

8. Hänsel R, Sticher O, Steinegger E. In: Pharmakognosie - Phytopharmazie, 6th ed. Berlin: Springer-Verlag, 1999:907-9.

9. Sonnenberg A, Sonnenberg GS. Epidemiologie der Obstipation. In: Müller-Lissner SA, Ackermans LMA, editors. Chronische Obstipation und Stuhlinkontinenz. Berlin: Springer-Verlag, 1989:141-56.

10. Preston DM, Lennard-Jones JE. Severe chronic

constipation of young women: 'Idiopathic slow transit constipation'. Gut 1986;27:41-8.

11. Sweetman SC, editor. Frangula Bark. In: Martindale - The complete drug reference, 33rd edition. London: Pharmaceutical Press 2002:1227 and 1248.

12. Klauser A, Peyerl C, Schindlbeck N, Müller-Lissner S. Obstipierte unterscheiden sich nicht von Gesunden hinsichtlich Ernährung und körperlicher Aktivität [Abstract]. Z Gastroenterol 1990;28:494.

13. Müller-Lissner SA. Effect of wheat bran on weight of stool and gastrointestinal transit time: a meta analysis. Br Med J 1988;296:615-7.

14. Klauser A, Beck A, Schindlbeck N, Müller-Lissner S. Dursten beeinflußt die Colonfunktion bei Probanden [Abstract]. Z Gastroenterol 1990;28:493.

15. Coenen C, Schmidt G, Wegener M, Hoffmann S, Wedmann B. Beeinflußt körperliche Aktivität den oro-analen Transit? - Eine prospektive, kontrollierte Studie [Abstract]. Z Gastroenterol 1990;28:469.

16. Bingham SA, Cummings JH. Effect of exercise and physical fitness on large intestinal function. Gastroenterology 1989;97:1389-99.

17. Bingham S. Does exercise affect large gut function? J Hum Nutr Diet 1991;4:281-5.

18. Klauser AG, Flaschenträger J, Gehrke A, Müller-Lissner SA. Abdominal wall massage: effect on colonic function in healthy volunteers and in patients with chronic constipation. Z Gastroenterol 1992;30: 247-51.

19. Westendorf J. Anthranoid derivatives - general discussion. In: De Smet PAGM, Keller K, Hänsel R, Chandler RF, editors. Adverse effects of herbal drugs, Volume 2. Berlin: Springer-Verlag, 1993:105-18.

20. Schmidt L. Vergleichende Pharmakologie und Toxikologie der Laxantien. Arch Exper Path Pharmakol 1955;226:207-18.

21. Brown JP, Brown RJ. Mutagenesis by 9,10-anthraquinone derivatives and related compounds in Salmonella typhimurium. Mutat Res 1976;40:203-24.

22. Liberman DF, Schaefer FL, Fink RC, Ramgopal M, Ghosh AC, Mulcahy RJ. Mutagenicity of islandicin and chrysophanol in the Salmonella/microsome system. Appl Environ Microbiol 1980;40:476-9.

23. Westendorf J, Marquardt H, Poginsky B, Dominiak M, Schmidt J, Marquardt H. Genotoxicity of naturally occurring hydroxyanthraquinones. Mutat Res 1990; 240:1-12.

24. Tikkanen L, Matsushima T, Natori S. Mutagenicity of anthraquinones in the Salmonella preincubation test. Mutat Res 1983;116:297-304.

25. Bruggeman IM, von der Hoeven JCM. Lack of activity of the bacterial mutagen emodin in HGPRT and SCE assay with V79 Chinese hamster cells. Mutat Res 1984; 138:219-24.

26. Poth A. Salmonella typhimurium reverse mutation assay with EX FR 10. Roßdorf, Germany: Cytotest Cell Research Report 17.09.1992, unpublished.

27. Heidemann A. Chromosome aberration assay in Chinese hamster ovary (CHO) cells in vitro with EX FR 10. Roßdorf, Germany: Cytotest Cell Research Report 14.09.1992, unpublished.

28. Faber P, Strenge-Hesse A. Relevance of rhein excretion into breast milk. Pharmacology 1988;36(Suppl 1):212-20.

29. Cooke WT. Laxative abuse. Clin Gastroenterol 1977; 6:659-73.

30. Tedesco FJ. Laxative use in constipation. Am J Gastroenterol 1985;80:303-9.

31. Ewe K, Karbach U. Factitious diarrhoea. Clin Gastroenterol 1986;15:723-40.

32. Cresseri A, Peruto I, Longo R. Biologische Wert-bestimmung der laxativen Wirkung der Polyhydroxy-Anthrachinone aus der Rinde von Rhamnus frangula L. Arch Pharm (Berlin) 1966;299:615-8.

33. Longo R. Attività e metabolismo nel topo di componenti la corteccia di Rhamnus frangula e di prodotti sintetici a struttura anthrachinonica. Boll Chim Farm 1980;119: 669-89.

34. Fairbairn JW, Moss MJR. The relative purgative activities of 1,8-dihydroxyanthracene derivatives. J Pharm Pharmacol 1970;22:584-93.

35. Ferguson NM. Synthetic laxative drugs. J Am Pharm Assoc (Sci. Ed.) 1956;45:650-3.

36. van Os FHL. Some aspects of the pharmacology of anthraquinone drugs. Pharmacology 1976;14(Suppl.1): 18-29.

37. Fairbairn JW. Biological assay and its relation to chemical structure. Pharmacology 1976;14(Suppl.1): 48-61.

38. Casparis P, Maeder R. Studien über die Anthrachinondrogen II. Pharmakochemische und physiologische Untersuchung der Cortex Frangulae unter besonderer Berücksichtigung des wirksamen Hauptbestandteils, des Glucofrangulins. Schweiz Apoth Ztg 1925;63:313-20.

39. Schultz OE. Konstitution und Wirkung dickdarm-wirksamer Laxantien. Arzneim-Forsch/Drug Res 1952; 2:49-55.

40. Lemmens L, Borja E. The influence of dihydroxy-anthracene derivatives on water and electrolyte movement in rat colon. J Pharm Pharmacol 1976; 28:498-501.

41. de Witte P. Metabolism and pharmacokinetics of anthranoids. Pharmacology 1993;47(Suppl.1):86-97.

42. Teng CM, Lin CH, Lin CN, Chung MI, Huang TF. Frangulin B, an antagonist of collagen-induced platelet

aggregation and adhesion, isolated from *Rhamnus formosana*. Thrombosis Haemostasis 1993;70:1014-8.

43. Wei BL, Lu CM, Tsao LT, Wang JP, Lin CN. *In vitro* anti-inflammatory effect of quercetin 3-O-methyl ether and other constituents from *Rhamnus* species. Planta Med 2001;67:745-7.

44. Liang JW, Hsiu SL, Wu PP, Chao PDL. Emodin pharmacokinetics in rabbits. Planta Med 1995;61:406-8.

45. Müllerschön H. Gene mutation assay in Chinese hamster V79 cells in vitro with EX FR 10. Roßdorf, Germany: Cytotest Cell Research Report 10.09.1992, unpublished.

46. NTP Technical Report 493. Toxicology and carcino-genesis studies of emodin (CAS No. 518-82-1) in F344/N rats and B6C3F$_1$ mice. NIH Publication No. 99-3952, 1999.

47. Loew D, Bergmann U, Schmidt M, Überla KH. Anthranoidlaxantien. Ursache für Kolonkarzinom? Dtsch Apoth Ztg 1994;134:3180-3.

48. Loew D, Bergmann U, Dirschedl P, Schmidt M, Überla K. Anthranoidlaxanzien. Dtsch Apoth Ztg 1997;137:2088-92.

49. Van Gorkom BAP, De Vries EGE, Karrenbeld A, Kleibeuker H. Review article: anthranoid laxatives and their potential carcinogenic effects. Aliment Pharmacol Ther 1999;13:443-52.

GENTIANAE RADIX

Gentian Root

DEFINITION

Gentian root consists of the dried, fragmented underground organs of *Gentiana lutea* L.

The material complies with the monograph of the European Pharmacopoeia [1].

CONSTITUENTS

Secoiridoid bitter glycosides including gentiopicroside (1-4%) and extremely bitter amarogentin (0.025-0.4%) [2-12]; oligosaccharides including bitter-tasting gentianose and gentiobiose [6-11,13]; xanthones (ca. 0.1%), mainly gentisin, isogentisin and gentioside [14-16]; and traces of essential oil [17].

CLINICAL PARTICULARS

Therapeutic indications
Anorexia [9,11,18-20] e.g. after illness [9,20,21]; dyspeptic complaints [9,18-22].

Posology and method of administration

Dosage
Adult single dose: 0.1-2 g of drug in 150 ml of water in infusion, decoction or maceration, up to 3 times daily [8,11,19,23]. Tincture (1:5, ethanol 45-70 % V/V) [19,23]: average single dose of 1 ml, up to 3 times daily [11,19]. Hydroethanolic extracts of equivalent bitterness value [1,20,22].
Elderly: dose as for adults.
Children, average daily dose: 4-10 years of age, 1-2 g of drug; *10-16 years of age*, 2-4 g [24]; in ethanol-free dosage forms.

The dosage may be adjusted according to the bitterness sensitivity of the individual [19,25].

Method of administration
For oral use in liquid preparations; in anorexia a single dose administered half to one hour before a meal [8,9,19]; in dyspeptic complaints, a single dose after the meal [9].

Duration of administration
No restriction. If symptoms persist, consult your doctor.

Contra-indications
Gastric or duodenal ulcers [9,19]; hyperacidity [19,20].

E/S/C/O/P
MONOGRAPHS
Second Edition

Special warnings and special precautions for use
None required.

Interaction with other medicaments and other forms of interaction
None reported.

Pregnancy and lactation
In accordance with general medical practice, the product should not be used during pregnancy without medical advice [19,26]

Effects on ability to drive and to use machines
None known.

Undesirable effects
Occasional headaches may occur [9,11,19].

Overdose
Overdose may lead to nausea or even vomiting [19,20].

PHARMACOLOGICAL PROPERTIES

Pharmacodynamic properties

In vitro experiments
An aqueous extract from gentian root appeared to directly stimulate acid secretion in cultured cells from rat gastric mucosa, causing a concentration-dependent 1.7-fold acid increase at 100 µg/ml (p<0.01) [27].

Selective antifungal activity of gentian root extracts has been reported [19].

Gentian root extract was reported to stimulate phagocytic activity of human leukocytes [28], indicating possible immunostimulatory activity.

In vivo experiments
The bitter principles of gentian root reflexively stimulate secretion of gastric juice and bile and thereby enhance appetite and digestion [29,30]. Gentian tincture administered orally to dogs, in an experiment which prevented the tincture reaching the stomach, caused secretion of gastric juice in amounts elevated by 30% in comparison with untreated animals [19].

An ethanolic gentian extract was administered intraduodenally to rats at 500 mg/kg body weight daily for 2 days prior to and 1 day after intraperitoneal administration of carbon tetrachloride. Bile flow impaired by carbon tetrachloride significantly increased in comparison with control rats treated with carbon tetrachloride only (p<0.005) and also in comparison with those which received neither carbon tetrachloride nor the extract (p<0.01), suggesting that the extract had high choleretic activity [31].

Gentian root extract (equivalent in bitterness value to 200 Ph. Helv. VI units/g), perfused into the stomach of anaesthetized rats, increased gastric secretion in a dose-dependent fashion (12%, 27% and 37% higher than controls). It also had an unexpected effect on pH (no change at lower doses, an increase from pH 4.25 to pH 4.85 at the highest dose) at concentrations of 0.25%, 1% and 4% of the extract. A dose of 0.5 ml/kg of the same gentian preparation did not affect the incidence of gastric ulceration in pyloric ligation tests in rats [32].

Gentian root infusion, administered orally to sheep as a daily dose of 5 g before feeding, produced a stimulant effect on secretion of enzymes in the small intestine [33].

Bronchosecretion in rabbits was elevated in comparison with control animals after administration of gentian root extract directly to the stomach by gavage for 3 days at the equivalent of 12.6 mg/kg/day of dried root [34].

Gentiopicroside significantly inhibited the production of tumour necrosis factor in models of hepatic injury in mice after intraperitoneal administration at 30 mg/kg body weight/day (p<0.05) or 60 mg/kg body weight/day (p<0.01) for 5 days [35].

Pharmacological studies in humans
Patients with inflammatory conditions of the gastro-intestinal tract, colitis ulcerosa (n = 8), morbus Crohn (n = 2) and non-specific inflammatory disorders (n = 9), all of whom had elevated secretory immuno-globulin (sIgA) levels (20-200 mg/dl) in their saliva, were treated with gentian root tincture (3 × 20 drops/day) for 8 days. A group of 8 healthy individuals (sIgA levels of 3-25 mg/dl) was treated in the same way. Apart from two patients in whom sIgA increased, sIgA levels steadily declined in both groups. This was stated to correlate with clinical findings in the patients, but no clinical data were reported [36].

Secretion of gastric juice in 10 healthy individuals was stimulated after one oral dose of alcoholic gentian root extract equivalent to 0.2 g of dried root. In the same experiment emptying of the gall bladder, observed using X-ray contrast, was increased and prolonged; this was interpreted as a cholagogic effect [37].

Clinical studies
In an open study, 205 patients with various dyspeptic symptoms (heartburn, vomiting, stomach aches, nausea, loss of appetite, constipation, flatulence) were treated with a dry hydroethanolic extract (5:1) of gentian root at a dosage of 240 mg twice or three times daily (average daily dose 576 mg of extract, equivalent to 2.9 g of dried root) for about 15 days. Improvements in symptoms were evident after 5 days

in most cases and by the end of the study the average level of improvement was 68%. The efficacy of the preparation was assessed by the doctors as excellent (symptoms eliminated) in 31% of patients, good in a further 55%, moderate in 9% and inadequate in 5% of cases [22].

Pharmacokinetic properties

Metabolic conversion of gentiopicroside was demonstrated *in vitro*, using human intestinal bacteria. Gentiopicroside anaerobically incubated with *Veillonella parvula* ssp. *parvula,* produced five metabolites which were identified as erythrocentaurin, gentiopicral, 5-hydroxymethyl-isochroman-1-one, 5-hydroxymethyl-isochromen-1-one and *trans*-5,6-dihydro-5-hydroxymethyl-6-methyl-1*H*,3*H*-pyrano[3,4-c]pyran-1-one [38].

Preclinical safety data

Gentian root extracts show no toxicity and are generally well tolerated [19]. The acute oral LD_{50} in mice of 25 ml/kg of gentian extract (37% ethanol and a bitterness value of 200 Ph. Helv. units/g) was the same as that of 30% ethanol [32].

Rabbits treated with 12.6 mg/day of gentian extract for 3 days did not exhibit symptoms of toxicity nor abnormal clinical serum parameters with the exception of slightly lower erythrocyte levels in the treatment group compared to a control group [34].

No treatment-related adverse effects were observed in rats treated orally for 13 weeks with 1.6 ml/kg of a combination product containing alcoholic extracts of gentian root, chamomile and liquorice. No effect was observed on reproduction, fertility or mating performance in female rats, and no teratogenic effect was observed in rabbits [39].

Gentian root extracts and isolated minor constituents showed weak mutagenicity in the Ames test with *Salmonella typhimurium* strains TA 97, 98, 100 and 2637 activated with S9 enzyme mixture [19,40-42]. Mutagenic activity of the extract was attributed to low levels of the xanthones gentisin and isogentisin. Isogentisin and other xanthones in gentian root have a striking structural resemblance to, and may react analogous to, quercetin, a well known mutagen in food, which is reported to be non-carcinogenic and considered to be safe [19,43,44].

Clinical safety data

From a total of 205 patients who received on average 576 mg of a dry hydroethanolic extract, equivalent to 2.9 g of dried gentian root, for 15 days, only 5 (2.4%) reported mild adverse effects such as flatulence, stomach cramp, nausea or headache [22].

REFERENCES

1.   Gentian Root - Gentianae radix. European Pharmacopoeia, Council of Europe.

2.   Sticher O, Meier B. Quantitative Bestimmung der Bitterstoffe in Wurzeln von *Gentiana lutea* und *Gentiana purpurea* mit HPLC. Planta Med 1980;40:55-67.

3.   Takino Y, Koshioka M, Kawaguchi M, Miyahara T, Tanizawa H, Ishii Y et al. Quantitative determination of bitter components in Gentianaceous plants. Planta Med 1980;38:344-50.

4.   Bricout J. Identification et dosage des constituants amers des racines de *Gentiana lutea* L. Phytochemistry 1974;13:2819-23.

5.   Quercia V, Battaglino G, Pierini N, Turchetto L. Determination of the bitter constituents of the Gentiana root by high-performance liquid chromatography. J Chromatogr 1980;193:163-9.

6.   Rossetti V, Lombard A, Sancin P, Buffa M, Menghini A. Composition of *Gentiana lutea* L. dried roots harvested at different altitudes. Plant Méd Phytothér 1984;18:15-23.

7.   Franz C, Fritz D. Anbauversuche mit *Gentiana lutea* und Inhaltsstoffe einiger Ökotypen. Planta Med 1975; 28:289-300.

8.   Wichtl M, Schäfer-Korting M. Enzianwurzel - Gentianae radix. In: Hartke K, Hartke H, Mutschler E, Rücker G and Wichtl M, editors. Kommentar zum Europäischen Arzneibuch. Stuttgart: Wissenschaftliche Verlagsgesellschaft, 1999 (11. Lfg.):E 8.

9.   Steinegger E, Hänsel R. Enzianwurzel. In: Pharmakognosie, 5th ed. Berlin-Heidelberg: Springer-Verlag, 1992:595-9.

10. Franz C, Fritz D. Cultivation aspects of *Gentiana lutea* L. Acta Horticulturae 1978;73:307-14.

11. Bisset NG, editor (translated from Wichtl M, editor. Teedrogen). Gentianae radix. In: Herbal Drugs and Phytopharmaceuticals. Stuttgart: Medpharm, Boca Raton-London: CRC Press, 1994:233-5.

12. Krupinska A, Segiet-Kujawa E, Skrypczak L, Ellnain-Wojtaszek M. Quantitative determination of amarogentin by TLC-densitometry. Sci Pharm 1991; 59:135-8.

13. Buffa M, Rossetti V, Lombard A, Sancin P, Bosia PD. *Gentiana lutea* L. fresh roots: variations in composition as a function of harvest location. Acta Pharm Jugosl 1991;41:67-73.

14. Atkinson JE, Gupta P, Lewis JR. Some phenolic constituents of *Gentiana lutea*. Tetrahedron 1969; 24:1507-11.

15. Nikolaeva GG, Glyzin VI, Mladentseva MS, Sheichenko VI, Patudin AV. Xanthones of *Gentiana lutea*. Khim Prir Soedin 1983:107-8, translated into English as: Chem Nat Compd 1983;19:106-7.

16. Hayashi T and Yamagishi T. Two xanthone glycosides from *Gentiana lutea*. Phytochemistry 1988;27:3696-9.

17. Chialva F, Frattini C, Martelli A. Unusual essential oils with aromatic properties. III. Volatile components of gentian roots. Z Lebensm Unters Forsch 1986;182:212-4.

18. Gentiana. In: British Herbal Pharmacopoeia 1983. Bournemouth: British Herbal Medicine Association, 1983:99-100.

19. Meier B, Meier-Liebi M. Gentiana. In: Hänsel R, Keller K, Rimpler H, Schneider G, editors. Hagers Handbuch der Pharmazeutischen Praxis, 5th ed. Volume 5: Drogen E-O. Berlin: Springer-Verlag, 1993:227-47.

20. Weiß RF. In: Lehrbuch der Phytotherapie, 7th ed. Stuttgart: Hippokrates Verlag, 1991:74-9.

21. Benigni R, Capra C, Cattorini PE. Genziana maggiore. In: Piante Medicinali: Chimica, farmacologia e terapia, Volume 1. Milano: Inverni & Della Beffa, 1962:646-53.

22. Wegener T. Anwendung eines Trockenextraktes aus Gentianae luteae radix bei dyspeptischem Symptomcomplex. Z Phytotherapie 1998;19:163-4.

23. Tisanes: Gentiane (racine). In: Pharmacopée Française, Xᵉ. 1989.

24. Dorsch W, Loew D, Meyer-Buchtela E, Schilcher H. In: Kinderdosierung von Phytopharmaka, 3rd ed. Teil I. Empfehlungen zur Anwendung und Dosierung von Phytopharmaka, monographierte Arzneidrogen und ihren Zubereitungen in der Pädiatrie: Gentianae radix (Enzianwurzel). Bonn: Kooperation Phytopharmaka, 2000:72.

25. Henschler D. Genetische Besonderheiten zur Wahrnehmung von Bitterstoffen. Planta Med 1966;15(Suppl):42-5.

26. Duke JA. *Gentiana lutea* L. In: Handbook of medicinal herbs. Boca Raton, Florida: CRC Press, 1985:207-8.

27. Gebhardt R. Stimulation of acid secretion by extracts of *Gentiana lutea* L. in cultured cells from rat gastric mucosa. Pharm Pharmacol Lett 1997;7:106-8.

28. Schmolz M. Immunological features of extracts from Radix Gentianae, Flores Primulae, Flores Sambuci, Herba Verbenae and Herba Rumicis as well as from a combination thereof (Sinupret®). In: Abstracts of 4th and International Congress on Phytotherapy. Munich, 10-13 September 1992 (Abstract SL 36).

29. Paris RR, Moyse H. Gentianaceae. In: Précis de matière médicale, 2nd ed. Volume III. Paris: Masson, 1971:100-6.

30. Schmid W. Zur Pharmakologie der Bittermittel. Planta Med 1966;14(Suppl):34-41.

31. Öztürk N, Herekman-Demir T, Öztürk Y, Bozan B, Baser KHC. Choleretic activity of *Gentiana lutea* ssp. *symphyandra* in rats. Phytomedicine 1998;5:283-8.

32. Leslie GB. A pharmacometric evaluation of nine Bio-Strath herbal remedies. Medita 1978;8:31-47.

33. Kazakov BN. The effect of plant bitters on the secretion of enzymes in the small intestine of sheep. Materialy 8-oi Nauchn Konf po Farmakol, Moscow Sb, 1963:63-5; through Chem Abstr 1964:16389.

34. Chibanguza G, März R, Sterner W. Zur Wirksamkeit und Toxizität eines pflanzlichen Sekretolytikums und seiner Einzeldrogen. Arzneim Forsch/Drug Res 1984; 34:32-6.

35. Kondo Y, Takano F, Hojo H. Suppression of chemically and immunologically induced hepatic injuries by gentiopicroside in mice. Planta Med 1994;60:414-6.

36. Zimmermann W, Gaisbauer G, Gaisbauer M. Wirkung von Bitterstoff-Drogen auf das darmassoziierte Immunsystem. Z Phytotherapie 1986;7:59-64.

37. Glatzel H, Hackenberg K. Röntgenologische Untersuchungen der Wirkungen von Bittermitteln auf die Verdauungsorgane. Planta Med 1967;15:223-32.

38. El-Sedawy AI, Hattori M, Kobashi K, Namba T. Metabolism of gentiopicroside (gentiopicrin) by human intestinal bacteria. Chem Pharm Bull 1989;37:2435-7.

39. Leslie GB, Salmon G. Repeated dose toxicity studies and reproductive studies on nine Bio-Strath herbal remedies. Swiss Med 1979;1:43-5.

40. Morimoto I, Nozaka T, Watanabe F, Ishino M, Hirose Y, Okitsu T. Mutagenic activities of gentisin and isogentisin from Gentianae radix (Gentianaceae). Mutation Res 1983;116:103-17.

41. Göggelmann W, Schimmer O. Mutagenic activity of phytotherapeutical drugs. In: Knudsen I, editor. Genetic Toxicology of the Diet. New York: Alan R Liss, 1986:63-72.

42. Matsushima T, Araki A, Yagame O, Muramatsu M, Koyama K, Ohsawa K et al. Mutagenicities of xanthone derivatives in *Salmonella typhimurium* TA100, TA98, TA97 and TA2637. Mutation Res 1985;150:141-6.

43. Bertram B. Flavonoide - Eine Klasse von Pflanzeninhaltsstoffen mit vielfältigen biologischen Wirkungen, auch mit karzinogener Wirkung? Dtsch Apoth Ztg 1989;129:2561-71.

44. Fintelmann V. Johanniskraut weiterhin unbedenklich. Dtsch Apoth Ztg 1988;128:1499-1500.

GINKGO FOLIUM

Ginkgo Leaf

E/S/C/O/P
MONOGRAPHS
Second Edition

DEFINITIONS

Ginkgo Leaf

Ginkgo leaf consists of the dried leaves of *Ginkgo biloba* L. It contains not less than 0.5 per cent of flavonoids, expressed as flavone glycosides (M_r 757) and calculated with reference to the dried drug.

The material complies with the monograph of the European Pharmacopoeia [1].

Standardized Ginkgo Dry Extract

Standardized ginkgo dry extract consists of an extract produced from ginkgo leaf. It contains 22.0 to 27.0 per cent of flavonoids, expressed as flavone glycosides (M_r 756.7), and 5.0 to 7.0 per cent of terpene lactones including 2.8 to 3.4 per cent of ginkgolides A, B and C, and 2.6 to 3.2 per cent of bilobalide.

The material complies with the monograph of the Deutsches Arzneibuch [2]. A draft monograph intended for the European Pharmacopoeia has been published [3].

CONSTITUENTS of Ginkgo Leaf

The characteristic constituents are terpenes and flavonoids. The principal terpenes are diterpene trilactones called ginkgolides (A, B, C and J), which differ in the number and position of their hydroxyl groups, and by the sesquiterpene trilactone bilobalide [4-6]. Terpenes are present in amounts of less than 0.1% up to 0.9% [4,7-12]. Pharmaceutical dried leaf should contain not less than 0.1% of terpene lactones, calculated as the sum of bilobalide and ginkgolides A, B and C.

The main flavonoids are mono-, di- and triglycosides of the flavonols quercetin, kaempferol and isorhamnetin. Diglycosides esterified with *p*-coumaric acid are also present [13-16]. Other flavonoids include biflavones, notably amentoflavone and its methylated derivatives [17-19], monomeric flavan-3-ols such as (+)-catechin, (–)-epicatechin, (–)-epigallocatechin and (+)-gallocatechin, and oligomeric and polymeric procyanidins [20,21].

Long-chain alkylphenolic acids (ginkgolic acids, also called anacardic acids) and alkylphenols (cardanols and urushiols) [22,23], organic acids, phytosterols, polysaccharides, cyclitols and carotenoids [23] are also present.

CLINICAL PARTICULARS

Note: Unless stated otherwise, wherever the term "extract" is used under Clinical Particulars and Pharmacological Properties it refers to a standardized ginkgo dry extract as described under Definitions.

Therapeutic indications

Preparations based on standardized extracts
Symptomatic treatment of: mild to moderate dementia syndromes including primary degenerative dementia, vascular dementia and mixed forms [24-29]; cerebral insufficiency [30-37].
Neurosensory disturbances such as dizziness/vertigo [38,39] and tinnitus [40,41].
Enhancement of cognitive performance [42-48].

Symptomatic treatment of peripheral arterial occlusive disease (intermittent claudication) [49-52].

Posology and method of administration

Dosage

Preparations based on standardized extracts
Adult daily dose: 120-240 mg of standardized ginkgo dry extract (as described under Definitions), divided into 2-3 doses [53-57]; equivalent preparations.

Elderly: dose as for adults.

No data available for children.

Method of administration
For oral administration.

Duration of administration
No restriction [27].

In cases of dementia, treatment should be maintained for at least 12 weeks [26,27]. After this period an evaluation should be carried out to determine whether the patient is a responder or a non-responder; treatment should be continued only in the case of a responder.

Contra-indications
Hypersensitivity or intolerance to ginkgo leaf preparations [56].

Special warnings and special precautions for use
None known.

Interaction with other medicaments and other forms of interaction
An interaction with substances that inhibit blood coagulation cannot be excluded [58,59]. However, no such interactions have been observed in controlled studies [60,61].

Pregnancy and lactation
No data in humans available. In accordance with general medical practice the product should not be used during pregnancy or lactation without careful consideration of the risk/benefit ratio.

Effects on ability to drive and use machines
None reported.

Undesirable effects
In rare cases, mild gastrointestinal disorders, headache or allergic skin reactions have been reported [4,55,62].

Overdose
No significant adverse reactions have been reported in patients ingesting up to 600 mg of dry extract in single doses [55,62-65].

PHARMACOLOGICAL PROPERTIES

Pharmacodynamic properties
The principal studies performed between 1980 and 1997 on the effects of a standardized dry extract and certain active components of ginkgo leaf on the cardiovascular system and/or central nervous system have been reviewed by DeFeudis [62].

Pharmacological studies on ginkgo leaf extracts are a very active field of research and the results of recent studies are summarized below. They relate mainly to vaso- and tissue-protective effects and cognition-enhancing effects.

In vitro experiments

Antioxidant activity
The free radical-scavenging activity of a ginkgo leaf extract against hydroxyl radical and superoxide anion has been demonstrated in several experimental models. Antioxidant properties have been demonstrated by membrane microrheological changes and also by inhibition of lipoperoxidation induced by exposure of human erythrocytes to hydrogen peroxide [66,67]. More recently, a ginkgo leaf extract was found to attenuate oxidative stress in macrophages and endothelial cells induced by zymosan and *tert*-butylhydroperoxide [68].

A ginkgo leaf extract inhibited the endothelium-derived relaxing factor (EDRF; thought to be nitric oxide) mechanism in acellular systems [69] and competed with oxyhaemoglobin for nitric oxide (NO) generated during the interaction of hydroxylamine with Complex I of catalase. It caused a concentration-dependent decrease (IC_{50}: 20 ng/ml) in the amount of nitrite formed in the reaction of O_2 with NO produced from a solution of 5 mM sodium nitroprusside [70]. An extract concentration-dependently inhibited nitrite and nitrate production (taken as an index for NO synthesis) in macrophages activated by lipopoly-saccharide plus γ-interferon. Inhibition of induction of the enzymic activity of inducible NO synthase (iNOS) was also reported [71].

The scavenging activity of a ginkgo leaf extract on peroxyl radicals has been demonstrated in both aqueous and lipid environments by the protection of human low-density lipoproteins (LDL) against oxidative damage induced by water- and lipid-soluble peroxyl radical generators [72]. Ginkgo leaf extracts also proved to be strongly antioxidant against copper-mediated human LDL oxidative damage [73] and, at 100 µg/ml, capable of preventing apoptosis and DNA fragmentation induced by exposure of rat cerebellar neurones to hydroxyl radicals [74].

The effects of a ginkgo leaf extract and quercetin on isolated rat thoracic aorta has been investigated. The extract produced concentration-dependent relaxation of the aortic ring precontracted with noradrenaline and the relaxation was suppressed by L-N(G)-nitroarginine methyl ester (L-NAME). Quercetin produced a similar relaxation, which was also suppressed by L-NAME. Furthermore, both the extract and quercetin caused significant increases in the intracellular calcium level $[Ca^{2+}]i$ in the endothelial cells. The increase in $[Ca^{2+}]i$ produced by quercetin at 10^{-6} M was suppressed by removing the extracellular Ca^{2+}, but was not affected by thapsigargin, a calcium pump inhibitor. These findings suggest that vaso-dilation can be produced by activation of nitric oxide synthesis and release by increasing $[Ca^{2+}]i$ in vascular endothelial cells [75].

In another study the effect of isolated bilobalide on reactive oxygen species (ROS)-induced apoptosis in PC12 cells was investigated. When cells were treated simultaneously with ROS and bilobalide (25-100 µM) a concentration-dependent reduction in the apoptic rate was observed. The percentage of cells with positive staining for c-Myc and p53 decreased from 27.8 and 50.1% to 16.7 and 23.2% respectively when bilobalide (25 µM) was added. Bilobalide also effectively reduced ROS-induced elevation of Bax and activation of caspase-3. These results showed that bilobalide may block apoptosis in the early stage and then attenuate the elevation of c-Myc, p53 and Bax, and activation of caspase-3 in cells [76].

The antioxidant properties of isolated terpenes and flavonoids have been evaluated in isolated rat liver cells treated with tert-butyl hydrogen peroxide. Terpenes did not show the high antioxidant activity typical for amentoflavone, luteolin and some flavonols, the antioxidant activities of which are related to the presence of free phenolic hydroxy groups; myricetin with five hydroxy groups was the most effective, followed by quercetin with four and then kaempferol

and rutin with three [77].

Protection from ischaemia-reperfusion induced damage
On isolated rat heart a ginkgo leaf extract at 200 mg/litre showed anti-arrhythmic effects on post-ischaemic arrhythmia and a protective action against cardiac ischaemia-reperfusion oxidative injury, inhibiting the formation of oxygen radicals during reperfusion and preventing leakage and oxidation of ascorbate, a myocardial endogenous antioxidant [78,79]. In the presence of superoxide dismutase (SOD) the extract at 50 mg/litre completely inhibited oxygen radical formation [78].

When infused at concentrations of 1 and 10 µg/ml into isolated rat heart subjected to ischaemia-reperfusion, a ginkgo leaf extract improved haemodynamic parameters and partially reduced the hydroxyl radical in coronary effluents. Ginkgolides A and B (0.05 µg/ml) and bilobalide (0.15 µg/ml) also showed cardio-protective effects [80].

The protective effect of a ginkgo leaf extract has been investigated in an *in vitro* model in which human endothelial cells were exposed to hypoxia-reoxygenation or hypoxia alone, mimicking *in vivo* models of ischaemia-reperfusion or ischaemia respectively. The extract and bilobalide delayed the onset of glycolysis activation during hypoxia on endothelial cells and also protected mitochondrial respiratory activity during the first 60 minutes [81].

Ventricular myocytes of guinea pig heart were used to examine the effects of a ginkgo leaf extract on the action potential and individual transmembrane ionic currents. Ginkgo leaf extract (5-50 µm/ml) did not affect the normal action potential or the various ionic currents involved in its generation. However, exposure to the ginkgo leaf extract (> 5 µg/ml) elicited a marked concentration-dependent inhibition of isoproterenol-induced Cl- current, the maximal effect being observed at 50 µg/ml [82].

Haemodynamic and electron spin resonance (ESR) analyses were performed on isolated ischaemic and reperfused rat hearts to assess the activity of a ginkgo leaf extract (5, 50 or 200 µg/ml), its terpenoid constituents (ginkgolide A, 0.05 µg/ml; ginkgolide B, 0.05, 0.25 or 0.50 µg/ml), and a terpene-free fraction (5 or 50 µg/ml). Test substances were added to the perfusion fluid during the last 10 minutes of control perfusion, low-flow ischaemia and the first 10 minutes of reperfusion. The results showed that the extract (5 or 50 µg/ml) and ginkgolides A and B (both at 0.05 µg/ml) had delayed the onset of contraction during ischaemia at the lowest concentrations used [83].

Platelet-activating factor antagonism
Ginkgolides are PAF-antagonists, the most potent

being ginkgolide B in tests using a PAF-induced platelet aggregation assay [84]. Ginkgolide B was effective in improving blood rheology and micro-circulation. It also inhibited superoxide generation induced by PAF and cytokines such as tumour necrosis factor in isolated human neutrophils [85] and modulated the effect of PAF on vascular flow [86,87].

PAF formation is probably involved in the pathogenesis of neuronal degeneration induced by excitatory amino acids. The PAF-antagonists ginkgolides A and B (1-100 μM) elicited concentration-dependent protective activity against glutamate-induced neuronal injury in cultured neurons from embryonic chick telencephalon [88]. Bilobalide (10 μM), which is devoid of PAF-antagonistic properties, also protected cultured rat hippocampal neurons against glutamate-induced damage [89].

Activity on the central nervous system
Peroxidation of neuronal membrane lipids induced by ascorbic acid/Fe^{2+} is associated with a decrease in membrane fluidity, which then diminishes the efficiency of the dopamine transporter to take up dopamine. The decrease in membrane fluidity of mouse striatal synaptosomes was prevented by a ginkgo leaf extract (2-16 μg/ml) as well as by desferrioxamine (0.1 mM) and trolox C (0.1 mM) [90].

The effect of a ginkgo leaf extract on the uptake of biogenic amines has been investigated. The extract had a biphasic effect on [^{3}H]5-hydroxytryptamine (5-HT) uptake in a synaptosomal fraction of mouse cerebral cortex; uptake was significantly increased by 23% at 4-16 μg/ml (p<0.05), whereas at 32 μg/ml and higher concentrations 5-HT uptake was inhibited (p<0.01 at 500 μg/ml) [91]. Incubation of mouse brain synaptosomes in oxygenated Krebs-Ringer medium at 37°C in the presence of ascorbic acid (0.1 mM) led to decreases in striatal [^{3}H]dopamine uptake and cerebral cortical [^{3}H]5-HT uptake after 20 minutes, and uptake was essentially suppressed after 60 minutes; a ginkgo leaf extract prevented the loss of synaptosomal amine uptake [92]. In a similar experiment, the decrease in synaptosomal dopamine uptake that occurred during a 60-minute incubation in the presence of ascorbic acid (0.1 mM) was prevented by a ginkgo leaf extract (4-16 μg/ml) [93].

A marked increase in choline release from rat hippocampal slices was observed when the slices were superfused with oxygen-free buffer, indicating hypoxia-induced hydrolysis of choline-containing phospholipids. This increase in choline release was suppressed by bilobalide but not by a mixture of ginkgolides. The EC_{50} for bilobalide was 0.38 μM [94].

Another study investigated the effect of flavonoids and terpenoids in a ginkgo leaf extract against toxicity induced by nitric oxide generators on cells of the hippocampus. The effects of sodium nitroprusside (SNP, 100 μM) were blocked by either the extract (10-100 μg/ml) or its flavonoid fraction (25 μg/ml), as well as by inhibitors of protein kinase C (PKC; chelerythrine) and L-type calcium channel blockers (nitrendipine). In contrast, bilobalide and ginkgolide B failed to display any significant effects. Furthermore, at 50 μg/ml the extract was able to rescue hippocampal cells pre-exposed to SNP (up to 1 mM), and at 100 μg/ml blocked the activation of PKC induced by SNP (100 μM) [95].

The potential effectiveness of a ginkgo leaf extract against toxicity induced by β-amyloid (Aβ)-derived peptides ($Aβ_{25-35}$, $Aβ_{1-40}$ and $Aβ_{1-42}$) on hippocampal primary cultured cells was also investigated. Co-treatment with the extract concentration-dependently (10-100 μg/ml) protected hippocampal neurones against toxicity induced by Aβ fragments, with complete protection at the highest concentration tested. Similar, albeit less potent, protective effects were seen with the flavonoid fraction of the extract, while the terpenes were ineffective. The ginkgo leaf extract (100 μg/ml) was also able to protect hippocampal cells after pre-exposure to $Aβ_{25-35}$ and $Aβ_{1-40}$, and it protected and rescued hippocampal cells from toxicity induced by hydrogen peroxide (50-150 μM) [96].

Changes in the susceptibility of apoptotic cells to death due to oxidative stress in ageing and its inhibition by a ginkgo leaf extract were evaluated by investigation of basal and reactive oxygen species (ROS)-induced levels of apoptotic lymphocytes derived from the spleen in young (3 months) and old (24 months) mice. ROS were induced by 2-deoxy-D-ribose (dRib), which depletes the intracellular pool of reduced glutathione. Lymphocytes from aged mice accumulate apoptotic cells to a significantly greater extent under basal conditions compared to cells from young mice. Treatment with dRib enhanced this difference, implicating a higher sensitivity to ROS in ageing. Apoptosis can be reduced *in vitro* by treatment with the ginkgo leaf extract. Furthermore, ROS-induced apoptosis was significantly reduced in mice by daily oral treatment with 100 mg/kg of the extract for 2 weeks. Interestingly, this effect seemed to be more pronounced in old mice [97].

In another study, lipid peroxidation (LPO) and the activity of the antioxidant enzymes catalase (CAT) and superoxide dismutase (SOD) were evaluated in the hippocampus, striatum and substantia nigra (SN) of rats treated with a ginkgo leaf extract. An increase in CAT and SOD activities in the hippocampus, striatum and SN, and a decrease in LPO in the hippocampus were observed [98].

The ability of a ginkgo leaf extract and isolated

terpene lactones to inhibit neuronal apoptosis has also been investigated. Apoptosis was induced in cultured chick embryonic neurons, and in mixed cultures of neurons and astrocytes from neonatal rat hippocampus, by serum deprivation or treatment with staurosporine. An increase in the level of apoptotic chick neurons from 12% in controls to 30% after 24 hours of serum deprivation was reduced to the control level by a ginkgo leaf extract (10 mg/litre), ginkgolide B (10 µM), ginkgolide J (100 µM) and bilobalide (1 µM). After treatment with staurosporine (200 nM) for 24 hours 74% of the chick neurons were apoptotic. This level of apoptotic neurons was reduced to 24%, 62% and 31% in the presence of the ginkgo leaf extract (100 mg/litre), ginkgolide J (100 µM) and ginkgolide B (10 µM) respectively. Bilobalide (10 µM) decreased apoptotic damage induced by staurosporine treatment for 12 hours nearly to the control level. In mixed neuronal/glial cultures, the extract (100 mg/litre) and bilobalide (100 µM) rescued rat neurons from apoptosis caused by serum deprivation, while bilobalide (100 µM) and ginkgolide B (100 µM) reduced staurosporine-induced apoptotic damage. Ginkgolide A revealed no anti-apoptotic effect in either serum-deprived or staurosporine-treated neurons [99].

In vivo experiments

Activity on myocardial ischaemia and cardiac function
The cardioprotective activity of a ginkgo leaf extract against ischaemic damage induced by oxygen-derived free radicals, previously demonstrated *in vitro* in isolated heart preparations, was confirmed *ex vivo*. Prolonged oral administration of the extract to rats at 25-200 mg/kg daily for 10 days before ischaemia-reperfusion in their isolated hearts dose-dependently reduced the incidence of reperfusion-induced arrhythmias (at 200 mg/kg, $p<0.01$ for ventricular fibrillation and $p<0.05$ for ventricular tachycardia); the extract administered orally at 50 mg/kg in combination with intravenous superoxide dismutase for 10 days had a similar effect [78].

Another *ex vivo* study was performed on non-diabetic and streptozotocin-induced diabetic rats, which received 25 or 50 mg/kg/day of a ginkgo leaf extract orally for 10 days. Their isolated hearts were non-preconditioned or preconditioned by short periods of ischaemia and reperfusion before induction of prolonged ischaemia. Preconditioning is reported to have a cardioprotective effect. The extract improved cardiac function in ischaemic non-preconditioned and preconditioned hearts from both the non-diabetic and diabetic rats, and it reduced by 50-70% the amount of free radicals during reperfusion. Preconditioning alone did not protect diabetic hearts against ischaemia-reperfusion-induced arrhythmias [100].

The effect of ginkgo leaf extract treatment on early

arrhythmia, induced by 30 minutes of coronary occlusion followed by 5 minutes of reperfusion, was studied in anaesthetised dogs. The extract was administered intravenously at 1 mg/kg five minutes before coronary occlusion, then continuously infused at 0.1 mg/kg/min until five minutes after reperfusion, and an additional 1 mg/kg was injected immediately prior to reperfusion. Compared to controls, dogs treated with the extract had less ventricular premature beats during coronary occlusion and they were protected against ventricular fibrillation during reperfusion [101].

An experimental study was carried out on the cardio-protective mechanism of a ginkgo leaf extract on myocardial ischaemia-reperfusion injury in the rabbit. When injected into the coronary artery at 10 mg/kg, the extract inhibited lipid peroxidation and prevented CuZn-SOD depletion in both plasma and tissue during and at the end of the reperfusion period. Furthermore, less severe histological lesions were observed on myocytes of the treated heart following ischaemia-reperfusion in comparison with the control heart. The extract also suppressed changes in fibrinolytic activity that occur during the reperfusion phase [102].

Oral treatment of rats with a ginkgo leaf extract at 60 mg/kg/day or ginkgolide A at 4 mg/kg/day for 15 days produced anti-ischaemic effects, improving myocardial functional recovery of their excised and perfused hearts in comparison with placebo-treated rats. A decrease in post-ischaemic levels of hydroxyl radicals in coronary effluents was also reported [80]. The protective effect of a ginkgo leaf extract (100 mg/kg daily for 3 months in drinking water) against hypoxic damage in old rats has been demonstrated by ultrastructural-morphometric analysis of cardio-myocytes and microvascular endothelium [103,104].

Activity on liver ischaemia
The ability of a ginkgo leaf extract to prevent post-ischaemic reperfusion injury in the liver was investigated in rats. Left hepatic lobar ischaemia was induced by clamping the left hepatic artery and the left portal branch. The ischaemic period of 60 minutes was followed by reperfusion for 120 minutes. After ischaemia, the left lobe of the liver was exteriorized on a mechanical stage for IVM. Animals of group A (n = 10) received the extract (20 mg/kg) intravenously 20 minutes before reperfusion. Group B (n = 10) served as control, with an identical experimental protocol except without administration of the extract. Hepatic oxygen saturation and haemoglobin concentration decreased equally in both groups during ischaemia of the left liver lobe, which returned to normal values within 2 hours of reperfusion. In the early reperfusion period (15-45 minutes after reperfusion) quantitative investigation of the hepatic microcirculation revealed significantly better sinusoidal perfusion rates (peri-portal, midzonal and pericentral) of 83.3%, 88.8%

and 92.1% in group A compared to 70.7%, 76.7% and 78.3% in group B (p = 0.001). Sinusoidal perfusion rates improved in both groups after 90 minutes of reperfusion, but still with a significant difference (p<0.05) in the midzonal area of the acini. The number of sticking leukocytes in post-sinusoidal venules in group B was twice that in group A after 15 minutes and after 90 minutes of reperfusion (p<0.001). Blood samples after 2, 4 and 6 hours of ischaemia/reperfusion showed increasing serum transaminase activities, reaching their peak values within 6 hours; compared to group B, the values in group A were slightly higher during the first 4 hours, but without significant difference. Post-ischaemic bile production was similar in both groups. Reflectance spectroscopy revealed no difference between groups with respect to parenchymal oedema formation after ischaemia and reperfusion [105].

Activity on the central nervous system
The neuroprotective effects of a ginkgo leaf extract and some of its constituents have been investigated in rodent models of focal and global cerebral ischaemia. Some experiments were carried out to determine whether treatment with the extract modified convulsion-induced activation of phospholipase A_2 and C in the hippocampus (a structure known to be highly vulnerable to ischaemia and convulsion) and the cerebral cortex. Oral treatment of rats with the extract at 100 mg/kg/day for 14 days decreased their neurochemical responses to electroconvulsive shock (ECS), indicating neuroprotection. These effects were consistent with modulation of ECS-induced, phospholipase C-mediated degradation of polyphosphoinositides in the hippocampus [106]. In another study, bilobalide administered subcutaneously to mice at 5-20 mg/kg 60 minutes before induction of focal cerebral ischaemia dose-dependently reduced the infarct area on the brain. At 10 mg/kg, bilobalide administered to rats before focal cerebral ischaemia reduced cortical and total infarct volume, whereas a lack of activity was observed in the rat model of global ischaemia. Ginkgolide A (50 mg/kg, s.c.) and ginkgolide B (100 mg/kg, s.c.) also showed protective activity against focal cerebral ischaemia in mice. Ginkgo leaf extract administered intravenously to rats at 2 × 100 mg/kg improved cerebral blood flow after 10 minutes of global ischaemia, but did not show neuroprotective activity [89].

In vitro and *ex vivo* experiments have demonstrated that bilobalide and ginkgo leaf extract inhibit hypoxia-induced, phospholipase A_2-dependent release of choline from rat hippocampal slices. Oral administration of 2-20 mg/kg of bilobalide 1 hour prior to decapitation and slice preparation is, in fact, capable of suppressing hypoxia-induced choline release. Half-maximal effects were noted at 6 mg/kg, while 20 mg/kg led to complete inhibition of the hypoxic effect. Administration of a ginkgo leaf extract (200 mg/kg, containing approximately 3% of bilobalide) reduced the release of choline to about 50%, indicating that the efficiency of the extract is exclusively due to its bilobalide content. In another experiment the effect of bilobalide on basal brain choline concentrations was tested *in vivo*. Rats were treated with bilobalide at 20 mg/kg by gavage and 1 hour later blood and cerebrospinal fluid were obtained and analyzed for choline. Total brain choline was determined following microwave fixation of the brain. Choline concentrations found in arterial blood (12.2 µM), cerebrospinal fluid (8.9 µM) and brain (31.9 nmol/g) from bilobalide-treated animals were not significantly different from control values [94].

A ginkgo leaf extract was shown to be effective against bromethalin-induced cerebral oedema in rats. Given by gavage at 100 mg/kg immediately after administration of bromethalin at 1.0 mg/kg, the extract caused a statistically significant decrease (p<0.05) in clinical sign severity compared to bromethalin-treated, saline-treated rats [107].

Beneficial effects of a ginkgo leaf extract on functional recovery from hemiplegia induced in young rats by motor cortex ablation have been reported. The active substances producing the beneficial effect were traced to the non-terpenic fraction of the extract [108,109].

Oral administration of a ginkgo leaf extract to aged (22-month-old) rats at 50-100 mg/kg/day for 30 days increased Na$^+$-dependent high-affinity [^{3}H]choline uptake into hippocampal synaptosomes [110].

A ginkgo leaf extract, administered at 50 mg/kg daily for 7 months in drinking water to old mice of three inbred strains, exerted a neuroprotective and/or neurotropic action in the hippocampus. The extract seemed to protect the intra- and interpyramidal mossy fibers (iipMF) against age-related damage and to stimulate compensatory processes of synaptic plasticity. When subjected to a Morris water navigation memory test the chronically treated mice performed better in spatial learning in comparison with controls. The antioxidant activity of the extract may inhibit oxidative events that seem to be involved in age-related degenerative processes on iipMF [111].

Age-related decrease in the density of hippocampal α_2-adrenoceptors (determined by [^{3}H] rauwolscine binding) in 24-month-old rats was significantly reversed (p<0.05) by intraperitoneal administration of a ginkgo leaf extract at 5 mg/kg/day for 21 days [112]. In a study of the effects of a ginkgo leaf extract on brain 5-HT$_{1A}$ receptors in relation to ageing, intraperitoneal administration of the extract at 5 mg/kg/day for 21 days did not alter receptor binding in young rats, but significantly increased the number of binding sites in aged rats (p<0.005 compared to vehicle controls) [113].

An extract administered orally at 50 mg/kg for 14 days was also able to prevent cold stress-induced desensitization of hippocampal serotonergic receptors in old, isolated rats exposed to a low room temperature of 4-5°C for 5 days; this indicated that the extract may restore age-related decreased capacity to adapt to sub-chronic stress [114]. In a study of anti-stress activity using a discrimination learning task in young (4-month-old) and old (20-month-old) rats, repeated oral treatment with a ginkgo leaf extract at 50 or 100 mg/kg/day for 20 days suppressed auditory stress-induced disruption of learning significantly by the third day of learning ($p \leq 0.01$ for young rats, $p \leq 0.05$ for old rats, compared to stressed but untreated controls) [115].

The social interaction test was used to determine the anxiolytic/anxiogenic potential of a ginkgo leaf extract and its interaction with diazepam (an anxiolytic drug) and ethyl β-carboline-3-carboxylate (β-CCE, an anxiogenic substance). When administered alone, the extract elicited an anxiogenic-like effect, decreasing social behaviour in rats. However, it enhanced the anxiolytic effect of diazepam and neutralized the anxiogenic effect of β-CCE. The molecular mechanisms underlying interactions of the extract with diazepam and β-CCE seemed to involve a similar site or distinct sites of action at central $GABA_A$/benzodiazepine/Cl$^-$ channel receptor complexes [116].

The effects of daily oral treatment with a ginkgo leaf extract at 100 mg/kg daily for 3 weeks on passive avoidance learning and brain membrane fluidity were tested in young, middle-aged and aged mice. Short-term (but not long-term) memory significantly improved ($p < 0.03$) and age-related changes in membrane fluidity were attenuated ($p < 0.01$) in aged animals. However, no significant correlation was found between cognitive function and improvements in brain membrane fluidity [117].

In tests on rats using an eight-arm radial maze, chronic post-session oral administration of a ginkgo leaf extract at 50 mg/kg had no effect on continuous learning, but the same dose given pre-session resulted in a trend toward fewer sessions to reach criterion performance, as well as fewer errors. Treatment and testing were continued for 24 months. Rats treated with the extract lived significantly longer than vehicle-treated control rats. Since no changes in cognitive behaviour were observed at 50 mg/kg, the pre-session extract dose was increased to 200 mg/kg in a second series of experiments; under these conditions significant decreases in both retroactive and proactive errors ($p < 0.01$) was observed during a post-delay sub-session [118].

High-density oligonucleotide microarrays were applied to define transcriptional effects in the cortex and hippocampus of mice on diets supplemented with a ginkgo leaf extract. Gene expression analysis focused on mRNAs that showed a more than 3-fold change in their expression. In the cortex, mRNAs for neuronal tyrosine/threonine phosphatase 1 and microtubule-associated tau were significantly enhanced. Expression of the genes coding alpha-amino-3-hydroxy-5-methyl-4-isoxazolepropionic acid (AMPA)-2, calcium and chloride channels, prolactin and growth hormone (GH), all of which are associated with brain function, were also upregulated. In the hippocampus, only transthyretin mRNA was upregulated. Transthyretin plays a role in hormone transport in the brain and possibly a neuroprotective role by amyloid-beta sequestration [119].

The effects of a ginkgo leaf extract on cerebral oedema were studied in rats intoxicated with triethyltin chloride (TET). The brains of TET-treated rats showed elevated water and sodium levels and a significant increase in the sodium/potassium ratio, whereas animals treated with TET plus the extract (100 mg/kg) did not show water and electrolyte changes. Using light and electron microscopy to follow the course of intoxication and treatment, severe oedema with extensive vacuolization was seen in the cerebral and cerebellar white matter. Morphometric measurements revealed a significant decrease in these manifestations of cytotoxic oedema in animals treated with the extract [120].

Na,K-ATPase activity and expression, fatty acid content and malondialdehyde content (an index of lipid peroxidation) were compared in ipsilateral (ischaemic) and contralateral (unlesioned) cortices in the mouse after 1 hour of unilateral focal cortical cerebral ischaemia. For 10 days before ischaemia a ginkgo leaf extract (110 mg/kg) was administered daily to 50% of the animals. Ischaemia significantly reduced Na,K-ATPase activity by about 40% and increased malondialdehyde content; pretreatment with the extract suppressed these effects. The free radical scavenging properties of the extract are a potential mechanism by which Na,K-ATPase injury and lipoperoxidation are prevented [121].

Computerized EEG analysis was used to investigate the effects of preventive treatment with a ginkgo leaf extract in cerebral global ischaemia and reperfusion in rats. The extract was administered at 100 mg/kg over 24 hours, for 5 days before and 5 days after cerebral ischaemia-reperfusion. The onset of isoelectric EEG (flat-line) following 4-vessel occlusion was observed after a mean time of 25 seconds in extract-treated rats and after 18 seconds in control rats ($p < 0.0015$). Spectral analysis of EEG showed that the percentage of slow waves 10 minutes after reperfusion was 117% higher in the control group than in the ginkgo group ($p < 0.015$) and the percentage of slow waves after 15 minutes of reperfusion was

100% higher in the control group than in the ginkgo group (p<0.02). Five days after cerebral ischaemia-reperfusion the percentage of slow waves was insignificantly higher in the control group than in the ginkgo group (p>0.05) [122].

A cranial window (intravital videomicroscopy), for observation of the capillary network on the cerebral cortex, was surgically inserted into 20 normotensive and 24 spontaneously hypertensive (SHR) rats to investigate the effects of a ginkgo leaf extract on hypertension. The rats received orally either ginkgo leaf extract at 100 mg/kg/day or placebo for 9 days and measurements were taken of arterial blood pressure, red cell velocity (V), microvascular diameter (D), number of open capillaries (OCN), circulating endothelial cells (CEC) in blood, relative blood flow (Flow) and frequency (Fc), and amplitude (AMP) of vasomotion. Untreated SHR rats showed very severe dysfunction in microcirculation with high systolic blood pressure (213 mm Hg). Systolic blood pressure dropped significantly to 153 mm Hg in the ginkgo-treated SHR group compared with that of untreated rats. Blood flow velocity and laser Doppler flow increased in both normotensive and hypertensive rats after ginkgo treatment. The vasomotor property, CEC and OCN improved in ginkgo-treated SHR rats, but no significant difference was observed in normotensive rats. It was suggested that the ginkgo leaf extract had a therapeutic effect on SHR rats by increasing perfusion, regulating vasomotion function, opening capillaries efficiently and reducing peripheral resistance. The injured vascular endothelium of SHR rats was also partly repaired by ginkgo treatment. It was concluded that the extract could be used to regulate hypertension and to protect cerebral microcirculatory function [123].

The effect of a ginkgo leaf extract on experimental vasospasm and vasculopathy was evaluated in a double haemorrhage model of chronic cerebral vasospasm involving 14 dogs, randomly assigned to one of two groups. The ginkgo group received the extract at 100 mg/kg, while saline was administered to the control group in an equal volume. In the ginkgo group the diameter of the basilar artery decreased from 2.01 mm at day 0 to 1.72 mm at day 8, whereas in the control group the vessel diameter decreased from 1.95 mm at day 0 to 1.11 mm at day 8. Thus the decreases in vessel diameter were 14.4% in the ginkgo group and 43.1% in the control group (p<0.05). Histopathological studies of specimens obtained from basilar arteries revealed pathological signs of proliferative vasculopathy, including narrowing of the vessel lumen, corrugation of the lamina elastica and subendothelial thickening in all animals of the control group, but not in the ginkgo group. The results suggested that ginkgo leaf extract may have a protective effect against subarachnoid haemorrhage-induced vasospasm and vasculopathy as a result of

antioxidant properties [124].

The animal model of intracerebroventricular strepto-zotocin (i.c.v. STZ) treatment was used to test the effects of a ginkgo leaf extract on memory enhancing properties and metabolic brain parameters. After a 1-week training period on the holeboard, improvements in learning, memory and cognition were seen in all animals and the improvement was maintained over the investigation period of 12 weeks in the control group, in which the energy pool in the cerebral parietotemporal cortex was found to be large and the energy turnover high. After triplicate i.c.v. STZ injection, working memory (WM), reference memory (RM) and passive avoidance (PA) behaviour fell off and continued to deteriorate throughout the investigation period. Otherwise there were no significant differences in locomotor activity, excluding the possibility that activity per se might have contributed to the behavioural abnormalities, which were accompanied by a permanent deficit in cerebral energy metabolism. The progressive deterioration in behaviour and maintained deficit in cerebral energy metabolism occurring after triplicate i.c.v. STZ injection were significantly slowed down by ginkgo leaf extract at 50 mg/day. Deficits in learning, memory and cognition were partially compensated, and disturbances in cerebral energy metabolism returned to almost normal values [125].

Using a spontaneous recognition procedure, the effects on olfactory short-term memory of chronic treatment with a ginkgo leaf extract at 30 or 60 mg/kg/day for 30 days were evaluated in young male rats (Experiment 1), while the effects of a single injection of the extract were assessed either in young male rats at 60 or 120 mg/kg (Experiment 2) or in aged female rats at 60 mg/kg (Experiment 3). Chronic treatment at the higher dose (60 mg/kg), enhanced recognition performance, allowing recognition following delays after which control animals showed none. Acute treatment enhanced recognition at both doses tested. The results of Experiment 3 showed that the ginkgo extract had an overall enhancement effect on the performance of aged rats [126].

In an experimental model of acute encephalopathy, 90 four-month-old rats received 4.5 Gy of total body irradiation (TBI) on day 1 while 15 rats received sham irradiation. Oral treatment was started 1 day (study A) or 22 days (study B) after irradiation and repeated daily for 12 days. In the irradiated groups, three subgroups were defined according to the treatment received: a ginkgo leaf extract at 50 or 100 mg/kg, or water. A behavioural study based on a conditioning test of negative reinforcement, the one-way avoidance test, was performed after irradiation (in study A daily from day 7 to day 14; in study B from day 28 to day 35). In study A (three groups of 15 rats), irradiated rats treated with water showed a significant delay in learning the one-way avoidance test in comparison with sham-irradiated rats ($p<0.0002$) or irradiated rats treated with the ginkgo leaf extract at 50 mg/kg ($p<0.0017$) or 100 mg/kg ($p<0.0002$). Irradiated rats treated with the extract (50 or 100 mg/kg) did not differ from the sham-irradiated controls. In study B (three groups of 15 rats), irradiated rats treated with water or the extract (50 or 100 mg/kg) did not differ from the sham-irradiated controls. The results indicated that a relatively low dose of total body irradiation induced substantial acute learning dysfunction in the rat, which persisted for 14 days after TBI. The effect was prevented by administration of ginkgo leaf extract (50 or 100 mg/kg) starting 24 hours after irradiation [127].

Effects on the visual, vestibular and auditory system
Rats treated orally with chloroquine at 75 mg/kg daily for 20 days developed abnormalities in their electro-retinograms in comparison with control animals. However, no chloroquine-induced retinopathy was observed in animals treated orally with a ginkgo leaf extract, alone at 100 mg/kg daily for 10 days and then at 100 mg/kg simultaneously with chloroquine at 75 mg/kg daily for 20 days [128].

Oral administration of a ginkgo leaf extract at 100 mg/kg for 10 days protected the retina of rats against lipoperoxidation induced by $FeSO_4$ and Na ascorbate, and against oxidative damage induced by ischaemia-reperfusion, reducing the decrease in electro-retinogram (ERG) b-wave amplitude, oedema, necrosis and ion imbalance. At 100 mg/kg daily for 15-18 days the extract also attenuated ERG changes induced by chloroquine both *ex vivo* (in isolated retina from treated rats) and *in vivo* [129].

By an analytical method using the fluorescent dye monochlorobimane it was demonstrated that a ginkgo leaf extract, administered orally to guinea pigs at 40 mg/kg body weight for 2 months, prevented age-related reduction of the intracellular glutathione 'reserve' in Mueller (retinal glial) cells [130].

Daily oral treatment of rats with either a ginkgo leaf extract at 100 mg/kg or superoxide dismutase (SOD) for 10 days significantly reduced the development of reperfusion-induced retinal oedema ($p<0.001$), occurring after 90 minutes of ischaemia followed by 4 or 24 hours of reperfusion, and significantly prevented neutrophil infiltration ($p<0.05$ to $p<0.01$). Both treatments also protected against reperfusion-induced injury when administered just before reperfusion [131,132]. Other experiments showed that both ginkgo leaf extract and SOD significantly inhibited increases in Na^+ and Ca^{2+} and loss of K^+ occurring in the retina of rats subjected to ischaemia [133,134]. These findings have been confirmed in streptozotocin-induced diabetic rats by the same authors. A ginkgo leaf extract administered orally to diabetic rats at 25-100 mg/kg/day for 10 days before induction of retinal ischaemia and reperfusion exerted dose-dependent protection against reperfusion-induced ion imbalance directly in retinal cells without influencing blood glucose content [135].

Oral administration of a ginkgo leaf extract to adult guinea pigs at 100 mg/kg daily for 4-6 weeks partly counteracted sodium salicylate-induced decreases in cochlear blood flow (CBF) and enhanced CBF increases induced by hypoxia [136].

In an experimental model of CNS plasticity, daily postoperative administration to cats which had undergone unilateral vestibular neurectomy of a ginkgo leaf extract (intraperitoneally at 25 or 50 mg/kg; orally at 40 or 80 mg/kg) or a terpene-free ginkgo leaf extract (intraperitoneally at 10 or 25 mg/kg) accelerated locomotor balance recovery compared to control groups. This activity of the extract appeared to be localised in the non-terpenic fraction and was significantly greater by the intraperitoneal route than by the oral route [137].

Using a model of tinnitus in rats, daily oral administration of a ginkgo leaf extract at 10-100 mg/kg began 2 weeks before behavioural procedures and continued until the end of the experiment. Tinnitus was induced by daily subcutaneous administration of sodium salicylate (corresponding to 275 mg/kg of salicylic acid) to 14 groups of pigmented rats, 6 animals per group. The results from salicylate- and ginkgo-treated animals were compared to control groups receiving salicylate, saline or ginkgo extract only (at 100 mg/kg). Administration of the ginkgo leaf extract at 25, 50 or 100 mg/kg/day resulted in a significant decrease in behavioral manifestations of tinnitus [138].

Pharmacological studies in humans

Antioxidant activity
A study was carried out in patients undergoing cardiopulmonary bypass surgery (CPB) to evaluate whether or not a ginkgo leaf extract could reduce the extent of CPB- and reperfusion-induced lipid peroxidation, ascorbate depletion, tissue necrosis and cardiac dysfunction. Patients received orally either 320 mg of a ginkgo leaf extract (n = 8) or placebo (n = 7) daily for 5 days before surgical intervention. Plasma samples were obtained from the peripheral circulation and the coronary sinus at crucial stages of the operation (before incision, during ischaemia and within the first 30 minutes post-unclamping) and up to 8 days postoperatively. Upon aortic unclamping, the ginkgo leaf extract inhibited transcardiac release of thiobarbituric acid-reactive species ($p<0.05$) and attenuated the early (5-10 minute) decrease in dimethylsulfoxide/ascorbyl free radical levels ($p<0.05$). The extract also significantly reduced

the more delayed leakage of myoglobin (p = 0.007) and had an almost significant effect on ventricular myosin leakage (p = 0.053, 6 days postoperatively). The results demonstrated the usefulness of adjuvant ginkgo leaf extract therapy in limiting oxidative stress in cardiovascular surgery [139].

Anti-ischaemic activity; haemorheological effects
Oral and intravenous administration of a ginkgo leaf extract to healthy volunteers has been reported to improve the membrane properties of erythrocytes and impede spontaneous and platelet activating factor-induced platelet aggregation. In patients with disorders of arterial blood flow, administration of the extract improved elevated whole blood and plasma viscosity, and inhibited red cell and platelet aggregation and caused a decrease in hyperfibrinogenaemia. Cutaneous blood flow was increased by infusion of the extract [140].

In a randomized, open, placebo-controlled trial, 48 patients with vascular dementia received over a period of 1 hour an infusion of 250 ml of 0.9% saline containing 50, 100 or 200 mg of a ginkgo leaf extract, or saline only (placebo). Extract doses of 100 or 200 mg increased microperfusion of the skin (p<0.05 vs. placebo, from 30 minutes after commencement) and the highest dose significantly decreased whole blood viscosity (p<0.05 vs. placebo, 60 minutes after commencement) [141].

Effects on high altitude sickness
A randomized, controlled study was carried out on 44 healthy male mountaineers who had experienced acute altitude sickness on previous climbs; they received 160 mg of a ginkgo leaf extract or placebo daily for 8 days during ascension to a Himalayan base camp. None of the climbers in the ginkgo group experienced acute mountain sickness (headache, dizziness, shortness of breath, nausea, vomiting etc.) compared to 41% of the placebo group. From assessment of respiratory parameters, 14% of climbers in the ginkgo group experienced altitude sickness compared to 82% in the placebo group. The ginkgo leaf extract was also rated as significantly more effective in preventing cold-related circulatory problems (numbness, tingling, aching, swelling of extremities) based on evaluation of functional disabilities and results obtained by plethysmography (measurement of extremity circulation). Furthermore, only 18% of climbers in the ginkgo group reported moderate or severe impairment of diuresis compared to 77% on placebo [142].

A randomized, double-blind, placebo-controlled study evaluated whether ginkgo leaf extract is an effective prophylactic against acute mountain sickness (AMS) if begun 1 day prior to rapid ascent; 26 participants, who normally resided at sea level, received the extract (3 × 60 mg daily; n =12) or placebo (n =14),

starting 24 hours before ascending Mauna Kea, Hawaii. They were transported from sea level to the summit (4205 m) over a period of 3 hours, including 1 hour at 2835 m. The Lake Louise Self-report Questionnaire constituted the primary outcome measure at baseline, at 2835 m, and after 4 hours at 4205 m. AMS was defined as a Lake Louise Self-report Score (LLSR) >/= 3 with headache. Subjects who developed severe AMS were promptly transported to a lower altitude for the remainder of the study. The ginkgo and placebo groups were well matched: 58% vs. 50% female; median age 28 (range 22-53) vs. 33 years (range 21-53); 58% vs. 57% Caucasian. Two subjects (17%) on ginkgo leaf extract and nine (64%) on placebo developed severe AMS and required descent for their safety (p = 0.021); all recovered without sequelae. The median LLSR score at 4205 m was significantly lower (p = 0.03) in the ginkgo group than in the placebo group: 4 (range 1-8) vs. 5 (range 2-9). With respect to lowering the incidence of AMS, results in the ginkgo group did not quite reach statistical significance (p = 0.07 compared to placebo): ginkgo group 7/12 (58.3%) vs. placebo 13/14 (92.9%). This was the first study to demonstrate that 1 day of pretreatment with ginkgo leaf extract may significantly reduce the severity of AMS prior to rapid ascent from sea level to over 4000 m [143].

Effects on ocular blood flow
Since glaucoma patients may benefit from improvements in ocular blood flow, the effect of a ginkgo leaf extract was evaluated in a phase I, placebo-controlled, cross-over trial; 3 × 40 mg of the extract or placebo was administered orally for 2 days to 11 healthy volunteers (aged 34 ± 3 years) with a 2-week washout period between treatment phases. Ocular blood flow before and after treatment was measured by Colour Doppler imaging. The ginkgo leaf extract significantly increased end diastolic velocity in the ophthalmic artery to 7.7 cm/sec compared to 6.5 cm/sec at baseline (23% change, p = 0.023), while no significant change was observed in the placebo group. No side effects related to the extract were observed and it did not alter arterial blood pressure, heart rate or intraocular pressure. It was concluded that ginkgo deserves further investigation in ocular blood flow and neuroprotection for possible application to the treatment of glaucomatous optic neuropathy and other ischaemic ocular diseases [144].

Effects on the central nervous system (CNS)

Exploratory data
The effects of a ginkgo leaf extract on the CNS were evaluated in a double-blind, placebo-controlled, cross-over study using the Quantitative Pharmacoelectro-encephalogram method. Twelve healthy male volunteers aged 18-65 years received one of three different single oral doses of the extract (40, 120 and 240 mg) or placebo at minimum intervals of 3 days.

Pharmacological effects of the extract on the CNS (increases in alpha activity and cognitive activating type response) were significantly different from those of placebo and more evident at the higher doses (p = 0.002 and p = 0.008 respectively with 240 mg), the electroencephalogram profile being comparable to those of well-known cognitive activators [145].

Using long-latency auditory event-related potentials (ERPs), the effects of a ginkgo leaf extract (120 mg daily for 57 days) on cognitive information processing were investigated in a double-blind, placebo-controlled study involving 48 patients (aged 51-79 years) suffering from age-associated memory impairment. ERP investigations were performed on days 1 and 57, before the daily dose and 3 hours after, to evaluate acute, chronic and superimposed effects of the drug. In comparison with placebo the extract reduced latency of the ERP component P300, which may reflect shorter stimulus-evaluation time [146].

The effects of acute doses of a ginkgo leaf extract on memory and psychomotor performance were investigated in 31 healthy volunteers aged 30-59 years using a randomized, double-blind, placebo-controlled, 5-way cross-over design. The volunteers received 3 × 50 mg, 3 × 100 mg, 1 × 120 mg or 1 × 240 mg of the extract, or placebo, daily for 2 days (separated by 5-day wash-out periods). Following baseline measurements, medication was administered at 09.00 for single doses and 09.00, 15.00 and 21.00 hours for multiple doses. The psychometric test battery was administered pre-dose at 08.30 and then at frequent intervals until 11 hours post-dose. The results showed that effects of the extract on aspects of cognition in asymptomatic volunteers are more pronounced for memory, particularly working memory. They also showed that these effects may be dose-dependent, although not in a linear dose-related manner, and that 120 mg of extract produced the most evident effects of the doses examined. Additionally, the results suggested that cognition-enhancing effects of the extract are more likely to be apparent in individuals aged 50-59 years [42].

In an open, uncontrolled, cross-over study, the effects of a single oral dose of 240 mg of a ginkgo leaf extract or, separated by a 3-7 day interval, 40 mg of tacrine (a drug used in the treatment of Alzheimer's disease) were investigated in 18 elderly patients (mean age 67.4 years) suffering from possible or probable Alzheimer's disease with mild to moderate dementia. Results from computer-analyzed, quantitative electro-encephalograms (EEGs) recorded before, and at 1- and 3-hour intervals after, drug administration indicated that within 3 hours ginkgo leaf extract induced pharmacological effects (a relative increase in alpha wave activity and decrease of slow waves) similar to those induced by responders to tacrine as well as other "cognitive activators" and anti-dementia drugs. 240 mg of ginkgo leaf extract produced characteristic cognitive activator EEG profiles in more responders (8 of 18) than 40 mg tacrine (3 of 18 subjects); 2 of them responded to both of the drugs [147].

Effects on cognition and memory

In a randomized, double-blind, placebo-controlled trial, 61 healthy participants (aged 18-40 years) received either 120 mg of ginkgo leaf extract or placebo daily for 30 days. Validated neuropsychological tests were conducted before and after treatment to assess a wide range of cognitive variables. The results indicated that ginkgo leaf extract improves memory processes, particularly working memory processes (digit span backwards and working memory speed, p<0.05) and memory consolidation (p<0.01), and executive functioning (a trail making test, p<0.01) [43].

Another recent study on healthy volunteers evaluated dose-dependent effects of acute administration of a ginkgo leaf extract on coherent cognitive domains, assessing the four Cognitive Drug Research (CDR) factors: speed of attention, accuracy of attention, speed of memory and quality of memory. In a placebo-controlled, double-blind, multi-dose, balanced cross-over design, 20 participants (mean age 20 years) received on different days 120 mg, 240 mg and 360 mg of the extract or placebo. Cognitive performance was assessed using the CDR computerised test battery immediately prior to dosing and 1, 2.5, 4 and 6 hours thereafter. The primary outcome measures, the four aspects of cognitive performance, were previously derived by factor analysis of CDR subtests. Compared to placebo, the ginkgo leaf extract produced a number of significant changes in performance measures, the most striking being a dose-dependent improvement in the 'speed of attention' factor following 240 mg or 360 mg of the extract, evident after 2.5 hours and still present after 6 hours [44].

In a 6-week, double-blind, placebo-controlled study, the relatively short-term efficacy of a ginkgo leaf extract on neuropsychological functioning of cognitively intact older adults (aged 55-86 years) was evaluated using a battery of neuropsychological tests and measures. Participants were randomly assigned to either the extract at 180 mg/day or placebo. To evaluate the participants' cognitive and behavioural functioning, testing was carried out prior to initiation of therapy (pre-treatment baseline) and again just prior to termination of treatment after 6 weeks. By the end of treatment participants who received the extract showed significantly greater improvement in a task assessing speed of processing abilities (the Stroop Colour and Word Test) compared to the placebo group. Improved performance trends in favour of the ginkgo group were also demonstrated in three of the four remaining tasks involving a timed, speed of processing component, although they did not reach statistical significance. Furthermore, a significant relationship was found between the treatment and participants' ratings of overall ability to remember; compared to the placebo group, more participants in the ginkgo group rated their overall ability to remember as "improved" by the end of treatment. In contrast, no significant differences were found between groups in any of the four objective memory tests [45].

In a larger randomized, double-blind, placebo-controlled study by the same authors to evaluate the effect of ginkgo leaf on neuropsychological functioning, 262 community-dwelling, cognitively intact volunteers aged 60 years or older (mean 66.7 years) with unremarkable medical histories (no dementia or significant neurocognitive impairment and a score of at least 26 in the Mini-Mental State Examination) were assigned to treatment with 180 mg of a ginkgo leaf dry extract or matched placebo daily for 6 weeks. Efficacy was assessed by changes from baseline in a battery of neuropsychological tests. Compared to the placebo group, patients in the ginkgo group achieved significantly greater improvement in Selective Reminding tasks involving 30-minute-delayed free recall (p<0.04) and recognition (p<0.01) of non-contextual verbal material, and in the Wechsler Memory Scale III-FII subtest of 30-minute-delayed recognition of visual material (human faces; p<0.025), although the last result should be treated with caution since there was a significant difference at baseline (p<0.03 in favour of the placebo group). The ginkgo group also showed more improvement than the placebo group, albeit below the significance level, in 8 out of the 10 other neuropsychological tests employed in the study. In a self-reporting questionnaire significantly more participants in the ginkgo group subjectively rated their overall ability to remember as improved (p<0.05). An overall conclusion was drawn that the results provided complementary evidence of the potential efficacy of relatively short-term use of the ginkgo leaf extract in enhancing certain memory functions in cognitively intact older adults [46].

Following administration of a single 360 mg dose of a ginkgo leaf extract to 20 healthy young adults, modulation of cognition and mood was demonstrated using a randomized placebo-controlled, double-blind, balanced, cross-over design. Cognitive testing comprised completion of the Cognitive Drug Research (CDR) computerized assessment battery and two serial subtraction mental arithmetic tasks; mood was assessed with Bond-Lader visual analogue scales. After baseline cognitive assessment, further test sessions took place 1, 2.5, 4 and 6 hours after ingestion of the extract. Improvements in secondary memory performance (in the CDR battery), subtraction tasks and self-rated mood were reported [47].

Healthy, capable, community-dwelling volunteers over 60 years of age (average 69 years), recruited through newspaper advertisements, participated in a randomized, double-blind, placebo-controlled study to evaluate whether a ginkgo leaf extract improved memory in elderly adults. The 230 participants (132 women, 98 men) were assigned to treatment with either 3 × 40 mg of the extract (as marketed film-coated tablets) or placebo (lactose gelatin capsules) daily for 6 weeks. The main outcome measures were standardized neuropsychological tests of verbal and non-verbal learning and memory, attention and concentration, naming and expressive language, participant self-reporting in a memory questionnaire and clinical global impression of change documented by a spouse, relative or friend in regular contact with the participant. Analysis of the modified intent-to-treat population (the 291 participants who returned for evaluation) indicated no significant differences between treatment groups on any outcome measure; this was also the case from analysis of the fully evaluable population (the 203 participants who complied with the protocol and returned for evaluation). The data suggested that, at the recommended dosage, ginkgo leaf extract provided no measurable benefit in memory or related cognitive function to adults with healthy cognitive function [148]. The use of non-matching placebos (with a different dosage form) in this study has been criticized [149].

Clinical studies
Various controlled studies assessing the efficacy of standardized ginkgo leaf extracts are described in the following text under headings of Dementia, Cerebral insufficiency, Neurosensory disturbances and Peripheral arterial occlusive disease, and summarized in corresponding Tables 2-5. Published critical reviews and meta-analyses of clinical studies are summarized in Table 1.

DEMENTIA (Table 2)

The efficacy of standardized ginkgo leaf extracts in dementia has been assessed in numerous controlled, double-blind studies and confirmed in three systematic reviews [150-152] and a meta-analysis [153].

In a randomized, double-blind, placebo-controlled study the efficacy of a ginkgo leaf extract, administered at 120 mg/day over a period of 1-3 months, was investigated in 40 patients (average age 72 years) with mild to moderate primary degenerative dementia. Compared to placebo the extract significantly improved both psychometric test performance and clinical assessment. After 3 months of treatment with the extract a mean improvement of 23.5 % compared to baseline was found on the Crichton scale (p<0.0001). The SCAG (Sandoz Clinical Assessment: Geriatric) total score improved by approximately

33% compared to baseline values (p<0.0001). No adverse reactions were reported [24].

In another randomized, double-blind study, 40 patients (aged 50-75 years) diagnosed as suffering from senile dementia of the Alzheimer type received either 3 × 80 mg of a ginkgo leaf extract or placebo daily for 3 months. The patients were assessed by a battery of tests at baseline and after 1, 2 and 3 months. Results in the Syndrom-Kurztest (a brief cognitive test of memory and attention) improved significantly (p<0.001) as did psychopathology, psychomotoric performance, functional dynamics and neurophysiology. No adverse events were observed [25].

The efficacy of a ginkgo leaf extract was investigated in outpatients with presenile and senile primary degenerative dementia of the Alzheimer type and multi-infarct dementia, diagnosed in accordance with DSM-III-R, in a prospective, randomized, double-blind, placebo-controlled, multicentre study. After a 4-week placebo run-in period, 216 patients aged over 55 years received orally 240 mg of extract or placebo daily for 24 weeks. In accordance with the recommended multi-dimensional evaluation approach, three primary variables were chosen: Clinical Global Impressions (CGI) for psycho-pathological assessment, the Syndrom-Kurztest (SKT) for assessment of memory and attention, and the Nürnberger Alters-Beobachtungsskala (NAB) for behavioural assessment of activities in daily life. Clinical efficacy was assessed by means of a responder analysis, with therapy response defined as response in at least two of the three primary variables. Data from the 156 patients who complied with the protocol were used for the confirmatory analysis of valid cases. The frequency of therapy responders in the two treatment groups differed significantly in favour of the ginkgo leaf extract (p<0.005); intent-to-treat analysis of 205 patients gave similar results [26].

In another randomized, double-blind, placebo-controlled, multicentre study, patients with Alzheimer's disease or multi-infarct dementia diagnosed in accordance with DSM-III-R and ICD-10 were assigned to treatment with 3 × 40 mg of a ginkgo leaf extract or placebo daily for 52 weeks. Three primary outcome measures were evaluated at 12, 26 and 52 weeks: cognitive impairment, objectively assessed by the Alzheimer's Disease Assessment Scale cognitive subscale (ADAS-Cog); daily living and social behaviour, assessed by the total score of the Geriatric Evaluation by Relative's Rating Instrument (GERRI, completed by the caregiver); and general psychology, assessed by the Clinical Global Impression of Change rating (CGIC, completed by the physicians). From 309 patients included in the intention-to-treat analysis, 202 provided evaluable data for the 52-week end-point analysis. In the intention-to-treat analysis, the ADAS-Cog and GERRI scores of the ginkgo group

were superior by 1.4 points (p = 0.04) and 0.14 points (p = 0.004) respectively to those of the placebo group. The same patterns were observed in the evaluable data set: 27% of patients in the ginkgo group achieved at least a 4-point improvement on the ADAS-Cog, compared to 14% in the placebo group (p = 0.005); GERRI scores of 37% of patients were considered improved after ginkgo treatment, compared to 23% in the placebo group (p = 0.003). No difference was found in CGIC ratings. It was concluded that the ginkgo leaf extract was safe and appeared capable of stabilizing and, in a substantial number of cases, improving the cognitive performance and social functioning of demented patients for 6 months to 1 year. Changes induced by the extract were of sufficient magnitude to be recognized by caregivers in the GERRI scores [27].

Subsequently, to facilitate comparison with ginkgo clinical studies of 6 months duration, a full analysis was carried out of 26-week results from the above study. It showed that, among the 244 patients (from the initial 309) who completed 26-week evaluation, the placebo group showed a significant worsening in all domains of assessment compared to baseline values, while the ginkgo group slightly improved on cognitive assessment and daily living/social behaviour; ADAS-Cog (p = 0.04) and GERRI (p = 0.007) scores were in favour of the ginkgo leaf extract. In the ginkgo group 26% of patients achieved at least a 4-point improvement in ADAS-Cog score, compared to 17% in the placebo group (p = 0.04). With respect to GERRI scores, 30% of the ginkgo group improved and 17% worsened, while the placebo group showed an opposite trend with 25% of patients improved and 37% worsened (p = 0.006). Thus, compared to placebo, significant benefit from use of the ginkgo leaf extract was evident after 26 weeks [28].

In a randomized, double-blind, placebo-controlled study, 20 outpatients suffering from mild to moderate dementia of the Alzheimer type were assigned to oral treatment with either 3 × 80 mg of a ginkgo leaf extract or placebo daily for 3 months. Scores at the end of treatment in the primary variable, the SKT test for objective assessment of attention and memory, had improved from 19.67 to 16.78 in the ginkgo group compared to a deterioration from 18.11 to 18.89 in the placebo group, the results being significant in favour of the ginkgo leaf extract (p<0.013) [29].

In a 24-week double-blind, placebo-controlled, multicentre study, 214 elderly patients of average age 83 years (all of whom were in residential care homes for the elderly), with mild to moderate dementia of the Alzheimer or vascular type (n = 63) or age-associated memory impairment (n = 151), were randomly assigned to daily oral treatment with 160 mg (standard dose) or 240 mg (high dose) of a ginkgo leaf extract, or placebo. After 12 weeks, both ginkgo groups were randomly divided to continue on ginkgo leaf extract or change to placebo, while the original placebo group continued with placebo, for a further 12 weeks. This resulted in 5 groups of approximately equal size: ginkgo 160 mg (24 weeks), ginkgo 240 mg (24 weeks), placebo (24 weeks), ginkgo 160 mg (12 weeks) + placebo (12 weeks) and ginkgo 240 mg (12 weeks) + placebo (12 weeks). The allocation of the 63 participants with dementia to the 5 different treatment groups was not stated. Outcome measures assessed after 12 and 24 weeks included psychometric tests [digit memory span G (NAI-ZN-G), verbal learning (NAI-WL) and a trail-making, cognitive speed test (NAI-ZVT-G)], clinical assessment [presence and severity of geriatric symptoms (SCAG), depressive mood (GDS), self-perceived health and memory status (report marks)], and behavioural assessment (self-reported level of instrumental daily life activities). Intention-to-treat analysis showed no effect on any of the outcome measures for participants assigned to the ginkgo leaf extract (n = 79) compared to placebo (n = 44) over the 24-week period. After 12 weeks, the total performance of the combined standard dose and high dose ginkgo groups (n = 166) was slightly better with regard to self-reported activities of daily life, but slightly worse with regard to self-perceived health status compared to the placebo group (n = 48). No beneficial effects were evident from the higher dose or longer treatment. The results suggested that ginkgo leaf extract is not effective as a treatment for elderly people with mild to moderate dementia or age-associated memory impairment and are in sharp contrast with results from other studies [154].

The unconventional and complex design of the above study [154] has received adverse comment [155], not least in terms of the composite patient population, with a broad and heterogeneous spectrum of cognitive decline (some patients suffering from either Alzheimer or vascular type dementia and others non-demented, with age-associated memory impairment), of high average age (83 years) and high comorbidity, and living in the non-challenging environment of care-assisted homes for the elderly, which is less sensitive than daily living in open society for the detection of treatment effects. Questions have also been raised with respect to the adequacy of procedures applied to selection of participants (particularly since they did not include physicians to perform clinical screening examinations and differential diagnosis supported by concomitant laboratory and neuroimaging work), the nature of the outcome measurements and the statistical power of the study in relation to sample size. It was suggested [155] that these and other limitations preclude comparison with the effects of ginkgo in out-patient populations with Alzheimer's disease or vascular dementia as reported, for example, in the studies by Kanowski [26] and Le Bars [27,28]

CEREBRAL INSUFFICIENCY (Table 3)

The term "cerebral insufficiency" does not denote a precise syndrome, but a number of cerebral disturbances such as impairment of recent memory, confusion, change in social behaviour, lack of initiative, and affective and somatic troubles. Cerebral insufficiency symptoms have been associated with impaired cerebral circulation; sometimes they are considered to be early signs of dementia. In a 1992 critical review [156] of 40 controlled studies in cerebral insufficiency (involving a somewhat wider range of disorders than described above), 8 studies [30-34,39,40,48] were considered to have been conducted in accordance with standards that allowed reliable conclusions to be drawn; these and more recently published controlled studies are described in this section (or, where appropriate, under Neurosensory disturbances).

The therapeutic effectiveness of standardized ginkgo leaf extracts in the treatment of cerebral insufficiency has been confirmed in a meta-analysis [157].

In a randomized, double-blind, placebo-controlled, multicentre study, 166 patients (average age 82 years) with cerebral disorders due to ageing were assigned to 160 mg of ginkgo leaf extract or placebo daily for 12 months. Using a specially devised geriatric clinical evaluation scale, improvement was shown in both groups after 3, 6, 9 and 12 months but the results were significantly in favour of the ginkgo leaf extract after 3 months (p<0.05) and the difference increased at each assessment (p<0.01 after 12 months). These results were in accord with overall clinical assessment by the physicians [30].

In another randomized, double-blind study, 60 in-patients with cerebral insufficiency, the leading symptom being depressive mood, were treated daily for 6 weeks with 160 mg of a ginkgo leaf extract or placebo. After 2, 4 and 6 weeks, changes in 12 typical symptoms were evaluated and compared to results of the previous examination. Minor but progressive improvements were observed in the placebo group. However, the total number of improvements was significantly larger in the ginkgo group; after 2 weeks the differences were marked for only a few of the symptoms; after 4 and 6 weeks, in 11 of the 12 symptoms (p<0.001 for all 11 symptoms after 6 weeks). The largest number of improvements in the ginkgo group was observed between the 2nd and 4th weeks of treatment. In this period, about two-thirds of the patients on ginkgo leaf extract and about one-fifth of patients on placebo showed improvements [31].

In a double-blind, placebo-controlled, multicentre study the efficacy of a ginkgo leaf extract was investigated in 303 elderly out-patients with cerebral insufficiency, who received either 3 × 50 mg of the extract or placebo daily for 12 weeks. Data from 209 patients (110 verum, 99 placebo) were available for the statistical evaluation. Compared to the placebo group, the ginkgo group showed significant improvements (p<0.05 to p<0.001) after 6 weeks for 3 out of 11, and after 12 weeks for 8 out of 11, typical symptoms of cerebral insufficiency. In a number connection test, the time period for number connection improved by 25% in the ginkgo group and only 14% in the placebo group (p<0.01). At the end of therapy, both the doctors' and patients' assessments of efficacy showed highly significant differences between the two groups in favour of the ginkgo leaf extract (p<0.001) [32].

In a randomized, double-blind, placebo-controlled study, 99 out-patients (aged 51-68 years) with typical symptoms of cerebral insufficiency were assigned to treatment with 150 mg of a ginkgo leaf extract or placebo daily for 12 weeks. Compared to the placebo group after 12 weeks, 10 out of 12 typical symptoms in the ginkgo group were clearly improved (p<0.01 for each of 7 symptoms) [33].

In a randomized, double-blind, placebo-controlled study, 100 patients (aged 55-85 years) with at least 4 out of 6 symptoms of cerebral insufficiency were treated with 3×15 ml of a solution corresponding to a daily dose of 112 mg of a ginkgo leaf extract (containing 30 mg of flavone glycosides and 1-2% of terpene lactones) or placebo for 12 weeks. Average scores for severity of symptoms decreased by more than 50% in the verum group and about 25% in the placebo group. Compared to the placebo group, significant reductions in scores were achieved in the verum group for the following symptoms: memory deficiencies, poor concentration (both p<0.001 at 4, 8 and 12 weeks), anxiety, dizziness and headaches (all three p<0.001 at 8 and 12 weeks) [34].

The efficacy of 120 mg of a ginkgo leaf extract daily for 3 months on relevant symptoms of mild to medium cerebrovascular insufficiency was tested on 40 out-patients in a randomized, double-blind, placebo-controlled study. In the ginkgo group the total SCAG score (Sandoz Clinical Assessment - Geriatric) dropped by 9 points on average, whereas it remained unchanged in the placebo group (p = 0.00005). Evaluation of individual SCAG components revealed favourable effects of the extract, particularly on disturbances of short-term memory, mental awareness and dizziness; superior effects were also evident with respect to headaches and tinnitus, and in results of the Syndrome Kurztest [35].

The effects of 160 mg of a ginkgo leaf extract daily for 24 weeks on basic parameters of mental performance were evaluated in 72 out-patients with cerebral insufficiency using a randomized, double-blind, placebo-controlled design. Computer-aided psycho-metric assessment of short-term memory and basic learning rate was carried out. Significant improvements in short-term memory after 6 weeks and learning rate after 24 weeks were evident in the ginkgo group, but not in the placebo group (longitudinal analysis). The difference between the ginkgo and placebo groups attained statistical significance by the 24th week (horizontal analysis) [36].

The efficacy of 150 mg of a ginkgo leaf extract daily for 12 weeks was evaluated in a randomized, double-blind, placebo-controlled study involving 90 outpatients (average age 62.7 years) with cerebral insufficiency. In a range of psychometric tests, significant improvements were observed in the performance of patients in the ginkgo group compared to those in the placebo group. Continuous positive changes were observed in the ginkgo group, particularly with regard to tests of speed and comprehension level (basic reaction time and quick learning time) [37].

In a randomized, double-blind study the effect of 120 mg of ginkgo leaf extract daily for 3 months on cognitive function and quality of life was evaluated in comparison with placebo in 54 elderly patients, living at home and showing mild signs of impairment in everyday function on the Crichton Geriatric Rating Scale. Cognitive function was measured before, and at monthly intervals during, the trial using a battery of tests of mental ability comprising both computerized and pencil-and-paper tasks. Quality of life was assessed using a behavioural questionnaire before and after the study. Individual analyses of cognitive test results showed some advantage of ginkgo leaf extract over placebo. When accuracy scores from all eight tests were combined using two different techniques, both groups improved over time but improvement in the ginkgo group at week 12 was significantly greater than in the placebo group. No signs of improvement were detected under placebo treatment when reaction time (speed) measures were combined, whereas by week 4 the ginkgo group reacted significantly faster than at baseline (p = 0.0082 and p = 0.005 by different data analysis techniques), and was superior to placebo throughout the study. These improvements in mental efficiency were accompanied by a significant increase in the interest taken in everyday activities in the ginkgo group (p = 0.015 compared to baseline), but not in the placebo group (p = 0.43) [48].

In a randomized, double-blind, placebo-controlled, three-armed study, 241 out-patients (aged 55-86 years, mean 68.9 years) with age-related cognitive impair-ment (difficulties of memory and/or concentration) were assigned to treatment with 2.85 ml (low dose, LD; n = 82) or 5.7 ml (high dose, HD; n = 77) of a 70%-ethanolic extract from fresh ginkgo leaf (drug to ex-tract ratio 1:4, total flavone glycosides, 0.20 mg/ml; total ginkgolides, 0.34 mg/ml) or placebo (PL; n = 82) daily for 24 weeks. A battery of psychometric tests was used to assess the patients at 0, 12 and 24 weeks. 197 patients completed the study. In objective tests the scores of all three groups improved over the study period, probably due to a learning effect. In the Benton test of short term visual memory, increases from baseline scores of 18%, 26% and 11% were observed in the HD, LD and PL groups respectively, the contrast analysis showing significant differences between groups: PL < HD < LD (MANOVA: p = 0.0076). No significant differences between groups were observed after 24 weeks in results of the Expanded Mental Control Test (EMCT; measuring attention and concentration) or Rey word tests 1 (short-term verbal memory and learning) and 2 (long-term memory by recognition), nor in subjective parameters (patients' perception of memory and concentration, and physicians' assessment of the severity of memory complaints). Since the baseline scores for EMCT and Rey tests were already high, the study authors suggested that the patients were simply "too good" overall for measurement of differences. In the subgroup (n = 44) with lower baseline scores in EMCT and Rey tests, improvement in the Rey 2 test (but not in EMCT or Rey 1) was significantly greater in patients treated with the extract (p<0.02) than in those treated with placebo. The efficacy of the treatment was judged as low by both patients and physicians [158]. In terms of flavone glycosides and ginkgolides content, it should be noted that the dosages used in this study were very low compared to those normally used for standardized ginkgo dry extracts; the "high" daily dose of 5.7 ml per day contained 1.14 mg of flavone glycosides and 1.94 mg of ginkgolides, compared to approx. 29.4 mg and 3.72 mg respectively in 120 mg of a standardized ginkgo dry extract.

NEUROSENSORY DISTURBANCES (Table 4)

Neurosensory disturbances involving the vestibular and auditory systems, such as vertigo and dizziness, tinnitus, idiopathic hearing loss and nystagmus, may be regarded as symptoms associated with disturbances of CNS function. Damage to vestibular mechanisms, interference with blood supply to the internal ear and/or alterations in the function of the autonomic nervous system, the acoustic nerve or more central auditory pathways, as well as age-associated arthrosis of the cervical vertebrae, have been associated with such neurosensory disturbances. Other neurosensory problems, such as retinal ischaemia and degeneration, are related more specifically to dysfunctions of the visual system and its associated neural pathways. Beneficial effects which a ginkgo leaf extract may have on neurosensory disturbances are considered to be due to a vasoregulatory action [62].

Vestibular/auditory disturbances
(vertigo, tinnitus, sudden hearing loss)
In a randomized, double-blind study, 35 patients with

vestibular vertigo were treated by a course of physical training; additionally they were assigned to treatment with 160 mg of a ginkgo leaf extract or placebo daily for 4 weeks. Compared to the placebo group, clear amelioration of vertigo was evident and a greater diminution in body sway amplitude was observed in the verum group (22.2 mm vs. 10.3 mm in the placebo group) [38].

A randomized, double-blind, multicentre study involved 70 patients with vertiginous syndrome of recent onset and unclear origin, who were treated with either 160 mg of a ginkgo leaf extract or placebo daily for 3 months. The effectiveness of the extract on the intensity, frequency and duration of the disorder was significant (p<0.05). By the end of the study, symptoms had resolved in 47% of patients in the ginkgo group compared to 18% in the placebo group [39].

In a randomized, double-blind, placebo-controlled, multicentre study, 103 out-patients with tinnitus (which had started during the past 12 months) were assigned to treatment with 2 × 80 mg (as 2 × 2 ml of solution) of a ginkgo leaf extract or placebo daily for 3 months. The results were significant in favour of the extract with respect to improvement in the intensity (p<0.03) and rapidity of disappearance (p<0.03) of tinnitus, and global comparison of the groups (p<0.05). From the results it was possible to determine the prognostic value of different parameters, among which the site and periodicity of the disease were of special importance, However, treatment with ginkgo leaf extract improved the condition of all patients, irrespective of the prognostic factor [40].

A randomized, double-blind, placebo-controlled study evaluated the effect of 120 mg of a ginkgo leaf extract daily on tinnitus intensity in 99 patients who had suffered from tinnitus for at least 2 years (mean duration 4.5 years). During 12 weeks of treatment sound (tinnitus) intensity, determined by audiometry in the initially more severely affected ear, decreased from 42.3 to 39.0 dB in the ginkgo group compared to a slight increase from 44.1 to 45.1 dB in the placebo group (p = 0.015). Subjective improvement was reported by 15 patients in the ginkgo group and 7 in the placebo group [41].

To assess whether a ginkgo leaf extract was effective in treating tinnitus, a double-blind, placebo-controlled study was based on mailed questionnaires and telephone interviews with 1,121 people aged between 18 and 70 years, who were assigned to treatment with 150 mg of the extract or placebo daily for 12 weeks. From these participants 360 matched pairs, having completed the treatment and questionnaires, were included in the 12-week comparison. Medical diagnoses and monitoring were not possible due to the design of this study. No significant differences were evident between the two groups in primary or secondary outcome measures. 34 of 360 participants who received active treatment reported that their tinnitus was less troublesome after 12 weeks compared to 35 of 360 who took placebo [159].

A study aimed at evaluating the efficacy of an undefined ginkgo extract in tinnitus was carried out in two phases. In an open phase without placebo control, 80 patients with persistent severe tinnitus were treated with only 29.2 mg of ginkgo leaf extract daily for 2 weeks. This was followed by a randomized, double-blind, placebo-controlled, crossover study, using the same dosage, in 20 patients from the 21 who had reported a positive effect on tinnitus in the open phase. The primary outcome measures were subjective complaints and treatment preferences of the patients; 7 patients preferred ginkgo extract to placebo, 7 placebo to ginkgo extract and 6 patients had no preference. Statistical analysis between groups gave no support to the hypothesis that ginkgo extract has any effect on tinnitus at the very low dose level used [160].

From a systematic review of 5 randomized, controlled clinical studies (of which 4 were placebo-controlled) carried out up to 1998 in which ginkgo leaf extracts were used as a treatment for tinnitus, the authors found the overall results to be favourable but considered that a firm conclusion about efficacy was not yet possible due to the small body of available evidence [161].

A randomized reference-controlled study involving 80 patients with idiopathic sudden hearing loss, existing no longer than 10 days, evaluated the effects of a ginkgo leaf extract (175 mg in infusion + 160 mg orally) in comparison with those of naftidrofuryl (400 mg intravenous + 400 mg orally), a reference drug with antiserotonergic and vasodilatory properties. After one week of observation, 40% of the patients in each group showed a complete remission of hearing loss, which the authors attributed primarily to spontaneous recovery. After 2 and 3 weeks of observation, however, there was a borderline benefit in relative hearing gain in the ginkgo group (p = 0.06) without any side effects. Some patients in the naftidrofuryl group developed side effects such as orthostatic dysregulation, headache or sleep disturbances [162].

Visual dysfunction

In a double-blind, placebo-controlled study, the effects of a ginkgo leaf extract on senile macular degeneration were evaluated by fundoscopy and measurement of visual acuity and visual field in out-patients who received 160 mg of the extract (n = 10) or placebo (n = 10) daily for 6 months. In spite of the small population sample, a significant improvement in long distance visual acuity was observed in the ginkgo group (p<0.05

compared to the placebo group). From global clinical assessment the physicians found improvement in the condition of 9 out of 10 patients in the ginkgo group (p<0.01 compared to the placebo group) [163].

A double-blind study involving 29 diabetic subjects with early diabetic retinopathy (evidenced by angiography and associated with a blue-yellow dyschromatopsia) evaluated the effects on colour vision of 160 mg of a ginkgo leaf extract or placebo daily for 6 months. In the ginkgo group there was a significant improvement with respect to Desaturated Panel D-15 results in subjects without retinal ischaemia, whereas the condition was aggravated in the placebo group. These results on visual function corroborate pharmacological effects of ginkgo leaf extract observed on the diabetic retina [164].

The efficacy of a ginkgo leaf extract in chronic retinal insufficiency, an organ-specific expression of generalized vascular cerebral deficiency, was evaluated in two groups of 12 elderly patients (mean age 75 years) in a randomized, double-blind study comprising two consecutive 4-week phases: phase 1 (extract at 80 mg/day in group A, 160 mg/day in group B); phase 2 (extract at 160 mg/day in both groups). Automated perimetry (an indirect non-invasive technique) was used to evaluate the effect of the extract on reversibility of visual field disturbances, the main parameter investigated being the change in luminous density difference threshold. At 160 mg/day the extract significantly increased retinal sensitivity within 4 weeks (p<0.05). At the lower dose of 80 mg/day, retinal sensitivity did not change until the dose was increased to 160 mg/day in the second 4-week phase (p<0.01). The relative sensitivity of damaged retinal areas was more strongly influenced than that of healthy-looking areas. Assessment of the general condition of patients by both physicians and patients indicated significant improvement after therapy (p<0.01 to p<0.001 compared to initial data) [165].

PERIPHERAL ARTERIAL OCCLUSIVE DISEASE (Table 5)

A recent meta-analysis of randomized, double-blind, placebo-controlled studies on the symptomatic treatment of intermittent claudication concluded that standardized ginkgo leaf extracts are superior to placebo and confirmed a significant difference in the increase in pain-free walking distance [166]. The results corroborated a previous evaluation of less extensive data [167].

A randomized, double-blind, placebo-controlled study was conducted on 79 patients suffering from peripheral arteriopathy (Fontaine stage IIb), who were assigned to 3 × 40 mg of a ginkgo leaf extract or placebo daily for 24 weeks. The ginkgo leaf extract was significantly superior to placebo with respect to pain-free (p<0.05) and maximum walking (p<0.001) distances, and in plethysmography results (p<0.01). Overall assessment of efficacy by the physicians and patients correlated well with the clinical findings [49].

A randomized, double-blind, placebo-controlled study was carried out to assess the efficacy of a ginkgo leaf extract on objective and subjective parameters of walking performance in trained patients suffering from peripheral arterial occlusive disease (Fontaine stage IIb). Following a 2-week placebo run-in phase, 60 patients (aged 47-82 years), with angiographically proven peripheral arterial occlusive disease of the lower extremities and an intermittent claudication for at least 6 months, were assigned to daily treatment with either 3 × 40 mg of a ginkgo leaf extract or placebo for 24 weeks. No improvement had been observed with other measures despite consistent walking training. A maximum pain-free walking distance on the treadmill of less than 150 m was recorded for all subjects at the beginning of the study. The main outcome measure was the difference between the initial walking distance and the distance after 8, 16 and 24 weeks of treatment, measured on a treadmill (walking speed 3 km/hour and slope of 12%). Secondary parameters were the corresponding differences for the maximum walking distance, the relative increase of pain-free walking distance, the Doppler index and subjective evaluation of the patients. In the ginkgo group, absolute median changes in pain-free walking distance at weeks 8, 16 and 24 compared to the initial distance (95% confidence interval in parentheses) were 19 m (14, 33), 34 m (18, 50) and 41 m (26, 64) respectively. Corresponding values in the placebo group were 7 m (−4, 12), 12 m (5, 22) and 8 m (−1, 21). Compared to the placebo group the changes in pain-free walking distance in the ginkgo group were superior at all 3 time points (p<0.0001, p = 0.0003 and p<0.0001 respectively). A clinically relevant difference of 20% between the two groups was also significant (p = 0.008). The Doppler index remained unchanged in both groups. Subjective assessments by the patients correlated with the clinical findings. The results demonstrated that treatment with ginkgo leaf extract produced significant and clinically relevant improvements in walking performance in trained patients suffering from intermittent claudication [50].

In a similar study, with a randomized, double-blind, placebo-controlled, multicentre design, 111 patients with a mean age of 62 years, suffering from angiographically proven peripheral occlusive arterial disease (Fontaine stage IIb) and intermittent claudication (pain-free walking distance of less than 150 m on the treadmill) were treated, following a 2-week placebo run-in period, with either 3 × 40 mg of a ginkgo leaf extract or placebo daily for 24 weeks. The primary variable was the difference in pain-free walking distance between the end of the run-in

period and 8, 16 and 24 weeks later, measured on a treadmill (walking speed 3 km/hour and slope of 12%). Initially, the mean pain-free walking distances were very similar: 108.5 m in the ginkgo group and 105.2 m in the placebo group. At the end of treatment, they had increased to 153.2 m and 126.6 m, respectively, the differences between groups being significant at all three time points: p = 0.017 after 8 weeks, p = 0.007 after 16 weeks and p = 0.016 after 24 weeks. Differences for maximum walking distance, and relative increases in pain-free walking distance and maximum distance, were also significantly higher in the ginkgo group (p<0.05 in each case). Subjective assessments by the patients indicated improvement in both groups. The results showed that treatment with ginkgo leaf extract caused a significant and therapeutically relevant increase in the patients' walking distance [51].

Another randomized, double-blind, placebo-controlled study in patients suffering from peripheral arterial occlusive disease of the lower extremities (Fontaine stage IIb) involved 40 out-patients, who were assigned to daily treatment with either 2 × 80 mg of a ginkgo leaf extract or placebo for 24 weeks. In terms of pain-free walking distance, the results demonstrated significant superiority of the ginkgo leaf extract over placebo after 8, 16 and 24 weeks (p<0.001 in each case). At the end of treatment, the mean pain-free walking distance had increased by 37.7 m (47.7%) in the ginkgo group and by 3.7 m (14.3%) in the placebo group. The maximum walking distance also increased significantly in the ginkgo group compared to the placebo group (p = 0.002 after 8 weeks, p<0.001 after 16 weeks and p = 0.007 after 24 weeks). Subjective evaluation of the treatment by patients was significantly in favour of the ginkgo leaf extract (p = 0.006) [52].

A ginkgo leaf extract in injectable form was evaluated as a pre-operative treatment for chronic occlusive arterial disease of the lower limbs (Fontaine stage III). In the randomized, double-blind, placebo-controlled, multicentre study, 64 patients of average age 64.6 years, with an educational and intellectual level as well as a physical condition allowing them to play an active role in the experiment (self-evaluation of pain) were assigned to receive daily for 8 days two infusions of 500 ml of physiological saline containing either 100 mg of the ginkgo leaf extract (a lyophilizate for parenteral use) or a placebo (32 patients per group). During the treatment period, anticoagulant therapy was authorized and pentazocine (an opioid analgesic) was allowed at the patient's request, but haemodilution and vasoactive or platelet anti-aggregating drugs were forbidden. Pain was rated using a visual analogue scale, with each patient marking a point between two extremes, "maximum imaginable pain" and "total absence of pain". A questionnaire based on the McGill Pain Questionnaire completed the qualitative as well as quantitative self-evaluation of pain; the results being assessed on the basis of 4 scores, each determined by the patient's choice among 3 evaluation figures. Analysis of the results, based on 26 observations in the extract group and 29 in the placebo group), showed significant superiority of the ginkgo leaf extract (p<0.04) [168].

Pharmacokinetic properties

Pharmacokinetics in animals

After oral administration of ^{14}C-labelled ginkgo leaf extract to rats at 380 mg/kg body weight, about 16% of the administered dose was recovered as ^{14}C-carbon dioxide in exhaled air within the first 3 hours and about 38% after 72 hours, while 22% was excreted in the urine and 29% in the faeces. Therefore, at least 60% of the radiolabelled extract was absorbed. The largest amount of radioactivity was detected in glandular, neuronal and ocular tissues and was more rapidly eliminated in the stomach and small intestine than in plasma. After 72 hours, only 2.5% of the dose was detected in tissues. The pharmacokinetics are best described by a two-compartment model with an apparent first order phase and a biological half-life of about 4.5 hours [169].

The bioavailability of ginkgolides A and B and bilobalide was studied in rats after single oral administration of 30, 55 and 100 mg/kg of a standardized ginkgo leaf extract. The pharmacokinetics of these substances were found to be dose-linear. At the lowest dose, maximum concentrations were 68, 40 and 159 ng/ml and half-lives were 1.7, 2.0 and 2.2 hours for ginkgolides A and B and bilobalide respectively. Clearance values ranged from 24.2 to 37.6 ml/min/kg [170].

Pharmacokinetics in humans

After oral administration (on separate occasions) of 50, 100 and 300 mg of a standardized ginkgo leaf extract to 2 healthy volunteers, flavonol glycosides reached dose-dependent peak plasma concentrations within 2-3 hours and had half-lives of between 2 and 4 hours. Plasma concentrations returned to baseline levels within 24 hours [171].

The pharmacokinetics and bioavailability of ginkgolides A and B and bilobalide were studied in 12 healthy young volunteers following oral (in fasting conditions and after a standard meal) and intravenous single-dose administration of a standardized ginkgo leaf extract. The oral dose (120 mg of extract) corresponded to 1.44 mg of ginkgolide A, 1.03 mg of ginkgolide B and 3.36 mg of bilobalide. Plasma and urine samples collected for up to 36 and 48 hours were evaluated. When taken orally in fasting conditions, ginkgolides A and B and bilobalide showed a high bioavailability of 80, 88 and 79% respectively.

After food intake the bioavailability of the three compounds was unchanged, except for the lag time in reaching peak concentration. Peak concentrations in blood ranged from 16.5 to 33.3 ng/ml in fasting conditions, and from 11.5 to 21.1 ng/ml after a standard meal. The mean plasma elimination half-life was in the range of 9.5-10.6 hours for ginkgolide B and 3.2-4.5 hours for the other two compounds. After intravenous administration the elimination half-lives of ginkgolide A and bilobalide were comparable to those obtained after oral administration, while ginkgolide B had a shorter elimination half-life. Urinary excretion of ginkgolides A and B and bilobalide accounted for 72, 41 and 31% respectively of the administered oral dose in fasting conditions [172].

In a study involving subjects with mild to moderate dementia, an oral dose of 240 mg of a standardized ginkgo leaf extract induced EEG changes (decrease in slow wave activity and increase in alpha activity) within 3 hours, suggesting that it was adequately absorbed and metabolized, and had crossed the blood-brain barrier [173].

Preclinical safety data

All of the following data relate to standardized extracts of ginkgo leaf.

Acute toxicity

LD_{50} values of an extract in mice were determined as 7.7 g/kg (oral), 1.9 g/kg (intraperitoneal) and 1.1 g/kg (intravenous); LD_{50} values in rats were found to be 2.1 g/kg (intraperitoneal) and 1.1 g/kg (intravenous), with no lethal effect after oral administration of up to 10 g/kg [12,53,62,174].

Chronic toxicity

When an extract was administered orally to dogs and rats for 6 months in daily doses of up to 400 mg/kg and 500 mg/kg respectively, dogs proved to be more sensitive than rats. At 100 mg/kg in dogs, mild and transient vasodilatatory effects were seen in the cranial vessel after 60 days of treatment; at 400 mg/kg these disturbances were stronger and occurred after 35 days. No biochemical, haematological or histological abnormalities were observed, and liver and kidney function remained unaltered [4,12,53,174,175].

Mutagenicity, carcinogenicity, teratogenicity and embryotoxicity

In toxicity testing of a ginkgo leaf extract, no mutagenic potential was detected in the Ames test or in three other tests and no carcinogenic effects were observed after oral administration to rats for 104 weeks at 4, 20 and 100 mg/kg/day [174]. Oral administration of an extract at up to 1.6 g/kg/day in rats and 0.9 g/kg/day in rabbits did not cause any embryotoxic or teratogenic effects and reproduction was not affected [12,174, 176,177].

Clinical safety data
All of the following data relate to standardized extracts of ginkgo leaf.

Exposure to ginkgo leaf extracts in clinical studies
Ginkgo leaf extracts have very rarely been associated with adverse events [57,62].

In human pharmacological studies with ginkgo leaf extracts, healthy volunteers were exposed to single doses of 360 mg [44] and 600 mg [63-65] and 18 elderly subjects with benign memory deficits (mean age 69 years) received a single dose of 600 mg [178]; no adverse effects were observed in any of these studies.

Kleijnen and Knipschild reviewed 40 clinical studies involving two different ginkgo leaf extracts and more than 2,000 patients; no serious side effects were noted [156]. These findings were corroborated by a subsequent review of more than 50 clinical studies involving patients with dementia or cognitive impairment, which revealed no significant adverse effects from the same two extracts [153]. In very rare cases, mild gastrointestinal complaints, headache, and allergic skin reactions have been reported [156,179].

A large drug monitoring study with a ginkgo leaf extract involved 13,565 patients with vascular-type dementia (40%), Alzheimer-type dementia (28%) or mixed forms (32%), of whom 10,815 received 120 mg of the extract daily for a minimum of 3 months. Adverse events were observed in 183 patients (1.69%), the more important being headache (0.22%), nausea (0.34%), gastrointestinal complaints (0.14%), diarrhoea (0.14%) and allergic reactions (0.09%); no cases of therapy discontinuation due to the extract were reported [180].

This finding is consistent with pharmacovigilance data collected systematically in Germany from 1982 to 1994. The rates of adverse effects per million packages sold of a ginkgo leaf extract preparation were 0.35 for gastrointestinal disturbances, 0.19 for headaches and 0.8 for allergic reactions [181]. A similar finding was observed in a 12-month clinical study involving 309 patients with dementia, who received 120 mg of an extract or placebo daily. The final analysis revealed that adverse events were equally distributed between the two treatment groups with the exception of gastrointestinal symptoms, which were more often attributed to the active drug group (18 out of 29 events) [27].

In contrast, in a clinical study during which 216 patients with dementia received either 240 mg of a ginkgo leaf extract or placebo daily for 24 weeks, conspicuous differences in adverse events were observed in relation to two WHO-defined organo-physical systems: adverse effects in skin and its appendages were observed more frequently in the ginkgo group, whereas gastrointestinal disorders occurred more often under placebo. No specific substance-related changes were evident in laboratory parameters [26].

Specific safety issues
Generally, no serious adverse events during treatment with standardized ginkgo extracts have been published in the literature. Five cases of bleeding have been reported, two of them under co-medication with acetylsalicylic acid or warfarin [58,59,182-186]. However, four of the cases involved dietary supplements, the identity, purity and content of which could not be established. Lewis and Rowin concluded that these cases did not prove that ginkgo leaf extracts contributed to haemorrhages in these patients [59].

Fifty healthy male subjects were enrolled in a randomized, controlled, cross-over, safety study to investigate whether a ginkgo leaf extract could amplify the known effects of acetylsalicylic acid (ASA) on platelet aggregation, bleeding time, or other coagulation parameters. The volunteers received either 500 mg of ASA or 500 mg of ASA + 240 mg of ginkgo leaf extract daily for 7 days. ASA and the combination of ASA + extract exerted similar effects on all coagulation parameters measured, including bleeding time and PAF-induced platelet aggregation. These findings suggest that there is no risk of interaction from concomitant intake of ASA and ginkgo leaf extract [60].

The potential interaction of a ginkgo leaf extract with warfarin was tested in a randomized, placebo-controlled, cross-over study involving 24 patients (aged 33-79 years) on long-term warfarin for recurrent venous thromboembolism, mechanical heart valves or chronic atrial fibrillation. The patients received 100 mg of the extract or placebo daily for 4 weeks. The target range for INR (International Normalised Ratio) was 2.0-4.0 and was adjusted weekly if necessary. Mean doses of warfarin did not change during either treatment period (p = 0.77 for the extract vs. placebo) [61].

The influence of a ginkgo leaf extract (2 × 120 mg daily for 7 days) on bleeding time, coagulation parameters, platelet aggregation and platelet morphology was evaluated in 50 healthy male volunteers in a randomized, placebo-controlled, crossover study with a wash-out interval of at least 3 weeks. Among 29 coagulation and bleeding parameters assessed, none showed any evidence of inhibition of blood coagulation by the extract [187].

A prospective, randomized, double-blind, placebo-controlled study was carried out in 32 healthy male volunteers (aged 18-45 years), allocated to four parallel groups, to evaluate the effects on haemostasis, coagulation and fibrinolysis of three dose levels of a ginkgo leaf extract: 120, 240 or 480 mg/day for 14 days in comparison with placebo. This study did not reveal any alteration of platelet function or coagulation [188].

ABBREVIATIONS used in the following tables

ADAS-Cog	Alzheimer's Disease Assessment Scale - Cognitive subscale
CGI	Clinical Global Impression rating
EACG	Echelle d'Appréciation Clinique en Geriatrie (Geriatric Clinical Evaluation Scale)
GERRI	Geriatric Evaluation by Relative's Rating Instrument
SCAG	Sandoz Clinical Assessment: Geriatric scale
SGDE	Standardized Ginkgo Dry Extract
SKT	Syndrom Kurztest (Syndrome Short Test)
NAB	Nürnberger Alters-Beobachtungsskala

STUDY First author/year and ref. no.	NUMBER OF STUDIES DESIGN	DIAGNOSES	DOSAGE and duration of treatment	EFFICACY Main results
Letzel 1996 [150]	25 studies (dementia 8, cerebral function impairment 17); randomized, double-blind, placebo-controlled	Dementia, or cerebral function impairment not explicitly diagnosed as dementia	SGDE (oral) Dosage and duration of treatment not stated	Efficacy of SGDE in 23 of the 25 studies was similar to that of nimodipine and tacrine
Oken 1998 [153]	4 studies; randomized, double-blind, placebo-controlled	Alzheimer's disease	SGDE 120-240 mg/day (oral) 3-6 months	Meta-analysis indicated a small but significant effect of SGDE on objective measures of cognitive function
Ernst 1999 [151]	9 studies; randomized, double-blind, placebo-controlled	Dementia	SGDE 120-240 mg/day (oral in 8 studies; intravenous in 1 study) 6 weeks to 12 months	SGDE more effective than placebo
Wettstein 1999 [152]	Comparison of 2 studies on SGDE with 4 studies on cholinesterase inhibitors	Dementia	SGDE 120-240 mg/day (oral) 6-13 months	No major differences in efficacy between SGDE and four cholinesterase inhibitors (tacrine, donepezil, rivastigmine, metrifonate)
Kleijnen 1992 [156] Same studies reviewed in Kleijnen 1992 [54]	40 controlled studies (of which 8 considered to be well-performed)	Cerebral insufficiency	SGDE In 8 well-performed studies: 112-160 mg/day (oral) 6 weeks to 12 months	39 out of 40 studies showed positive effects of SGDE. Further studies needed, with larger numbers of patients and improved procedures.
Hopfenmüller 1994 [157]	11 studies; 10 randomized, double-blind, placebo-controlled; 1 comparative	Cerebral insufficiency	SGDE 112-160 mg/day (oral) 6-12 weeks	Meta-analysis of 8 studies indicated significant superiority of SGDE compared to placebo; 7 studies confirmed effectiveness, 1 inconclusive.
Ernst 1999 [161]	5 studies; randomized, double-blind; 4 placebo-controlled, 1 comparative vs. two reference medications.	Tinnitus	SGDE 120-240 mg/day, except 29.2 mg/day in one study (oral) 4 weeks to 3 months	Significantly better results with SGDE than with placebo (except in one under-dosed study) or reference medications. However, the body of evidence is small; further studies needed for firm conclusion on efficacy.
Ernst 1996 [167]	6 studies; 5 double-blind; 4 placebo-controlled, 2 comparative vs. reference medication	Intermittent claudication	SGDE 120-160 mg/day (oral) 1 month to 24 weeks	The studies were heterogeneous. All implied that SGDE is an effective therapy for intermittent claudication, but this hypothesis requires confirmation in further trials using meticulous methodology.
Pittler 2000 [166]	8 studies; randomized, double-blind, placebo controlled	Intermittent claudication	SGDE 120-240 mg/day (oral) 3-6 months	Meta-analysis suggested SGDE superior to placebo in symptomatic treatment of intermittent claudication.

TABLE 1: CRITICAL REVIEWS AND META-ANALYSES OF CLINICAL STUDIES

STUDY First author/year, ref. no. and design	NUMBER OF PATIENTS (verum/control)	DIAGNOSES	DOSAGE and duration of treatment	EFFICACY Main results
Weitbrecht 1986 [24] Double-blind, placebo-controlled	40 (20/20)	Primary degenerative dementia	SGDE 120 mg/day (oral) 3 months	Crichton scale $p<0.0001$ SCAG: $p<0.0001$
Hofferberth 1994 [25] Double-blind, placebo-controlled	40 (21/19)	Alzheimer's disease	SGDE 240 mg/day (oral) 3 months	SKT: $p = 0.00043$ SCAG: $p<0.05$ overall, $p<0.01$ in 6 single items
Kanowski 1996 [26] Double-blind, placebo-controlled	156 (79/77)	Dementia of Alzheimer- and multi-infarct types	SGDE 240 mg/day (oral) 24 weeks	Responder rates (%): CGI: 32/17, $p<0.05$ SKT: 38/18, $p<0.05$ NAB: 33/23, $p<0.095$ (n.s.) Proportion of therapy responders: 28% vs 10% ($p<0.005$)
Le Bars 1997 [27] Double-blind, placebo-controlled Analysis after 26 weeks: Le Bars 2000 [28]	309 (155/154)	Alzheimer's disease Multi-infarct dementia	SGDE 120 mg/day (oral) 52 weeks	ADAS-Cog: $p = 0.04$ GERRI: $p = 0.004$ CGI: no significant difference
Maurer 1997 [29] Double-blind, placebo-controlled	20 (10/10)	Dementia of the Alzheimer type	SGDE 240 mg/day (oral) 3 months	SKT: $p<0.013$ CGI: $p = 0.069$ (n. s.)
van Dongen 2000 [154] Double-blind, placebo-controlled	214 (166 verum in 4 groups; placebo 48)	Dementia (Alzheimer's, vascular or a mixed type; n = 68) or age-associated memory impairment (n = 151)	SGDE 160 or 240 mg/day (oral) 24 weeks	SGDE not effective

TABLE 2: CLINICAL STUDIES IN DEMENTIA

STUDY: First author/year, ref. no. and design	NUMBER OF PATIENTS (verum/control)	DIAGNOSES	DOSAGE and duration of treatment	EFFICACY Main results
Taillandier 1986 [30] Double-blind, placebo-controlled	166 (80/86)	Cerebral insufficiency	SGDE 160 mg/day (oral) 12 months	EACG: p = 0.01
Eckmann 1990 [31] Double-blind, placebo-controlled	60 (30/30)	Cerebral insufficiency	SGDE 160 mg/day (oral) 6 weeks	11 typical symptoms: $p<0.001$
Brüchert 1991 [32] Double-blind, placebo-controlled	303 (153/150)	Cerebral insufficiency	SGDE 150 mg/day (oral) 12 weeks	Global assessment of efficacy: $p<0.001$
Schmidt 1991 [33] Double-blind, placebo-controlled	99 (50/49)	Cerebral insufficiency	SGDE 150 mg/day (oral) 12 weeks	Global assessment of efficacy: $p<0.01$
Vorberg 1989 [34] Double-blind, placebo-controlled	100 (50/50)	Cerebral insufficiency	SGDE 112 mg/day (oral) 12 weeks	Memory: $p<0.001$ Concentration: $p<0.001$ Anxiety: $p<0.001$ Dizziness: $p<0.001$ Headaches: $p<0.001$ Ear noise: not significant
Halama 1988 [35] Double-blind, placebo-controlled	40 (20/20)	Mild to medium cerebral insufficiency	SGDE 120 mg/day (oral) 12 weeks	SCAG: $p = 0.00005$
Gräsel 1992 [36] Double-blind, placebo-controlled	72 (29/24)	Cerebral insufficiency	SGDE 160 mg/day (oral) 6 months	Short-term memory capacity: IQ: + 13 vs + 1 Long-term memory capacity: MQ: + 10 vs 0
Vesper 1994 [37] Double-blind, placebo-controlled	86 (42/44)	Cerebral insufficiency	SGDE 150 mg/day (oral) 12 weeks	Computer-aided psychometric tests: $p<0.05$
Wesnes 1987 [48] Double-blind, placebo-controlled	54 (27/27)	Mild idiopathic cognitive impairment	SGDE 120 mg/day (oral) 12 weeks	Combined scores from cognitive test battery for accuracy and reaction time indicated superiority of SGDE over placebo.
Brautigam 1998 [158] Double-blind, placebo-controlled	241 (82-77/82)	Age-related mild cognitive impairment	70%-ethanolic liquid extract (1:4) from fresh ginkgo leaf, 2.85 or 5.7 ml/day (oral) 24 weeks	Short-term visual memory: placebo < 5.7 ml < 2.85 ml (MANOVA; p = 0.0076). No significant differences in other tests of memory and concentration.

TABLE 3: CLINICAL STUDIES IN CEREBRAL INSUFFICIENCY

STUDY: (First author/year, ref. no. and design)	NUMBER OF PATIENTS (verum/control)	DIAGNOSES	DOSAGE and duration of treatment	EFFICACY Main results
Hamann 1985 [38] Double-blind, placebo-controlled	40 (20/20)	Vertigo	SGDE 160 mg/day (oral) 1 month	Combination of physical training and SGDE treatment led to significant diminution in body sway amplitude: (p<0.0001)
Haguenauer 1986 [39] Double-blind, placebo-controlled	70 (35/35)	Vertiginous syndrome	SGDE 160 mg/day (oral) 3 months	Intensity, frequency and duration of the disorder: p<0.05. Global assessment: p<0.001
Meyer 1986 [40] Double-blind, placebo-controlled	103 (58/45)	Tinnitus and associated symptoms	SGDE 160 mg/day (oral) 3 months	Global assessment of change in clinical signs: p = 0.05
Morgenstern 1997 [41] Double-blind, placebo-controlled	99 (49/50)	Tinnitus	SGDE 120 mg/day (oral) 12 weeks	Reduction in intensity of tinnitus substantially greater in SGDE group (p = 0.015)
Drew 2001 [159] Double-blind, placebo-controlled	1121 (559/562)	Tinnitus	SGDE 150 mg/day (oral) 12 weeks	No significant differences vs placebo
Holgers 1994 [160] Open phase followed by double-blind, placebo-controlled phase	80 (open phase) 20 (placebo crossover)	Severe tinnitus	Undefined dry extract 29.2 mg/day (oral) for 2 weeks 29.2 mg/day (oral) for 2 weeks	No significant difference vs placebo
Hoffmann 1994 [162] Comparative study vs naftidrofuryl	80 (40/40)	Sudden hearing loss	SGDE 175 mg in 500 ml solution + 80 mg/day (oral) 3 weeks	Gain in hearing capacity: SGDE + 23% vs naftidrofuryl + 13% (p = 0.06)
Lebuisson 1986 [163] Double-blind, placebo-controlled	20 (10/10)	Senile macular degeneration	SGDE 160 mg/day (oral) 6 months	Improvement in long distance visual acuity: p<0.05 Global assessment: p<0.01
Lanthony 1988 [164] Double-blind, placebo-controlled	29	Early diabetic retinopathy	SGDE 160 mg/day (oral) 6 months	Significant improvement in colour vision
Raabe 1991 [165] Double-blind, Two dose levels	24	Chronic cerebral retinal insufficiency syndrome	SGDE 160 mg/day (8 weeks; oral) or 80 mg/day (4 weeks) + 160 mg/day (4 weeks)	Increase in retinal sensitivity after 160 mg/day (p<0.05 to p<0.01)

TABLE 4: CLINICAL STUDIES IN NEUROSENSORY DISTURBANCES

STUDY First author/year, ref. no. and design	NUMBER OF PATIENTS (verum/control)	DIAGNOSES	DOSAGE and duration of treatment	EFFICACY Main results
Bauer 1984 [49] Double-blind, placebo-controlled	79 (44/35)	Peripheral arteriopathy Fontaine stage IIb	SGDE 120 mg/day (oral) 24 weeks	Increase in pain-free walking distance: p<0.05 Increase in maximum walking distance: p<0.001 Decrease in pain: p<0.001
Blume 1996 [50] Double-blind, placebo-controlled	60 (30/30)	Peripheral arteriopathy Fontaine stage IIb (fully trained patients)	SGDE 120 mg/day (oral) 24 weeks	Increase in pain-free walking distance: p<0.0001 Increase in maximum walking distance: p<0.0001
Peters 1998 [51] Double-blind, placebo-controlled	111 (53/58)	Peripheral arteriopathy Fontaine stage IIb	SGDE 120 mg/kg (oral) 24 weeks	Increase in pain-free walking distance: p = 0.016 Increase in maximum walking distance: p<0.05
Blume 1998 [52] Double-blind, placebo-controlled	41 (21/20)	Peripheral arteriopathy Fontaine stage IIb	SGDE 160 mg/day (oral) 24 weeks	Increase in pain-free walking distance: p = 0.021 Increase in maximum walking distance: p<0.007
Saudreau 1989 [168] Double-blind, placebo-controlled	64 (32/32)	Peripheral arteriopathy Fontaine stage III	SGDE 200 mg/day (intravenous) 8 days	Pain intensity: p = 0.04

TABLE 5: CLINICAL STUDIES IN PERIPHERAL ARTERIAL OCCLUSIVE DISEASE

REFERENCES

1. Ginkgo Leaf - Ginkgo folium. European Pharmacopoeia. Council of Europe.

2. Eingestellter Ginkgotrockenextrakt - Ginkgo extractum siccum normatum. Deutsches Arzneibuch.

3. Ginkgo Dry Extract, Standardised - Ginkgo extractum siccum normatum. Pharmeuropa 1999;11:333-7.

4. Woerdenbag HJ, Van Beek TA. *Ginkgo biloba*. In: De Smet PAGM, Keller K, Hänsel R, Chandler RF, editors. Adverse Effects of Herbal Drugs, Volume 3. Berlin-Heidelberg: Springer-Verlag, 1997:51-66.

5. Boralle N, Braquet P, Gottlieb OR. *Ginkgo biloba*: a review of its chemical composition. In: Braquet P, editor. Ginkgolides - Chemistry, Biology, Pharmacology and Clinical Perspectives, Volume 1. Barcelona: JR Prous Science Publishers, 1988:9-25.

6. Nakanishi K, Habaguchi K, Nakadaira Y, Woods MC, Maruyama M, Major RT et al. Structure of bilobalide, a rare *tert*-butyl containing sesquiterpenoid related to the C_{20}-ginkgolides. J Am Chem Soc 1971;93:3544-6.

7. van Beek TA, Scheeren HA, Rantio T, Melger WC, Lelyveld GP. Determination of ginkgolides and bilobalide in *Ginkgo biloba* leaves and phyto-pharmaceuticals. J Chromatogr 1991;543:375-87.

8. Hasler A, Meier B. Determination of terpenes from *Ginkgo biloba* L. by capillary gas chromatography. Pharm Pharmacol Lett 1992;2:187-90.

9. van Beek TA, Lelyveld GP. Concentration of ginkgolides and bilobalide in *Ginkgo biloba* leaves in relation to the time of year. Planta Med 1992;58:413-6.

10. Flesch V, Jacques M, Cosson L, Teng BP, Petiard V, Balz JP. Relative importance of growth and light level on terpene content of *Ginkgo biloba*. Phytochemistry 1992;31:1941-5.

11. Teng BP. Chemistry of ginkgolides. In: Braquet P, editor. Ginkgolides - Chemistry, Biology, Pharmacology and Clinical Perspectives, Volume 1. Barcelona: JR Prous Science Publishers, 1988:37-42.

12. O'Reilly J. *Ginkgo biloba* - cultivation, extraction and therapeutic use of the extract. In: van Beek TA, Breteler H, editors. Phytochemistry and Agriculture, Volume 34. Oxford: Clarendon Press, 1993:253-70.

13. Victoire C, Haag-Berrurier M, Lobstein-Guth A, Balz JP, Anton R. Isolation of flavonol glycosides from *Ginkgo biloba* leaves. Planta Med 1988:54:245-7.

14. Hasler A, Gross G-A, Meier B, Sticher O. Complex flavonol glycosides from the leaves of *Ginkgo biloba*. Phytochemistry 1992;31:1391-4.

15. Hasler A, Sticher O, Meier B. High-performance liquid chromatographic determination of five widespread flavonoid aglycones. J Chromatogr 1990;508:236-40.

16. Hasler A, Sticher O, Meier B. Identification and determination of the flavonoids from *Ginkgo biloba* by high-performance liquid chromatography. J Chromatogr 1992;605:41-8.

17. Baker W, Finch ACM, Ollis WD, Robinson KW. The structures of the naturally occurring biflavonyls. J Chem Soc 1963;1477-90.

18. Joly M, Haag-Berrurier M, Anton R. Le 5'-méthoxy-bilobétine, une biflavone extraite du *Ginkgo biloba*. Phytochemistry 1980;19:1999-2002.

19. Miura H, Kihara T, Kawano N. Studies on bisflavones in the leaves of *Podocarpus macrophylla* and *P. nagi*. Chem Pharm Bull 1969;17:150-4.

20. Weinges K, Bähr W, Kloss P. Übersicht über die Inhaltsstoffe aus den Blättern des Ginkgo-Baumes (*Ginkgo biloba* L.). Arzneim-Forsch 1968;18:537-9.

21. Weinges K, Bähr W, Theobald H, Wiesenhütter A, Wild R, Kloss P. Über das Vorkommen von Proantho-cyanidinen in Pflanzenextrakten. Arzneim-Forsch 1969;19:328-30.

22. Schötz K. Detection of allergenic urushiols in *Ginkgo biloba* leaves. Pharmazie 2002;57:508-10.

23. Hasler A. Chemical constituents of *Ginkgo biloba*. In: van Beek TA, editor. *Ginkgo biloba*. (Medicinal and Aromatic Plants - Industrial Profiles series). Amsterdam: Harwood Academic, 2000:109-42.

24. Weitbrecht W-U, Jansen W. Primär degenerative Demenz. Therapie mit *Ginkgo biloba*-Extrakt. Fortschr Med 1986;104:199-202.

25. Hofferberth B. The efficacy of EGb 761 in patients with senile dementia of the Alzheimer type, a double-blind, placebo-controlled study on different levels of investigation. Hum Psychopharmacol 1994;9:215-22.

26. Kanowski S, Hermann WM, Stephan K, Wierich W, Hörr R. Proof of efficacy of the *Ginkgo biloba* special extract EGb 761 in outpatients suffering from mild to moderate primary degenerative dementia of the Alzheimer type or multi-infarct dementia. Pharmaco-psychiatry 1996;29:47-56. *Republished in*: Phytomedicine 1997;4:3-13.

27. Le Bars PL, Katz MM, Berman N, Itil TM, Freedman AM, Schatzberg AF. A placebo-controlled, double-blind, randomized trial of an extract of *Ginkgo biloba* for dementia. JAMA 1997;278:1327-32.

28. Le Bars PL, Kieser M, Itil KZ. A 26-week analysis of a double-blind, placebo-controlled trial of the *Ginkgo biloba* extract EGb 761® in dementia. Dement Geriatr Cogn Disord 2000;11:230-7.

29. Maurer K, Ihl R, Dierks T, Frölich L. Clinical efficacy of *Ginkgo biloba* special extract EGb 761 in dementia of the Alzheimer type. J Psychiat Res 1997;31:645-55. *Republished in*: Phytomedicine 1998;5:417-24.

30. Taillandier J, Ammar A, Rabourdin JP, Ribeyre JP, Pichon J, Niddam S, Pierart H. Traitement des troubles du vieillissement cérébral par l'extrait de *Ginkgo biloba*.

Etude longitudinale multicentrique à double insu face au placebo. Presse Méd 1986;15:1583-7.

31. Eckmann F. Hirnleistungsstörungen - Behandlung mit Ginkgo-biloba-Extrakt. Zeitpunkt des Wirkungseintritts in einer Doppelblindstudie mit 60 stationären Patienten. Fortschr Med 1990;108:557-60.

32. Brüchert E, Heinrich SE, Ruf-Kohler P. Wirksamkeit von LI 1370 bei älteren Patienten mit Hirnleistungs-schwäche. Multizentrische Doppelblindstudie des Fachverbandes Deutscher Allgemeinärzte. Münch med Wschr 1991;133(Suppl 1):S9-S14.

33. Schmidt U, Rabinovici K, Lande S. Einfluß eines Ginkgo-Spezial-extraktes auf die Befindlichkeit bei zerebraler Insuffizienz. Münch med Wschr 1991;133:(Suppl 1): S15-S18.

34. Vorberg G, Schenk N, Schmidt U. Wirksamkeit eines neuen Gingko-biloba-Extraktes bei 100 Patienten mit zerebraler Insuffizienz. Herz + Gefässe 1989;9:936-41.

35. Halama P, Bartsch G, Meng G. Hirnleistungsstörungen vaskulärer Genese. Randomisierte Doppelblindstudie zur Wirksamkeit von Ginkgo-biloba-Extrakt. Fortschr Med 1988;106:408-12.

36. Gräßel E. Effect of Ginkgo biloba extract on mental performance. Double-blind study using computerized measurement conditions in patients with cerebral insufficiency. Fortschr Med 1992;110(5):73-6.

37. Vesper J, Hänsgen K-D. Efficacy of Ginkgo biloba in 90 outpatients with cerebral insufficiency caused by old age. Results of a placebo-controlled double-blind trial. Phytomedicine 1994;1:9-16.

38. Hamann K-F. Physikalische Therapie des vestibulären Schwindels in Verbindung mit Ginkgo-biloba-Extrakt. Eine posturografische Studie. Therapiewoche 1985; 35:4586-4590.

39. Haguenauer JP, Cantenot F, Koskas H, Pierart H. Traitement des troubles de l'équilibre par l'extrait de Ginkgo biloba. Etude multicentrique à double insu face au placebo. Presse Méd 1986;15:1569-72.

40. Meyer B. Etude multicentrique randomisée à double insu face au placebo du traitement des acouphènes par l'extrait de Ginkgo biloba. Presse Méd 1986;15:1562-4.

41. Morgenstern C, Biermann E. Ginkgo-Spezialextrakt EGb 761 in der Behandlung des Tinnitus aurium. Fortschr Med 1997;115 (Originalien IV):7-11.

42. Rigney U, Kimber S, Hindmarch I. The effects of acute doses of standardized Ginkgo biloba extract on memory and psychomotor performance in volunteers. Phyto-therapy Res 1999;13:408-15.

43. Stough C, Clarke J, Lloyd J, Nathan PJ. Neuro-psychological changes after 30-day Ginkgo biloba administration in healthy participants. Internat J Neuropsychopharmacol 2001;4:131-4.

44. Kennedy D, Scholey AB, Wesnes K. Enhancement of

45. Mix JA, Crews WD. An examination of the efficacy of Ginkgo biloba extract EGb761 on the neuropsychologic functioning of cognitively intact older adults. J Alternative Complement Med 2000;6:219-29.

46. Mix JA, Crews WD. A double-blind, placebo-controlled, randomized trial of Ginkgo biloba extract EGb761® in a sample of cognitively intact older adults: neuro-psychological findings. Hum Psychopharmacol Clin Exp 2002;17:267-77.

47. Kennedy DO, Scholey AB, Wesnes KA. Modulation of cognition and mood following administration of single doses of Ginkgo biloba, ginseng and a ginkgo/ginseng combination to healthy young adults. Physiol Behav 2002;75:739-51.

48. Wesnes K, Simmons D, Rook M, Simpson P. A double-blind placebo-controlled trial of Tanakan in the treatment of idiopathic cognitive impairment in the elderly. Hum Psychopharmacol 1987;2:159-69.

49. Bauer U. 6-Month double-blind randomised clinical trial of Ginkgo biloba extract versus placebo in two parallel groups in patients suffering from peripheral arterial insufficiency. Arzneim-Forsch/Drug Res 1984; 34:716-20.

50. Blume J, Kieser M, Hölscher U. Placebokontrollierte Doppelblindstudie zur Wirksamkeit von Ginkgo-biloba-Spezialextrakt EGb 761 bei austrainierten Patienten mit Claudicatio intermittens. VASA 1996;25:265-74.

51. Peters H, Kieser M, Holscher U. Demonstration of the efficacy of Ginkgo biloba special extract EGb 761® on intermittent claudication - A placebo-controlled, double-blind multicenter trial. VASA 1998;27:106-10.

52. Blume J, Kieser M, Hölscher U. Ginkgo-Spezialextrakt EGb 761® bei pAVK. Plazebokontrollierte Doppel-blindstudie bei Patienten mit pAVK im Stadium IIb nach Fontaine. Fortschr Med 1998;116:36-7.

53. Juretzek W. Recent advances in Ginkgo biloba extract (EGb 761). In: Hori T, Ridge RW, Tulecke W, Del Tredici P, Trémouillaux-Guiller J, Tobe H, editors. Ginkgo biloba - A global treasure. From biology to medicine. Tokyo: Springer-Verlag, 1997:341-58.

54. Kleijnen J, Knipschild P. Ginkgo biloba. Lancet 1992: 1136-9.

55. Barnes J, Anderson LA, Phillipson JD. Ginkgo. In: Herbal Medicines - A guide for healthcare professionals, 2nd ed. London-Chicago: Pharmaceutical Press, 2002: 250-63.

56. Cuccinelli JH. Alternative Medicine: Ginkgo biloba. Clinician Rev 1999;9(8):93-4 and 97.

57. Folium Ginkgo. In: WHO monographs on selected medicinal plants, Volume 1. Geneva: World Health Organization, 1999:154-67.

58. Rosenblatt M, Mindel J. Spontaneous hyphema

cognitive performance by single doses of Ginkgo biloba. J Psychopharmacol 2000;14(Suppl):A45.

associated with ingestion of *Ginkgo biloba* extract. New Engl J Med 1997;336:1108.

59. Matthews MK. Association of *Ginkgo biloba* with intracerebral hemorrhage [*Comment on Rowin J, Lewis SL. 1996*]. Neurology 1998;50:1933.
Reply from the authors: Lewis SL, Rowin J. Neurology 1998;50:1933-4.

60. Wolf HRD. Effect of EGb 761® and ASA on coagulation and bleeding. Innere Medizin, Diakonie Krankenhaus, Bad Kreuznach, Germany (submitted for publication, 2003).

61. Engelsen J, Nielsen JD, Winther K. Effect of coenzyme Q_{10} and *Ginkgo biloba* on warfarin dosage in stable, long-term warfarin treated outpatients. A randomised, double blind, placebo-crossover trial. Thromb Haemost 2002;87:1075-6.

62. DeFeudis FV. *Ginkgo biloba* extract (EGb 761): from chemistry to the clinic. ISBN 3-86126-173-1. Wiesbaden: Ullstein Medical, 1998.

63. Hindmarch I. Activity of *Ginkgo biloba* extract on short-term memory. In: Fünfgeld EW, editor. Rökan (*Ginkgo biloba*). Recent results in pharmacology and clinic. Berlin: Springer-Verlag, 1988:321-6.

64. Guinot P, Caffrey E, Lambe R, Darragh A. Tanakan inhibits platelet-activating-factor-induced platelet aggregation in healthy male volunteers. Haemostasis 1989;19:219-23.

65. Lacomblez L, Warot D, Tarrade T, Puech AJ. Psychopharmacological effects of *Ginkgo biloba* extract (EGb 761) in healthy volunteers. Eur J Pharmacol 1990; 183:1460.

66. Köse K, Dogan P. Lipoperoxidation induced by hydrogen peroxide in human erythrocyte membranes. 1. Protective effect of *Ginkgo biloba* extract (EGb 761). J Int Med Res 1995;23:1-8.

67. Artmann GM, Schikarski C. *Ginkgo biloba* extract (EGb 761) protects red blood cells from oxidative damage. Clin Hemorheol 1993;13:529-39.

68. Rong Y, Geng Z, Lau BHS. *Ginkgo biloba* attenuates oxidative stress in macrophages and endothelial cells. Free Radical Biol Med 1996;20:121-7.

69. Marcocci L, Maguire JJ, Droy-Lefaix MT, Packer L. The nitric oxide-scavenging properties of *Ginkgo biloba* extract EGb 761. Biochem Biophys Res Commun 1994; 201:748-55.

70. Marcocci L, Packer L, Droy-Lefaix M-T, Sekaki A, Gardès-Albert M. Antioxidant action of *Ginkgo biloba* extract EGb 761. Methods Enzymol 1994;234:462-75.

71. Kobuchi H, Droy-Lefaix MT, Christen Y, Packer L. *Ginkgo biloba* extract (EGb 761): inhibitory effect on nitric oxide production in the macrophage cell line RAW 264.7. Biochem Pharmacol 1997;53:897-903.

72. Maitra I, Marcocci L, Droy-Lefaix MT, Packer L. Peroxyl radical scavenging activity of *Ginkgo biloba* extract EGb 761. Biochem Pharmacol 1995;49:1649-55.

73. Yan L-J, Droy-Lefaix MT, Packer L. *Ginkgo biloba* extract (EGb 761) protects human low density lipoproteins against oxidative modification mediated by copper. Biochem Biophys Res Commun 1995;212: 360-6.

74. Ni Y, Zhao B, Hou J, Xin W. Preventive effect of *Ginkgo biloba* extract on apoptosis in rat cerebellar neuronal cells induced by hydroxyl radicals. Neurosci Lett 1996; 214:115-8.

75. Kubota Y, Tanaka N, Umegaki K, Takenaka H, Mizuno H, Nakamura K et al. *Ginkgo biloba* extract-induced relaxation of rat aorta is associated with increase in endothelial intracellular calcium level. Life Sci 2001; 69:2327-36.

76. Zhou L-J, Zhu X-Z. Reactive oxygen species-induced apoptosis in PC12 cells and protective effect of bilobalide. J Pharmacol Exp Therap 2000;293:982-8.

77. Joyeux M, Lobstein A, Anton R, Mortier F. Comparative antilipoperoxidant, antinecrotic and scavenging properties of terpenes and biflavones from *Ginkgo* and some flavonoids. Planta Med 1995;61:126-9.

78. Tosaki A, Droy-Lefaix M-T, Pali T, Das DK. Effects of SOD, catalase and a novel antiarrhythmic drug, EGb 761, on reperfusion-induced arrhythmias in isolated rat hearts. Free Rad Biol Med 1993;14:361-70.

79. Haramaki N, Aggarwal S, Kawabata T, Droy-Lefaix M-T, Packer L. Effects of natural antioxidant *Ginkgo biloba* extract (EGb 761) on myocardial ischemia-reperfusion injury. Free Rad Biol Med 1994;16:789-94.

80. Pietri S, Maurelli E, Drieu K, Culcasi M. Cardioprotective and anti-oxidant effects of the terpenoid constituents of *Ginkgo biloba* extract (EGb 761). J Mol Cell Cardiol 1997;29:733-42.

81. Janssens D, Michiels C, Delaive E, Eliaers F, Drieu K, Remacle J. Protection of hypoxia-induced ATP decrease in endothelial cells by *Ginkgo biloba* extract and bilobalide. Biochem Pharmacol 1995;50:991-9.

82. Masson F, Néliat G, Drieu K, DeFeudis FV, Jean T. Effects of an extract of *Ginkgo biloba* on the action potential and associated transmembrane ionic currents in mammalian cardiac myocytes: Inhibition of isoproterenol-induced chloride current. Drug Dev Res 1994; 32:29-41.

83. Liebgott T, Miollan M, Berchadsky Y, Drieu K, Culcasi M, Pietri S. Complementary cardioprotective effects of flavonoid metabolites and terpenoid constituents of *Ginkgo biloba* extract (EGb 761) during ischemia and reperfusion. Basic Res Cardiol 2000;95:368-77.

84. Braquet P, Esanu A, Buisine E, Hosford D, Broquet C, Koltai M. Recent progress in ginkgolide research. Med Res Rev 1991;11:295-355.

85. Braquet P, Hosford D, Koltz P, Guilbaud J, Paubert-Braquet M. Effect of platelet-activating factor on tumor necrosis factor-induced superoxide generation from

human neutrophils. Possible involvement of G proteins. Lipids 1991;26:1071-5.

86. Koltai M, Hosford D, Guinot P, Esanu A, Braquet P. Platelet activating factor (PAF): A review of its effects, antagonists and possible future clinical implications (Part I). Drugs 1991;42:9-29.

87. Koltai M, Hosford D, Guinot P, Esanu A, Braquet P. PAF: A review of its effects, antagonists and possible future clinical implications (Part II). Drugs 1991;42:174-204.

88. Prehn JHM, Krieglstein J. Platelet-activating factor antagonists reduce excitotoxic damage in cultured neurons from embryonic chick telencephalon and protect the rat hippocampus and neocortex from ischemic injury in vivo. J Neurosci Res 1993;34:179-88.

89. Krieglstein J, Ausmeier F, El-Abhar H, Lippert K, Welsch M, Rupalla K, Henrich-Noack P. Neuroprotective effects of Ginkgo biloba constituents. Eur J Pharm Sci 1995; 3:39-48.

90. Ramassamy C, Girbe F, Christen Y, Costentin J. Ginkgo biloba extract (EGb 761) or trolox C prevent the ascorbic acid/Fe^{2+} induced decrease in synaptosomal membrane fluidity. Free Rad Res Commun 1993;19:341-50.

91. Ramassamy C, Christen Y, Clostre F, Costentin J. The Ginkgo biloba extract, EGb 761, increases synaptosomal uptake of 5-hydroxytryptamine: in vitro and ex-vivo studies. J Pharm Pharmacol 1992;44:943-5.

92. Ramassamy C, Naudin B, Christen Y, Clostre F, Costentin J. Prevention by Ginkgo biloba extract (EGb 761) and trolox C of the decrease in synaptosomal dopamine or serotonin uptake following incubation. Biochem Pharmacol 1992;44:2395-401.

93. Ramassamy C, Girbe F, Pincemail J, Christen Y, Costentin J. Modifications of the synaptosomal dopamine uptake and release by two systems generating free radicals: ascorbic acid/Fe^{2+} and L-arginine/NADPH. Ann NY Acad Sci 1994;738:141-51.

94. Klein J, Chatterjee SS, Löffelholz K. Phospholipid breakdown and choline release under hypoxic conditions: inhibition by bilobalide, a constituent of Ginkgo biloba. Brain Res 1997;755:347-50.

95. Bastianetto S, Zheng W-H, Quirion R. The Ginkgo biloba extract (EGb 761) protects and rescues hippocampal cells against nitric oxide-induced toxicity: involvement of its flavonoid constituents and protein kinase C. J Neurochem 2000;74:2268-77.

96. Bastianetto S, Ramassamy C, Doré S, Christen Y, Poirier J, Quirion R. The Ginkgo biloba extract (EGb 761) protects hippocampal neurones against cell death induced by β-amyloid. Eur J Neurosci 2000;12:1882-90.

97. Schindowski K, Leutner S, Kressmann S, Eckert A, Müller WE. Age-related increase of oxidative stress-induced apoptosis in mice: prevention by Ginkgo biloba extract (EGb 761). J Neural Transm 2001;

108:969-78.

98. Bridi R, Crossetti FP, Steffen VM, Henriques AT. The antioxidant activity of standardized extract of Ginkgo biloba (EGb 761) in rats. Phytother Res 2001;15:449-51.

99. Ahlemeyer B, Möwes A, Krieglstein J. Inhibition of serum deprivation- and staurosporine-induced neuronal apoptosis by Ginkgo biloba extract and some of its constituents. Eur J Pharmacol 1999;367:423-30.

100. Tosaki A, Pali T, Droy-Lefaix M-T. Effects of Ginkgo biloba extract and preconditioning on the diabetic rat myocardium Diabetologia 1996;39:1255-62.

101. Lo H-M, Lin F-Y, Tseng C-D, Chiang F-T, Hsu K-L, Tseng Y-Z. Effect of EGb 761, a Ginkgo biloba extract, on early arrhythmia induced by coronary occlusion and reperfusion in dogs. J Formos Med Assoc 1994; 93:592-7.

102. Shen J-G, Zhou D-Y. Efficiency of Ginkgo biloba extract (EGb 761) in antioxidant protection against myocardial ischemia and reperfusion injury. Biochem Molec Biol Int 1995;35:125-34.

103. Fitzl G, Welt K, Schaffranietz L. Myocardium-protective effects of Ginkgo biloba extract (EGb 761) in old rats against acute isobaric hypoxia. An electron microscopic morphometric study. I. Protection of cardiomyocytes. Exp Toxic Pathol 1996;48:33-9.

104. Welt K, Fitzl G, Schaffranietz L. Myocardium-protective effects of Ginkgo biloba extract (EGb 761) in old rats against acute isobaric hypoxia. An electron microscopic morphometric study. II. Protection of microvascular endothelium. Exp Toxic Pathol 1996;48:81-6.

105. Topp S, Knoefel WT, Schutte A, Brilloff S, Rogiers X, Gundlach M. Ginkgo biloba (EGb 761) improves microcirculation after warm ischemia of the rat liver. Transplantation Proc 2001;33:979-81.

106. Rodriguez de Turco EB, Droy-Lefaix MT, Bazan NG. Decreased electroconvulsive shock-induced diacylglycerols and free fatty acid accumulation in the rat brain by Ginkgo biloba extract (EGb 761): selective effect in hippocampus as compared with cerebral cortex. J Neurochem 1993;61:1438-44.

107. Dorman DC, Côté LM, Buck WB. Effects of an extract of Ginkgo biloba on bromethalin-induced cerebral lipid peroxidation and edema in rats. Am J Vet Res 1992;53:138-42.

108. Brailowsky S, Montiel T, Hernández-Echeagaray E, Flores-Hernández J, Hernández-Pineda R. Effects of a Ginkgo biloba extract on two models of cortical hemiplegia in rats. Restorative Neurol Neurosci 1991;3:267-74.

109. Brailowsky S, Montiel T, Medina-Ceja L. Acceleration of functional recovery from motor cortex ablation by two Ginkgo biloba extracts in rats. Restorative Neurol Neurosci 1995;8:163-7.

110. Kristofiková Z, Benesová O, Tejkalová H. Changes of

high-affinity choline uptake in the hippocampus of old rats after long-term administration of two nootropic drugs (tacrine and *Ginkgo biloba* extract). Dementia 1992;3:304-7.

111. Barkats M, Venault P, Christen Y, Cohen-Salmon C. Effect of long-term treatment with EGb 761 on age-dependent structural changes in the hippocampi of three inbred mouse strains. Life Sci 1995;56:213-22.

112. Huguet F, Tarrade T. α_2-Adrenoceptor changes during cerebral ageing. The effect of *Ginkgo biloba* extract. J Pharm Pharmacol 1992;44:24-7.

113. Huguet F, Drieu K, Piriou A. Decreased cerebral 5-HT_{1A} receptors during ageing: reversal by *Ginkgo biloba* extract (EGb 761). J Pharm Pharmacol 1994;46:316-8.

114. Bolaños-Jiménez F, Manhães de Castro R, Sarhan H, Prudhomme N, Drieu K, Fillion G. Stress-induced 5-HT_{1A} receptor desensitization: protective effects of *Ginkgo biloba* extract (EGb 761). Fundam Clin Pharmacol 1995;9:169-74.

115. Rapin JR, Lamproglou I, Drieu K, DeFeudis FV. Demonstration of the "anti-stress" activity of an extract of *Ginkgo biloba* (EGb 761) using a discrimination learning task. Gen Pharmacol 1994;25:1009-16.

116. Chermat R, Brochet D, DeFeudis FV, Drieu K. Interactions of *Ginkgo biloba* extract (EGb 761), diazepam and ethyl β-carboline-3-carboxylate on social behavior of the rat. Pharmacol Biochem Behav 1997; 56:333-9.

117. Stoll S, Scheuer K, Pohl O, Müller WE. *Ginkgo biloba* extract (EGb 761) independently improves changes in passive avoidance learning and brain membrane fluidity in the aging mouse. Pharmacopsychiatry 1996;29:144-9.

118. Winter JC. The effects of an extract of *Ginkgo biloba*, EGb 761, on cognitive behavior and longevity in the rat. Physiol Behavior 1998;63:425-33.

119. Watanabe CM, Wolffram S, Ader P, Rimbach G, Packer L, Maguire JJ et al. The *in vivo* neuromodulatory effects of the herbal medicine *Ginkgo biloba*. Proc Natl Acad Sci USA 2001;98:6577-80.

120. Otani M, Chatterjee SS, Gabard B, Kreutzberg GW. Effect of an extract of *Ginkgo biloba* on triethyltin-induced cerebral edema. Acta Neuropathol 1986;69:54-65.

121. Pierre S, Jamme I, Droy-Lefaix MT, Nouvelot A, Maixent JM. *Ginkgo biloba* extract (EGb 761) protects Na,K-ATPase activity during cerebral ischemia in mice. Neuroreport 1999;10(1):47-51.

122. Zâgrean L, Vâtâsescu R, Munteanu AM, Moldovan M, al Nità D, Coculescu M. Preliminary EEG study of protective effects of Tebonin in transient global cerebral ischemia in rats. Romanian J Physiol 1998;35:161-8.

123. Zhang J, Fu S, Liu S, Mao T, Xiu R. The therapeutic effect of *Ginkgo biloba* extract in SHR rats and its possible mechanisms based on cerebral microvascular flow and vasomotion. Clin Hemorheol Microcirc 2000;23:133-8.

124. Kurtsoy A, Canbay S, Oktem IS, Akdemir H, Koç RK, Menkü A, Tucer B. Effect of EGb 761 on vasospasm in experimental subarachnoid hemorrhage. Research Exp Med 2000;199:207-15.

125. Hoyer S, Lannert H, Nöldner M, Chatterjee SS. Damaged neuronal energy metabolism and behavior are improved by *Ginkgo biloba* extract (EGb 761). J Neural Transm 1999;106:1171-88.

126. Wirth S, Stemmelin J, Will B, Christen Y, Di Scala G. Facilitative effects of EGb 761 on olfactory recognition in young and aged rats. Pharmacol Biochem Behav 2000;65:321-6.

127. Lamproglou I, Boisserie G, Mazeron JJ, Bok B, Baillet F, Drieu K. Effet de l'extrait de *Ginkgo biloba* (EGb 761) chez le rat sur un modèle expérimental d'encéphalopathie aiguë après irradiation corporelle totale. Cancer/Radiother 2000;4:202-6.

128. Droy-Lefaix MT, Vennat JC, Besse G, Doly M. Effect of *Ginkgo biloba* extract (EGb 761) on chloroquine induced retinal alterations. Lens Eye Toxicity Res 1992; 9:521-8

129. Droy-Lefaix MT, Cluzel J, Menerath JM, Bonhomme B, Doly M. Antioxidant effect of a *Ginkgo biloba* extract (EGb 761) on the retina. Int J Tiss Reac 1995;17:93-100.

130. Paasche G, Huster D, Reichenbach A. The glutathione content of retinal Müller (glial) cells: the effects of aging and application of free-radical scavengers. Ophthalmic Res 1998;30:351-60.

131. Szabo ME, Droy-Lefaix MT, Doly M, Braquet P. Free radical-mediated effects in reperfusion injury: a histologic study with superoxide dismutase and EGb 761 in rat retina. Ophthalmic Res 1991;23:225-34.

132. Szabo ME, Droy-Lefaix MT, Doly M, Carré C, Braquet P. Ischemia and reperfusion-induced histologic changes in the rat retina. Invest Ophthalmol Vis Sci 1991; 32:1471-8.

133. Szabo ME, Droy-Lefaix MT, Doly M. Modification of reperfusion-induced ionic imbalance by free radical scavengers in spontaneously hypertensive rat retina. Free Radical Biol Med 1992;13:609-20.

134. Szabo ME, Droy-Lefaix MT, Doly M, Braquet P. Ischaemia- and reperfusion-induced Na$^+$, K$^+$, Ca^{2+} and Mg^{2+} shifts in rat retina: effects of two free radical scavengers, SOD and EGb 761. Exp Eye Res 1992;55:39-45.

135. Szabo ME, Droy-Lefaix M-T, Doly M. EGb 761 and the recovery of ion imbalance in ischemic reperfused diabetic rat retina. Ophthalmic Res 1995;27:102-9.

136. Didier A, Droix-Lefaix M-T, Aurousseau C, Cazals Y. Effects of *Ginkgo biloba* extract (EGb 761) on cochlear vasculature in the guinea pig: morphometric measurements and laser Doppler flowmetry. Eur Arch

Otorhinolaryngol 1996;253:25-30.

137. Tighilet B, Lacour M. Pharmacological activity of the *Ginkgo biloba* extract (EGb 761) on equilibrium function recovery in the unilateral vestibular neurectomized cat. J Vestibular Res 1995;5:187-200.

138. Jastreboff PJ, Zhou S, Jastreboff MM, Kwapisz U, Gryczynska U. Attenuation of salicylate-induced tinnitus by *Ginkgo biloba* extract in rats. Audiol Neurootol 1997;2:197-212.

139. Pietri S, Séguin JR, d'Arbigny P, Drieu K, Culcasi M. *Ginkgo biloba* extract (EGb 761) pretreatment limits free radical-induced oxidative stress in patients undergoing coronary bypass surgery. Cardiovasc Drugs Ther 1997;11:121-31.

140. Witte S. Klinische Ergebnisse über hämorheologische Wirkungen von Ginkgo-biloba-extrakt. Hämostaseologie 1993;13:35-42.

141. Költringer P, Langsteger W, Eber O. Dose-dependent hemorheological effects and microcirculatory modifications following intravenous administration of *Ginkgo biloba* special extract EGb 761. Clin Hemorheol 1995;15:649-56.

142. Roncin JP, Schwartz F, d'Arbigny P. EGb 761 in control of acute mountain sickness and vascular reactivity to cold exposure. Aviat Space Environ Med 1996;67:445-52.

143. Gertsch JH, Seto TB, Mor J, Onopa J. *Ginkgo biloba* for the prevention of severe acute mountain sickness (AMS) starting one day before rapid ascent. High Alt Med Biol 2002;3:29-37.

144. Chung HS, Harris A, Kristinsson JK, Ciulla TA, Kagemann C, Ritch R. *Ginkgo biloba* extract increases ocular blood flow velocity. J Ocul Pharmacol Ther 1999;15:233-40.

145. Itil TM, Eralp E, Tsambis E, Itil KZ, Stein U. Central nervous system effects of *Ginkgo biloba*, a plant extract. Am J Therapeut 1996;3:63-73.

146. Semlitsch HV, Anderer P, Saletu B, Binder GA, Decker KA. Cognitive psychophysiology in nootropic drug research: effects of *Ginkgo biloba* on event-related potentials (P300) in age-associated memory impairment. Pharmacopsychiatry 1995;28:134-42.

147. Itil TM, Eralp E, Ahmed I, Kunitz A, Itil KZ. The pharmacological effects of *Ginkgo biloba*, a plant extract, on the brain of dementia patients in comparison with tacrine. Psychopharmacol Bull 1998;34:391-7.

148. Solomon PR, Adams F, Silver A, Zimmer J, DeVeaux R. Ginkgo for memory enhancement. A randomized controlled trial. JAMA 2002;288:835-40.

149. Bruhn C. Ginkgo in der Kritik: neue Studie bleibt umstritten. Z Phytotherapie 2002;23:238-9.

150. Letzel H, Haan J, Feil WB. Nootropics: efficacy and tolerability of products from three active substance classes. J Drug Dev Clin Pract 1996;8:77-94.

151. Ernst E, Pittler MH. *Ginkgo biloba* for dementia. A systematic review of double-blind, placebo-controlled trials. Clin Drug Invest 1999;17:301-8.

152. Wettstein A. Cholinesterase inhibitors and gingko extracts - are they comparable in the treatment of dementia? Comparison of published placebo-controlled efficacy studies of at least six months' duration. Phytomedicine 1999;6:393-401.

153. Oken BS, Storzbach DM, Kaye JA. The efficacy of *Ginkgo biloba* on cognitive function in Alzheimer disease. Arch Neurol 1998;55:1409-15.

154. van Dongen MCJM, van Rossum E, Kessels AGH, Sielhorst HJG, Knipschild PG. The efficacy of ginkgo for elderly people with dementia and age-associated memory impairment: New results of a randomized clinical trial. J Am Geriatr Soc 2000;48:1183-94.

155. Le Bars P. Conflicting results on ginkgo research. Forsch Komplementärmed Klass Naturheilkd 2002; 9:19-20.

156. Kleijnen J, Knipschild P. *Ginkgo biloba* for cerebral insufficiency. Br J Clin Pharmacol 1992;34:352-8.

157. Hopfenmüller W. Nachweis der therapeutischen Wirksamkeit eines *Ginkgo biloba*-Spezialextraktes. Meta-Analyse von 11 klinischen Studien bei Patienten mit Hirnleistungsstörungen im Alter. Arzneim-Forsch/ Drug Res 1994;44:1005-13.

158. Brautigam MRH, Blommaert FA, Verleye G, Castermans J, Jansen Steur ENH, Kleijnen J. Treatment of age-related memory complaints with *Ginkgo biloba* extract: a randomized double blind placebo-controlled study. Phytomedicine 1998;5:425-34.

159. Drew S, Davies E. Effectiveness of *Ginkgo biloba* in treating tinnitus: double blind, placebo controlled trial. BMJ 2001;322:1-6.

160. Holgers KM, Axelsson A, Pringle I. *Ginkgo biloba* extract for the treatment of tinnitus. Audiology 1994; 33:85-92.

161. Ernst E, Stevinson C. Ginkgo biloba for tinnitus: a review. Clin Otolaryngol 1999;24:164-7.

162. Hoffmann F, Beck C, Schutz A, Offermann P. Ginkgoextrakt EGb 761 (Tebonin®)/HAES versus Naftidrofuryl (Dusodril®)/HAES. Eine randomisierter Studie zur Hörsturztherapie. Laryngo-rhino-otologie 1994;73:149-52.

163. Lebuisson DA, Leroy L, Rigal G. Traitement des dégénérescences "maculaire séniles" par l'extrait de *Ginkgo biloba*. Etude préliminaire à double insu face au placebo. Presse Méd 1986;15:1556-8.

164. Lanthony P, Cosson JP. Evolution de la vision des couleurs dans la rétinopathie diabétique débutante traitée par extrait de Ginkgo biloba. Etude préliminaire à double insu contre placebo. J Fr Ophtalmol 1988; 11:671-4.

165. Raabe A, Raabe M, Ihm P. Therapieverlaufskontrolle

mittels automatisierter Perimetrie bei chronischer zerebroretinaler Mangelversorgung älterer Patienten. Prospektive randomisierte Doppelblinduntersuchung mit dosisgestaffelter Ginkgo biloba-Behandlung (EGb 761). Klin Monatsbl Augenheilkunde 1991;199:432-8.

166. Pittler MH, Ernst E. Ginkgo biloba extract for the treatment of intermittent claudication: a meta-analysis of randomized trials. Am J Med 2000;108:276-81.

167. Ernst E. Ginkgo biloba in der Behandlung der Claudicatio intermittens. Eine systematische Recherche anhand kontrollierter Studien in der Literatur. Fortschr Med 1996;114:85-7

168. Saudreau F, Serise JM, Pillet J, Maiza D, Mercier V, Kretz JG, Thibert A. Efficacité de l'extrait de Ginkgo biloba dans le traitement des artériopathies oblitérantes chroniques des membres inférieurs au stade III de la classification de Fontaine. J Malad Vasc 1989;14:177-82.

169. Moreau JP, Eck CR, McCabe J, Skinner S. Absorption, distribution et élimination de l'extrait marqué de feuilles de Ginkgo biloba chez le rat. Presse Méd 1986;15:1458-61.

170. Biber A, Koch E. Bioavailability of ginkgolides and bilobalide from extracts of Ginkgo biloba using GC/MS. Planta Med 1999;65:192-3.

171. Nieder M. Pharmakokinetik der Ginkgo-Flavonole im Plasma. Münch med Wschr 1991;133(Suppl 1):S61-S62.

172. Fourtillan JB, Brisson AM, Girault J, Ingrand I, Decourt JP, Drieu K et al. Propriétés pharmacocinétiques du bilobalide et des ginkgolides A et B chez le sujet sain après administrations intraveineuses et orales d'extrait de Ginkgo biloba (EGb 761). Thérapie (Paris) 1995; 50:137-44.

173. Itil T, Martorano D. Natural substances in psychiatry (Ginkgo biloba in dementia). Psychopharmacol Bull 1995;31:147-58.

174. Hänsel R, Keller K, Rimpler H, Schneider G, editors. Ginkgo. In: Hagers Handbuch der Pharmazeutischen Praxis, 5th ed. Volume 5: Drogen E-O. Berlin: Springer-Verlag, 1993:269-92.

175. Schilcher H. Ginkgo biloba L. Untersuchungen zur Qualität, Wirkung, Wirksamkeit und Unbedenklichkeit. Z Phytotherapie 1988;9:119-27.

176. Herrschaft H. Zur klinischen Anwendung von Ginkgo biloba bei dementiellen Syndromen. (Hirnleistungsstörungen bei vasculärer oder degenerativer ZNS-Erkrankung). Pharm unserer Zeit 1992;21:266-75.

177. Woerdenbag HJ, De Smet PAGM. Adverse effects and toxicity of Gingko extracts. In: van Beek TA, editor. Ginkgo biloba (Medicinal and Aromatic Plants - Industrial Profiles). Amsterdam: Harwood Academic, 2000:443-51.

178. Allain H, Raoul P, Lieury A, LeCoz F, Gandon J-M. Effect of two doses of Ginkgo biloba extract (EGb 761) on the dual-coding test in elderly subjects. Clin Ther 1993;15:549-58

179. Vorberg G. Gingko biloba extract (GBE): a long-term study of chronic cerebral insufficiency in geriatric patients. Clin Trials J 1985;22:149-57.

180. Burkard G, Lehrl S. Verhältnis von Demenzen vom Multiinfarkt- und vom Alzheimertyp in ärztlichen Praxen. Diagnostische und therapeutische Konsequenzen am Beispiel eines Ginkgo-biloba-Präparates. Münch Med Wochenschr 1991;133(Suppl 1):S38-S43.

181. Habs M, Meyer B. Demenz: Phytotherapeutische Möglichkeiten mit Ginkgo biloba. Geriatrie Praxis 1997;1:24-31.

182. Rowin J, Lewis SL. Spontaneous bilateral subdural hematomas associated with chronic Ginkgo biloba ingestion. Neurology 1996;46:1775-6.

183. Odawara M, Tamaoka A, Yamashita K. Ginkgo biloba [Comment on Rowin J, Lewis SL. 1996]. Neurology 1997;48:789-90.
Reply from the authors: Rowin J, Lewis SL. Neurology 1997;48:790.

184. Gilbert GJ. Ginkgo biloba [Comment on Rowin J, Lewis SL. 1996]. Neurology 1997;48:1137.
Reply from the authors: Lewis SL, Rowin J. Neurology 1997;48:1137.

185. Vale S. Subarachnoid haemorrhage associated with Ginkgo biloba. Lancet 1998;352:36.

186. Skogh M. Extracts of Ginkgo biloba and bleeding or haemorrhage [Comment on Vale S. 1998]. Lancet 1998;352:1145-6.
Reply from the author: Vale S. Lancet 1998;352:1146.

187. Köhler S. Influence of Gingko biloba extract versus placebo on coagulation. Clinical Research Department, Dr. Willmar Schwabe Pharmaceuticals, 76227 Karlsruhe (submitted for publication, 2003).

188. Bal dit Sollier C, Caplain H, Drouet L. No alteration in platelet function or coagulation induced by EGb761 in a controlled study. Clin Lab Haem 2003;25:251-3.

GINSENG RADIX

Ginseng

E/S/C/O/P
MONOGRAPHS
Second Edition

DEFINITION

Ginseng consists of the whole or cut dried root of *Panax ginseng* C.A. Meyer (Araliaceae). It contains not less than 0.4 per cent of combined ginsenosides Rg$_1$ (C$_{42}$H$_{72}$O$_{14}$.2H$_2$O; M$_r$ 837) and Rb$_1$ (C$_{54}$H$_{92}$O$_{23}$. 3H$_2$O; M$_r$ 1163), calculated with reference to the dried drug.

The material complies with the monograph of the European Pharmacopoeia [1].

CONSTITUENTS

Triterpene saponins of the dammarane type, as derivatives of either protopanaxadiol or protopanaxatriol. Examples of protopanaxadiol saponins are: ginsenosides Ra$_1$, Ra$_2$ and Ra$_3$; ginsenosides Rb$_1$, Rb$_2$ and Rb$_3$; ginsenosides Rc and Rd; and malonyl-ginsenosides Rb$_1$, Rb$_2$, Rc and Rd. Examples of protopanaxatriol saponins are: ginsenosides Re and Rf; 20-gluco-ginsenoside Rf; ginsenosides Rg$_1$, Rg$_2$ and Rh$_1$. Ginsenoside Ro is a derivative of oleanolic acid.

The ginsenosides considered the more important are ginsenosides Rb$_1$, Rb$_2$, Rc, Rd, Re, Rf, Rg$_1$ and Rg$_2$, with Rb$_1$, Rb$_2$, Re and Rg$_1$ being the most abundant. The total ginsenoside content of a 6-year-old main root varies between 0.7 and 3%. The lateral roots can contain two to three times more saponins than the main root while the slender roots can contain up to 10 times more [2-10].

Other constituents include peptidoglycans called panaxans, acetylenic compounds such as panaxynol, pyrazine derivatives such as 3-*sec*-butyl-2-methoxy-5-pyrazine, oligo- and polysaccharides, phenolic compounds such as vanillic acid and salicylates, and traces of essential oil containing sesquiterpenes such as eremophilene [8,9].

CLINICAL PARTICULARS

Therapeutic indications
Decreased mental and physical capacities such as weakness, exhaustion, tiredness and loss of concentration, as well as during convalescence [11-16].

Posology and method of administration

Dosage
Adult daily dose: 0.5 g up to a maximum of 2 g of dried root; equivalent preparations [2,11,13,14].

Method of administration
For oral administration.

Duration of administration
If symptoms persist or worsen after one month, medical advice should be sought.

Contra-indications
None known.

Special warnings and precautions for use
Do not exceed the recommended dose.
Diabetics should consult a physician prior to taking ginseng root [17].

Interaction with other medicaments and other forms of interaction
Ginseng intake may slightly reduce blood glucose levels [17].

A case of possible interaction of ginseng with warfarin anticoagulant therapy has been reported, but the mechanism remains unknown; studies are needed to verify this potential interaction and the underlying mechanism [18]. In rats, concomitantly administered ginseng had no significant effect on the pharmacokinetics or pharmacodynamics of warfarin [19].

Pregnancy and lactation
In animals, no effect on fetal development has been observed. No human data are available [20].

In accordance with general medical practice, ginseng should not be used during pregnancy or lactation without medical advice.

Effects on ability to drive and use machines
None known.

Undesirable effects
On the basis of ginseng's long-term usage and the relative infrequency of significant demonstrable side effects, it has been concluded that the use of ginseng is not associated with serious adverse effects if taken at the recommended dose level [20,21].

Oestrogenic-like side effects have been reported in both pre- and post-menopausal women following the use of ginseng. Seven cases of mastalgia in post-menopausal women after ingestion of ginseng products of unspecified botanical origin have been reported [22-24]. However, in clinical studies with more than 100 patients to whom a standardized ginseng extract had been given, no oestrogenic-like side effects have been observed and only normal hormone blood levels have been found in the specific tests carried out in these studies [25,26].

An *in vitro* study showed that the concentration of ginseng extract or ginsenosides needed for competitive inhibition of the binding of promegestone to the cytosolic progesterone receptor of human myometrium is far higher than the ginsenoside concentrations which can be reached after oral administration [27].

Overdose
Critical analysis of a report on a so-called Ginseng Abuse Syndrome [28] has shown that there were no controls or analysis to determine the type of ginseng ingested or the constituents of the preparation taken, and that some of the amounts ingested were clearly excessive (as much as 15 g, whereas the recommended daily dose is 0.5 to 2 g daily) [20,29,30]. The only conclusion that can validly be drawn from the above report is that excessive and uncontrolled intake of ginseng products should be avoided [20].

One case of ginseng-associated cerebral arteritis has been reported in a patient consuming 200 ml of a preparation made from 12.5 g (dry weight) of ginseng and 200 ml of rice wine [31].

PHARMACOLOGICAL PROPERTIES

Pharmacodynamic properties

A review of the major findings of pharmacological tests and human studies carried out with a number of plant drugs including ginseng supported the view that ginseng enhances physical performance and learning capacities and has immunomodulatory properties [32].

In vitro experiments

Cell proliferation
In experiments with human male fetal lung fibroblasts (MRC-5), addition of ginseng extract (dialyzed or heat treated to inactivate protein-precipitating activity) to the culture medium resulted in the following:
- up to 100% increase in cell density at concentrations equivalent to 0.05-2.0 mg whole root/ml medium and decreased cell density at more than 5.0 mg/ml.
- 0.75 mg extract/ml had an effect on cell density equivalent to that of 5 µg hydrocortisone/ml.
- faster growth rate, smaller and more mitotic cells and longer survival time without media change after addition of 0.75 mg/ml or after addition of 5 µg hydrocortisone/ml [33].

Activation of biosynthesis
Addition of a fraction from a ginseng extract to a homogenate of rat testes stimulated DNA and protein synthesis. The effect was reduced by addition of the enzyme inhibitor cycloheximide [34].

A standardized ginseng extract stimulated D-glucose transport in Ehrlich ascites tumour cells and D-glucose uptake in rabbit cerebral cortical tissue [35,36].

Hormone receptor binding
Binding of the radioactive-labelled sex hormone promegestone to the cytosolic progesterone receptor of human myometrium in the presence or absence of ginseng extract or pure ginsenosides was investigated. The results demonstrated that the concentration of ginseng extract or ginsenosides needed for competitive inhibition of the binding of promegestone to the receptor were far higher than the concentrations which can be reached after oral administration [31].

Immunomodulation
Peripheral blood mononuclear cells from healthy volunteers (n = 20) or from patients with chronic fatigue syndrome (n = 20) or AIDS (n = 20) were tested, in the presence or absence of varying concentrations of ginseng extract, for natural killer cell activity against K562 cells and for antibody-dependent cellular cytotoxicity against human herpes virus 6-infected H9 cells. Ginseng extract in concentrations of 1, 10 and 100 μg/ml significantly (p<0.05 to p<0.001) enhanced cellular immune function of peripheral blood mononuclear cells from all groups [37].

The mitogenic activity and anticomplement activity of a standardized ginseng extract and several fractions from it were tested in mice spleen cell cultures. It was found that the extract possessed anticomplement and mitogenic activities, the strongest anticomplement activity being observed in a crude polysaccharide fraction. The polysaccharide with the major anticomplement activity consisted of arabinose, galactose and glucose with small amounts of galacturonic acid, glucuronic acid and rhamnose; its molecular weight was estimated to be 3.68×10^5 kD [38].

An acidic polysaccharide fraction from ginseng containing galactose, arabinose and uronic acids inhibited *Helicobacter pylori*-induced haem-agglutination with a minimum inhibitory concentration of 250 μg/ml. Digestion of the fraction with pectinase resulted in a lower molecular weight oligosaccharide fraction which was non-inhibitory at 4 mg/ml [39].

Ex vivo experiments

Antioxidant properties
Two groups of 5 rats were given ginseng extract as 10 mg/ml in drinking water (corresponding to 1.6 g/kg/day) for one week then one group was exposed to hyperbaric 100% oxygen (HBO) for 6 hours; two control groups (no ginseng extract) drank an equal amount of water and one control group was exposed to HBO. Isolated perfused hearts from the rats were subjected to mild ischaemia and then reperfused. The results indicated that the ginseng extract prevented myocardial ischaemia/reperfusion damage and the impairment of endothelial functionality induced by reactive oxygen species arising from HBO exposure, through an antioxidant intervention [40].

In experiments with perfused rabbit lungs, a ginseng extract inhibited vasoconstriction induced by the thromboxane analogue U46619 or by acetylcholine after exposure to free radicals generated by electrolysis. This effect appeared to be due to the release of nitric oxide from the pulmonary endothelium. The extract had activities superior to pure ginsenosides. Moreover, pure ginsenosides at higher concentrations appeared to have a negative effect rather than a protective one [41,42].

Immunomodulation
After oral administration of a standardized ginseng extract to mice at 10 mg/day for 4 consecutive days the effect on immune response was investigated. The extract enhanced antibody plaque forming cell response and circulating antibody titre against sheep erythrocytes [43].

The above finding was confirmed by experiments involving oral administration to mice of a ginseng extract with defined ginsenoside content. Oral administration at 10, 50 or 250 mg/kg body weight daily for 5-6 days resulted in enhanced immune responses in a battery of 6 *ex vivo* tests which included primary and secondary immune response against sheep red cells, natural killing activity, mitogen-induced proliferation, interferon production and T-cell mediated cytotoxicity [44].

In vivo experiments

Humoral effects
Intraperitoneal administration of ginseng saponin fractions to rats stimulated adrenocorticotrophic hormone (ACTH) secretion from the hypothalamus/hypophysis, leading to increased corticosterone synthesis and excretion [45,46].

Effects on performance
Intraperitoneal administration to rats of a 1% ginseng extract (20 mg extract/kg body weight twice with a 24-hour interval) led to significant differences in energy metabolism after exercise (swimming for 60 minutes) as measured by determination of plasma concentrations of relevant metabolites. Glucose was higher (p<0.01) and free fatty acids were lower (p<0.01) after 30 minutes, whereas pyruvic acid (p<0.05) and lactic acid (p<0.01) were lower after 60 minutes compared to saline treated controls. It was concluded that ginseng extract shifted the skeletal muscle energy metabolism towards oxidation of fatty acids, thereby conserving carbohydrate stores [47].

The effects of a standardized dry ginseng extract

administered intraperitoneally to rabbits were investigated using electrocorticograms. The results indicated that the extract stimulated metabolic activity of cerebral tissue. Incubation of sliced rabbit brain tissue with the same extract (23 and 46 µg/ml) led to highly significant metabolic changes (p<0.0005 compared to control values): glucose uptake increased, while lactate and pyruvate production and the lactate/pyruvate ratio decreased. The effects appeared to be dose-dependent [36].

Oral administration of a standardized ginseng extract to rats for 3 months at 3, 10 or 100 mg/kg body weight per day produced dose-dependent, significant increases in performance in the treadmill test and diminished hepatic lipid peroxidation compared to controls (p<0.05) [48,49].

After oral administration of a standardized ginseng extract, rats were subjected to learning and memory retention tests and ^{14}C-phenylalanine transport across the blood-brain barrier was also determined. After intraperitoneal injection of rats with the extract the brain stem and brain cortex were analysed for concentrations of monoamines and 3',5'-cyclic adenosine monophosphate (AMP), and for the activity of phosphodiesterase and adenylate cyclase. The following results were obtained:

- Improved learning and memory retention (5 of 7 tests) after oral administration of the extract at 20 mg/kg body weight for 3 days, but unchanged or even decreased learning and memory retention (4 of 7 tests) after 100 mg/kg orally for 3 days.
- Increased ^{14}C-phenylalanine transport across the blood-brain barrier after 30 mg extract/kg orally for 5 days.
- Unchanged phosphodiesterase activity in brain stem and cortex after 50 mg extract/kg intraperitoneally for 5 days.
- Decreased adenylate cyclase activity (with or without NaF-activation) after 30 mg and 200 mg extract/kg intraperitoneally for 5 days, except after 30 mg extract without NaF-activation when adenylate cyclase activity was increased.
- Decreased 3',5'-cyclic AMP concentration in brain stem and cortex after 200 mg extract/kg intraperitoneally for 5 days.
- Increased dopamine and noradrenaline concentrations in brain stem, whereas the serotonin concentration was decreased in brain stem and increased in brain cortex, after 50 mg extract/kg intraperitoneally for 5 days.

This study thus revealed the influence of ginseng extract on complex neurological processes such as learning and memory as well as on several aspects of brain metabolism [50].

Oral versus intraperitoneal administration of a standardized ginseng extract was compared in a study involving tests for exhaustion by swimming in mice and cold stress resistance in rats. Physiological and biochemical tests (body weight increase, food and water consumption, urine analysis for sodium, potassium and chloride, liver total cholesterol, total lipids and triglycerides, adrenal total cholesterol, blood and serum glucose, triglyceride and cholesterol values) were also carried out. Significant effects (p<0.05) seen in this study were:

- A prolongation of time to exhaustion in mice after a single intraperitoneal administration of ginseng extract. Oral administration of a daily dose corresponding to 37.5 mg/kg body weight for 15 days also produced an effect.
- Body temperature under cold stress in rats was higher after intraperitoneal administration of ginseng extract or 5 mg ACTH per kg body weight compared to controls receiving saline solution. Hydrocortisone (10 mg/kg) did not have this cold-protective activity. In adrenalectomized rats on the other hand, ginseng extract did not have cold-protective activity whereas hydrocortisone did.
- In a study in weanling rats the fresh weight of thymus was reduced after intraperitoneal administration of ginseng extract for 4 days in doses corresponding to 1.5-30 mg of ginsenosides/kg. The magnitude of effect was dose-dependent.
- Liver protein, total cholesterol and total lipids were reduced in male and female rats after 15 days of intraperitoneal administration of extract in doses corresponding to 3 or 30 mg ginsenosides/kg body weight/day. Such changes were not seen after 15 days oral administration of extract doses corresponding to 1.87 or 37.5 mg ginsenosides/kg body weight/day except for a reduction of liver protein in female rats receiving the higher oral dose. Adrenal total cholesterol was markedly reduced only in orally treated animals. Furthermore, body weight increase was monitored weekly in a prolongation of the same experiment comparing 5 weeks oral administration with 4 weeks intraperitoneal administration. Growth retardation was seen in male rats both after oral and intraperitoneal treatment but was stronger and dose-dependent after intraperitoneal treatment. In female rats weak and non-dose-dependent growth retardation was only seen after intraperitoneal treatment. It was concluded that ginseng acts indirectly on the level of central humoral regulation via the adrenocortical system [51].

Groups of 7-week-old male Swiss mice (15 per group) received, as their only liquid for up to 96 days, either distilled water or an infusion from ginseng corresponding to 33 mg of dry root powder/ml. The average consumption per mouse corresponded to daily ingestion of 274 mg of root powder. No significant differences between treatments were seen in weight gain or in the cold swimming test after 35, 46 or 96 days [52].

In another study rats received by stomach tube, 48 hours and 1 hour before a warm water swimming test, crude saponins from 6 different types of ginseng at 50 mg/kg body weight. Swimming time until drowning, plasma levels of lactic acid, glucose, insulin and glucagon, and liver glycogen, were measured in both resting and drowned animals. The only significant differences (p<0.05) were an increased plasma level of glucose in drowned rats that had received ginseng. Plasma glucose levels were higher in all resting rats that had received saponins but the differences were within normal biological variability [53].

In a study of antioxidant activity, liver lipid peroxide levels following ethanol intoxication were determined in mice which had received oral doses of various ginseng root constituents (maltol, salicylic acid, vanillic acid, coumaric acid and ginsenosides Rb_1, Rb_2, Rc, Re, Rg_1) at 0.001-1 mg per 30 g body weight for 3 days before the test. Maltol, salicylic acid and vanillic acid decreased liver lipid peroxide levels strongly while saponins had a weaker effect and coumaric acid was inactive [54].

Immunomodulation
Daily subcutaneous administration to thymectomized rats of an extract corresponding to 25 mg ginseng/kg body weight for 10 days gave significant protection (p<0.04 to p<0.004) against intratracheal challenge with alginate-embedded *Pseudomonas aeruginosa* [55].

Anti-ulcer effects
Oral administration to rats of 50, 200 or 500 mg/kg body weight of a 70%-methanol extract from ginseng inhibited in a dose-dependent manner gastric ulceration induced by pyloric ligation, serotonin or endotoxin, but did not inhibit stress-induced ulceration. Serotonin- or endotoxin-induced effects on gastric mucosal tissue blood flow were reduced. Most effects observed after doses of 200 mg/kg or 500 mg/kg were statistically significant (p<0.05 or p<0.01) [56].

Hepatoprotective effects
Intraperitoneal administration of a single dose of a ginseng extract to rats at 50 mg/kg body weight did not protect the animals against CCl_4-induced hepatotoxicity [57].

Subcutaneous injection of rats with dexamethasone (0.5 mg and 1.0 mg/day) for 7 days, alone or in combination with a ginseng extract (corresponding to 100 mg of root/day) for 5 days, demonstrated that the extract reduced dexamethasone-elevated alanine amino transferase (ALAT) and aspartate amino transferase (ASAT) levels to normal [58].

Pharmacological studies in humans

Performance
In a double-blind crossover study, 12 student nurses working night shifts (3-4 consecutive nights followed by 3 days of rest) were given 1.2 g of ginseng or placebo for the first three consecutive nights of night work and tested on the morning after the third night. Crossover medication was given after an interval of at least 2 weeks. A third series of tests was carried out during normal daytime working, after no medication and following a good night's sleep (GNS). The subjects assessed their mood, physical well-being and degree of lethargy by means of linear self-rating scales; two psychophysiological performance tests and haematological tests were also carried out. The detrimental effects of night shifts on mood and performance were clearly seen. A constant trend in favour of ginseng compared to placebo was noted. Ginseng ratings were favourable for mood criteria, but unfavourable for physical well-being criteria. Ginseng restored blood glucose levels raised by night shift stress to the GNS level. It was concluded that ginseng had a small but consistent anti-fatigue effect [11].

Various tests of psychomotor performance were carried out in a group of 16 healthy male volunteers given a standardized ginseng extract (2 × 100 mg daily for 12 weeks) and in a similar group given placebo under double-blind conditions. A favourable effect of ginseng relative to baseline performance was observed in attention (cancellation test), processing (mental arithmetic, logical deduction), integrated sensory-motor function (choice reaction time) and auditory reaction time. However, end performance of the ginseng group was statistically superior (p<0.05) to the placebo group only in mental arithmetic. No difference between ginseng and placebo was found in tests of pure motor function (tapping test), recognition (digit symbol substitution) and visual reaction time [12].

In a double-blind, placebo-controlled, crossover study, 43 top triathletes received either 200 mg of a standardized ginseng extract or placebo daily for periods of 10 weeks. Significant differences (p<0.05) in various endurance parameters were seen only after the second treatment phase. It was concluded that ginseng improved endurance (resistance to end of season stress) but did not improve optimum performance [13].

Twenty top class male athletes received 200 mg of a standardized ginseng extract daily for 9 weeks. In the bicycle ergometer exercise test lasting 8 minutes, post-treatment values were higher for maximal oxygen absorption and lower for blood lactate level and heart rate during exercise compared to pretreatment values. The differences were significant (p<0.001) [14].

In a double-blind study athletes were given 200 mg of ginseng extract standardized to 7% ginsenosides (n = 10) or 200 mg of ginseng extract standardized to 4% ginsenosides + 400 mg of vitamin E (n = 10) or placebo (n = 10) daily for 9 weeks. Using the same bicycle ergometer test, significant differences were observed in favour of either of the two ginseng preparations compared to placebo with respect to heart rate (p<0.05), blood lactate (p<0.01) and maximal oxygen absorption (p<0.01) after exercise. Differences between the two ginseng preparations were not significant. Levels of testosterone and luteinising hormone in plasma and of free cortisol in urine were unchanged after all treatments [14,15].

A double-blind, placebo-controlled study involving 28 trained male athletes examined the persistence of effects of a 9-week treatment (200 mg of ginseng extract with 4% ginsenosides, or placebo) beyond the treatment period. Compared to placebo the ginseng extract produced significant improvements in maximal oxygen uptake during exercise (p<0.01), heart rate at maximal exercise (p<0.001), forced expiratory volume (p<0.01), forced vital lung capacity (p<0.05) and visual reaction time (p<0.01). These positive effects lasted for at least 3 weeks after treatment. It was concluded that the effects of ginseng are based on clinically relevant metabolic changes, which persist for a certain period after treatment [16].

In a double-blind, placebo-controlled study involving 50 ambulant patients suffering from asthenia, depressive syndrome or neurovegetative disorders, the effects of 8 weeks of daily treatment with 200 mg of a standardized ginseng extract on performance were evaluated by two psychometric tests and from the results of a comprehensive psychological questionnaire (Sandoz Clinical Assessment Geriatric). Significant improvement (p<0.05 and p<0.01) was seen in most of the parameters [59].

In a randomized, double-blind study, healthy male volunteers received 200 mg (n = 11) or 400 mg (n = 10) of a ginseng extract, or placebo (n = 10), daily for 8 weeks. The extract had no effect on oxygen consumption, respiratory exchange ratio, minute ventilation, blood lactic acid concentration, heart rate or perceived exertion [60].

In another randomized, double-blind study, healthy female volunteers received 200 mg of a ginseng extract (n = 10) or placebo (n = 9) daily for 8 weeks. Ginseng had no effect on maximal work performance or on resting, exercise and recovery oxygen uptake, respiratory exchange ratio, minute ventilation, heart rate or blood lactic acid levels [61].

In a double-blind, placebo-controlled, crossover study involving 8 healthy volunteers (mean age 25 years) who regularly practised physical activities, 30 days of oral treatment with 400 mg of a standardized ginseng extract per day did not improve performance in supramaximal exercise (125% of the maximum aerobic power on a bicycle ergometer), nor did it influence blood lactate or blood testosterone [62].

In a study of the blood oxygenation status of 8 male and 2 female middle-aged subjects (average age 50 years), a significant increase (p<0.05) in resting arterial pO_2 was observed after 4 weeks of daily oral treatment with 200 mg of a standardized ginseng extract; the resting arterial pO_2 increased by 4.5 mm Hg. In synergy with oxygen treatment the increase was 10.1 mm Hg. Venous pO_2 decreased (4.3 mm Hg) [63].

The effects of 400 mg/day of a ginseng extract for 8-9 weeks on a variety of cognitive functions were compared with placebo treatment in a randomized, double-blind study involving 112 healthy volunteers older than 40 years (55 verum, 57 placebo). The ginseng group showed a tendency to faster simple reactions and significantly better abstract thinking than the controls. However, there was no significant difference between groups in concentration, memory or subjective experience [64].

The effects of a standardized ginseng extract on psychological mood states and perceptual response to submaximal and maximal exercise stress were evaluated in a study involving 19 young adult females who received either 200 mg of a standardized ginseng root extract (n = 10) or placebo (n = 9) daily. The results did not support claims that ginseng can enhance psychological function characteristics at rest and during exercise stress [65].

The effects of a standardized ginseng extract (300 mg/day) on healthy, untrained male students and on healthy male students who received regular bicycle ergometer training were compared to placebo in an 8-week randomized, double-blind study (n = 41). Administration of the ginseng extract produced training-like effects on VO_2 max. and on anaerobic power and leg muscle strength, but no synergistic effect on these fitness variables occurred when administration of ginseng extract was combined with exercise training [66].

Immunomodulation
The effects of ginseng on immune parameters were studied in a randomized, double-blind study in which groups of healthy volunteers of both sexes, aged between 18 and 50 years, were treated orally with 2 × 100 mg of a standardized ginseng extract (n = 20) or 2 × 100 mg of a dry aqueous extract from ginseng (n = 20) or placebo (n = 20) daily for 8 weeks.

- Standardized ginseng extract increased the chemotaxis of circulating polymorphonuclear leucocytes (p<0.05 at week 4 and p<0.001 at week 8), increased the phagocytosis index and phagocytosis fraction (p<0.001 at weeks 4 and 8), increased total lymphocytes (T3) (p<0.05 at week 4 and p<0.001 at week 8), increased the T-helper subset (T4) (p<0.05 at week 4 and p<0.001 at week 8), increased the helper/suppressor (T4/T8) ratio (p<0.05 at weeks 4 and 8), enhanced induction of blastogenesis in circulating lymphocytes (p<0.05 at weeks 4 and 8 after induction by cocanavalin A and pokeweed mitogen; p<0.001 at weeks 4 and 8 after induction by lipopolysaccharide) and enhanced natural killer cell activity (p<0.05 at week 4 and p<0.001 at week 8).

- Aqueous ginseng extract increased the chemotaxis of circulating polymorphonuclear leucocytes (p<0.05 at weeks 4 and 8), increased the phagocytosis index and phagocytosis fraction (p<0.05 at week 8), increased total lymphocytes (T3) (p<0.05 at week 4 and p<0.001 at week 8), increased the T-helper subset (T4) (p<0.05 at week 8), enhanced induction of blastogenesis in circulating lymphocytes (p<0.05 at week 8 after induction by cocanavalin A and pokeweed mitogen) and enhanced natural killer cell activity (p<0.05 at week 8).

- With placebo, only enhancement of natural killer cell activity was significant (p<0.05) after 8 weeks.

It was concluded that ginseng extracts act as immunostimulants in man and that the standardized extract was more active than the aqueous extract [67,68].

Healthy volunteers enrolled in a multicentre, randomized, double-blind, placebo-controlled study to investigate potential effects of ginseng on resistance to influenza and the common cold were treated with 200 mg of a standardized ginseng extract (n = 114) or placebo (n = 113) daily for 12 weeks. All participants received an anti-influenza polyvalent vaccine at week 4. Results from examinations at weeks 4, 8 and 12 showed highly significant differences (p<0.0001) between the ginseng extract and placebo with regard to the frequency of influenza or colds between weeks 4 and 12 (15 cases in the verum group versus 42 cases in the placebo group). Antibody titres at week 8 were also much higher after verum treatment (272 units versus 171 units after placebo) and natural killer cell activity in the verum group was almost twice as high as in the placebo group [69].

In a controlled single-blind study to investigate the effects of a standardized ginseng extract (200 mg/day) in 40 patients suffering from chronic bronchitis the extract significantly (p<0.001) improved

alveolar macrophage activity compared to baseline [70].

In a pilot study involving 15 patients with severe chronic respiratory diseases, a standardized ginseng extract was administered orally at 200 mg/day for 3 months and respiratory parameters such as vital capacity, expiratory volume and flow, ventilation volume and walking distance were evaluated. The results led to the conclusion that ginseng extract improved pulmonary function and oxygenation capacity, which seemed to be the reason for improved walking capacity [71].

A study in two groups of 10 healthy young Thai males evaluated the effects of 300 mg of a standardized ginseng extract daily for 8 weeks in comparison with placebo on peripheral blood leukocytes and lymphocyte subsets. No significant differences were observed [72].

In a first attempt at a systematic review of some of these studies it was suggested that further investigations are needed to conclusively establish the efficacy of ginseng [73].

Pharmacokinetic properties

Pharmacokinetics in animals

A study involving intravenous, intraperitoneal and oral administration of purified or semipurified ginsenosides Rg_1, Rb_2, Rd and Re in rabbits gave the following results:

- The pharmacokinetic behaviour of some ginsenosides is best described by a one-compartment open model.
- Ginsenoside Rb_2 had a longer elimination half-life (445 minutes) and lower metabolic and renal clearance than ginsenosides Rg_1 and Re, obviously due to a higher rate of plasma protein binding.
- Absorption into the systemic circulation after intraperitoneal administration was slow for all the ginsenosides studied.
- No ginsenosides were found in plasma or urine samples after oral administration; analysis of faecal samples for ginsenoside Rg_1 also gave a negative result [74].

The pharmacokinetics of ginsenoside Rg_1 were studied in rats, comparing oral and intravenous administration. Rapid absorption of 1.9-20.0% of orally administered Rg_1 (t_{max} 30 minutes) and rapid excretion of intravenous Rg_1 (almost 60% of the dose in bile within 4 hours and 24% in urine within 12 hours) were detected by TLC [75].

The pharmacokinetics of ginsenoside Rb_1 were studied

in rats after oral or intravenous administration. Orally administered Rb_1 was very poorly absorbed (approx. 0.1%) from rat intestine. Excretion of Rb_1 after intravenous administration was biphasic with a half-life of 11.6 minutes for the α-phase and 14.6 hours for the β-phase. Excretion was mainly in the urine (44% within 120 hours) and poorly in bile (0.8% within 24 hours) [76].

Decomposition products of ginsenosides Rb_1 and Rg_1 in the rat gastro-intestinal tract have been investigated. The pattern of decomposition products in rat stomach was similar to hydrolysis products under mild acidic conditions except for one compound. Decomposition products in the large intestine were due to the activitiy of enteric bacteria and an enteric enzyme [77].

The metabolites of ginsenosides are poorly investigated with regard to pharmacokinetics as there are more than 10 ginsenosides, each giving rise to at least 5 different metabolites. A study in mini-pigs following intravenous administration of Rb_1 and Rg_1 confirmed findings in rats and rabbits. Rb_1 was excreted biexponentially (two-compartment open model) with a half-life of 16 hours in the β-phase (20 minutes in the α-phase). Rg_1 pharmacokinetics are best explained by a one-compartment model, the elimination half-life being 27 minutes [78].

A study in mice involving intravenous or oral administration of tritiated [^{3}H]ginsenoside Rg_1 indicated rapid absorption after oral administration (appr. 30% after 1 hour). Relatively high concentrations were found in blood, liver, bile, subcutis, conjunctiva and epithelia of oral and nasal cavities and oesophagus, whereas the concentration in muscle and endocrine organs was low. Addition of total ginseng extract or of a purified ginsenoside fraction to oral administration of tritiated Rg_1 did not change the distribution pattern of Rg_1. Excretion of intact Rg_1 in faeces and urine was low, whereas excretion of metabolites was high [79].

After oral administration of ginsenoside Rb_2 to rats, six decomposition products were found in the large intestine by TLC. On the basis of ^{13}C-NMR, five decomposition products resulted from stepwise cleavage of sugar moieties [80].

The decomposition of ginsenoside Rb_2 in rat stomach was compared to its decomposition in 0.1N HCl. There was little decomposition in the stomach with only small amounts of 24- and 25-hydroxy- and -hydroperoxy-derivatives being found. Decomposition in 0.1 N HCl solution yielded two main derivatives due to cleavage of a sugar moiety [81].

A further study investigated the decomposition of ginsenosides Rb_1 and Rb_2 in rat stomach and large intestine, in 0.1 N HCl and in crude hesperidinase solution. The results confirmed a quantitatively small

decomposition to hydroxy- and hydroperoxy-derivatives in rat stomach, whereas decomposition in 0.1 N HCl yielded derivatives arising from cleavage of sugar moieties. It was also found that the decomposition of Rb_1 and Rb_2 by cleavage of sugar moieties in rat large intestine was partly due to bacteria and partly due to enteric enzymes such as β-glucosidase. Different decomposition products were found in rat large intestine compared to those found after treatment with hesperidinase [82].

Pharmacokinetics in humans
Dose-dependent urinary excretion of 20(S)-protopanaxatriol glycosides (1.5% of the dose) was observed in 4 healthy volunteers after oral ingestion of ginseng powder and ginseng extract preparations corresponding to 6.2-27.6 mg of ginsenosides per day [83].

Using selective ion-monitoring GC-MS, ginsenoside aglycones were quantified in urine from athletes who claimed to have consumed ginseng preparations for at least 10 days before urine collection. Aglycone concentrations of 2-35 ng/ml were found in 60 out of 65 urine samples [84].

Cleavage of sugar moieties from ginsenosides Rb_1, Rb_2, Rc and Rd by intestinal bacteria isolated from human faecal samples has been demonstrated. *Prevotella oris* was identified as the major bacterial species with this ability [85].

Preclinical safety data
A 1984 review [20] summarized the results of several toxicity studies of a standardized ginseng root extract in animals:

Single dose toxicity
- The oral LD_{50} was determined as > 5 g/kg body weight in the rat, > 2 g/kg in the guinea pig and > 1 g/kg in mice.
- The intraperitoneal LD_{50} was > 1 g/kg in rats and mice.
- After oral administration of the ginseng extract to mini-pigs at 0.25, 0.5 or 2.0 g/kg body weight no noticeable changes were observed in cardiovascular parameters such as ECG, pulse, blood pressure, cardiac output and stroke volume.

Repeated dose toxicity
- No haematological or histological abnormalities were observed in rats after oral administration of the extract at 4.0 g/kg/day for 20 days.
- No treatment-related haematological or histo-pathological findings were observed in beagle dogs after oral administration of the extract at 1.5, 5.0 and 15 mg/kg/day for 90 days.

- An additional study showed no changes in haematological parameters in rats following subcutaneous injection of a ginseng extract (corresponding to 100 mg of root) daily for 5 days [52].

Reproductive toxicity
- No decrease in growth rate or reproduction and no treatment-related haematological or histopathological findings were observed in rats during a 33-week two-generation study with the ginseng extract administered orally at 1.5, 5.0 or 15 mg/kg body weight/day.

Embryo, foetal and perinatal toxicity
- No abnormalities of foetal development were found after oral administration of the ginseng extract to rats at 40 mg/kg/day during days 1-15 after mating or to rabbits at 20 mg/kg/day during days 7-15 after mating.

Genotoxicity
- In the hepatocyte-DNA repair test no genotoxicity of the ginseng extract was observed at concentrations of 0.1-10 mg/ml, with or without ginsenosides, or of ginsenoside Rg_1 at 1-50 µg/ml.

In a study involving intraperitoneal administration of ginsenosides Rb_1 and Rg_1 to mice at 25, 50 or 100 mg/kg body weight, neither single nor repeated large doses of 100 mg/kg caused any toxic symptoms or adverse behavioural effects such as ataxia or sedation [86].

Clinical safety data

In a double-blind, placebo-controlled study involving 60 females and 60 males, daily oral administration of 200 mg of a standardized ginseng extract for 12 weeks did not cause any significant differences in blood levels of sex hormones (luteinizing hormone, follicle-stimulating hormone, testosterone, oestradiol) in comparison with placebo groups [25].

In an open study of 49 menopausal women (33 of whom had undergone a hysterectomy) regular speculum examinations and cytological smears from the cervix and vaginal wall did not reveal any changes during 3 months of oral treatment with 200 mg of a standardized ginseng extract per day [26].

REFERENCES

1. Ginseng - Ginseng radix. European Pharmacopoeia, Council of Europe.

2. Schweins S, Sonnenborn U. *Panax*. In Hänsel R, Keller K, Rimpler H, Schneider G, editors. Hagers Handbuch der Pharmazeutischen Praxis, 5th ed. Volume 6: Drogen P-Z. Berlin: Springer-Verlag, 1994:12-34.

3. Shibata S, Tanaka O, Shoji J, Saito H. Chemistry and pharmacology of *Panax*. In Wagner H, Hikino H, Farnsworth NR, editors. Economic and Medicinal Plant Research, Volume 1. London: Academic Press, 1985: 217-84.

4. Sticher O, Soldati F. HPLC separation and quantitative determination of ginsenosides from *Panax ginseng, Panax quinquefolium* and from ginseng drug preparations. 1. Planta Medica 1979;36:30-42.

5. Soldati F, Sticher O. HPLC separation and quantitative determination of ginsenosides from *Panax ginseng, Panax quinquefolium* and from ginseng drug preparations. 2. Planta Medica 1979;39:348-57.

6. Bruneton J. Ginseng, *Panax ginseng* C.A. Meyer, Araliaceae. In: Pharmacognosy, Phytochemistry, Medicinal Plants. Paris: Lavoisier, 1995:563-5.

7. Cui JF. Identification and quantification of ginsenosides in various commercial ginseng preparations. Eur J Pharm Sci 1995;3:77-85.

8. Sprecher E. Ginseng - Wunderdroge oder Phytopharmakon? Dtsch Apoth Ztg 1987;9:52-61.

9. Tang W, Eisenbrand G. *Panax ginseng* C.A. Mey. In: Chinese Drugs of Plant Origin. Berlin: Springer-Verlag, 1992:711-37.

10. Corthout J, Naessens T, Apüers S, Vlietinck AJ. Quantitative determination of ginsenosides from *Panax ginseng* roots and ginseng preparations by thin layer chromatography-densitometry. J Pharmaceut Biomed Analysis 1999;21:187-92.

11. Hallstrom C, Fulder S, Carruthers M. Effects of ginseng on the performance of nurses on night duty. Compar Med East West 1982;6:277-82.

12. D'Angelo L, Grimaldi R, Caravaggi M, Marcoli M, Perucca E, Lecchini S, Frigo GM, Crema A. A double-blind, placebo-controlled clinical study on the effect of a standardized ginseng extract on psychomotor performance in healthy volunteers. J Ethnopharmacol 1986;16:15-22.

13. Van Schepdael P. Les effets du ginseng G115 sur la capacité physique de sportifs d'endurance. Acta Ther 1993;19:337-47.

14. Forgo I, Kirchdorfer AM. Ginseng steigert die körperliche Leistung. Kreislaufphysiologische Untersuchungen an Spitzensportlern beweisen: Der Stoffwechsel wird aktiviert. Ärztl Praxis 1981;33:1784-6.

15. Forgo I. Wirkung von Pharmaka auf körperliche Leistung und Hormonsystem von Sportlern. Munch med Wochenschr 1983;125:822-4.

16. Forgo I, Schimert GC. Zur Frage der Wirkungsdauer des standardisierten Ginseng-Extraktes G115 bei gesunden Leistungssportlern. Notabene Medici 1985;15:636-40.

17. Sotaniemi EA, Haapakoski E, Rautio A. Ginseng therapy in non-insulin-dependent diabetic patients. Diabetes Care 1995;18:1373-5.

18. Janetzki K, Morreale AP. Probable interaction between warfarin and ginseng. Am J Health Syst Pharm 1997;54: 692-3.

19. Zhu M, Chan KW, Ng LS, Chang Q, Chang S, Li RC. Possible influences of ginseng on the pharmacokinetics and pharmacodynamics of warfarin in rats. J Pharm Pharmacol 1999;51:175-80.

20. Soldati F. Toxicological studies on ginseng. Proceedings of the 4th International Ginseng Symposium, September 18-20, 1984. Daejon, Korea.

21. Sonnenborn U, Hänsel R. Panax ginseng. In: De Smet PAGM, Keller K, Hänsel R, Chandler RF, editors. Adverse Effects of Herbal Drugs, Volume 1. Berlin: Springer-Verlag, 1992:179-92.

22. Palmer BV, Montgomery ACV, Monteiro JCMP: Gin Seng and mastalgia. Br Med J 1978;279:1284.

23. Koriech OM. Ginseng and mastalgia. Br Med J 1978; 297:1556.

24. Punnonen R, Lukola A. Oestrogen-like effect of ginseng. Br Med J 1980;281:1110.

25. Forgo I, Kayasseh L, Staub JJ. Einfluß eines standardisierten Ginseng-Extraktes auf das Allgemein-befinden, die Reaktionsfähigkeit, Lungenfunktion und die gonadalen Hormone. Med Welt 1981;32:751-6.

26. Reinhold E. Der Einsatz von Ginseng in der Gynä-kologie. Natur- und GanzheitsMedizin 1990;4:131-4.

27. Büchi K, Jenny E. On the interference of the standardized ginseng extract G115 and pure ginsenosides with agonists of the progesterone receptor of the human myometrium. Pharmaton Report. 18 January 1984:3-11.

28. Siegel RK. Ginseng abuse syndrome. Problems with the panacea. JAMA 1979;241:1614-5.

29. Sonnenborn U. Ginseng-Nebenwirkungen: Fakten oder Vermutungen? Med Mo Pharm 1989;12:46-53.

30. Tyler V, editor. Chapter 12. Performance and immune deficiencies; performance and endurance enhancers; the ginsengs. In: Herbs of Choice. The Therapeutic Use of Phytomedicinals. Pharmaceutical Products Press: New York, 1994:171-4.

31. Ryu SJ, Chien YY. Ginseng-associated cerebral arteritis. Neurology 1995;45:829-30.

32. Wagner H, Nörr H, Winterhoff H. Plant adaptogens. Phytomedicine 1994;1:63-76.

33. Fulder S. The growth of cultured human fibroblasts treated with hydrocortisone and extracts of the medicinal plant Panax ginseng. Exp Gerontol 1977; 12:125-31.

34. Yamamoto M, Kumagai A, Yamamura Y. Stimulatory effect of Panax ginseng principles on DNA and protein synthesis in rat testes. Arzneim-Forsch/Drug Res 1977; 27:1404-5.

35. Yamasaki K, Murakami C, Ohtani K, Kasai R, Kurokawa T, Ishibashi S et al. Effects of the standardized Panax ginseng extract G115 on the D-glucose transport by Ehrlich ascites tumour cells. Phytotherapy Res 1993; 7:200-2.

36. Hassan Samira MM, Attia Attia M, Allam M, Elwan O. Effect of the standardized ginseng extract G115 on the metabolism and electrical activity of the rabbit's brain. J Int Med Res 1985;13:342-8.

37. See DM, Broumand N, Sahl L, Tilles JG. In vitro effects of echinacea and ginseng on natural killer and antibody-dependent cell cytotoxicity in healthy subjects and chronic fatigue syndrome or acquired immuno-deficiency syndrome patients. Immunopharmacology 1997;35:229-35.

38. Yamada H, Otsuka H, Kiyohara H. Fractionation and characterization of anticomplementary and mitogenic substances from Panax ginseng extract G 115. Phyto-therapy Res 1995;9:264-9.

39. Belogortseva NI, Yoon JY, Kim KH. Inhibition of Helicobacter pylori hemagglutination by poly-saccharide fractions from roots of Panax ginseng. Planta Med 2000;66:217-20.

40. Maffei Facino R, Carini M, Aldini G, Berti F, Rossoni G. Panax ginseng administration in the rat prevents myocardial ischemia-reperfusion damage induced by hyperbaric oxygen: evidence for an antioxidant intervention. Planta Med 1999;65:614-9.

41. Rimar S, Lee-Mengel M, Gillis CN. Pulmonary protective and vasodilator effects of a standardized Panax ginseng preparation following artificial gastric digestion. Pulmonary Pharmacol 1996;9:205-9.

42. Gillis N. Panax ginseng pharmacology: a nitric oxide link? Biochem Pharmacol 1997;54:1-8.

43. Singh VK, Agarwal SS, Gupta BM. Immunomodulatory activity of Panax ginseng extract. Planta Med 1984; 50:462-5.

44. Jie YH, Cammisuli S, Baggiolini M. Immunomodulatory effects of Panax ginseng C.A. Meyer in the mouse. Agents Actions 1984;15:386-91.

45. Hiai S, Yokoyama H, Oura H, Yano S. Stimulation of pituitary-adrenocortical system by ginseng saponin. Endocrinol Jpn 1979;26:661.

46. Hiai S, Sasaki S, Oura H. Effect of ginseng saponin on rat adrenal cyclic AMP. Planta Med 1979;37:15-9.

47. Avakian EV, Sugimoto RB, Taguchi S, Horvath SM. Effect of Panax ginseng extract on energy metabolism during exercise in rats. Planta Med 1984;50:151-4.

48. Alvarez AI, Voces J, Ferrando A, Vila L, Prieto JG. Muscle antioxidant response to ginseng extract G115 administration: Effects on different oxidative and glycolytic muscles in exhaustive exercise. XXXIII.

International Congress of Physiological Sciences IUPS. St. Petersburg, Russia, 30 June-5 July 1997.

49. Prieto JG, Voces J, Ferrando A, Vila L, Alvarez AI. Effects of extract G115 administration on antioxidant hepatic function after exhaustive exercise. XXXIII. International Congress of Physiological Sciences IUPS. St. Petersburg, Russia, 30 June-5 July 1997.

50. Petkov V. Effect of ginseng on the brain biogenic monoamines and $3',5'$-AMP system. Experiments on rats. Arzneim-Forsch 1978;28:338-9.

51. Bombardelli E, Cristoni A, Lietti A. The effect of acute and chronic ginseng saponins treatment on adrenals function: Biochemical and pharmacological aspects. In Korea Ginseng Research Inst., editor, Proceedings of 3rd International Ginseng Symposium. Seoul, Korea 1980:9-16.

52. Lewis WH, Zenger VE, Lynch RG. No adaptogen response of mice to *Ginseng* and *Eleutherococcus* infusions. J Ethnopharmacol 1983;8:209-14.

53. Martinez B, Staba, EJ. The physiological effects of *Aralia, Panax* and *Eleutherococcus* on exercised rats. Jap J Pharmacol 1984;35:79-85.

54. Han BH, Han YN, Park MH. Chemical and biochemical studies on antioxidant components of ginseng. In: Chang HM, Tso WW, Koo A, editors. Advances in Chinese Medicinal Materials Research. Singapore-Philadelphia: World Scientific, 1985:485-98.

55. Song ZJ, Johansen HK, Faber V, Høiby N. Ginseng treatment enhances bacterial clearance and decreases lung pathology in athymic rats with chronic *P. aeruginosa* pneumonia. APMIS (Copenhagen) 1997;105:438-44.

56. Matsuda H, Kubo M. Pharmacological study on *Panax ginseng* C.A. Meyer. II. Effect of red ginseng on the experimental gastric ulcer. Yakugaku Zasshi 1984; 104:449-53.

57. Kumazawa N, Ohta S, Ishizuka O, Sakurai N, Kamogawa A, Shinoda M. Protective effects of various methanol extracts of crude drugs on experimental hepatic injury induced by carbon tetrachloride in rats. Yakugaku Zasshi 1990;110:950-57.

58. Lin JH, Wu LS, Tsai KT, Leu SP, Jeang YF, Hsieh MT. Effects of *Ginseng* on the blood chemistry profile of dexamethasone-treated male rats. Am J Chin Med 1995;23:167-72.

59. Rosenfeld MS, Nachtajler SP, Schwartz TG, Sikorsky NM. Evaluation of the efficacy of a standardized ginseng extract in patients with psychophysical asthenia and neurological disorders. La Semana Médica 1989; 173:148-54.

60. Engels H-J, Wirth JC. No ergogenic effects of ginseng (*Panax ginseng* C.A. Meyer) during graded maximal aerobic exercise. J Am Diet Assoc 1997;97:1110-5.

61. Engels H-J, Said JM, Wirth JC. Failure of chronic ginseng supplementation to affect work performance

and energy metabolism in healthy adult females. Nutr Res 1996;16:1295-305.

62. Collomp K, Wright F, Collomp R, Shamari K, Bozzolan F, Préfaut C. Ginseng et exercice supramaximal. Science & Sports 1996;11:250-1.

63. Von Ardenne M, Klemm W. Measurements of the increase in the difference between the arterial and venous Hb-O_2 saturation obtained with daily administration of 200 mg standardized ginseng extract G115 for four weeks. Panminerva Med 1987;29:143-50.

64. Sørensen H, Sonne J. A double-masked study of the effects of ginseng on cognitive functions. Curr Ther Res 1996;57:959-68.

65. Smith K, Engels HJ, Martin J, Wirth JC. Efficacy of a standardized ginseng extract to alter psychological function characteristics at rest and during exercise stress. Med Sci Sports Exerc 1995;27(5,Suppl):S147.

66. Cherdrungsi P, Rungroeng K. Effects of standardized ginseng extract and exercise training on aerobic and anaerobic exercise capacities in humans. Korean J Ginseng Sci 1995;19:93-100.

67. Scaglione F, Ferrara F, Dugnani S, Falchi M, Santoro G, Fraschini F. Immunomodulatory effects of two extracts of *Panax ginseng* C.A. Meyer. Drugs Exptl Clin Res 1990;16:537-42.

68. Soldati F. Immunological studies of ginseng. Proceedings of 5th International Ginseng Symposium. Seoul, Korea. 1988:108-14.

69. Scaglione F, Cattaneo G, Alessandria M, Cogo R. Efficacy and safety of the standardized ginseng extract G115 for potentiating vaccination against common cold and/or influenza syndrome. Drugs Exptl Clin Res 1996;22:65-72.

70. Scaglione F, Cogo R, Cocuzza C, Arcidiano M, Beretta A. Immunomodulatory effects of *Panax ginseng* C.A. Meyer (G115) on alveolar macrophages from patients suffering with chronic bronchitis. Int J Immunotherapy 1994;10:21-4.

71. Gross D, Krieger D, Efrat R, Dayan M. Ginseng extract G115 for the treatment of chronic respiratory diseases. Schweiz Zschr GanzheitsMedizin 1995:29-33.

72. Srisurapanon S, Rungroeng K, Apibal S, Cherdrugsi P, Siripol R, Vanich-Angkul V, Timvipark C. The effect of standardized ginseng extract on peripheral blood leukocytes and lymphocyte subsets: a preliminary study in young healthy adults. J Med Assoc Thai 1997;80 (Suppl 1):S81-S85.

73. Vogler BK, Pittler MH, Ernst E. The efficacy of ginseng. A systematic review of randomised clinical trials. Eur J Clin Pharmacol 1999;55:567-75.

74. Chen SE, Sawchuk RJ, Staba EJ. American ginseng. III. Pharmacokinetics of ginsenosides in the rabbit. Eur J Drug Metab Pharmacokinet 1980;5:161-8.

75. Odani T, Tanizawa H, Takino Y. Studies on the

absorption, distribution, excretion and metabolism of ginseng saponins. II. The absorption, distribution and excretion of ginsenoside Rg_1 in the rat. Chem Pharm Bull 1983;31:292-8.

76. Odani T, Tanizawa H, Takino Y. Studies on the absorption, distribution, excretion and metabolism of ginseng saponins. III. The absorption, distribution and excretion of ginsenoside Rb_1 in the rat. Chem Pharm Bull 1983;31:1059-66.

77. Odani T, Tanizawa H, Takino Y. Studies on the absorption, distribution, excretion and metabolism of ginseng saponins. IV. Decomposition of ginsenoside-Rg_1 and -Rb_1 in the digestive tract of rats. Chem Pharm Bull 1983;31:3691-7.

78. Jenny E, Soldati F. Pharmacokinetics of ginsenosides in the mini-pig. In: Chang HM, Tso WW, Koo A, editors. Advances in Chinese Medicinal Materials Research. Singapore-Philadelphia: World Scientific, 1985.

79. Strömbom J, Sandberg F, Dencker L. Studies on absorption and distribution of ginsenoside Rg_1 by whole-body autoradiography and chromatography. Acta Pharm Suec 1985;22:113-22.

80. Karikura M, Miyase T, Tanizawa H, Takino Y, Taniyama T, Hayashi T. Studies on absorption, distribution, excretion and metabolism of ginseng saponins. V. The decomposition products of ginsenoside Rb_2 in the large intestine of rats. Chem Pharm Bull 1990;38:2859-61.

81. Karikura M, Miyase T, Tanizawa H, Taniyama T, Takino Y. Studies on absorption, distribution, excretion and metabolism of ginseng saponins. VI. The decomposition products of ginsenoside Rb_2 in the stomach of rats. Chem Pharm Bull 1991;39:400-4.

82. Karikura M, Miyase T, Tanizawa H, Taniyama T, Takino Y. Studies on absorption, distribution, excretion and metabolism of ginseng saponins. VII. Comparison of the decomposition modes of ginsenoside-Rb_1 and -Rb_2 in the digestive tract of rats. Chem Pharm Bull 1991;39:2357-61.

83. Cui JF, Björkhem I, Eneroth P. Dose-dependent urinary excretion of 20(S)-protopanaxadiol and 20(S)-protopanaxatriol glycosides in man after ingestion of ginseng preparations - a pilot study. In: Cui JF: Analysis of Ginsenosides [Thesis]. Stockholm: Karolinska Institute, 1995.

84. Cui JF, Garle M, Björkhem I, Eneroth P. Determination of aglycones of ginsenosides in ginseng preparations sold in Sweden and in urine samples from Swedish athletes consuming ginseng. Scand J Clin Lab Invest 1996;56:151-60.

85. Hasegawa H, Sung J-H, Benno Y. Role of human intestinal *Prevotella oris* in hydrolyzing ginseng saponins. Planta Med 1997;63:436-40.

86. Kim H-S, Hong Y-T, Jang C-G. Effects of the ginsenosides Rg_1 and Rb_1 on morphine-induced hyperactivity and reinforcement in mice. J Pharm Pharmacol 1998;50:555-60.

HAMAMELIDIS AQUA

Hamamelis Water

DEFINITION

Hamamelis water is a clear, colourless distillate prepared from recently cut and partially dried dormant twigs of *Hamamelis virginiana* L.

The material complies with the monograph of the United States Pharmacopeia [1].

CONSTITUENTS

From 1 kg of partially dried dormant twigs the USP method of preparation yields approximately 1 litre (980 g) of hamamelis water containing 14-15% of ethanol (added after distillation) [1]. Since it is obtained by a distillation process, the constituents are those of the volatile fraction, devoid of tannins [2].

Distillation of fresh twigs yielded 0.09% of volatile fraction on the dry weight basis, consisting of aliphatic hydrocarbons (45.4%, predominantly alkanes), terpenes (approx. 30%; mainly sesquiterpenes such as α-ylangene and monoterpenes such as linalool), phenylpropanoids (7.5%) such as *trans*-anethole and eugenol, and aliphatic aldehydes (6.1%) and alcohols (5.3%); over 160 compounds were detected [3,4].

Distillation of fresh leaves yielded 0.13% of volatile fraction on the dry weight basis consisting of aliphatic hydrocarbons (62.8%, predominantly alkanes), terpenes (21.1% including 3.7% of linalool and 9.8% of the acyclic diterpene *trans*-phytol), aliphatic aldehydes (3.8%) and fatty acids and fatty acid esters (3.6%); over 170 compounds were detected [3,4].

CLINICAL PARTICULARS

Therapeutic indications

External use
Treatment of bruises, skin irritations, sunburn, insect bites, external haemorrhoids [2,5-11]. Minor inflammatory conditions of the skin and mucosa [2,5-8].

Posology and method of administration

Dosage

External use
For compresses: Hamamelis water undiluted or diluted 1:3 with water; in semi-solid preparations, 20-30% [2,6-12]. Apply as often as required [5].

E/S/C/O/P
MONOGRAPHS
Second Edition

For mucosa: Hamamelis water undiluted or diluted with water, several times daily [2].

Method of administration
For local application.

Duration of administration
No restriction.

Contra-indications
None known.

Special warnings and special precautions for use
None required.

Interaction with other medicaments and other forms of interaction
None reported.

Pregnancy and lactation
No data available.

Effects on ability to drive and use machines
None known.

Undesirable effects
Although the content of volatile fraction is very low, allergic reactions of the skin may occur in very rare cases [2,5].

Overdose No toxic effects reported.

PHARMACOLOGICAL PROPERTIES

Pharmacodynamic properties
In the following text, material prepared by distillation of partially dried dormant twigs of *Hamamelis virginiana* and complying with the monograph for Witch Hazel USP [1] (or Hamamelis Water BPC 1973 [13], which is essentially similar) is described as 'hamamelis water'. Material prepared by distillation of fresh leaves and twigs of *Hamamelis virginiana* is described as 'hamamelis distillate'.

Pharmacological studies in humans

Anti-inflammatory effect
The activity of hamamelis distillate against erythema was evaluated in creams with two concentrations of the drug (standardized to 0.64 mg or 2.56 mg of hamamelis ketones per 100 g) and two different vehicles: oil-in-water emulsions, with or without phosphatidylcholine (PC). The effects were compared with those of hydrocortisone 1% cream, four base preparations and an untreated control area in two randomized, double-blind studies, each involving 24 healthy volunteers; in one study erythema was induced by UV irradiation, in the other by repeated stripping of the horny layer with adhesive tape. 24 hours after

UV-irradiation noteworthy reductions in erythema were observed only after use of low dose hamamelis-PC cream and hydrocortisone 1% cream, more pronounced from the latter. Erythema 4-8 hours after stripping of the horny layer was significantly suppressed by hydrocortisone cream, while less pronounced but noteworthy reductions were observed with low and high dose hamamelis-PC creams. The results demonstrated some anti-inflammatory activity of hamamelis distillate in a PC-containing vehicle. A four-fold increase of drug concentration did not, however, increase activity [6].

The anti-inflammatory effects of an aftersun lotion containing 10% of hamamelis water, in comparison with the corresponding vehicle, were tested in 30 healthy volunteers using a UV-B erythema test at four different UV-B intensities. Chromametry was used to compare the degrees of erythema in treated areas of skin with those in irradiated but untreated control areas 7, 24 and 48 hours after irradiation. Erythema suppression ranged from approx. 20% at 7 hours to 27% after 48 hours in the hamamelis water-treated areas, and from 10% at 7 hours to 12% after 48 hours in areas treated with the vehicle. Hamamelis water led to a highly significant reduction in erythema compared to the vehicle ($p = 0.00001$) and untreated, irradiated skin ($p = 0.00001$) [8].

Hamamelis distillate ointment applied to the skin of 22 healthy volunteers, and also 5 patients suffering from atopic neurodermitis and psoriasis, had a mild anti-inflammatory effect, causing a decrease in blood circulation as indicated by measurements of the thermal conductivity of the skin (fluvography) [7].

Clinical studies

Analgesic effect
In a randomised, open study involving 300 postnatal mothers, three topical agents were evaluated for their efficacy in achieving analgesia for episiotomy pain following instrumental (forceps) vaginal delivery: hamamelis water, or ice or a foam containing hydro-cortisone acetate 1% and pramoxine hydrochloride 1%. Oral analgesics were permitted and taken to the same extent in all three groups. According to data collected from 266 women, the three topical agents were equally effective in achieving analgesia, with no significant differences on day 1, although from subjective and professional assessment about one-third of all mothers derived little benefit from any agent. On days 3 and 5 ice tended to be better. 126 mothers were further assessed after 6 weeks; no differences were found between the three groups in terms of healing, pain and intercourse patterns [12].

Dermatological conditions
In a randomized, double-blind study, 22 patients suffering from atopic dermatitis were treated on one

forearm with an ointment containing hamamelis distillate (25 g/100 g) and on the other forearm with bufexamac ointment (50 mg/g) three times daily for 3 weeks. From assessment of symptoms such as reddening, scaling, lichenification, itching and infiltration no statistical difference was observed between the two treatments; both forearms showed clear improvements [9].

In a randomized, double-blind, paired trial, 72 patients suffering from moderately severe atopic eczema were treated for 2 weeks with a cream containing hamamelis distillate (5.35 g/100g), or the corresponding vehicle-only cream, or hydrocortisone 0.5% cream. The reduction in total scores for three basic criteria, itching, erythema and scaling, was significantly greater (p<0.0001) following application of hydrocortisone in comparison with hamamelis distillate, while the score for the hamamelis preparation did not differ from that of the vehicle [10].

In another double-blind study, 116 patients with eczema of different aetiologies were treated with either ointment A containing hamamelis distillate (25 g/100g) or hamamelis preparation B (not defined, but presumed to contain distillate) as a control, or both preparations (applied to different hands), several times daily for 4-6 weeks. Improvements in the symptoms of itching, burning sensations, infiltration, reddening and scaling were observed in the majority of cases with both preparations; ointment A gave superior results with endogenous eczema but not with toxic-degenerative eczema [11].

REFERENCES

1.   Witch Hazel. United States Pharmacopeia.

2.   Hoffmann-Bohm K, Ferstel W, Aye R-D. Hamamelis. In: Hänsel R, Keller K, Rimpler H, Schneider G, editors. Hagers Handbuch der pharmazeutischen Praxis, 5th ed, Volume 5: Drogen E-O. Berlin: Springer-Verlag, 1993:367-84.

3.   Engel R, Gutmann M, Hartisch C, Kolodziej H, Nahrstedt A. Study on the composition of the volatile fraction of Hamamelis virginiana. Planta Med 1998;64:251-8.

4.   Hartisch C. Isolierung, Strukturaufklärung und antiinflammatorische Wirksamkeit von Polyphenolen aus Hamamelis virginiana L. sowie Analyse der wasserdampfflüchtigen Fraktion aus dem Cortexmaterial [Dissertation]. Freie Universität Berlin, 1996.

5.   Witch Hazel. Federal Register 1982;47:180-1.

6.   Korting HC, Schäfer-Korting M, Hart H, Laux P, Schmid M. Anti-inflammatory activity of hamamelis distillate applied topically to the skin. Influence of vehicle and dose. Eur J Clin Pharmacol 1993;44:315-8.

7.   Sorkin B. Hametum Salbe, eine kortikoidfreie anti-inflammatorische Salbe. Phys Med Rehab 1980;21:53-7.

8.   Hughes-Formella BJ, Bohnsack K, Rippke F, Benner G, Rudolph M, Tausch I, Gassmueller J. Anti-inflammatory effect of hamamelis lotion in a UVB erythema test. Dermatology 1998;196:316-22.

9.   Swoboda M, Meurer J. Therapie von Neurodermitis mit Hamamelis-virginiana-Extrakt in Salbenform. Eine Doppelblindstudie. Z Phytotherapie 1991;12:114-7.

10. Korting HC, Schäfer-Korting M, Klövekorn W, Klövekorn G, Martin C, Laux P. Comparative efficacy of hamamelis distillate and hydrocortisone cream in atopic eczema. Eur J Clin Pharmacol 1995;48:461-5.

11. Pfister R. Zur Problematik der Behandlung und Nachbehandlung chronischer Dermatosen. Eine klinische Studie über Hametum Salbe. Fortschr Med 1981;99:1264-8.

12. Moore W, James DK. A random trial of three topical analgesic agents in the treatment of episiotomy pain following instrumental vaginal delivery. J Obstet Gynaecol 1989;10:35-9.

13. Pharmaceutical Society of Great Britain. Hamamelis Water. In: British Pharmaceutical Codex 1973, London: Pharmaceutical Press, 1973:825.

HAMAMELIDIS CORTEX

Hamamelis Bark

DEFINITION

Hamamelis bark consists of the dried bark from stems and branches of *Hamamelis virginiana* L., collected in spring. It contains not less than 4.0% of hide powder-precipitable tannins, expressed as pyrogallol ($C_6H_6O_3$; M_r 126.1) and calculated with reference to the dried drug.

The material complies with the monograph of the Deutscher Arzneimittel-Codex [1] or the British Herbal Pharmacopoeia [2].

CONSTITUENTS

The main characteristic constituent is hamameli-tannin, a mixture of the α- and β-forms of 2',5-di-O-galloyl-hamamelose [1-8]. Proanthocyanidins are also present including: procyanidin dimers such as catechin-(4α→8)-catechin, 3-O-galloyl-epicatechin-(4β→8)-catechin [6-9] and epicatechin-(4β→8)-catechin-3-O-(4-hydroxy)benzoate; prodelphinidins such as epigallocatechin-(4β→8)-catechin, 3-O-galloyl epigallocatechin-(4β→8)-catechin and 3-O-galloyl epigallocatechin-(4β→8)-gallocatechin [9]; and proanthocyanidin oligomers consisting of 4-9 catechin/gallocatechin units, some of which are 3-O-galloylated [9-11].

Other constituents include flavan-3-ols such as (+)-catechin, (+)-gallocatechin, (–)-epicatechin-3-O-gallate, and (–)-epigallocatechin-3-O-gallate [6,8]; di-and tri-O-galloyl-hamameloses and related 4-hydroxybenzoates [5,8,9], pentagalloyl glucose [6], gallic acid [6,7] and about 0.1% of volatile oil [3].

CLINICAL PARTICULARS

Therapeutic indications

Internal use
Inflammation of mucous membranes of the oral cavity [2-3,12,13].
Short-term symptomatic treatment of diarrhoea [2,13].

External use
Haemorrhoids [2-3,12-16], minor injuries and local inflammations of the skin [3,12,13,16].
Symptomatic treatment of problems related to varicose veins, such as painful and heavy legs [3,12,15].

E/S/C/O/P
MONOGRAPHS
Second Edition

Posology and method of administration

Dosage

Internal use

2-10 g of the drug daily as a decoction, used as a mouthwash [3,12,15], or 2-3 g daily as a tea [12]. 2-4 ml of tincture, used diluted as a mouthwash 3 times daily [2].
Other preparations: the equivalent of 0.1-1 g of the drug, 1-3 times daily [3,12].

External use

5-10 g of the drug as a decoction in 250 ml of water [3].
Extracts in semi-solid or liquid preparations corresponding to 20-30% of the drug [3].

Method of administration

For oral administration or local application.

Duration of administration

No restriction. Medical advice should be sought if diarrhoea persists for more than 4 days.

Contra-indications

None known.

Special warnings and special precautions for use

None required.

Interaction with other medicaments and other forms of interaction

None reported.

Pregnancy and lactation

No data available. In accordance with general medical practice, the product should not be used internally during pregnancy and lactation without medical advice.

Effects on ability to drive and use machines

None known.

Undesirable effects

None known from topical application [17]. In sensitive persons, stomach irritation may occasionally occur after intake of hamamelis bark preparations [3].

Overdose

No toxic effects reported.

PHARMACOLOGICAL PROPERTIES

Pharmacodynamic properties

In vitro experiments

Astringent effect
The astringent effect of a tincture (1:3; 62% ethanol)

prepared from fresh hamamelis bark was demonstrated with hide powder [18].

Cytotoxic activity
After 4 days of incubation, polyphenols isolated from hamamelis stem and twig bark showed moderate cytotoxicity to GLC_4 lung carcinoma and COLO 320 cells. The 3-O-galloyl compounds were more effective than other compounds. IC_{50} values of galloyl compounds were between 38 μM and 110 μM for GLC_4 and between 18.3 μM and 90.8 μM for COLO 320 cells; almost complete inhibition of growth was observed at 200 μM [8].

Anti-inflammatory effects
In the lyso-PAF:acetyl-CoA acetyltransferase assay, hamamelitannin proved to be ineffective [10], but in the same assay a proanthocyanidin oligomer isolated from hamamelis bark showed inhibitory potential [8,10]. A range of compounds from hamamelis bark had an inhibitory effect on 5-lipoxygenase (from a cytosol fraction of RBL-1 cells), galloyl compounds showing greater potency than other substances; hamamelitannin had the strongest effect with an IC_{50} of 1.0 μM [8,10].

Anti-inflammatory effects of polyphenols isolated from hamamelis stem and twig bark were evaluated in human polymorphonucleocytes (PMNs) and human macrophages. With the exception of hamamelitannin, all the tested substances inhibited the synthesis of platelet activating factor (PAF) in human PMNs. Dimeric galloylated proanthocyanidins showed the strongest effects with IC_{50} values of 7.8 and 6.4 μM. The synthesis of leukotriene B_4 (LTB_4) in PMNs was inhibited by the tested substances. Oligomeric proanthocyanidins had stronger activity (IC_{50}: 1.5 μM) than hamamelitannin, which had the weakest effect (IC_{50}: 12.5 μM). The polyphenols were shown to inhibit zymosan-induced luminol-dependent chemiluminescence in human macrophages, with galloylated proanthocyanidins having stronger effects (IC_{50}: 2.3 and 2.0 μM) than hamamelitannin (IC_{50}: 10.5 μM) [8].

Antiviral activity
Hamamelitannin and fractions obtained by ultrafiltration from a hydroethanolic extract of hamamelis bark exhibited antiviral activity against *Herpes simplex* virus type 1 (HSV-1) in monkey kidney cells. After 2-3 days the ED_{50} of hamamelitannin for antiviral activity was 26 μg/ml, compared to 6.3 μg/ml for a fraction consisting mainly of oligomeric to polymeric proanthocyanidins and 0.42 μmol/ml for acyclovir as a positive control [19].

Radical-scavenging effects
A dry 50%-ethanolic extract from hamamelis bark exhibited active-oxygen scavenging activity, determined by an electron spin resonance (ESR) spin-

trapping technique, with IC_{50} values of 0.17 µg/ml for superoxide anions, 7.79 µg/ml for hydroxyl radicals and 44.08 µg/ml for singlet oxygens, compared to 4.10, 3.30 and 21.18 µg/ml respectively for ascorbic acid. The extract at 50 µg/ml also protected murine dermal fibroblasts from cell damage induced by active-oxygen, increasing the survival rate to 69.0% (p<0.01) compared to about 15% for the control [20].

A suppressive effect of hamamelitannin against depolymerization of hyaluronic acid (induced by a xanthine/xanthine oxidase system) was demonstrated by measuring the viscosity of a 0.9 mg/ml solution; the inhibitory rate was 73.8% for hamamelitannin compared to 24.7% for ascorbic acid and 84.4% for superoxide dismutase [21].

The radical scavenging properties of hamamelitannin and gallic acid were evaluated in further experiments using ESR spin-trapping. For superoxide anion scavenging, the IC_{50} values were 1.31 µM for hamamelitannin and 1.01 µM for gallic acid, compared to 23.31 µM for ascorbic acid [21-23]. In hydroxyl radical scavenging, hamamelitannin gave the lowest IC_{50} of 5.46 µM, compared to 78.04 µM for gallic acid and 86.46 µM for propyl gallate (a well-known anti-oxidant). In singlet oxygen scavenging, the IC_{50} values of hamamelitannin and gallic acid were 45.51 µM and 69.81 µM respectively, compared to 66.66 µM for propyl gallate [22].

Hamamelitannin was also found to have antioxidative and scavenging activities against organic radicals such as 1,1-diphenyl-2-picrylhydrazyl (DPPH). Expressed as an index number (the number of mol required to scavenge one mol of DPPH), hamamelitannin and gallic acid gave results of 9.4 and 8.8 respectively, compared to 2.2 for DL-α-tocopherol and 2.0 for ascorbic acid [22].

The protective activities of hamamelitannin and gallic acid on cell damage induced by superoxide anion radicals, were evaluated in a cell-culture system using murine fibroblasts. Hamamelitannin and gallic acid showed significant protective activity against superoxide radicals at minimum concentrations of 50 µM and 100 µM respectively (p<0.01) [22,23]; at 50 µM, hamamelitannin enhanced the survival of fibroblasts to 52.4% compared to 36.9% for the control [23]. Pre-treatment of fibroblasts with hamamelitannin at 200 µM for 24 hours at 37°C before exposure to superoxide anions increased cell survival to 63.8%, compared to 25.4% for gallic acid and 19.0% for the control. Further observations confirmed that hamamelitannin is superior to gallic acid in protecting against cell damage induced by superoxide anions and suggested that the high affinity of hamamelitannin for cells or membranes may be an important factor for protecting cells against active oxygen species [23].

In contrast, against cell damage induced in murine fibroblasts by hydroxyl radicals, hamamelitannin showed protective activity at a minimum concentration of 500 µM whereas gallic acid was effective at 50 µM. Against cell damage induced by singlet oxygens hamamelitannin at 100 µM enhanced survival to 80.6% (p<0.01), while gallic acid had no significant effect at 100 µM and required 500 µM to enhance survival to 98.6% (p<0.01) compared to 60.4% survival for controls [22].

Hamamelitannin and a fraction of molecular weight < 3 kDa obtained by ultrafiltration from a hydroethanolic hamamelis bark extract were found to have greater radical scavenging activity (ED_{50} values of 29 and 80 ng/ml respectively) than a higher molecular weight procyanidin fraction (≥ 3 kDa; ED_{50} 160 ng/ml) as quantified by the emission of chemiluminescence during autoxidation of mouse brain lipids [19].

Antimutagenic activity
In the Ames mutagenicity test, a tincture (1:5) and a methanolic extract (1:5) of hamamelis bark dose-dependently inhibited 2-nitrofluorene-induced mutagenicity in *Salmonella typhimurium* TA98, by 60% and 54% respectively at 100 µl/plate. It was demonstrated that the antimutagenic effect increased with increasing degree of polymerisation of pro-anthocyanidins, the most active fraction consisting of catechin and gallocatechin oligomers with an average degree of polymerization of 9.2 [11].

In vivo experiments

Anti-inflammatory effect
A hydroethanolic extract of hamamelis bark showed a significant anti-inflammatory effect (43% inhibition of oedema; p<0.05) in the croton oil ear oedema test in mice when applied topically at 250 µg per ear. After ultrafiltration of the crude extract, this effect was shown to be mainly due to proanthocyanidins of molecular weight ≥ 3 kDa (69% inhibition at 250 µg per ear; p<0.05); proanthocyanidins of lower molecular weight had no effect and hamamelitannin produced only 7% inhibition [19].

Clinical studies
In a double-blind, three-arm comparative study, 90 patients with first-degree haemorrhoids were treated for 14-21 days with an ointment containing hamamelis bark fluid extract (3% m/m) and basic bismuth gallate (n = 30), or metacresolsulphonic acid-formaldehyde ointment (n = 30) or ointment containing the corticosteroid fluocinolone acetonide (n = 30); all three preparations also contained a local anaesthetic. Follow-up examinations were performed on days 3, 7, 14 and 21 of treatment. At the end of treatment, the levels of improvement in four target criteria (pruritus, bleeding, burning sensation and pain) assessed by both physicians and patients were 73.9-94.4% in

patients using the ointment containing hamamelis bark, compared to 76.2-89.5% in those treated with metacresol-sulphonic acid-formaldehyde and 72.0-81.8% in those treated with fluocinolone acetonide. All three preparations were considered highly effective with no major differences between groups [14].

REFERENCES

1. Hamamelisrinde - Hamamelidis cortex. In: Deutscher Arzneimittel-Codex.

2. Hamamelis Bark. In: British Herbal Pharmacopoeia.

3. Hänsel R, Keller K, Rimpler H, Schneider G, editors. Hamamelis. In: Hagers Handbuch der pharmazeutischen Praxis, 5th ed. Volume 5: Drogen E-O. Berlin: Springer-Verlag, 1993:367-84.

4. Mayer W, Kunz W, Loebich F. Die Struktur des Hamamelitannins. Liebigs Ann Chem 1965;688:232-8.

5. Haberland C, Kolodziej H. Novel galloylhamameloses from Hamamelis virginiana. Planta Med 1994;60:464-6.

6. Friedrich H, Krüger N. Neue Untersuchungen über den Hamamelis-Gerbstoff. I. Der Gerbstoff der Rinde von H. virginiana Planta Med 1974;25:138-48.

7. Vennat B, Pourrat H, Pouget MP, Gross D, Pourrat A. Tannins from Hamamelis virginiana: Identification of proanthocyanidins and hamamelitannin quantification in leaf, bark and stem extracts. Planta Med 1988;54: 454-7.

8. Hartisch C. Isolierung, Strukturaufklärung und antiinflammatorische Wirksamkeit von Polyphenolen aus Hamamelis virginiana L. sowie Analyse der wasserdampfflüchtigen Fraktion aus dem Cortexmaterial [Dissertation]. Freien Universität Berlin, 1996.

9. Hartisch C, Kolodziej H. Galloylhamameloses and proanthocyanidins from Hamamelis virginiana. Phytochemistry 1996;42:191-8.

10. Hartisch C, Kolodziej H, von Bruchhausen F. Dual inhibitory activities of tannins from Hamamelis virginiana and related polyphenols on 5-lipoxygenase and lyso-PAF:acetyl-CoA acetyltransferase. Planta Med 1997;63:106-10.

11. Dauer A, Metzner P, Schimmer O. Proanthocyanidins from the bark of Hamamelis virginiana exhibit antimutagenic properties against nitroaromatic compounds. Planta Med 1998;64:324-7.

12. Czygan F-C. Hamamelidis cortex. Hamamelisrinde. In: Wichtl M, editor. Teedrogen und Phytopharmaka, 3rd ed. Stuttgart: Wissenschaftliche Verlagsgesellschaft, 1997:270-2.

13. Laux P, Oschmann R. Die Zaubernuß - Hamamelis virginiana L. Z. Phytotherapie 1993;14:155-66.

14. Knoch H-G, Klug W, Hübner W-D. Salbenbehandlung von Hämorrhoiden ersten Grades. Wirksamkeitsvergleich eines Präparats auf pflanzlicher Grundlage mit zwei nur synthetische Wirkstoffe enthaltenden Salben. Fortschr Med. 1992;110:135-8.

15. Van Hellemont J. In: Fytotherapeutisch compendium. Utrecht: Bohn, Scheltema & Holkema, 1988:284-6.

16. Reynolds JEF, editor. Hamamelis Bark. In: Martindale - The Extra Pharmacopoeia, 28th ed. London: Pharmaceutical Press, 1982:265.

17. Hörmann HP, Korting HC. Evidence for the efficacy and safety of topical herbal drugs in dermatology. Part I: Anti-inflammatory agents. Phytomedicine 1994; 1:161-71.

18. Gracza L. Adstringierende Wirkung von Phytopharmaka. Dtsch Apoth Ztg 1987;127:2256-8.

19. Erdelmeier CAJ, Cinatl J, Rabenau H, Doerr HW, Biber A, Koch E. Antiviral and antiphlogistic activities of Hamamelis virginiana bark. Planta Med 1996;62:241-5.

20. Masaki H, Sakaki S, Atsumi T, Sakurai H. Active-oxygen scavenging activity of plant extracts. Biol Pharm Bull 1995;18:162-6.

21. Masaki H, Atsumi T, Sakurai H. Evaluation of superoxide scavenging activities of Hamamelis extract and hamamelitannin. Free Rad Res Comms 1993;19:333-40.

22. Masaki H, Atsumi T, Sakurai H. Hamamelitannin as a new potent active oxygen scavenger. Phytochemistry 1994;37:337-43.

23. Masaki H, Atsumi T, Sakurai H. Protective activity of hamamelitannin on cell damage induced by superoxide anion radicals in murine dermal fibroblasts. Biol Pharm Bull 1995;18:59-63.

HAMAMELIDIS FOLIUM

Hamamelis Leaf

E/S/C/O/P
MONOGRAPHS
Second Edition

DEFINITION

Hamamelis leaf consists of the whole or cut, dried leaf of *Hamamelis virginiana* L. It contains not less than 3 per cent of tannins, expressed as pyrogallol ($C_6H_6O_3$; M_r 126.1) and calculated with reference to the dried drug.

The material complies with the monograph of the European Pharmacopoeia [1].

CONSTITUENTS

The main characteristic constituents are tannins (5-10%) [2], including condensed tannins (mainly proanthocyanidin oligomers with catechin and/or gallocatechin units) and hydrolysable gallotannins, notably a small amount of hamamelitannin [3-5]. (+)-Catechin, (+)-gallocatechin, (–)-epicatechin-gallate and (–)-epigallocatechingallate are also present [6].

Other constituents include flavonoids such as kaempferol, quercetin, quercitrin, isoquercitrin and myricetin; phenolic acids such as caffeic acid and gallic acid [3,7-9]; and a volatile fraction, 0.04-0.14% [10], containing aliphatic hydrocarbons (63%), mono- and sesquiterpenes (11%) and aldehydes and ketones (4.6%) among over 170 compounds detected [11].

CLINICAL PARTICULARS

Therapeutic indications

Internal use
Symptomatic treatment of complaints related to varicose veins, such as painful and heavy legs, and of haemorrhoids [7-9,12,13].

External use
Bruises, sprains and minor injuries of the skin [7,8,14].
Local inflammations of the skin and mucosa [7-9].
Haemorrhoids [7,8,15].
Relief of the symptoms of neurodermitis atopica [16] and feeling of heavy legs [7].

Posology and method of administration

Dosage

Internal use
Adults: 2-3 g of drug as infusion [7] or 2-4 ml of liquid extract (1:1, 45% ethanol), three times daily [15].

External use

Extracts in semisolid or liquid preparations, containing 5-10% of drug [7].

Decoctions, 5-10 g of drug per 250 ml water for compresses or washes [7].

Suppositories containing 200 mg of dried extract, 1-2 per day [14].

Ointment containing 10% of liquid extract [14].

Method of administration

For oral administration and topical application.

Duration of administration

If symptoms persist or worsen, medical advice should be sought.

Contra-indications

None known.

Special warnings and special precautions for use

None required.

Interaction with other medicaments and other forms of interaction

None reported.

Pregnancy and lactation

No data available. In accordance with general medical practice, the drug should not be used internally during pregnancy without medical advice.

Effects on ability to drive and use machines

None known.

Undesirable effects

In sensitive patients there is a possibility of stomach upsets after taking hamamelis leaf preparations [7].

Overdose

No toxic effects reported.

PHARMACOLOGICAL PROPERTIES

Pharmacodynamic properties

In vivo experiments

Venotonic activity was demonstrated in experiments where the dried residue (300 mg) from aqueous or various hydroethanolic extracts of hamamelis leaf was added to one litre of an isotonic dextran/water (60 g/litre) solution. This was perfused at constant pressure into the arteries of the hind quarters of rabbits (45-100 drops/min). Venoconstriction, measured in terms of output on the venous side, was reduced by up to 60-70% depending on the type of extract [17].

A dry 70%-ethanolic extract of hamamelis leaf, administered orally to rats at 200 mg/kg daily for 19 days, significantly inhibited paw swelling (p<0.05) in the chronic phase of adjuvant-induced arthritis but was not active against the acute phase of oedema [18].

Pharmacological studies in humans

In a study conducted on 30 human volunteers, topical application of a hydroglycolic extract of hamamelis leaf produced a significant reduction in skin temperature (p<0.001 after 5 min; p<0.03 after 60 min), which was interpreted as a vasoconstrictor effect [19].

Clinical studies

In a pilot study involving cases of neurodermitis atopica, hamamelis leaf extract incorporated into a cream was applied twice daily for 2 weeks in six groups of patients:

- Group I consisted of 7 children aged from 6 to 14 years with atopic neurodermitis on the feet (chilblains). After treatment the condition had considerably improved in all the patients.

- Group II consisted of 5 children with eczema in the flexure of the joints in subacute and chronic forms. After treatment 3 children were completely cured; in 2 children a considerable reduction of the inflamed condition and a clear reduction of the itch was noted.

- In Group III, which consisted of 10 adults with eczema in the flexure of the joints, 7 cases showed a good response and in three cases there was reasonable improvement.

- Group IV consisted of 5 adults with eczema of the neck and throat. 3 cases were completely cured and a remarkable reduction in symptoms was noted in the remaining 2 cases.

- Group V consisted of 3 adults with atopic eczema of the trunk. In one patient there was extensive healing and in the others a noticeable reduction of symptoms.

- Group VI consisted of 2 cases of atopic xerodermia. Following twice daily application of the cream, there was an improvement of the skin barrier situation and a clear diminution of desquamating pruritus in both cases [16].

Pharmacokinetic properties

No data available.

Preclinical safety data

Carcinogenicity

15 male and 15 female NIH black rats, 1-2 months old, were injected subcutaneously with a lyophilised aqueous leaf extract at a dosage of 10 mg (dissolved in 0.5 ml of normal saline solution) weekly for a period of 78 weeks; 30 animals were injected with normal saline solution only. The animals were observed for a period of 90 weeks. After about 73 weeks, three of the male rats developed malignant mesenchymoma, while in the control animals no tumours developed. The tumour rate was not considered to be significant [7].

REFERENCES

1. Hamamelis Leaf - Hamamelidis folium. European Pharmacopoeia, Council of Europe.

2. Wichtl M and Egerer HP. Hamamelisblätter. In: Hartke K, Hartke H, Mutschler E, Rücker G and Wichtl M, editors. Arzneibuch-Kommentar. Wissenschaftliche Erläuterungen zum Europäischen Arzneibuch und zum Deutschen Arzneibuch. Stuttgart: Wissenschaftliche Verlagsgesellschaft, 1999 (11 Lfg):H 6/1.

3. Vennat B, Gross D, Pourrat A, Pourrat H. *Hamamelis virginiana*: Identification and assay of proanthocyanidins, phenolic acids and flavonoids in leaf extracts. Pharm Acta Helv 1992;67:11-4.

4. Vennat B, Pourrat H, Pouget MP, Gross D, Pourrat A. Tannins from *Hamamelis virginiana*: Identification of proanthocyanidins and hamamelitannin quantification in leaf, bark and stem extracts. Planta Med 1988;54:454-6.

5. Scholz E. Pflanzliche Gerbstoffe. Pharmakologie und Toxikologie. Dtsch Apoth Ztg 1994;134:3167-79.

6. Friedrich H, Krüger N. Neue Untersuchungen über den Hamamelis-Gerbstoff. II. Der Gerbstoff der Blätter von *H. virginiana*. Planta Med 1974;26:327-32.

7. Hänsel R, Keller K, Rimpler H, Schneider G, editors. Hamamelis. In: Hagers Handbuch der Pharmazeutischen Praxis, 5th ed. Volume 5: Drogen E-O. Berlin-Heidelberg: Springer-Verlag, 1993:367-84.

8. Laux P, Oschmann R. Die Zaubernuß - *Hamamelis virginiana* L. Z Phytotherapie 1993;14:155-66.

9. Bernard P. Les feuilles d'hamamélis. Plantes Méd Phytothér 1977;11(Spécial):184-8.

10. Messerschmidt W. Zur Kenntnis des Wasserdampf-destillats der Blätter von *Hamamelis virginiana* L. 4. Mitteilung: Charakterisierung von Blattdroge und Destillat. Dtsch Apoth Ztg 1971; 111:299-301.

11. Engel R, Gutmann M, Hartisch C, Kolodziej H, Nahrstedt A. Study on the composition of the volatile fraction of *Hamamelis virginiana*. Planta Med 1998;64:251-8.

12. Hörmann HP, Korting HC. Evidence for the efficacy and safety of topical herbal drugs in dermatology: Part 1: Anti-inflammatory agents. Phytomedicine 1994; 1:161-71.

13. Van Hellemont J. Hamamelis virginiana L. In: Fytotherapeutisch compendium, 2nd ed. Houten, Netherlands: Bohn Stafleu Van Loghum, 1988:284-6.

14. Pharmaceutical Society of Great Britain. Hamamelis. In: British Pharmaceutical Codex 1973. London: Pharmaceutical Press 1973:218.

15. Hamamelis Leaf. In: British Herbal Pharmacopoeia 1983. Bournemouth: British Herbal Medicine Association, 1983:110.

16. Wokalek H. Zur Bedeutung epidermaler Lipide und des Arachidonsäurestoffwechsels bei Neurodermitis atopica. Deutsche Dermatologe 1993;5:498-506.

17. Bernard P, Balansard P, Balansard G, Bovis A. Valeur pharmacodynamique toniveineuse des préparations galéniques à base de feuilles d'hamamélis. J Pharm Belg 1972;27:505-12.

18. Duwiejua M, Zeitlin IJ, Waterman PG, Gray AI. Anti-inflammatory activity of *Polygonum bistorta*, *Guaiacum officinale* and *Hamamelis virginiana* in rats. J Pharm Pharmacol 1994;46:286-90.

19. Diemunsch A-M, Mathis C. Effet vasoconstricteur de l'hamamélis en application externe. STP Pharma 1987; 3:111-4.

HARPAGOPHYTI RADIX

Devil's Claw Root

E/S/C/O/P
MONOGRAPHS
Second Edition

DEFINITION

Devil's claw root consists of the cut and dried tuberous, secondary roots of *Harpagophytum procumbens* D.C. It contains not less than 1.2 per cent of harpagoside ($C_{24}H_{30}O_{11}$; M_r 494.5), calculated with reference to the dried drug [1].

The material complies with the monograph of the European Pharmacopoeia [1].

CONSTITUENTS

The characteristic constituents are iridoid glucosides, principally harpagoside (1-3%) [2-5] together with small amounts of harpagide, 8-*p*-coumaroylharpagide (0.03-0.13%), procumbide and its 6'-*p*-coumaroyl ester [3-7]. The phenolic glycosides acteoside (verbascoside) and isoacteoside [8], and sugars, mainly the tetrasaccharide stachyose (up to 46%) with smaller amounts of raffinose, sucrose and monosaccharides [9], are also present.

CLINICAL PARTICULARS

Therapeutic indications

Symptomatic treatment of painful osteoarthritis [10-18], relief of low back pain [19-23], loss of appetite and dyspepsia [24-30].

Posology and method of administration

Dosage

Painful osteoarthritis
Adult daily dose: 2-5 g of the drug or equivalent aqueous or hydroalcoholic extracts [11,13-15,17, 18].

Relief of low back pain
Adult daily dose: 4.5-9 g of the drug as dry extract equivalent to 30-100 mg of harpagoside [19-23].

Loss of appetite or dyspeptic complaints
Adult dose: 0.5 g of the drug in decoction, three times daily, or preparations with equivalent bitterness value [10,24]; tincture (1:10, 25% ethanol), 3 ml [10,25].

Elderly: dose as for adults.
Not recommended for children.

Method of administration
For oral administration.

Duration of administration

Treatment for at least 2-3 months is recommended in cases of painful osteoarthritis [11,14,16]. If symptoms persist consult a doctor.

Contra-indications

Gastric and duodenal ulcers [24,30].

Special warnings and special precautions for use

None required.

Interaction with other medicaments and other forms of interaction

None reported.

Pregnancy and lactation

No data available. In accordance with general medical practice, the product should not be used during pregnancy and lactation without medical advice.

Effects on ability to drive and use machines

None known.

Undesirable effects

Mild gastro-intestinal disturbances (e.g. diarrhoea, nausea, stomach upset) may occur in sensitive individuals especially at higher dosage levels [14,16,19].

Overdose

No toxic effects reported.

PHARMACOLOGICAL PROPERTIES

Pharmacodynamic properties

The anti-inflammatory, analgesic, antiarrhythmic and hypotensive effects of devil's claw root and the iridoid glucoside harpagoside have been extensively investigated.

In vitro experiments

A crude methanolic extract of devil's claw root (1 mg and 2 mg, containing 0.085 mg and 0.17 mg of harpagoside respectively) and, to a lesser extent, pure harpagoside (0.085 mg and 0.17 mg) showed a significant, dose-dependent, protective action against arrhythmias induced by reperfusion in isolated rat hearts [31]. The same methanolic extract (1 mg) showed a protective effect against arrhythmias induced by calcium chloride and epinephrine-chloroform in isolated rabbit heart [32].

Following oral administration to 6 volunteers of 600 mg of devil's claw root extract containing ca. 25% harpagoside, the effect on biosynthesis of eicosanoids was studied ex vivo in samples of their blood. After stimulation with ionophore A23187 for 60 minutes, the synthesis of thromboxane B_2 (an indicator of the cyclooxygenase metabolic pathway) and leukotriene

C_4 (an indicator of the 5-lipoxygenase metabolic pathway) were measured by radio-immunoassay. Blood samples of all subjects revealed a time-dependent reversible inhibition of leukotriene C_4 biosynthesis with maximum inhibition of 50% after ca. 3 hours. The biosynthesis of thromboxane B_2 was not inhibited [33,34].

Human whole blood samples from healthy young males were pretreated with devil's claw root extracts containing 7.3% and 2.07% of harpagoside respectively, or pure harpagoside or BAY X1005 (a synthetic 5-lipoxygenase inhibitor used as a reference substance), stimulated with ionophore A23187 and incubated, then analyzed to compare their effects on the biosynthesis of cysteinyl leukotrienes (metabolites of the 5-lipoxygenase metabolic pathway) and thromboxane B_2 (metabolite of the cyclooxygenase metabolic pathway). BAY X1005 or harpagoside at 1-100 μM concentration-dependently inhibited the biosynthesis of cysteinyl leukotrienes with IC_{50} values of ca. 6.5 μM and 39.0 μM respectively. The devil's claw root extracts showed similar inhibition in proportion to their harpagoside contents (7.3% and 2.07%), with calculated harpagoside IC_{50} values of 9.2 μM and 61.7 μM respectively. Thus the extract with a harpagoside content of 7.3% produced more effective inhibition than pure harpagoside. With respect to the biosynthesis of thromboxane B_2 BAY X1005 did not show significant inhibition ($IC_{50} > 100$ μM); harpagoside and devil's claw root extract (7.3% harpagoside) gave harpagoside IC_{50} values of 48.6 μM and 55.3 μM respectively, while devil's claw root extract (2.07% harpagoside) gave a harpagoside IC_{50} of > 100 μM. An explanation of the observed effects could be that harpagoside effectively inhibits the biosynthesis of both cysteinyl leukotrienes and thromboxane B_2 in eicosanoid metabolic processes, but that devil's claw root extracts contain other substances which may, directly or indirectly, inhibit the biosynthesis of cysteinyl leukotrienes [34,35].

An endotoxin-free dry extract of devil's claw root, prepared with ethanol 60% V/V and containing 2.9% harpagoside, prevented lipopolysaccharide (LPS)-induced synthesis of tumour necrosis factor alpha (TNF-α) in stimulated primary human monocytes in a dose-dependent manner with an IC_{50} of about 100 μg/ml. Harpagoside and harpagide had no effect on LPS-induced TNF-α release between 0.01 μg/ml and 10 μg/ml [36].

In vivo experiments

Anti-inflammatory effects

In repeated dose studies (formaldehyde-, Freund adjuvant- and granuloma-induced experimental arthritis), extracts of devil's claw root appeared to be effective [37,38] although other studies have not confirmed these results [39-41]. In the croton oil-induced granuloma pouch test in rats the reduction in inflammation produced by 12-day intraperitoneal administration of harpagoside (20 mg/kg/day) [37] and by oral administration of aqueous and methanolic extracts of devil's claw root (200 mg/kg/day) [38] was similar to that of phenylbutazone. In the formaldehyde-induced arthritis test an effect comparable to that of phenylbutazone (40 mg/kg/day) was demonstrated with an aqueous extract of devil's claw root (20 mg/kg/day) after 10-day intraperitoneal administration, but no effect was apparent with harpagoside (50 mg/kg/day) [37]. Daily oral treatment with devil's claw root at a high dose level of 2 g/kg for 7 days produced no significant effect on secondary inflammatory reaction in the rat [41]. Adjuvant (*M. tuberculosis*)-induced arthritis was also unresponsive to treatment with a dry aqueous extract of devil's claw root (100 mg/kg/day) administered orally for 21 days in the rat [39].

No, or only slight, activity of devil's claw root or harpagoside in acute conditions (carrageenan-induced oedema etc.) has been found by several authors [37-42]. On the other hand, a 48% reduction in adriamycin-induced oedema in rats was obtained after oral administration of 37 mg/kg of powdered root containing 3.0% of iridoid glucosides [43].

Intraperitoneal pre-treatment of rats with a dry aqueous extract (2.2% harpagoside) of devil's claw root significantly reduced carrageenan-induced hind paw oedema, in a dose-dependent manner. Doses of 400 and 1200 mg/kg, corresponding to 665 and 2000 mg/kg of dried root, reduced oedema 3 hours after administration by 43% and 64% respectively. The efficacy of the 1200 mg/kg dose was similar to that of indometacin 10 mg/kg [4]. In the same model, a dry ethanolic extract (400 mg/kg) had an anti-inflammatory effect (68.8% inhibition) similar to that of phenyl-butazone (150 mg/kg) 4 hours after oedema induction [44]. Significant, dose-dependent, anti-inflammatory effects in the carrageenan-induced paw oedema test have also been demonstrated following intraperitoneal pre-treatment of rats with devil's claw root aqueous extract with a harpagoside content of 1.8% at dose levels of 100 mg/kg (38% inhibition) to 400 mg/kg (72% inhibition). The highest dose tested (400 mg/kg) was more effective than pre-treatment with 10 mg/kg of indometacin (58% inhibition). Pure harpagoside was ineffective in these experiments [45].

Another study using the carrageenan-induced rat paw oedema test assessed the anti-inflammatory activity of devil's claw root extracts when administered by different routes: dry aqueous extracts, prepared by lyophilization from cryoground fresh plant, without cyclodextrin (intraperitoneal administration) or with cyclodextrin (oral and intraduodenal administration). The results indicated that intraperitoneal pre-treatment of rats with doses of 200 and 400 mg of extract

significantly reduced carrageenan-induced oedema (p<0.001). Similarly, intraduodenal pre-treatment with 200, 400 and 1600 mg of extract significantly reduced oedema (p<0.01). In contrast, when administered orally (by gavage), the extracts were ineffective regardless of the dose used (200, 400, 800 and 1600 mg/kg) [46]. This is consistent with the results of an earlier study [45], which showed absence of activity after treating the extract with 0.1N hydrochloric acid, simulating acid conditions in the stomach.

Since these results support the inference that gastric degradation of active principles may occur, the use of oral preparations protected against degradation by stomach acid has been suggested [45,46].

Analgesic effects
A devil's claw root aqueous extract with a harpagoside content of 1.8% exhibited dose-dependent peripheral analgesic effects in the writhing test after intra-peritoneal administration to mice (47% protection at 100 mg/kg to 78% at 400 mg/kg). 53% protection at 200 mg/kg was similar to the 59% result obtained with acetylsalicylic acid at 68 mg/kg; pure harpagoside at 10 mg/kg produced 42% protection [45]. In earlier work using the rabbit ear test, intraperitoneal admin-istration of harpagoside (20 mg/kg) produced an analgesic effect comparable to that of phenylbutazone (50 mg/kg), but harpagoside (20 mg/kg) hydrolysed to its aglycone by emulsin and an aqueous extract of devil's claw root (20 mg/kg) showed no statistically significant effects [37]. The number of writhings and stretchings induced in rats by 1.2% acetic acid was significantly and dose-dependently reduced after intraperitoneal administration of devil's claw root dry aqueous extract (2.2% harpagoside); the protective effect was 35% at 400 mg/kg and reached 62% at 1200 mg/kg, compared to 59% with acetylsalicylic acid at 68 mg/kg [4].

In a Randall-Soletto test, the threshold of pain induced in rats by subplantar injection of 0.1 ml of 20% yeast solution was measured just before, 30 minutes after and 60 minutes after intraperitoneal administration of a devil's claw root dry ethanolic extract of undefined potency. 200 and 400 mg/kg of extract dose-dependently increased the pain threshold, the effect after 30 minutes (28.5% and 61.5% respectively) being greater than that after 60 minutes; 800 mg/kg produced no further increase. The effects were superior to those of diclofenac sodium at 80 mg/kg (11.1% increase after 30 minutes) [44].

Other workers found no consistent analgesic effects in mice after oral administration of various extracts and fractions from devil's claw root at 20 and 200 mg/kg [38].

Other effects
A dry 53%-ethanolic extract of devil's claw root was

administered intraperitoneally to rats at 100 mg/kg and 200 mg/kg bodyweight daily for 1, 7 or 14 days to investigate its antioxidant activity in comparison with selegiline (2 mg/kg). The extract induced an increase in brain frontal cortex and striatum superoxide dismutase, catalase and glutathione peroxidase activities, and decreased lipid peroxidation, in a dose-related manner. The effects, evident only after 7 days of treatment and accentuated after 14 days, were similar to responses induced by selegiline [47].

Both oral and intraperitoneal treatment of rats with a dry methanolic extract of devil's claw root containing 8.5% of harpagoside gave considerable protection against arrhythmias induced by calcium chloride or epinephrine-chloroform. An oral dose of 400 mg/kg of extract produced 50% more effective protection against calcium chloride-induced arrhythmia than an oral dose of 100 mg/kg of lidocaine. Pure harpagoside gave much weaker protection than extract containing equivalent amounts of harpagoside [32].

Pharmacological studies in humans

No significant effects on mediators of acute inflammation (prostaglandin E_2, thromboxane B_2, 6-ketoprostaglandin $F_1\alpha$ and leukotriene B_4) were evident in 25 healthy volunteers after a 3-week daily intake of 4 × 500 mg capsules of powdered devil's claw root containing 3% of iridoid glucosides. The subjects served as their own control and were also compared with a separate control group. It was concluded that devil's claw root does not produce the biochemical effects on arachidonic acid metabolism characteristic of anti-arthritic drugs of the non-steroidal anti-inflammatory type [48].

Clinical studies

Relief of arthrosic and arthritic conditions
In a double-blind, placebo-controlled study on ambulant volunteers with articular pains of rheumatic origin, the efficacy and tolerability of capsules containing 335 mg of powdered devil's claw root (3.0% iridoid glucosides) were assessed at a dosage of 3 × 2 capsules daily for 2 months. Clinical parameters measured on days 0, 30 and 60, severity of pain on a 0-10 scale and joint mobility determined by finger-to-floor distance during anteflexion of the trunk, revealed a significant drop in the intensity of pain (p<0.05) and a significant increase in spinal and coxofemoral mobility (p<0.05) in the verum group (n = 45) compared to the placebo group (n = 44) after 30 and 60 days. Neither side effects nor changes in biological parameters (including blood tests) were observed during the study [11].

In a double-blind, placebo-controlled study, 50 volunteers suffering from arthrosis were given 3-week courses of daily treatment with 3 × 2 capsules, each containing 400 mg of devil's claw root hydro-ethanolic extract (1.5% iridoid glucosides), or placebo. Assessments were carried out 10 days after completion of treatment, with evaluation of the severity of pain in 5 conditions on a 0-4 scale. Individual patients were given from one to three courses of treatment. Compared to placebo, the extract produced a statistically significant decrease in the severity of pain. Improvements were more frequent in moderately invaliding arthrosis than in more severe cases [12].

46 patients suffering from osteoarthritis of the hip participated in a 20-week, double-blind, placebo-controlled study as two randomized groups. Patients in one group (n = 24) were treated with 2 tablets per day containing a 60% ethanolic dry extract of devil's claw root (480 mg, drug to extract ratio 4.4-5.0:1); those in the second group received placebo tablets. Both groups also received identical, stepwise-reducing daily doses of ibuprofen: 2 × 400 mg for the first 8 weeks, 1 × 400 mg for a further 8 weeks and none in the last 4 weeks of the study. Efficacy was evaluated from osteoarthritis scores reported by the patients, using the Western Ontario and McMaster Universities Arthrosis Index (WOMAC). WOMAC scores decreased in both groups over the study period, despite the reducing dosage of ibuprofen. WOMAC sub-scores for stiffness, pain and dysfunction decreased similarly in both groups. In the final, ibuprofen-free period, an increase of 20% or less in the pain score was considered a clinically relevant response rate; 71% of devil's claw patients, but only 41% of placebo patients, fulfilled this criterion (p = 0.04). 52% of patients in the devil's claw group, compared to 36% in the placebo group, were able to complete the study without using rescue therapy in the ibuprofen-free period. From evaluation by both patients and physicians, the tolerability of devil's claw root extract was comparable to that of placebo in the final, mono-therapy phase. Devil's claw root extract accompanied by reducing dosages of ibuprofen therefore appeared to be a possible substitution therapy in about 70% of the patients [13].

In a 4-month randomized comparative study, the effects of powdered devil's claw root at a daily dosage of 3 × 2 capsules, providing a total of 2610 mg of root containing 57 mg of harpagoside (n = 62), were compared with those of a symptomatic slow-acting drug for osteoarthritis, diacerhein at 100 mg/day (n = 60), in patients suffering from osteoarthritis of the knee and hip. Spontaneous pain and severity of osteoarthritis evaluated by Lequesne's index were significantly improved during the course of the study and there was no difference in the efficacy of the two treatments. On completion of the study, patients taking devil's claw root were using significantly less NSAIDs or other analgesics (p = 0.002). The most frequently reported adverse event was diarrhoea, which occurred in 8.1% and 26.7% of devil's claw root and diacerhein patients respectively. A global tolerance assessment by patients at the end of treatment favoured devil's claw root [14].

In a comparative study, patients suffering from articular pains of rheumatic origin (n = 40) and from gout (n = 10) were randomized into two identical groups of 25. The efficacy and tolerability of 1230 mg of devil's claw root dry aqueous extract (drug to extract ratio 2:1), divided into three oral daily doses, was compared to phenylbutazone (300 mg daily during the first four days, then 200 mg daily; tablets assumed to have the standard potency of 100 mg). After 28 days, from assessment of a range of clinical parameters including pain, stiffness and mobility, devil's claw root extract was found to have been equally as effective as, or even superior to, phenylbutazone. No adverse events were recorded in the devil's claw group whereas 6 patients taking phenylbutazone reported one or more adverse events [15].

In a large open study on 630 arthrosic cases, 42% to 85% of the patients, grouped according to the site of arthroses, showed improvements after 6 months of treatment with devil's claw root dry aqueous extract (drug to extract ratio ca. 3:1) containing 2.5% of iridoid glucosides at daily dosages of 3 g to 9 g, divided into three doses. No side effects other than mild gastro-intestinal disturbances were reported, even at the highest dosage level [16].

In a 30-day controlled pilot study involving 100 patients with varied rheumatic indications (activated arthrosis, chronic low back pain, non-articular rheumatic conditions), the pain-relieving effect of a devil's claw root dry extract (2:1; ethanol 40% V/V) at a daily dose of 2460 mg (n = 50), was compared with placebo (n = 50). Favourable effects of verum medication were clearly evident after 10 days. By the end of the study, the greatest therapeutic improvement was achieved in the verum subgroup suffering from low back pain [17].

In a drug monitoring study, 675 patients (mean age: 58.1 years) with painful osteoarthritis, spondyl-arthropathies or fibromyalgic complaints were treated daily for 8 weeks with 2 × 480 mg of a devil's claw root dry extract (4.4-5.0:1, ethanol 60% V/V). The main outcome criteria were the Clinical Global Impressions (CGI) score and reduction in a symptom severity score (from 0 = no pain to 3 = strong pain). The extent of use of non-steroidal anti-inflammatory drugs (NSAIDs) or corticosteroids as comedication for the underlying disease was assessed as a secondary parameter. Marked therapeutic effects were observed during the study period, the mean time to onset of action being 13 days. Due to the chronicity and phasic pattern of the disease, treatment with devil's claw root extract was continued after the monitoring phase in 79% of patients. Efficacy assessed by CGI scores was rated good or very good in 82% of cases.

The symptom score for painful motion decreased by 53% from 2.23 (indicating moderate pain) to 1.04 (indicating slight pain) after 8 weeks of treatment. Over the same period, previously prescribed comedication was successfully reduced or even discontinued in 60.3% of the 464 patients taking NSAIDs and 56% of the 50 patients taking corticosteroids. A clear improvement in quality of life was evident in so far as the devil's claw root extract was rated better than their previous antirheumatic treatment by 62.4% of patients in terms of efficacy and 80% in terms of tolerability [18].

On the other hand, no significant improvements were reported in 13 patients, suffering mainly from rheumatoid arthritis, after 6 weeks of daily treatment with 3 × 410 mg of devil's claw root dry aqueous extract [40].

Relief of back pain
Daily doses of 600 mg (n = 65) or 1200 mg (n = 66) of devil's claw root dry extract (6-9:1), providing 51 mg and 102 mg of harpagoside respectively, were compared to placebo (n = 66) in a 4-week randomized, double-blind study in patients suffering for longer than 6 months from chronic low back pain (worse than 5 on a 0-10 visual analogue scale) not readily attributable to identifiable causes. 3 patients in the placebo group, 6 in the devil's claw 600 mg group and 10 in the devil's claw 1200 mg group were pain-free without rescue medication (tramadol) for at least 5 days in the last week of treatment (p = 0.027). Subsidiary analyses of pain experienced by individual patients suggested a significant effect of devil's claw root extract only in patients with non-radiating and less severe pain. The only side effects related to devil's claw root were infrequent and mild gastro-intestinal disturbances [19].

In a randomized, double-blind, placebo-controlled study, 118 patients with chronic low back pain were treated daily for 4 weeks with 3 × 800 mg of a devil's claw root dry aqueous extract (2.5:1) providing 50 mg of harpagoside, or placebo. At the end of treatment, 9 out of 54 patients in the verum group and 1 out of 55 in the placebo group were pain-free (p = 0.008). Improvement of the overall Arhus low back pain index was 20% in the verum group compared to 8% in the placebo group (p<0.059); although this was not statistically significant, the pain index component of the Arhus index was significant (p = 0.016). However, the principal outcome measure, use of supplementary analgesic (tramadol) during the final 3 weeks, did not differ between the two groups. Only minor and non-specific adverse effects occurred during treatment with devil's claw root extract [20].

In a randomized, double-blind, placebo-controlled study, 63 patients with slight to moderate muscular tension or slight muscular pain of the back, shoulder and neck received 960 mg of devil's claw root dry extract (4.4-5.0:1, ethanol 60 % V/V), or placebo, for 4 weeks. The efficacy of verum treatment was clear from the clinical global score and patient and physician ratings. Significant effects were observed in the visual analogue scale, pressure algometer test, muscle stiffness test and muscular ischaemia test, but there were no differences from placebo in antinociceptive muscular reflexes or electromyogram activity. No serious adverse events occurred. The results imply that devil's claw root may have a beneficial effect on sensory and vascular muscle response. No evidence of CNS effects was observed [21].

In an open prospective study, 102 patients suffering from acute non-pseudoradiating low back pain for more than 6 months received either 3 × 600 mg/day of a devil's claw root dry aqueous extract (2.5:1) providing 30 mg/day of harpagoside, as a mono-therapy or combined with other therapies if needed (group J: n = 51), or conventional therapy only, mainly oral non-steroidal anti-inflammatory drugs (NSAIDs), physical exercises or paravertebral injections (group K: n = 51). The number of pain-free patients after 4 and 6 weeks of treatment was comparable between the groups (group J: 16 and 20; group K: 12 and 23, respectively). After 6 weeks of therapy, the Arhus low back pain index had improved in both groups by about 20%; the relative change in single components of the index (pain, invalidity and physical impairment) did not differ between the groups. The subgroup (n = 17) of group J receiving devil's claw root extract as mono-therapy showed improvement similar to that of groups J and K [22].

In an 8-week open study, 130 patients suffering from non-radiating chronic back pain for at least 6 months were treated daily with 960 mg of devil's claw root dry extract (4.4-5.0:1, ethanol 60% V/V). Rescue medication in the form of paracetamol was available for the first 4 weeks. Subjective perceptions of pain, evaluated by validated pain scales (the Multi-dimensional pain scale and the Arhus back pain index), decreased significantly (p<0.001) during treatment. The mobility of the spinal column, determined by the average finger-to-floor distance and using Schober's sign, also improved significantly (p<0.001). The average score obtained using the first subscale of Clinical Global Impressions decreased from 4.6 at the start of the study to 2.9 after 8 weeks of treatment. No serious adverse effects were observed; one gastro-intestinal complaint (bloating sensation) was reported [23].

Other effects
From experience of digestive disorders in a medical practice over a 3-year period, based on subjective assessment and on evaluation of clinical and biochemical parameters, the following results were obtained using decoctions of devil's claw root (1 teaspoonful to 2 cups of water): improvement in small

intestine complaints, normalization of constipation and diarrhoea, elimination of flatulence and stimulation of appetite [25].

Although pharmacological experiments in rodents [45,46] indicated that enteric coated dosage forms of devil's claw root might be necessary, clinical studies [11-23] do not support this contention. Furthermore, pure harpagoside and the harpagoside (2% and 7.3%) in two devil's claw root extracts were found to be chemically stable during incubation with simulated gastric and intestinal juices at 37°C for 90-120 minutes [33,49].

Pharmacokinetic properties
In whole human blood taken from one subject after ingestion of devil's claw root extract containing 44 mg of harpagoside, the level of harpagoside after 2 hours was found to be 15.4 ng/ml [49]. After oral administration to 6 volunteers of 600 mg of devil's claw root extract containing 25% harpagoside, maximum plasma harpagoside levels were observed after 1.3 hours (32.2 ng/ml), followed by a rapid decrease. A second peak observed after 8 hours indicated enterohepatic circulation. The elimination half-life of harpagoside was 5.6 hours [34].

The iridoid glycosides harpagoside, harpagide and 8-*p*-coumaroylharpagide from devil's claw root were transformed into the pyridine monoterpene alkaloid aucubinine B by human faecal flora and by bacteria isolated from the flora. Small amounts of aucubinine B were also obtained from these iridoid glycosides by incubation with β-glucosidase in the presence of ammonium ion [50].

Preclinical safety data
Aqueous and ethanolic extracts of devil's claw root and the isolated compounds harpagoside and harpagide have shown very low toxicity in rodents during acute and subacute tests [3,38,41].

In male and female Swiss Webster mice the acute oral LD_0 of devil's claw root was greater than 13.5 g/kg [41]. The acute intraperitoneal LD_{50} of pure constituents in mice was shown to be 1 g/kg for harpagoside and greater than 3.2 g/kg for harpagide [3].

The acute oral LD_0 and intravenous LD_0 in mice of aqueous, methanolic and butanolic dry extracts of devil's claw root were found to be greater than 4.6 g/kg and 1.0 g/kg respectively [38]. A purified extract containing 85% of harpagoside showed an acute oral LD_0 greater than 4.6 g/kg and acute intravenous LD_0 and LD_{50} of 395 mg/kg and 511 mg/kg respectively [38].

In male Wistar rats, no significant haematological or

gross pathological findings were evident following 21 days of subacute oral treatment with 7.5 g/kg of devil's claw root. No hepatotoxic effects were observed with respect to liver weight or levels of microsomal protein and six liver enzymes after 7 days of oral treatment with 2.0 g/kg [41].

Because of the lack of inhibitory effects of devil's claw root on the biosynthesis of prostanoids [41,48], it has been emphasized that adverse effects often associated with non-steroidal anti-inflammatory and gluco-corticoid drugs are not to be expected, even during long-term therapy [51].

REFERENCES

1. Devil's Claw Root - Harpagophyti radix. European Pharmacopoeia, Council of Europe.

2. Lichti H, von Wartburg A. Die Struktur des Harpagosids. Helv Chim Acta 1966;49:1552-65.

3. Van Haelen M, van Haelen-Fastré R, Samaey-Fontaine J, Elchamid A, Niebes P, Matagne D. Aspects botaniques, constitution chimique et activité pharmacologique d'Harpagophytum procumbens. Phytotherapy 1983;(5):7-13.

4. Baghdikian B, Lanhers MC, Fleurentin J, Ollivier E, Maillard C, Balansard G, Mortier F. An analytical study, anti-inflammatory and analgesic effects of Harpagophytum procumbens and Harpagophytum zeyheri. Planta Med 1997;63:171-6.

5. Eich J, Schmidt M, Betti G. HPLC analysis of iridoid compounds of Harpagophytum taxa: Quality control of pharmaceutical drug material. Pharm Pharmacol Lett 1998;8:75-8.

6. Bendall MR, Ford CW, Thomas DM. The structure of procumbide. Aust J Chem 1979;32:2085-91.

7. Kikuchi T, Matsuda S, Kubo Y, Namba T. New iridoid glucosides from Harpagophytum procumbens DC. Chem Pharm Bull 1983;31:2296-301.

8. Burger JFW, Brandt EV, Ferreira D. Iridoid and phenolic glycosides from Harpagophytum procumbens. Phytochemistry 1987;26:1453-7.

9. Ziller KH, Franz G. Analysis of the water soluble fraction from the roots of Harpagophytum procumbens. Planta Med 1979;37:340-8.

10. Bradley PR, editor. Devil's claw. In: British Herbal Compendium, Volume 1. Bournemouth: British Herbal Medicine Association, 1992:78-80.

11. Lecomte A, Costa JP. Harpagophytum dans l'arthrose. Etude en double insu contre placebo. 37°2 Le Magazine 1992;(15):27-30.

12. Guyader M. Les plantes antirhumatismales. Etude historique et pharmacologique, et étude clinique du nébulisat d'Harpagophytum procumbens D.C. chez 50 patients arthrosiques suivis en service hospitalier [Thesis]. Paris: Université Pierre et Marie Curie, 1984.

13. Frerick H, Biller A, Schmidt U. Stufenschema bei Coxarthrose: Doppelblindstudie mit Teufelskralle. Der Kassenarzt 2001;5:34-41.

14. Chantre P, Cappelaere A, Leblan D, Guédon D, Vandermander J, Fournié B. Efficacy and tolerance of Harpagophytum procumbens versus diacerhein in treatment of osteoarthritis. Phytomedicine 2000;7:177-83.
   Also published as:
   Leblan D, Chantre P, Fournié B. Harpagophytum procumbens in the treatment of knee and hip osteoarthritis. Four-month results of a prospective, multicenter, double-blind trial versus diacerhein. Joint Bone Spine 2000;67:462-7.

15. Schrüffler H. Salus Teufelskralle-Tabletten. Ein Fortschritt in der nichtsteroidalen antirheumatischen Therapie. Die Medizinische Publikation 1980:1-8.

16. Belaiche P. Etude clinique de 630 cas d'arthrose traités par le nébulisat aqueux d'Harpagophytum procumbens (Radix). Phytotherapy 1982;(1):22 8.

17. Schmelz H, Hämmerle HD, Springorum HW. Analgetische Wirkung eines Teufelskrallenwurzel-Extraktes bei verschiedenen chronisch-degenerativen Gelenkerkrankungen. In: Chrubasik S, Wink M, editors. Rheumatherapie mit Phytopharmaka. Stuttgart: Hippokrates, 1997:86-9.

18. Ribbat JM, Schakau D. Behandlung chronisch aktivierter Schmerzen am Bewegungsapparat. NaturaMed 2001;16:23-30.

19. Chrubasik S, Junck H, Breitschwerdt H, Conradt C, Zappe H. Effectiveness of Harpagophytum extract WS 1531 in the treatment of exacerbation of low back pain: a randomized, placebo-controlled, double-blind study. Eur J Anaesthesiol 1999;16:118-29.

20. Chrubasik S, Zimpfer C, Schütt U, Ziegler R. Effectiveness of Harpagophytum procumbens in treatment of acute low back pain. Phytomedicine 1996;3:1-10.

21. Göbel H, Heinze A, Ingwersen M, Niederberger U, Gerber D. Harpagophytum-Extrakt LI 174 (Teufelskralle) bei der Behandlung unspezifischer Rückenschmerzen. Effekte auf die sensible, motorische und vaskuläre Muskelreagibilität. Schmerz 2001;15:10-8.

22. Chrubasik S, Schmidt A, Junck H, Pfisterer M. Wirksamkeit und Wirtschaftlichkeit von Teufelskrallen-wurzelextrakt bei Rückenschmerzen: Erste Ergebnisse einer therapeutischen Kohortenstudie. Forsch Komplementärmed 1997;4:332-6.

23. Laudahn D, Walper A. Efficacy and tolerance of Harpagophytum extract LI 174 in patients with chronic non-radicular back pain. Phytother Res 2001;15:621-4.

24. Hänsel R, Keller K, Rimpler H, Schneider G, editors. Harpagophytum. In: Hagers Handbuch der Pharmazeutischen Praxis, 5th ed. Volume 5: Drogen E-O. Berlin: Springer-Verlag, 1993:384-90.

25. Zimmerman W. Pflanzliche Bitterstoffe in der Gastro-enterologie. Z Allgemeinmed 1976;54:1178-84.

26. Schilcher H. Teufelskralle. In: Kleines Heilkräuter-lexikon, 4th ed. Weil der Stadt: Haedecke, 1999:187-8.

27. Braun H, Frohne D. Harpagophytum procumbens DC. Teufelskralle. In: Heilpflanzen-Lexikon für Ärzte und Apotheker, 5th ed. Stuttgart: Gustav Fischer, 1987:129.

28. Czygan F-C. Harpagophytum - Teufelskralle. Z Phyto-therapie 1987;8:17-20.

29. Bisset NG, editor (translated from Wichtl M, editor. Teedrogen). Harpagophyti radix. In: Herbal Drugs and Phytopharmaceuticals. Stuttgart: Medpharm, Boca Raton-London, CRC Press, 1994:248-50.

30. Weiss RF. Harpagophytum procumbens, Teufelskralle. In: Lehrbuch der Phytotherapie, 7th ed. Stuttgart: Hippokrates, 1991:86 and 340-2.

31. Costa de Pasquale R, Busa G, Circosta C, Iauk L, Ragusa S, Ficarra P, Occhiuto F. A drug used in traditional medicine: Harpagophytum procumbens DC. III. Effects on hyperkinetic ventricular arrhythmias by reperfusion. J Ethnopharmacol 1985;13:193-9.

32. Circosta C, Occhiuto F, Ragusa S, Trovato A, Tumino G, Briguglio F, De Pasquale A. A drug used in traditional medicine: Harpagophytum procumbens DC. II. Cardiovascular activity. J Ethnopharmacol 1984; 11:259-74.

33. Loew D, Puttkammer S. Pharmacological and pharmacokinetic studies with Harpagophytum extracts. In: Chrubasik S, Roufogalis BD, editors. Herbal medicinal products for the treatment of pain. Lismore, Australia: Southern Cross University Press, 2000:56-62.

34. Loew D, Möllerfeld J, Schrödter A, Puttkammer S, Kaszkin M. Investigations on the pharmacokinetic properties of Harpagophytum extracts and their effects on eicosanoid biosynthesis in vitro and ex vivo. Clin Pharm Ther 2001;69:356-64.

35. Tippler B, Syrovets T, Loew D, Simmet T. Harpagophytum procumbens: Wirkung von Extrakten auf die Eicosanoidbiosynthese in Ionophor A23187-stimuliertem menschlichem Vollblut. In: Loew D, Rietbrock N, editors. Phytopharmaka II. Forschung und klinische Anwendung. Darmstadt: Steinkopff, 1996:95-100.

36. Fiebich BL, Heinrich M, Hiller K-O, Kammerer N. Inhibition of TNF-α synthesis in LPS-stimulated primary human monocytes by Harpagophytum extract SteiHap 69. Phytomedicine 2001;8:28-30.

37. Eichler O, Koch C. Über die antiphlogistische, analgetische und spasmolytische Wirksamkeit von Harpagosid, einem Glykosid aus der Wurzel von Harpagophytum procumbens DC. Arzneim-Forsch/Drug Res 1970;20:107-9.

38. Erdös A, Fontaine R, Friehe H, Durand R, Pöppinghaus T. Beitrag zur Pharmakologie und Toxikologie verschiedener Extrakte, sowie des Harpagosids aus Harpagophytum procumbens DC. Planta Med 1978; 34:97-108.

39. McLeod DW, Revell P, Robinson BV. Investigations of Harpagophytum procumbens (Devil's claw) in the treatment of experimental inflammation and arthritis in the rat. Brit J Pharmacol 1979;66:140P-1P.

40. Grahame R, Robinson BV. Devil's claw (Harpagophytum procumbens): pharmacological and clinical studies. Ann Rheum Dis 1981;40:632.

41. Whitehouse LW, Znamirowska M, Paul CJ. Devil's claw (Harpagophytum procumbens): no evidence for anti-inflammatory activity in the treatment of arthritic disease. Can Med Assoc J 1983;129:249-51.

42. Recio MC, Giner RM, Máñez S, Ríos JL. Structural considerations on the iridoids as anti-inflammatory agents. Planta Med 1994;60:232-4.

43. Jadot G, Lecomte A. Activité anti-inflammatoire d'Harpagophytum procumbens DC. Lyon Méditerranée Médical Médecine du Sud-Est 1992;28:833-5.

44. Morgenstern E, Pollex S. Antiphlogistische und analgetische Wirkung von Teufelskrallenextrakt LI 174 [Poster]. In: Abstracts of Gesellschaft für Phytotherapie Symposium (Phytopharmakaforschung 2000). Bonn, 27-28 November 1998:92-3 (Poster P18).

45. Lanhers MC, Fleurentin J, Mortier F, Vinche A, Younos C. Anti-inflammatory and analgesic effects of an aqueous extract of Harpagophytum procumbens. Planta Med 1992;58:117-23.

46. Soulimani R, Younos C, Mortier F, Derrieu C. The role of stomachal digestion on the pharmacological activity of plant extracts, using as an example extracts of Harpagophytum procumbens. Can J Physiol Pharmacol 1994;72:1532-6.

47. Bhattacharya A, Bhattacharya SK. Anti-oxidant activity of Harpagophytum procumbens (Devil's claw). Br J Phytother 1998;5:68-71.

48. Moussard C, Alber D, Toubin M-M, Thevenon N, Henry J-C. A drug used in traditional medicine, Harpagophytum procumbens: no evidence for NSAID-like effect on whole blood eicosanoid production in human. Prostagland Leukotr Essent Fatty Acids 1992;46:283-6.

49. Loew D, Schuster O, Möllerfeld J. Stabilität und biopharmazeutische Qualität. Voraussetzung für Bioverfügbarkeit und Wirksamkeit von Harpagophytum procumbens. In: Loew D, Rietbrock N, editors. Phytopharmaka II. Forschung und Klinische Anwendung. Darmstadt: Steinkopff, 1996:83-93.

50. Baghdikian B, Guiraud-Dauriac H, Ollivier E, N'Guyen A, Dumenil G, Balansard G. Formation of nitrogen-containing metabolites from the main iridoids of Harpagophytum procumbens and H. zeyheri by human intestinal bacteria. Planta Med, 1999;65:164-6.

51. Loew D. Harpagophytum procumbens DC - Eine Übersicht zur Pharmakologie und Wirksamkeit. Erfahrungsheilkunde 1995;(2):74-9.

HEDERAE HELICIS FOLIUM

Ivy Leaf

E/S/C/O/P
MONOGRAPHS
Second Edition

DEFINITION

Ivy leaf consists of the dried leaves of *Hedera helix* L. It contains three main saponins: hederasaponin C (hederacoside C), hederasaponin B and hederasaponin D (saponin k10), with not less than 2.5% of hederasaponin C.

The material complies with the monograph of the Pharmacopée Française [1].

Fresh material may also be processed provided that when dried it complies with the monograph of the Pharmacopée Française.

CONSTITUENTS

Triterpene saponins (2.5-6%), predominantly bisdesmosidic glycosides of hederagenin with hederasaponin C (hederacoside C) as the main saponin, and a small amount of the monodesmosidic saponin α-hederin [2,3]. Other saponins present, in decreasing order of concentration, are hederasaponins B,D,F,G,E,H and I.

Other constituents include phytosterols, polyines such as falcarinol and didehydrofalcarinol, essential oil, flavonoids and other phenolic compounds such as caffeoylquinic acids [2,3].

CLINICAL PARTICULARS

Therapeutic indications
Coughs, particularly when associated with hypersecretion of viscous mucus; as adjuvant treatment of inflammatory bronchial diseases [4-11].

Posology and method of administration

Dosage
Note: Most preparations from ivy leaf contain hydroethanolic dry extracts incorporated into ethanol-containing or ethanol-free oral liquids, or suppositories. The following recommendations are:

Daily doses expressed as the corresponding amounts of dried ivy leaf

ORAL USE

Ethanol-containing preparations
Adults: 250-420 mg [5].
Children 4-12 years: 150-210 mg [8,9].
Children 1-4 years: 50-150 mg [12].

Children 0-1 year: 20-50 mg [12].

Ethanol-free preparations
Adults: 300-945 mg [10,11,13].
Children 4-12 years: 200-630 mg [6,7,10,11,13,14].
Children 1-4 years: 150-300 mg [10,11,14].
Children 0-1 years: 50-200 mg [10-12].

RECTAL USE

Suppositories
Children 4-10 years: 960 mg [8].

Method of administration
For oral administration in liquid or solid dosage forms; for rectal application as suppositories.

Duration of administration
If symptoms persist or worsen medical advice should be sought.

Contra-indications
None known.

Special warnings and special precautions for use
None required.

Interaction with other medicaments and other forms of interaction
None reported.

Pregnancy and lactation
No human data available. In accordance with general medical practice, the product should not be used during pregnancy or lactation without medical advice.

Effects on ability to drive and use machines
None known.

Undesirable effects
Fresh ivy leaf and the leaf sap can cause allergic contact dermatitis [15-17]. Falcarinol and didehydro-falcarinol have been reported to be allergenic [18,19].

Overdose
Overdosage can provoke nausea, vomiting, diarrhoea and excitation [20]. In these cases a physician should be consulted immediately.

PHARMACOLOGICAL PROPERTIES

Pharmacodynamic properties

In vitro experiments

Spasmolytic activity
Saponins and phenolic compounds isolated from a 30%-ethanolic extract of ivy leaf (6:1) exhibited spasmolytic activity against acetylcholine-induced contractions of isolated guinea pig ileum. Spasmolytic activity equivalent to that of 1 mg of papaverine was exerted by 169 mg of hederacoside C, 18 mg of α-hederin and 21 mg of their aglycone, hederagenin, which was not present in the extract (p<0.05 for all three compounds); 7 mg of kaempferol and 18 mg of quercetin (p<0.01, although less than 0.01% of each of these flavonol glycosides was present in the extract); and 46 mg of 3,5-dicaffeoylquinic acid (p<0.05; about 0.5% present in the extract). Taking into account the amounts of such constituents present in the extract in relation to their activity, the saponins α-hederin and hederacoside C appeared to contribute most of the spasmolytic activity, with α-hederin the more prominent in this respect. Each of 5 fractions of the extract, in total representing over 90% of the original extract, had spasmolytic activity (all p<0.05) [21,22].

Antimicrobial activity
A saponin mixture (predominantly hederacoside C) from ivy leaf exhibited antibacterial activity against Gram-positive bacteria (*Bacillus* spp., *Staphylococcus* spp., *Enterococcus* spp., *Streptococcus* spp.) with minimum inhibitory concentrations (MICs) of 0.3-1.25 mg/ml and against Gram-negative bacteria (*Salmonella* spp., *Shigella* spp., *Pseudomonas* spp., *Escherichia coli*, *Proteus vulgaris*) with MICs of 1.25-5 mg/ml [23]. An ethanolic extract from ivy leaf completely inhibited the growth of *Staphylococcus aureus* and *Pseudomonas aeruginosa* and partially inhibited the growth of *E. coli* [24].

α-Hederin at 0.5 mg/ml exhibited antifungal activity against *Candida albicans* and the dermatophyte *Microsporum canis* (0.05 mg/ml), but hederacoside C and crude saponin mixtures from ivy leaf were ineffective against these and other dermatophytic fungi [25]. Other experiments confirmed the antifungal activity of α-hederin (MIC: 0.25 mg/ml) [26].

Hederacoside C has been reported to have antiviral activity against influenza virus A2/Japan-305 [27].

Other activities
In vitro experiments have demonstrated inhibition of hyaluronidase activity by hederagenin (but not by hederacoside C or α-hederin) [28], anthelminthic activity of ivy leaf extracts [29], antileishmanial activity of ivy leaf saponins [30-32] and anti-trypanosomial activity of α-hederin and hederagenin (but not hederasaponin C) [33]

In vivo experiments

Spasmolytic activity
In the compressed air model in conscious guinea pigs, an orally administered ethanolic extract from ivy leaf at 50 mg/kg body weight dose-dependently inhibited bronchoconstriction induced by inhalation of ovalbumin (57% inhibition, p = 0.01) or platelet

activating factor (43% inhibition, p = 0.03) [34].

Anti-inflammatory activity
An orally administered ethanolic extract from ivy leaf at 162 mg/kg body weight inhibited carrageenan-induced rat paw oedema by 39% after 1 hour and by 5% after 5 hours [34]. A saponin mixture isolated from ivy leaf, administered intravenously, inhibited ovalbumin-induced rat paw oedema with an ED_{50} of 0.32 mg/kg [35].

Antifungal activity
Candida albicans infections, as abscesses on the backs of mice, were eliminated after oral administration of a saponin mixture (60% hederasaponin C) from ivy leaf at 50 mg/kg body weight for 10 days. At the same dose level and duration, α-hederin eliminated the infection in 90% of animals and hederasaponin C in 40% of animals. In comparison, the infections were eliminated by oral amphotericin B at 2.5 mg/kg within 6 days [25].

Other effects
Anthelmintic properties of ivy leaf [29] and hepato-protective properties of α-hederin [36,37] have been demonstrated in mice.

Clinical studies
In early clinical studies, ivy leaf extracts were used in the treatment of children and adults suffering from various respiratory complaints involving coughing. Reductions were observed in the frequency of coughs [38-44].

In a randomized, double-blind, comparative study, 99 patients (aged from 25 to 70 years) with mild to moderate, simple or obstructive, chronic bronchitis were treated daily for 4 weeks with either an oral liquid containing ivy leaf dry extract (5-7.5:1, ethanol 30% m/m; 2 g of dry extract per 100 ml) [3-5 × 20 drops of the oral liquid and 3 × 1 placebo tablet] or ambroxol [3-5 × 20 drops placebo and 3 × 1 ambroxol 30 mg tablet]. Improvements in spirometric and auscultation parameters were observed in both groups with no significant differences between groups. The patients' diaries indicated a tendency towards greater decreases in frequency of coughing, sputum production and dyspnoea in the ivy leaf extract group [5].

In a randomized, comparative, crossover study, 26 children (aged 5 to 11 years) suffering from bronchial asthma were treated for 3 days with preparations containing a 30%-ethanolic dry extract (5-7.5:1) from ivy leaf: 2 × 25 drops of an oral liquid preparation daily (= 35 mg of the extract daily) and then, after a wash-out interval, 2 suppositories daily (= 160 mg of the extract daily), or vice versa. Compared to initial values, reductions of 31% (oral liquid) and 23% (suppositories) in obstruction of the airways was observed. Both dosage forms were well tolerated [8].

In a randomized, double-blind, placebo-controlled, crossover study, 24 patients aged 4-12 years suffering from bronchial asthma were treated with an oral liquid containing ivy leaf dry extract (2 × 25 drops, corresponding to 35 mg of the extract or 210 mg of crude drug daily) for 3 days and, over a separate 3-day period, with placebo drops. A significant reduction in airway resistance was observed in the verum group (p = 0.0361) in comparison with the placebo group [9].

In an open multicentre study involving 52 children (aged up to 12 years) suffering from bronchial complaints, the above-mentioned oral liquid preparation containing ivy leaf dry extract (5-7.5:1; ethanol 30% m/m) was compared with another containing ivy leaf dry extract (3-6:1; ethanol 60%; 200 mg of hederacoside C per 100 ml). The daily dose was: children up to 4 years, 2 × 5 ml daily; 4-10 years, 2 × 7.5 ml daily; 10-12 years, 2 × 10 ml daily. Treatment for 10 days led to improvement of symptoms in both groups with no significance differences between groups [14].

In a open pilot study, 26 children (aged 4-10 years) with chronic, obstructive bronchitis were treated with an ethanol-free oral preparation of ivy leaf extract (4 × 1-2 teaspoonsful daily) for 4 weeks. Spirometry results, auscultatory findings and symptoms such as cough, sputum and dyspnoea improved after the first week in most of the children. Good to very good efficacy was reported in more than two-thirds of the children and no adverse reactions were reported [4].

In a multicentre surveillance study, 113 children (aged 6-15 years) suffering from recurrent obstructive respiratory complaints were treated with an ethanol-free oral preparation of ivy leaf extract for up to 20 days (in some cases up to 30 days). As the daily dose the majority took 6 × 2.5 ml, one-third took 8-10 × 2.5 ml and a few took only 3-4 × 2.5 ml. Compared to baseline, improvements were observed in lung function and accompanying symptoms of coughing and expectoration. The physicians concluded that the optimal daily dosage was 6 × 2.5 ml [6].

In a randomized, double-blind, crossover study involving 25 children (aged 10-15 years) with chronic obstructive pulmonary complaints, changes in lung function were examined after treatment over separate 10-day periods with two oral liquid preparations based on the same ivy leaf dry extract: an ethanol-free preparation (3 × 5 ml daily, corresponding to 3 × 35 mg of dry extract or 630 mg of crude drug daily) and an ethanol-containing preparation (3 × 20 drops daily, corresponding to 3 × 14 mg of dry extract or 252 mg of crude drug daily). Comparable improvements in spirometric and body-plethysmographic parameters were observed after both treatments. However, higher dosages of the ethanol-free preparation were required to achieve a therapeutic effect equivalent to that of the ethanol-containing preparation [7].

In an open comparative study, children aged 10-14 years suffering from chronic obstructive bronchitis were treated daily for 3 days with two different oral liquid preparations containing ivy leaf dry extract, both dosages corresponding to 250 mg of dried ivy leaf per day: an ethanolic preparation and an ethanol-free preparation. The spirometry results showed that, despite identical dosages in terms of crude drug, improvements in lung function after taking the ethanolic preparation were clearly superior to those after the ethanol-free preparation, with increases in 1-second capacity (FEV$_1$) of 18% and 8.2% respectively (p<0.05) [13].

In an open study 372 children (aged from 2 months to over 10 years, average 5.7 years) suffering from respiratory tract infections were treated for 7 days with an ethanol-free oral liquid preparation containing a dry extract from ivy leaf (6-7:1, ethanol 40%; 2 ml of preparation contained 18 mg of extract corresponding to 108-126 mg of crude drug). Depending on age, average daily doses ranged from 2.8 ml to 6.7 ml. Compared to baseline, substantial improvements were observed in lung function and cough symptoms, and the physicians rated efficacy as good to very good in 94.4% of patients [10].

In an open study, 1024 children suffering from acute infections of the upper respiratory tract (52.4%), acute bronchitis/bronchiolitis (26.6%) or bronchitis (not further specified, 22.2%) were treated with an ivy leaf dry extract. Compared to initial values, significant reductions were observed in coughing, expectoration and airway resistance (p<0.01) [11].

Pharmacokinetic properties
No data available.

Preclinical safety data

Single dose toxicity
The oral LD$_{50}$ of several ivy leaf extracts in mice was determined as > 3 g/kg body weight [45]. Oral administration of a dry extract of ivy leaf (ethanol 66% V/V) to rats at up to 4.1 g/kg body weight caused no deaths within 72 hours; only diarrhoea was observed [3,46].

Oral LD$_{50}$ values in mice of saponin mixtures from ivy leaf containing 60% and 90% of hederacoside C, and of hederasaponin C and α-hederin, were all > 4 g/kg body weight; the intraperitoneal LD$_{50}$ values for α-hederin and the saponin mixture containing 60% of hederacoside C were 1.8 and 2.3 g/kg respectively [25]. In an earlier study, oral and intravenous LD$_{50}$

values in rats for crude saponins from ivy leaf were reported as > 100 mg/kg and 13 mg/kg respectively [35].

Repeated dose toxicity
Daily oral administration of an ivy leaf dry extract to rats at 1.5 g/kg body weight for 100 days caused no toxic effects; haematological and biochemical parameters, histological findings and kidney and liver weights were normal compared to those of control animals [47]. Haemolytic effects were detected after oral administration of a hydroethanolic dry extract from ivy leaf to rats at 4 g/kg body weight for 90 days [45].

Mutagenicity and cytotoxicity
α-hederin, β-hederin and δ-hederin isolated from ivy leaf showed no mutagenic potential in the Ames test using *Salmonella typhimurium* strain TA 98, with or without S9 activation. These three saponins showed dose-dependent antimutagenic effects against benz[a]pyrene at levels between 80 and 200 µg/plate in the Ames test [48]. In another study, α-hederin prevented gene mutations caused by doxorubicin in human lymphocytes [49].

Cytotoxic properties of α and β-hederin have been demonstrated in mouse 3T3 non-cancer fibroblasts, mouse B16 melanoma cells and human HeLa tumour cells [50,51]. In the presence of serum albumin, the cytotoxic effect decreased. α-Hederin also induced vacuolisation of the cytoplasma and membrane alterations leading to cell death [51].

Reproductive toxicity
No data available on ivy leaf or extracts from it.

Intoxication of the maternal animal causes an acute phase reaction characterized by redistribution of the trace elements zinc, copper and iron, and by an increase in various plasma and liver proteins (e.g. metallothionein, α$_1$-acid glycoprotein and cerulo-plasmin), associated with non-specific malformations in the embryo. Subcutaneous administration of α-hederin at 3 to 300 µmol/kg body weight to pregnant rats on gestation days 8 and/or 11 induced an acute phase response indicated by decreased concentrations of Fe and Zn and increased concentrations of Cu, α$_1$-acid glycoprotein and ceruloplasmin in plasma along with a dose-dependent increase in the concentration of maternal hepatic metallothionein (MT). The maximum induction of MT was 11- to 15-fold greater than in controls after doses of 30 µmol/kg or higher. Doses of both 30 and 300 µmol/kg significantly increased resorption incidence (p = 0.05), and 300 µmol/kg body weight also decreased fetal weight and increased the incidence of abnormal fetuses [52].

In another study α-hederin was subcutaneously administered to rats at 20 and 30 µmol/kg body weight daily on gestation days 6-15, resulting in sustained elevation of hepatic metallothionein and subsequent redistribution of zinc. This led to a decrease in the zinc available to the embryo and ultimately to adverse development of the offspring. Repeated dosing throughout organogenesis increased the severity of the effects previously observed with single large doses of α-hederin administered during mid-gestation [53].

Addition of α-hederin to an embryo culture, directly (300 μmol) or as serum collected 2 hours after administration of α-hederin to the maternal rat (i.e. before the onset of MT synthesis), had no embryotoxic effect. However, after addition of serum obtained at the peak of metallothionein synthesis (18 hours after application of α-hederin to the maternal animals), the embryos developed normally only after addition of zinc [52].

The above studies showed that single high toxic doses, or repeated low doses, of α-hederin alter (as do many other substances) systemic zinc distribution in the pregnant rat, which is associated with abnormal embryo development. Abnormalities of embryogenesis due to the amount of α-hederin orally administered in therapeutic doses of ivy leaf extracts (with absorption to a lesser extent) cannot be deduced from these results.

REFERENCES

1. Lierre grimpant - Hedera helix. Pharmacopée Française.

2. Willuhn G. Hederae folium - Efeublätter. In: Wichtl M, editor. Teedrogen und Phytopharmaka. Ein Handbuch für die Praxis auf wissenschaftlicher Grundlage, 4th ed. Stuttgart: Wissenschaftliche Verlagsgesellschaft, 2002: 274-7.

3. Horz KH, Reichling J. Hedera. In: Hänsel R, Keller K, Rimpler H, Schneider G, editors. Hagers Handbuch der Pharmazeutischen Praxis, 5th ed. Volume 5: Drogen E-O. Berlin: Springer-Verlag, 1993:398-407.

4. Gulyas A, Lämmlein MM. Zur Behandlung von Kindern mit chronisch-obstruktiver Bronchitis. Prospan-Kindersaft, ein altbewährtes Produkt in neuer Darreichungsformen - Ergebnisse einer klinischen Prüfung. Sozialpädiatrie 1992;14:632-4.

5. Meyer-Wegener J, Liebscher K, Hettich M, Kastner H-G. Efeu versus Ambroxol bei chronischer Bronchitis. Eine Doppelblindstudie zum Vergleich der klinischen Wirksamkeit und Verträglichkeit von Efeublätter-trockenextrakt und Ambroxol. Z Allg Med 1993;69:61-6.

6. Lässig W, Generlich H, Heydolph F, Paditz E. Wirksamkeit und Verträglichkeit efeuhaltiger Husten-mittel. Prospan® Kindersaft bei rezidivierenden obstructiven Atemwegserkrankungen. TW Pädiatrie 1996;9:489-91.

7. Gulyas A, Repges R, Dethlefsen U. Konsequente Therapie chronisch-obstruktiver Atemwegser-krankungen bei Kindern. Atemw-Lungenkrkh 1997; 23:291-4.

8. Mansfeld H-J, Höhre H, Repges R, Dethlefsen U. Sekretolyse und Bronchospasmolyse. Klinische Studie: Behandlung von Kindern mit chronisch obstruktiven Atemwegserkrankungen mit Prospan®. TW Pädiatrie 1997;10:155-7.

9. Mansfeld H-J, Höhre H, Repges R, Dethlefsen U. Therapie des Asthma bronchiale mit Efeublätter-Trockenextrakt. Münch Med Wschr 1998;140:26-30.

10. Jahn E, Müller B. Efeublättertrockenextrakt. Pädiatrische Therapie-studie zur Wirksamkeit und Verträglichkeit. Dtsch Apoth Ztg 2000;140:1349-52.

11. Roth R. Anwendungsbeobachtung bestätigt Wirksam-keit der Behandlung mit Efeublätter-Trockenextrakt. Efeublätter wirken sekretolytisch und broncho-spasmolytisch. Pädiatrische Nachrichten, September 2000.

12. Dorsch W, Loew D, Meyer-Buchtela E, Schilcher H. Hederae helicis folium (Efeublätter). In: Kooperation Phytopharmaka, editor. Kinderdosierung von Phytopharmaka, 3rd ed. Teil I. Empfehlungen zur Anwendung und Dosierung von Phytopharmaka, monographierte Arzneidrogen und ihren Zubereitungen in der Pädiatrie. Bonn: Kooperation Phytopharmaka, 2002:76-7.

13. Hecker M. Efeublättertrockenextract: Hustentropfen mit Ethanol - deutlich bessere Wirksamkeit; Verschie-dene Zubereitungen von Efeublättertrockenextract. Dosisanpassung erforderlich. T & E (Therapie & Erfolg) Pädiatrie 1997;10:648-50.

14. Unkauf M, Friederich M. Bronchitis bei Kindern: klinische Studie mit Efeublätter Trockenextrakt. Der Bayerische Internist 2000;(4)(Beilage, 29 June 2002):1-4.

15. Boyle J, Harman RM. Contact dermatitis to Hedera helix (common ivy). Contact Dermatitis 1985;12:111-2.

16. García M, Fernández E, Navarro JA, del Pozo MD, Fernández de Corrès L. Allergic contact dermatitis from Hedera helix L. Contact Dermatitis 1995;33:133-4.

17. Sánchez-Pérez J, Córdoba S, Hausen BM, Moreno de Vega MJ, Aragüés M, García-Díez A. Allergic contact dermatitis from common ivy confirmed with stored allergens. Contact Dermatitis 1998;39:259-60.

18. Hausen BM, Bröhan J, König WA, Faasch H, Hahn H, Bruhn G. Allergic and irritant contact dermatitis from falcarinol and didehydrofalcarinol in common ivy (Hedera helix L.). Contact Dermatitis 1987;17:1-9.

19. Gafner F, Epstein W, Reynolds G, Rodriguez E. Human maximization test of falcarinol, the principal contact allergen of English ivy and Algerian ivy (Hedera helix, H. canariensis). Contact Dermatitis 1988;19:125-8

20. Von Mühlendahl KE, Oberdisse U, Bunjes R, Ritter S, editors. Vergiftungsunfälle mit pflanzen. In: Vergiftungen im Kindesalter, 3rd ed. Stuttgart: Ferdinand Enke Verlag, 1995:347.

21. Trute A, Groß J. Mutschler E, Nahrstedt A. In vitro spasmolytic principle of commercial dry extract from Hedera helix L. In: Abstracts of 2nd International Congress on Phytomedicine. Munich, 11-14 September 1996. Published as: Phytomedicine 1996;3(Suppl 1):248 (Abstract P-73).

22. Trute A, Gross J, Mutschler E, Nahrstedt A. In vitro antispasmodic compounds of the dry extract obtained from Hedera helix. Planta Med 1997;63:125-9.

23. Cioacá C, Margineanu C, Cucu V. The saponins of Hedera helix with antibacterial activity. Pharmazie 1978;33:609-10.

24. Ieven M, Vanden Berghe DA, Mertens F, Vlietinck A, Lammens E. Screening of higher plants for biological activities. I. Antimicrobial activity. Planta Med 1979; 36:311-21.

25. Timon-David P, Julien J, Gasquet M, Balansard G, Bernard P. Recherche d'une activité antifongique de plusieurs principes actifs. Extraits du lierre grimpant: Hedera helix L. Ann Pharm Fr 1980;38:545-52.

26. Moulin-Traffort J, Favel A, Elias R, Regli P. Study of the action of α-hederin on ultrastructure of Candida albicans. Mycoses 1998;41:411-6.

27. Rao GS, Sinsheimer JE, Cochran KW. Antiviral activity of triterpenoid saponins containing acylated β-amyrin aglycones. J Pharm Sci 1974;63:471-3.

28. Maffei Facino R, Carini M, Stefani R, Aldini G, Saibene L. Anti-elastase and anti-hyaluronidase activities of saponins and sapogenins from Hedera helix, Aesculus hippocastanum and Ruscus aculeatus: Factors contributing to their efficacy in the treatment of venous insufficiency. Arch Pharm (Weinheim) 1995;328:720-4.

29. Julien J, Gasquet M, Maillard C, Balansard G, Timon-David P. Extracts of the ivy plant, Hedera helix, and their anthelmintic activity on liver flukes. Planta Med 1985;51:205-8.

30. Majester-Savornin B, Elias R, Diaz-Lanza AM, Balansard G, Gasquet M, Delmas F. Saponins of the ivy plant, Hedera helix, and their leishmanicidic activity. Planta Med 1991;57:260-2.

31. Delmas F, Di Giorgio C, Elias R, Gasquet M, Azas N, Mshvildadze V et al. Antileishmanial activity of three saponins isolated from ivy, α-hederin, β-hederin and hederacolchiside A₁, as compared to their action on mammalian cells cultured in vitro. Planta Med 2000;66:343-7.

32. Ridoux O, Di Giorgio C, Delmas F, Elias R, Mshvildadze V, Dekanosidze G et al. In vitro antileishmanial activity of three saponins isolated from ivy, α-hederin, β-hederin and hederacolchiside A₁, in association with pentamidine and amphotericin B. Phytother Res 2001; 15:298-301.

33. Tedlaouti F, Gasquet M, Delmas F, Timon-David P, Elias R, Vidal-Ollivier E et al. Antitrypanosomial activity of some saponins from Calendula arvensis, Hedera helix and Sapindus mukurossi. Planta Med 1991; 57(Suppl 2):A78.

34. Haen E. Pharmacological activities of Thymus vulgaris and Hedera helix. In: Abstracts of 2nd International Congress on Phytomedicine. Munich, 11-14 September 1996. Published as: Phytomedicine 1996;3(Suppl 1):144 (Abstract SL-115).

35. Vogel G, Marek M-L. Zur Pharmakologie einiger Saponine. Arzneim-Forsch 1962;12:815-25.

36. Liu J, Choudhuri S, Liu Y, Kreppel H, Andrews GK, Klaassen CD. Induction of metallothionein by α-hederin. Toxicol Appl Pharmacol 1993;121:144-51.

37. Liu J, Liu Y, Bullock P, Klaassen CD. Suppression of liver cytochrome P450 by α-hederin: relevance to hepatoprotection. Toxicol Appl Pharmacol 1995; 134:124-31.

38. Stöcklin P. Klinische Erfahrungen mit dem Hustenmittel "Prospan". Schweiz Rundschau Med (Praxis) 1959;48: 934-8.

39. Rath F. Klinische Prüfung der Wirksamkeit des Hustenmittels Prospan. Fortschr Med 1968;86:1015-6.

40. Arch F. Erfahrungsbericht über die Aerosol-Behandlung der Bronchitis mit Prospan®. Notabene Medici 1974;4(6):2-8.

41. Düchtel-Brühl A. Ergebnisse der Behandlung spastischer Bronchitiden im Kindesalter mit Prospan. Med Welt 1976;27:481.

42. Böhlau V. Therapeutische Erfahrungen mit Prospan® bei chronisch-obstruktiven Atemwegserkrankungen. Notabene Medici 1977;7(11):26-9.

43. Rudkowski Z, Latos T. Inhalationsbehandlung chronischer Bronchitiden im Kindesalter mit Prospan®. Ärztliche Praxis 1979;31:342-6.

44. Leskow P. Behandlung bronchialer Erkrankungen mit dem Phytotherapeutikum Prospan®. Z Phytotherapie 1985;6:61-4.

45. Bucher K. Pharmakologische und toxikologische Untersuchungen mit Extrakten aus Hedera helix. Internal report for Karl Engelhard Fabrik, Frankfurt, October 1969.

46. Lanza JP, Steinmetz MD, Pellegrin E, Mourgue M. Actions toxique et pharmacodynamique sur le rat d'extraits de lierre grimpant (Hedera helix L.). Plantes Méd Phytothér 1980;14:221-9.

47. Kramer H. Untersuchungen zur chronischen Toxizität eines Efeu-Trockenextraktes an Ratten. Battelle-Institut, Frankfurt: Internal report for Hausheer AG, Wettingen, Switzerland, April 1968.

48. Elias R, De Méo M, Vidal-Ollivier E, Laget M, Balansard G, Duménil G. Antimutagenic activity of some saponins

isolated from *Calendula officinalis* L., *C. arvensis* L. and *Hedera helix* L. Mutagenesis 1990; 5:327-31.

49. Amara-Mokrane YA, Lehucher-Michel MP, Balansard G, Duménil G, Botta A. Protective effects of α-hederin, chlorophyllin and ascorbic acid towards the induction of micronuclei by doxorubicin in cultured human lymphocytes. Mutagenesis 1996; 11:161-7.

50. Quetin-Leclercq J, Elias R, Balansard G, Bassleer R, Angenot L. Cytotoxic activity of some triterpenoid saponins. Planta Med 1992;58:279-81.

51. Danloy S, Quetin-Leclercq J, Coucke P, De Pauw-

Gillet M-C, Elias R, Balansard G et al. Effects of α-hederin, a saponin extracted from *Hedera helix*, on cells cultured *in vitro*. Planta Med 1994;60:45-9.

52. Daston GP, Overmann GJ, Baines D, Taubeneck MW, Lehmann-McKeeman LD, Rogers JM, Keen CL. Altered Zn status by α-hederin in the pregnant rat and its relationship to adverse development outcome. Reproductive Toxicol 1994;8:15-24.

53. Duffy JY, Baines D, Overmann GJ, Keen CL, Daston GP. Repeated administration of α-hederin results in alterations in maternal zinc status and adverse developmental outcome in the rat. Teratology 1997;56:327-34.

HIPPOCASTANI SEMEN

Horse-chestnut Seed

DEFINITION

Horse-chestnut seed consists of the dried seeds of *Aesculus hippocastanum* L. containing not less than 3.0 per cent of triterpene glycosides, expressed as anhydrous aescin ($C_{55}H_{86}O_{24}$; M_r 1131) and calculated with reference to the dried drug.

The material complies with the monographs of the French [1] and German [2] pharmacopoeias.

Draft monographs on Horse-chestnut [3] and Standardised Horse-chestnut Dry Extract [4], intended for the European Pharmacopoeia, have been published.

CONSTITUENTS

The characteristic constituents, collectively known as aescin (3-10%), are a mixture of acylated triterpene glycosides (saponins) based on two main aglycones, protoaescigenin and barringtogenol C, which differ only in that protoaescigenin has a hydroxyl group on C-24. All the saponins have a trisaccharide group at C-3, comprising glucuronic acid with substituent sugars (glucose, galactose or xylose) at the 2- and 4-positions. The two major saponins, both arising from protoaescigenin, are esterified at the 21β-position, one with angelic acid, the other with tiglic acid, and with acetic acid at the 22α-position [5-11].

More than 30 different saponins have been identified in aescin. They can be fractionated into: β-aescin, containing only 22-*O*-acetyl compounds; crypto-aescin, containing only 28-*O*-acetyl compounds; and α-aescin, which is a mixture of β-aescin and cryptoaescin [6,8,11,12].

Other constituents include flavonoids, principally di- and triglycosides of quercetin and kaempferol (0.3%) [13], sterols [14,15], essential oil [16] and a high proportion of starch (30-60%) [11].

The seed pericarp contains saponins based on two aglycones, barringtogenol C and R_1-barrigenol [17], and proanthocyanidins [18-20].

E/S/C/O/P
MONOGRAPHS
Second Edition

CLINICAL PARTICULARS

Therapeutic indications
Chronic venous insufficiency, varicosis [11,21-33].

Posology and method of administration

Dosage

Adult daily dose: drug or hydroalcoholic extract containing 50-150 mg of triterpene glycosides (calculated as aescin), usually in divided doses [21-33].
Elderly: dose as for adults.

Not recommended for children.

Method of administration
For oral administration in solid or liquid preparations.

Duration of administration
No restriction.

Contra-indications
None known.

Special warnings and special precautions for use.
None required.

Interactions with other medicaments and other forms of interaction
None reported.

Pregnancy and lactation
Horse-chestnut seed extracts have been used in clinical studies involving pregnant women [21,25,27,28], with some studies excluding those in the third trimester [25,28]. No adverse effects have been reported but, in accordance with general medical practice, the drug should not be used during pregnancy or lactation without medical advice.

Effects on ability to drive and use machines
None known.

Undesirable effects
In rare cases gastric irritation or pruritus may occur [11,27,33,34].

Overdose
No toxic effects reported.

PHARMACOLOGICAL PROPERTIES

Note: HCSE is used as an abbreviation for "horse-chestnut seed extract" in the following text.

Pharmacodynamic properties

Anti-inflammatory and anti-oedematous effects

In vitro experiments
A saponin fraction from horse-chestnut seed inhibited the activity of prostaglandin synthetase [35].

In vivo experiments
Aescin significantly inhibited egg albumin-induced rat paw oedema (p<0.001) when administered intravenously at 0.2 and 2.5 mg/kg body weight [36].

Aescin administered intraperitoneally at 4 mg/kg body weight completely inhibited dextran-induced exudative oedema on rat paw skin; the effect was considered to be due primarily to the potent vaso-constrictive activity of aescin [37].

In carrageenan-induced rat paw oedema a saponin fraction from horse-chestnut seed, administered intravenously at 3.75 mg/kg body weight, inhibited inflammation; it also showed significant analgesic activity when administered orally at 7.5 mg/kg or intravenously at 3.75 mg/kg (p<0.001) [35].

When aescin was injected at 2.5 mg/kg into the tail veins of rats, which were subsequently treated intra-peritoneally with 50% egg white solution (24 ml/kg) and 1% Evans Blue (5 ml/kg, intravenously), the dye remained mainly in the mesenteric vessels, whereas in control animals a high concentration of dye was found in the abdominal cavity. Thus aescin effectively prevented an increase in vascular permeability caused by egg white injection [36].

Pharmacological studies in humans
The effect of HCSE on transcapillary filtration has been assessed by measuring capillary filtration co-efficients in two randomized, placebo-controlled studies [38,39]. In the first study, oral administration of a single dose of HCSE (300 mg; n = 12) or placebo (n = 14) to healthy volunteers produced a significantly lower capillary filtration coefficient in the verum group [38]. In the second study, which had a double-blind, crossover design and involved 22 patients with chronic venous insufficiency, 3 hours after oral admin-istration of a single dose of HCSE (600 mg, standardized to 100 mg of aescin) the capillary filtration coefficient had decreased significantly by 22% (p = 0.006), compared to a slight increase with placebo [39]. Both studies demonstrated the oedema-protective effect of HCSE, induced by an increase in capillary resistance.

Effects on venous tone

In vitro experiments
HCSE (standardized to 16% aescin) and pure aescin in concentrations of 5-150 µg/ml had no effect on the tone of isolated veins from cows (vena metacarpalis) or humans (vena saphena). However, higher concentrations of the extract (0.2 mg/ml) and aescin (0.1 mg/ml) slowly induced a contraction, which was irreversible even 3 hours after exposure. The effect was comparable to that of a standard saponin (Merck) tested in the same experiment [40].

Similar effects on venous tone were observed with

HCSE at 0.2-1 mg/ml on isolated veins of rabbits [41] and with aescin at 1 ng/ml to 1 mg/ml on human vein (vena saphena) preparations [42]. The effects were comparable to those of essential phospholipids [41], serotonin or dihydroergotamine [43], and significantly greater than those of acetylcholine or vasopressin [42].

The above results could be reproduced on isolated human vein (vena saphena) and rabbit portal vein with aescin at 5-10 mg/ml; these lower concentrations increased the tonus of the veins [44]. The effect is partly explained by the ability of aescin to enhance $PGF_{2\alpha}$ generation in the veins. It has been suggested that the prostaglandins act primarily as local hormones in the regulation of vascular reactivity [44].

In the isolated canine saphenous vein, HCSE induced concentration-dependent contractions at concentrations above 5×10^{-5} mg/ml; the contraction at 5×10^{-4} mg/ml reached a maximum in 15 minutes and lasted more than 5 hours [45].

In vivo experiments
HCSE administered intravenously at 50 mg significantly increased femoral venous pressure (p<0.001) in anaesthetized dogs [45].

In the canine saphenous vein perfused in the opposite direction to blood flow, HCSE decreased the flow in a dose-dependent manner, 100 mg producing an effect comparable to that of 10 µg of noradrenaline, demonstrating that it can ensure closure of valves [45].

HCSE orally administered to rats at 200 mg/kg significantly decreased cutaneous capillary hyperpermeability induced by histamine or serotonin (p<0.001) [45].

Pharmacological studies in humans
In a study of venous tone, a single dose of 150 mg of HCSE was administered orally to 23 healthy young subjects. A further 14 subjects received either 80 mg of HCSE or identical placebo capsules in a double-blind, crossover design. Plethysmographic measurements taken before and 2 hours after administration showed that both dosages of HCSE significantly increased venous tone and decreased venous capacity [46].

Comparable results were obtained from a further study in which 12 healthy volunteers firstly received placebos and then a single oral dose of HCSE (360 mg, standardized to 90 mg of aescin). In contrast, intravenous administration of 20 mg of aescin had no effect on venous tone [47].

Effects on lysosymal enzymes

In vitro experiments
Aescin showed inhibitory activity (IC_{50}: 149.9 µM) on hyaluronidase, which promotes the degradation of hyaluronic acid, the main component of the extravascular matrix surrounding capillary walls; its activity was considerably greater than that of its genin, aescinol (IC_{50}: 1.65 mM) [48].

Pharmacological studies in humans
Three hydrolases, β-N-acetylglucosaminidase, β-glucuronidase and arylsulphatase, catalyze the breakdown of proteoglycans, which constitute part of capillary walls. In the serum of varicose in-patients the activity of these enzymes has been found to be markedly increased (by 60-120%) compared to healthy subjects; this may render the capillaries more permeable and fragile [49]. In two studies, one with 10 patients [49] and the other with 15 patients [50], oral administration of HCSE (900 mg, standardized to 150 mg of aescin) daily for 12 consecutive days led to significant reductions in the activity of these enzymes (p<0.01 and p<0.05 respectively), of the same order of magnitude (about 30%) for each enzyme. It was hypothesized that HCSE does not inhibit the individual enzymes but has a protective action towards the site of enzyme release, the fragile lysosomal membrane. The observed enzyme inhibition should reduce degradation of the proteoglycans, providing an explanation for the effect of HCSE on capillary permeability and capillary resistance [51].

Effects on blood flow

Pharmacological studies in humans
Treatment of 30 varicosis patients with oral HCSE (1800 mg daily) for 12 days led to a 30% increase in flow velocity of venous blood between the instep and groin, as quantitatively determined by the "133Xe appearance method". Blood viscosity was reduced at the same time. The favourable effects on haemodynamics correlated with improvements in subjective complaints in 73% of the cases [43].

Effects on haematoma

Pharmacological studies in humans
The efficacy of a topically applied gel containing 2% of aescin in reducing the tenderness to pressure of haematoma (experimentally induced by injection) was demonstrated in a randomized, double blind, placebo-controlled, single dose study involving 70 healthy subjects (34 verum, 36 placebo). Based on tonometric sensitivity measurements, the aescin gel significantly reduced tenderness to pressure (p<0.001) and this effect was observed from 1 hour after treatment until the end of the 9-hour study period [52].

Clinical studies

Anti-inflammatory and anti-oedematous effects
The anti-oedematous effect of various HCSE preparations, standardized on aescin and administered

orally, has been proven in a number of clinical studies on patients suffering from chronic venous insufficiency or varicosis [21-33].

In three double-blind, placebo-controlled, crossover studies [21-23], twice daily oral administration of a preparation containing HCSE (300 mg, standardized to 50 mg of aescin) for 20-21 days produced significant improvement in symptoms compared to placebo.

In the first crossover study, based on objective and subjective assessments on 96 female patients with varicosis of varying etiology, significant improvements (p<0.001) were noted over a range of symptoms such as oedema, inflammation, pruritus, tenderness and pigmentation [21].

In the second crossover study, subjective assessment of 226 predominantly female patients with varicosis showed significant improvements in symptoms of oedema, pain and pruritus (p<0.01 or 0.05) [22].

In the third crossover study, on 95 patients with varicosis or chronic venous insufficiency, subjective assessments revealed significant improvements in oedema, systremma, pain and fatigue or heaviness of the legs (p<0.01 or p<0.05), but not in pruritus [23].

Measurements of leg or foot volume (with a hydro-plethysmometer) and/or circumferences, in some cases accompanied by assessment of subjective symptoms, were used to demonstrate the anti-oedematous and oedema-protective effects of oral treatment with HCSE in the following studies [24-33].

39 patients with venous oedema attributed to chronic venous insufficiency were treated with either HCSE (standardized to 150 mg of aescin; n = 20) or placebo (n = 19) daily for 6 weeks in a randomized, double-blind study. Leg volume before and after oedema provocation, i.e. subjecting the leg to stress in the form of a haemostatic load, was measured at 2-week intervals. A significant reduction in average leg volume from 1565 ml to 1481 ml was observed in the verum group (p<0.01) over the 6-week period. The results were more discernible after oedema provocation, demonstrating that the extract has a venoprotective effect under practical conditions of daily activity. These observations were corroborated by auxiliary tests and subjective assessments [24].

In a randomized, double-blind, crossover study, 20 female patients between 20 and 40 years of age with varicosis during pregnancy (excluding patients in their third trimester) or attributed to chronic venous insufficiency stage I received either HCSE (600 mg extract, standardized to 100 mg of aescin) or placebo daily for 2 weeks. A reduction in leg volume after verum treatment was significant (p = 0.009); improvements in the patients who received verum treatment

first were eliminated in the subsequent placebo phase. Leg circumferences and subjective symptoms were also significantly reduced during verum therapy (p<0.05). In assessment of efficacy the verum treatment was rated as significantly better than placebo by both the physicians (p<0.01) and the patients (p<0.05) [25].

30 outpatients with symptoms of chronic venous insufficiency including peripheral oedema received either HCSE (600 mg, standardized to 100 mg of aescin; n = 15) or placebo (n =15) daily for 20 days in a randomized, double-blind study. A significant reduction in leg circumference (p<0.05), and hence in oedema, was observed in the verum group [26].

In a randomized, double-blind, crossover study, 50 pregnant women (stage of pregnancy not stated) with oedema due to chronic venous insufficiency received either HCSE (480-580 mg, standardized to 100 mg of aescin) or placebo daily for 20 days. Significant reductions in foot volume (p<0.01) before and after oedema provocation were observed after verum treatment; the circumferences at heel, ankle and calf paralleled these changes. Subjective symptoms (pain, fatigue, swelling, itching) were also less severe after verum treatment [27].

In a randomized, double-blind, crossover study, 20 patients with pregnancy-related varicosis (excluding patients in their third trimester) or chronic venous insufficiency received, in two 14-day treatment phases separated by a 5-day wash-out period, HCSE (480-580 mg daily, standardized to 100 mg of aescin) and then placebo, or vice versa. Significant reductions in leg volume (p = 0.0009) were observed after verum treatment. Decreases in leg circumference and improvements in subjectively assessed symptoms correlated with this finding [28].

In a randomized, double-blind comparative study 40 patients suffering from chronic venous insufficiency and peripheral venous oedema received, after a one-week placebo run-in period, either HSCE (standard-ized to 150 mg of aescin; n = 20) or a preparation pro-viding 2000 mg of O-(β-hydroxyethyl)-rutoside (n = 20) daily for 8 weeks. Based on leg circumferences (measured both before and after an oedema-provoking procedure with legs hanging free), the two preparations had a similar and favourable effect in reducing oedema over 8 weeks of treatment, but the HSCE preparation had a more pronounced effect [29].

Patients with chronic venous insufficiency received either HCSE (standardized to 100 mg of aescin; n = 19) or placebo (n = 20) daily for 4 weeks in a double-blind study. Foot and lower leg volume was signifi-cantly reduced in the verum group (p<0.01 after 14 days, p<0.001 after 28 days); this was the case both in normal blood flow and in pronounced ischaemia. Subjective symptoms (pain, tiredness, feeling of tension and pruritus in the legs) and global assessment of the treatment by physicians and patients also showed significant improvement in the verum group. There were no differences between verum and placebo with regard to venous capacity or venous drainage when the leg was elevated [30].

In a randomized study, 240 patients with substantial lower leg oedema due to chronic venous insufficiency received, after a 2-week placebo run-in period, one of three treatments daily for 12 weeks: HCSE providing 100 mg of aescin (n = 95), compression therapy with elastic compression stockings (n = 99) or placebo (n = 46). The study was blinded in the HCSE and placebo groups. Patients allocated to compression treatment received a diuretic daily during the first 7 days and thereafter were provided with individually fitted class II compression stockings. Based on measurement of lower leg volumes in the more severely affected leg, significant oedema reductions were achieved in the HCSE (p = 0.005) and compression therapy (p = 0.002) groups compared to the placebo group, and the two verum therapies were shown to be equivalent (p<0.001). It was concluded that HCSE offers an alternative to compression for the treatment of oedema resulting from chronic venous insufficiency; a 12-week course of HCSE may provide a 25% reduction in mean oedema volume [31].

In a randomized, double-blind, crossover study, 50 patients with varicosis and oedema attributed to chronic venous insufficiency received, after a one-week placebo run-in phase, an unspecified HCSE preparation (one sustained release tablet twice daily) for 2 weeks and then, after a one-week wash-out phase, placebo, or vice versa. A significant decrease in leg volume (p<0.01) was achieved after verum treatment compared to placebo [32].

In a randomized, double-blind study, 137 female postmenopausal patients with chronic venous insufficiency were given one of the following treat-ments (plus placebo tablets and/or capsules of identical appearance to the alternative treatments):
a) 600 mg of HCSE standardized to 100 mg of aescin, daily for 12 weeks (n = 51),
   or
b) a standardized mixture of oxerutins, 1000 mg daily for 12 weeks (OX1000; n = 51),
   or
c) a standardized mixture of oxerutins, 1000 mg (loading dose) daily for 4 weeks, followed by 500 mg (maintenance dose) daily for 8 weeks (OX1000-500; n = 35).

After a one-week placebo run-in and 12 weeks of treatment, there was a follow-up period of 6 weeks without treatment. Reductions in mean leg volumes after 18 weeks, expressed as area under baseline (ml.d), were 3004 for HCSE, 5273 for OX1000 and 3187 for OX1000-500. The numerical superiority of

oxerutins seemed to be based not on a higher intrinsic potency but on a higher responder fraction of the study population. It was concluded that 600 mg of HCSE or 1000 mg of oxerutins daily are effective in treatment of chronic venous insufficiency and able to produce a mean reduction in leg volume of about 100 ml after 12 weeks in responding patients. This represents a therapeutically relevant reduction in oedema, comparable to values reported for com-pression therapy [33].

The conclusions from a criteria-based systematic review of 13 randomized, double-blind, controlled clinical studies (8 placebo-controlled and 5 controlled against reference medications) were that the evidence implied that:
- HCSE is superior to placebo and as effective as reference medications in alleviating the objective signs and subjective symptoms of chronic venous insufficiency.
- HCSE is safe and effective as a symptomatic, short-term treatment of chronic venous insufficiency.

Publication bias and methodological shortcomings were considered important caveats to these con-clusions, with more rigorous randomized controlled trials required to verify the usefulness of the treatment, especially for long term use and as an adjunct to compression therapy [53].

Pharmacokinetic properties

Pharmacokinetics in animals
After intravenous administration of ^{3}H-aescin to rats and mice the concentrations in blood declined rapidly during the first few hours and more slowly thereafter. Elimination took place via the liver and kidneys. One hour after injection about 30% of the dose had been excreted, two thirds in bile and one third in urine, mostly as the parent drug. Organ distribution studies showed higher concentrations than in the blood only in the excretion organs, while the CNS was almost free from aescin [54,55].

After oral administration to rats and mice ^{3}H-aescin was absorbed to the extent of 10-15% of the dose, measured by the amounts of aescin and metabolites excreted in bile and urine. Aescin seemed to be absorbed mainly from the duodenum. The percentage of metabolites was higher than after intravenous injection; their chromatographic profile appeared partly aescinol-like and partly as aglycones [54,55].

Pharmacokinetics in humans
After intravenous administration the pharmacokinetics of aescin correspond to an open three compartment model. With an intravenous dose of 5 mg of aescin (infusion rate: 718 µg/min) the elimination half-life $t_{0.5}\alpha$ was 6.6 minutes; $t_{0.5}\beta$ was 1.74 hours and $t_{0.5}\gamma$ was 14.36 hours. The distribution volume under

steady state conditions was 100.9 litres, total plasma clearance 21.8 ml/min and renal clearance 1.7 ml/min. Urinary excretion from 0 to 120 hours after injection comprised 8.2% of the dose [34].

After oral administration of an aescin solution the absolute bioavailability was determined as only 1.5%. This low bioavailability is due to a pronounced first pass effect (metabolism and biliary excretion). The relative bioavailability of aescin from a horse-chestnut seed extract was 100% compared to an aescin solution [34].

No significant differences in relative bioavailability between rapid and slow release oral dosage forms of HCSE were seen by Kunz et al. [56,57] whereas Schrader et al. [58] and Dittgen et al. [59] noted higher bioavailability with the rapid release form. Maximum plasma concentrations were found between 1.8 and 3.3 hours [57-61] irrespective of the type of preparation. Terminal plasma half-lives were calculated as 17.8-21.2 hours [60] and 18.5-24.0 hours [59] respectively. Only 0.1% of the dose could be detected in urine [34]. The pharmacokinetics and bioavailability of aescin in various extract preparations have been reviewed by Loew et al. [62,63].

In a recent randomized, open, crossover study, 18 healthy volunteers received an oral rapid-release tablet formulation (2 × 300 mg of HCSE, providing 2 × 50 mg of aescin, daily for 7 days) and subsequently, without a wash-out period, a prolonged-release capsule formulation as a reference preparation (2 × 240-290 mg of HCSE, providing 2 × 50 mg of aescin, daily for 7 days), or vice versa. Blood samples covering a full 24-hour cycle were taken on the 7th day in each test period for steady-state pharmacokinetic profiling using a specific radioimmunoassay for serum concentrations of β-aescin. With both formulations, C_{max} after the first dose of the day was in the range 16.7-18.5 ng/ml, t_{max} was 2.1 hours and $C_{average}$ 9.9-10.6 ng/ml. Somewhat lower values for C_{max} (10.2-11.7 ng/ml) and $C_{average}$ (7.0-7.1 ng/ml) after the second dose of the day were attributed to the effects of food. The two formulations proved bioequivalent with respect to the extent of absorption of aescin; AUC values (0-24 hours) ranged from 84% to 114% (90% confidence interval; point estimate 98%) [57].

Plasma protein binding of aescin was determined to be 84% [34]; binding to erythrocytes can be ignored [64]. In agreement with the animal studies [54] a blood-brain barrier for aescin was also apparent in humans [64].

Preclinical safety data

Acute toxicity
LD_{50} values for HCSE determined in various laboratory

animals are given in Table 1. Dogs were also tested but the oral LD_{50} could not be established since doses of more than 130 mg/kg body weight caused vomiting of the substance shortly after administration [65].

TABLE 1
LD_{50} values of horse-chestnut seed extract in mg/kg body weight [65]

Animal	Mode of Administration		
	Oral	Intra-peritoneal	Intra-venous
Mouse	990	342	138
Rat	2150		165
Guinea pig	1120		465
Rabbit	1530		180

The oral LD_{50} of an aqueous extract (1:1) from horse-chestnut seed was determined as 10.7 and 10.6 g/kg body weight in adult Syrian hamsters and two-week-old chicks respectively [66].

Sub-acute intravenous toxicity
Daily intravenous doses of HCSE at 9, 30 or 90 mg/kg body weight were administered to rats for 8 weeks. With the 90 mg/kg dose, 8 out of 30 animals died during the first few days but the others developed normal body weights; 9 mg/kg was tolerated virtually without symptoms [65]. The no-effect intravenous dose level was considered to be around 30 mg/kg body weight, approximately 7 times the daily therapeutic dose given orally to humans [34].

Chronic oral toxicity
Neither toxic effects nor organ damage were observed after 34-week oral administration of HCSE to dogs (2 male, 2 female per dose and control group) at 20, 40 or 80 mg/kg body weight daily (5 days per week) and to rats (20 male, 20 female per dose and control group) at 100, 200 and 400 mg/kg body weight daily [65].

The highest dose level used in dogs corresponds to 8 times, and that used in rats to 40 times, the usual daily therapeutic dose in humans.

Teratogenicity
No significant effects compared to control animals were observed in teratogenicity studies involving daily oral administration of HCSE at 100 mg/kg body weight to rats and rabbits or at 300 mg/kg to rats. At

300 mg/kg in rabbits a significant reduction (p<0.001) was apparent in the mean body weight of foetuses, 25.2 g compared to 31.2 g in control animals [65]. However, 300 mg/kg body weight is approximately 30 times the recommended therapeutic dose in humans [34].

Mutagenicity
In the Ames mutagenicity test, using *Salmonella typhimurium* strain TA98, HCSE gave a negative response without activation, but a weakly positive response (factor 2-3) with S9 activation. Fluid extracts of horse-chestnut seed gave a weakly positive response (factor 2-3) without activation and a negative response with activation. The authors suggested that quercetin is possibly the main mutagenic principle in these extracts [67]. However, the potential genotoxicity of quercetin, an ubiquitous substance found in many fruits and vegetables (daily intake from food estimated as at least 25 mg), has been extensively studied and the results have been interpreted as not relevant to humans [68].

Clinical safety data
From controlled studies in patients with chronic venous insufficiency the rate of adverse reactions from HCSE has ranged from 0.9 to 3.0%, mainly involving gastrointestinal complaints, dizziness, headache or itching. In a large observational study, only 0.6% of patients reported adverse events, consisting mainly of gastrointestinal disturbances. Horse-chestnut seed preparations and aescin are therefore considered to have excellent tolerability [69].

REFERENCES

1. Marron d'Inde - Aesculus hippocastanum. Pharmacopée Française.

2. Roßkastaniensamen - Hippocastani semen. Deutsches Arzneibuch.

3. Horse-chestnut - Hippocastani semen. Pharmeuropa 1995;7:519-21.

4. Horse-chestnut Dry Extract, Standardised - Hippocastani extractum siccum normatum. Pharmeuropa 1996;8;7-9.

5. Wulff G, Tschesche R. Über Triterpene. XXVI. Über die Struktur des Rosskastaniensaponine (Aescin) und die Aglykone verwandter Glykoside. Tetrahedron 1969; 25:415-36.

6. Wagner J, Schlemmer W, Hoffmann H. Über Inhaltsstoffe des Roßkastaniensamens. IX. Struktur und Eigenschaften der Triterpenglykoside. Arzneim-Forsch/ Drug Res 1970;20:205-9.

7. Bogs U, Bremer D. Über Roßkastaniensamen und daraus hergestellte Auszüge. Pharmazie 1971;26:410-8.

8. Wagner H, Reger H, Bauer R. Saponinhaltige Drogen und Fertigarzneimittel. HPLC-Analyse am Beispiel von Roßkastaniensamen. Dtsch Apoth Ztg 1985;125:1513-8.

9. Profumo P, Gastaldo P, Martinucci R. Variations in escin content in Aesculus hippocastanum seeds during the year. Fitoterapia 1987;58:184-6.

10. Yoshikawa M, Harada E, Murakami T, Matsuda H, Wariishi N, Yamahara J et al. Escins-Ia, Ib, IIa, IIb, and IIIa, bioactive triterpene oligoglycosides from the seeds of Aesculus hippocastanum L.: their inhibitory effects on ethanol absorption and hypoglycemic activity on glucose tolerance test. Chem Pharm Bull 1994;42:1357-9.

11. Beck M. Aesculus. In: Hänsel R, Keller K, Rimpler H, Schneider G, editors. Hagers Handbuch der Pharmazeutischen Praxis, 5th ed. Volume 4: Drogen A-D. Berlin: Springer-Verlag, 1992:108-22.

12. Wagner J, Hoffmann H, Löw I. Über Inhaltsstoffe des Roßkastaniensamens. VIII. Die Acylaglyka des Kryptoäscins und α-Äscins. Hoppe-Seyler's Z Physiol Chem 1970;351:1133-40.

13. Hübner G, Wray V, Nahrstedt A. Flavonol oligosaccharides from the seeds of Aesculus hippocastanum. Planta Med 1999;65:636-42.

14. Stankovic SK, Bastic MB, Jovanovic JA. 4α-Methylergosta-8,24(28)-dien-3β-ol, a minor sterol in the seed of horse-chestnut. Phytochemistry 1985;24:2466-9.

15. Stankovic SK, Bastic MB, Jovanovic JA. Composition of the sterol fraction in horse-chestnut. Phytochemistry 1984;23:2677-9.

16. Buchbauer G, Jirovetz L, Wasicky M. Volatiles of common horsechestnut (Aesculus hippocastanum L.) (Hippocastanaceae) peels and seeds. J Essent Oil Res 1994;6:507-11.

17. Vadkerti A, Proksa B, Voticky Z. Structure of hippocastanoside, a new saponin from the seed pericarp of horse-chestnut (Aesculus hippocastanum L.). I. Structure of the aglycone. Chem Papers 1989;43:783-91.

18. Mayer W, Goll L, Moritz von Arndt E, Mannschreck A. Procyanidino-(−)-epicatechin, ein zweiarmig verknüpftes, kondensiertes Proanthocyanidin aus Aesculus hippocastanum. Tetrahedron Letters 1966; 4:429-35.

19. Morimoto S, Nonaka G-I, Nishioka I. Tannins and related compounds. LIX. Aesculitannins, novel proanthocyanidins with doubly-bonded structures from Aesculus hippocastanum L. Chem Pharm Bull 1987; 35:4717-29.

20. Santos-Buelga C, Kolodziej H, Treutter D. Procyanidin trimers possessing a doubly linked structure from Aesculus hippocastanum. Phytochemistry 1995;38: 499-504.

21. Alter H. Zur medikamentösen Therapie der Varikosis. Z Allg Med 1973;49:1301-4.

22. Neiss A, Böhm C. Zum Wirksamkeitsnachweis von Roßkastaniensamenextrakt beim varikösen Symptomenkomplex. Münch med Wschr 1976;118:213-6.

23. Friederich HC, Vogelsberg H, Neiss A. Ein Beitrag zur Bewertung von intern wirksamen Venenpharmaka. Z Hautkr 1978;53:369-74.

24. Diehm C, Vollbrecht D, Hübsch-Müller C, Müller-Bühl U. Clinical efficacy of edema protection in patients with venous edema due to chronic venous insufficiency. In: Davy A and Stemmer R, editors. *Phlébologie '89*, Volume 2. London-Paris: John Libbey Eurotext. 1989: 712-5. (Actes de 10ᵉ Congrès Mondial, Union Internationale de Phlébologie. Strasbourg 25-29 September 1989).
Also published in modified form as:
Diehm C, Vollbrecht D, Amendt K, Comberg HU. Medical edema protection - clinical benefit in patients with chronic deep vein incompetence. A placebo controlled double blind study. VASA 1992;21:188-92.

25. Steiner M. Untersuchung zur ödemvermindernden und ödemprotektiven Wirkung von Roßkastaniensamenextrakt. Phlebol Proktol 1990;19:239-42.

26. Pilz E. Ödeme bei Venenerkrankungen. Med Welt 1990;41:1143-4.

27. Steiner M, Hillemanns HG. Venostasin retard in the management of venous problems during pregnancy. Phlebology 1990;5:41-4.

28. Steiner M, Hillemanns HG. Untersuchung zur ödemprotektiven Wirkung eines Venentherapeutikums. Münch med Wschr 1986;128:551-2.

29. Erler M. Roßkastaniensamenextrakt bei der Therapie peripherer venöser Ödeme. Med Welt 1991;42:593-6.

30. Rudofsky G, Neiß A, Otto K, Seibel K. Ödemprotektive Wirkung und klinische Wirksamkeit von Roßkastaniensamenextrakt im Doppelblindversuch. Phlebol Proktol 1986;15:47-54.

31. Diehm C, Trampisch HJ, Lange S, Schmidt C. Comparison of leg compression stocking and oral horse-chestnut seed extract therapy in patients with chronic venous insufficiency. Lancet 1996;347:292-4.
Comments and authors' reply published as:
Vayssairat M, Debure C, Maurel A, Gaitz JP; Simini B; Diehm C, Trampisch HJ, Lange S, Schmidt C. Horse-chestnut seed extract for chronic venous insufficiency [Letters]. Lancet 1996;347:1182-3.

32. Steiner M. Clinical efficacy of edema protection in peripheral venous edemas due to CVI. In: Davy A and Stemmer R, editors. *Phlébologie '89*, Volume 2. London-Paris: John Libbey Eurotext. 1989:734-7. (Actes du 10ᵉ Congrès Mondial, Union Internationale de Phlébologie. Strasbourg 25-29 September 1989).

33. Rehn D, Unkauf M, Klein P, Jost V, Lücker PW. Comparative clinical efficacy and tolerability of oxerutins and horse chestnut extract in patients with chronic venous insufficiency. Arzneim-Forsch/Drug Res 1996; 46:483-7.

34. Hitzenberger G. Die therapeutische Wirksamkeit des Roßkastaniensamenextraktes. Wien med Wschr 1989: 385-9.

35. Cebo B, Krupinska J, Sobanski H, Mazur J, Czarnecki R. Pharmacological properties of saponin fractions obtained from domestic crude drugs: *Saponaria officinalis*, *Primula officinalis* and *Aesculus hippocastanum*. Herba Polonica 1976;22:154-62 [Polish, with English summary].

36. Girerd RJ, Di Pasquale G, Steinetz BG, Beach VL, Pearl W. The anti-edema properties of aescin. Arch Int Pharmacodyn 1961;133:127-37.

37. Damas P, Volon G, Damas J, Lecomte J. Sur l'action antioedème de l'escine. Bull Soc Roy Sci Liège 1976; 45:436-42.

38. Pauschinger P, Wörz E, Zwerger E. Die Messung des Filtrationskoeffizienten am menschlichen Unterschenkel und seine pharmakologische Beeinflussung. Med Welt 1981;32:1953-5.

39. Bisler H, Pfeifer R, Klüken N, Pauschinger P. Wirkung von Roßkastaniensamenextrakt auf die transkapilläre Filtration bei chronischer venöser Insuffizienz. Dtsch med Wschr 1986;111:1321-9.

40. Lochs H, Baumgartner H, Konzett H. Zur Beeinflussung des Venentonus durch Roßkastanienextrakte. Arzneim-Forsch/Drug Res 1974;24:1347-50.

41. Balansard P, Joanny P, Bouyard P. Comparaison de l'activité toniveineuse de l'extrait sec de marron d'Inde et de l'association phospholipides essentiels et extrait sec de marron d'Inde. Thérapie 1975;30:907-17.

42. Annoni F, Mauri A, Marincola F, Resele LF. Venotonic activity of escin on the human saphenous vein. Arzneim-Forsch/Drug Res 1979;29:672-5.

43. Klemm J. Strömungsgeschwindigkeit von Blut in varikösen Venen der unteren Extremitäten. Einfluß eines Venentherapeutikums (Venostasin®). Münch med Wschr 1982;124:579-82.

44. Longiave D, Omini C, Nicosia S, Berti F. The mode of action of aescin on isolated veins: relationship with $PGF_{2\alpha}$. Pharmacol Res Commun 1978;10:145-52.

45. Guillaume M, Padioleau F. Veinotonic effect, vascular protection, antiinflammatory and free radical scavenging properties of horse chestnut extract. Arzneim-Forsch/Drug Res 1994;44:25-35.

46. Nehring U. Zum Nachweis der Wirksamkeit von Roßkastanienextrakt auf den Venentonus nach oraler Applikation. Med Welt 1966;17:1662-5.

47. Ehringer H. Zum venentonisierenden Prinzip des Roßkastanienextraktes. Wirkung von reinem Roßkastanienextrakt und von Aescin auf Venenkapazität, Venentonus und Durchblutung der Extremitäten. Med Welt 1968;19:1781-5.

48. Maffei Facino R, Carini M, Stefani R, Aldini G, Saibene L. Anti-elastase and anti-hyaluronidase activities of

saponins and sapogenins from *Hedera helix, Aesculus hippocastanum* and *Ruscus aculeatus*: factors contributing to their efficacy in the treatment of venous insufficiency. Arch Pharm (Weinheim) 1995;328:720-4.

49. Kreysel HW, Nissen HP, Enghofer E. Erhöhte Serumaktivitäten lysosomaler Enzyme bei Varikosis. Beeinflussung durch einen Roßkastaniensamenextrakt. Therapiewoche 1983;33:1098-104.

50. Kreysel HW, Nissen HP, Enghofer E. A possible role of lysosomal enzymes in the pathogenesis of varicosis and the reduction in their serum activity by Venostasin®. VASA 1983;4:377-82.

51. Enghofer E, Seibel K, Hammersen F. Die antiexsudative Wirkung von Roßkastaniensamenextrakt. Neue Ergebnisse zu ihrem Mechanismus. Therapiewoche 1984;34:4130-44.

52. Calabrese C, Preston P. Report of the results of a double-blind, randomized, single-dose trial of a topical 2% escin gel versus placebo in the acute treatment of experimentally-induced hematoma in volunteers. Planta Med 1993;59:394-7.

53. Pittler MH, Ernst E. Horse-chestnut seed extract for chronic venous insufficiency. A criteria-based systematic review. Arch Dermatol 1998;134:1356-60. *Also published in German as:* Pittler MH, Ernst E. Rosskastaniensamen-Extrakt zur Behandlung der chronisch-venösen Insuffizienz. Ein systematischer Review. In: Loew D, Blume H, Dingermann T, editors. Phytopharmaka V. Forschung und klinische Anwendung. Darmstadt: Steinkopff, 1999:127-34.

54. Lang W, Mennicke WH. Pharmakokinetische Untersuchungen mit tritiiertem Aescin an Maus und Ratte. Arzneim-Forsch/Drug Res 1972;22:1928-32.

55. Henschler D, Hempel K, Schultze B, Maurer W. Zur Pharmakokinetic von Aescin. Arzneim-Forsch/Drug Res 1971;21:1682-92.

56. Kunz K, Schaffler K, Biber A, Wauschkuhn CH. Bioverfügbarkeit von β-Aescin nach oraler Gabe zweier Aesculus-Extrakt enthaltender Darreichungsformen an gesunden Probanden. Pharmazie 1991;46:145.

57. Kunz K, Lorkowski G, Petersen G, Samcova E, Schaffler K, Wauschkuhn CH. Bioavailability of escin after administration of two oral formulations containing *Aesculus* extract. Arzneim-Forsch/Drug Res 1998;48:822-5.

58. Schrader E, Schwankl W, Sieder Ch, Christoffel V. Vergleichende Untersuchung zur Bioverfügbarkeit von β-Aescin nach oraler Einmalverabreichung zweier Roßkastaniensamenextrakt enthaltender, galenisch unterschiedlicher Darreichungsformen. Pharmazie 1995;50:623-7.

59. Dittgen M, Zimmermann H, Wober W, Höflich C, Breitbarth H, Timpe C. Untersuchung der Bioverfügbarkeit von β-Aescin nach oraler Verabreichung verschiedener Darreichungsformen. Pharmazie 1996;51:608-10.

60. Oschmann R, Biber A, Lang F, Stumpf H, Kunz K. Pharmakokinetik von β-Aescin nach Gabe verschiedener Aesculus-Extrakt enthaltender Formulierungen. Pharmazie 1996;51:577-81.

61. Schrödter A, Loew D, Schwankl W, Rietbrock N. Zur Validität radioimmunologisch bestimmter Bioverfügbarkeitsdaten von β-Aescin in Roßkastaniensamenextrakten. Arzneim-Forsch/Drug Res 1998;48:905-10.

62. Loew D, Schrödter A, Schwankl W, März RW. Measurement of the bioavailablity of aescin-containing extracts. Methods Findings Exp Clin Pharmacol 2000;22:537-42.

63. Loew D, Schrödter A. Pharmakokinetik und Äquivalenz von Zubereitungen aus Hippocastani semen. In: Loew D, Blume H, Dingermann T, editors. Phytopharmaka V. Forschung und klinische Anwendung. Darmstadt: Steinkopff, 1999:135-43.

64. Ascher PW, Paltauf F. Klinische Untersuchungen über die Pharmakodynamik von tritiummarkierten Aescin. Ärztl Forsch 1970;24:294-8.

65. Liehn HD, Franco PA, Hampel H, Hofrichter G. A toxicological study of extractum Hippocastani semen (EHS). Panminerva Med 1972;14:84-91.

66. Williams MC, Olsen JD. Toxicity of seeds of three *Aesculus* spp to chicks and hamsters. Am J Vet Res 1984;45:539-42.

67. Schimmer O, Krüger A, Paulini H, Haefele F. An evaluation of 55 commercial plant extracts in the Ames mutagenicity test. Pharmazie 1994;49:448-51.

68. Ito N; Hirono I. Is quercetin carcinogenic? [Letters]. Jpn J Cancer Res 1992;83:312-4.

69. Sirtori CR. Aescin: pharmacology, pharmacokinetics and therapeutic profile. Pharmacol Res 2001;44:183-93.

HYPERICI HERBA

St. John's Wort

DEFINITION

St. John's wort consists of the whole or cut, dried flowering tops of *Hypericum perforatum* L., harvested during flowering time. It contains not less than 0.08 per cent of total hypericins, expressed as hypericin ($C_{30}H_{16}O_8$; M_r 504.4) and calculated with reference to the dried drug.

The material complies with the monograph of the European Pharmacopoeia [1].

CONSTITUENTS

The characteristic constituents are naphthodianthrones and phloroglucinols. Naphthodianthrones (0.05-0.3%), consisting mainly of hypericin and pseudo-hypericin, accumulate primarily in the flowers and buds [2,3]; lower levels than 0.1% may result from harvesting of lower parts of the herb. Other naphtho-dianthrones present, and included in the term 'total hypericins', are the biosynthetic precursors proto-hypericin and protopseudohypericin (which are transformed into hypericin and pseudohypericin respectively on exposure to light), and a small amount of cyclopseudohypericin [4-6].

The principal phloroglucinols are hyperforin (2-4.5%) and adhyperforin (0.2-1.8%) [7-9]. Both compounds have limited stability [10-14] and their oxidated derivatives are also present [9].

Quercetin glycosides (2-4%), including hyperoside, quercitrin, isoquercitrin and rutin, are the main flavonoids [2,15-17]; a small amount of free quercetin is also found [17]. Biflavonoids such as I3,II8-biapigenin (0.1-0.5%) and I3',II8-biapigenin (amentoflavone, 0.01-0.05%) occur exclusively in the flowers [2,17-19].

Other constituents include phenylpropanoids, such as chlorogenic acid and other caffeoylquinic and *p*-coumaroylquinic esters [2,20]; condensed tannins and oligomeric proanthocyanidins [2,3] including procyanidins A2, B1, B2, B3, B5, B7 and C1 [21,22], together with catechin and epicatechin monomers [2,21]; trace amounts of xanthones such as 1,3,6,7-tetrahydroxyxanthone (0.0004% in the leaves and stems) [2,23]; and essential oil (0.1-0.25%), containing mainly higher n-alkanes and monoterpenes [2].

E/S/C/O/P
MONOGRAPHS
Second Edition

CLINICAL PARTICULARS

Therapeutic indications

Preparations based on hydroalcoholic extracts (50-60% ethanol or 80% methanol) and tinctures (49-50% ethanol)
Episodes of mild depressive disorders [24-31] or mild to moderate depressive episodes in accordance with ICD-10 categories F32.0, F32.1, F33.0 and F33.1 (see the boxes below) [32-45].

Other preparations
Mild depression [46]; support of emotional balance [47].

Posology and method of administration

Dosage

Preparations based on hydroalcoholic extracts (50-60% ethanol or 80% methanol)
Adults and children from 12 years: 450-1050 mg daily of hydroalcoholic dry extracts with drug-to-extract ratios of 2.5-5:1, 4-7:1 or 5-7:1 [28-31,34-41, 43-45, 50,51].

Herbal tinctures and teas
3-4.5 ml daily of tincture (1:5, ethanol 60 % V/V) [24-27,32,33,52,53].
2-4 g of the drug daily for tea infusions [47].

Elderly: dose as for adults

Children from 6 to 12 years under medical supervision only: half the adult dose.

Method of administration
For oral administration.

Duration of administration
No restriction. If symptoms persist for more than 4-6 weeks, seek medical advice.

Contra-indications
Not to be used after organ transplants [54] or by HIV-antibody positive individuals treated with protease-1 inhibitors (e.g. indinavir) [55].

Special warnings and special precautions for use
As with all antidepressant treatments, full manifestation of the therapeutic effect may take 3-4 weeks;

Classification of severity of depression based on ICD-10 criteria [48]

Mild depressive episode: [F32.0/F33.0] — Mild first manifestation or mild recurrence of at least two target signs and at least two associated symptoms

Moderate depressive episode: [F32.1/F33.1] — Two or three target signs and at least three or four associated symptoms (first manifestation or recurrent episode)

Severe depressive episode: [F32.2/F33.2/F32.3/F33.3] — All three target signs and at least four associated symptoms, some particularly pronounced (first manifestation or recurrent, without or with psychotic symptoms)

Diagnostic features of depressive disorders according to ICD-10 Chapter V Primary Care Version [49]

Target signs
Low or sad mood
Loss of interest or pleasure
Fatigue or loss of energy

Associated symptoms
Disturbed sleep
Feelings of guilt and unworthiness
Reduced self-esteem and self confidence
Poor concentration
Disturbed appetite
Decreased libido
Suicidal throughts or acts
Agitation or slowing of movement or speech
Weight loss

Symptoms of anxiety or nervousness are also frequently present there is a risk of suicide, particularly at the beginning of treatment, due to the delay between treatment and clinical improvement. If a significant treatment response in depressive disorders is not apparent after 4 weeks, the medication should be discontinued.

Clinical data on the efficacy of St. John's wort do not support its use in patients with severe major depression or with acute severe depressive disorders [56-58].

It appears advisable to discontinue therapy with St. John's wort in patients to be treated with ciclosporin or indinavir or other antiretroviral substances, and to take particular care in patients on other medication such as antidepressants, anticoagulant therapy (monitoring of clotting time) or therapy with digoxin or theophylline (monitoring of blood levels).

Interaction with other medicaments and other forms of interaction
A number of interactions with preparations of St. John's wort have been reported [7,59,60]. Several types of interaction are involved, such as the so-called serotonin syndrome in cases of concomitant use of St. John's wort preparations with certain antidepressants [61,62] or reductions in blood levels and hence efficacy of other medications. Reduced blood levels have been reported with respect to ciclosporin [54,63,64], indinavir and potentially other antiretroviral protease and transcriptase inhibitors [55], the anticoagulants phenprocoumon and warfarin [65,66], theophylline [67] and digoxin [68].

Induction of several subtypes of the enzyme cytochrome P450 has been discussed as a potential mechanism of the interactions [69-75], but increased expression of the P-glycoprotein drug transporter has also been reported [76].

It remains an open question whether St. John's wort preparations also interact with oral contraceptives, particularly low dose contraceptives (< 50 μg of oestrogen) but a clinical study with a St. John's wort preparation and a contraceptive containing 0.15 mg of desogestrel and 20 μg of ethinylestradiol did not show any sign of an interaction [77].

Pregnancy and lactation
No human data available. In accordance with general medical practice, the product should not be used during pregnancy and lactation without medical advice.

Effects on ability to drive and use machines
Clinical studies indicate no negative influence on general performance or the ability to drive [78,79].

Undesirable effects
At therapeutic dose levels (up to the equivalent of 6 g of drug), occasional mild gastrointestinal disturbances, nausea, restlessness, fatigue, headache or allergic reactions have been reported [24-47,50-53,56-58,80-93]. Onset of mania was reported in 2 patients with latent bipolar disorders [94]. In one patient taking 500 mg of powdered St. John's wort daily for 4 weeks, stinging pain was experienced on the face, the dorsum of both hands and on arms and legs after exposure to sunlight; the symptoms, which disappeared after discontinuation of the product, were restricted to areas of skin exposed to sunlight; no motor or other sensory disturbances were noted [95]. In another patient, who had ingested 240 mg of St. John's wort extract daily for 3 years, an itchy rash developed on skin areas exposed to light; after discontinuation the symptoms disappeared completely within 2 weeks [96].

In healthy subjects treated with 1800 mg of hydromethanolic extract (containing 5.6 mg of total hypericin) daily for 15 days a slight increase in dermal light sensitivity, evidenced by a change in skin pigmentation, was observed. This could be compensated by reducing light exposure time by 21% [97].

Overdose
Serious phototoxic reactions may occur at much higher dosages than used therapeutically [98]. In healthy subjects, photosensitivity occurred after ingestion of a single dose of 3600 mg (but not after 900 mg or 1800 mg) of a hydromethanolic extract of St. John's wort containing 11.25 mg of total hypericin and experimental exposure to UV-A light, but with only marginal significance (p<0.03) compared to placebo [97]. Typical phototoxic symptoms include rash, pruritus and erythema. Treatment consists of avoiding exposure to direct sunlight [99].

PHARMACOLOGICAL PROPERTIES

Pharmacodynamics

In vitro experiments

Effects on enzyme activity
Hydroethanolic extracts of *Hypericum perforatum* have shown inhibition of type A monoamine oxidase (MAO) [100]. Hypericin and St. John's wort preparations have rather low MAO inhibiting activity, whereas xanthones, which are present only in minor quantities (up to 10 ppm) appear to have high MAO-inhibiting activity [101,102].

Inhibition of the enzyme catechol-O-methyl-transferase (COMT) is reported in St. John's wort fractions containing mainly flavonoids [101].

A hydroethanolic extract of St. John's wort, as well as pure hypericin, inhibited the enzyme dopamine-β-hydroxylase *in vitro* [103]. Dopamine-β-hydroxylase was inhibited by an ethanolic extract from St. John's wort with an IC_{50} of 0.1 μmol/litre (molarity referring to total hypericin content) and by commercially available hypericin with an IC_{50} of 21 μmol/litre; tyrosinase and tyrosine decarboxylase were not influenced by hypericin at 1-10 μmol/litre [104]. In another investigation, dopamine-β-hydroxylase was inhibited by pseudohypericin with an IC_{50} of 3 μmol/litre and by hypericin with an IC_{50} of 5 μmol/litre, whereas the IC_{50} values of various flavonoids were 50 μmol/litre and higher [105].

Receptor binding
Depression has been attributed to reduced availability of serotonin (5-HT), norepinephrine or dopamine in the CNS. Consequently, antidepressants increase the levels of neurotransmitters, e.g. by reuptake inhibition or by inhibiting the degradation. N-Methyl-D-aspartate (NMDA) receptor-mediated processes or binding to opioid receptors have also been considered to be involved in the mechanism of action of conventional antidepressants.

Receptor binding studies with a hydroethanolic extract containing approx. 0.15% of total hypericin revealed moderate interactions with the GABA$_A$/benzodiazepine receptor/chloride-ionophore complex: displacement of ^{3}H-muscimol, ^{3}H-flunitrazepam and ^{35}S-TBPS (t-butyl-bicyclo-phosphorothionate) binding. Pure hypericin resulted in increased binding at the GABA$_A$ and benzodiazepine receptors and at the 5-HT$_1$ receptor [106].

The biflavonoid amentoflavone has binding activity at the benzodiazepine receptor [107]. A hydromethanolic extract caused reduced expression of serotonin receptors in a neuroblastoma cell line model [108]. Binding to benzodiazepine binding sites in rat brain was inhibited with an IC_{50} of 6.8 μg/ml by a flower extract from St. John's wort, obtained by extraction with methanol followed by acetone, whereas leaf extracts up to 200 μg/ml caused only 25% inhibition of flumazenil binding. The IC_{50} of amentoflavone was 14.9 nM ≅ 7.45 ng/ml, whereas hypericin, flavones and glycosylated flavonoids at concentrations up to 1 μM did not inhibit binding [109].

A St. John's wort extract showed receptor affinity for adenosine (non-specific), GABA$_A$, GABA$_B$, benzodiazepine, inositol triphosphate and MAO-A and –B, whereas pure hypericin had affinity only for NMDA receptors. Only the concentrations required at the GABA$_A$ and GABA$_B$ receptors (between 0.005 and 0.5 μg/ml) were in a relevant dose range. The involvement of GABA in affective disorders is under discussion [110].

The affinity of 1 μM hypericin was determined at 30 receptors or binding sites; more than 40% inhibition was found for non-selective muscarinic cholinergic receptors and for non-selective σ-opioid receptors. Opioid receptor binding of hypericin might be linked to clinical efficacy [111]. Binding of [^{3}H]naloxone to human μ- and rat κ-opioid receptors was inhibited by St. John's wort extracts with IC_{50} values of 25 and 90 μg/ml respectively. Up to a concentration of 10 μM (≅ 5 μg/ml) quercetin, kaempferol and quercitrin were ineffective [112].

Ethanolic extracts produced relatively weak inhibition of binding to μ-, κ- and δ-opioid, GABA$_A$ and oestrogen-α receptors; the opioid binding was inhibited approximately 10 times more potently by methanolic extracts. A hexane fraction strongly inhibited binding to μ-, κ- and δ-opioid receptors and to 5-HT$_6$ and 5-HT$_7$ serotonin receptors. Hypericin, pseudohypericin and hyperforin inhibited binding to both opioid and serotonin receptors in the low micromolar range (the naphthodianthrones at 1-4 μM at opioid receptors and 1, 6 or 10 μM at serotonin receptors; hyperforin at 0.4-1 μM at opioid receptors and 2-3 μM at serotonin receptors). Oestrogen binding was inhibited by biapigenin at a low micromolar concentration. The inhibitory effect of the ethanolic extract on GABA$_A$ binding at about 3 μg/ml was not considered to be correlated to antidepressant activity since extracts of *Valeriana officinalis* and *Passiflora incarnata* were similarly active [113].

Reuptake inhibition
A methanolic extract of St. John's wort inhibited serotonin uptake by rat synaptosomes with an IC_{50} of 6.2 μg/ml [114]. A methanolic extract, a CO_2 extract and pure hyperforin were compared for reuptake inhibition in synaptosomal preparations. Pronounced reuptake inhibition for serotonin, noradrenaline, dopamine, GABA and glutamate was shown for the CO_2 extract (38.8% hyperforin) and for pure hyperforin. IC_{50} values of the methanolic extract (1.5% hyperforin) were about 10 times higher than those of the CO_2 extract, indicating that other constituents besides hyperforin must cause reuptake inhibition [115].

A hydromethanolic extract of St. John's wort (hyperforin content < 5%) inhibited the accumulation of [^{3}H]serotonin (5-HT) in rat brain cortical synaptosomes with an IC_{50} of 7.9 μg/ml, compared to 1.8 μg/ml for pure hyperforin. Thus the activity of the extract cannot be explained solely by its hyperforin content. The same extract at 3-10 μg/ml and hyperforin at 0.3-1 μg/ml induced marked tritium release from synaptosomes preloaded with [^{3}H]5-HT. This indicates reserpine-like properties and excludes marked serotonin uptake inhibition as the mode of action of a hydromethanolic extract of St. John's wort [116].

A hydromethanolic extract from St. John's wort (0.3% hypericin, 4.9% hyperforin) inhibited serotonin and norepinephrine uptake in astrocytes in a dose-dependent manner with IC_{50} values of 25 μg/ml and 10 μg/ml respectively [117]. A hydromethanolic extract from St. John's wort showed only weak inhibitory activity on MAO-A and MAO-B, but effectively inhibited synaptosomal uptake of serotonin, dopamine and norepinephrine with IC_{50} values of 2.43, 0.85 and 4.47 μg/ml respectively [118].

Hyperforin inhibited the reuptake of serotonin, dopamine, noradrenaline and GABA with IC_{50} values of 0.05-0.1 μg/ml and of glutamate with an IC_{50} of 0.5 μg/ml in rat synaptosomal preparations [115]. Elevation of free intracellular Na^+ seems to be responsible for the reuptake inhibition of hyperforin [119]. Hyperforin was tested on voltage- and ligand-gated ionic conductances to measure neuronal responses on stimulation of NMDA (N-methyl-D-aspartate) or AMPA (α-amino-3-hydroxy-5-methylisoxazole-4-propionic acid) receptors. At concentrations between 3 and 100 μM antagonistic effects on the NMDA receptor and on responses mediated by AMPA or GABA were seen [120]. Hyperforin was found to non-competitively inhibit the synaptosomal uptake of ^{3}H-glutamate and ^{3}H-GABA [121].

Immunological parameters
A hydromethanolic extract of St. John's wort caused pronounced suppression of interleukin-6 release in human blood samples after stimulation with phytohaemagglutinin [122]. Hypericin in the micromolar range inhibited phorbol myristate acetate (PMA)- and TNF-α-induced activation of NF-κB, whereas hyperforin or a St. John's wort extract containing 0.15% hypericin and 5% hyperforin were inactive [123]. The myeloperoxidase-catalyzed dimerization of enkephalins was inhibited by St. John's wort extracts [124].

Mononuclear cells from healthy donors were incubated overnight with a hydromethanolic extract from St. John's wort or serotonergic antidepressant drugs (selective serotonin reuptake inhibitors, SSRIs). Cells were tested for natural killer cell activity, since serotonergic pharmacotherapy is associated with an increase in natural killer cell activity. The extract was tested at very low concentrations (0.5-20 ng/ml), paroxetine at 120 ng/ml and norfluoxetine at 100 ng/ml. In contrast to the SSRIs, St. John's wort extract failed to enhance natural killer cell activity at the concentrations studied [125].

In vivo experiments

Behavioural studies
Hydroethanolic preparations of St. John's wort containing known amounts of hypericin (equivalent to 2-12 mg/kg, administered orally) showed CNS activities in mice which can be interpreted as an antidepressant effect. Aggressive behaviour was significantly reduced after 3 weeks of daily oral treatment with extract equivalent to 6 or 12 mg/kg of hypericin. Physical activity was enhanced and no undesired anticholinergic effect was found. A significant increase in physical activity was also observed after intraperitoneal administration of pure hypericin at 20 mg/kg. The same extract significantly increased ethanol-induced sleeping time after oral doses equivalent to 2.4 or 6 mg/kg of hypericin. Oral administration of the extract to mice at doses equivalent to 1, 2 or 3 mg/kg (but not 6 mg/kg) of hypericin resulted in weak reserpine antagonism, indicated by reductions in reserpine-induced hypothermia [126].

A hydromethanolic extract of St. John's wort (0.24-0.32% total hypericin) was studied in a rat model for antidepressant activity, the Porsolt forced-swimming test. At doses of 125-1000 mg/kg body weight the extract significantly reduced the duration of immobility; lower and higher doses were ineffective, indicating a U-shaped dose-activity relationship. As motor activity was not increased in this dose range and the activity was confirmed by repeated application, these findings indicate antidepressant activity. The extract also reduced ketamine-induced sleeping time and increased body temperature in mice. The effects of this extract on immobility time in the Porsolt test, on sleeping time and on body temperature were eliminated by dopamine D_2 antagonists, indicating dopaminergic activity of the extract [127].

After acute oral administration to rats at 250-500 mg/kg, a St. John's wort extract enriched in flavonoids (0.3% hypericin, 4.5% hyperforin and 50% flavonoids) significantly and dose-dependently decreased immobility time in the Porsolt forced-swimming test (p<0.001 compared to saline). Compared to the effect of the extract alone at 500 mg/kg, concomitant treatment of the rats with sulpiride (a dopamine receptor antagonist) or metergoline (a serotonin receptor antagonist) or 6-hydroxydopamine (which destroys noradrenaline-containing neurons) significantly increased the period of immobility by 22-57%, the largest effect being with metergoline (57%; p<0.001). The results indicated that the neurotransmitters studied could be involved in the anti-immobility effects of St. John's wort and suggest that its antidepressant action is probably mediated by serotonergic, noradrenergic and dopaminergic system activation; an increase in serotonergic tone is probably predominant [128].

A hydroethanolic extract proved to be active in three animal models of depression: an acute form of escape deficit (ED), a subacute form of ED and a model of anhedonia. Oral dosages between 250 and 1000 mg/kg body weight were used. The activity of the extract was clearly reduced by antagonists at the dopamine D_1 receptor or the serotonin 5-HT$_{1A}$ receptor [129].

Adaptive changes

Following subacute treatment of rats with 240 mg/kg of a methanolic St. John's wort extract, β-adreno-receptor down-regulation was observed in the frontal cortex, a common characteristic finding for many anti-depressant drugs. The simultaneous up-regulation of $5-HT_2$ receptors observed was in contrast to the $5-HT_2$ down-regulation observed with many classic anti-depressants [118].

Activity of constituents

Chromatographic fractionation of a methanolic St. John's wort extract yielded two fractions with high activity in the Porsolt test, one containing mainly flavonoids, the other naphthodianthrones. Pure hypericin was inactive in the Porsolt test at a dose of 0.8 mg/kg body weight, but procyanidins present in the naphthodianthrones fraction, namely procyanidin B2, markedly increased solubility as well as bioactivity; in combination with B2 even 0.009 mg/kg hypericin was significantly active. Comparable results were obtained with pseudohypericin. Activity due to procyanidin B2 alone could be excluded [130].

In addition to hypericins, a flavonoid fraction from a methanolic extract of St. John's wort and the isolated flavonoids hyperoside, isoquercitrin and miquelianin (0.6 mg/kg) showed significant activity in the Porsolt test after acute and subacute administration [131].

A supercritical carbon dioxide extract from St. John's wort (38.8% hyperforin) was compared to an ethanolic extract (4.5% hyperforin) for activity in the Porsolt test and the learned helplessness paradigm in rats. Both extracts were active, the effect of 5, 15 and 30 mg/kg body weight of the CO_2 extract being comparable to that of 50, 150 or 300 mg/kg of the ethanolic extract [115]. A hydromethanolic and a hydroethanolic extract were compared for activity in the Porsolt test after acute administration. Both extracts, injected intraperitoneally, reduced immobility time in the dose range of 5-40 mg/kg body weight. The effect was more pronounced after one week of pretreatment [132]. After 3 days of pre-treatment, a 50% ethanolic extract of St. John's wort, administered orally at 100 and 200 mg/kg, was as effective as an antidepressant drug (imipramine at 15 mg/kg intraperitoneally) in the Porsolt test, the learned helplessness paradigm and the tail suspension test [133].

Biochemical findings in vivo

St. John's wort extracts

After acute oral administration (24 hours and 1 hour before testing) of a methanolic St. John's wort extract (62.5-500 mg/kg; 0.3% hypericin, 6% flavonoids) or an extract enriched in flavonoids (62.5-500 mg/kg; 0.3% hypericin, 50% flavonoids) their effects on levels of tryptophan, serotonin (5-HT), 5-hydroxy-indolacetic acid (5-HIAA), noradrenaline and dopamine in the cortex, diencephalon and brainstem of rats were evaluated. Results with respect to 5-HT turnover were compared with the effects of fluoxetine (10-80 mg/kg), a selective serotonin reuptake inhibitor with antidepressant activity. The two St. John's wort extracts and fluoxetine increased 5-HT levels in the cortex. The flavonoid-enriched extract increased 5-HT and 5-HIAA levels in the diencephalon, and 5-HT and noradrenaline levels in the brainstem. Both the St. John's wort extracts increased noradrenaline and dopamine levels in the diencephalon [134]. Comparable results for the flavonoid-enriched extract were obtained in a subsequent study using similar techniques; it did not modify tryptophan content, but significantly enhanced 5-HT and 5-HIAA levels in the cortex, diencephalon and brainstem at 125-500 mg/kg, and increased noradrenaline and dopamine in the diencephalon and noradrenaline in the brainstem at 250-500 mg/kg [128].

Rats were treated orally with 300 mg/kg of a hydro-methanolic extract of St. John's wort three times (23.5 hours, 5 hours and 1 hour before the experimental period), then tested in the Porsolt forced swimming test; the extract significantly reduced immobility time (p<0.01), confirming antidepressant-like properties. However, in rats treated with the same extract by the same schedule, no significant changes in monoamine levels were detected in cortical or hippocampal brain regions 1 hour and 24 hours after the last dose [116].

Following long term administration (26 weeks) of a hydromethanolic extract of St. John's wort to rats at 2700 mg/kg/day, the number of serotonin receptors $(5-HT_{1A}$ and $5-HT_{2A})$ in the brain had increased by 50%; the affinity was unaltered [135]. After acute and repeated treatment of mice with as little as 10 mg/kg of St. John's wort extract, the levels of serotonin and the serotonin metabolite 5-hydroxyindolacetic acid were increased in hypothalamus and hippocampus indicating increased turnover; 5-hydroxyindolacetic acid levels were also increased in other regions of the brain [136].

Effects on the levels of serotonin (5-HT), nor-epinephrine, dopamine and their metabolites in the hypothalamus and hippocampus of rat brain were investigated after short-term (2 weeks) and long-term (8 weeks) daily oral administration to rats of the tricyclic antidepressant imipramine (15 mg/kg) or St. John's wort extract (500 mg/kg) or hypericin (0.2 mg/kg). All three treatments significantly increased 5-HT levels in the hypothalamus (p<0.05) after 8 weeks, but not after 2 weeks; levels in the hippocampus were unchanged. 5-HT turnover (the ratio of 5-HIAA to 5-HT) was significantly reduced in both brain regions (both p<0.05) after 8 weeks of treatment with the St. John's wort extract (but not with hypericin); imipramine reduced 5-HT turnover only in the hippocampus. Consistent changes in catecholamine levels were only detected in hypothalamic tissues after long-term treatment. Comparable to imipramine, St. John's wort extract and hypericin significantly decreased 3,4-dihydroxyphenylacetic acid and homovanillic acid levels in the hypothalamus (p<0.01). The data showed that long-term, but not short-term, administration of St. John's wort and its active constituent hypericin modified levels of neurotransmitters in brain regions involved in the pathophysiology of depression [137].

Activity of constituents
The effects of an ethanolic extract containing 4.5% of hyperforin (50, 150 and 300 mg/kg) were compared to those of a supercritical carbon dioxide extract with 38.8% of hyperforin but devoid of hypericins (5, 15 and 30 mg/kg) after oral administration to rodents on three consecutive days. Differences in activity became obvious. The ethanolic extract increased dopamin-ergic behavioural responses, e.g. in the DOPA-potentiation test and the apomorphine-induced stereotypy, whereas the CO_2 extract exerted more pronounced serotoninergic responses, e.g. 5-hydroxy-tryptophan-induced increase in the number of head twitches [138].

Microdialysis probes were implanted into the left nucleus accumbens, in the left striatum or in the ventral hippocampus of rats. After oral administration of 1 mg/kg of a CO_2 extract a slight but significant increase of dopamine outflow was observed in both the nucleus accumbens and the striatum, whereas serotonin release remained unchanged [139].

Using the push-pull superfusion technique, neuro-transmitter concentrations in the locus coeruleus of rats were studied after intraperitoneal injection of hyperforin at 10 mg/kg. Extracellular concentrations of dopamine, noradrenaline, serotonin and glutamate had increased, whereas 5-HIAA, GABA, taurine, aspartate, serine and arginine remained unchanged [140].

A methanolic (4.67% hyperforin) and a CO_2 (30.14% hyperforin) extract of St. John's wort, administered orally in amounts providing equal hyperforin content, were compared for their effects on the "tele-stereo-EEG" of freely moving rats. At first both extracts produced increases in the alpha-1 band of the striatum; later only the methanolic extract caused an increase in delta activity [141].

Using the resources of the National Institute of Mental Health Psychoactive Drug Screening Program (USA), the *in vitro* pharmacology of various pure constituents of St. John's wort (hypericin, pseudohypericin, hyper-forin, quercetin, isoquercitrin, quercitrin, miquelianin, rutin, hyperoside and amentoflavone) has been characterized at 42 biogenic amine receptors and transporters using radioligand binding assays. The compounds were screened for activity at G-protein-coupled receptors (GPCRs) including 5-HT, adrenergic, opioid, histamine, metabotropic glutamate and muscarinic acetylcholine, and ligand-gated ion channels including $GABA_{A/B}$ receptors as well as various neurotransmitter transporters. The data clearly demonstrated that some of the investigated compounds showed unanticipated binding inhibition in several receptor assays, whereas most were inactive. The most potent binding activities were observed for amentoflavone, hypericin and pseudohypericin; these showed distinct spectra of activity across receptor assays such as dopaminergic, adrenergic or opioid systems. In contrast, hyperforin and the flavonoids showed only relatively weak binding inhibition in the same systems. Amentoflavone significantly inhibited binding at serotonin ($5-HT_{1D}$, $5-HT_{2C}$), dopamine D3, δ-opioid and benzodiazepine receptors. Hypericin and pseudohypericin had significant activity at dopamine D3 and D4 receptors, and hypericin (but not pseudohypericin) at β-adrenergic receptors. With the exception of dopamine D1 and D5 receptors, hyperforin was less active than the other tested constituents on all screened receptors. Taken together, these data revealed novel interactions of St. John's wort constituents with a number of GPCRs, but further studies are necessary to establish their *in vivo* pharma-cological relevance to therapeutic effects [142].

In summary, *in vitro* and *in vivo* experiments have demonstrated relevant activity of naphthodianthrones, hyperforin and flavonoids. Although the mode of action of St. John's wort extracts is still under discussion, activity comparable to that of synthetic antidepressants has been observed in diverse test systems.

Effects on ethanol preference
Ethanol preference and ethanol intake in two strains of alcohol-preferring rats were significantly reduced by a methanolic extract containing 0.22% of naphtho-dianthrones and 4.05% of hyperforin. No tolerance developed during 2 weeks of oral treatment with 400 mg/kg/day of the extract; the reduction in ethanol preference remained unchanged [143]. A hydro-ethanolic extract of St. John's wort (0.3% hypericin, 3.8% hyperforin), injected intraperitoneally at 10-40 mg/kg, reduced both ethanol intake and ethanol preference [132]. The same St. John's wort extract, administered intragastrically at 250 mg/kg, was active in the Porsolt test and reduced ethanol intake in alcohol-preferring rats. Since the anti-immobility effect was abolished by σ-receptor blockade and diminished in the presence of experimentally lowered serotonin levels, whereas the ethanol intake remained un-changed under these conditions, both activities seem to be caused by other mechanisms [144].

Other pharmacological effects
Externally applied St. John's wort preparations have been reported to have anti-inflammatory and anti-

bacterial effects [145].The antibiotic effect has been attributed to the presence of hyperforin [146]. A hydroethanolic extract reduced croton oil-induced ear oedema in rodents by 50% (p<0.05); from fractionation experiments it was concluded that the anti-inflammatory principle is concentrated in the lipophilic fractions [147].

In vitro antibacterial activity of hyperforin against Gram-positive bacteria and multiresistant *Staphylococcus aureus* has been reported [148]. However, this activity was obvious only at high concentrations [149,150].

Strong antiviral effects of hypericin have been demonstrated *in vitro* [151-158]. Antiviral activity of hypericin and pseudohypericin has also been demonstrated *in vivo*; a single intravenous 50 µg dose completely inhibited splenomegaly (enlargement of the spleen) induced in mice by Friend leukaemia virus (FV), an aggressive retrovirus [156], and a single intravenous 150 µg dose enabled survival of FV-inoculated mice for at least 240 days compared to 23 days for untreated FV-inoculated animals, hypericin being the more potent antiretroviral agent [155].

A dry ethanolic extract of St. John's wort showed strong antioxidant activity *in vitro* and, when administered orally to rats at 250 mg/kg/day, significantly reduced immobilization stress-induced lipid peroxidation (measured *ex vivo* in liver homogenate; 42% protection after 30 days, p<0.001) [159].

Clinical studies

The efficacy and safety of standardized hydroalcoholic St. John's Wort extracts have been assessed in 31 controlled, double-blind [24-47,50,53,56-58,92,93] and 2 open [51,52] studies, involving more than 3900 patients and 13 different preparations; drug monitoring studies and numerous case reports have involved a further 10,000 patients [80-91,160]. The major indication in most of the studies was mild or mild to moderate depressive disorders. Three studies were designed for treatment of severe depressive disorders [56-58]. A significant improvement in main symptoms (mood, loss of interest and activity) and other symptoms of the depressive syndrome (sleep, concentration, somatic complaints) has been demonstrated in many of these trials. The activity was studied against placebo and against different antidepressants (amitriptyline, imipramine, maprotiline, fluoxetine), and in two studies simultaneously against placebo and imipramine or placebo and sertraline. Three meta-analyses [161-163] and six systematic reviews [164-169] of clinical trials with different selection criteria, have confirmed the efficacy of various St. John's wort extracts in mild to moderate depression, but not in severe depression.

The studies summarized below are grouped according to the preparations tested. Essential similarity is assumed for hydroalcoholic dry extracts within the range 60% ethanol to 80% methanol on the basis of their similar active constituents profiles [170]. An overview of the controlled studies is given in Table 1.

ABBREVIATIONS used in the summaries of clinical studies

CGI	Clinical Global Impressions scale [172]
DSM-III-R	Diagnostic and Statistical Manual of Mental Disorders, 3rd ed., revised [173]
DSM-IV	Diagnostic and Statistical Manual of Mental Disorders, 4th ed. [174]
HAMA	Hamilton Anxiety Scale [175]
HAMD	Hamilton Depression Scale [176,177]
ICD-09	International Classification of Diseases, Ninth Revision: Mental Disorders [178]
ICD-10	International Statistical Classification of Diseases and Related Health Problems, Tenth Revision [48,49].

TABLE 1: OVERVIEW OF CONTROLLED CLINICAL STUDIES

First Author Year Reference number	Number of patients	Type of preparation Extraction solvent	Daily dosage	Reference therapy	Duration (days)	Mean intial HAMD	Severity of depression
Sommer 1994 [29]	105	Dry extract, 80% methanol	3 × 300 mg*	Placebo	28	15.8	Mild
Hänsgen 1996 [38]	102	Dry extract, 80% methanol	3 × 300 mg	Placebo	42	20.7	Mild to moderate
Häring 1996 [31]	28	Dry extract, 80% methanol	3 × 300 mg	Placebo	Not stated	Not stated	Mild
Martinez 1994 [51]	20	Dry extract, 80% methanol	3 × 300 mg	Phototherapy	28	21.3	Mild to moderate
Hübner 1994 [30]	40	Dry extract, 80% methanol	3 × 300 mg	Placebo	28	12.5	Mild
Harrer 1994 [39]	102	Dry extract, 80% methanol	3 × 300 mg	Maprotiline	28	21.0	Mild to moderate
Vorbach 1994 [40]	135	Dry extract, 80% methanol	3 × 300 mg	Imipramine	42	19.8	Mild to moderate
Wheatley 1997 [41]	165	Dry extract, 80% methanol	3 × 300 mg	Amitriptyline	42	20.7	Mild to moderate
Vorbach 1997 [58]	209	Dry extract, 80% methanol	3 × 600 mg	Imipramine	42	25.7	Severe
Shelton 2001 [56]	200	Dry extract, 80% methanol	3 × 300-400 mg	Placebo	56	22.5	Severe
Davidson 2002 [57]	340	Dry extract, 80% methanol	3 × 300-500 mg	Sertraline; Placebo	56	22.8	Moderate to severe
Lehrl 1993 [50]	50	Dry extract, 80% methanol	3 × 300 mg*	Placebo	28	22.7	Mild to moderate
Halama 1991 [34]	50	Dry extract, 80% methanol	3 × 300 mg*	Placebo	28	18.3	Mild to moderate
Laakmann 1998 [35]	147	Dry extract, 60% ethanol	3 × 300 mg	Different St. John's wort extract; Placebo	42	20.8	Mild to moderate
Kalb 2001 [36]	72	Dry extract, 60% ethanol	3 × 300 mg	Placebo	42	19.9	Mild to moderate
Philipp 1999 [37]	263	Dry extract, 60% ethanol	3 × 350 mg	Imipramine; Placebo	56	22.6	Moderate
Harrer 1999 [28]	149	Dry extract, 60% ethanol	2 × 400 mg	Fluoxetine	42	16.9	Mild
Witte 1995 [42]	97	Dry extract, 50% ethanol	2 × 100-120 mg	Placebo	42	23.6	Moderate
Schrader 1998 [43]	162	Dry extract, 50% ethanol	2 × 250 mg	Placebo	42	19.5	Mild to moderate
Schrader 2000 [44]	240	Dry extract, 50% ethanol	2 × 250 mg	Fluoxetine	42	19.6	Mild to moderate
Woelk 2000 [45]	324	Dry extract, 50% ethanol	2 × 250 mg	Imipramine	42	22.3	Mild to moderate
Warnecke 1986 [52]	60	Tincture, 50% ethanol	3 × 1.5 ml	Diazepam	94	---	Mild
Hoffmann 1979 [24]	60	Tincture, 50% ethanol	3 × 1.5 ml	Placebo	42	---	Mild
Schlich 1987 [25]	49	Tincture, 49% ethanol	3 × 1 ml	Placebo	28	23.5	Mild
Schmidt 1989 [32]	40	Tincture, 49% ethanol	3 × 1.5 ml	Placebo	28	29.4	Mild to moderate
Harrer 1991 [33]	120	Tincture, 49% ethanol	3 × 1.5 ml	Placebo	42	21.3	Mild to moderate
Quandt 1993 [27]	88	Tincture, 49% ethanol	3 × 1.5 ml	Placebo	28	17.6	Mild
Werth 1989 [53]	30	Tincture, 49% ethanol	3 × 1.5 ml	Imipramine	23	---	Mild
Kugler 1990 [26]	80	Tincture, 49% ethanol	3 × 1.5 ml	Bromazepam	28	---	Mild
Lenoir 1999 [46]	348	Dry ethanolic extract fromfresh shoot tips	3 × 60 mg	Different dose levels of same extract	42	16.5	Mild
Engesser 1996 [47]	19	Tea preparation	Not stated	Milfoil tea	14	---	Mild

*Daily dosage was up to 50% lower due to up to 50% of excipients in the amount stated [171].

Clinical studies and drug surveillance studies
*in **mild to moderate depression** performed*
with hydro-methanolic extracts (80% methanol)

In 102 outpatients (mean age 52 years) with depression of mild or moderate severity (DSM-III-R: 296.2, 296.3), 3 × 300 mg of a St. John's wort extract (4-7:1, methanol 80%) daily over a period of 4 weeks was compared to placebo. Average HAMD scores at baseline were 21 in the verum group and 20.4 in the placebo group. After 4 weeks the average score was significantly lower (p<0.001) in the verum group (8.9) than in the placebo group (14.4). Similar results were obtained on the von Zerssen self-rating depression scale (p<0.001). Responder rates, defined as at least 50% reduction in initial HAMD score or a final score of less than 10, were 70% under verum and 24% under placebo (p<0.001). This randomized, double-blind period was followed by a further 2-week period during which all patients were treated openly with the St. John's wort extract; HAMD scores decreased further, to 6 in the former verum group and more substantially to 8.7 in the former placebo group [38].

In a placebo-controlled, randomized, double-blind study, 40 patients (mean age 51 years) suffering from mild depression with somatic symptoms (ICD-09: 300.4, neurotic depression; 309.0, brief depressive reaction) were treated with 3 × 300 mg of a St. John's wort extract (4-7:1, methanol 80%) or placebo daily for 4 weeks. Initial mean HAMD scores of 12.5 dropped to 5.5 in the St. John's wort group compared to 10.8 in the placebo group (p<0.05). Patients in the placebo group had an improved score of 9 after 2 weeks, but this subsequently increased. Responder rates, defined by an endpoint score of less than 10 or a drop of at least 50% from baseline value, were 70% and 47% respectively [30].

In a prospective, placebo-controlled, double-blind pilot study, 28 outpatients undergoing a chemotherapy regimen for solid tumours were randomly assigned to 3 × 300 mg of a St. John's wort extract (4-7:1, methanol 80%) or placebo daily for 2-3 chemotherapy treatment cycles. Although the average HAMD score in the St. John's wort group showed a slight trend towards improvement, results from the two treatment groups were comparable with respect to a quality of life analysis, the von Zerssen self-rating depression scale and the CGI scale [31].

In an open, randomized, single-blind study involving patients (mean age 46 years) suffering from seasonal affective disorder (major depression with a seasonal pattern diagnosed in accordance with DSM-III-R), daily treatment for 4 weeks with 3 × 300 mg of a St. John's wort extract (4-7:1, methanol 80%) was combined with phototherapy: either bright light (3000 lux; n = 10) or dim light (< 300 lux, n = 10) for 2 hours per day. Average HAMD scores at baseline (21.9 in the

bright light group and 20.6 in the dim light group) decreased significantly in both groups, to 6.1 and 8.2 respectively (p<0.001). Due to the small sample size, the difference between groups was not statistically significant [51].

In a 4-week randomized, double-blind, comparative study (no placebo group), the efficacy and tolerability of 3 × 300 mg daily of a St. John's wort extract (4-7:1, methanol 80%) was compared with 3 × 75 mg daily of the antidepressant maprotiline in 102 patients of mean age 46 years with a diagnosis of moderate depression (ICD-10: F 32.1). Initial HAMD scores fell from 20.5 to 12.2 in the St. John's wort group and from 21.5 to 10.5 in the maprotiline group. Responder rates, defined by an endpoint score of less than 10 or a drop of at least 50% from the baseline, were 61% and 67% respectively. Overall, there were no significant differences between groups [39].

In a 6-week multicentre, randomized, double-blind, comparative study without placebo control, 3 × 300 mg daily of a St. John's wort extract (4-7:1, methanol 80%) was compared to 3 × 25 mg daily of the antidepressant imipramine. The 135 patients (mean age 53 years) had diagnoses in accordance with DSM-III-R criteria of depression with a single episode (296.2), several episodes (296.3), depressive neurosis (300.4) or adjustment disorder with depressed mood (309.0). The main outcome criteria were HAMD scores, the von Zerssen depression scale (D-S) and CGI. Initial HAMD scores declined from 20.2 to 8.8 in the St. John's wort group and from 19.4 to 10.7 points in the imipramine group. Group comparisons showed no significant differences. Analysis of D-S and CGI patterns in the two groups also revealed comparable results. Subgroups with initial HAMD scores of 21 or more performed significantly better (p<0.05) after St. John's wort extract (n = 26) than after imipramine (n = 25) with regard to HAMD score and CGI [40].

In a 6-week multicentre, randomized, double-blind, comparative study without placebo group, 165 mildly to moderately depressed outpatients (mean age 40 years) diagnosed in accordance with DSM-IV were treated with 3 × 300 mg daily of a St. John's wort extract (4-7:1, methanol 80%) or 3 × 25 mg daily of the sedative tricyclic antidepressant amitriptyline. Initial HAMD scores were between 17 and 24 (mean 20.7). No statistically significant difference between groups was observed with respect to the primary outcome parameter, the response rate (defined as an endpoint HAMD score of less than 10, or a drop of at least 50% from baseline values). 59.7% of patients in the St. John's wort group were classified as responders compared to 77.8% in the amitriptyline group (p = 0.064). HAMD scores had dropped to 10 in the St. John's wort group and to 6 in the amitriptyline group after 6 weeks, a difference significantly in favour of amitriptyline (p<0.05). Analysis of another secondary efficacy parameter, the Montgomery-Asberg rating scale for depression (MADRS), also favoured amitriptyline (p<0.05) [41].

In a multicentre drug surveillance study 3250 patients (mean age 51 years), of whom 49% had mild, 46% moderate and 3% severe depressive symptoms, were monitored for 4 weeks while taking 3 × 300 mg daily of a St. John's wort extract (4-7:1, methanol 80%). Scores using the von Zerssen Depression Scale dropped from 23.2 to 11.8 over the 4-week period. At the end of treatment, 82% of patients were assessed as improved or symptom-free by the physicians and 79% by the patients. Although efficacy was only slightly dependent on age, the therapeutic effect was better in patients younger than 50 years. Cases with mild or moderate depression responded to treatment to the same extent, while severe cases improved somewhat less [85].

In a multicentre drug surveillance study, 1060 patients (mean age 51 years) with mild to moderate depressive symptoms were assessed over a 4-week period of treatment with 3 × 300 mg daily of a St. John's wort extract (4-7:1, methanol 80%). By the end of the study, the average HAMD score had dropped from 18.4 to 5.4 and the von Zerssen self-rating depression score from 21.1 to 7.3. According to CGI evaluation, 66% of patients had improved and 27% were symptom-free after 4 weeks [86].

In a 5-week drug monitoring study, the efficacy of a St. John's wort extract (3 × 135-225 mg of extract, providing 900 μg of total hypericin daily) was assessed in 114 patients (mean age 48 years) with mild depressive symptoms. The treatment was evaluated by the von Zerssen self-rating depression scale (D-S), the distribution of characteristic psychic and somatic symptoms, and a global rating by the physician. From an initial 21 the D-S score dropped to 15 after 2 weeks and to 2 after 5 weeks. The physicians rated 39% of patients as improved and 35% as symptom-free after 5 weeks [87].

In a 12-week drug-monitoring study the efficacy of a St. John's wort extract (3 × 135-225 mg of extract, providing 900 μg of total hypericin daily) was assessed in 111 women (mean age 52 years) with menopausal symptoms. Women who had received hormone replacement therapy with oestrogens or oestrogen-progestogen combinations were excluded from the study. Treatment was evaluated by the menopause rating scale (MRS), a questionnaire for assessing sexuality, and the CGI scale. Climacteric complaints diminished or disappeared completely in 79% of the women as rated by the physician (CGI rating better or symptom-free). Sexual well-being was favourably affected in approximately 60% of the women. The average MRS total score dropped from an initial 63.4 (corresponding to a marked intensity of symptoms) to

23.5 (slight intensity) after 12 weeks [88].

In another drug-surveillance study 647 patients with mild to moderate depression were treated daily for 6 weeks with 3 × 300 mg of a St. John's wort extract (4-7:1, methanol 80%). In 75% of the patients the condition improved. The von Zerssen self-rating depression score dropped from 19.8-21.2 at baseline to 8.1-9.3 after 6 weeks. In patients older than 65 years the condition improved at a somewhat slower rate but the severity of depression did not appear to affect the outcome [89].

In a multicentre drug monitoring study with 1606 patients (mean age 52 years) suffering from typical depressive symptoms such as low mood, loss of interest and energy, and disturbed sleep, more than 90% were treated 2-3 times daily with 300 mg of a St. John's wort extract (4-7:1, methanol 80%; standardized to 900 μg of total hypericin). After a mean treatment period of 5 weeks, the intensity of dominating symptoms was markedly reduced. The efficacy was rated as very good or good by 81% of the physicians and 76% of patients. No age-dependent correlation of efficacy was reported [90].

Older clinical studies in
mild to moderate depression *performed with hydromethanolic extracts (80% methanol) at lower daily dosages (see the footnote to Table 1).*

In a multicentre, randomized, double-blind study, 105 patients (mean age 45 years) with depressive symptoms (ICD-09: 300.4, neurotic depression; or 309.0, brief depressive reaction) were allocated to 3 × 300 mg of a St. John's wort extract (4-7:1, 80% methanol), or placebo daily for 4 weeks. By the end of the study initial HAMD scores (15.8 points in both groups) had dropped to 7.2 in the St. John's wort group and 11.3 in the placebo group, a statistically significant difference (p<0.01). Responder rates, defined by a total endpoint score of less than 10 or a drop of at least 50% from baseline values, were 67% and 28% respectively [29].

In a multicentre, placebo-controlled study, 50 patients (mean age 49 years) with depressive symptoms (ICD-09: 300.4 and 309.0) were treated daily for 4 weeks with either 3 × 300 mg of a St. John's wort extract (4-7:1, methanol 80%) or placebo. HAMD scores improved from 23.7 to 17.4 in the verum group and from 21.6 to 16.8 in the placebo group, the difference not being significant. In an evaluation of cognitive performance using the short test for general basic capacities of information processing (KAI), patients on St. John's wort extract showed slightly better improvement than those on placebo (p<0.1) [50].

In a randomized, placebo-controlled study involving 50 patients suffering from psychovegetative depressive symptoms (ICD-09: neurotic depression or depressive mood of short duration), 3 × 300 mg daily, in some cases reduced to 2 × 300 mg after week 2, of a St. John's wort extract (4-7:1, methanol 80%) led to a substantial improvement after 4 weeks of therapy. A reduction of at least half from their initial HAMD total score or a score below 10 after 4 weeks was achieved by 50% of patients in the St. John's wort group (p<0.01), but by none in the placebo group. Other parameters, such as the von Zerssen Complaint Score and CGI score, showed similar differences between verum and placebo [34].

Clinical studies in **major depression** *or* **severe, recurrent depressive episodes** *in accordance with ICD-10 F33.2, performed with hydromethanolic extracts (80% methanol)*

Two hundred adult outpatients (mean age 42 years) with a DSM-IV diagnosis of major depression and an initial HAMD total score of at least 20 participated in a randomized, double-blind, placebo-controlled study conducted in 11 academic medical centres in the USA. The patients were suffering from recurrent depression (64%) or a single episode of depression (35%) and around 40% were melancholic. The duration of the current major depressive disorder was more than 2 years on average and onset of the initial major depressive disorder was more than 10 years ago. Initial HAMD total scores were about 22.5 (estimated from a graph). After a 1-week, single-blind run-in with placebo, patients were treated for 8 weeks with either a St. John's wort extract (4-7:1, methanol 80%), 3 × 300 mg daily for 4 weeks, increased thereafter to 4 × 300 mg daily in the absence of adequate response, or placebo. The primary outcome measure was the rate of change in HAMD score over the treatment period. Random coefficient analyses for the HAMD showed significant effects for time (p<0.001) but not for treatment (p = 0.16) or time-by-treatment interaction (p = 0.58). Similar results were obtained for the secondary outcome measures, HAMA and CGI. 26.5% of patients in the St. John's wort group and 18.6% in the placebo group were responders (defined a priori as HAMD score of 12 or less and CGI Intensity score of 1 or 2); these proportions were not statistically different. A significantly higher (p = 0.02) remission rate (remission being defined as an endpoint HAMD score of 7 or less and CGI-I score of 1 or 2) was estimated for St. John's wort (14.3%) than for placebo (4.9%), but both rates were low. In this study St. John's wort was not effective for the treatment of rather severe depression [56].

In a multicentre, randomized, placebo-controlled, double-blind, three-armed study, 340 outpatients (mean age 42 years) with major depression of moderate severity (DSM-IV: maximum score of 60 on Global Assessment of Functioning) and a baseline HAMD score of at least 20 were assigned to one of three treatments daily for 8 weeks: 3 × 300 mg of a St. John's wort extract standardized to 0.12-0.28% hypericin and containing 3.1% of hyperforin (although not stated, the identified extract is assumed to have had a drug-to-extract ratio of 4-7:1, extracted with methanol 80%) or 50 mg of sertraline (divided into 3 doses) or placebo. Daily dosage could be increased after week 3 to 1500 mg of St. John's wort extract or to 100 mg of sertraline if warranted; the mean highest daily doses prescribed during the 8-week period were 1299 mg of St. John's wort extract, 75 mg of sertraline or placebo equivalent. With respect to the two primary efficacy parameters, change from HAMD baseline and full response rates, defined as an endpoint HAMD score of 8 or less and a CGI-I score of 1 (very much improved) or 2 (much improved), neither St. John's wort extract nor sertraline were significantly different from placebo over the 8-week period. Mean reductions in HAMD scores were 8.7 for St. John's wort extract, 10.5 for sertraline and 9.2 for placebo. Full response rates were 23.9% for St. John's wort extract, 24.8% for sertraline and 31.9% for placebo. The results did not therefore support efficacy of St. John's wort extract in moderately severe major depression [57].

In a 6-week multicentre, randomized, double-blind comparative trial without placebo group, 209 patients with a mean age of 49 years (38 hospitalized and 171 outpatients treated by psychiatrists) were allocated to 3 × 600 mg daily of a St. John's wort extract (4-7:1, methanol 80%) or 3 × 50 mg daily of imipramine. The inclusion criteria were defined in accordance with ICD-10 F33.2: a severe episode of a major depressive disorder, recurrent, without psychotic symptoms. The primary target parameter, mean HAMD scores, dropped from 25.3 to 14.4 points in the St. John's wort group and from 26.1 to 13.4 points in the imipramine group, the difference between groups being significant in favour of imipramine (p = 0.021). Equivalence of the two treatments could be shown with respect to response rates, defined as the percentage of patients showing a reduction of at least 50% in HAMD total score over the study period: 35.3% in the St. John's wort group, 41.2% in the imipramine group [58].

Clinical studies and drug surveillance studies in **mild to moderate depression** *performed with hydro-ethanolic extracts (ethanol 60%)*

In a multicentre, randomized, double-blind, placebo-controlled study, 147 outpatients (mean age 49 years) suffering from depression of mild or moderate severity in accordance with DSM-IV criteria, and with initial HAMD scores of at least 17, were treated daily for 6 weeks with placebo or 3 × 300 mg of one of two St. John's wort extracts (4:1, no data on naphthodianthrones): one extract contained 5% hyperforin, the other 0.5% hyperforin. The average HAMD score at baseline was 20.8. At the end of the study, the extract group receiving the 10-fold higher content of hyperforin had the largest reduction in HAMD score from baseline (10.3 ± 4.6), followed by the extract group with a lower content of hyperforin (8.5 ± 6.1) then the placebo group (7.9 ± 5.2). After 6 weeks the proportions of responders (defined as a reduction of at least 50% from initial HAMD scores) were 49% in the 5% hyperforin group, 39% in the 0.5% hyperforin group and 33% in the placebo group. HAMD score reduction was statistically superior to placebo only in the 5% hyperforin group (p = 0.004, Mann-Whitney U-test). Results were similar for other outcome measures (CGI scale and von Zerssen self-rating depression scale). The important contribution of hyperforin to the antidepressant activity of St. John's wort was deduced from this study [35].

Another 6-week multicentre, randomized, double-blind, placebo-controlled study was carried out with a St. John's wort extract (2.5-5:1, ethanol 60%; 5% hyperforin, no data on naphthodianthrones) in 72 patients with mild to moderate major depressive disorder in accordance with DSM-IV criteria. The daily dose was 3 × 300 mg of extract or placebo. Group differences in favour of the verum group were statistically significant after 4 weeks (p = 0.011) and 6 weeks (p<0.001). Average HAMD scores decreased from 19.7 to 8.9 in the St. John's wort group and from 20.1 to 14.4 in the placebo group. Analysis of responders showed a reduction of at least 50% from HAMD baseline scores in 62.2% of the St. John's wort group and 42.9% of the placebo group (p = 0.10). The difference was larger when '60%-responders' were considered (51.4% vs. 17.1%). Based on an adaptive interim analysis, the study was stopped after 6 weeks because convincing efficacy had already been demonstrated; however, according to an exponential regression model, the data suggested considerable potential for further HAMD reduction if treatment were continued with the St. John's wort extract, but not with placebo [36].

In a multicentre, randomized, double-blind, three-armed study, 263 primary care patients (mean age 47 years) with a diagnosis of moderate depression (ICD-10: F32.1 and F33.1) were allocated to 3 × 350 mg of a St. John's wort extract (5-7:1, 60% ethanol; 0.2-0.3% of total hypericin and 2-3% of hyperforin by HPLC) or 100 mg of imipramine (50 mg + 25 mg + 25 mg) or placebo daily for 8 weeks. The primary endpoint was the change from baseline in HAMD scores (mean initial score 22.6 points). The St. John's wort extract more effectively reduced HAMD scores than placebo (mean decrease after 6 weeks of 13.4 versus 10.3). Mean decreases in scores from baseline at 8 weeks were similar for St. John's wort extract and imipramine (15.4 versus 14.2). More patients receiving St. John's wort extract had ≥ 50% improvement in HAMD scores than did patients receiving placebo (p = 0.027); the proportions did not differ between St. John's wort and imipramine (p = 0.14). Comparable results were

found for HAMA and CGI scores, and were most pronounced for the Zung self-rating depression (SDS) score. Quality of life as measured by the SF-36 standardized mental component scale was more improved by both active treatments than by placebo (40.5% more by St. John's wort extract, 30% more by imipramine). Using the SF-36 physical component scale, quality of life compared with placebo was markedly improved only by St. John's wort extract (74.5% more by St. John's wort extract, 23% by imipramine) [37].

The effects of 2 × 400 mg of a St. John's wort extract (5-7:1, ethanol 60%) or 2 ×10 mg of fluoxetine daily were compared in a 6-week randomized, double-blind, comparative trial (without a placebo group) involving 149 elderly outpatients (mean age 69 years) suffering from a first episode of mild or moderate depression (ICD-10: F32.0 or F32.1). Over the study period average HAMD scores decreased from 16.6 to 7.9 in the St. John's wort group and from 17.2 to 8.1 in the fluoxetine group. The efficacy of the two medications was found to be equivalent in both mild and moderate depressive episodes (no statistical confirmation of equivalence; no data on standard deviation or confidence intervals). Responder rates after 6 weeks (defined by a total HAMD score of not more than 10 or a reduction of at least 50% from initial score) were 71% in the St. John's wort group and 72% in the fluoxetine group [28].

In a drug surveillance study, 2404 patients (mean age 50 years) with depressive symptoms of varying severity were treated with a St. John's wort extract (5-7:1, 60% ethanol). The average dose was 120-180 mg of extract twice daily and the average treatment period 5 weeks. Typical symptoms of depression decreased in both frequency and intensity, the response rates (defined by the proportion of patients showing marked improvement or a symptom-free condition) with respect to individual symptoms being: depressed mood (73%), loss of interest (81%), reduced self-esteem and self-confidence (66%), lack of concentration (69%) and anxiety symptoms (68%). Overall, 90% of patients responded to treatment and more than 50% noticed an improvement in symptoms 2 weeks after commencement of therapy. Using the CGI scale, the investigators rated efficacy as good or very good in 77% of patients (about 80% for patients younger than 54 years, decreasing to 73% with older patients). A correlation was evident between severity of condition and response rates (82% for mild, over 79% for moderate, 64% for marked severity) [82].

In another drug monitoring study, 607 patients (mean age 50.5 years) with depressive symptoms were treated once or twice daily for 6 weeks with 425 mg of a St. John's wort extract (5-7:1; ethanol 60%). The initial mean HAMD score of 19.2 had dropped to 7.4 points by the end of the treatment. Similar results were obtained using the von Zerssen self-rating depression scale, the score decreasing from 22.2 to 8.9 points. Core symptoms such as low mood, lack of energy and concentration improved by 50% [83].

*Clinical studies and drug surveillance studies in **mild to moderate depression** performed with hydroethanolic extracts (50% ethanol)*

In a randomized, double-blind, multicentre trial, 97 outpatients (mean age 43 years) with a moderate depressive episode (ICD-10, F32.1) were allocated to receive 2 × 100-120 mg of a St. John's wort extract (5-8:1; ethanol 50%) or placebo daily for 6 weeks. By the end of the study initial HAMD scores had dropped from 24.6 to 7.9 points in the St. John's wort group and from 22.6 to 10.3 in the placebo group, a statistically significant difference (p = 0.019). Responder rates (defined by a total score at the endpoint of less than 10 or a drop of at least 50% from initial score) were 79% and 56% respectively [42].

In a randomized, double-blind, multicentre trial with 162 outpatients (mean age 43 years) suffering from mild to moderate depression (ICD-10: F32.0, F32.1) the treatment was either 2 × 250 mg of a St. John's wort extract (4-7:1, 50% ethanol; 0.2% total hypericin) or placebo daily for 6 weeks. Over the course of the study HAMD scores dropped from 20.1 to 10.5 in the St. John's wort group and from 18.8 to 17.9 in the placebo group, a significant difference (p<0.001). Responder rates (defined by an endpoint score of not more than 10 or a drop of at least 50% from initial score) were 56% and 15% respectively [43].

In another randomized, double-blind, multicentre study, involving 240 subjects (mean age 47 years) with mild to moderate depression (ICD-10: F32.0, F32.1) and HAMD scores in the range 16-24 (mean initial score 19.6), the treatment was either 2 × 250 mg of a St. John's wort extract (4-7:1, 50% ethanol; 0.2% total hypericin) or 1 × 20 mg of fluoxetine daily for 6 weeks. No placebo group was included. After 6 weeks, HAMD scores had dropped from 19.65 to 11.5 in the St. John's wort group and from 19.5 to 12.2 in the fluoxetine group. Statistical analysis of the main outcome variable, the change in mean HAMD score, confirmed the equivalence of the two treatments with regard to overall antidepressant effect. In analysis of secondary variables, there was a trend in favour of St. John's wort in improving the absolute HAMD score (p = 0.09). Responder rates (defined by an endpoint score of not more than 10 or a drop of at least 50% from initial score) were 60% for the St. John's wort extract and 40% for fluoxetine (p = 0.05) [44].

In a randomized, double-blind, multicentre study with 324 outpatients (mean age 46 years) with mild to moderate depression (ICD-10: F32.0, F32.1, F33.0, F33.1), the treatment was either 2 × 250 mg of a St. John's wort extract (4-7:1, 50% ethanol; 0.2% total hypericins) or 2 × 75 mg of imipramine daily for 6 weeks. No placebo group was included. By the end of the study, HAMD scores had dropped from 22.4 to 12.0 in the St. John's wort group and from 22.1 to 12.75 in the imipramine group. Neither this difference nor differences between treatment groups in pre-defined secondary efficacy parameters were statistically significant, except for a difference in HAMD anxiety-somatisation subscale scores in favour of St. John's wort (p = 0.03). Responder rates, defined by a drop of at least 50% of the baseline HAMD values, were 43% in the St. John's wort group and 40% in the imipramine group [45].

In an open, multicentre drug surveillance study, 170 patients (mean age 49 years) with masked, mild, moderately severe or severe depression received 2 × 250 mg of a St. John's wort extract (4-7:1, 50% ethanol; 0.2% total hypericin) daily for an average treatment period of 66 days and were monitored with regard to efficacy and safety. HAMD scores were evaluated in 84 patients at the beginning and end of the study. Treatment response was satisfactory in patients with masked, mild and moderate depression but not in those with severe depression. Typical depressive symptoms, summarized in an unvalidated complaint score, decreased by 40% in the former group but by only 12.5% in the subgroup with severe depression. In the subgroup of patients whose HAMD scores were evaluated, the mean initial score of 36.3 dropped to 27.2 by the end of therapy. Again in a subgroup analysis, severe cases did not significantly benefit from the treatment (descriptive p-value of 0.46). Global efficacy, judged in 94 patients, was rated as good or very good in 78%, slight in 3% and insufficient in 19% of this subgroup [91].

Clinical studies performed with tinctures (49-50% ethanol)

In the first randomized, double-blind, placebo-controlled study of a St. John's wort preparation, 60 depressive patients (mean age 49 years) were treated daily for 6 weeks with 3 × 1.5 ml of a St. John's wort tincture (50% ethanol, daily dose equivalent to 0.9 mg of total hypericins) or placebo. The types of depression were classified as psychogenic, climacteric, somato-genic, involutional or juvenile. Using a self-developed, graded scale with 52 symptoms, the authors demonstrated a considerable reduction of 61.4% in the total score in the St. John's wort group compared to only 15.8% in the placebo group. Responder rates, defined by the investigators' assessment of good or very good improvement, were 63% in the St. John's wort group and 10% in the placebo group. Statistical parameters were not reported [24].

In another randomized, double-blind, placebo-controlled study, 49 patients (mean age 42.3 years) with mild to moderate depressive symptoms were treated with 3 × 1 ml of a St. John's wort tincture (49% ethanol, 0.4:1) or placebo daily for 4 weeks. In the placebo group the mean number of symptoms had increased from 24 to 29.6 after 4 weeks, whereas patients treated with St. John's wort experienced an average reduction from 22.9 to 16.4 symptoms (p<0.05) [25].

In a two-centre, double-blind, placebo-controlled study, 40 patients (mean age 47 years) with depressive symptoms received daily either 3 × 1.5 ml of a St. John's wort tincture (49% ethanol, 0.4:1) or placebo. After 4 weeks, results from 16 patients in the St. John's wort group and 12 in the placebo group showed that initial HAMD total scores had decreased from 29.25 to 9.75 in the St. John's wort group and from 29.5 to 19.5 in the placebo group. Responder rates (defined by a drop of at least 50% from baseline HAMD scores or an endpoint score of 10 or less) were 62.5% in the St. John's wort group and 33.3% in the placebo group [32].

In a multicentre, double-blind, placebo-controlled study, 120 outpatients (mean age 48.5 years) suffering from mild depressive symptoms (ICD-09: 304.4 and 309.9; initial HAMD scores of 16-20) were treated with 3 × 1.5 ml of a St. John's wort tincture (49% ethanol; 0.25 mg of total hypericins per ml) or placebo daily for 6 weeks. Results from 116 patients are presented for quantitative analysis. In terms of overall symptomatology, there was a marked reduction of 57.9% in HAMD total scores in the St. John's wort group (from 21.6 to 8.9) compared to only 18.1% in the placebo group (from 20.9 to 16.1). Comparable results were obtained using the HAMA scale and von Zerssen's self-rating scale depression scale. Responder rates (defined by a total HAMD score of not more than 10 at endpoint or a drop of at least 50% from baseline scores) were 65.9% in the St. John's wort group and 25% in the placebo group [33].

In another randomized, double-blind, placebo-controlled, multicentre study, 88 outpatients (mean age 43.3 years) suffering from mild to moderate depressive symptoms (ICD-09: 300.4; HAMD score at least 16) were treated with either 3 × 1.5 ml of a St. John's wort tincture (49% ethanol; 0.25 mg of total hypericins per ml) or placebo daily for 4 weeks. HAMD scores dropped from 17.8 to 5.2 in the St. John's wort group (p<0.001) and from 17.3 to 15.5 in the placebo group. Responder rates, defined by a total HAMD score at endpoint of not more than 10 or a drop of at least 50% from baseline scores, were 70.7% in the St. John's wort group and only 7.1% in the placebo group [27].

In other studies, the same preparation at the same daily dosage was compared to 50 mg of imipramine daily in 30 patients with depressive states after surgery

[53], and to 6 mg of bromazepam daily in 80 patients suffering from psychogenic depressive symptoms [26]. Comparable efficacy results for the St. John's wort tincture and the reference medication were reported in both studies.

In an open, comparative study in a gynaecological practice, patients (mean age 52.9 years) with climacteric complaints were treated daily with either 3 × 1.5 ml of a St. John's wort tincture (50% ethanol; daily dose equivalent to 0.9 mg of total hypericins; n = 40) or 3 × 2 mg of diazepam (n = 20). Treatment response was evaluated after 1 and 3 months using the CGI scale for overall efficacy, the HAMA scale and the Zung Self Rating Depression Scale (SDS). Subjective data on hot flushes, increased perspiration and general well-being were recorded in patient's diaries. In the investigator's judgement, 77.5% of patients treated with St. John's wort and 50% of patients treated with diazepam were fully remitted after 3 months. The score for the depression component of the HAMA scale (no HAMA total scores reported) dropped from 2.80 to 1.73 after 1 month and to 0.79 after 3 months in the St. John's wort group, and from 2.95 to 1.86 after 3 months in the diazepam group. Similar results were obtained from SDS score evaluation. No quantitative data from the patients' diaries were reported [52].

Clinical studies performed with other preparations

In a randomized, double-blind, multicentre, three-armed study involving 348 outpatients (mean age not reported) suffering from mild to moderate depression diagnosed in accordance with ICD-10, three preparations containing a dry extract (4-5:1) from fresh shoot tips of St. John's wort (standardized to 0.17 mg, 0.33 mg or 1 mg of total hypericins per day) were assessed for efficacy and safety over a treatment period of 6 weeks. The highest daily dose corresponded to 3 × 60 mg of the extract. Mainly for ethical reasons, no placebo group was included. In the per protocol analysis of the main outcome measure, initial average HAMD scores of 16-17 dropped to 8-9 after 6 weeks in all three groups. Response rates (defined by a decrease in the score to below 10 or a reduction of at least 50% from the initial score) were 62%, 65% and 68% respectively in the intention to treat analysis. No statistically significant differences between the three groups were detected [46].

In a randomized, double-blind, crossover study, the antidepressant effect of a St. John's wort tea taken twice daily (at least 0.28 mg of total hypericins per day) was assessed in 19 patients (at least 60 years old) and compared to milfoil tea (*Achillea millefolium*) as a control. Each treatment period lasted 14 days, separated by a wash-out period of 3 days. Thirteen patients reported better results with St. John's wort tea, while five patients had better results with milfoil tea and one patient showed no difference. The pilot study indicated a trend towards a better mood in patients treated with St. John's wort tea (p = 0.06) [47].

Pharmacokinetic properties

Pharmacokinetics in animals
A study of the absorption and distribution of orally administered radioactively labelled ^{14}C-hypericin and ^{14}C-pseudohypericin in mice showed that 6 hours after administration 80% of hypericin and 60% of pseudohypericin had been absorbed. The distribution was not indicative of selective accumulation in certain organs. Most radioactivity was found in the blood, but radioactivity was also present in the brain [179].

The tissue uptake and distribution of hypericin was measured in rabbits and nude mice transplanted with P3 human squamous cell carcinoma. Maximum levels were attained 4 hours after intravenous administration to rabbits. The lungs had 5-fold higher levels than the spleen followed by liver, blood and kidney. Mice were investigated after acute administration and after 3 and 7 days of treatment. Peak concentrations were reached in murine organs after 4 hours. After 7 days of treatment elimination was rapid in most organs with a residue of < 10%, although 25-30% was retained in squamous cell tumours and in the brain, stomach and skin [180]. The tissue distribution of hypericin (2, 5 or 20 mg/kg, administered intra-peritoneally) was studied in DBA/2 mice bearing subcutaneously implanted P388 lymphoma cells. Uptake was very high in the liver and spleen. Clearance of hypericin from plasma occurred at a fairly high rate and followed a two-phase exponential decay: a first phase of rapid clearance (half-life 6.9 hours) was followed by a slower phase (half-life 37.9 hours) [181].

After oral administration of an ethanolic extract containing 5% hyperforin to rats at 300 mg/kg, maximum plasma levels of 370 ng/ml hyperforin were reached after 3 hours. Estimated half-life and clearance values were 6 hours and 70 ml/min/kg [182].

Pharmacokinetics in humans
A study of the bioavailability of hypericin in 2 healthy volunteers after oral administration of a St. John's wort extract (300, 600 and 1200 mg at intervals of 7 days) demonstrated that plasma levels of hypericin were dose-dependent. After ingestion of a single dose of 600 mg of the extract by 12 volunteers, the following parameters were determined for hypericin: t_{max} 2.5 hours, c_{max} 4.3 ng/ml and a plasma half-life of about 6 hours [183].

Oral administration to 12 healthy volunteers (at intervals of at least 10 days) of single doses of a methanolic extract of St. John's wort containing 250, 750 and 1,500 µg of hypericin and 526, 1,578 and 3,135 µg of pseudohypericin respectively gave peak plasma levels of 1.3, 7.2 and 16.6 µg/litre for hypericin and 3.3, 12.2 and 29.7 µg/litre for pseudohypericin. C_{max} and AUC values for the lowest dose were disproportionately lower than those for the higher doses. Lag times were determined as 1.9 hours for hypericin and 0.4 hours for pseudohypericin. Mean half-lives for absorption, distribution and elimination were 0.6, 6.0 and 43.1 hours after 750 µg of hypericin, and 1.3, 1.4 and 24.8 hours after 1,578 µg of pseudo-hypericin. After 14 days of oral treatment with 250 µg of hypericin and 526 µg of pseudohypericin, steady state levels of 7.9 µg/litre for hypericin and 4.8 µg/litre for pseudohypericin were achieved. Kinetic para-meters in two subjects after intravenous administration resembled those after oral administration. Hypericin and pseudohypericin were initially distributed into volumes of 4.2 and 5.0 litres respectively; at steady state the mean distribution volumes were 19.7 litres for hypericin and 39.3 litres for pseudohypericin; systemic bioavailability from the methanolic extract was about 14 and 21% respectively [184].

A methanolic St. John's wort extract was administered orally as single doses of 900, 1,800 and 3,600 mg, containing 2.81, 5.62 and 11.25 mg of total hypericins. Maximum plasma concentrations of total hypericin, observed about 4 hours after administration, were 0.028, 0.061 and 0.159 mg/litre. Phototoxic reactions could not be excluded for hypericin doses above 11.25 mg of total hypericin and plasma levels above 100 µg/litre [97].

Hypericin levels in serum and skin blister fluid were determined in volunteers after oral administration of a hydromethanolic extract as a single dose of 6 tablets or 3 × 1 tablet daily for 7 days. Each tablet contained 300 mg of St. John's wort extract, standardized to 900 µg of total hypericins. Six hours after the single high dose, mean levels of total hypericin were 43 ng/ml in serum and 5.3 ng/ml in skin blister fluid. After 3 tablets daily for one week, mean levels were 12.5 ng/ml in serum and 2.8 ng/ml in skin blister fluid. Hypericin levels in skin of >100 ng/ml are considered to be phototoxic [185].

Plasma levels of hyperforin were measured over a 24-hour period in volunteers treated with 300 mg of an ethanolic extract of St. John's wort containing 14.8 mg of hyperforin. Maximum plasma levels of about 150 ng/ml were reached 3.5 hours after oral admin-istration. Half-life and mean residence time of hyper-forin were 9 and 12 hours respectively. Up to 600 mg of the extract, hyperforin kinetics were linear [182].

Preclinical safety data
Systematic studies on single dose toxicity, reproductive toxicity and carcinogenicity of St. John's wort extracts

have been carried out by major manufacturers, but not published.

In vitro experiments

Hamster oocytes were incubated in St. John's wort extract before sperm/oocyte interaction. Penetration was prevented by a very high dose of 0.6 mg/ml, but 0.06 mg/ml had no effect [186]. Apparently this can be easily explained by the tannin content of the drug and does not indicate an antifertility effect.

Foetal calf serum or albumin strongly inhibited the photocytotoxic effects of pseudohypericin, but not those of hypericin, in A431 tumour cells. The authors concluded that hypericin is likely to be the constituent responsible for hypericism [187]. Human keratinocytes were cultured in the presence of different concentrations of St. John's wort extract and irradiated with UV-A or UV-B. A phototoxic effect was seen only on irradiation with UV-A at high hypericin concentrations (≥ 50 μg/ml) [188].

In vivo experiments

Effects on offspring

20 female mice were treated orally with 180 mg/kg/day of St. John's wort extract containing 0.3% of hypericin for 2 weeks before conception and throughout gestation. Perinatal outcomes, growth and physical milestones of the offspring were compared to a control group. Gestational ages at delivery and litter sizes did not differ between the groups. Body weight, body length and head circumference from postnatal day 3 to adulthood did not differ regardless of gender. The only difference between the groups was a temporary delay in the eruption of upper incisors in male offspring exposed to St. John's wort. Reproductive capacity, perinatal outcomes and growth and development of second-generation offspring were unaffected by treatment with St. John's wort extract [189].

Human studies

An experimental, double-blind, placebo-controlled study with 40 volunteers showed that photosensitivity was not induced by therapeutically relevant dosages of total hypericin, i.e. up to 1 mg daily for 8 days [190]. In a study involving intravenous administration of synthetic hypericin to HIV-infected patients, (reversible) symptoms of phototoxicity were observed at the highest dosage regime, which was 35 times higher than the highest oral dosage of total hypericin used in the therapy of depressive disorders [191].

Following administration of a methanolic extract to human volunteers as single doses of 900, 1800 and 3600 mg (containing 2.81, 5.62 and 11.25 mg of total hypericins respectively) and subsequent irradiation with solar-simulated irradiation or UV-A only, sensitivity to UV-A light increased slightly at the highest dose, but no correlation was found between plasma total hypericins levels and photosensitivity. After 15 days of treatment with 3×600 mg of the extract (5.6 mg total hypericins/day) sensitivity to both forms of irradiation had increased significantly; this effect could be compensated by reducing irradiation time by 21% [97].

Hypericin levels in skin of more than 100 ng/ml are considered to be phototoxic [184].

Photosensitization caused by St. John's wort has mainly been reported in veterinary studies, especially in unpigmented skin of grazing animals [192,193]. Dose-dependent phototoxic symptoms were observed in calves within 4 hours after single oral doses of dried St. John's wort at 3-5 g/kg body weight [194]. Merino ewes (an unpigmented breed, freshly shorn of wool), dosed orally with 5.7, 4.0 or 2.85 g/kg of dried St. John's wort (corresponding to 5.3, 3.7 or 2.65 mg/kg of hypericin) and then exposed to bright sunlight, had a tolerance level for hypericin of less than 2.65 mg/kg [192].

Clinical safety data

St. John's wort extracts have a particularly high level of clinical safety. Preparations have been studied in more than 13,900 patients, in whom good tolerability has generally been proven.

In 17 randomized, placebo-controlled clinical studies of St. John's wort, the few adverse effects noted were mainly headache, dizziness, sleep disorders, itching or non-specific gastrointestinal disturbances [24,25, 27,29-36,38,42,43,50,57,92].

In comparative clinical studies against synthetic antidepressants, the incidence of adverse events reported for St. John's wort preparations is generally higher than in placebo-controlled studies; this is considered a psychodynamic phenomenon resulting from the informed consent instructions in the double-blind design, in which the clinical investigator has to mention all possible side effects which might occur with both treatments offered. However, the overall rate of side-effects is still more favourable for St. John's wort than for synthetic antidepressants [60]. Pooled data from 8 studies representing more than 1,400 patients show that the proportions of patients reporting "any" side effects were 23.9% with St. John's wort preparations compared to 40.5% with standard antidepressants [28,39-41,44,45,56,93].

Two three-armed studies have compared a St. John's wort extract with both a synthetic antidepressant and placebo. In the first study, the rate of adverse events was 46% in an imipramine group, 22% in the St. John's wort group and 19% in the placebo group [37]. In the second study, the absolute rates of adverse events were not stated but, from the adverse events that differed significantly by treatment, the average rates for the events were 25% in a sertraline group (with diarrhoea occurring in 38% of the patients), 22% in the St. John's wort group (with frequent urination occurring in 27%) and 15% in the placebo group (with forgetfulness in 22%) [57].

In more naturalistic settings such as drug monitoring studies, subjective adverse events may be assessed in a more suitable quantitative and qualitative way. From these studies, the incidence of total adverse events among treated patients was 1-3% [81-91]. For comparison, the rate of adverse events in observational studies with tricyclic antidepressants is between 30 and 60% and with selective serotonin reuptake inhibitors (SSRIs) between 15 and 30% [60]. The most frequent side effects in the two largest St. John's wort studies, covering a total of 5,654 patients [82,85], were reported as mild gastrointestinal symptoms (0.42% [82], 0.55% [85]) such as stomach-ache, nausea, diarrhoea or constipation; allergic reactions such as pruritus and exanthema (0.52% [85]); fatigue (0.4% [85]); anxiety and restlessness (0.21% [82], 0.26% [85]); dizziness (0.12% [82], 0.15% [85]) and headache (0.12% [82]). According to an official Adverse Drug Reactions recording system, reversible skin reactions (photosensitization) have been reported in 1 per 300,000 cases treated with St. John's wort preparations [60], which is very rare. Significant phototoxicity occurred only in HIV-infected persons after administration of intravenous hypericin, 0.25-0.5 mg/kg twice weekly or 0.25 mg three times daily, or oral hypericin 0.25 mg/kg daily [98].

Systematic studies evaluating long-term side effects of St. John's wort are not available.

A detailed overview of the pharmacological, toxicological and clinical literature on St. John's Wort is given in two recent reviews [7,195].

REFERENCES

1. St. John's Wort - Hyperici herba. European Pharmacopoeia, Council of Europe.

2. Nahrstedt A, Butterweck V. Biologically active and other chemical constituents of the herb of *Hypericum perforatum* L. Pharmacopsychiatry 1997;30(Suppl 2): 129-34.

3. Brantner A, Kartnig T, Quehenberger F. Vergleichende phytochemische Untersuchungen an *Hypericum perforatum* L. und *Hypericum maculatum* Crantz. Sci Pharm 1994;62:261-76.

4. Schütt H, Hölzl J. Vergleichende Qualitätsuntersuchung von Johanniskraut-Fertigarzneimitteln unter Verwendung verschiedener quantitativer Bestimmungsmethoden. Pharmazie 1994;49:206-9.

5. Krämer W, Wiartalla R. Bestimmung von Naphthodianthronen (Gesamthypericin) in Johanniskraut (*Hypericum perforatum* L.). Pharm Ztg Wiss 1992;137: 202-7.

6. Häberlein H, Tschiersch KP, Stock S, Hölzl J. Johanniskraut (*Hypericum perforatum* L.). Teil 1: Nachweis eines weiteren Naphthodianthrons. Pharm Ztg Wiss 1992;137:169-74.

7. Greeson JM, Sanford B, Monti DA. St. John's wort (*Hypericum perforatum*): a review of the current pharmacological, toxicological and clinical literature. Psychopharmacology 2001;153:402-14.

8. Maisenbacher P, Kovar K-A. Adhyperforin: a homologue of hyperforin from *Hypericum perforatum*. Planta Med 1992;58:291-3.

9. Bergonzi MC, Bilia AR, Gallori S, Guerrini D, Vincieri FF. Variability in the content of the constituents of *Hypericum perforatum* L. and some commercial extracts. Drug Dev Indust Pharm 2001;27:491-7.

10. Orth HCJ, Rentel C, Schmidt PC. Isolation, purity analysis and stability of hyperforin as a standard material from *Hypericum perforatum* L. J Pharm Pharmacol 1999;51:193-200.

11. Orth HCJ, Hauer H, Erdelmeier CAJ, Schmidt PC. Orthoforin: the main degradation product of hyperforin from *Hypericum perforatum* L. Pharmazie 1999;54:76-7.

12. Fuzzati N, Gabetta B, Strepponi I, Villa F. High-performance liquid chromatography-electrospray ionization mass spectrometry and multiple mass spectrometry studies of hyperforin degradation products. J Chromatogr A 2001;926:187-98.

13. Bilia AR, Bergonzi MC, Morgenni F, Mazzi G, Vincieri FF. Evaluation of chemical stability of St. John's wort commercial extract and some preparations. Internat J Pharmaceut 2001;213:199-208.

14. Trifunovic S, Vajs V, Macura S, Juranic N, Djarmati Z, Jankov R, Milosavljevic S. Oxidation products of hyperforin from *Hypericum perforatum*. Phytochemistry 1998;49:1305-10.

15. Hölzl J, Ostrowski E. Johanniskraut (*Hypericum perforatum* L.). HPLC-Analyse der wichtigen Inhaltsstoffe und deren Variabilität in einer Population. Dtsch Apoth Ztg 1987;127:1227-30.

16. Girzu-Amblard M, Carnat A, Fraisse D, Carnat A-P, Lamaison J-L. Flavonoid and dianthranoid levels of St. John's wort flowering tops. Ann Pharm Fr 2000;58:341-5.

17. Tekel'ová D, Repcák M, Zemková E, Tóth J. Quantitative changes of dianthrones, hyperforin and flavonoids content in the flower ontogenesis of *Hypericum perforatum*. Planta Med 2000;66:778-80.

18. Berghöfer R, Hölzl J. Biflavonoids in *Hypericum perforatum*. Part 1. Isolation of I3, II8-biapigenin. Planta Med 1987;53:216-7.

19. Berghöfer R, Hölzl J. Isolation of I3´,II8-biapigenin (amentoflavone) from *Hypericum perforatum*. Planta Med 1989;55:91.

20. Jürgenliemk G and Nahrstedt A. Phenolic compounds from *Hypericum perforatum*. Planta Med 2002;68:88-91.

21. Ploss O, Petereit F, Nahrstedt A. Procyanidins from the herb of *Hypericum perforatum*. Pharmazie 2001;56:509-11.

22. Melzer R, Fricke U, Hölzl J. Vasoactive properties of procyanidins from *Hypericum perforatum* L. in isolated porcine coronary arteries. Arzneim-Forsch/Drug Res 1991;41:481-3.

23. Sparenberg B, Demisch L, Hölzl J. Untersuchungen über antidepressive Wirkstoffe von Johanniskraut. Pharm Ztg Wiss 1993;138:50-4.

24. Hoffmann J, Kühl E-D. Therapie von depressiven Zuständen mit Hypericin. Z Allg Med 1979;55:776-82.

25. Schlich D, Braukmann F, Schenk N. Behandlung depressiver Zustandsbilder mit Hypericinium. Doppelblindstudie mit einem pflanzlichen Antidepressivum. psycho 1987;13:440-7.

26. Kugler J, Weidenhammer W, Schmidt A, Groll S. Therapie depressiver Zustände. Hypericum-Extrakt Steigerwald als Alternative zur Benzodiazepin-Behandlung. Z Allg Med 1990;66:21-9.

27. Quandt J, Schmidt U, Schenk N. Ambulante Behandlung leichter und mittelschwerer depressiver Verstimmungen. Allgemeinarzt 1993;15:97-102.

28. Harrer G, Schmidt U, Kuhn U, Biller A. Comparison of equivalence between the St. John's wort extract LoHyp-57 and fluoxetine. Arzneim-Forsch/Drug Res 1999;49:289-96.

29. Sommer H, Harrer G. Placebo-controlled double-blind study examining the effectiveness of a hypericum preparation in 105 mildly depressed patients. J Geriatr Psychiatry Neurol 1994;7(Suppl 1):S9-S11.
Also published as:
Harrer G, Sommer H. Treatment of mild/moderate depressions with Hypericum. Phytomedicine 1994;1:3-8.
Previously published in German as:
Harrer G, Sommer H. Therapie leichter/mittel-schwerer Depressionen mit Hypericum. Münch med Wschr 1993;135:305-9.
Also published in German as:
Sommer H, Harrer G. Placebo-kontrollierte Studie zur Wirksamkeit eines Hypericum-Präparates bei 105 Patienten mit Depressionen. Nervenheilkunde 1993;12:274-7.
Previously published in German, with data on fewer patients, as:
Sommer H. Besserung psychovegetativer Beschwerden durch Hypericum im Rahmen einer multizentrischen Doppelblindstudie. Nervenheilkunde 1991;10:308-10.

30. Hübner W-D, Lande S, Podzuweit H. Hypericum treatment of mild depressions with somatic symptoms.

J Geriatr Psychiatry Neurol 1994;7(Suppl. 1):S12-S14.
Previously published in German as:
Hübner W-D, Lande S, Podzuweit H. Behandlung larvierter Depressionen mit Johanniskraut. Nervenheilkunde 1993;12:278-80.

31. Häring B, Hauns B, Hermann C, Hübner W-D, Maier-Lenz H, Marschner N. A double-blind, placebo-controlled pilot study of LI 160 in combination with chemotherapy in patients with solid tumors. In: Abstracts of 2nd International Congress on Phytomedicine. Munich, 11-14 September 1996. *Published as*: Phytomedicine 1996;3 (Suppl. 1):113 (Abstract SL-88).

32. Schmidt U, Schenk N, Schwarz I, Vorberg G. Zur Therapie depressiver Verstimmungen. Hypericin-Applikation. psycho 1989;15:665-71.

33. Harrer G, Schmidt U, Kuhn U. "Alternative" Depressionsbehandlung mit einem Hypericum-Extrakt. TW Neurol Psychiatr 1991;5:710-6.

34. Halama P. Wirksamkeit des Hypericum-Extraktes LI 160 bei 50 Patienten einer psychiatrischen Fachpraxis. Nervenheilkunde 1991;10:305-7.
Also published as:
Halama P. Wirksamkeit des Johanniskrautextraktes LI 160 bei depressiver Verstimmung. Plazebokontrollierte Doppelblindstudie mit 50 Patienten. Nervenheilkunde 1991;10:250-3.

35. Laakmann G, Schüle C, Baghai T, Kieser M. St. John's wort in mild to moderate depression: the relevance of hyperforin for the clinical efficacy. Pharmacopsychiatry 1998;31(Suppl 1):54-9.
Also published as:
Laakmann G, Dienel A, Kieser M. Clinical significance of hyperforin for the efficacy of *Hypericum* extracts on depressive disorders of different severities. Phytomedicine 1998;5:435-42.

36. Kalb R, Trautmann-Sponsel RD, Kieser M. Efficacy and tolerability of *Hypericum* extract WS 5572 versus placebo in mildly to moderately depressed patients. A randomized double-blind multicenter clinical trial. Pharmacopsychiatry 2001;34:96-103.

37. Philipp M, Kohnen R, Hiller K-O. Hypericum extract versus imipramine or placebo in patients with moderate depression: randomised multicentre study of treatment for eight weeks. Br Med J 1999;319:1534-9.

38. Hänsgen K-D, Vesper J. Antidepressive Wirksamkeit eines hochdosierten Hypericumextraktes. Münch med Wschr 1996;138:29-33.
Previously published, with data on fewer patients, as:
Hänsgen K-D, Vesper J, Ploch M. Multicenter double-blind study examining the antidepressant effectiveness of the hypericum extract LI 160. J Geriatr Psychiatry Neurol 1994;7(Suppl 1):S15-S18.
Previously published in German, with data on fewer patients, as:
Hänsgen KD, Vesper J, Ploch M. Multizentrische Doppelblindstudie zur antidepressiven Wirksamkeit des Hypericum-Extraktes LI 160. Nervenheilkunde 1993;12:285-9.

39. Harrer G, Hübner W-D, Podzuweit H. Effectiveness

and tolerance of the hypericum extract LI 160 compared to maprotiline: A multicenter double-blind study. J Geriatr Psychiatry Neurol 1994;7(Suppl. 1):S24-S28.
Previously published in German as:
Harrer G, Hübner W-D, Podzuweit H. Wirksamkeit und Verträglichkeit des Hypericum-Präparates LI 160 im Vergleich mit Maprotilin. Multizentrische Doppelblindstudie mit 102 depressiven Patienten. Nervenheilkunde 1993;12:297-301.

40. Vorbach E-U, Hübner W-D, Arnoldt K-H. Effectiveness and tolerance of the hypericum extract LI 160 in comparison with imipramine: Randomized double-blind study with 135 outpatients. J Geriatr Psychiatry Neurol 1994;7(Suppl. 1):S19-S23.
Previously published in German as:
Vorbach E-U, Hübner W-D, Arnoldt K-H. Wirksamkeit und Verträglichkeit des Hypericum-Extraktes LI 160 im Vergleich mit Imipramin. Randomisierte Doppelblindstudie mit 135 ambulanten Patienten. Nervenheilkunde 1993;12:290-6.

41. Wheatley D. LI 160, an extract of St. John's wort, versus amitriptyline in mildly to moderately depressed outpatients - A controlled 6-week clinical trial. Pharmacopsychiatry 1997;30(Suppl 2):77-80.

42. Witte B, Harrer G, Kaptan T, Podzuweit H, Schmidt U. Behandlung depressiver Verstimmungen mit einem hochkonzentrierten Hypericumpräparat. Eine multizentrische plazebokontrollierte Doppelblindstudie. Fortschr Med 1995;113:404-8.

43. Schrader E, Meier B, Brattström A. Hypericum treatment of mild-moderate depression in a placebo-controlled study. A prospective, double-blind, randomized, placebo-controlled, multicentre study. Human Psychopharmacol 1998;13:163-9.

44. Schrader E. Equivalence of St. John's wort extract (Ze 117) and fluoxetine: a randomized, controlled study in mild-moderate depression. Internat Clin Psychopharmacol 2000;15:61-8.

45. Woelk H. Comparison of St. John's wort and imipramine for treating depression: randomised controlled trial. Br Med J 2000;321:536-9.

46. Lenoir S, Degenring FH, Saller R. A double-blind randomised trial to investigate three different concentrations of a standardised fresh plant extract obtained from the shoot tips of *Hypericum perforatum* L. Phytomedicine 1999;6:141-6.

47. Engesser A, Christe C, Dean-Romano A, Ellgehausen K, Frey P, Gallacchi P et al. St. John's Wort tea against depressed mood in old age - a pilot study. In: Abstracts of 2nd International Congress on Phytomedicine. Munich, 11-14 September 1996. *Published as:* Phytomedicine 1996;3 (Suppl 1):265 (Poster P-86).

48. World Health Organisation. ICD-10: International Statistical Classification of Diseases and Related Health Problems. Tenth Revision. Geneva: WHO, 1992.

49. World Health Organization. Diagnostic and Management Guidelines for Mental Disorders in Primary Care: ICD-10, Chapter V. Primary Care Version. Göttingen:

WHO/Hogrefe & Huber, 1996.

50. Lehrl S, Willemsen A, Papp R, Woelk H. Ergebnisse von Messungen der kognitiven Leistungsfähigkeit bei Patienten unter der Therapie mit Johanniskraut-Extrakt. Nervenheilkunde 1993;12:281-4.

51. Martinez B, Kasper S, Ruhrmann S, Moeller H-J. Hypericum in the treatment of seasonal affective disorders. J Geriatr Psychiatry Neurol 1994;7(Suppl 1):S29-S33.
Previously published in German as:
Martinez B, Kasper S, Ruhrmann S, Moeller H-J. Hypericum in der Behandlung von saisonal abhängigen Depressionen. Nervenheilkunde 1993;12:302-7.

52. Warnecke G. Beeinflussung klimakterischer Depressionen. Therapieergebnisse mit Hypericin (Johanniskraut-Extrakt). Z Allg Med 1986;62:1111-3.

53. Werth W. Psychotonin® M versus Imipramin in der Chirurgie. Vergleichende klinische Prüfung bei Patienten mit Amputationen. Kassenarzt 1989;(15):64-8.

54. Ruschitzka F, Meier PJ, Turina M, Lüscher TF, Noll G. Acute heart transplant rejection due to Saint John's wort. Lancet 2000;355:548-9.

55. Piscitelli SC, Burstein AH, Chaitt D, Alfaro RM, Falloon J. Indinavir concentrations and St. John's wort. Lancet 2000;355:547-8.

56. Shelton RC, Keller MB, Gelenberg A, Dunner DL, Hirschfeld R, Thase ME et al. Effectiveness of St John's wort in major depression. A randomized controlled trial. JAMA 2001;285:1978-86.

57. Davidson JRT/Hypericum Depression Trial Study Group. Effect of *Hypericum perforatum* (St John's wort) in major depressive disorder. A randomized controlled trial. JAMA 2002;287:1807-14.

58. Vorbach EU, Arnoldt KH, Hübner W-D. Efficacy and tolerability of St. John's wort extract LI 160 versus imipramine in patients with severe depressive episodes according to ICD-10. Pharmacopsychiatry 1997;30 (Suppl 2):81-5.

59. Bon S, Hartmann K, Kuhn M. Johanniskraut: Ein Enzyminduktor? Schweiz Apothekerzeitung 1999; 16:535-6.

60. Schulz V. Incidence and clinical relevance of the interactions and side effects of hypericum preparations. Phytomedicine 2001;8:152-60.

61. Gordon JB. SSRIs and St. John's wort: Possible toxicity? American Family Physician, March 1, 1998.

62. Prost N, Tichadou L, Rodor F, Nguyen N, David JM, Jean-Pastor MJ. Interaction millepertuis-venlafaxine. Presse Méd 2000;29:1285-6.

63. Breidenbach T, Hoffmann MW, Becker T, Schlitt H, Klempnauer J. Drug interaction of St John's wort with ciclosporin. Lancet 2000,355:1912.

64. Mai I, Krüger H, Budde K, Johne A, Brockmöller J,

Neumayer H-H, Roots I. Hazardous pharmacokinetic interaction of Saint John's wort (*Hypericum perforatum*) with the immunosuppressant cyclosporin. Internat J Clin Pharmacol Ther 2000;38:500-2.

65. Maurer A, Johne A, Bauer S, Brockmöller J, Donath F, Roots I et al. Interaction of St. John's wort extract with phenprocoumon. Eur J Clin Pharmacol 1999;55:A22.

66. Yue Q-Y, Bergquist C, Gerdén B. Seven cases of decreased effect of warfarin during concomitant treatment with St John's wort. Lancet 2000;355:576-7.

67. Nebel A, Schneider BJ, Baker RK, Kroll DJ. Potential metabolic interaction between St. John's wort and theophylline. Ann Pharmacother 1999;33:502.

68. Johne A, Brockmöller J, Bauer S, Maurer A, Langheinrich M, Roots I. Pharmacokinetic interaction of digoxin with an herbal extract from St John's wort (*Hypericum perforatum*). Clin Pharmacol Ther 1999;66:338-45.

69. Obach RS. Inhibition of human cytochrome P450 enzymes by constituents of St. John's wort, an herbal preparation used in the treatment of depression. J Pharmacol Exp Ther 2000;294:88-95.

70. Markowitz JS, DeVane CL, Boulton DW, Carson SW, Nahas Z, Risch SC. Effect of St. John's wort (*Hypericum perforatum*) on cytochrome P-450 2D6 and 3A4 activity in healthy volunteers. Life Sci 2000;66(9):PL133-9.

71. Wentworth JM, Agostini M, Love J, Schwabe JW, Chatterjee VKK. St John's wort, a herbal antidepressant, activates the steroid X receptor. J Endocrinol 2000; 166:R11-R16.

72. Moore LB, Goodwin B, Jones SA, Wisely GB, Serabjit-Singh CJ, Willson TM et al. St. John's wort induces hepatic drug metabolism through activation of the pregnane X receptor. Proc Natl Acad Sci USA 2000; 97:7500-2.

73. Roby CA, Anderson GD, Kantor E, Dryer DA, Burstein AH. St John's wort: Effect on CYP3A4 activity. Clin Pharmacol Ther 2000;67:451-6.

74. Nöldner M, Chatterjee S. Effects of two different extracts of St John's wort and some of their constituents on cytochrome P450 activities in rat liver microsomes. Pharmacopsychiatry 2001;34(Suppl 1):S108-S110.

75. Wang Z, Gorski JC, Hamman MA, Huang S-M, Lesko LJ, Hall SD. The effects of St John's wort (*Hypericum perforatum*) on human cytochrome P450 activity. Clin Pharmacol Ther 2001;70:317-26.

76. Hennessy M, Kelleher D, Spiers JP, Barry M, Kavanagh P, Back D et al. St John's Wort increases expression of P-glycoprotein: implications for drug interactions. Br J Clin Pharmacol 2002;53:75-82.

77. Käufeler R, Meier B, Brattström A. Der Johannis-krautextrakt Ze 117 - ein hyperforinarmer Extrakt: Belege zur klinischen Wirksamkeit und Verträglichkeit. Phytotherapie 2001;1:13-6.

78. Schmidt U, Sommer H. Johanniskraut-Extrakt zur ambulanten Therapie der Depression. Aufmerksamkeit und Reaktionsvermögen bleiben erhalten. Fortschr Med 1993;111:339-42.

79. Herberg KW. Psychotrope Phytopharmaka im Test. Alternative zu synthetischen Psychopharmaka? Therapiewoche 1994;44:704-13.

80. Pieschl D, Angersbach P, Toman M. Zur Behandlung von Depressionen. Verbundstudie mit einem pflanzlichen Extrakt aus Johanniskraut. Therapiewoche 1989;39:2567-71.

81. Maisenbacher H-J, Kuhn U. Therapie von Depressionen in der Praxis. Ergebnisse einer Anwendungs-beobachtung mit Herba Hyperici. natura med 1992; 7:394-9.

82. Schakau D, Hiller K-O, Schultz-Zehden W, Teschner F. Nutzen/Risiko-Profil von Johanniskrautextrakt STEI 300 bei 2404 Patienten mit psychischen Störungen unterschiedlicher Schweregrade. Psychopharmako-therapie 1996;3:116-22.

83. Mueller BM. St. John's wort for depressive disorders: results of an outpatient study with the hypericum preparation HYP 811. Adv Ther 1998;15:109-16.

84. Bernhardt M, Liske E. Antidepressive Therapie mit Johanniskraut-Extrakt unter besonderer Berücksichti-gung von zwei unterschiedlichen Dosierungsschemata. Jatros Neurologie 1996;12:43-8.

85. Woelk H, Burkard G, Grünwald J. Benefits and risks of the hypericum extract LI 160: drug monitoring study with 3250 patients. J Geriatr Psychiatry Neurol 1994;7 (Suppl 1):S34-S38.

86. Albrecht M, Hübner W-D, Podzuweit H, Schmidt U. Johanniskraut-Extrakt zur Behandlung der Depression. Therapiebegleitende Anwendungsbeobachtung mit Jarsin® Dragees. Der Kassenarzt 1994;41:45-54.

87. Grube B, Grünwald J, Walper A, Hopfenmüller W. Johanniskraut bei leichten temporären Verstimmungen. Anwendungsbeobachtung belegt Behandlungserfolg. naturamed 1996;11:21-7.

88. Grube B, Walper A, Wheatley D. St. John's wort extract: efficacy for menopausal symptoms of psychological origin. Adv Ther 1999;16:177-86.

89. Holsboer-Trachsler E, Vanoni C. Clinical efficacy and tolerance of the hypericum special extract LI 160 in depressive disorders - a drug monitoring study [Article in German]. Schweiz Rundsch Med Prax 1999;88:1475-80.

90. Sepehrmanesh M. Johanniskrautextrakt in der ärztlichen Praxis. Erfahrungen anhand einer Anwendungs-beobachtung mit Texx® 300. Z Allg Med 1999;75:170-3.

91. Meier B, Liske E, Rosinus V. Wirksamkeit und Verträglichkeit eines standardisierten Johanniskraut-Vollextraktes (Ze 117) bei Patienten mit depressiver Symptomatik unterschiedlicher Schweregrade - eine Anwendungsbeobachtung. Forsch Komplementärmed

1997;4:87-93.

92. Reh C, Laux P, Schenk N. Hypericum-Extrakt bei Depressionen - eine wirksame Alternative. Therapie-woche 1992;42:1576-81.

93. Bergmann R, Nüßner J, Demling J. Behandlung leichter bis mittelschwerer Depressionen. Vergleich von Hypericum perforatum mit Amitriptylin. TW Neurol Psychiatr 1993;7:235-40.

94. Nierenberg AA, Burt T, Matthews J, Weiss P. Mania associated with St. John's wort. Biol Psychiatry 1999; 46:1707-8.

95. Bove GM. Acute neuropathy after exposure to sun in a patient treated with St. John's wort. Lancet 1998;352: 1121-2.

96. Golsch S, Vocks E, Rakoski J, Brockow K, Ring J. Reversible Erhöhung der Photosensitivität im UV-B-Bereich durch Johanniskraut-Präparate. Der Hautarzt 1997;48:249-52.

97. Brockmöller J, Reum T, Bauer S, Kerb R, Hübner W-D, Roots I. Hypericin und pseudohypericin: pharmaco-kinetics and effects on photosensitivity in humans. Pharmacopsychiatry 1997;30(Suppl 2):94-101.

98. Gulick RM, McAuliffe V, Holden-Wiltse J et al. Phase I studies of hypericin, the active compound in St. John's wort, as an antiretroviral agent in HIV-infected adults. Ann Intern Med 1999;130:510-4.

99. Hänsel R, Keller K, Rimpler H, Schneider G, editors. Hypericum. In: Hagers Handbuch der Pharma-zeutischen Praxis, 5th ed. Volume 5: Drogen E-O. Berlin-Heidelberg-New York-London: Springer-Verlag, 1993:474-95.

100. Demisch L, Hölzl J, Gollnik B, Kaczmarczyk P. Identification of selective MAO-type-A inhibitors in Hypericum perforatum L. (Hyperforat®). Pharmaco-psychiatry 1989;22:194.

101. Thiede H-M, Walper A. MAO- und COMT-Hemmung durch Hypericum-Extrakte und Hypericin. Nerven-heilkunde 1993;12:346-8.

102. Bladt S, Wagner H. MAO-Hemmung durch Fraktionen und Inhaltsstoffe von Hypericum-Extrakt. Nerven-heilkunde 1993;12:349-52.

103. Obry T. Einfluß eines ethanolischen Auszuges aus Hypericum perforatum auf die Enzyme der Nor-adrenalinsynthese und auf die Diaphorase [Diploma study]. München: Maximilians-Universität, 1991.

104. Kleber E, Obry T, Hippeli S, Schneider W, Elstner EF. Biochemical activities of extracts from Hypericum perforatum L. 1st communication: Inhibition of dopamine-β-hydroxylase. Arzneim-Forsch/Drug Res 1999;49:106-9.

105. Denke A, Schempp H, Weiser D, Elstner EF. Biochemical activity of extracts from Hypericum perforatum L. 5th communication: Dopamine-β-hydroxylase-product quantification by HPLC and inhibition by hypericins and flavonoids. Arzneim-Forsch/Drug Res 2000;50:415-9.

106. Curle P, Kato G, Hiller K-O. Neurochemical studies on Valeriana and Hypericum. Battelle-Europe Report Nr. 2107 (1988); unpublished.

107. Nielsen M, Frøkjær S, Braestrup C. High affinity of the naturally-occurring biflavonoid, amentoflavon, to brain benzodiazepine receptors in vitro. Biochem Pharmacol 1988;37:3285-7.

108. Müller WEG, Rossol R. Einfluß von Hypericum-Extrakt auf die Expression von Serotonin-Rezeptoren. Nervenheilkunde 1993;12:357-8.

109. Baureithel KH, Büter KB, Engesser A, Burkard W, Schaffner W. Inhibition of benzodiazepine binding in vitro by amentoflavone, a constituent of various species of Hypericum. Pharm Acta Helv 1997;72:153-7.

110. Cott JM. In vitro receptor binding and enzyme inhibition by Hypericum perforatum extract. Pharmacopsychiatry 1997;30(Suppl 2):108-12.

111. Raffa RB. Screen of receptor and uptake-site activity of hypericin component of St. John's wort reveals σ receptor binding. Life Sciences 1998;62:265-70.

112. Simmen U, Schweitzer C, Burkhard W, Schaffner W, Lundstrom K. Hypericum perforatum inhibits the binding of μ- and κ-opioid receptor expressed with the Semliki Forest virus system. Pharm Acta Helv 1998;73:53-6.

113. Simmen U, Burkard W, Berger K, Schaffner W, Lundstrom K. Extracts and constituents of Hypericum perforatum inhibit the binding of various ligands to recombinant receptors expressed with the Semliki Forest virus system. J Recept Signal Transduct Res 1999;19:59-74.

114. Perovic S, Müller WEG. Pharmacological profile of hypericum extract. Effect on serotonin uptake by post-synaptic receptors. Arzneim-Forsch/Drug Res 1995; 45:1145-8.

115. Chatterjee SS, Bhattacharya SK, Wonnemann M, Singer A, Müller WE. Hyperforin as a possible antidepressant component of hypericum extracts. Life Sciences 1998; 63:499-510.

116. Gobbi M, Dalle Valle F, Ciapparelli C, Diomede L, Morazzoni P, Verotta L et al. Hypericum perforatum L. extract does not inhibit 5-HT transporter in rat brain cortex. Naunyn-Schmiedeberg's Arch Pharmacol 1999; 360:262-9.

117. Neary JT, Bu Y. Hypericum LI 160 inhibits uptake of serotonin and norepinephrine in astrocytes. Brain Res 1999;816:358-63.

118. Müller WE, Rolli M, Schäfer C, Hafner U. Effects of hypericum extract (LI 160) in biochemical models of antidepressant activity. Pharmacopsychiatry 1997;30 (Suppl 2):102-7.

119. Singer A, Wonnemann M, Müller WE. Hyperforin, a major antidepressant constituent of St. John's wort,

inhibits serotonin uptake by elevating free intracellular Na+. J Pharmacol Exp Ther 1999;290:1363-8.

120. Chatterjee S, Filippov V, Lishko P, Maximyuk O, Nöldner M and Krishtal O. Hyperforin attenuates various ionic conductance mechanisms in the isolated hippocampal neurons of rat. Life Sciences 1999; 65:2395-405.

121. Wonnemann M, Singer A, Müller WE. Inhibition of synaptosomal uptake of ^{3}H-L-glutamate and ^{3}H-GABA by hyperforin, a major constituent of St. John's wort: the role of amiloride sensitive sodium conductive pathways. Neuropsychopharmacology 2000;23:188-97.

122. Thiele B, Brink I, Ploch M. Modulation der Zytokin-Expression durch Hypericum-Extrakt. Nervenheilkunde 1993;12:353-6.

123. Bork PM, Bacher S, Schmitz ML, Kaspers U, Heinrich M. Hypericin as a non-antioxidant inhibitor of NF-κB. Planta Med 1999;65:297-300.

124. Denke A, Schneider W, Elstner EF. Biochemical activities of extracts from Hypericum perforatum L. 2nd communication: Inhibition of metenkephaline- and tyrosine-dimerization. Arzneim-Forsch/Drug Res 1999; 49:109-14.

125. Helgason CM, Wieseler Frank JL, Johnson DR, Frank MG, Hendricks SE. The effects of St. John's wort (Hypericum perforatum) on NK cell activity in vitro. Immunopharmacology 2000;46:247-51.

126. Okpanyi SN, Weischer ML. Tierexperimentelle Untersuchungen zur psychotropen Wirksamkeit eines Hypericum-Extraktes. Arzneim-Forsch/Drug Res 1987; 37:10-3.

127. Winterhoff H, Butterweck V, Nahrstedt A, Gumbinger HG, Schulz V, Erping S et al. Pharmakologische Untersuchungen zur antidepressiven Wirkung von Hypericum perforatum L. In: Loew D, Rietbrock N, editors. Phytopharmaka in Forschung und klinischer Anwendung. Darmstadt: Steinkopff, 1995:39-56.

128. Calapai G, Crupi A, Firenzuoli F, Inferrera G, Squadrito F, Paris A et al. Serotonin, norepinephrine and dopamine involvement in the antidepressant action of Hypericum perforatum. Pharmacopsychiatry 2001;34:45-9.

129. Gambarana C, Ghiglieri O, Tolu P, De Montis MG, Giachetti D, Bombardelli E, Tagliamonte A. Efficacy of a Hypericum perforatum (St. John's wort) extract in preventing and reverting a condition of escape deficit in rats. Neuropsychopharmacology 1999;21:247-57.

130. Butterweck V, Petereit F, Winterhoff H, Nahrstedt A. Solubilized hypericin and pseudohypericin from Hypericum perforatum exert antidepressant activity in the forced swimming test. Planta Med 1998;64:291-4.

131. Butterweck V, Jürgenliemk G, Nahrstedt A, Winterhoff H. Flavonoids from Hypericum perforatum show antidepressant activity in the forced swimming test. Planta Med 2000;66:3-6.

132. De Vry J, Maurel S, Schreiber R, de Beun R, Jentzsch KR. Comparison of hypericum extracts with imipramine and fluoxetine in animal models of depression and alcoholism. Eur Neuropsychopharmacol 1999;9:461-8.

133. Kumar V, Singh PN, Jaiswal AK, Bhattacharya SK. Antidepressant activity of Indian Hypericum perforatum Linn in rodents. Indian J Exp Biol 1999;37:1171-6.

134. Calapai G, Crupi A, Firenzuoli F, Costantino G, Inferrera G, Campo GM, Caputi AP. Effects of Hypericum perforatum on levels of 5-hydroxytryptamine, noradrenaline and dopamine in the cortex, diencephalon and brainstem of the rat. J Pharm Pharmacol 1999;51: 723-8.

135. Teufel-Mayer R, Gleitz J. Effects of long-term administration of hypericum extracts on the affinity and density of the central serotonergic 5-HT1 A and 5-HT2 A receptors. Pharmacopsychiatry 1997;30(Suppl 2):113-6.

136. Yu PH. Effect of the Hypericum perforatum extract on serotonin turnover in the mouse brain. Pharmacopsychiatry 2000;33:60-5.

137. Butterweck V, Böckers T, Korte B, Wittkowski W, Winterhoff H. Long-term effects of St. John's wort and hypericin on monoamine levels in rat hypothalamus and hippocampus. Brain Res 2002;930:21-9.

138. Bhattacharya SK, Chakrabarti A, Chatterjee SS. Activity profiles of two hyperforin-containing hypericum extracts in behavioral models. Pharmacopsychiatry 1998;31 (Suppl 1):22-9.

139. Di Matteo V, Di Giovanni G, Di Mascio M, Esposito E. Effect of acute administration of Hypericum perforatum-CO_2 extract on dopamine and serotonin release in the rat central nervous system. Pharmacopsychiatry 2000; 33:14-8.

140. Kaehler ST, Sinner C, Chatterjee SS, Philippu A. Hyperforin enhances the extracellular concentrations of catecholamines, serotonin and glutamate in the rat locus coeruleus. Neurosci Lett 1999;262:199-202.

141. Dimpfel W, Schober F, Mannel M. Effects of a methanolic extract and a hyperforin-enriched CO_2 extract of St. John's wort (Hypericum perforatum) on intracerebral field potentials in the freely moving rat (tele-stereo-EEG). Pharmacopsychiatry 1998;31(Suppl 1):30-5.

142. Butterweck V, Nahrstedt A, Evans J, Hufeisen S, Rauser L, Savage J et al. In vitro receptor screening of pure constituents of St. John's wort reveals novel interactions with a number of GPCRs. Psychopharmacology 2002; 162:193-202.

143. Rezvani AH, Overstreet DH, Yang Y, Clark E. Attenuation of alcohol intake by extract of Hypericum perforatum (St. John's wort) in two different strains of alcohol-preferring rats. Alcohol & Alcoholism 1999; 34:699-705.

144. Panocka I, Perfumi M, Angeletti S, Ciccocioppo R, Massi M. Effects of Hypericum perforatum extract on ethanol intake and on behavioral despair: a search for

the neurochemical systems involved. Pharmacol Biochem Behav 2000;66:105-11.

145. Hölzl J. Inhaltsstoffe und Wirkmechanismen des Johanniskrautes. Z Phytother 1993;14:255-64.

146. Brondz I, Greibrokk T, Groth PA, Aasen AJ. The relative stereochemistry of hyperforin - an antibiotic from *Hypericum perforatum* L. Tetrahedron Lett 1982; 23:1299-300.

147. Brantner A, Della Loggia R, Sosa S, Kartnig T. Untersuchungen zur antiphlogistischen Wirkung von *Hypericum perforatum* L. Sci Pharm 1994;62:97-8.

148. Schempp CM, Pelz K, Wittmer A, Schöpf E, Simon JC. Antibacterial activity of hyperforin from St. John's wort against multiresistant *Staphylococcus aureus* and Gram-positive bacteria [Letter]. Lancet 1999;353:2129.

149. Voss A, Verweij PE. Antibacterial activity of hyperforin from St. John's wort. Lancet 1999;354:777.

150. Fiebich BL, Heinrich M, Langosch JM, Kammerer N, Lieb K. Antibacterial activity of hyperforin from St. John's wort [Letter]. Lancet 1999;354:777.

151. Andersen DO, Weber ND, Wood SG, Hughes BG, Murray BK, North JA. In vitro virucidal activity of selected anthraquinones and anthraquinone derivatives. Antiviral Res 1991;16:185-96.

152. Barnard DL, Huffman JH, Morris JLB, Wood SG, Hughes BG, Sidwell RW. Evaluation of the antiviral activity of anthraquinones, anthrones and anthraquinone derivatives against human cytomegalovirus. Antiviral Res 1992;17:63-77.

153. Hudson JB, Lopez-Bazzocchi I, Towers GHN. Antiviral activities of hypericin. Antiviral Res 1991;15:101-12.

154. Kraus GA, Pratt D, Tossberg J, Carpenter S. Antiretroviral activity of synthetic hypericin and related analogs. Biochem Biophys Res Commun 1990;172:149-53.

155. Lavie G, Valentine F, Levin B, Mazur Y, Gallo G, Lavie D et al. Studies of the mechanisms of action of the antiretroviral agents hypericin and pseudohypericin. Proc Natl Acad Sci USA 1989;86:5963-7.

156. Meruelo D, Lavie G, Lavie D. Therapeutic agents with dramatic antiretroviral activity and little toxicity at effective doses: aromatic polycyclic diones hypericin and pseudohypericin. Proc Natl Acad Sci USA 1988; 85:5230-4.

157. Schinazi RF, Chu CK, Babu JR, Oswald BJ, Saalmann V, Cannon DL et al. Anthraquinones as a new class of antiviral agents against human immunodeficiency virus. Antiviral Res 1990;13:265-72.

158. Takahashi I, Nakanishi S, Kobayashi E, Nakano H, Suzuki K, Tamaoki T. Hypericin and pseudohypericin specifically inhibit protein kinase C: possible relation to their antiretroviral activity. Biochem Biophys Res Commun 1989;165:1207-12.

159. Tripathi YB, Pandey E. Role of alcoholic extract of shoot

of *Hypericum perforatum* Linn on lipid peroxidation and various species of free radicals in rats. Indian J Exp Biol 1999;37:567-71.

160. Daniel K. Kurze Mitteilung über 12jährige therapeutische Erfahrungen mit Hypericin. Klin Wschr 1951; 29:260-2.

161. Linde K, Ramirez G, Mulrow CD, Pauls A, Weidenhammer W, Melchart D. St John's wort for depression - an overview and meta-analysis of randomised clinical trials. Br Med J 1996;313:253-8.

162. Linde K, Mulrow CD. St. John's wort for depression. The Cochrane Library: 2000 Issue 1.

163. Kim HL, Streltzer J, Goebert D. St. John's wort for depression. A meta-analysis of well-defined clinical trials. J Nerv Ment Dis 1999;187:532-8.

164. Volz H-P. Controlled clinical trials of hypericum extracts in depressed patients - an overview. Pharmacopsychiatry 1997;30(Suppl 2):72-6.

165. Hippius H. St. John's wort (*Hypericum perforatum*) - a herbal antidepressant. Curr Med Res Opin 1998;14:171-84.

166. Wheatley D. Hypericum extract. Potential in the treatment of depression. CNS Drugs 1998;9:431-40.

167. Stevinson C, Ernst E. Hypericum for depression. An update of the clinical evidence. Eur Neuropsychopharmacol 1999;9:501-5.

168. Vitiello B. *Hypericum perforatum* extracts as potential antidepressants. J Pharm Pharmacol 1999;51:513-7.

169. Gaster B, Holroyd J. St. John's wort for depression. A systematic review. Arch Intern Med 2000;160:152-6.

170. Gaedcke F. In: Gaedcke F, Steinhoff B, editors. Phytopharmaka - Wissenschaftliche und rechtliche Grundlagen für die Entwicklung, Standardisierung und Zulassung in Deutschland und Europa. Stuttgart: Wissenschaftliche Verlagsgesellschaft, 2000:49 and 74.

171. Schulz V, Hänsel R, Tyler VE. St. John's wort as an antidepressant. In: Rational Phytotherapy: A physicians' guide to herbal medicine, 3rd ed. Berlin-Heidelberg-New York: Springer-Verlag, 1998:50-65.

172. Guy W. Clinical global impressions. In: ECDEU assessment manual for psychopharmacology, revised. Rockville MD: US Department of Health, Education and Welfare, National Institute of Mental Health, 1967:217-22.

173. American Psychiatric Association. Diagnostic and statistical manual of mental disorders, 3rd ed. revised. Washington DC: American Psychiatric Association Press, 1987.

174. American Psychiatric Association. Diagnostic and statistical manual of mental disorders, 4th ed. Washington DC: American Psychiatric Association Press, 1994.

175. Hamilton M. The assessment of anxiety states by rating. Brit J Med Psychol 1959;32:50-5.

176. Hamilton M. A rating scale for depression. J Neurol Neurosurg Psychiatry 1960;23:56-62.

177. Williams JBW. A structured interview guide for the Hamilton depression rating scale. Arch Gen Psychiatry 1988;45:742-7.

178. World Health Organisation. International Statistical Classification of Diseases and Related Health Problems. Ninth Revision. Geneva: WHO, 1975.

179. Stock S, Hölzl J. Pharmacokinetic test of [^{14}C]-labelled hypericin and pseudohypericin from *Hypericum perforatum* and serum kinetics of hypericin in man. Planta Med 1991;57(Suppl 2):A61-2.

180. Chung P-S, Saxton RE, Paiva MB, Rhee C-K, Soudant J, Mathey A et al. Hypericin uptake in rabbits and nude mice transplanted with human squamous cell carcinomas: study of a new sensitizer for laser photo-therapy. Laryngoscope 1994;104:1471-6

181. Chen B, de Witte PA. Photodynamic therapy efficacy and tissue distribution of hypericin in a mouse P388 lymphoma tumor model. Cancer Lett 2000;150:111-7.

182. Biber A, Fischer H, Römer A, Chatterjee SS. Oral bioavailability of hyperforin from hypericum extracts in rats and human volunteers. Pharmacopsychiatry 1998;31(Suppl 1):36-43.

183. Weiser D. Pharmakokinetik von Hypericin nach oraler Einnahme des Johanniskraut-Extraktes LI 160. Nervenheilkunde 1991;10:318-9.

184. Kerb R, Brockmöller J, Staffeldt B, Ploch M, Roots I. Single-dose and steady-state pharmacokinetics of hypericin and pseudohypericin. Antimicrob Agents Chemother 1996;40:2087-93.

185. Schempp CM, Winghofer B, Langheinrich M, Schopf E, Simon JC. Hypericin levels in human serum and interstitial skin blister fluid after oral single-dose and steady-state administration of *Hypericum perforatum* extract (St. John's wort). Skin Pharmacol Appl Skin Physiol 1999;12:299-304.

186. Ondrizek RR, Chan PJ, Patton WC, King A. An alternative medicine study of herbal effects on the penetration of zona-free hamster oocytes and the integrity of sperm deoxyribonucleic acid. Fertil Steril 1999;71:517-22.

187. Vandenbogaerde AL, Kamuhabwa A, Delaey E, Himpens BE, Merlevede WJ, de Witte PA. Photo-cytotoxic effect of pseudohypericin versus hypericin. J Photochem Photobiol B: Biology 1998;45:87-94.

188. Bernd A, Simon S, Ramirez-Bosca A, Kippenberger S, Diaz Alperi J, Miquel J et al. Phototoxic effects of hypericum extract in cultures of human keratinocytes compared with those of psoralen. Photochem Photobiol 1999;69:218-21.

189. Rayburn WF, Gonzalez CL, Christensen D, Stewart JD. Effect of prenatally administered hypericum (St. John's wort) on growth and physical maturation of mouse offspring. Am J Obstet Gynecol 2001;184:191-5.

190. Wienert V, Claßen R, Hiller K-O. Zur Frage der Photosensibilisierung von Hypericin in einer Baldrian-Johanniskraut-Kombination - klinisch-experimentelle, plazebokontrollierte Vergleichsstudie [Poster abstract]. In: Abstracts of 3. Phytotherapie-Kongreß, Lübeck-Travemünde, 3-6 October 1991 (Poster P23).

191. James JS. Hypericin, February 1992. AIDS Treatment News (San Francisco) 1992; (6 March, No. 146):1-4.

192. Bourke CA. Sunlight associated hyperthermia as a consistent and rapidly developing clinical sign in sheep intoxicated by St. John's wort (*Hypericum perforatum*). Aust Vet J 2000;78:483-8.

193. Giese AC. Hypericism. Photochem Photobiol Rev 1980;5;229-55.

194. Araya OS, Ford EJH. An investigation of the type of photosensitization caused by the ingestion of St. John's wort (*Hypericum perforatum*) by calves. J Comp Pathol 1981;91;135-41.

195. Nathan PJ. *Hypericum perforatum* (St. John's wort): a non-selective reuptake inhibitor? A review of the recent advances in its pharmacology. J Psychopharmacol 2001;5:47-54.

281

JUNIPERI PSEUDO-FRUCTUS

Juniper

DEFINITION

Juniper consists of the dried ripe cone berry of *Juniperus communis* L. It contains not less than 10 ml/kg of essential oil, calculated with reference to the anhydrous drug.

The material complies with the monograph of the European Pharmacopoeia [1].

CONSTITUENTS

Essential oil (up to 3.0% V/m) [2] of very variable composition depending on the source but consisting mainly of monoterpene hydrocarbons, principally α-pinene. Monoterpene alcohols including terpinen-4-ol and sequiterpenes such as β-caryophyllene are also present [2-6]. About 105 constituents occur in the oil [2]. Analysis of essential oil from 15 batches of juniper from various sources gave results in the ranges: α-pinene (24.1-55.4%), β-pinene (2.1-6.0%), myrcene (7.3-22.0%), sabinene (1.4-28.8%), limonene (2.3-10.9%), terpinen-4-ol (0.7-17.0%), α-terpineol (up to 1.7%), terpinolene (0.7-1.9%), γ-terpinene (0.5-5.8%), α-terpinene (0.5-2.6%), α-thujene (0.6-1.9%) and caryophyllene (1.3-2.3%) [5].

Other constituents include condensed tannins [7], flavonoids [8,9], diterpene acids, aldehydes and alcohols [10,11], fatty alcohols [11] and about 30% of glucose and fructose [12].

CLINICAL PARTICULARS

Therapeutic indications

Juniper has widely documented uses as a remedy to enhance the renal elimination of water [12-15] and for dyspeptic complaints [12-14]. Published scientific evidence does not yet adequately support these therapeutic indications.

Posology and method of administration

Dosage

Adults: 2-3 g of dried berries as an infusion in 150 ml of hot water, 3-4 times daily [13]. Tincture (1:5 in ethanol 45%), 1-2 ml three times daily [14].

Method of administration

For oral administration.

E/S/C/O/P
MONOGRAPHS
Second Edition

Duration of administration
Juniper should not be used for more than 4 weeks without consulting a doctor [13].

Contra-indications
Acute or chronic inflammation of the kidney [13,16].

Special warnings and special precautions for use
None required.

Interaction with other medicaments and other forms of interaction
Juniper may influence glucose levels in diabetics [17].

Pregnancy and lactation
Should not be used during pregnancy and lactation [18,19]. Abortifacient activity of juniper has been observed in rats after oral administration of a 50% ethanolic extract at 300 mg/kg bodyweight [19].

Effects on ability to drive and use machines
None known.

Undesirable effects
None for juniper.

In the past, based on very old reports (1937 and earlier, but still reiterated in secondary literature), adverse effects such as kidney irritation have been associated with juniper and juniper oil. However, a comprehensive review of the literature concluded that such reports are unreliable; they related only to juniper oil and adverse effects were probably due to contamination with turpentine oil [16,20].

Overdose
No toxic effects reported for juniper.

PHARMACOLOGICAL PROPERTIES

Pharmacodynamic properties

In vivo experiments

Diuretic effects
A 10% aqueous infusion of juniper or a 0.1% aqueous solution of juniper oil (with 0.2% of Tween 20 solubilizer) or a 0.01% aqueous solution of terpinen-4-ol were orally administered to groups of rats at 5 ml/100 g body weight; control groups were given water or water + 0.2 % Tween orally and reference groups were given antidiuretic hormone (ADH; vasopressin) intraperitoneally at 0.004, 0.04 or 0.4 IU/100 g. Compared to water, the 10% aqueous infusion of juniper and the 0.1% aqueous solution of juniper oil (in which the ratio of pinene fraction to terpinen-4-ol was 5:1) caused reductions of only 6% in diuresis over a 24-hour period, equivalent to the effect of

0.004 IU/100 g of ADH, while the 0.01% solution of terpinen-4-ol caused a reduction of 30% in diuresis (p<0.01), equivalent to 0.4 IU/100 g i.p. of ADH. However, after continued daily administration at the same dose levels, the two juniper preparations and terpinen-4-ol stimulated diuresis on days 2 and 3, although only the 10% aqueous infusion of juniper exerted significant diuretic activity (+ 43% on day 2; + 44% on day 3; p<0.05), suggesting that the diuretic effect is due partly to the essential oil and partly to hydrophilic constituents [21].

After oral administration to rats of a lyophilised aqueous extract of juniper at 1000 mg/kg body weight, no increase in urine volume or excretion of Na^+, K^+ or Cl^- ions could be demonstrated over a 6-hour period compared to the effect of the same volume of water [22].

Oral administration to rats of an aqueous infusion equivalent to 125 mg of juniper increased urine amount by 36% and chloride excretion by 119% compared to animals given water only [23]. In similar experiments, urine volume increased by 20% in rabbits after the equivalent of 750 mg of juniper and by 38% in mice after the equivalent of 50 mg of juniper [24]. However, in all cases, twice or half these doses had much less or no effect [23,24].

No significant diuresis was observed in rats after oral administration of juniper oil at 100 or 333 mg/kg/day for 28 days [25].

Subcutaneous injection of juniper oil (1 ml/kg) into rats produced significant levels of diuresis after 4 and 24 hours compared to a control (sodium chloride solution). Terpinen-4-ol isolated from the oil and injected subcutaneously at a dose of 0.1 ml/kg showed almost twice the diuretic activity of the oil [26]; increased amounts of K^+, Na^+ and Cl^- were also excreted [27].

Anti-inflammatory effects
A dry 80%-ethanolic extract of juniper, administered orally at 100 mg/kg, reduced carrageenan-induced rat paw oedema by 60% (p<0.001) compared to 45% for indometacin at 5 mg/kg (p<0.01) [28].

Hypoglycemic effects
An orally administered decoction of juniper showed significant hypoglycemic activity in normal rats after single doses equivalent to 250-500 mg juniper/kg and in streptozotocin-induced diabetic rats after 24-day treatment with doses equivalent to 125 mg juniper/kg. The effects were attributed to an increase in peripheral absorption of glucose, independent of plasma insulin levels [17]. However, a subsequent study failed to show an antihyperglycaemic effect of juniper in streptozotocin-induced diabetic mice [29].

Other effects

Intravenous administration of a lyophilised aqueous extract of juniper (25 mg/kg body weight) to normotensive rats produced an initial transient rise in arterial pressure followed by a reduction of 27%. A dose of 1.2 g/kg of the same extract produced an analgesic response of 178% as measured by thermal stimuli in mice [22].

Pharmacokinetic properties

No data available.

Preclinical safety data

Acute toxicity

The intraperitoneal LD_{50} of a lyophilized aqueous extract of juniper was calculated as 3 g/kg body weight in mice [22]. No mortality occurred and no side effects were apparent in rats after a single oral dose of 2.5 g/kg body weight of a dry 80%-ethanolic extract of juniper [28].

Juniper oil had an oral LD_{50} of 6.28 g/kg in the rat [30]. The acute dermal LD_{50} of the oil exceeded 5 g/kg in rabbits [31].

The LD_{50} of terpinen-4-ol was 0.75 ml/kg in mice after subcutaneous injection and 0.78 ml/kg after intramuscular injection; in rats, the LD_{50} after intramuscular injection was 1.5 ml/kg [27].

Chronic toxicity

Chronic administration of terpinen-4-ol at therapeutic dose levels caused no pathological changes in the rat [27].

Nephrotoxicity

The oral toxicity, especially possible nephrotoxicity, of two juniper oils of good pharmaceutical quality were tested in rats for 28 days in two series of experiments. In the first series, rats were treated with 100, 333 or 1000 mg of oil/kg body weight/day with an α-pinene + β-pinene to terpinen-4-ol ratio of 3:1. In the second series, rats received 100, 300 or 900 mg of oil/kg/day with an α-pinene + β-pinene to terpinen-4-ol ratio of 5:1; an additional group received 400 mg/kg/day of terpinen-4-ol, a constituent of the oil with postulated diuretic effects. From biochemical, pathological and histological investigations, neither of the juniper oils nor terpinen-4-ol produced nephrotoxic effects and they were considered non-toxic at therapeutic dose levels [25].

Juniper oils with a relatively low content of pinenes (monoterpene hydrocarbons less than 60%) and a high terpinen-4-ol content have been recommended for pharmaceutical use [16,20].

Teratogenicity

No evidence of teratogenicity was observed in rats after oral administration of a dry 50% ethanolic extract of juniper at 300-500 mg/kg bodyweight [19].

REFERENCES

1. Juniper - Iuniperi pseudo-fructus. European Pharmacopoeia, Council of Europe.

2. Chatzopoulou PS, Katsiotis ST. Study of the essential oil from *Juniperus communis* "berries" (cones) growing wild in Greece. Planta Med 1993;59:554-6.

3. Chatzopoulou PS, Katsiotis ST. Procedures influencing the yield and the quality of the essential oil from *Juniperus communis* L. berries. Pharm Acta Helv 1995; 70:247-53.

4. Koukos PK, Papadopoulou KI. Essential oil of *Juniperus communis* L. grown in northern Greece: variation of fruit oil yield and composition. J Essent Oil Res 1997; 9:35-9.

5. Schilcher H, Emmrich D, Koehler C. Gaschromatographischer Vergleich von ätherischen Wacholderölen und deren toxikologischer Bewertung. Pharm Ztg Wiss 1993;138:85-91.

6. Formácek V, Kubeczka K-H. Juniper berry oil. In: Essential oils analysis by capillary gas chromatography and carbon-13 NMR spectroscopy. Chichester-New York: John Wiley, 1982:125-9.

7. Schulz JM and Herrmann K. Vorkommen von Catechinen und Proanthocyanidinen in Gewürzen. V. Über Gewürzphenole. Z Lebensm Unters Forsch 1980; 171:278-80.

8. Hiermann A, Kompek A, Reiner J, Auer H, Schubert-Zsilavecz M. Untersuchung des Flavonoidmusters in den Früchten von *Juniperus communis* L. Sci Pharm 1996;64:437-44.

9. Lamer-Zarawska E. Phytochemical studies on flavonoids and other compounds of juniper fruits (*Juniperus communis* L.). Pol J Chem 1980;54:213-9; through Chem Abstr 1980;93:128746.

10. De Pascual Teresa J, San Feliciano A, Barrero AF. Composition of *Juniperus communis* (common juniper) fruit. An Quim 1973;69:1065-7; through Chem Abstr 1974;81:74847.

11. De Pascual Teresa J, Barrero AF, San Feliciano A, Sanchez Bellido I. Componentes de las arcestidas de *Juniperus communis* L. IV. Fracción neutra. An Quim 1977;73:568-73.

12. Wichtl M, Henke D. Wacholderbeeren - Juniperi fructus. In: Hartke K, Hartke H, Mutschler E, Rücker G, Wichtl M, editors. DAB-Kommentar: Wissenschaftliche Erläuterungen zum Deutschen Arzneibuch. Stuttgart: Wissenschaftliche Verlagsgesellschaft, Frankfurt: Govi-Verlag, 1997 (8. Lfg.):W1.

13. Bisset NG, editor (translated from Wichtl M, editor. Teedrogen, 2nd ed.). Juniperi fructus. In: Herbal Drugs and Phytopharmaceuticals. A handbook for practice on a scientific basis. Stuttgart: Medpharm, Boca Raton-London, CRC Press, 1994:283-5.

14. Juniperus. In: British Herbal Pharmacopoeia 1983. Bournemouth: British Herbal Medicine Association, 1983.

15. Schilcher H. Juniperi fructus (Wacholderbeeren). In: Phytotherapie in der Urologie. Stuttgart: Hippokrates, 1992:114-5.

16. Schilcher H, Heil BM. Nierentoxizität von Wacholder-beerzubereitungen. Eine kritische Literaturauswertung von 1844 bis 1993. Z Phytotherapie 1994;15:205-13.

17. Sánchez de Medina F, Gámez MJ, Jiménez I, Jiménez J, Osuna JI, Zarzuelo A. Hypoglycemic activity of juniper "berries". Planta Med 1994;60:197-200.

18. Prakash AO. Potentialities of some indigenous plants for antifertility activity. Int J Crude Drug Res 1986;24:19-24.

19. Agrawal OP, Santosh B, Mathur R. Antifertility effects of fruits of Juniperus communis. Planta Med 1980;(Suppl):98-101.

20. Schilcher H. Wacholderbeeröl bei Erkrankungen der ableitenden Harnwege? Med Monatsschr Pharm 1995;18:198-9.

21. Stanic G, Samarzija I, Blazevic N. Time-dependent diuretic response in rats treated with juniper berry preparations. Phytother Res 1998;12:494-7.

22. Lasheras B, Turillas P, Cenarruzabeitia E. Étude pharmacologique préliminaire de Prunus spinosa L.

Amelanchier ovalis Medikus, Juniperus communis L. et Urtica dioica L. Plant Méd Phytothér 1986;20:219-26.

23. Vollmer H, Hübner K. Untersuchungen über die diuretische Wirkung der Fructus juniperi, Radix levistici, Radix ononidis, Folia betulae, Radix liquiritiae und Herba equiseti an Ratten. Naunyn-Schmiedebergs Arch Exp Path Pharmakol 1937;186:592-605.

24. Vollmer H, Weidlich R. Untersuchungen über die diuretische Wirkung der Fructus juniperi, Radix levistici, Radix liquiritiae und Herba violae tricoloris an Kaninchen und Mäusen. Naunyn-Schmiedebergs Arch Exp Path Pharmakol 1937;186:574-83.

25. Schilcher H, Leuschner F. Untersuchungen auf mögliche nephrotoxische Wirkungen von aetherischem Wacholderbeeröl. Arzneim-Forsch/Drug Res 1997;47:855-8.

26. Janku I, Háva M, Motl O. Ein diuretisch wirksamer Stoff aus Wacholder (Juniperus communis L.). Experientia 1957;13:255-6.

27. Janku I, Háva M, Kraus R, Motl O. Das diuretische Prinzip des Wacholders. Naunyn-Schmiedebergs Arch Exp Path Pharmakol 1960;238:112-3.

28. Mascolo N, Autore G, Capasso F, Menghini A, Fasulo MP. Biological screening of Italian medicinal plants for anti-inflammatory activity. Phytother Res 1987;1:28-31.

29. Gray AM, Flatt PR. Nature's own pharmacy: the diabetes perspective. Proc Nutr Soc 1997;56:507-17.

30. Von Skramlik E. Über die Giftigkeit und Verträglichkeit von ätherischen Ölen. Pharmazie 1959;14:435-45.

31. Opdyke DLJ. Monographs on fragrance raw materials: Juniper berry oil. Food Cosmet Toxicol 1976;14:333.

285

LICHEN ISLANDICUS

Iceland Moss

DEFINITION

Iceland moss consists of the whole or cut dried thallus of *Cetraria islandica* (L.) Acharius s.l.

The material complies with the monograph of the European Pharmacopoeia [1].

CONSTITUENTS

Polysaccharides (over 50%), principally lichenan (or lichenin), a hot water-soluble, linear β-D-glucan with 1→4 and 1→3 links (ratio greater than 2:1) [2-4] and isolichenan (or isolichenin), a cold water-soluble, linear α-D-glucan with 1→3 and 1→4 links (ratio approx. 55:45) [5,6]. An α-D-glucan (denoted as Ci-3) resembling isolichenan but with a much higher degree of polymerization [7], a branched galacto-mannan [8,9] and an acidic, branched polysaccharide containing D-glucose and D-glucuronic acid units [10] are also present.

Other characteristic constituents are bitter-tasting lichen acids including the depsidones fumarproto-cetraric acid (2.6-11.5%) [11,12] and protocetraric acid (0.2-0.3%) [12], and the aliphatic lactone protolichesterinic acid (0.1-0.5%) [11].

CLINICAL PARTICULARS

Therapeutic indications
Dry cough; irritation or inflammation of the oral and pharyngeal mucosa [13-18].

Iceland moss is also widely documented as a bitter remedy for lack of appetite [15-18].

Posology and method of administration

Dosage

For upper respiratory tract ailments
Adult daily dose: 3-8 g of the drug as a decoction or equivalent liquid preparation [15-20], taken in small amounts as required. In the form of pastilles containing aqueous extract from 50-300 mg of the drug, 10 or more daily [13].

As a bitter
Adult single dose: 1-2 g of the drug [15] as a cold macerate, infusion, tincture or other bitter-tasting preparation [15-18, 21].
Elderly: dose as for adults.

E/S/C/O/P
MONOGRAPHS
Second Edition

Children, average daily dose: 1-4 years of age, 1-2 g; 4-10 years, 2-4 g; 10-16 years, 4-6 g [22].

Method of administration
For oral administration in liquid or solid dosage forms. In the treatment of respiratory tract ailments, the addition of sweetener to liquid preparations is recommended to mask the bitter taste [17]; pastilles should be sucked slowly in the mouth [14].

Duration of administration
No restriction.
If symptoms persist or worsen, medical advice should be sought.

Contra-indications
None known.

Special warnings and special precautions for use
None required.

Interaction with other medicaments and other forms of interaction
None reported.

Pregnancy and lactation
No data available. In accordance with general medical practice, the product should not be used during pregnancy or lactation without medical advice.

Effects on ability to drive and use machines
None known.

Undesirable effects
None reported.

Overdose
No toxic effects reported.

PHARMACOLOGICAL PROPERTIES

Pharmacodynamic properties

In vitro experiments

Immunomodulatory effects
Immunostimulating activity, demonstrated by enhancement of phagocytosis using human granulocytes, was exhibited by two polysaccharides isolated from Iceland moss, an alkali-soluble galactomannan denoted as KI-M-7 [9] and a water-soluble neutral α-D-glucan denoted as Ci-3 [7], as well as by a hot water extract of Iceland moss and polysaccharide fractions from it [23].

Anti-inflammatory activity
A hot water extract of Iceland moss, and also the α-D-glucan Ci-3, showed activity in a haemolytic anti-complementary assay [7].

The activity of 5-lipoxygenase in porcine leucocytes was inhibited by protolichesterinic acid with an IC_{50} of 20 μM [24]. Leukotriene B_4 biosynthesis in stimulated bovine polymorphonuclear leukocytes was inhibited by protolichesterinic acid with an IC_{50} of 9 μM (p<0.05) [25].

Antiproliferative activity
Antiproliferative and cytotoxic effects exhibited by protolichesterinic acid may be related to its inhibitory activity on 5-lipoxygenase. At an ED_{50} between 1.1 and 24.6 μg/ml protolichesterinic acid caused a significant reduction in DNA synthesis in three malignant human cell lines (T-47D and ZR-75-1 from breast carcinomas and K-562 from erythroleukaemia); significant cell death occurred in all three cell lines at concentrations above 20 μg/ml. The proliferative response of mitogen-stimulated peripheral blood lymphocytes was also inhibited with a mean ED_{50} of 8.4 μg/ml. In contrast, DNA synthesis, proliferation and survival of normal skin fibroblasts were not affected at doses of up to 20 μg/ml [26].

Antibacterial activity
Inhibitory activity of protolichesterinic acid against 35 strains of *Helicobacter pylori* has been demonstrated. The MIC_{90} was 32 μg/ml, considerably higher than that of ampicillin (0.125 μg/ml) and erythromycin (0.25 μg/ml) but only twice as high as that of metronidazole (16 μg/ml) [27].

In a study of the activity of protolichesterinic acid against *Mycobacterium aurium*, a non-pathogenic organism with a similar sensitivity profile to *M. tuberculosis*, the MIC was found to be too high (250 μg/ml compared to 0.25 μg/ml for streptomycin) to merit further investigation of antimycobacterial potential [28].

Antiviral activity
Protolichesterinic acid has been shown to be a potent inhibitor of human immunodeficiency virus-1 reverse transcriptase with an IC_{50} of 24 μM [29].

Other effects
In a study of the bioadhesive effects of purified (> 95%) polysaccharides from medicinal plants on porcine buccal membranes, polysaccharides from Iceland moss showed only slight adhesion to epithelial tissue whereas moderate adhesion was observed with polysaccharides from *Althaea officinalis* and *Plantago lanceolata* and strong adhesion with polysaccharides from *Fucus vesiculosus* and *Calendula officinalis* [30].

In vivo experiments

Immunomodulatory effects
A hot water extract at 1 mg/kg body weight [23] and

an alkali-soluble galactomannan (isolated from Iceland moss) at 10 mg/kg [9], administered intra-peritoneally, exhibited marked immunomodulating activity in the carbon clearance assay in mice, sub-stantially increasing the rate of reticuloendothelial phagocytosis. Both substances stimulated the rate of removal of injected colloidal carbon particles from the bloodstream by a mean ratio of 1.9 compared to controls.

Cognitive effects

Synaptic plasticity in the hippocampal area of the brain is important in the initial storage of certain forms of memory. Isolichenan isolated from Iceland moss and administered intravenously to rats at 1 mg/kg body weight significantly enhanced short-term potentiation of hippocampal synaptic plasticity (p<0.05), evoked by high-frequency sub-threshold tetanic stimulation (20 pulses at 60 Hz) as an approximation to learning stimulus [31,32].

When isolichenan was orally administered to rats at 100 mg/kg it significantly repaired the effect of β-amyloid peptide-induced memory impairment (p<0.05) in the Morris water maze test, which depends heavily on intact hippocampal function. Similarly, in mice with learning ability impaired by pretreatment with 30% ethanol, oral isolichenan significantly improved memory acquisition in passive-avoidance tests (p<0.01 at 100 mg in step-through tests, p<0.01 at 400 mg/kg in step-down tests). No effect was observed on the cognitive performance of healthy rats or mice [31,32].

Clinical studies

In a comparative double-blind study, 63 patients with inflammation and dryness of the oral cavity due to breathing only through the mouth after nasal surgery were divided into three random groups and treated daily with 10 pastilles, each containing aqueous extract equivalent to: 0.048 g (n = 23) or 0.3 g (n = 18) or 0.5 g (n = 22) of Iceland moss. Treatment comm-enced on the day after surgery and continued for 5 days. Assessments by physicians, using biometric observations on a 0-3 scale, of coating, dryness and inflammation of the mucosa, conspicuousness of lymph nodes, tongue coating and symptoms such as hoarseness and sore throat revealed a similar and substantial degree of improvement in all three groups over the 5-day treatment, indicating that the lowest dosage, equivalent to 10 × 0.048 g (approximately 0.5 g) of Iceland moss daily, was sufficient [13].

In an open study, 100 patients aged between 7 and 85 years with pharyngitis, laryngitis or acute/chronic bronchial ailments were treated with pastilles (1-2 pastilles every 2-3 hours), each containing aqueous extract from 160 mg of Iceland moss, for between 4 days and 3 weeks. The results were assessed as positive in 86 cases [14].

Pharmacokinetic properties

No data available

Preclinical safety data

Protolichesterinic acid showed no appreciable cytotoxic activity in *in vitro* tests with a variety of cultured mammalian cells [29].

Clinical safety data

In two clinical studies, involving the treatment of a total of 163 patients for 4-5 days (in some cases 3 weeks) with pastilles containing Iceland moss aqueous extracts in amounts corresponding to 0.5-5 g of crude drug daily, the preparations were well tolerated with an absence of side effects [13,14].

REFERENCES

1. Iceland Moss - Lichen islandicus. European Pharmacopoeia, Council of Europe.

2. Peat S, Whelan WJ, Roberts JG. The structure of lichenin. J Chem Soc 1957:3916-24.

3. Perlin AS, Suzuki S. The structure of lichenin: selective enzymolysis studies. Can J Chem 1962;40:50-6.

4. Cunningham WL, Manners DJ. Studies on carbohydrate-metabolizing enzymes. 11. The hydrolysis of lichenin by enzyme preparations from malted barley and *Rhizopus arrhizus*. Biochem J 1964;90:596-602.

5. Peat S, Whelan WJ, Turvey JR, Morgan K. The structure of isolichenin. J Chem Soc 1961:623-9.

6. Krämer P, Wincierz U, Grübler G, Tschakert J, Voelter W, Mayer H. Rational approach to fractionation, isolation and characterization of polysaccharides from the lichen *Cetraria islandica*. Arzneim-Forsch/Drug Res 1995;45:726-31.

7. Olafsdottir ES, Ingólfsdottir K, Barsett H, Smestad Paulsen B, Jurcic K, Wagner H. Immunologically active (1→3)-(1→4)-α-D-glucan from *Cetraria islandica*. Phyto-medicine 1999;6:33-9.

8. Gorin PAJ, Iacomini M. Polysaccharides of the lichens *Cetraria islandica* and *Ramalina usnea*. Carbohydr Res 1984;128:119-32.

9. Ingolfsdottir K, Jurcic K, Fischer B, Wagner H. Immunologically active polysaccharide from *Cetraria islandica*. Planta Med 1994;60:527-31.

10. Hranisavljevic-Jakovljevic M, Miljkovic-Stojanovic J, Dimitrijevic R, Micovic VM. An alkali-soluble polysaccharide from the oak lichen, *Cetraria islandica* (L.) Ach. Carbohydr Res 1980;80:291-5.

11. Gudjónsdóttir GA, Ingólfsdóttir K. Quantitative deter-mination of protolichesterinic and fumarprotocetraric acids in *Cetraria islandica* by high-performance liquid chromatography. J Chromatogr A 1997;757:303-6.

12. Huovinen K, Härmälä P, Hiltunen R, v Schantz M. Variation of fumarprotocetraric and protocetraric acids in *Cetraria islandica* and *C. ericetorum*. Planta Med 1986;52:508.

13. Kempe C, Grüning H, Stasche N, Hörmann K. Isländisch-Moos-Pastillen zur Prophylaxe bzw. Heilung von oralen Schleimhautirritationen und ausgetrockneter Rachen-schleimhaut. Laryngo-Rhino-Otol 1997;76:186-8.

14. Vorberg G. Flechtenwirkstoffe lindern Reizzustände der Atemwege. Neben den entzündungshemmenden Eigenschaften wirkt sich der Schleimhautschutz besonders günstig aus. Ärztl Praxis 1981;33:3068.

15. Cetraria. In: British Herbal Pharmacopoeia 1983. Bournemouth: British Herbal Medicine Association, 1983:58-9.

16. Wichtl M, Henke D. Isländisches Moos/Isländische Flechte. In: Hartke K, Hartke H, Mutschler E, Rücker G, Wichtl M, editors. Kommentar zum Europäischen Arzneibuch. Stuttgart: Wissenschaftliche Verlags-gesellschaft, 2001 (14 Lfg):I 31/05.

17. Bisset NG (translated from Wichtl M, editor. Teedrogen, 2nd ed.). Cetrariae lichen. In: Herbal Drugs and Phytopharmaceuticals: a handbook for practice on a scientific basis. Boca Raton-London: CRC Press, Stuttgart: Medpharm, 1994:137-9.

18. Kartnig T. *Cetraria islandica* - Isländisches Moos. Z Phytotherapie 1987;8:127-30.

19. Todd RG, editor. Iceland Moss. In: Martindale - The Extra Pharmacopoeia, 25th ed. London: Pharmaceutical Press, 1967:80.

20. Cetraria. In: British Pharmaceutical Codex 1934. London: Pharmaceutical Press, 1934:307-8.

21. Weiss RF, Fintelmann V. *Cetraria islandica*, Iceland Moss. In: Herbal Medicine, 2nd ed. (translated from 9th German ed. of Lehrbuch der Phytotherapie). Stuttgart-New York: Thieme, 2000:61-2.

22. Dorsch W, Loew D, Meyer-Buchtela E, Schilcher H. In: Kooperation Phytopharmaka, editor. Kinderdosierung von Phytopharmaka, 3rd ed. Teil 1 Empfehlungen zur Anwendung und Dosierung von Phytopharmaka, mono-graphierte Arzneidrogen und ihren Zubereitungen in der Pädiatrie: Lichen islandicus (Isländisch Moos).

Bonn: Kooperation Phytopharmaka, 2002:83.

23. Ingólfsdóttir K, Jurcic K, Wagner H. Immunomodulating polysaccharides from aqueous extracts of *Cetraria islandica* (Iceland moss). Phytomedicine 1998;5:333-9.

24. Ingolfsdottir K, Breu W, Huneck S, Gudjonsdottir GA, Müller-Jakic B, Wagner H. In vitro inhibition of 5-lipoxygenase by protolichesterinic acid from *Cetraria islandica*. Phytomedicine 1994;1:187-91.

25. Kumar KCS, Müller K. Lichen metabolites. 1. Inhibitory action against leukotriene B_4 biosynthesis by a non-redox mechanism. J Nat Prod 1999;62:817-20.

26. Ögmundsdóttir HM, Zoëga GM, Gissurarson SR, Ingólfsdóttir K. Anti-proliferative effects of lichen-derived inhibitors of 5-lipoxygenase on malignant cell-lines and mitogen-stimulated lymphocytes. J Pharm Pharmacol 1998;50:107-15.

27. Ingolfsdottir K, Hjalmarsdottir MA, Sigurdsson A, Gudjonsdottir GA, Brynjolfsdottir A, Steingrimsson O. In vitro susceptibility of *Helicobacter pylori* to protolichesterinic acid from the lichen *Cetraria islandica*. Antimicrob Agents Chemother 1997;41:215-7.

28. Ingólfsdóttir K, Chung GAC, Skúlason VG, Gissurarson SR, Vilhelmsdóttir M. Antimycobacterial activity of lichen metabolites in vitro. Eur J Pharm Sci 1998;6:141-4.

29. Pengsuparp T, Cai L, Constant H, Fong HHS, Lin L-Z, Kinghorn AD et al. Mechanistic evaluation of new plant-derived compounds that inhibit HIV-1 reverse transcriptase. J Nat Prod 1995;58:1024-31.

30. Schmidgall J, Schnetz E, Hensel A. Evidence for bio-adhesive effects of polysaccharides and polysaccharide-containing herbs in an *ex vivo* bioadhesion assay on buccal membranes. Planta Med 2000;66:48-53.

31. Smriga M, Chen J, Zhang J-T, Narui T, Shibata S, Hirano E, Saito H. Isolichenan, an α-glucan isolated from lichen *Cetrariella islandica*, repairs impaired learning behaviors and facilitates hippocampal synaptic plasticity. Proc Japan Acad Ser B. 1999;75:219-23.

32. Smriga M, Saito H. Effect of selected thallophytic glucans on learning behaviour and short-term potentiation. Phytother Res 2000;14:153-5.

LINI
SEMEN

Linseed

DEFINITION

Linseed consists of the dried ripe seeds of *Linum usitatissimum* L.

The material complies with the monograph of the European Pharmacopoeia [1].

CONSTITUENTS

The seeds contain 3-9% of mucilage polysaccharides composed mainly of galacturonic acid, xylose, galactose and rhamnose units [2-4,5]; 30-45% of fixed oil [4] mainly consisting of triglycerides of linolenic (40-60% [6]), linoleic and oleic acids [2,7,8]; approx. 25% of protein [2,3]; and 0.1-1.5% of cyanogenic glycosides such as the diglucosides linustatin and neolinustatin (the glucosides of linamarin and lotaustralin respectively) [2-4,9,10]. Other constituents include secoisolariciresinol diglucoside, a precursor of lignans in mammals [11-14], and a serine proteinase inhibitor (LUTI = *Linum usitatissimum* trypsin inhibitor) [15].

CLINICAL PARTICULARS

Therapeutic indications

Internal use
Constipation [2-4,16-21].
Irritable bowel syndrome [17,18].
Diverticular disease [17,18].
Symptomatic short-term treatment of gastritis and enteritis [2-4,16,19,22].

External use
Painful skin inflammations [4,19,23].

Posology and method of administration

Dosage and method of administration

Adults and children over 12 years of age

Internal use
As a laxative: 5 g of whole, finely-cracked or freshly crushed seeds, soaked in water and taken with a glassful of liquid three times daily. The effect starts 18-24 hours later [3,4,16,19,24].

E/S/C/O/P
MONOGRAPHS
Second Edition

As a demulcent for gastritis and/or enteritis: for a mucilaginous preparation soak 5-10 g of whole linseed in 150 ml water and strain after 20-30 minutes [2,4,19].

External use
30-50 g of crushed or powdered seed (may be defatted) as a warm poultice or warm compress [4,19].

Children from 6 to 12 years of age: half the adult dose [25].
Children under 6 years of age: to be treated under medical supervision only.

Duration of administration
Because of the gradual mode of action of bulk-forming laxatives, treatment should be continued for a minimum of 2-3 days to ensure optimum benefit [26].

If abdominal pain occurs, or if there is no response after 48 hours, use of linseed should be discontinued and medical advice must be sought.

Contra-indications
Atonic and obstructive ileus, subileus or conditions likely to lead to intestinal obstruction. Acute abdominal pain of any origin (e.g. appendicitis) [2,18].

Special warnings and special precautions for use
Linseed (whole, finely-cracked or freshly crushed) should be soaked and taken with at least 10 times the amount of fluid, otherwise bezoar formation and intestinal obstruction may occur [27,28].

Persons with weight problems should take linseed whole, not cracked, because of its rich energy content of about 470 kcal (1960 kJ)/100 g [2].

Interaction with other medicaments and other forms of interaction
The absorption of other medications taken at the same time may be delayed [15,29].
Diabetics should be aware of a potential delay in glucose absorption [29-33].

Pregnancy and lactation
There are no reports of any harmful or deleterious effects during pregnancy and lactation [34].

Effects on ability to drive and use machines
None known.

Undesirable effects
None reported.

Overdose
In spite of its content of cyanogenic glycosides, single doses of up to 150-300 g of powdered linseed are not toxic. Health risks are not to be expected [2-4,6,16,19,35-38].

PHARMACOLOGICAL PROPERTIES

Pharmacodynamic properties

Laxative effect
Dietary fibre such as linseed binds with water and swells to form a demulcent gel in the intestine. As water bound to the fibre is prevented from being absorbed in the colon, the faeces are softened and the volume of bowel contents increases [2,4,16-18].

A decrease in transit time and increase of stool weight by physical stimulation of intestinal peristalsis have been demonstrated in two multicentric studies (n = 108 and n = 114) in patients suffering from constipation [20,21].

Effect on gastro-intestinal complaints
The mucilage has been reported to have a palliative effect in patients with pain associated with gastro-intestinal problems [2,4,16].

Clinical studies
In an open pilot study 70 patients suffering from various functional upper abdominal complaints such as sensations of pressure and repletion, loss of appetite, nausea, vomiting and heartburn were treated with an aqueous linseed mucilage preparation (1:10) at a dosage of 8 × 25 g (including a small amount of excipients) per day. All except three patients experienced improvements. After 3 days the total symptom score had significantly decreased (p<0.01). Each individual symptom score decreased on average, the largest reductions being observed for the sensation of pressure (41.5%) and the sensation of repletion (36.8%). In global assessments by both patients and physicians the efficacy was rated as good or very good in most cases [22].

Effect on blood glucose levels

Pharmacological studies in humans
Viscous types of dietary fibre may cause a delay in gastric emptying as shown in two studies with 11 and 7 healthy volunteers [29,30]. In these studies [29,30], and in one involving 8 non-insulin-dependent diabetic volunteers [31], it could be demonstrated that addition of certain types of dietary fibre to the diet significantly decreased postprandial hyperglycaemia. Thus an improvement in the control of blood-glucose concentration might be expected [31].

Effect on blood lipid levels

In vivo experiments
The effect of secoisolariciresinol diglucoside (SDG) was investigated in rabbits receiving either their normal diet (chow pellets, control group, n = 8), a control diet supplemented with SDG (15 mg/kg body weight/day, n = 5), a diet containing cholesterol (1%, n = 6) or

cholesterol + SDG (1% cholesterol + SDG 15 mg/kg body weight/day, n = 5). Blood samples were collected before the experiment, and after 4 and 8 weeks, then the aorta was removed for assessment of atherosclerotic plaques, malondialdehyde (an aortic tissue lipid peroxidation product) and aortic tissue chemiluminescence (a marker for antioxidant reserve). Serum total cholesterol (TC), LDL-cholesterol (LDL-C) and the ratio LDL-C/HDL-C and TC/HDL-C increased in the 3rd and 4th group. SDG significantly reduced TC and LDL-C by 33 and 35% respectively at week 8 (p<0.05), and significantly increased HDL-C by >140% at week 4 (p<0.05). It also decreased TC/HDL-C and LDL-C/HDL-C ratios significantly by approx. 64% (p<0.05). Comparing atherosclerotic plaques in the 3rd and 4th groups, it was found that SDG significantly reduced hypercholesterolaemic atherosclerosis by 73% (p<0.05). There were increases in aortic malondialdehyde and chemiluminescence in the 3rd group, but they were significantly lower in the 4th than in the 3rd group (p<0.05) [39].

Clinical studies
In a randomized, cross-over trial, 22 men and 7 postmenopausal women with hyperlipidaemia who followed a National Cholesterol Education Program (NCEP) Step II diet received fibre-rich muffins containing either partially defatted linseed (approx. 50g daily) or wheat bran as a control, both corresponding to approx. 20 g of fibre daily, for 3 weeks, the treatment phases being separated by at least 2 weeks. Linseed supplementation significantly reduced total cholesterol by 4.6% (p = 0.001), LDL cholesterol by 7.6% (p<0.001), apolipoprotein B by 5.4% (p = 0.001) and apolipoprotein A-I by 5.8% (p = 0.070) compared to the control, but had no effect on serum lipoprotein ratios. No significant effects were observed on serum HDL cholesterol, serum protein carbonyl content or *ex vivo* androgen and progestin activity [40].

Oestrogenic effects

In vitro experiments
Lignan precursors present in linseed are converted by bacteria present in the colon to metabolites interfering with metabolism and activity of oestrogens [13].

In vivo experiments
Experiments in pigs demonstrated the capacity of various fibres to bind to oestrogens [41]. It has therefore been suggested that linseed may lower the risk of oestrogen dependent tumours, e.g. some colon and mammary carcinomas [11-13,42].

Pharmacological studies in humans
Quantitative urine assays in 62 women studied 4 times during one year showed a significant positive correlation between the intake of fibre and urinary excretion of lignans and phytoestrogens and the concentration of plasma SHBG [42].

In an open randomized cross-over study involving 18 women with normal cycles, the effects of ingestion of linseed powder on the menstrual cycle was investigated. Each of them consumed her usual omnivorous, low fibre (control) diet for 3 cycles and her usual diet supplemented with linseed (10 g/day) for another 3 cycles. The second and third linseed cycles were compared to the corresponding control cycles. During these 36 control cycles, 3 anovulatory cycles occurred, compared to none during the 36 linseed cycles. Compared to ovulatory control cycles, the ovulatory linseed cycles were consistently associated with longer luteal phase (LP) lengths (mean 12.6 vs. 11.4 days; p = 0.002). There were no significant differences between linseed and control cycles in concentrations of oestradiol or oestrone during the early follicular phase, midfollicular phase or LP. Although linseed ingestion had no significant effect on LP progesterone concentrations, LP progesterone/oestradiol ratios were significantly higher during the linseed cycles. Midfollicular phase testosterone concentrations were slightly higher during the linseed cycles. Linseed ingestion had no effect on early follicular phase concentrations of DHEA-S, PRL or sex hormone-binding globulin [43].

Effects on β-glucuronidase activity

In vivo experiments
Six groups of Sprague-Dawley rats were fed one of the following diets for 100 days: a basal high-fat diet (20% fat), the basal diet supplemented with 2.5 or 5% of linseed, the basal diet supplemented with 2.5 or 5% of defatted linseed, or the basal diet with a daily dose of 1.5 mg of secoisolariciresinol diglucoside isolated from linseed. All rats were injected with a single dose of azoxymethane (15 mg/kg body weight) one week before treatment. Urinary lignan excretion, an indicator of mammalian lignan production, significantly increased in both the linseed groups and in the low-dose defatted linseed group (p<0.0003, p<0.0001 and p<0.0001 respectively) compared to the control. The total activity of caecal β-glucuronidase significantly increased in a dose-dependent manner in both the defatted linseed groups and in the high-dose linseed group (p<0.01, p<0.047 and p<0.0004 respectively). Compared to control the number of aberrant crypts per focus was significantly reduced (p<0.01 to p<0.04) in the distal colon of the five groups of treated rats. Four microadenomas and two polyps were observed in the control group but none in the treated groups. The total activity of β-glucuronidase was positively correlated with total urinary lignan excretion (r = − 0.280, p<0.036, n = 60), and negatively with the total number of aberrant crypts (r = − 0.330, p<0.010, n = 57) and the total number of aberrant crypt foci (r = − 0.310, p<0.018, n = 57) in the distal colon. There were no significant differences between linseed and corresponding defatted linseed groups. It was concluded that linseed

has a colon cancer protective effect, partly due to secoisolariciresinol, and that the protective effect is associated with increased β-glucuronidase activity [44].

Anti-tumour effects

In vivo experiments

The effects of linseed oil fed to female mice as 10% of their diet were compared to corn oil, which contains much less α-linolenic acid (18:3n-3) than linseed oil. The respective diets were fed for 3-8 weeks prior to subcutaneous injections of one of two syngeneic mammary tumour cell types (410 and 410.4). The growth of 410.4 mammary tumours was significantly lower in mice given linseed oil than in animals given corn oil (p<0.05). Linseed oil also significantly enhanced incorporation of n-3 fatty acids into tumours (p<0.005) and significantly reduced tumour prostaglandin E production (p<0.005) compared to corn oil. These data suggested an inhibitory effect of dietary α-linolenic acid on mammary tumour growth and metastasis [45].

Supplementation of a high-fat diet (20% corn oil) fed to 70 female rats for 4 weeks with either linseed flour or defatted linseed meal (5% and 10%) reduced epithelial cell proliferation by 38.8-55.4% and nuclear aberrations by 58.8-65.9% in mammary glands, optimum effects being observed with 5% linseed flour [46].

Five groups of 7 male rats were fed the same diet supplemented in the same manner for 4 weeks following a single injection of azoxymethane at 15 mg/kg body weight. In the descending colon of the supplemented groups, the total number of aberrant crypts and foci were significantly reduced (p≤0.05), by 41-53% and 48-57% respectively. The labelling index (the number of labelled cells, or cells undergoing DNA synthesis, per 100 cells in the epithelia of crypts from each section of the rat colon) was 10-22% lower in these groups, except for the 5% linseed meal group [47].

In a long-term experiment, two groups of 60 female rats were fed the same high-fat diet, one group having the diet supplemented with 5% linseed flour. After 4 weeks, tumours were induced in 44 rats by a single dose of 5 mg of 7,12-dimethylbenz[a]-anthracene. After an additional week, half of the the group fed the basal diet received the supplemented diet for 20 weeks, while half of the group previously supplemented received the basal diet only, in order to differentiate between initiation and promotional effects of supplementation. The group fed a linseed-supplemented diet only during the promotional stage of mammary carcinogenesis had significantly smaller (p≤0.05) tumour volume (66.7%) than all other groups, but also had an increased tumour burden and number

of tumours per group compared with the group fed the supplemented diet throughout the experiment. Feeding the basal diet at the initiation stage of tumour development resulted in a greater number of tumours occurring consistently over time. However, linseed supplementation at initiation and throughout the experimental period tended to reduce the number of tumours per tumour-bearing rat [48].

After administration of a single dose of 5 mg of 7,12-dimethylbenz[a]anthracene, 5 groups of female rats (n = 19-21) received either a basal diet or a diet supplemented with secoisolariciresinol diglycoside (SD, 2200 nmol/day), 1.82% of linseed oil or 2.5 or 5% of linseed. After 7 weeks of treatment, the volume of established tumours was over 50% smaller in all treatment groups (p<0.08, p<0.04, p<0.04, p<0.04 respectively) whereas there was no change in the basal diet group. The number and volume of new tumours were lowest in the SD (p<0.02) and 2.5% linseed (p<0.07) groups. Combined established and new tumour volumes were smaller in the SD, 2.5 and 5% linseed groups (p<0.02) than in the linseed oil and basal diet groups [49].

Antibacterial activity

In vitro experiments

Hydrolysed linseed oil and linolenic acid showed 100% antibacterial activity against methicillin-resistant strains of *Staphylococcus aureus* at concentrations of 0.025% (30°C and 37°C) and 0.01% (37°C) respectively [50].

Pharmacokinetic properties

The breakdown of non-cellulosic polysaccharides takes place mainly in the colon, where anaerobic fermentation yields volatile fatty acids (acetate, propionate and butyrate) and carbon dioxide, hydrogen and methane [51].

Since lignans and isoflavonoid phyto-oestrogens, produced from plant precursors by colonic bacteria, may protect against certain cancers, the effects of ingestion of linseed powder on urinary lignans and isoflavonoids were investigated in 18 premenopausal women in a randomized crossover study. Each consumed her usual omnivorous diet, except avoiding foods containing linseed (high in lignan precursors) or soy (high isoflavone content), for 3 cycles and her usual diet supplemented with linseed (10 g/day) for another 3 cycles, or vice versa. Three-day urine samples from follicular and luteal phases were analysed for lignans and isoflavonoids. Excretion of the two major mammalian lignans, enterodiol and enterolactone, increased with linseed supplementation from 1.09 ± 1.08 and 3.16 ± 1.47 to 19.48 ± 1.10 and 27.79 ± 1.50 μmol/day respectively (p<0.0002). Enterodiol and enterolactone excretion in response to linseed varied widely among the subjects (3- to 285-fold increase). There were no differences in excretion of isoflavonoids or the lignan matairesinol with linseed. Excretion was not altered by phase of the menstrual cycle or duration of linseed consumption [52].

As a sub-study of the above larger study, involving 13 women from the original 18 and the same dietary design, faeces were collected on days 7-11 of the last menstrual cycle in each diet period. Excretion of lignans (nmol/day) increased significantly with linseed intake, from 80.0 ± 80.0 to 2560 ± 3100 for enterodiol (p<0.01), from 640 ± 480 to $10,300 \pm 7580$ for entero-lactone (p<0.01), and from 7.33 ± 10.0 to 11.9 ± 8.06 nmol/day for matairesinol (p<0.05). There were no differences in faecal excretion of isoflavonoids [53].

In a randomized cross-over study, 9 healthy young women supplemented their diets with 5, 15 or 25 g of raw or 25 g of processed (as muffin or bread) linseed for 7 days during the follicular phase of their menstrual cycles. Urine samples (24-hours) were collected at baseline and on the final day of supplementation. As an adjunct to the 25 g raw linseed arm, they consumed 25g for an additional day. Blood and urine samples were collected at specific intervals and analysed for enterolactone and enterodiol. A dose-dependent increase in urinary lignan excretion in response to linseed was observed ($r = 0.72$, p≤0.001) and processing did not affect the quantity of lignan excretion. Plasma lignan concentrations were significantly greater than baseline (p≤0.001) by 9 hours after linseed in-gestion (29.35 and 51.75 nmol/litre respectively). The total plasma AUC was higher on the 8th than on the 1st day (1840 and 1027 nmol.h/litre respectively) [54].

Preclinical safety data
No toxic effects of linseed were observed in a brine shrimp lethality bioassay [55].

Linseed did not show any mutagenic activity in the Ames test using *Salmonella typhimurium* strains TA 98 and TA 102 [55].

Clinical safety data
No drug-related adverse effects were observed from treatment of 70 patients with functional upper abdominal complaint with an aqueous linseed mucilage preparation (1:10) at a dosage of 8×25 g (including a small amount of excipients) daily for 3 days [22].

REFERENCES

1. Linseed - Lini semen. European Pharmacopoeia, Council of Europe.

2. Willuhn G. Lini semen - Leinsamen. In: Wichtl M, editor. Teedrogen und Phytopharmaka. Ein Handbuch für die Praxis auf wissenschaftlicher Grundlage. 4th ed. Stuttgart: Wissenschaftliche Verlagsgesellschaft, 2002: 342-6.

3. Wagner H. In: Pharmazeutische Biologie, Volume 2: Arzneidrogen und ihre Inhaltsstoffe. 6th ed. Stuttgart: Wissenschaftliche Verlagsgesellschaft, 1999:357.

4. Franz G, Alban S. Leinsamen (Lini semen Ph.Eur. 1997). In: Hänsel R, Sticher O, Steinegger E. Pharma-kognosie - Phytopharmazie, 6th ed. Berlin-Heidelberg: Springer-Verlag, 1999:370-1.

5. Fedeniuk RW, Biliaderis CG. Composition and physicochemical properties of linseed (*Linum usitatissimum* L.) mucilage. J Agric Food Chem 1994; 42:240-7.

6. Leng-Peschlow E. Linum. In: Hänsel R, Keller K, Rimpler H, Schneider G, editors. Hagers Handbuch der Pharmazeutischen Praxis, 5th ed. Volume 5: Drogen E-O. Berlin-Heidelberg: Springer-Verlag, 1993:670-86.

7. El-Shattory Y. Chromatographic column fractionation and fatty acid composition of different lipid classes of linseed oil. Die Nahrung 1976;20:307-11.

8. Schilcher H, Nissler A. Pflanzliche Öle - ihre Analytik und diätetische Verwendung. Phys Med u Reh 1980; 21:141-56.

9. Smith CR, Weisleder D, Miller RW, Palmer IS, Olson OE. Linustatin and neolinustatin: cyanogenic glycosides of linseed meal that protect animals against selenium toxicity. J Org Chem 1980;45:507-10.

10. Schilcher H, Wilkens-Sauter M. Quantitative Bestimmung cyanogener Glykoside in *Linum usitatissimum* mit Hilfe der HPLC. Fette Seifen Anstrichmittel 1986;88:287-90.

11. Axelson M, Sjövall J, Gustafsson BE, Setchell KDR. Origin of lignans in mammals and identification of a precursor from plants. Nature 1982;298:659-60.

12. Adlercreutz H. Does fiber-rich food containing animal lignan precursors protect against both colon and breast cancer? An extension of the "fiber hypothesis". Gastroenterology 1984;86:761-4.

13. Borriello SP, Setchell KDR, Axelson M, Lawson AM. Production and metabolism of lignans by the human faecal flora. J Appl Bacteriol 1985;58:37-43.

14. Johnsson P, Kamal-Eldin A, Lundgren LN, Åman P. HPLC method for analysis of secoisolariciresinol diglucoside in flaxseeds. J Agric Food Chem 2000; 48:5216-9.

15. Lorenc-Kubis I, Kowalska J, Pochron B, Zuzlo A, Wilusz T. Isolation and amino acid sequence of a serine proteinase inhibitor from common flax (*Linum usitatissimum*) seeds. Chembiochem 2001;2:45-51.

16. Schilcher H, Schulz V, Nissler A. Zur Wirksamkeit und

Toxikologie von Semen Lini. Z Phytotherapie 1986; 7:113-7.

17. Kay RM, Strasberg SM. Origin, chemistry, physiological effects and clinical importance of dietary fibre. Clin Invest Med 1978;1:9-24.

18. Brunton LL. Laxatives. In: Gilman AG, Rall TW, Nies AS, Taylor P, editors. Goodman and Gilman's The Pharmacological Basis of Therapeutics. New York-Oxford: Pergamon Press, 1990:915-8.

19. Weiß RF, Fintelmann V. In: Lehrbuch der Phytotherapie, 8th ed. Stuttgart: Hippokrates, 1997:69,108 and 340.

20. Kurth W. Therapeutische Wirksamkeit, Verträglichkeit und Akzeptabilität von Linusit® in der Praxis. Der Kassenarzt 1976;16:3546-53.

21. Jens R, Nitsch-Fitz R, Wutzl H, Maruna H. Ergebnisse einer Praxisstudie mit einer Leinsamen/Molke-Kombination zur Behebung der chronischen Obstipation bei 114 Patienten aus dem Raum Wien. Der Praktische Arzt 1981;35:80-96.

22. Grützner KI, Müller A, Schöllig HP. Wirksamkeit einer Schleimzubereitung aus Leinsamen bei funktionellen Oberbauchbeschwerden. Z Phytotherapie 1997;18: 263-9.

23. Evans WC. In: Trease and Evans' Pharmacognosy. 14th ed. London: WB Saunders 1996:498.

24. Schilcher H. Phytopharmaka bei Magen- und Darmer-krankungen. Dtsch Apoth Ztg 1990;130:555-60

25. Kooperation Phytopharmaka (editor). Kinderdosier-ungen von Phytopharmaka. 2nd ed. Bonn: Kooperation Phytopharmaka 1998:80-1.

26. Reynolds JEF, editor. Martindale - The Extra Pharmacopoeia. 30th ed. London: The Pharmaceutical Press, 1993:886.

27. Van Olffen GH, Tytgat GNJ. De buik vol van zemelen. Ned T Geneesk 1982;126:1993-5.

28. Hardt M, Geisthövel W. Schwerer Obstruktionsileus durch Leinsamenbezoar. Kasuistik mit kritischer Bestandsaufnahme der Anwendung von Ballaststoffen. Med Klin 1986;81:541-3.

29. Jenkins DJA, Wolever TMS, Leeds AR, Gassull MA, Haisman P, Dilawari J et al. Dietary fibres, fibre analogues and glucose tolerance: importance of viscosity. Br Med J 1978;1:1392-4.

30. Holt S, Heading RC, Carter DC, Prescott LF, Tothill P. Effect of gel fibre on gastric emptying and absorption of glucose and paracetamol. Lancet 1979;i:636-9.

31. Jenkins DJA, Goff DV, Leeds AR, Alberti KGMM, Wolever TMS, Gassull MA, Hockaday TDR. Unabsorbable carbohydrates and diabetes: decreased post-prandial hyperglycaemia. Lancet 1976;ii:172-4.

32. Munoz JM, Sandstead HH, Jacob RA, Johnson L, Mako ME. Effects of dietary fiber on glucose tolerance of normal men. Diabetes 1979;28:496-502.

33. Vaaler S, Hanssen KF, Aagenaes O. Effects of different kinds of fibre on postprandial blood glucose in insulin-dependent diabetics. Acta Med Scand 1980;208:389-91.

34. Lewis JH, Weingold AB. The use of gastrointestinal drugs during pregnancy and lactation. Am J Gastroenterol 1985; 80:912-23.

35. Anon. Leinsamen - Blausäurevergiftung nicht zu befürchten. Dtsch Apoth Ztg 1983;123:876.

36. Czygan F-C. Leinsamen (Semen Lini) ist ungiftig! Z Phytotherapie 1984;5:770-1.

37. Schilcher H. Zyanidvergiftung durch Leinsamen? Dtsch Ärzteblatt 1979;76:955-6.

38. Schulz V, Löffler A, Gheorghiu T. Resorption von Blau-säure aus Leinsamen. Leber Magen Darm 1983; 13:10-4.

39. Prasad K. Reduction of serum cholesterol and hypercholesterolemic atherosclerosis in rabbits by secoisolariciresinol diglucoside isolated from flaxseed. Circulation 1999;99:1355-62.

40. Jenkins DJA, Kendall CWC, Vidgen E, Agarwal S, Rao AV, Rosenberg RS et al. Health aspects of partially defatted flaxseed, including effects on serum lipids, oxidative measures, and ex vivo androgen and progestin activity: a controlled crossover trial. Am J Clin Nutr 1999;69:395-402.

41. Arts CJM, Govers CARL, van den Berg H, Wolters MGE, van Leeuwen P, Thijssen JHH. In vitro binding of estrogens by dietary fiber and the in vivo apparent digestibility tested in pigs. J Steroid Biochem Molec Biol 1991;38:621-8.

42. Adlercreutz H, Höckerstedt K, Bannwart C, Bloigu S, Hämäläinen E, Fotsis T, Ollus A. Effect of dietary components, including lignans and phytoestrogens, on enterohepatic circulation and liver metabolism of estrogens and on sex hormone binding globulin (SHBG). J Steroid Biochem 1987;27:1135-44.

43. Phipps WR, Martini MC, Lampe JW, Slavin JL, Kurzer MS. Effect of flax seed ingestion on the menstrual cycle. J Clin Endocrinol Metab 1993;77:1215-9.

44. Jenab M, Thompson LU. The influence of flaxseed and lignans on colon carcinogenesis and β-glucuronidase activity. Carcinogenesis 1996;17:1343-8.

45. Fritsche KL, Johnston PV. Effect of dietary α-linolenic acid on growth, metastasis, fatty acid profile and prostaglandin production of two murine mammary adenocarcinomas. J Nutr 1990;120:1601-9.

46. Serraino M, Thompson LU. The effect of flaxseed supplementation on early risk markers for mammary carcinogenesis. Cancer Lett 1991;60:135-42.

47. Serraino M, Thompson LU. Flaxseed supplementation and early markers of colon carcinogenesis. Cancer Lett 1992;63:159-65.

48. Serraino M, Thompson LU. The effect of flaxseed supplementation on the initiation and promotional stages of mammary carcinogenesis. Nutr Cancer 1992; 17:153-9.

49. Thompson LU, Rickard SE, Orcheson LJ, Seidl MM. Flaxseed and its lignan and oil components reduce mammary tumor growth at a late stage of carcinogenesis. Carcinogenesis 1996;17:1373-6.

50. McDonald MI, Graham I, Harvey KJ, Sinclair A. Antibacterial activity of hydrolysed linseed oil and linolenic acid against methicillin-resistant *Staphylococcus aureus*. Lancet 1981;ii:1056.

51. Cummings JH. Dietary fibre. Br Med Bull 1981;37:65-70.

52. Lampe JW, Martini MC, Kurzer MS, Adlercreutz H, Slavin JL. Urinary lignan and isoflavonoid excretion in premenopausal women consuming flaxseed powder. Am J Clin Nutr 1994;60:122-8.

53. Kurzer MS, Lampe JW, Martini MC, Adlercreutz H. Fecal lignan and isoflavonoid excretion in premenopausal women consuming flaxseed powder. Cancer Epidemiol Biomark Prev 1995;4:353-8.

54. Nesbitt PD, Lam Y, Thompson LU. Human metabolism of mammalian lignan precursors in raw and processed flaxseed. Am J Clin Nutr 1999;69:549-55.

55. Mahmoud I, Alkofahi A, Abdelaziz A. Mutagenic and toxic activities of several spices and some Jordanian medicinal plants. Int J Pharmacognosy 1992;30:81-5.

LIQUIRITIAE RADIX

Liquorice Root

DEFINITION

Liquorice root consists of the dried unpeeled or peeled, whole or cut root and stolons of *Glycyrrhiza glabra* L. It contains not less than 4.0 per cent of glycyrrhizic acid ($C_{42}H_{62}O_{16}$; M_r 823), calculated with reference to the dried drug.

The material complies with the monograph of the European Pharmacopoeia [1].

CONSTITUENTS

The main characteristic constituents are triterpene glycosides (saponins, 2-15%), principally glycyrrhizic acid, the 3β-diglucuronide of glycyrrhetic acid, which occurs as a mixture of potassium and calcium salts known as glycyrrhizin [2-5].

Other constituents include flavonoids (1-2%) such as liquiritin (a flavanone glucoside) and glabrol (a flavanone); isoflavonoids such as glabrene and glabridin (isoflavans); chalcones such as isoliquiritin; coumarins such as liqcoumarin; polysaccharides and essential oil (approx. 0.05%) [2-5].

Note: The names glycyrrhizic acid and glycyrrhetic acid are used in this text, as in the European Pharmacopoeia. In the literature the names glycyrrhizinic acid and glycyrrhetinic acid respectively are often used for these substances; in some texts the term glycyrrhizin is used synonymously with glycyrrhizic acid.

CLINICAL PARTICULARS

Therapeutic indications
Adjuvant therapy of gastric and duodenal ulcers and gastritis [2,6-11].
Coughs and bronchial catarrh, as an expectorant [2,6-8].

Posology and method of administration

Dosage

Gastric and duodenal ulcers and gastritis
Adult daily dose, taken in divided doses: 5-15 g of liquorice root, equivalent to 200-600 mg of glycyrrhizic acid; equivalent aqueous preparations [2,12] or 5-15 ml of Standardised Liquorice Ethanolic Liquid Extract Ph. Eur. (containing 4.0% m/m of glycyrrhizic acid and 52-65% V/V of ethanol).

E/S/C/O/P
MONOGRAPHS
Second Edition

Coughs and bronchial catarrh
Adult daily dose, taken in divided doses when required: 1.5-5 g of liquorice root, equivalent to 60-200 mg of glycyrrhizic acid; equivalent aqueous preparations [2,12] or 1.5-5 ml of Standardised Liquorice Ethanolic Liquid Extract Ph. Eur. (containing 4.0% m/m of glycyrrhizic acid and 52-65% V/V of ethanol).

Elderly: dose as for adults.

Children 4 years of age and older as an expectorant only, in aqueous preparations: proportion of adult dose according to age or body weight [13].

Method of administration
For oral administration.

Duration of administration
Preparations of liquorice root should not be taken for more than 4-6 weeks without medical advice [2,7, 14,15].

Contra-indications
Cardiovascular-related disorders such as hypertension [2,7,8,14], renal disorders, cholestatic or inflammatory liver disorders [2,7,14], hypokalaemia [2,7] and severe obesity [14].

Special warnings and special precautions for use
The maximum daily dose of 15 g of liquorice root (or a content of 600 mg of glycyrrhizin) should never be exceeded [15].

Consumption of glycyrrhizin as a taste modifier should be limited to 100 mg/day and, for example, not more than 50 g of liquorice confections (with an average glycyrrhizin content of 0.2%) should be consumed daily [15]. However, individual tolerance varies widely and regular daily intake of even this amount may cause adverse effects in the most sensitive individuals [14,16].

Interaction with other medicaments and other forms of interaction
Hypokalaemia (resulting from excessive use of liquorice root) may potentiate the action of cardiac glycosides and interact with antiarrhythmic drugs or with drugs which induce reversion to sinus rhythm (e.g. quinidine). Concomitant use with other drugs inducing hypokalaemia (e.g. thiazide or loop diuretics, adrenocorticosteroids and stimulant laxatives) may aggravate electrolyte imbalance.

Glycyrrhizic acid has been reported to decrease plasma clearance and increase the AUC of prednisolone [17], and to potentiate hydrocortisone activity in human skin [17,18].

Pregnancy and lactation
Liquorice root should not be used during pregnancy and lactation [2,7].

Effects on ability to drive and use machines
None known.

Undesirable effects
High or prolonged intake may lead to mineralocorticoid effects in the form of electrolyte imbalance (sodium retention and potassium loss) accompanied by hypertension, oedema and suppression of the renin-angiotensin-aldosterone system [2,14,16,19-26]. In rare cases hypokalaemic myopathy may occur [27,28].

Overdose
Prolonged use of excessive doses (preparations equivalent to more than 20 g of liquorice root per day) [14] can cause hypermineralocorticoidism [16,19,21] with various clinical symptoms from hypertension [22-25,29-35], headache [21,36], lethargy, oedema [21] and muscle weakness [30-32] to temporary paralysis [27,32,34], hypertensive encephalopathy and retinopathy [35], and even heart failure or cardiac arrest [2,29,37]. Rare cases of hyperprolactinaemia have also been reported [14,36].

In most cases, after discontinuation of liquorice root the symptoms of overdose revert to normal within a few weeks or several months [8,16].

PHARMACOLOGICAL PROPERTIES

Pharmacodynamic properties

In vitro experiments

Inhibitory effects on enzymes
Glycyrrhetic acid inhibited 11β-hydroxysteroid dehydrogenase, an enzyme that converts hydrocortisone (cortisol) to its inactive product cortisone (by converting its 11-hydroxyl group to a ketonic group), in human placental homogenate [38] and rat liver and kidney preparations [39].

Isolated glycyrrhetic acid also potently inhibited Δ^4-5β-reductase activity ($p < 0.001$), and to a small extent inhibited Δ^4-5α-reductase activity, in rat liver preparations. Thus it inhibited the inactivation by these two enzymes of Δ^4-3-keto-steroidal hormones such as hydrocortisone (cortisol) and aldosterone through reduction of the C4-C5 double bond to yield dihydroderivatives, which have no hormonal activity [40-42]. Similar inhibition of Δ^4-5β-reductase was observed in liver preparations from rats to which glycyrrhetic acid or glycyrrhizic acid had previously been administered intramuscularly at 50 mg/100 g body weight for 7 and 14 days respectively [40].

Glycyrrhizic acid was found to be a potent inhibitor of the activity of β-glucuronidase activity in rat liver microsome and a β-glucuronidase-producing strain of *Escherichia coli* with IC_{50} values of 0.08 and 0.01 mg/ml respectively. 18β-Glycyrrhetic acid was also a potent inhibitor with IC_{50} values of 0.02 and 0.24 mg/ml respectively [43].

Expectorant activity
Due to its saponin content liquorice root decreases surface tension, a mechanism for decreasing the viscosity of mucus and thus increasing secretolytic and expectorant activity. It has no effect on mucociliary transport in the trachea [2,42,44].

Anti-inflammatory and anti-allergic activities
An aqueous extract from *Glycyrrhiza uralensis* root (0.01-1 mg/ml) inhibited tube formation from cultured aortic endothelial cells of rats in the angiogenic phase of the inflammatory process in a concentration-dependent manner (IC_{50}: 0.5 mg/ml). Isolated isoliquiritin had a potency 44-fold greater than that of the liquorice extract and appeared to play a major role in the inhibition of tube formation in angiogenesis; in contrast, glycyrrhizic acid and glycyrrhetic acid increased tube formation [45].

Isolated glycyrrhizic acid had no effect on human neutrophil chemotaxis or phagocytosis. However, it significantly decreased generation of the reactive oxygen species O_2^- (IC_{50}: 0.5 μg/ml), $OH^{\bullet}$ (IC_{50}: 5 μg/ml) and H_2O_2 (IC_{50}: 5 μg/ml) by human neutrophils [46].

Antiviral activity
When added to infected cultures of human aneuploid HEp2 cells, glycyrrhizic acid (4-8 mM) showed strong inhibitory activity on the growth of vaccinia, herpes simplex, Newcastle disease and vesicular stomatitis viruses [47]. The same compound at 3×10^{-3} M caused complete disappearance of hemagglutinating activity of influenza viruses A and B and Newcastle disease virus in infected embryonated hen eggs [48] and, with an ED_{50} of less than 400 μg/ml, inhibited hepatitis A virus antigen expression in human hepatoma PLC/PRF/5 cells [49].

Glycyrrhizic acid completely inhibited HIV-induced plaque formation in MT-4 cells at a concentration of 0.6 mM (IC_{50}: 0.15 mM). It also completely inhibited the cytopathic effect of HIV and the HIV-specific antigen expression in MT-4 cells at concentrations of 0.3 and 0.6 mM respectively, but had no direct effect on the reverse transcriptase of HIV [50]. Based on subsequent work, the same authors suggested that the inhibitory effect of glycyrrhizic acid on HIV-1 replication may result from a specific inhibition and also from a non-specific inhibition of virus adsorption to the cells complemented by an inhibitory effect on protein kinase C [51].

Antimicrobial effects
Glabrene, glabrol and glabridin showed antimicrobial

activity against *Staphylococcus aureus* and *Mycobacterium smegmatis* with MICs of 25, 1.56 and 6.25 μg/ml respectively [52].

In vivo experiments

Anti-inflammatory activity
In the adjuvant-induced granuloma pouch test in mice, isolated isoliquiritin administered intraperitoneally at 0.31-3.1 mg/kg body weight dose-dependently inhibited granuloma angiogenesis with an ID_{50} of 1.46 mg/kg, a potency 50-fold greater than that of liquorice root extract (typical isoliquiritin content: 0.8-1.6%), whereas glycyrrhizic acid had an effect weaker than that of the extract; the results indicated that the antiangiogenic effect of liquorice depended on the effect of isoliquiritin. The weight of pouch fluid was also inhibited by isoliquiritin with a potency 18-fold greater than that of the extract [45].

Antiulcerogenic effects
Granules of ibuprofen (60 mg/kg), alone or coated with liquorice containing more than 6.8% of glycyrrhizic acid or deglycyrrhized liquorice or highly glycyrrhized liquorice containing 15% of glycyrrhizic acid (30 mg/kg of coating in each case), were administered orally to rats as a single dose and mucosal damage was assessed 4 hours later. Compared to treatment with ibuprofen only, the additional liquorice extract (p<0.05) or deglycyrrhized liquorice (p<0.02) significantly reduced the size and number of mucosal lesions and ulcers in the rat gastric mucosa; highly glycyrrhized liquorice was less effective [53]. In a similar experiment with aspirin at 266 mg/kg, coating with liquorice, deglycyrrhized liquorice or highly glycyrrhized liquorice (133 mg/kg of coating in each case) significantly reduced the ulcer index (p<0.001 in each case), liquorice being the most effective in reducing the incidence of ulcers (46% incidence compared to 96% with aspirin alone) [54].

A liquid alcoholic extract of liquorice root (16 mg of glycyrrhizic acid per ml), administered orally to rats at 2.5-10 ml/kg body weight, had a histologically-confirmed, dose-dependent protective effect against indometacin-induced ulcers; about 95% protection at 10 ml/kg was comparable to the effect of oral cimetidine at 100 mg/kg. Oral pre-treatment of rats with the same extract (but lyophilized and reconstituted with water only) at 5 ml/kg significantly reduced gastric juice acidity, increased mucin concentration, and increased the prostaglandin E_2 content but reduced the leukotriene content of the gastric juice compared to indometacin-treated animals [55].

A decoction from 2 g of liquorice root, orally administered to rats daily for 15 days, did not significantly reduce total gastric acid secretion but significantly lowered free hydrochloric acid (p<0.05) by about 50% compared to the control group [11].

Effect on pancreatic secretion
Intraduodenal administration to dogs of a dry fraction from a methanolic extract of liquorice root containing 13-19% of glycyrrhizic acid and 4-13% of iso-flavonoids at three different doses (0.5, 1 and 2 g) induced significant increases in both plasma secretin concentration and pancreatic bicarbonate secretion in a dose-related manner. Intragastric administration of the liquorice fraction (2 g) in 5% liver extract meal also resulted in significant increases in both plasma secretin levels and pancreatic bicarbonate output [42,56].

Anti-tumour activity
Initiation with 7,12-dimethylbenzen[a]anthracene (DMBA, one application) followed by promotion with 12-O-tetradecanoylphorbol-13-acetate (TPA, twice weekly for 15 weeks) of tumours on the depil-ated skin of mice were significantly inhibited by topical pretreatment with 18α- or 18β-glycyrrhetic acid (GA) over a 16-week period. As total number of tumours per mouse, α-GA pretreatment resulted in 20% inhibition (p<0.05) and β-GA in 50% inhibition (p<0.001) [57].

Hepatoprotective activity
Glycyrrhizic acid administered orally to rats at 100 mg/kg had a preventive effect, attributed to its β-glucuronidase-inhibiting activity, on carbon tetra-chloride-induced hepatotoxicity (p<0.01). When glycyrrhizic acid was administered intraperitoneally at 100 mg/kg no significant effect was observed, but glycyrrhetic acid showed significant hepatoprotective activity at 50 mg/kg (p<0.05) and 100 mg/kg (p<0.01) [43].

Pharmacological studies in humans
Daily doses of dried aqueous extract of liquorice root containing 108, 217, 380 or 814 mg of glycyrrhizic acid were administered for 4 weeks to similar groups 1, 2, 3 and 4 respectively of healthy volunteers, each comprising 3 males and 3 females (aged from 22 to 39 years). Parameters evaluated before the study and after 1, 2 and 4 weeks involved anthropometric measurements, heart rate, mean arterial pressure, renal function, serum electrolytes, renin-aldosterone axis, blood glucose and haematocrit. No significant effects were observed in groups 1 and 2. Depression of plasma renin activity occurred in groups 3 (p = 0.024) and 4 (p = 0.049), and of plasma aldosterone concentration in group 4 (p = 0.019). In group 4, transient reduction in kalaemia (p = 0.014) and increase in body weight (p = 0.041) were noted after 1 and 2 weeks respectively, but had returned towards the baseline by the end of week 4.

Administration was stopped after 2 weeks in three subjects due to side effects: a female in group 3 (continuous headache), a male in group 4 with a family history of hypertension (arterial hypertension) and a female in group 4 who was also taking an oral contraceptive (headache, borderline arterial hyper-tension, hypokalaemia and peripheral oedema). In each case, the side effects disappeared within 24-48 hours after discontinuation.

Overall, the intake of up to 217 mg of glycyrrhizic acid per day (as liquorice extract) led to neither clinical effects nor changes in laboratory parameters, suggesting the absence of mineralocorticoid-like activity. Only the two highest doses of extract led to adverse effects in healthy subjects, in particular those with subclinical diseases or in situations favouring sodium retention, such as in the premenstrual period or when taking oral contraceptives. The effects were less common and less pronounced than those reported after comparable intake of isolated glycyrrhizic acid, as such or as a flavouring in food. Clinical symptoms disappeared promptly on discontinuation of the extract. The metabolic effects of liquorice root extract were dose-related and more frequent in women than in men [58].

In another study, 14 healthy volunteers ate 100 g or 200 g of confectionery liquorice (equivalent to 0.7-1.4 g of glycyrrhizic acid) daily for 1-4 weeks. Plasma potassium levels fell by over 0.3 mM in 11 subjects, including 4 who had to be withdrawn from the study because of hypokalaemia. Sodium retention, with concomitant weight gain was also evident, but blood pressure did not rise significantly in any of the subjects. One or more values of the renin-angiotensin-aldost-erone axis, especially plasma renin activity and urinary aldosterone levels, were considerably depressed in all subjects. The results demonstrated that potentially serious metabolic effects may occur in some persons after intake of modest amounts of liquorice daily for less than one week [21].

Glycyrrhetic acid, administered orally to 10 healthy, normotensive volunteers for 8 days at 500 mg/day (in two divided doses), exerted pronounced mineralo-corticoid activity as shown by significant increases in plasma sodium (p<0.01) and urinary potassium, significant decreases in plasma potassium (p<0.01) and aldosterone (p<0.05), and changes in other parameters. Urinary excretion of free hydrocortisone was elevated and plasma hydrocortisone levels virtually unchanged in the presence of markedly decreased levels of both plasma cortisone and urinary free cortisone. The results provided direct clinical support for the hypothesis that glycyrrhetic acid induces inhibition of the activity of 11β-hydroxy-steroid dehydrogenase, resulting in a blockade in the conversion of hydrocortisone (cortisol) to cortisone [20].

Clinical studies

Anti-ulcer activity
In an open study, 15 patients with radiologically proven peptic ulcer were treated with 3 × 3 g of powdered

liquorice root daily for 1-3 months. Evaluation after 2 months suggested that liquorice root produced beneficial effects, relieving pain in the epigastrium (56% of cases) and burning in the epigastric/retrosternal regions (78% of cases). Radiological evidence showed complete or near complete healing in 50% of cases and partial healing in a further 40% [11].

Although some studies using deglycyrrhizinated liquorice showed apparent beneficial effects on ulcers [59], placebo-controlled studies involving a total of 271 patients and daily dosages of 2.3-5 g of deglycyrrhizinated liquorice for 4-6 weeks revealed no clinical advantage over placebo in the treatment of gastric [60,61] or duodenal [62,63] ulcers.

Pharmacokinetic properties

Pharmacokinetics in vitro
Under anaerobic conditions, human intestinal bacteria hydrolyzed glycyrrhizic acid to its aglycone, glycyrrhetic acid, which was then isomerized through 3-dehydro-glycyrrhetic acid to 3-*epi*-glycyrrhetic acid and *vice versa* [64,65].

Pharmacokinetics in animals
The mechanism of gastrointestinal absorption of glycyrrhizic acid in rats was investigated using an *in situ* loop technique. Glycyrrhizic acid was poorly absorbed from the gut of rats (with a bioavailability of about 4%), but after oral administration at 200 mg/kg it was detected in rat plasma together with glycyrrhetic acid. Glycyrrhizic acid was hydrolysed to glycyrrhetic acid by rat gastric and large-intestinal (but not small-intestinal) contents. The glycyrrhetic acid formed was absorbed mainly from the large intestine, with a bioavailability of 14% and a peak plasma concentration 12 hours after oral dosing. After intravenous administration of glycyrrhizic acid, no glycyrrhetic acid could be detected in the plasma, suggesting that systemic hydrolysis is low, and 80% of the dose was excreted unchanged in the bile [66]. When glycyrrhizic acid (100 mg/kg) was administered orally to germ-free rats, no glycyrrhetic acid was detected in the plasma, caecal contents or faeces, indicating that hydrolysis to glycyrrhetic acid depends on bacteria [67].

After bolus injection of glycyrrhizic acid into the portal vein, its plasma level fell rapidly within 30 minutes, but at 60 minutes it had fallen only slightly further. This suggested that glycyrrhizic acid is distributed in the tissues then eliminated from the blood and excreted only slowly [68]. From studies on enterohepatic recycling of glycyrrhizic acid in rats following intravenous administration (100 mg/kg) it was concluded that glycyrrhizic acid was predominantly secreted from the liver into the bile (80.6 ± 9.9% of the administered dose) [69].

The effects of other components of aqueous liquorice root extract on the pharmacokinetics of glycyrrhizic acid and glycyrrhetic acid were investigated in rats. Lower plasma levels of glycyrrhizic acid and glycyrrhetic acid were found in rats treated orally with the aqueous extract compared to those treated with a corresponding amount of pure glycyrrhizic acid [70,71]. After complete removal of glycyrrhizic acid from a liquorice root extract and separation of the remainder into lipophilic and hydrophilic components, the lipophilic components were found to reduce absorption of glycyrrhizic acid; in contrast, the hydrophilic components increased the bioavailability of glycyrrhizic acid as glycyrrhetic acid [72].

Pharmacokinetics in humans
Plasma levels of glycyrrhetic acid after oral administration of an aqueous liquorice root extract to healthy volunteers were found to be lower than those observed after oral administration of a corresponding amount of pure glycyrrhizic acid [70,71]. The lower absorption and bioavailability from liquorice root extract could explain the various adverse clinical effects resulting from chronic oral administration of pure glycyrrhizic acid as opposed to the extract [70].

After oral administration of a liquorice root decoction containing 133 mg of glycyrrhizic acid to 5 healthy volunteers the peak serum concentration of glycyrrhizic acid occurred less than 4 hours after administration and was not detectable after 96 hours. In contrast, the serum concentration of glycyrrhetic acid reached a maximum after about 24 hours and remained detectable in the urine for approx. 130 hours. The low urinary concentrations of both compounds suggested excretion via the gastrointestinal route [73]. In another study, after oral administration of 100 mg of glycyrrhizic acid to 3 healthy volunteers none was detected in plasma but 1-3% was detected in the urine, suggesting partial absorption intact from the gastrointestinal tract; glycyrrhetic acid appeared in the plasma at < 200 ng/ml but was not detected in the urine [74].

A comparison study in which glycyrrhizic acid was administered orally to 10 healthy men before or after breakfast showed that maximum plasma concentrations and areas under curves of glycyrrhizic acid and glycyrrhetic acid were not significantly influenced by consumption of food [75].

The glycyrrhetic acid level in blood of 10 patients with, and 11 patients without, liquorice-induced pseudoaldosteronism was comparable. On the other hand, the level of another metabolite, 3β-mono-glucuronyl-glycyrrhetic acid, was elevated in patients with pseudoaldosteronism but not in patients without this syndrome. It is likely that in certain patients, especially older ones, longer administration of glycyrrhizic acid may induce an enzyme in intestinal bacterial flora which results in increased production of 3β-monoglucuronyl-glycyrrhetic acid and that this metabolite causes pseudoaldosteronism [76].

Preclinical safety data

Acute toxicity

For a liquorice root dry extract containing 48-58% of glycyrrhizic acid the oral, intraperitoneal and subcutaneous LD_{50} values in rats and mice were determined as 14.2-18.0 g/kg, 1.42-1.70 g/kg and 4.0-4.4 g/kg respectively [77]. The oral LD_{50} of glycyrrhetic acid was determined as 560 mg/kg in mice [41].

Subacute toxicity

Oral administration of a liquorice root dry extract containing 48-58% of glycyrrhizic acid to rats at 0.31-0.63 g/kg/day for 90 days had no toxic effect, whereas 2.5 g/kg/day over the same period led to decreases in body weight gain, blood cell count and thymus weight, and also atrophic cortex and sporadic lymphofollicle formation in the medulla of the thymus gland. All these changes disappeared after discontinuation of the drug [77].

Subchronic toxicity

Rats fed on a diet containing 1.2-2.6 g/kg/day of the ammonium salt of glycyrrhizic acid for 4-6 months exhibited hypertension, increased relative weights of kidney and heart, and a slight decrease in body weight and growth as well as bradycardia and polydipsia [78].

Mutagenicity and carcinogenicity

An aqueous extract from liquorice root and various fractions from it showed no mutagenic potential in the Ames test using *Salmonella typhimurium* strains TA98 and TA100 [79]. In the *Salmonella*/microsome reversion assay using strain TA100 an ethanolic extract of liquorice root (0.8% glycyrrhizic acid) showed antimutagenic activity against ethyl methane-sulphonate and ribose-lysine [80].

REFERENCES

1. Liquorice Root - Liquiritiae radix. European Pharmacopoeia, Council of Europe.

2. Hänsel R, Keller K, Rimpler H, Schneider G, editors. Glycyrrhiza. In: Hagers Handbuch der Pharmazeutischen Praxis, 5th ed. Volume 5: Drogen E-O. Berlin: Springer-Verlag, 1993:311-36.

3. Wichtl M and Schäfer-Korting M. Süßholzwurzel. In: Hartke K, Hartke H, Mutschler E, Rücker G and Wichtl M, editors. Kommentar zum Europäischen Arzneibuch. Stuttgart: Wissenschaftliche Verlagsgesellschaft, 1999 (11 Lfg):S 62.

4. Tang W, Eisenbrand G. *Glycyrrhiza* spp. In: Chinese Drugs of Plant Origin - Chemistry, Pharmacology and Use in Traditional and Modern Medicine. Berlin-Heidelberg-New York-London: Springer-Verlag, 1992; 74:567-88.

5. Evans WC. Liquorice root. In: Trease and Evans' Pharmacognosy, 14th ed. London-Philadelphia: WB Saunders, 1996:305-8.

6. Bruneton J. Licorice, *Glycyrrhiza glabra* L., Fabaceae. In: Pharmacognosy - Phytochemistry - Medicinal Plants [English translation of 2nd French ed. of Pharmacognosie]. Paris: Lavoisier, Andover UK: Intercept, 1995:549-54.

7. Willuhn G. Liquiritiae radix - Süßholzwurzel. In: Wichtl M, editor. Teedrogen, 3rd ed. Stuttgart: Wissenschaftliche Verlagsgesellschaft, 1997: 351-5.

8. Barnes J, Anderson LA and Phillipson JD. Liquorice. In: Herbal Medicines - A guide for healthcare professionals, 2nd ed. London-Chicago: Pharmaceutical Press, 2002: 325-9.

9. Benigni R, Capra C, Cattorini PE. Liquerizia o Liquirizia. In: Piante Medicinali: Chimica, farmacologia e terapia, Volume 2. Milano: Inverni & Della Beffa 1964;2:840-66.

10. Davis EA, Morris DJ. Medicinal uses of licorice through the millennia: the good and plenty of it. Molec Cell Endocrinol 1991;78:1-6.

11. Chaturvedi GN, Prasad M, Agrawal AK, Gupta JP. Some clinical and experimental studies on whole root of *Glycyrrhiza glabra* Linn (Yashtimadhu) in peptic ulcer. Indian Medical Gazette 1979;(June):200-5.

12. Glycyrrhiza. In: British Herbal Pharmacopoeia 1983. Bournemouth: British Herbal Medicine Association, 1983:104-5.

13. Dorsch W, Loew D, Meyer-Buchtela E, Schilcher H. Liquiritiae radix - Süßholzwurzel. In: Kinderdosierung von Phytopharmaka, 3rd ed. Teil I. Empfehlungen zur Anwendung und Dosierung von Phytopharmaka, monographierte Arzneidrogen und ihren Zubereitungen in der Pädiatrie: Bonn: Kooperation Phytopharmaka, 2002:86-7.

14. Chandler RF. *Glycyrrhiza glabra*. In: De Smet PAGM, Keller K, Hänsel R, Chandler RF, editors. Adverse Effects of Herbal Drugs, Volume 3. Berlin-Heidelberg: Springer-Verlag, 1997:67-87.

15. Schilcher H, Kammerer S. Süßholzwurzel (Liquiritiae radix). In: Leitfaden Phytotherapie. München-Jena: Urban & Fischer, 2000:219-21.

16. Størmer FC, Reistad R, Alexander J. Glycyrrhizic acid in liquorice - evaluation of health hazard. Food Chem Toxicol 1993;31:303-12.

17. Fugh-Berman A. Herb-drug interactions. Lancet 2000; 355:134-8.

18. Teelucksingh S, Mackie ADR, Burt D, McIntyre MA, Brett L, Edwards CRW. Potentiation of hydrocortisone

activity in skin by glycyrrhetinic acid. Lancet 1990; 335:1060-3.

19. Stewart PM, Wallace AM, Valentino R, Burt D, Shackleton CHL, Edwards CRW. Mineralocorticoid activity of liquorice: 11-beta-hydroxysteroid dehydrogenase deficiency comes of age. Lancet 1987;II:821-4.

20. MacKenzie MA, Hoefnagels WHL, Jansen RWMM, Benraad TJ, Kloppenborg PWC. The influence of glycyrrhetinic acid on plasma cortisol and cortisone in healthy young volunteers. J Clin Endocrinol Metab 1990;70:1637-43.

21. Epstein MT, Espiner EA, Donald RA, Hughes H. Effect of eating liquorice on the renin-angiotensin-aldosterone axis in normal subjects. Br Med J 1977;1:488-90.

22. Scali M, Pratesi C, Zennaro MC, Zampollo V, Armanini D. Pseudohyperaldosteronism from liquorice-containing laxatives. J Endocrinol Invest 1990;13:847-8.

23. Beretta-Piccoli C, Salvadé G, Crivelli PL, Weidmann P. Body-sodium and blood volume in a patient with licorice-induced hypertension. J Hypertension 1985; 3:19-23.

24. Cuspidi C, Gelosa M, Moroni E, Sampieri L. Pseudo-sindrome di Conn da ingestione abituale di liquirizia. Rapporto su alcuni casi clinici. Minerva Med 1981; 72:825-30.

25. Farese RV, Biglieri EG, Shackleton CHL, Irony I, Gomez-Fontes R. Licorice-induced hypermineralocorticoidism. New Engl J Med 1991;325:1223-7.

26. Biglieri EG, Kater CE. Steroid characteristics of mineralocorticoid adrenocortical hypertension. Clin Chem 1991;37:1843-8.

27. Shintani S, Murase H, Tsukagoshi H, Shiigai T. Glycyrrhizin (licorice)-induced hypokalemic myopathy. Report of 2 cases and review of the literature. Eur Neurol 1992;32:44-51.

28. Sundaram MBM, Swaminathan R. Total body potassium depletion and severe myopathy due to chronic liquorice ingestion. Postgrad Med J 1981;57:48-9.

29. Haberer JP, Jouve P, Bedock B, Bazin PE. Severe hypokalaemia secondary to overindulgence in alcohol-free "pastis" [Letter]. Lancet 1984;I:575-6.

30. Cereda JM, Trono D, Schifferli J. Liquorice intoxication caused by alcohol-free pastis [Letter]. Lancet 1983;I: 1442.

31. Blachley JD, Knochel JP. Tobacco chewer's hypo-kalemia: licorice revisited. New Engl J Med 1980; 302:784-5.

32. Nielsen I, Pedersen RS. Life-threatening hypokalaemia caused by liquorice ingestion. Lancet 1984;I:1305.

33. Rosseel M, Schoors D. Chewing gum and hypokalaemia. Lancet 1993;341:175.

34. Caradonna P, Gentiloni N, Servidei S, Perrone GA, Greco AV, Russo MA. Licorice ingestion: reversible loss of myoadenylate deaminase activity. Ultrastruct Pathol 1992;16:529-35.

35. Garnier-Fabre A, Chaine G, Paquet R, Robert N, Fischbein L, Robineau M. Rétinopathie hypertensive et oedème papillaire. A propos d'un cas d'intoxication par la glycyrrhizine. J Fr Ophtalmol 1987;10:735-40.

36. Werner S, Brismar K, Olsson S. Hyperprolactinaemia and liquorice. Lancet 1979;I:319.

37. Bannister B, Ginsburg R, Shneerson J. Cardiac arrest due to liquorice-induced hypokalaemia. Br Med J 1977;(2):738-9.

38. Teelucksingh S, Benediktsson R, Lindsay RS, Burt D, Seckl JR, Edwards CRW et al. Liquorice [Letter]. Lancet 1991;337:1549.

39. Monder C, Stewart PM, Lakshmi V, Valentino R, Burt D, Edwards CRW. Licorice inhibits corticosteroid 11β-dehydrogenase of rat kidney and liver: in vivo and in vitro studies. Endocrinology 1989;125:1046-53.

40. Tamura Y, Nishikawa T, Yamada K, Yamamoto M, Kumagai A. Effects of glycyrrhetinic acid and its derivatives on Δ⁴-5α- and 5β-reductase in rat liver. Arzneim-Forsch/Drug Res 1979;29:647-9.

41. Takahashi K, Shibata S, Yano S, Harada M, Saito H, Tamura Y, Kumagai A. Chemical modification of glycyrrhetinic acid in relation to the biological activities. Chem Pharm Bull 1980;28:3449-52.

42. Hikino H. Recent research on oriental medicinal plants. In: Wagner H, Hikino H, Farnsworth NR, editors. Economic and Medicinal Plant Research, Volume 1. London: Academic Press, 1985:53-85.

43. Shim S-B, Kim N-J, Kim D-H. β-Glucuronidase inhibitory activity and hepatoprotective effect of 18β-glycyrrhetinic acid from the rhizomes of Glycyrrhiza uralensis. Planta Med 2000;66:40-3.

44. Müller-Limmroth W, Fröhlich H-H. Wirkungsnachweis einiger phytotherapeutischer Expektorantien auf den mukoziliaren Transport. Fortschr Med 1980;98:95-101.

45. Kobayashi S, Miyamoto T, Kimura I, Kimura M. Inhibitory effect of isoliquiritin, a compound in licorice root, on angiogenesis in vivo and tube formation in vitro. Biol Pharm Bull 1995;18:1382-6.

46. Akamatsu H, Komura J, Asada Y, Niwa Y. Mechanism of anti-inflammatory action of glycyrrhizin: effect on neutrophil functions including reactive oxygen species generation. Planta Med 1991;57:119-21.

47. Pompei R, Pani A, Flore O, Marcialis MA, Loddo B. Antiviral activity of glycyrrhizic acid. Experientia 1980; 36:304.

48. Pompei R, Paghi L, Ingianni A, Uccheddu P. Glycyrrhizic acid inhibits influenza virus growth in embryonated eggs. Microbiologica 1983;6:247-50.

49. Crance JM, Biziagos E, Passagot J, van Cuyck-Gandré H, Deloince R. Inhibition of hepatitis A virus replication in vitro by antiviral compounds. J Med Virol 1990; 31:155-60.

50. Ito M, Nakashima H, Baba M, Pauwels R, De Clercq E, Shigeta S, Yamamoto N. Inhibitory effect of glycyrrhizin on the in vitro infectivity and cytopathic activity of the human immunodeficiency virus [HIV (HTLV-III/LAV)]. Antiviral Res 1987;7:127-37.

51. Ito M, Sato A, Hirabayashi K, Tanabe F, Shigeta S, Baba M et al. Mechanism of inhibitory effect of glycyrrhizin on replication of human immunodeficiency virus (HIV). Antiviral Res 1988;10:289-98.

52. Mitscher LA, Park YH, Clark D, Beal JL. Antimicrobial agents from higher plants. Antimicrobial isoflavanoids and related substances from *Glycyrrhiza glabra* L. var. *typica*. J Nat Prod 1980;43:259-69.

53. Dehpour AR, Zolfaghari ME, Samadian T, Kobarfard F, Faizi M, Assari M. Antiulcer activities of liquorice and its derivatives in experimental gastric lesion induced by ibuprofen in rats. Int J Pharmaceut 1995;119:133-8.

54. Dehpour AR, Zolfaghari ME, Samadian T, Vahedi Y. The protective effect of liquorice components and their derivatives against gastric ulcer induced by aspirin in rats. J Pharm Pharmacol 1994;46:148-9.

55. Khayyal MT, El-Ghazaly MA, Kenawy SA, Seif-El-Nasr M, Mahran LG, Kafafi YAH, Okpanyi SN. Anti-ulcerogenic effect of some gastrointestinally acting plant extracts and their combination. Arzneim-Forsch/Drug Res 2001;51:545-53.

56. Watanabe S-I, Chey WY, Lee KY, Chang T-M. Release of secretin by licorice extract in dogs. Pancreas 1986; 1:449-54.

57. Wang ZY, Agarwal R, Zhou ZC, Bickers DR, Mukhtar H. Inhibition of mutagenicity in *Salmonella typhimurium* and skin tumor initiating and tumor promoting activities in SENCAR mice by glycyrrhetinic acid: comparison of 18α- and 18β-stereoisomers. Carcinogenesis 1991;12: 187-92.

58. Bernardi M, D'Intino PE, Trevisani F, Cantelli-Forti G, Raggi MA, Turchetto E, Gasbarrini G. Effects of prolonged ingestion of graded doses of licorice by healthy volunteers. Life Sci 1994;55:863-72.

59. Kassir ZA. Endoscopic controlled trial of four drug regimens in the treatment of chronic duodenal ulceration. Irish Med J 1985;78:153-6.

60. Bardhan KD, Cumberland DC, Dixon RA, Holdsworth CD. Clinical trial of deglycyrrhizinised liquorice in gastric ulcer. Gut 1978;19:779-82.

61. Engqvist A, von Feilitzen F, Pyk E, Reichard H. Double-blind trial of deglycyrrhizinated liquorice in gastric ulcer. Gut 1973;14:711-5.

62. Misiewicz JJ, Russell RI, Baron JH, Cox AG, Grayson MJ, Howel Jones J et al. Treatment of duodenal ulcer with glycyrrhizinic-acid-reduced liquorice. A multicentre trial. Br Med J 1971;3:501-3.

63. Feldman H, Gilat T. A trial of deglycyrrhizinated liquorice in the treatment of duodenal ulcer. Gut 1971;12:449-51.

64. Hattori M, Sakamoto T, Kobashi K, Namba T. Metabolism of glycyrrhizin by human intestinal flora. Planta Med 1983;48:38-42.

65. Hattori M, Sakamoto T, Yamagishi T, Sakamoto K, Konishi K, Kobashi K, Namba T. Metabolism of glycyrrhizin by human intestinal flora. II. Isolation and characterization of human intestinal bacteria capable of metabolizing glycyrrhizin and related compounds. Chem Pharm Bull 1985;33:210-7.

66. Wang Z, Kurosaki Y, Nakayama T, Kimura T. Mechanism of gastrointestinal absorption of glycyrrhizin in rats. Biol Pharm Bull 1994;17:1399-403.

67. Akao T, Hayashi T, Kobashi K, Kanaoka M, Kato H, Kobayashi M. Intestinal bacterial hydrolysis is indispensable to absorption of 18β-glycyrrhetic acid after oral administration of glycyrrhizin in rats. J Pharm Pharmacol 1994;46:135-7.

68. Sakiya Y, Akada Y, Kawano S, Miyauchi Y. Rapid estimation of glycyrrhizin and glycyrrhetinic acid in plasma by high-speed liquid chromatography. Chem Pharm Bull 1979;27:1125-9.

69. Ichikawa T, Ishida S, Sakiya Y, Sawada Y, Hanano M. Biliary excretion and enterohepatic cycling of glycyrrhizin in rats. J Pharm Sci 1986;75:672-5.

70. Cantelli-Forti G, Maffei F, Hrelia P, Bugamelli F, Bernardi M, D'Intino P et al. Interaction of licorice on glycyrrhizin pharmacokinetics. Environ Health Perspect 1994;102 (Suppl 9):65-8.

71. Raggi MA, Maffei F, Bugamelli F, Cantelli Forti G. Bioavailability of glycyrrhizin and licorice extract in rat and human plasma as detected by a HPLC method. Pharmazie 1994;49:269-72.

72. Wang Z, Nishioka M, Kurosaki Y, Nakayama T, Kimura T. Gastrointestinal absorption characteristics of glycyrrhizin from *Glycyrrhiza* extract. Biol Pharm Bull 1995;18:1238-41.

73. Terasawa K, Bandoh M, Tosa H, Hirate J. Disposition of glycyrrhetic acid and its glycosides in healthy subjects and patients with pseudoaldosteronism. J Pharmacobio-Dyn 1986;9:95-100.

74. Yamamura Y, Kawakami J, Santa T, Kotaki H, Uchino K, Sawada Y et al. Pharmacokinetic profile of glycyrrhizin in healthy volunteers by a new high-performance liquid chromatographic method. J Pharm Sci 1992;81:1042-6.

75. Nishioka Y, Kyotani S, Miyamura M, Kusunose M. Influence of time of administration of a Shosaiko-to extract granule on blood concentration of its active constituents. Chem Pharm Bull 1992;40:1335-7.

76. Kato H, Kanaoka M, Yano S, Kobayashi M. 3-Mono-

glucuronyl-glycyrrhetinic acid is a major metabolite that causes licorice-induced pseudoaldosteronism. J Clin Endocrinol Metab 1995;80:1929-33.

77. Komiyama K, Kawakubo Y, Fukushima T, Sugimoto K, Takeshima H, Ko Y et al. Acute and subacute toxicity test on the extract from *Glycyrrhiza*. Oyo Yakuri 1977; 14:535-48; through Chem Abstr 1978;88:69205.

78. Sobotka TJ, Spaid SL, Brodie RE, Reed GF. Neurobehavioral toxicity of ammoniated glycyrrhizin, a licorice component, in rats. Neurobehav Toxicol Teratol 1981;3:37-44.

79. Lee HK, Kim YK, Kim Y-H, Roh JK. Effect of bacterial growth-inhibiting ingredients on the Ames mutagenicity of medicinal herbs. Mutation Res 1987;192:99-104.

80. Zani F, Cuzzoni MT, Daglia M, Benvenuti S, Vampa G, Mazza P. Inhibition of mutagenicity in *Salmonella typhimurium* by *Glycyrrhiza glabra* extract, glycyrrhizinic acid, 18a- and 18ß-glycyrrhetinic acids. Planta Med 1993;59:502-7.

LUPULI FLOS

Hop Strobile

DEFINITION

Hop strobile consists of the dried, generally whole, female inflorescences of *Humulus lupulus* L.

The material complies with the monograph of the European Pharmacopoeia [1].

CONSTITUENTS

Bitter principles consisting mainly of prenylated phloroglucinol derivatives called α-acids or humulones (2-12% of dried strobile), principally humulone (35-70%), and β-acids or lupulones (1-10% of dried strobile), principally lupulone (30-55%) [2-6].

Essential oil, 0.5-1.5% [2] consisting mainly of myrcene, humulene and β-caryophyllene [2,7]. Although only a trace of 2-methyl-3-buten-2-ol is found in freshly-harvested hop strobile [8,9], the amount is higher in stored material, increasing to a maximum of approx. 0.15% of the dry weight (up to 20% of the volatiles) after 2 years due to degradation of humulones and lupulones [4,5,8,9].

Flavonoids (0.5-1.5%) including quercetin and kaempferol glycosides [10,11] and at least 22 prenylated (or geranylated) flavonoids [12], notably the chalcones xanthohumol (up to 1% of dried strobile and 80-90% of total flavonoids), desmethyl-xanthohumol and dehydrocycloxanthohumol, and the flavanones isoxanthohumol, 8-prenylnaringenin (25-60 mg/kg) and 6-prenylnaringenin [12-16].

Other constituents include proanthocyanidins, phenolic acids, proteins (15%), polysaccharides (40-50%) and minerals [2,3,5].

CLINICAL PARTICULARS

Therapeutic indications
Tenseness, restlessness and sleep disorders [4,17-20].

Posology and method of administration

Dosage

Internal use
Adults and children over 12 years of age: 0.5 g of the drug as an infusion, 2-4 times daily; 0.5-2 ml of liquid extract (1:1, 45% ethanol) or 1-2 ml of tincture (1:5,

E/S/C/O/P
MONOGRAPHS
Second Edition

60% ethanol), up to 3 times daily; other equivalent preparations [19,20].

External use
Infants and young children: Up to 500 g of dry hop strobile (previously stored for 1-2 years) in a hop pillow [21].

Method of administration
For oral administration; combination with other herbal sedatives may be beneficial [4]. Also externally in hop pillows for overnight use [21].

Duration of administration
No restriction.

Contra-indications
None known.

Special warnings and special precautions for use
None required.

Interaction with other medicaments and other forms of interaction
None reported.

Pregnancy and lactation
No data available. In accordance with general medical practice, hop strobile preparations should not be used internally during pregnancy and lactation without medical advice.

Effects on ability to drive and use machines
None reported.

Undesirable effects
None reported.

Overdose
No toxic effects reported.

PHARMACOLOGICAL PROPERTIES

Pharmacodynamic properties
Over the past decade considerable pharmacological research has been carried out on hop strobile and its constituents, particularly with respect to oestrogenic activity. However, no new studies relating to the sedative effects of hop strobile appear to have been published.

In vitro experiments

Oestrogenic activity of hop strobile
Circumstantial evidence over many years, including menstrual disturbances reported to be common among female hop pickers, linked hop strobile with potential oestrogenic activity [2,3]. However, early studies to confirm this activity experimentally were inconclusive

or contradictory due to methodology of inadequate sensitivity [3,22].

In recent screening of plant drugs for oestrogenic activity, a 50%-ethanolic extract (2 g of hop strobile to 10 ml) exhibited binding to oestrogen receptors in intact, oestrogen-dependent [ER(+)], human breast cancer MCF-7 cells with a potency equivalent to 0.5 µg of oestradiol per 2 g of dried strobile (for comparison, the potencies of 2 g of thyme or red clover were equivalent to 0.5 or 3 µg of oestradiol, respectively). The extract also showed significant ability to *stimulate* cell proliferation in ER(+) T47D, but not in ER(−) MDA 468, breast cancer cells [23]. In contrast, in a different series of experiments, a similarly-prepared extract of hop strobile at concentrations of 0.01-1.0% V/V was found to significantly *inhibit* serum-stimulated growth of ER(+) T47D breast cancer cells (p<0.001) [24].

Ovarian cells isolated from immature female rats, which 48 hours previously had been injected (primed) with pregnant mare's serum gonadotrophin, were incubated with follicle-stimulating hormone to induce oestradiol secretion. Addition to the culture medium of purified water-soluble fractions F_1 or F_2 from de-fatted hop strobile extract reduced the amounts of oestrogen E_2 released from the ovarian cells (p<0.01) with a probably related decrease in cAMP release (p<0.05) [25].

Oestrogenic activity of 8-prenylnaringenin
8-prenylnaringenin, a flavanone occurring in hop strobile at levels of 25-60 mg/kg [15], has been shown to be a potent phyto-oestrogen with activity greater than that of other established plant oestrogens [26]. Oestrogenic activity of a much lower order (less than one-hundredth of that of 8-prenylnaringenin) has also been detected in three other hop flavonoids, 6-prenylnaringenin, 8-geranylnaringenin and 6,8-diprenylnaringenin, while xanthohumol and isoxanthohumol were found inactive [16]. EC_{50} values for 17β-oestradiol, 8-prenylnaringenin, 6-prenyl-naringenin, coumestrol, genistein and daidzein were 0.3, 40, >4000, 70, 1200 and 2200 nM, respectively, in a screen using oestrogen-inducible yeast (*Saccharomyces cerevisiae*) expressing the human oestrogen receptor, and 0.8, 4, 500, 30, 200 and 1500 nM, respectively, for stimulation of alkaline phosphatase activity in a human endometrial cell line (Ishikawa Var I). The relative binding affinities of 17β-oestradiol, 8-prenylnaringenin, coumestrol and genistein with rat uterine cytosol containing soluble oestrogen receptor were 1, 0.023, 0.008 and 0.003, respectively [26].

The oestrogenic activity of 8-prenylnaringenin was confirmed in competitive binding assays using purified human recombinant oestrogen receptors α and β (ERα and ERβ). 8-prenylnaringenin competed strongly with 17β-oestradiol for binding to both receptors with a relative binding affinity of about 0.1, compared to 1.0 for 17β-oestradiol and 0.001 for 8-geranylnaringenin [16].

In another study, involving displacement of [^3H]-17β-oestradiol, 8-prenylnaringenin showed competitive binding affinity for the oestrogen receptor in bovine uterine cytosol with an IC_{50} of 140 nM, compared to 1.0 nM for oestradiol and 320 nM for genistein. 8-Prenylnaringenin also dose-dependently stimulated the proliferation of cultured, oestrogen-dependent, human breast cancer MCF-7 cells with an EC_{50} of 1.9 nM, compared to 0.0032 nM for oestradiol and 47 nM for genistein, suggesting that it was an oestrogen receptor agonist [27].

Antiproliferative activity of xanthohumols
Xanthohumol (XN), dehydrocycloxanthohumol (DX) and isoxanthohumol (IX) caused dose-dependent (0.1 to 100 µM) decreases in growth of human breast cancer MCF-7, colon cancer HT-29 and ovarian cancer A-2780 cells, xanthohumol being the most potent. With MCF-7 cells the IC_{50} values were 13.3, 15.7 and 15.3 µM after 2 days and 3.5, 6.7 and 4.7 after 4 days for XN, DX and IX, respectively. HT-29 cells were more resistant than MCF-7 cells. With A-2780 cells xanthohumol was highly antiproliferative with IC_{50} values of 0.5 and 5.2 µM after 2 and 4 days of exposure, respectively. At 100 µM all three compounds were cytotoxic to all three cell lines [28].

Spasmolytic activity
An alcoholic extract of hop strobile (1 g of dried drug in 10 ml of 70 % ethanol) produced a strong spasmolytic effect on isolated smooth muscle from guinea pig intestine with ED_{50} values equivalent to 37×10^{-6} g of hop strobile per ml for acetylcholine-induced contractions compared to 60×10^{-9} g/ml with atropine, and 39×10^{-6} of hop strobile per ml for barium chloride-induced contractions compared to 57×10^{-7} g/ml with papaverine. The extract also inhibited contractions of rat uterus with an ED_{50} equivalent to 31×10^{-6} g of hop strobile per ml [29].

Effect on calcium flux
A methanolic extract from hop strobile showed strong inhibitory activity on calcium fluxes, inhibiting depolarization-induced $^{45}Ca^{2+}$ uptake in clonal rat pituitary cells by 94.7% at 20 µg/ml (p<0.001). The activity was attributed to prenylated flavonoids, although individual compounds from hop strobile have not so far been tested in this way [30].

Other activities
A methanolic extract of hop strobile showed inhibitory activity against rat liver diacylglycerol acyltransferase (DGAT), which is involved in triacylglycerol formation. By fractionation, the activity was traced to xanthohumol and a related chalcone, xanthohumol B; they inhibited DGAT activity in rat liver microsomes dose-dependently with IC_{50} values of 50 and 194 µM, respectively, and also inhibited DGAT activity in intact Raji cells [31].

Using an *in vitro* 'pit formation assay' (formation of pits on dentine slices incubated with mouse bone cells), xanthohumol and humulone have been identified as inhibitors of bone resorption at concentrations at or above 10^{-6} and 10^{-11}, respectively (p<0.01); humulone showed remarkably high inhibitory activity with an IC_{50} of 5.9×10^{-9} M [32].

Several prenylated flavonoids from hop strobile, particularly xanthohumol, isoxanthohumol and 8-prenylnaringenin, were shown to be potent and selective inhibitors of certain cDNA-expressed human cytochrome P450 enzymes known to bioactivate carcinogens. At 10 µM, xanthohumol almost completely inhibited (2.5% of control) the 7-ethoxyresorufin O-deethylase (EROD) activity of CYP1A1 and completely eliminated EROD activity of CYP1B1, while other prenylated flavonoids showed somewhat less activity. In contrast, 8-prenylnaringenin (25 µM) and isoxanthohumol (100 µM) were the most effective inhibitors of CYP1A2 acetanilide 4-hydroxylase activity (> 90% inhibition) and also of CYP1A2 metabolism of the carcinogen aflatoxin B$_1$ [33].

In vivo experiments

Sedative effects
To assess effects on the central nervous system, an extract of hop strobile was administered intraperitoneally to mice before a series of behavioural tests. Spontaneous locomotor activity was dose-dependently suppressed by 100 mg/kg (p<0.05), 250 and 500 mg/kg (p<0.001); at 250 and 500 mg/kg the activity was 11% and 3% respectively of that of saline-treated mice in the first hour after administration. Pentobarbital-induced sleeping time increased dose-dependently; not significant at 100 mg/kg, by 1.9-fold at 250 mg/kg (p<0.05) and 2.6-fold at 500 mg/kg (p<0.01). In the hot plate test, latency time for licking the forepaws increased with doses of 100 and 250 mg/kg (p<0.01). Rotarod performance decreased by 59% and 65% respectively at 250 and 500 mg/kg (p<0.05). The time to onset of convulsion and survival time after administration of pentylenetetrazole were significantly lengthened by 500 mg/kg (p<0.001), but not by 250 mg/kg. A significant and time-dependent fall in rectal temperature was observed after a dose of 500 mg/kg (p<0.001 after 120 minutes). Thus hop strobile extract showed sedative and hypnotic properties at lower doses (100-250 mg/kg), and at a higher dose of 500 mg/kg it also produced anti-convulsive and hypothermic effects [34,35].

2-Methyl-3-buten-2-ol, given intraperitoneally to mice

at a high dose of 800 mg/kg, showed central nervous depressant activity, producing deep narcosis for about 8 hours, without subsequent abnormal behaviour [36]; in rats, intraperitoneal administration at 206.5 mg/kg caused a decline in motility of 50% [37]. Although 2-methyl-3-buten-2-ol is present only in small amounts in hop strobile, higher levels may be generated in vivo by metabolism of humulones and lupulones [8,9,38]. The sedative effect of this constituent is comparable, in the same dosage range, to that of the structurally-related drug methylpentynol [37].

Antigonadotrophic effects
Purified water-soluble fractions from de-fatted hop strobile extract were administered subcutaneously twice daily for 3 days to immature female rats primed with 25 IU of pregnant mare's serum gonadotrophin (PMSG). None of the fractions induced a change in uterine weights. However, fractions F_1 (20 mg/rat) and F_2 (50 mg/rat) significantly suppressed PMSG-induced gain in ovarian weights by about 25% (p<0.05) compared to controls. Under the same conditions, two further fractions (4 mg/rat) purified from F_1 suppressed gain in ovarian weights by 42% and 33% (p<0.01) compared to controls [39]. In further experiments on PMSG-primed immature rats, by comparison with saline-treated control animals, subcutaneously administered fractions F_1 and F_2 reduced the number of ovulations (p<0.05); suppressed levels of serum luteinizing hormone (p<0.001); suppressed thymidine kinase activity in uterine tissue (p<0.01); reduced oestradiol E_2 secretion in cultures of ovarian cells from the rats (p<0.001); and reduced progesterone production in cultures of luteal cells from the rats (p<0.05 to p<0.001) [25].

Oestrogenic effects of 8-prenylnaringenin
Ovariectomized rats, as a model for oestrogen deficiency-induced osteoporosis, were treated subcutaneously with racemic 8-prenylnaringenin (OVX + 8PN) at 30 mg/kg/day or with 17β-oestradiol (OVX + OE) at 0.01 mg/kg/day, or with vehicle only (OVX). Another group of rats was sham-operated, i.e. subjected to ovariectomy surgery without removing the ovaries, and treated with the vehicle only (sham). After 2 weeks of treatment, 24-hour urine samples were collected and body weight gain, uterine weight and bone mineral density were determined. The uterine weights of sham and OVX + 8PN rats were found to be 165% higher (p<0.001), and of OVX + OE rats 235% higher (p<0.001), than those of OVX rats. Body weight gains of sham, OVX + OE and OVX + 8PN were significantly lower (p<0.05) than those of OVX rats. Urinary excretion of hydroxyproline (a conventional marker of bone resorption) was 1.62 µg/g/day from OVX rats compared to 1.18 and 1.16 µg/g/day for sham and OVX + OE rats respectively (p<0.01), and 1.01 µg/g/day from OVX + 8PN rats (p<0.001). The levels of urinary hydroxypyridinium crosslinks (assayed as pyridinoline and deoxy-

pyridinoline), which are recognized to be directly related to bone matrix degradation, were significantly lower in sham rats (p<0.01), and in OVX + OE and OVX + 8PN rats (p<0.001), than in OVX rats. Bone mineral densities of 139.1, 141.9 and 141.9 mg/cm^2 in sham, OVX + OE and OVX + 8PN rats, respectively, were significantly higher (p<0.001) than that in OVX rats (132.1 mg/cm^2). It was concluded that 8-prenylnaringenin functions as an oestrogen receptor agonist in reproductive tissues and that the dosage used had completely prevented ovariectomy-induced bone loss [40].

It should be noted, however, that (as summarized in the *in vitro* section) xanthohumol and especially humulone, neither of which has oestrogenic activity, also appear to be inhibitors of bone resorption [32]. If this finding can be corroborated, it may indicate that the inhibition of bone resorption is not associated with oestrogenicity [3].

Anti-inflammatory effects
A dry methanolic extract of hop strobile, applied topically at 2 mg/ear, inhibited 12-O-tetradecanoyl-phorbol-13-acetate (TPA)-induced ear oedema in mice by 90% (p<0.01) six hours after TPA treatment. Humulone, isolated from hop strobile by bioassay-guided fractionation and identified as an anti-inflammatory constituent, inhibited the oedema with an ID_{50} of 0.2 mg/ear (ID = inhibitory dose) [41]. Topically-applied humulone also inhibited arachidonic acid-induced inflammatory ear oedema in mice with an ID_{50} of 2.2 mg/ear (p<0.01 against controls) compared to 0.4 mg/ear (p<0.01) for indometacin [42].

Inhibition of tumour promotion
Humulone applied topically at 1 mg/mouse to the backs of mice markedly inhibited the tumour-promoting effect of TPA on 7,12-dimethylbenz[a]-anthracene-initiated skin tumour formation. In the control group 100% of mice developed tumours (first tumour appeared in week 6), compared to only 7% in the humulone-treated group (first appearance in week 16). Humulone treatment resulted in a 99% reduction in the average number of tumours per mouse at week 18 (p<0.01) [42].

Clinical studies
In a placebo-controlled study, 20 patients experiencing hot flushes due to ovarian insufficiency (15 in the menopausal phase and 5 following ovariectomy) were treated with a dry aqueous extract of hop strobile (5:1), initially at 1.6-2.6 g/day, later reduced in some cases to 1.2-1.6 g/day. 5 other patients received placebo. Assessment was based on scores calculated by multiplying the intensity of hot flushes (scale of 1 to 3) by their frequency (scale of 1 to 9). In verum patients, the initial average score of 22.7 decreased to 8.2 after 30 days of treatment, whereas

in the placebo group the initial score of 20 decreased only to 18. Compared to the placebo group, 76% of the verum patients achieved a statistically significant improvement in scores and 7 out of 20 patients achieved a reduction in score of at least 15 points [43].

Pharmacokinetic properties
No data available.

Preclinical safety data
Toxicity data on hop strobile are unavailable but, as an ingredient extensively used in the brewing industry, it is generally considered to lack toxicity.

In the Ames mutagenicity test, a hydroethanolic extract of hop strobile showed weakly mutagenic potential in *Salmonella typhimurium* strains TA 98 and TA 100, with or without activation [44].

Oestrogenic effects of hop strobile, and particularly of the potent constituent 8-prenylnaringenin, have been demonstrated, as summarized above. If hop strobile or extracts were consumed in sufficient amount, these effects could potentially be beneficial or undesirable depending on the circumstances. The content of 8-prenylnaringenin has been determined as 26-58 ppm in hop strobile, 1-13 ppm in carbon dioxide extracts of hop strobile used in brewing, 0.009-0.021 ppm in ales, and undetectable to 0.009 ppm in lagers [15]. Subcutaneous administration of 8-prenylnaringenin to rats for 2 weeks at 30 mg/kg/day produced no overt signs of toxicity [40].

REFERENCES

1. Hop strobile - Lupuli flos. European Pharmacopoeia, Council of Europe.

2. Verzele M. Centenary review: 100 years of hop chemistry and its relevance to brewing. J Inst Brew 1986;92:32-48.

3. De Keukeleire D, De Cooman L, Rong H, Heyerick A, Kalita J, Milligan SR. Functional properties of hop polyphenols. In: Gross GG, Hemingway RW, Yoshida T, editors. Plant Polyphenols 2: Chemistry, Biology, Pharmacology, Ecology. New York: Kluwer Academic/ Plenum Publishers, 1999:739-60.

4. Wohlfart R. Humulus. In: Hänsel R, Keller K, Rimpler H, Schneider G, editors. Hagers Handbuch der pharmazeutischen Praxis, 5th ed. Volume 5, Drogen E-O. Berlin: Springer-Verlag, 1993:447-58.

5. Hölzl J. Inhaltsstoffe des Hopfens (*Humulus lupulus* L.). Z Phytotherapie 1992;13:155-61.

6. Hänsel R, Schulz J. Hopfen und Hopfenpräparate: Fragen zur pharmazeutischen Qualität. Dtsch Apoth Ztg 1986;126:2033-7.

7. Eri S, Khoo BK, Lech J, Hartman TG. Direct thermal desorption-gas chromatography and gas chromatography-mass spectrometry profiling of hop (*Humulus lupulus* L.) essential oils in support of varietal characterization. J Agric Food Chem 2000;48:1140-9.

8. Hänsel R, Wohlfart R, Schmidt H. Nachweis sedativ-hypnotischer Wirkstoffe im Hopfen. 3. Mitteilung: Der Gehalt von Hopfen und Hopfenzubereitungen an 2-Methyl-3-buten-2-ol. Planta Med 1982;45:224-8.

9. Wohlfart R, Wurm G, Hänsel R, Schmidt H. Nachweis sedativ-hypnotischer Wirkstoffe im Hopfen. 5. Mitteilung: Der Abbau der Bittersäuren zum 2-Methyl-3-buten-2-ol, einem Hopfeninhaltsstoff mit sedativ-hypnotischer Wirkung. Arch Pharm (Weinheim) 1983;316:132-7.

10. McMurrough I. High-performance liquid chromatography of flavonoids in barley and hops. J Chromatogr 1981;218:683-93.

11. De Cooman L, Everaert E, De Keukeleire D. Quantitative analysis of hop acids, essential oils and flavonoids as a clue to the identification of hop varieties. Phytochem Analysis 1998;9:145-50.

12. Stevens JF, Taylor AW, Nickerson GB, Ivancic M, Henning J, Haunold A, Deinzer ML. Prenylflavonoid variation in *Humulus lupulus*: distribution and taxonomic significance of xanthogalenol and 4'-O-methylxanthohumol. Phytochemistry 2000;53:759-75.

13. Stevens JF, Ivancic M, Hsu VL, Deinzer ML. Prenyl-flavonoids from *Humulus lupulus*. Phytochemistry 1997;44:1575-85.

14. Stevens JF, Taylor AW, Deinzer ML. Quantitative analysis of xanthohumol and related prenylflavonoids in hops and beer by liquid chromatography-tandem mass spectrometry. J Chromatogr A 1999;832:97-107.

15. Rong H, Zhao Y, Lazou K, De Keukeleire D, Milligan SR, Sandra P. Quantitation of 8-prenylnaringenin, a novel phytoestrogen in hops (*Humulus lupulus* L.), hop products and beers, by benchtop HPLC-MS using electrospray ionization. Chromatographia 2000; 51:545-52.

16. Milligan SR, Kalita JC, Pocock V, van de Kauter V, Stevens JF, Deinzer ML et al. The endocrine activities of 8-prenylnaringenin and related hop (*Humulus lupulus* L.) flavonoids. J Clin Endocrinol Metab 2000;85:4912-5.

17. Schilcher H. Pflanzliche Psychopharmaka. Eine neue Klassifizierung nach Indikationsgruppen. Dtsch Apoth Ztg 1995;135:1811-22.

18. Hänsel R. Pflanzliche Beruhigungsmittel. Möglichkeiten und Grenzen in der Selbstmedikation. Dtsch Apoth Ztg 1995;135:2935-43.

19. Wichtl M. Lupuli strobulus - Hopfenzapfen. In: Wichtl M, editor. Teedrogen, 3rd ed. Stuttgart: Wissenschaftliche Verlagsgesellschaft, 1997:356-9.

20. Humulus. In: British Herbal Pharmacopoeia 1983. Bournemouth: British Herbal Medicine Association, 1983:111-2.

21. Schilcher H. Sedatives. In: Phytotherapy in Paediatrics. Handbook for Physicians and Pharmacists (translation of Phytotherapie in der Kinderheilkunde, 2nd ed.). Stuttgart: Medpharm Scientific, 1997:58-62.

22. De Keukeleire D, Milligan SR, De Cooman L, Heyerick A. The oestrogenic activity of hops (*Humulus lupulus* L.) revisited. Pharm Pharmacol Lett 1997;2/3:83-6.

23. Zava DT, Dollbaum CM, Blen M. Estrogen and progestin bioactivity of foods, herbs and spices. Proc Soc Exp Biol Med 1998;217:369-78.

24. Dixon-Shanies D, Shaikh N. Growth inhibition of human breast cancer cells by herbs and phytoestrogens. Oncol Rep 1999;6:1383-7.

25. Okamoto R, Kumai A. Antigonadotropic activity of hop extract. Acta Endocrinol 1992;127:371-7.

26. Milligan SR, Kalita JC, Heyerick A, Rong H, De Cooman L, De Keukeleire D. Identification of a potent phytoestrogen in hops (*Humulus lupulus* L.) and beer. J Clin Endocrinol Metab 1999;63:2249-52.

27. Kitaoka M, Kadokawa H, Sugano M, Ichikawa K, Taki M, Takaishi S et al. Prenylflavonoids: a new class of non-steroidal phytoestrogen (Part 1). Isolation of 8-isopentenylnaringenin and an initial study on its structure-activity relationship. Planta Med 1998; 64:511-5.

28. Miranda CL, Stevens JF, Helmrich A, Henderson MC, Rodriguez RJ, Yang Y-H et al. Antiproliferative and cytotoxic effects of prenylated flavonoids from hops (*Humulus lupulus*) in human cancer cell lines. Food Chem Toxicol 1999;37:271-85.

29. Caujolle F, Pham Huu Chanh, Duch-Kan P, Bravo Diaz L. Etude de l'action spasmolytique du houblon (*Humulus lupulus*, Cannabinacées). Agressologie 1969;10:405-10.

30. Rauha J-P, Tammela P, Summanen J, Vuorela P, Kähkönen M, Heinonen M et al. Actions of some plant extracts containing flavonoids and other phenolic compounds on calcium fluxes in clonal rat pituitary GH_4C_1 cells. Pharm Pharmacol Lett 1999;9:66-9.

31. Tabata N, Ito M, Tomoda H, Omura S. Xanthohumols, diacylglycerol acyltransferase inhibitors from *Humulus lupulus*. Phytochemistry 1997;46:683-7.

32. Tobe H, Muraki Y, Kitamura K, Komiyama O, Sato Y,

Sugioka T et al. Bone resorption inhibitors from hop extract. Biosci Biotech Biochem 1997;61:158-9.

33. Henderson MC, Miranda CL, Stevens JF, Deinzer ML, Buhler DR. *In vitro* inhibition of human P450 enzymes by prenylated flavonoids from hops, *Humulus lupulus*. Xenobiotica 2000;30:235-51.

34. Lee KM, Jung JS, Song DK, Kim YH. Neuropharmacological activity of *Humulus lupulus* extracts. Korean J Pharmacogn 1993;24:231-4.

35. Lee KM, Jung JS, Song DK, Kräuter M, Kim YH. Effects of *Humulus lupulus* extract on the central nervous system in mice. Planta Med 1993;59 (Suppl):A691.

36. Hänsel R, Wohlfart R, Coper H. Versuche, sedativ-hypnotische Wirkstoffe im Hopfen nachzuweisen. II. Narcotic action of 2-methyl-3-butene-2-ol, contained in the exhalation of hops. Z Naturforsch 1980;35c:1096-7.

37. Wohlfart R, Hänsel R, Schmidt H. Nachweis sedativ-hypnotischer Wirkstoffe im Hopfen. 4. Mitteilung: Die Pharmakologie des Hopfeninhaltsstoffes 2-Methyl-3-buten-2-ol. Planta Med 1983;48:120-3.

38. Wohlfart R. Wirkstoffprobleme des Hopfens. Z Phytotherapie 1982;3:393-5.

39. Kumai A, Okamoto R. Extraction of the hormonal substance from hop. Toxicol Lett 1984;21:203-7.

40. Miyamoto M, Matsushita Y, Kiyokawa A, Fukuda C, Iijima Y, Sugano M, Akiyama T. Prenylflavonoids: A new class of non-steroidal phytoestrogen (Part 2). Estrogenic effects of 8-isopentenylnaringenin on bone metabolism. Planta Med 1998;64:516-9.

41. Yasukawa K, Yamaguchi A, Arita J, Sakurai S, Ikeda A, Takido M. Inhibitory effect of edible plant extracts on 12-*O*-tetradecanoylphorbol-13-acetate-induced ear oedema in mice. Phytother Res 1993;7:185-9.

42. Yasukawa K, Takeuchi M, Takido M. Humulon, a bitter in the hop, inhibits tumor promotion by 12-O-tetra-decanoylphorbol-13-acetate in two-stage carcinogenesis in mouse skin. Oncology (Basel) 1995;52:156-8.

43. Goetz P. Traitement des bouffées de chaleur par insuffisance ovarienne par l'extrait de houblon (Humulus lupulus). Revue de Phytothérapie Pratique 1990;(4):13-15.

44. Göggelmann W, Schimmer O. Mutagenic activity of phytotherapeutical drugs. In: Knudsen I, editor. Genetic Toxicology of the Diet. New York: Alan R. Liss, 1986:63-72.

MATRICARIAE FLOS

Matricaria Flower

DEFINITION

Matricaria flower consists of the dried flower-heads of *Matricaria recutita* L. [*Chamomilla recutita* (L.) Rauschert]. It contains not less than 4 ml/kg of blue essential oil.

The material complies with the monograph of the European Pharmacopoeia [1].

Fresh material may also be used provided that when dried it complies with the monograph of the European Pharmacopoeia.

CONSTITUENTS

The main characteristic constituents of matricaria flower are the essential oil (0.5-1.5%) and flavone derivatives [2-6] such as apigenin-7-glucoside (approx. 0.5%) [2].

The essential oil contains approximately 50% of the sesquiterpenes (–)-α-bisabolol and its oxides A, B and C [6], bisabolonoxide A, up to 25% of *cis*- and *trans*-en-yn-dicycloethers (or spiroethers) [2] and matricin, which is converted to chamazulene on distillation (up to 15%) [2].

Other constituents of matricaria flower include coumarins (herniarin and umbelliferone) [2-4,6], phenolic acids [2,3,6] and polysaccharides (up to 10%) [2,3,6,7].

CLINICAL PARTICULARS

Therapeutic indications

Internal use
Symptomatic treatment of gastrointestinal complaints such as minor spasms, epigastric distension, flatulence and belching [2,5,8-14].

External use
Minor inflammation and irritations of skin and mucosa, including the oral cavity and the gums (mouth washes), the respiratory tract (inhalations) and the anal and genital area (baths, ointments) [8,11,14-29].

Posology and method of administration

Dosage

Internal use
Adults: As a tea infusion: 3 g of the drug to 150 ml of hot water, three to four times daily.
Fluid extract (1:2; 50% ethanol as preferred extraction solvent): 3-6 ml daily [2,30].
Dry extract: 50-300 mg three times daily [31].
Elderly: dose as for adults.
Children: Proportion of adult dose according to age or body weight.

External use
For compresses, rinses or gargles: 3-10% m/V infusion or 1% V/V fluid extract or 5% V/V tincture [2,31].
For baths: 5 g of the drug, or 0.8 g of alcoholic extract, per litre of water [2].
For solid and semi-solid preparations: hydroalcoholic extracts corresponding to 3-10% m/m of the drug [4,5].
For vapour inhalation: 10-20 ml of alcoholic extract per litre of hot water [28].

Method of administration
For oral administration, local application and inhalation.

Duration of administration
No restriction.

Contra-indications
Sensitivity to *Matricaria* or other members of the Compositae.

Special warnings and special precautions for use
None required.

Interaction with other medicaments and other forms of interaction
None reported.

Pregnancy and lactation
No harmful effects reported.

Effects on ability to drive and use machines
None known.

Undesirable effects
Rare cases of contact allergy have been reported in persons with known allergy to *Artemisia* species [6]. Matricaria flower of the bisabolol oxide B-type can contain traces of the contact allergen anthecotulide [6,14,32]. Matricaria possesses a much lower allergenic potential than other chamomile species and therefore allergic reactions to matricaria must be considered as extremely rare. Most of the described allergic reactions to matricaria were due to contamination with *Anthemis cotula* or related species,

which contain high amounts of anthecotulide. However, in cases where matricaria contact allergy has been acquired, cross-reactions to other sesquiterpene lactone-containing plants are common [32,33].

Overdose
No toxic effects reported.

PHARMACOLOGICAL PROPERTIES

Pharmacodynamic properties

Anti-inflammatory effects

In vitro experiments
Ethanolic (48% V/V) and isopropanolic (48% V/V) extracts of matricaria flower inhibited 5-lipoxygenase, cyclooxygenase and the oxidation of arachidonic acid with IC_{50} values of 0.05-0.3%, while a super-critical carbon dioxide extract had an IC_{50} of 6-25 µg/ml for these activities [34]. Investigation of individual constituents revealed that apigenin inhibited 5- and 12-lipoxygenase (IC_{50}: 8 and 90 µM respectively); chamazulene and (–)-α-bisabolol inhibited only 5-lipoxygenase (IC_{50}: 13 and 40 µM respectively); apigenin, *cis*-en-yn-spiroether and (–)-α-bisabolol inhibited cyclooxygenase (IC_{50}: 70-80 µM); only chamazulene had antioxidative activity (IC_{50}: 2 µM) [34].

Trans-en-yn-dicycloether inhibited the provoked degranulation of rat mast cells in concentrations above 0.1 mM [35].

Apigenin markedly inhibited the transcriptional activation of cyclooxygenase (IC_{50}: 8.7 µM) and of nitric oxide synthase (IC_{50}: 3.1 µM) in lipo-polysaccharide-activated macrophages [36].

In vivo experiments
The anti-inflammatory effects of orally administered (–)-α-bisabolol have been demonstrated in carrageenan-induced rat paw oedema, adjuvant arthritis of the rat, ultraviolet-induced erythema of the guinea pig and yeast-induced fever of the rat [37]. In the carrageenan-induced rat paw oedema test the following ED_{50} values (mmol/kg) were obtained after oral administration: (–)-α-bisabolol 2.69, chamazulene 4.48, guaiazulene 4.59, matricin 2.69 and salicyl-amide 1.53 [38].

A dry extract prepared from infusion of 20 g of matricaria flower in 100 ml of 42% ethanol, applied topically at 750 µg/ear, inhibited croton oil-induced oedema of mouse ear by 23.4% compared to controls; benzydamine at 450 µg/ear showed comparable inhibition of 26.6% [39]. In the same test system, two polysaccharides from matricaria flower at 300 µg/ear inhibited oedema by 14% and 22% respectively [40].

Antispasmodic effects

In vitro experiments
A hydroethanolic extract of matricaria flower showed antispasmodic activity on isolated guinea pig ileum stimulated by various spasmogens. The ED_{50} (mg/ml) and the strength of activity relative to papaverine (= 1.0) respectively were 1.22 and 0.0011 with barium chloride, 1.15 and 0.0019 with histamine dihydrochloride, 2.24 and 0.00074 with bradykinin, and 2.54 and ca. 0.00062 with serotonin. Pure constituents were also investigated: with barium chloride, (–)-α-bisabolol (ED_{50}: 136 µg/ml) exhibited activity comparable to papaverine while apigenin (ED_{50}: 0.8 µg/ml) was more than 3 times as active [41].

Anti-ulcerogenic effect

In vivo experiments
The development of ulcers induced in rats by indometacin, stress or ethanol was inhibited by an orally administered extract of matricaria flower with an ED_{50} of 1 ml per rat and by (–)-α-bisabolol with an ED_{50} of 3.4 mg/kg body weight. These substances also reduced healing times for ulcers induced in rats by chemical stress (acetic acid) or heat coagulation [42].

Wound healing effects

In vivo experiments
The wound healing activity of azulene has been demonstrated in studies on the thermally damaged rat tail [43] and of matricaria flower constituents in accelerated healing of experimental injuries [44].

Sedative effects

In vitro experiments
Apigenin competitively inhibited the binding of flunitrazepam to the central benzodiazepine receptor (K_i = 4 µM) but had no effect on muscarinic receptors, $α_1$-adrenoreceptors or on the binding of muscimol to $GABA_A$ receptors [45].

HPLC fractions of a methanolic extract of matricaria flower were able to displace flunitrazepam from its receptors in rat cerebellar membranes, the ligand Ro 5-4864 from 'peripheral' benzodiazepine receptors in rat adrenal gland membranes and muscimol from GABA receptors in rat cortical membranes. This last activity is mainly due to GABA present in the fractions [46].

Apigenin inhibited the binding of Ro 15-1788, a specific ligand for central benzodiazepine receptors with an IC_{50} of 0.25 mM. Apigenin also reduced GABA-activated Cl^- currents on cultured cerebellar granule cells dose-dependently by 15 ± 3% (0.1 µM

apigenin), 24 ± 2% (1 µM apigenin) and 32 ± 4% (10 µM apigenin). This effect was blocked by co-application of Ro 15-1788 [47].

In vivo experiments
A sedative effect of matricaria flower was demonstrated through prolongation of hexobarbital-induced sleep, reduction of spontaneous mobility and reduction of explorative activity in mice [48,49].

Restriction stress-induced increases in plasma ACTH levels in normal and ovariectomized rats were decreased by administration of diazepam and inhalation of matricaria flower oil vapour. Inhaling the vapour induced greater decreases in plasma ACTH levels in ovariectomized rats than treatment with diazepam; this difference was not observed in normal rats. Furthermore, the inhalation of matricaria flower oil vapour induced a decrease in plasma ACTH level that was blocked by pretreatment with flumazenil, a potent and specific benzodiazepine receptor antagonist [50].

Apigenin (25 and 50 mg/kg) significantly reduced the time of latency ($p<0.05$) in the onset of picrotoxin-induced (6 and 8 mg/kg) convulsions [47]. Apigenin also reduced locomotor activity after intraperitoneal injection in rats (minimal effective dose: 25 mg/kg) but showed no anxiolytic, myorelaxant or anti-convulsant activity [51].

Antimicrobial effects
Matricaria flower oil exerted a bactericidal effect against Gram-positive bacteria and a fungicidal effect against *Candida albicans* at a concentration of 0.7% V/V. The oil was not active against Gram-negative bacteria even in concentrations as high as 8% V/V [52].

An infusion of matricaria flower, a hydroethanolic extract and pure herniarin exhibited antimicrobial activity against various bacteria and fungi in the presence of near UV light [53,54].

Pharmacological studies in humans

Anti-inflammatory effects
In a comparative open study involving 20 healthy volunteers with chemically-induced toxic dermatitis, the smoothing effect on the skin of an ointment containing matricaria flower extract was significantly superior ($p<0.01$) to that of 0.1% hydrocortisone acetate or the ointment base [55].

In an open study on 12 healthy subjects, a cream containing matricaria flower extract (20 mg/g) did not suppress UV-induced erythema but it reduced visual scores of skin redness in the adhesive tape stripping test (p = 0.0625) [56]. In an analogous study, the cream produced 69% of the effect of a hydrocortisone-

27-acetate ointment [57].

In a randomized, double-blind study, 25 healthy volunteers with UVB light-induced erythema were treated with various matricaria flower preparations, hydrocortisone cream or the respective vehicle. Ranking the preparations according to visual assessment scores and mean values from chromametry, a cream containing a hydroalcoholic extract of matricaria flower gave the best result [58].

Clinical studies

Anti-inflammatory effects
In a bilateral comparative study 161 patients with inflammatory dermatoses, who had been treated initially with 0.1% of diflucortolone valerate, were treated during maintenance therapy with a cream containing matricaria flower extract or one of three alternatives: 0.25% hydrocortisone, 0.75% fluocortin butyl ester or 5% bufexamac. The therapeutic results with the extract were equivalent to those of hydrocortisone and superior to those of fluocortin butyl ester and bufexamac [59].

In an open study involving 98 cancer patients, a matricaria flower extract preparation containing 50 mg of α-bisabolol and 150-300 mg of apigenin-7-glucoside per 100 g, applied three times daily, reduced oral mucositis caused by localized irradiation or systemic chemotherapy [60].

In a phase III double-blind, placebo-controlled study involving 164 patients, a mouth-wash containing matricaria flower extract did not decrease 5-fluorouracil-induced stomatitis [61].

In a randomized, partially double-blind, comparison study, 72 patients with medium-degree atopic eczema were treated with a cream containing a matricaria flower extract, or a 0.5% hydrocortisone cream or a placebo cream. After 2 weeks of treatment the matricaria cream proved superior to the hydrocortisone cream and marginally superior to the placebo cream with respect to the symptoms pruritus, erythema and desquamation [62].

Anti-inflammatory and antispasmodic effects
In an open multicentric study, 104 patients with gastrointestinal complaints such as gastritis, flatulence or minor spasms of the stomach were treated orally for 6 weeks with a matricaria flower extract preparation (standardized to 50 mg of α-bisabolol and 150-300 mg of apigenin-7-glucoside per 100 g) at a daily dose of 5 ml. Subjectively evaluated symptoms improved in all patients and disappeared in 44.2% of patients [63].

Wound healing effects
In an open study, 147 female patients episiotomized during childbirth were treated for 6 days with either an ointment containing matricaria flower extract or a 5% dexpanthenol cream. The healing effect of the two preparations was comparable [64].

In a randomized, double-blind, placebo-controlled study on 14 patients, weeping dermatoses following dermabrasion of tattoos were treated topically with a matricaria flower fluid extract preparation (standardized to 50 mg of α-bisabolol and 3 mg of chamazulene per 100 g). After 14 days the decrease in weeping wound area and the improvement in drying tendency were significant in the matricaria flower group (p<0.05) [15].

In a randomized, open, placebo-controlled study, 120 patients with second degree haemorrhoids were treated with rubber band ligature alone, rubber band ligature with anal dilator and vaseline, or rubber band ligature with anal dilator and an ointment containing matricaria flower extract. The last group showed the best results in amelioration of haemorrhage, itching, burning and oozing [29].

Pharmacokinetic properties
After cutaneous administration of $[^{14}C](-)-\alpha$-bisabolol on mice, 82% of the radioactivity was found in the urine [65,66].

Apigenin and luteolin are also readily absorbed by the skin. Skin penetration studies using hydroethanolic solutions of apigenin and luteolin on the upper arms of 9 healthy female volunteers gave steady state fluxes of 10.31 ng/min/cm^2 and 6.11 ng/min/cm^2 respectively [67].

After oral administration of apigenin-7-glucoside to rats, free apigenin was detected in the urine [68].

After oral administration of 40 ml of a hydroethanolic matricaria flower extract (containing 225.5 mg of apigenin 7-glucoside, 22.5 mg of apigenin and 15.1 mg of herniarin per 100 ml) to a female volunteer, no flavones could be detected in blood plasma nor in 24-hour urine, while herniarin was found in both (maximum plasma concentration of ca. 35 ng/ml; 0.324 mg in 24-hour urine) [69].

In germ-free rats no hydrolysis of flavone glycosides could be observed; obviously intestinal microflora can effect the cleavage of the glycosidic bonds [68,70]. Furthermore, orally administered apigenin was detected in the blood serum of animals [71].

Preclinical safety data
The acute oral LD_{50} of matricaria flower oil in rats and the acute dermal LD_{50} in rabbits exceeded 5 g/kg. No irritant effects of the oil were observed after application

to the skin of nude mice [72].

In a 48-hour patch test in volunteers, matricaria oil neither caused skin irritation nor were there any discernible sensitization reactions or phototoxic effects. Matricaria oil has been granted GRAS status by FEMA and is approved by the FDA for use in food and cosmetics [72].

The acute oral toxicity of $(-)$-α-bisabolol in mice and rats was found to be very low, the LD_{50} being about 15 ml/kg. A six-week subacute toxicity study showed that the lowest toxic oral dose of $(-)$-α-bisabolol in rats and dogs was between 1 and 2 ml/kg. Oral doses up to 1 ml/kg of $(-)$-α-bisabolol produced no discernible effects on the prenatal development of rats or rabbits. No malformations were found at any of the dose levels tested [73].

The acute intraperitoneal LD_{50} of *cis*- and *trans*-enyn-dicycloethers is 670 mg/kg [3]. In the Ames test, apigenin and an aqueous matricaria flower extract showed no mutagenic or toxic activity [74,75].

Allergenicity
Based on the fact that matricaria flower generally contains no, or only traces of, the sesquiterpene lactone anthecotulide and that millions of people come into contact with matricaria flower daily, allergic reactions due to matricaria flower can be considered to be extremely rare [32,76]. However, cross-reactions with other sesquiterpene lactone-containing plants are common [32]: 2 reports of a patient allergic to *Artemisia vulgaris* mention severe anaphylactic reactions following ingestion of matricaria flower infusions and after eye washing with similar infusions [77,78]; 18 of 24 patients with Compositae allergy were also allergic to an ether extract of matricaria flower [79]; 11 of 14 patients with Compositae allergy were allergic to an aqueous extract of matricaria flower [33]; 96 patients from 4800 showed contact hypersensitivity to an ethanolic matricaria flower extract [80]; 3 case reports mention an allergic reaction to matricaria flower and extract [81-83].

In a study of contact allergy performed with 540 type IV allergic patients, of whom some gave positive reactions to standard phytogenic allergens, none gave a positive reaction to an anthecotulide-free matricaria flower extract [84].

In a study with 830 patients with contact dermatitis only 1 patient gave a positive reaction to a matricaria flower extract and cream. Even a patient who was highly sensitive to *Anthemis cotula*, and another with oral allergy syndrome and hypersensitivity to many plants, tested negative [76].

These studies demonstrate the importance of using anthecotulide-free matricaria flower.

REFERENCES

1. Matricaria Flower - Matricariae flos. European Pharmacopoeia, Council of Europe.

2. Carle R. Chamomilla. In: Hänsel R, Keller K, Rimpler H, Schneider G, editors. Hagers Handbuch der Pharmazeutischen Praxis, 5th ed. Volume 4: Drogen A-D. Berlin: Springer-Verlag, 1992:817-31.

3. Ammon HPT, Kaul R. Kamille. Pharmakologie der Kamille und ihrer Inhaltsstoffe. Dtsch Apoth Ztg 1992;132 (Suppl.27):1-26.

4. Zwaving JH. Echte en roomse kamille, hun verschil en overeenkomst in samenstelling en toepassing. Pharm Weekbl 1982;117:157-65.

5. Hänsel R, Haas H. Kamillenblüten. In: Therapie mit Phytopharmaka. Berlin: Springer-Verlag, 1984:146-50, 270-1.

6. Schilcher H. Die Kamille - Handbuch für Ärzte, Apotheker und andere Naturwissenschaftler. Stuttgart: Wissenschaftliche Verlagsgesellschaft, 1987.

7. Fuller E, Franz G. Neues von den Kamillenpolysacchariden. Dtsch Apoth Ztg 1993;133:4224-7.

8. Weiß RF. Kamille - "Heilpflanze 1987". Kneipp-Blätter 1987;1:4-8.

9. Demling L. Erfahrungstherapie - späte Rechtfertigung. In: Demling L, Nasemann T, Rösch W, editors. Erfahrungstherapie - späte Rechtfertigung. Karlsruhe: G. Braun, 1975:1-8.

10. Hatzky K. Über die Anwendung der Kamille in der inneren Medizin als Chamomillysatum Bürger. Med Klin 1930;26:819-20.

11. Matzker J. Kamillentherapie - in der Praxis bewährt, naturwissenschaftlich begründet? In: Demling L, Nasemann T, Rösch W, editors. Erfahrungstherapie - späte Rechtfertigung. Karlsruhe: G. Braun, 1975:77-89.

12. Hoffmann HA. Kamillosan liquidum bei Dickdarmerkrankungen. Fortschritte der Therapie 1926; 5:156-7.

13. Reicher K. Zur Therapie der akuten und chronischen Dysenterie, Kolitis, Sigmoiditis und Proktitis. Münch Med Wschr 1925;7:261-2.

14. Willuhn G. Matricariae flos - Kamillenblüten. In: Wichtl M, editor. Teedrogen und Phytopharmaka. Ein Handbuch für die Praxis auf wissenschaftlicher Grundlage, 4th ed. Stuttgart: Wissenschaftliche Verlagsgesellschaft, 2002:369-73.

15. Glowania HJ, Raulin C, Swoboda M. Wirkung der Kamille in der Wundheilung - eine klinische Doppelblindstudie. Z Hautkr 1987;62:1262-71.

16. Isar HJ. Alte und neue Anwendungsmöglichkeiten der deutschen Kamille in der dermatologischen und urologischen Praxis. Dermatol Wschr 1930;21:712-5.

17. Katz R. Therapeutische Erfahrungen mit Kamillosan. Fortschr Med 1928;46:388-91.

18. Tissot HC. Über Kamillosan und Kamillosept. Schweiz Med Wschr 1929;39:992-3.

19. Schmid F. Kamillenwirkstoffe und deren Indikationen in der Kinderheilkunde. In: Demling L, Nasemann T, Rösch W, editors. Erfahrungstherapie - späte Rechtfertigung. Karlsruhe: G. Braun, 1975:43-6.

20. Riepelmeier F. Uber das Kamillenpräparat Kamillosan und seine Brauchbarkeit in der Hals-, Nasen- und Ohrenheilkunde. Monatsschr Ohrenheilkunde Laryngo-Rhinol 1933;67:483-7.

21. Münzel M. Okkulte Sinusitis des Kindes. Selecta 1975; 24:2258-60.

22. Nasemann T. Kamillosan in der Dermatologie. In: Demling L, Nasemann T, Rösch W, editors. Erfahrungstherapie - späte Rechtfertigung. Karlsruhe: G. Braun, 1975:49-53.

23. Latz B. Uber meine Erfahrungen mit Kamille in besonderer Anwendungsform. Fortschritte der Therapie 1927;22:796-9.

24. Borgatti E. Le emorroidi: considerazioni cliniche e terapeutiche. Clinica Terapeutica 1985;112:225-31.

25. Benetti C, Manganelli F. Esperienze cliniche sul trattamento farmacologico delle vaginiti con impiego di ECB lavanda vaginale. Minerva Ginecol 1985; 37:799-801.

26. Carle R, Isaac O. Die Kamille - Wirkung und Wirksamkeit. Ein Kommentar zur Monographie Matricariae flos (Kamillenblüten). Z Phytotherapie 1987;8:67-77.

27. Weiß RF. Moderne Pflanzenheilkunde. Neues über Heilpflanzen und ihre Anwendung in der Medizin, 7th ed. Bad Wörishofen: Kneipp-Verlag, 1982:15-21.

28. Saller R, Beschorner M, Hellenbrecht D, Bühring M. Dose-dependency of symptomatic relief of complaints by chamomile steam inhalation in patients with common cold. Eur J Pharmacol 1990;183:728-9.

29. Förster CF, Süssmann H-E, Patzelt-Wenczler R. Optimisierung der Barron-Ligaturbehandlung von Hämorrhoiden zweiten und dritten Grades durch therapeutische Troika. Schweiz Rundschau Med 1996; 85:1476-81.

30. Mills S, Bone K. German Chamomile - Matricaria recutita (L.) Rauschert. In: Principles and Practice of Phytotherapy. Edinburgh-London-New York: Churchill Livingstone, 2000:319-27.

31. van Hellemont J. In: Fytotherapeutisch compendium. Utrecht: Bohn, Scheltema & Holkema, 1988:369-73.

32. Hausen BM. Sesquiterpene lactones - Chamomilla recutita. In: De Smet PAGM, Keller K, Hänsel R, Chandler RF, editors. Adverse Effects of Herbal Drugs, Volume 1. Berlin: Springer-Verlag, 1992:243-8.

33. de Jong NW, Vermeulen AM, Gerth van Wijk R, de Groot H. Occupational allergy caused by flowers. Allergy 1998;53:204-9.

34. Ammon HPT, Sabieraj J. Mechanismus der antiphlogistischen Wirkung von Kamillenextrakten und -inhaltsstoffen. Dtsch Apoth Ztg 1996;136:1821-33.

35. Miller T, Wittstock U, Lindequist U, Teuscher E. Effects of some components of the essential oil of chamomile, Chamomilla recutita, on histamine release from rat mast cells. Planta Med 1996;62:60-1

36. Liang YC, Huang YT, Tsai SH, Lin-Shiau SY, Chen CF, Lin JK. Suppression of inducible cyclooxygenase and inducible nitric oxide synthase by apigenin and related flavonoids in mouse macrophages. Carcinogenesis 1999;20:1945-52.

37. Jakovlev V, Isaac O, Thiemer K, Kunde R. Pharmakologische Untersuchungen von Kamillen-Inhaltsstoffen. II. Neue Untersuchungen zur antiphlogistischen Wirkung des (–)-α-Bisabolols und der Bisabololoxide. Planta Med 1979;35:125-40.

38. Jakovlev V, Isaac O, Flaskamp E. Pharmakologische Untersuchungen von Kamillen-Inhaltsstoffen. VI. Untersuchungen zur antiphlogistischen Wirkung von Chamazulen und Matricin. Planta Med 1983;49:67-73.

39. Tubaro A, Zilli C, Redaelli C, Della Loggia R. Evaluation of antiinflammatory activity of a chamomile extract after topical application. Planta Med 1984; 51:359.

40. Füller E, Sosa S, Tubaro A, Franz G, Della Loggia R. Anti-inflammatory activity of Chamomilla polysaccharides. Planta Med 1993;59:A 666-7.

41. Achterrath-Tuckermann U, Kunde R, Flaskamp E, Isaac O, Thiemer K. Pharmakologische Untersuchungen von Kamillen-Inhaltsstoffen. V. Untersuchungen über die spasmolytische Wirkung von Kamillen-Inhaltsstoffen und von Kamillosan® am isolierten Meerschweinchen-Ileum. Planta Med 1980; 39:38-50.

42. Szelenyi I, Isaac O, Thiemer K. Pharmakologische Untersuchungen von Kamillen-Inhaltsstoffen. III. Tierexperimentelle Untersuchungen über die ulkusprotektive Wirkung der Kamille. Planta Med 1979;35:218-27.

43. Deininger R. Eine neue Methode zum Nachweis der entzündungswidrigen Wirkung des Azulens. Arzneim-Forsch/Drug Res 1956;6:394-5.

44. Zita C. Vliv cistých látek hermánkové silice na tepelné poáleniny. Cas Lek Cesk 1955;8:203-8.

45. Viola H, Wasowski C, Levi de Stein M, Wolfman C, Silveira R, Dajas F et al. Apigenin, a component of Matricaria recutita flowers, is a central benzodiazepine receptors-ligand with anxiolytic effects. Planta Med 1995;61:213-6.

46. Avallone R, Zanoli P, Corsi L, Cannazza G, Baraldi M. Benzodiazepine-like compounds and GABA in flower heads of Matricaria chamomilla. Phytotherapy Res

1996;10(Suppl.1):S177-9.

47. Avallone R, Zanoli P, Puia G, Kleinschnitz M, Schreier P, Baraldi M. Pharmacological profile of apigenin, a flavonoid isolated from *Matricaria chamomilla*. Biochem Pharmacol 2000;59:1387-94.

48. Della Loggia R, Tubaro A, Redaelli C. Valutazione dell'attività sul S.N.C. del topo di alcuni estratti vegetali e di una loro associazione. Riv Neurol 1981; 51:297-310.

49. Della Loggia R, Traversa U, Scarica V, Tubaro A. Depressive effects of *Chamomilla recutita* (L.) Rauschert, tubular flowers, on central nervous system in mice. Pharmacol Res Commun 1982;14:153-62.

50. Yamada K, Miura T, Mimaki Y, Sashida Y. Effect of inhalation of chamomile oil vapour on plasma ACTH level in ovariectomized rat under restriction stress. Biol Pharm Bull 1996;19:1244-6.

51. Zanoli P, Avallone R, Baraldi M. Behavioral characterisation of the flavonoids apigenin and chrysin. Fitoterapia 2000;71(Suppl 1):S117-23.

52. Aggag ME, Yousef RT. Study of antimicrobial activity of chamomile oil. Planta Med 1972;22:140-4.

53. Ceska O, Chaudhary SK, Warrington PJ, Ashwood-Smith MJ. Coumarins of chamomile, *Chamomilla recutita*. Fitoterapia 1992;63:387-94.

54. Mares D, Romagnoli C, Bruni A. Antidermatophytic activity of herniarin in preparations of *Chamomilla recutita* (L.) Rauschert. Plantes Méd Phytothér 1993; 26:91-100.

55. Nissen HP, Biltz H, Kreysel HW. Profilometry. A new method to evaluate the therapeutic efficacy of Kamillosan® ointment. Z Hautkr 1988;63:184-90.

56. Korting HC, Schäfer-Korting M, Hart H, Laux P, Schmid M. Anti-inflammatory activity of hamamelis distillate applied topically to the skin. Eur J Clin Pharmacol 1993;44:315-8.

57. Albring M, Albrecht H, Alcorn G, Lücker PW. The measuring of the antiinflammatory effect of a compound on the skin of volunteers. Meth Find Exp Clin Pharmacol 1983;5:575-7.

58. Kerscher MJ. Influence of liposomal encapsulation on the activity of a herbal non-steroidal anti-inflammatory drug. In: Braun-Falco O, Korting HC, Maibach HI, editors. Liposome Dermatics. Berlin: Springer-Verlag, 1992:329-37.

59. Aertgeerts P, Albring M, Klaschka F, Nasemann T, Patzelt-Wenczler R, Rauhut K, Weigl B. Vergleichende Prüfung von Kamillosan® Creme gegenüber steroidalen (0,25% Hydrocortison, 0,75% Fluocortinbutylester) und nichtsteroidalen (5% Bufexamac) Externa in der Erhaltungstherapie von Ekzemerkrankungen. Z Hautkr 1985;60:270-7.

60. Carl W. Oral complications of cancer treatment and their management. In: Rao RS, Deo MG, Sanghvi LD,

editors. Proceedings of International Cancer Congress, New Delhi, 1994:981-6.

61. Fidler P, Loprinzi CL, O'Fallon JR, Leitch JM, Lee JK, Hayes DL et al. Prospective evaluation of a chamomile mouthwash for prevention of 5-FU-induced oral mucositis. Cancer 1996;77:522-5.

62. Patzelt-Wenczler R, Ponce-Pöschl E. Proof of efficacy of Kamillosan cream in atopic eczema. Eur J Med Res 2000;5:171-5.

63. Stiegelmeyer H. Therapie unspezifischer Magenbeschwerden mit Kamillosan®. Kassenarzt 1978; 18:3605-6.

64. Kaltenbach F-J. Antiphlogistische Wirkung von Kamillosan® Salbe im Vergleich zu einer nichtsteroidalen Salbe bei Episiotomien. In: Nasemann T, Patzelt-Wenczler R, editors. Kamillosan® im Spiegel der Literatur. Frankfurt: pmi Verlag, 1991:85-6.

65. Hahn B, Hölzl J. Resorption, Verteilung und Metabolismus von [^{14}C]-Levomenol in der Haut. Arzneim-Forsch/Drug Res 1987;37:716-20.

66. Hölzl E, Hahn B. Präparation von [^{14}C](–)-α-Bisabolol mit *Chamomilla recutita* (L.) Rauschert. Einsatz zur Untersuchung der dermalen und transdermalen Absorption. Dtsch Apoth Ztg 1985;125(Suppl I):32-8.

67. Merfort I, Heilmann J, Hagedorn-Leweke U, Lippold BC. *In vivo* skin penetration studies of camomile flavones. Pharmazie 1994;49:509-11.

68. Griffiths LA, Smith GE. Metabolism of apigenin and related compounds in the rat. Metabolite formation *in vivo* and by the intestinal microflora *in vitro*. Biochem J 1972;128:901-11.

69. Tschiersch K, Hölzl J. Resorption und Ausscheidung von Apigenin, Apigenin-7-glucosid und Herniarin nach peroraler Gabe eines Extrakts von *Matricaria recutita* (L.) [syn. *Chamomilla recutita* (L.) Rauschert]. Pharmazie 1993;48:554-5.

70. Griffiths LA, Barrow A. Metabolism of flavonoid compounds in germ-free rats. Biochem J 1972;130: 1161-2.

71. Redaelli C, Formentini L, Santaniello E. HPLC-determination of apigenin in natural samples, chamomile extracts and blood serum [Poster]. Int. Res. Congress on Natural Products and Medicinal Agents, Strasbourg, 1980.

72. Opdyke DLJ. Monographs on fragrance raw materials: Chamomile oil, German. Food Cosmet Toxicol 1974; 12:851.

73. Habersang S, Leuschner F, Isaac O, Thiemer K. Pharmakologische Untersuchungen von Kamillen-Inhaltsstoffen. IV. Untersuchungen zur Toxizität des (–)-α-Bisabolols. Planta Med 1979;37:115-23.

74. Rivera IG, Martins MT, Sanchez PS, Sato MIZ, Coelho MCL, Akisue M, Akisue G. Genotoxicity assessment through the Ames test of medicinal plants commonly

used in Brazil. Environ Toxicol Water Quality 1994; 9:87-93.

75. Birt DF, Walker B, Tibbels MG, Bresnick E. Antimutagenesis and anti-promotion by apigenin, robinetin and indole-3-carbinol. Carcinogenesis 1986;7:959-63.

76. Rudzki E, Jablonska S. Kamillosan is a safe product of camomile for topical application: result of patch testing consecutive patients with contact dermatitis. J Dermatol Treatm 2000;11:161-3.

77. Sánchez Palacios A. Reacción anafiláctica tras infusión de manzanilla en una paciente con alergia a *Artemisia vulgaris*. Rev Esp Alergol Immunol Clin 1992;7:37-9.

78. Foti C, Nettis E, Panebianco R, Cassano N, Diaferio A, Pia DP. Contact urticaria from *Matricaria chamomilla*. Contact Dermatitis 2000;42:360-1.

79. Paulsen E, Andersen KE, Hausen BM. Compositae dermatitis in a Danish dermatology department in one year. I. Results of routine patch testing with sesquiterpene

lactone mix supplemented with aimed patch testing with extracts and sesquiterpene lactones of Compositae plants. Contact Dermatitis 1993;29:6-10.

80. Dastychová E, Záhejský J. Kontaktní precitlivelost na hermánek. Ceskosl Dermatol 1992;67:14-8.

81. Rudzki E, Rebandel P. Positive patch test with Kamillosan in a patient with hypersensitivity to camomile. Contact Dermatitis 1998;38:164.

82. Jensen-Jarolim E, Reider N, Fritsch R, Breiteneder H. Fatal outcome of anaphylaxis to camomile-containing enema during labor: a case study. J Allergy Clin Immunol 1998;102:1041-2.

83. Rodriguez-Serna M, Sánchez-Motilla JM, Ramón R, Aliaga A. Allergic and systemic contact dermatitis from *Matricaria chamomilla* tea. Contact Dermatitis 1998; 39:192-3.

84. Jablonska S, Rudzki E. Kamillosan® Konzentrat - ein nicht allergisierender Extrakt aus Kamille. Z Hautkr 1996;71:542-6.

MELILOTI HERBA

Melilot

DEFINITION

Melilot consists of the dried flowering tops of *Melilotus officinalis* Desr.

The material complies with the monograph of the Pharmacopée Française [1].

Fresh material may also be used provided that, when dried, it complies with the monograph of the Pharmacopée Française.

CONSTITUENTS

The main characteristic constituents are coumarin derivatives, especially melilotoside (*cis-o*-coumaric acid β-glucoside, approximately 0.5%) which lactonises to coumarin after hydrolysis [2,3,4]; free coumarin, 3,4-dihydrocoumarin (melilotin), scopoletin and umbelliferone are also present [5]. Other constituents include kaempferol and quercetin glycosides [5,6]; triterpene saponins based on soyasapogenols [6,7,8] and melilotigenin [9]; phenolic acids, principally melilotic acid (= *o*-dihydrocoumaric acid) and caffeic acid [10]; volatile compounds [11].

The pterocarpan medicarpin [12,13] and dicoumarol [5,13] are absent from properly dried melilot.

CLINICAL PARTICULARS

Therapeutic indications
Symptomatic treatment of problems related to varicose veins, such as painful and heavy legs, nocturnal cramps in the legs, itching and swelling [14,15].

Posology and method of administration

Dosage

Internal use
Drug or preparation corresponding to 3-30 mg of coumarin daily [16].

External use
Extracts in semi-solid preparations.

Method of administration
For oral administration and topical application.

Duration of administration
No restriction.
If symptoms persist or worsen, medical advice should

E/S/C/O/P
MONOGRAPHS
Second Edition

be sought.

Contra-indications
None known.

Special warnings and special precautions for use
None required.

Interaction with other medicaments and other forms of interaction
Internal use may potentiate the activity of anti-coagulants [17].

Pregnancy and lactation
No abnormalities have been observed [18]. In accordance with general medical practice, the product should not be used during pregnancy or lactation without medical advice.

Effects on ability to drive and use machines
None known.

Undesirable effects
In rare cases headaches have been reported after internal use [16].

Overdose
No toxic effects reported.

PHARMACOLOGICAL PROPERTIES

Pharmacodynamic properties

In vitro experiments
Experiments on isolated segments of lymph vessels from guinea pigs demonstrated that a preparation containing melilot extract (coumarin 1.5 mg/ml) and rutin (15 mg/ml) had a marked myotropic action at an optimal dilution of $1:10^8$; pure coumarin had a similar effect at a dilution of $1:10^7$. Rhythm and tone were activated so that pulse rate, vascular amplitude and tone of lymphatic vessels increased considerably; there was also a rhythmifying effect on hypotonic vessels [19].

In vivo experiments
In experiments on carrageenan-induced rat paw oedema, intraperitoneal pre-treatment of the animals with coumarin (50 mg/kg body weight) isolated from melilot reduced the oedema by 42% after 4 hours and 33% after 6 hours compared to normal saline solution. The anti-oedematous effect was comparable to that obtained with flufenamic acid (1.5 mg/kg, administered intraperitoneally) [20].

A purified aqueous fraction from melilot containing 76-82% of polysaccharides was administered orally to 55 male rats and 120 female mice. Two doses were tested: 50 and 500 µg/kg body weight, once daily for 30 days. Rats treated with the extract showed increases in physical work capacity, their swimming time increasing by 38.5% (p<0.001) as compared to control (being longest on day 10 after the start of treatment), and in body weight throughout the 30-day treatment period, at the end of which they weighed 19.8% more than the control (p<0.01). In mice treated with the extract, the state of the peripheral blood and immuno-competent organs (spleen and thymus) was examined in detail. Both extract doses (50 and 500 µg/kg) led to decreases in spleen weight and significant rises in thymus weight and in erythrocyte, leukocyte, and particularly lymphocyte counts in the peripheral blood [21].

Clinical studies

Venous insufficiency
A comparative study was conducted in three groups (20 persons receiving 200 mg of a dry extract of melilot daily, 15 persons treated by ozonotherapy and 20 treated by the combined therapy). Administration of the melilot extract for 15 days significantly reduced some symptoms of chronic venous insufficiency, such as oedema (p<0.0005), nocturnal cramps (p<0.05) and heavy legs (p<0.05) [15].

A number of studies involving a total of 1818 patients have shown positive effects in cases of venous insufficiency and phlebitis, with a standardised preparation containing a melilot extract (0.05% of coumarin) in combination with rutin [18,22,23].

Lymphoedema
A group of 25 women with lymphoedema of the upper limbs due to axillary lymphadenectomy for breast cancer received 20 mg/day of a melilot extract containing 20% of coumarin for 12 weeks. A marked decrease in limb volume was observed after 6 weeks [24].

Another clinical study included 21 patients according to the following scheme: 4 patients as controls, 3 patients dropped out, 14 received a dry extract of melilot containing 8 mg of coumarin daily for 6 months. The extract was effective in reducing lymphoedema in 11 patients. The median reduction in upper arm circumference was about 5% compared to initial values [25].

Mastalgia
A study in 31 women showed that a melilot extract (dose not stated), taken daily for two periods of 2 months with an interval of 1 month, was effective in the treatment of cyclic mastalgias in 23 of the cases [26].

Pharmacokinetic properties
In studies on human volunteers, coumarin admin-

istered orally as a dose of 0.857 mg/kg was rapidly absorbed, but only 2-6% reached systemic circulation in intact form. The rest of the dose appeared quantitatively in systemic circulation as the metabolites 7-hydroxycoumarin and its glucuronide, indicating an extensive first pass effect. The biological half-lives of coumarin and 7-hydroxycoumarin glucuronide were determined as 1.02 and 1.15 hours respectively. Approximately 90% of the dose was eliminated in the urine in the form of 7-hydroxycoumarin glucuronide [27].

It has been hypothesized that coumarin is the prodrug and 7-hydroxycoumarin (umbelliferone) the pharmacologically active moiety since the glucuronide, as a polar substance, should have no pharmacological activity [28].

Preclinical safety data

Acute toxicity
No data available for melilot. The intraperitoneal LD_{50} of a melilot/rutin preparation in mice was too high to be determined [29].
LD_{50} data for coumarin have been determined as follows:
In mice: oral, 196 mg/kg; intraperitoneal, 220 mg/kg; subcutaneous, 242 mg/kg.
In rats: oral, 293 mg/kg.
In guinea pigs: oral, 202 mg/kg [30].

Repeated dose toxicity
No data available.

Reproductive toxicity
The teratogenic effects of a combination of coumarin and rutin have been investigated in white New Zealand rabbits. Intravenous administration of either coumarin alone or a coumarin/rutin combination at 10 and 100 times the therapeutic dose during sensitive phases of foetal development did not result in any increase in malformation rates compared to controls. Treatment over a period of 13 days did not result in an increased number of resorptions or increased foetal mortality [31].

Clinical safety data
In a study in which 25 pregnant women were treated with a melilot/rutin preparation during their second and third trimesters, all the children were born normal [18].

REFERENCES

1.   Mélilot - Melilotus officinalis. Pharmacopée Française.

2.   Charaux MC. Sur le mélilotoside, glucoside générateur d'acide coumarique, extrait des fleurs de *Melilotus altissima* et de *Melilotus arvensis*. Bull Soc Chim Biol 1925;7:1056-9.

3.   Bézanger-Beauquesne L, Pinkas M, Torck M. *Melilotus officinalis* L. et autres espèces. In: Les plantes dans la thérapeutique moderne, 2nd ed. Paris: Maloine, 1986: 285.

4.   Galand N, Pothier J, Mason V, Viel C. Separation of flavonoids, coumarins and anthocyanins in plant extracts by overpressured layer chromatography. Pharmazie 1999;54:468-71.

5.   Hänsel R, Sticher O, Steinegger E. Steinkleekraut, Steinklee-Extrakte. In: Pharmakognosie - Phytopharmazie, 6th ed. Berlin: Springer-Verlag, 1999:802-4.

6.   Kang SS, Lim C-H, Lee SY. Soyasapogenols B and E from *Melilotus officinalis*. Arch Pharm Res 1987;10:9-13.

7.   Sutiashvili MG, Alaniya MD. Flavonoids of *Melilotus officinalis*. Khim Prir Soedin 1999:673-4 [Russian], translated into English as: Chem Nat Compd 1999; 35:584.

8.   Hirakawa T, Okawa M, Kinjo J, Nohara T. A new oleanene glucuronide obtained from the aerial parts of *Melilotus officinalis*. Chem Pharm Bull 2000;48:286-7.

9.   Kang SS, Woo WS. Melilotigenin, a new sapogenin from *Melilotus officinalis*. J Nat Prod 1988;51:335-8.

10. Dombrowicz E, Swiatek L, Guryn R, Zadernowski R. Phenolic acids in herb *Melilotus officinalis*. Pharmazie 1991;46:156-7.

11. Wörner M, Schreier P. Flüchtige Inhaltsstoffe aus Steinklee (*Melilotus officinalis* L. Lam.). Z Lebensm Unters Forsch 1990;190:425-8.

12. Ingham JL. Medicarpin as a phytoalexin of the genus *Melilotus*. Z Naturforsch 1977;32c:449-52.

13. Ingham JL. Phytoalexin production by high- and low-coumarin cultivars of *Melilotus alba* and *Melilotus officinalis*. Can J Bot 1978;56:2230-3.

14. Weiss RF, Fintelmann V. Lehrbuch der Phytotherapie, 8th ed. Stuttgart: Hippokrates, 1997:201-2.

15. Stefanini L, Gigli P, Galassi A, Pierallini F, Tillieci A, Scalabrino A. Trattamento farmacologico e/o balneoterapico dell'insufficienza venosa cronica. Gazz Med Ital 1996:155:179-85.

16. Bisset NG, editor (translated from Wichtl M, editor. Teedrogen). Meliloti herba. In: Herbal drugs and phytopharmaceuticals. A handbook for practice on a scientific basis. Stuttgart: Medpharm, Boca Raton-London: CRC Press, 1994: 326-8.

17. Arora RB, Mathur CN. Relationship between structure and anticoagulant activity of coumarin derivatives. Brit J Pharmacol 1963;20:29-35.

18. Leng JJ, Heugas-Darraspen JP, Fernon MJ. Le traitement

des varices au cours de la grossesse et dans le post-partum. Expérimentation clinique de l'Esberiven. Bordeaux med 1974;7:2755-6.

19. Mislin H. Die Wirkung von Cumarin aus *Melilotus officinalis* auf die Funktion des Lymphangions. Arzneim-Forsch/Drug Res 1971;21:852-3.

20. Földi-Börcsök E, Bedall FK, Rahlfs VW. Die antiphlogistische und ödemhemmende Wirkung von Cumarin aus *Melilotus officinalis*. Arzneim-Forsch/Drug Res 1971;21:2025-30.

21. Podkolzin AA, Dontsov VI, Sychev IA, Kobeleva GY, Kharchenko ON. Immunomodulating, anti-anemic and adaptogenic effects of polysaccharides from plaster clover (*Melilotus officinalis*). Byull Eksp Biol Med 1996;121:661-3, translated into English as: Bull Exp Biol Med 1996:597-9.

22. Babilliot J. Contribution au traitement de l'insuffisance veineuse par Esberiven. Etude multicentrique sur 385 cas. Gaz Med Fr 1980;87:3242-6.

23. Klein L. Tratamiento de las flebopatías con extracto de *Melilotus*. Pren méd argent 1967;54:1191-3.

24. Muraca MG, Baroncelli TA. I linfedemi degli arti superiori post-mastectomia. Trattamento con l'estratto di meliloto officinale. Gazz Med Ital - Arch Sci Med 1999;158:133-6.

25. Pastura G, Mesiti M, Saitta M, Romeo D, Settineri N,

Maisano R et al. Linfedema dell'arto superiore in pazienti operati per carcinoma della mamella: esperienza clinica con estratto cumarinico di Melilotus officinalis. Clin Ter 1999;150:403-8.

26. Mazzocchi B, Andrei A, Bonifazi VF, Algeri R. Trattamento con estratto di Melilotus officinalis della mastodinia ciclica e non ciclica delle donne afferenti presso un ambulatorio senologico. Gazz Med Ital - Arch Sci Med 1997;156:221-4.

27. Ritschel WA, Brady ME, Tan HSI, Hoffmann KA, Yiu IM, Grummich KW. Pharmacokinetics of coumarin and its 7-hydroxy-metabolites upon intravenous and peroral administration of coumarin in man. Eur J Clin Pharmacol 1977;12:457-61.

28. Ritschel WA, Brady ME, Tan HSI. First-pass effect of coumarin in man. Internat J Clin Pharmacol Biopharm 1979;17:99-103.

29. Shimamoto K, Takaori S. Pharmakologische Untersuchungen mit einem *Melilotus*-Extrakt. Arzneim-Forsch/Drug Res 1965;15:897-9.

30. Lewis RJ. Coumarin. In: Sax's Dangerous Properties of Industrial Materials, 8th ed. Volume 2. New York: Van Nostrand Reinhold, 1992:958.

31. Grote W, Weinmann I. Überprüfung der Wirkstoffe Cumarin und Rutin im teratologischen Versuch an Kaninchen. Arzneim-Forsch/Drug Res 1973;23:1319-20.

MELISSAE FOLIUM

Melissa Leaf

DEFINITION

Melissa leaf consists of the dried leaves of *Melissa officinalis* L. It contains not less than 4.0 per cent of total hydroxycinnamic derivatives expressed as rosmarinic acid ($C_{18}H_{16}O_8$; M_r 360.3), calculated with reference to the dried drug.

The material complies with the monograph of the European Pharmacopoeia [1].

Fresh material may be used provided that when dried it complies with the monograph of the European Pharmacopoeia.

CONSTITUENTS

The main constituents are: essential oil (0.06-0.375% V/m) [2] containing monoterpenoid aldehydes, mainly geranial (citral a), neral (citral b) and citronellal [3-6]; flavonoids including glycosides of luteolin, quercetin, apigenin and kaempferol [7-9]; monoterpene glycosides [10,11]; phenylpropanoids, including hydroxycinnamic acid derivatives such as caffeic and chlorogenic acids, and in particular rosmarinic acid (up to 4%) [12-15]; triterpenes including ursolic and oleanolic acids [9,14].

CLINICAL PARTICULARS

Therapeutic indications

Internal use
Tenseness, restlessness and irritability; symptomatic treatment of digestive disorders such as minor spasms [16,17].

External use
Herpes labialis (cold sores) [18-21].

Posology and method of administration

Dosage

Internal use
2-3 g of the drug as an infusion, two to three times daily [16,17]. Tincture (1:5 in 45% ethanol), 2-6 ml three times daily [20]. Other equivalent preparations.

External use
Cream containing 1% of a lyophilised aqueous extract (70:1) two to four times daily [18-21].

E/S/C/O/P
MONOGRAPHS
Second Edition

Method of administration
For oral administration or topical application.

Duration of administration

Internal use
No restriction.

External use in *Herpes labialis*
From prodromal signs to a few days after the healing of lesions.

Contra-indications
None reported.

Special warnings and special precautions for use
None required.

Interaction with other medicaments and other forms of interaction
None reported.

Pregnancy and lactation
No data available. In accordance with general medical practice the product should not be taken orally during pregnancy and lactation without medical advice.

Effects on ability to drive and use machines
None known.

Undesirable effects
None reported.

Overdose
No toxic effects reported.

PHARMACOLOGICAL PROPERTIES

Pharmacodynamic properties

In vitro experiments

Antispasmodic activity
Essential oil of melissa leaf showed spasmolytic activity when tested on isolated guinea pig ileum, rat duodenum and vas deferens, and on the jejunum and aorta of rabbits [22,23]. It also had relaxant effects on guinea pig tracheal muscle (EC_{50}: 22 mg/litre) and inhibited phasic contractions of an electrically-stimulated ileal myenteric plexus longitudinal muscle preparation (EC_{50}: 7.8 mg/litre) [24].

However, a hydroethanolic extract (1 part plant to 3.5 parts of ethanol 30% m/m) from melissa leaf at concentrations of 2.5 ml and 10 ml/litre did not show any significant antispasmodic activity when tested on acetylcholine- and histamine-induced contractions of guinea pig ileum [25].

Antiviral activity
Aqueous extracts exhibited antiviral activity against Newcastle disease virus, Semliki forest virus, influenza viruses, myxoviruses, vaccinia and *Herpes simplex* virus [26-29].

An aqueous extract from melissa leaf showed anti-HIV-1 activity (ED_{50}: 16 µg/ml). The active components in the extract were found to be polar substances. This extract also inhibited giant cell formation in co-culture of Molt-4 cells with and without HIV-1 infection and showed inhibitory activity against HIV-1 reverse transcriptase [30].

Anti-inflammatory activity
Rosmarinic acid has been shown to inhibit complement-dependent mechanisms of inflammatory reactions [31-33].

Antimicrobial activity
Melissa leaf essential oil was active against bacteria, filamentous fungi and yeasts [34].

Receptor-binding activity
Investigations were carried out to evaluate human CNS cholinergic receptor binding activity of an ethanolic extract of melissa leaf. The plant extract displaced [^{3}H]-(*N*)-nicotine and [^{3}H]-(*N*)-scopolamine from nicotinic and muscarinic receptors in homogenates of human cerebral cortical cell membranes ($IC_{50} < 1$ mg/ml). Choline, a weak nicotinic ligand (IC_{50}: 3×10^{-4} M), was found in melissa leaf extract at concentrations of 10^{-6} to 10^{-5} M. Melissa leaf extract had a high [^{3}H]-(N)-nicotine displacement value [35].

In a similar study in human occipital cortex tissue the IC_{50} for the displacement of [^{3}H]-(*N*)-nicotine and [^{3}H]-(*N*)-scopolamine from nicotinic and muscarinic receptors by a standardized extract (30% methanol; after evaporation the resulting soft extract was mixed with 10% of inert processing agents) were 11 mg/ml and 4 mg/ml respectively [36].

Antioxidant activity
Antioxidant and free radical scavenging properties have been reported for an aqueous extract [13,15,37-39]. 1,3-Benzodioxole isolated from a methanolic extract of melissa leaf has also been shown to have antioxidant activity [40].

In vivo experiments

Sedative effects
The sedative effect of a lyophilised hydroethanolic (30%) extract administered intraperitoneally to mice has been demonstrated by means of familiar (two compartment) and non-familiar (staircase) environment tests. The effect was dose-dependent up to 25 mg/kg body weight, the dose producing maximum

effects. Low doses (3-6 mg/kg) of the extract induced sleep in mice treated with an infra-hypnotic dose of pentobarbital and also prolonged pentobarbital-induced sleep. At high doses (400 mg/kg) a peripheral analgesic effect was noted in the acetic acid-induced writhing test, but no central analgesic effect was observed [41,42].

The essential oil administered intraperitoneally to mice had no effect in the staircase test nor was it active in prolonging pentobarbital-induced sleep [41]. When administered orally to mice it showed sedative and narcotic effects at doses of 3.16 mg/kg and higher [22].

Anti-inflammatory effects
Rosmarinic acid administered intravenously at 0.1-1 mg/kg inhibited cobra venom factor-induced rat paw oedema and exerted weak inhibition of carrageenan-induced paw oedema [32].

Other effects
An ethanolic liquid extract from melissa leaf was tested for its potential anti-ulcerogenic activity against indometacin-induced gastric ulcers in rats as well as for its antisecretory and cytoprotective activity. It showed dose-dependent anti-ulcerogenic activity at oral doses of 2.5-10 ml/kg associated with reduced acid output and increased mucin secretion, an increase in prostaglandin E_2 release and a decrease in leuko-trienes. The effect on pepsin content was rather variable and did not seem to bear a relationship to the anti-ulcerogenic activity. The anti-ulcerogenic activity of the extract was also confirmed histologically. Cytoprotective effects of the extract could be partly due to its flavonoid content and to its free radical scavenging activity [43].

Rosmarinic acid inhibited passive cutaneous anaphylaxis in the rat with ID_{50} values of 1 mg/kg (intravenous) and 10 mg/kg (intramuscular) [32].

When applied topically (5% in vehicle) to rhesus monkeys, rosmarinic acid reduced both gingival and plaque indices over a 3-week study compared to placebo (p<0.001) [44].

Pharmacological studies in humans
A randomized, double-blind, placebo-controlled, crossover study was carried out in 20 healthy volunteers (mean age 19.2 years). The participants attended 4 days of treatment, receiving a single dose of either placebo or 300, 600 or 900 mg of a standardized melissa leaf extract (30% methanol; after evaporation the resulting soft extract was mixed with 10% of inert processing agents). Each treatment day was followed by a 7-day wash-out period. On each treatment day cognitive performance was assessed in a pre-dose testing session (baseline) and 1, 2.5, 4 and 6 hours after treatment using the Cognitive

Drug Research computerised test battery and two serial subtraction tasks. Subjective mood was measured by Bond-Lader visual analogue scales. Significant improvement was observed for quality of attention at all times after a dose of 600 mg (p = 0.0001 to p = 0.049). Significant decreases in the quality of working memory and secondary memory were seen 2.5 and 4 hours after the higher doses (p = 0.0005 to p = 0.05). Reduction of working memory was more pronounced at 1 and 2.5 hours after the higher doses. Self-rated calmness was elevated significantly after 1 and 2.5 hours by the lowest dose (p = 0.01 to p = 0.05), while alertness was significantly reduced at all time points (p = 0.001 to p = 0.05) [36].

Clinical studies
A 4-week multicentre, double-blind, placebo-controlled study involved 72 patients of mean age 78.5 years with clinically significant agitation in the context of severe dementia. The patients were treated topically twice daily with a lotion containing 10% of melissa essential oil, providing a daily total of 200 mg of the oil (n = 36), or a placebo lotion (n = 36). Lotion was gently applied to the patient's face and both arms as an aromatherapy treatment. Changes in agitation were determined by the Cohen-Mansfield Agitation Inventory (CMAI) score. Improvements in the CMAI total score (35% reduction in the verum group and 11% in the placebo group) were significantly greater in the verum group (p<0.0001). A 30% improvement in CMAI score was attained by 21 subjects in the verum group compared to only 5 in the placebo group (p<0.0001). Quality of life indices measured by Dementia Care Mapping also improved significantly in the verum group; compared to the placebo group the percentage of time spent socially withdrawn was reduced (p<0.005) and time engaged in constructive activities increased (p<0.001) [45].

In a multicentre, open, controlled study involving 115 patients, a cream containing 1% of a lyophilised aqueous extract from melissa leaf (70:1) significantly reduced the healing time of cutaneous Herpes simplex lesions (p<0.01). It also significantly extended the intervals between recurrences of infection compared to other external virustatic preparations containing idoxuridine and tromantidine hydrochloride (p<0.01) [18,20]. These effects, particularly a significant reduction in the size of lesions within 5 days (p = 0.01), were confirmed in a multicentre, double-blind, placebo-controlled study on 116 patients [19,20].

A randomized, double-blind, placebo-controlled study was carried out using a cream containing 1% of a melissa leaf dry extract (70:1) standardized in terms of antiviral potency. Sixty-six patients with a history of recurrent Herpes simplex labialis (at least four episodes per year) were treated topically; 34 of them with verum cream and 32 with placebo. The cream was applied to the affected area 4 times daily over 5 days.

A symptom score (ranging between 0 and 9), derived by combination of the severity ratings for complaints, size of affected area and number of blisters on day 2 of therapy, was used as the primary target parameter. There was a significant difference ($p<0.05$) in scores for the primary target parameter between treatment groups: verum 4.03 ± 0.33 (3.0); placebo 4.94 ± 0.40 (5.0); values given are the mean $\pm$ SEM (median) of the symptom scores on day 2. The significant difference in symptom scores on the second day of treatment is of particular importance because the complaints in patients suffering from *Herpes labialis* are usually most intensive at that time [21].

Pharmacokinetic properties

No data available.

Preclinical safety data

Mutagenic activity

A tincture (ethanol 70%, 1:5) of melissa leaf gave negative results in the Ames test using *Salmonella typhimurium* TA 98 and TA 100 strains with or without metabolic activation [46]. No genotoxic effects from a 20% tincture of melissa leaf were detected in a somatic segregation assay using the diploid strain *Aspergillus nidulans* D-30 [47].

REFERENCES

1. Melissa Leaf - Melissae folium. European Pharmacopoeia, Council of Europe.

2. Tittel G, Wagner H, Bos R. Über die chemische Zusammensetzung von Melissenölen. Planta Med 1982;46:91-8.

3. Enjalbert F, Bessiere JM, Pellecuer J, Privat G, Doucet G. Analyse des essences de Mélisse. Fitoterapia 1983; 54:59-65.

4. Pellecuer J, Enjalbert F, Bessiere JM, Privat G. Contribution á l'étude de l'huile essentielle de mélisse: *Melissa officinalis* L. (Lamiacées). Plantes Méd Phytothér 1981;15:149-53.

5. Schultze W, Zänglein A, Klose R, Kubeczka K-H. Die Melisse. Dünnschichtchromatographische Untersuchung des ätherischen Öles. Dtsch Apoth Ztg 1989; 129:155-63.

6. Hänsel R, Sticher O, Steinegger E. Melissenblätter. In: Pharmakognosie - Phytopharmazie, 6th ed. Berlin-Heidelberg: Springer, 1999:708.

7. Mulkens A. Étude phytochimique des feuilles de *Melissa officinalis* L. (Lamiaceae) [Thesis]. Université de Genève: Faculté des Sciences, 1987: No. 2255.

8. Mulkens A, Kapetanidis I. Flavonoïdes des feuilles de *Melissa officinalis* L. (Lamiaceae). Pharm Acta Helv 1987;62:19-22.

9. Koch-Heitzmann I, Schultze W. 2000 Jahre *Melissa officinalis*. Von der Bienenpflanze zum Virustatikum. Z Phytotherapie 1988;9:77-85.

10. Mulkens A, Stephanou F, Kapetanidis I. Hétérosides á génines volatiles dans les feuilles de *Melissa officinalis* L. (Lamiaceae). Pharm Acta Helv 1985;60:276-8.

11. Baerheim Svendsen A, Merkx IJM. A simple method for screening of fresh plant material for glycosidic bound volatile compounds. Planta Med 1989;55:38-40.

12. Mulkens A, Kapetanidis I. Eugenylglucoside, a new natural phenylpropanoid heteroside from *Melissa officinalis*. J Nat Prod 1988;51:496-8.

13. Lamaison JL, Petitjean-Freytet C, Duband F, Carnat AP. Rosmarinic acid content and antioxidant activity in French Lamiaceae. Fitoterapia 1991;62:166-71.

14. Dorner WG. Die Melisse - immer noch zu Überraschungen fähig. Pharm unserer Zeit 1985;14:112-21.

15. Lamaison JL, Petitjean-Freytet C, Carnat A. Lamiacées médicinales á propriétés antioxydantes, sources potentielles d'acide rosmarinique. Pharm Acta Helv 1991;66:185-8.

16. Czygan FC. Melissenblätter. In: Wichtl M, editor. Teedrogen, 4th ed. Stuttgart: Wissenschaftliche Verlagsgesellschaft, 2002:382-6.

17. Weiss RF. Lehrbuch der Phytotherapie, 7th ed. Stuttgart: Hippokrates, 1991;66-9.

18. Wölbling RH, Milbradt R. Klinik und Therapie des Herpes simplex. Vorstellung eines neuen phytotherapeutischen Wirkstoffes. Therapiewoche 1984;34: 1193-1200.

19. Vogt H-J, Tausch I, Wölbling RH, Kaiser PM. Eine placebo-kontrollierte Doppelblind-Studie. Melissenextrakt bei Herpes simplex. Wirksamkeit und Verträglichkeit von Lomaherpan® Creme. Größte Effektivität bei frühzeitiger Behandlung. Der Allgemeinarzt 1991;13:832-41.

20. Wölbling RH, Leonhardt K. Local therapy of herpes simplex with dried extract from *Melissa officinalis*. Phytomedicine 1994;1:25-31.

21. Koytchev R, Alken RG, Dundarov S. Balm mint extract (Lo-701) for topical treatment of recurring Herpes labialis. Phytomedicine 1999;6:225-30.

22. Wagner H, Sprinkmeyer L. Über die pharmakologische Wirkung von Melissengeist. Dtsch Apoth Ztg 1973; 113:1159-66.

23. Debelmas AM, Rochat J. Étude pharmacologique des huiles essentielles. Activité antispasmodique etudiée sur une cinquantaine d'échantillons differents. Plantes Méd Phytothér 1967;1:23-7.

24. Reiter M, Brandt W. Relaxant effects on tracheal and

ileal smooth muscles of the guinea pig. Arzneim-Forsch/Drug Res 1985;35:408-14.

25. Forster HB, Niklas H, Lutz S. Antispasmodic effects of some medicinal plants. Planta Med 1980;40:309-19.

26. Vanden Berghe DA, Vlietinck AJ, Van Hoof L. Present status and prospects of plant products as antiviral agents. In: Vlietinck AJ, Dommisse RA, editors. Advances in Medicinal Plant Research. Stuttgart: Wissenschaftliche Verlagsgesellschaft, 1985,47-99.

27. König B, Dustmann JH. The caffeoylics as a new family of natural antiviral compounds. Naturwissenschaften 1985;72:659-61.

28. Kucera LS, Herrmann EC Jr. Antiviral substances in plants of the mint family (Labiatae). I. Tannin of *Melissa officinalis*. Proc Soc Exp Biol Med 1967;124: 865-9.

29. May G, Willuhn G. Antivirale Wirkung wäßriger Pflanzenextrakte in Gewebekulturen. Arzneim-Forsch/Drug Res 1978;28:1-7.

30. Yamasaki K, Nakano M, Kawahata T, Mori H, Otake T, Ueba N et al. Anti-HIV-1 activity of herbs in Labiatae. Biol Pharm Bull 1998;21:829-33.

31. Rampart M, Beetens JR, Bult H, Herman AG, Parnham MJ, Winkelmann J. Complement-dependent stimulation of prostacyclin biosynthesis; inhibition by rosmarinic acid. Biochem Pharmacol 1986;35:1397-1400.

32. Parnham MJ, Kesselring K. Rosmarinic acid. Drugs of the Future 1985;10:756-7.

33. Gracza L, Koch H, Löffler E. Isolierung von Rosmarinsäure aus *Symphytum officinale* und ihre anti-inflammatorische Wirksamkeit in einem In-vitro-Modell. Arch Pharm (Weinheim) 1985;318:1090-5.

34. Larrondo JV, Agut M, Calvo-Torras MA. Antimicrobial activity of essences from labiates. Microbios 1995; 82(332):171-2.

35. Wake G, Court J, Pickering A, Lewis R, Wilkins R, Perry E. CNS acetylcholine receptor activity in European medicinal plants traditionally used to improve failing memory. J Ethnopharmacol 2000;69:105-14.

36. Kennedy DO, Scholey AB, Tildesley NTJ, Perry EK, Wesnes KA. Modulation of mood and cognitive performance following acute administration of *Melissa officinalis* (lemon balm). Pharmacol Biochem Behav 2002;72:953-64.

37. Lamaison JL, Petitjean-Freytet C, Carnat A. Teneurs en acide rosmarinique, en dérivés hydroxycinnamiques totaux et activité antioxydante chez les Apiacées, les Borraginacées et les Lamiacées médicinales. Ann Pharm Fr 1990;48:103-8.

38. Van Kessel KPM, Kalter ES, Verhoef J. Rosmarinic acid inhibits external oxidative effects of human polymorphonuclear granulocytes. Agents Actions 1985; 17:375-6.

39. Verweij-van Vught AMJJ, Appelmelk BJ, Groeneveld ABJ, Sparrius M, Thijs LG, MacLaren DM. Influence of rosmarinic acid on opsonization and intracellular killing of *Escherichia coli* and *Staphylococcus aureus* by porcine and human polymorphonuclear leucocytes. Agents Actions 1987;22:288-94.

40. Tagashira M, Ohtake Y. A new antioxidative 1,3-benzodioxole from *Melissa officinalis* Planta Med 1998;64:555-8.

41. Soulimani R, Fleurentin J, Mortier F, Misslin R, Derrieu G, Pelt J-M. Neurotropic action of the hydroalcoholic extract of *Melissa officinalis* in the mouse. Planta Med 1991;57;105-9.

42. Soulimani R, Younos C, Fleurentin J, Mortier F, Misslin R, Derrieux G. Recherche de l'activité biologique de *Melissa officinalis* L. sur le système nerveux central de la souris in vivo et le duodenum de rat in vitro. Plantes Méd Phytothér 1993;26:77-85.

43. Khayyal MT, El-Ghazaly MA, Kenawy SA, Seif-El-Nasr M, Mahran LG, Kafafi YAH, Okpanyi SN. Anti-ulcerogenic effect of some gastrointestinally acting plant extracts and their combination. Arzneim-Forsch/Drug Res 2001;51:545-53.

44. Van Dyke TE, Braswell L, Offenbacher S. Inhibition of gingivitis by topical application of ebselen and rosmarinic acid. Agents Actions 1986;19:376-7.

45. Ballard CG, O'Brien JT, Reichelt K, Perry EK. Aroma-therapy as a safe and effective treatment for the management of agitation in severe dementia: the results of a double-blind, placebo-controlled trial with *Melissa*. J Clin Psychiatry 2002;63:553-8.

46. Schimmer O, Krüger A, Paulini H, Haefele F. An evaluation of 55 commercial plant extracts in the Ames mutagenicity test. Pharmazie 1994;49:448-51.

47. Ramos Ruiz A, De la Torre RA, Alonso N, Villaescusa A, Betancourt J, Vizoso A. Screening of medicinal plants for induction of somatic segregation activity in *Aspergillus nidulans*. J Ethnopharmacol 1996; 52:123-7.

MENTHAE PIPERITAE AETHEROLEUM

Peppermint Oil

DEFINITION

Peppermint oil is obtained by steam distillation from the fresh overground parts of the flowering plant of *Mentha × piperita* L.

The material complies with the monograph of the European Pharmacopoeia [1].

CONSTITUENTS

The main components of the oil are menthol, principally in the form of (–)-menthol (usually 35-55%) with smaller amounts of stereoisomers such as (+)-neomenthol (ca. 3%) and (+)-isomenthol (ca. 3%), and menthone (10-35%) [2-5].

Over 100 components have been identified in the oil including numerous other monoterpenes and small amounts of sesquiterpenes, notably viridiflorol (ca. 0.5%), which is characteristic of oil from *Mentha × piperita* [5].

To comply with the European Pharmacopoeia the oil must contain menthol (30-55%), menthone (14-32%), isomenthone (1.5-10%), menthyl acetate (2.8-10%), menthofuran (1-9%), cineole (3.5-14%), limonene (1-5%), not more than 4% of pulegone and not more than 1% of carvone, with a ratio of cineole content to limonene content greater than 2 [1].

CLINICAL PARTICULARS

Therapeutic indications

Internal use
Symptomatic treatment of digestive disorders, such as flatulence [6]; irritable bowel syndrome [6-10]; symptomatic treatment of coughs and colds [6,11-16].

External use
Relief of coughs and colds; symptomatic relief of rheumatic complaints [17]; tension-type headache [18]; pruritus, urticaria and pain in irritable skin conditions [19-22].

Posology and method of administration

Dosage

ADULTS
Internal use
For digestive disorders: 0.02-0.08 ml (1-4 drops) up to

E/S/C/O/P
MONOGRAPHS
Second Edition

329

three times daily [2,5,23] in dilute aqueous preparations (e.g. peppermint water or emulsion), or as drops on a lump of sugar [24].

For irritable bowel syndrome: 0.2-0.4 ml three times daily in enteric-coated capsules [2,6,7,25-30].

External use

As an inhalation (for coughs and colds): 3-4 drops added to hot water [5].

In dilute liquid or semi-solid preparations, as an anaesthetic or antipruritic (equivalent to 0.1-1.0% m/m menthol) or as a counter-irritant and analgesic (equivalent to 1.25-16% m/m menthol), rubbed on to the affected area [31].

Tension-type headache: as a 10% solution rubbed on to the skin of forehead and temples [18].

CHILDREN FROM 4-16 YEARS OF AGE
Internal use

For digestive disorders: proportion of adult dose according to body weight.

External use

Semi-solid preparations: *4-10 years*, 2-10%; *10-16 years*, 5-15% [32].

Hydroethanolic preparations: *4-10 years*, 2-4%; *10-16 years*, 3-6% [32].

Method of administration

For oral administration, local application or inhalation.

Duration of administration

If symptoms persist or worsen, medical advice should be sought.

Contra-indications

Contact sensitivity to peppermint oil or menthol [33-36].

Special warnings and special precautions for use

Direct application of peppermint oil preparations to the nasal area or chest of babies and small children must be avoided because of the risk of laryngeal and bronchial spasms [17,37-42].

Interaction with other medicaments and other forms of interaction

Patients with achlorhydria (caused, for example, by medication with H_2 receptor blockers) should use peppermint oil only in enteric-coated capsules [25].

Pregnancy and lactation

No data available. In accordance with general medical practice, peppermint oil should not be used during pregnancy or lactation without medical advice.

Effects on ability to drive and use machines

None known.

Undesirable effects

Internal use

The use of non-enteric-coated peppermint oil preparations occasionally causes heartburn, especially in persons suffering from reflux oesophagitis [25,28,30,43].

External use

Rare cases of skin irritation have been reported [44,45]. Inhalation of menthol can cause apnoea and laryngoconstriction in susceptible individuals [40]. Menthol can cause jaundice in newborn babies. In certain cases this has been related to glucose-6-phosphate dehydrogenase deficiency and other factors [46-48].

Overdose

Excessive inhalation of mentholated products has caused reversible, undesirable effects, such as nausea, anorexia, cardiac problems, ataxia and other CNS problems, probably due to the presence of volatile menthol [49-51].

PHARMACOLOGICAL PROPERTIES

Pharmacodynamic properties

In vitro experiments

Spasmolytic effects
Electrically-evoked contractions of isolated longitudinal smooth muscle from guinea pig ileum were inhibited by peppermint oil with IC_{50} values (concentrations which produced 50% inhibition) varying from 26 mg/litre [12,52] to 176 mg/litre [53], compared to 1.3-8 mg/litre for papaverine [12,52,53]. Chemically-evoked contractions of the guinea pig ileum were inhibited in the presence of increasing concentrations of peppermint oil (0.5×10^{-6} to 1×10^{-4}% V/V) [54].

Peppermint oil relaxed carbachol-contracted guinea pig taenia coli (IC_{50}: 22.1 µg/ml) and inhibited spontaneous activity in guinea pig colon (IC_{50}: 25.9 µg/ml) and rabbit jejunum (IC_{50}: 15.2 µg/ml) [55].

Peppermint oil also exhibited relaxant effects on tracheal smooth muscle of the guinea pig with an IC_{50} of 87 mg/litre [12]. The oil inhibited potential-dependent calcium currents in a concentration-dependent manner (IC_{50}: 15.2 µg/ml); this was recorded using the whole cell clamp configuration in rabbit jejunum smooth muscle cells [55].

More detailed studies on the mode of action of peppermint oil in the guinea-pig ileum revealed that the spasmolytic effect is post-synaptic and not atropine-like. Adrenoreceptors were also not involved. Using a phosphodiesterase inhibitor, it was suggested that peppermint oil acts via a rise in intracellular cAMP, and not through cGMP, as shown by using a selective guanyl cyclase inhibitor. Peppermint oil was not considered to be acting as a potassium channel activator or a calcium channel blocker [56]. The latter is in contrast with other studies, which suggest that a reduction in calcium influx is involved. These differences might be due to different modes of action in different animal tissues (guinea pig taenia coli, rabbit jejunum) [54,55,57].

Other effects
Peppermint oil at concentrations of 20-50 µg/ml evoked ion permeability of heart cell membranes [57].

Menthol (10-30 µg/g tissue) antagonized contractions of the isolated frog rectum evoked by chemical and electrical stimulation. Vasodilatation was caused by the direct application of menthol to isolated ear vessels of rabbits [58].

Menthol has been reported to show antibacterial activity [20] and similarly peppermint oil showed antimicrobial activity [59]. Peppermint oil and 53 of its constituents were evaluated against *E. coli* in a preliminary screening test. It was found that peppermint oil and 3 of its constituents, menthol, menthone and neomenthol, had a bactericidal effect within 1 hour at concentrations of 400 µg/ml [60].

In vivo experiments
In experiments with anaesthetized guinea pigs, peppermint oil emulsified with tween 80 (0.1% in aqueous solution) caused resolution of a morphine-induced spasm of Oddi's sphincter. The oil administered intravenously at 1 mg/kg body weight partially unblocked Oddi's sphincter, which returned to normal in 17 minutes, whereas 3 mg/kg caused immediate total unblocking [61].

Peppermint oil appears to enhance production of bile [11]. In an anaesthetized, bile duct-cannulated dog, a peppermint leaf infusion (0.4 g/kg) strongly enhanced bile production [62]. Menthol also enhanced bile production: 0.06 g/kg in 1 dog [61] and 0.1-1.0 g/kg in rats [63].

Menthol dispersed in air, at concentrations of 140 ng/ml in cold air and 390 ng/ml in warm air, stimulated cold receptors in the respiratory tracts of 11 dogs and produced easier respiration [64]. Respiration was also facilitated when menthol was administered intravenously to 23 cats at 34.2 mg/kg [65].

Menthol inhibits hepatic HMGCoA reductase activity. Both menthol (468 mg/kg) and cineole (a minor constituent of peppermint oil; 262 mg/kg), separately administered orally to male rats, inhibited hepatic

HMGCoA reductase activity by approximately 70% [66,67].

Pharmacological studies in humans
Peppermint oil (dose not stated) injected into the colon of 20 patients (through the biopsy channel of a colonoscope), relieved colonic spasms within 30 seconds [68], while 0.2 ml of peppermint oil in 50 ml of 0.9% sodium chloride with 0.01% polysorbate as suspending agent, injected into the colon of 6 subjects, relieved colonic spasms within 2 minutes, the effect lasting for about 12 minutes [69].

Two actions of peppermint oil on secretion in the respiratory tract have been reported: secretolytic in the bronchi [11,15,16,31] and decongestant in the nose [12].

Studies to assess the decongestant action of menthol have been carried out: on 62 volunteers with common cold, of whom 30 received a lozenge containing 11 mg of menthol [13]; on 29 healthy subjects breathing through an inhaler containing 125 mg of menthol dissolved in 1 ml of liquid paraffin [14]; and on 31 subjects receiving for 5 minutes menthol-containing air produced by passing the air through a flask containing approximately 1 g of menthol at 80°C [70,71]. All these studies showed that inhalation of menthol causes a subjective sensation of improved nasal air flow or 'easier breathing'. However, in subjects with common cold suffering from nasal congestion, inhalation of menthol produces no objective reduction in nasal airway resistance as measured by rhinomanometry [13,72].

The analgesic effect of peppermint oil (10% in ethanol) was investigated in 32 healthy subjects in a randomized, double-blind, placebo-controlled, four-arm crossover study. The peppermint oil preparation significantly reduced sensitivity to pain in experimentally-induced headache (p<0.01-0.001, depending on the method of induction used) when applied externally to the forehead and temples [73].

Menthol moderated oral sensations of warmth and coldness, as shown by an experiment on 31 young adults receiving a 0.02% aqueous solution of menthol in the mouth for 5 seconds [74].

Clinical studies

Irritable bowel syndrome
In an open, multicentre trial, 50 patients suffering from irritable bowel syndrome received an enteric-coated peppermint oil (0.2 ml) capsule 3 times per day, administered orally 30 minutes before a meal. Evaluation of all signs and symptoms confirmed a significant decrease in symptoms (p<0.005) after 4 weeks of treatment compared to initial values. No toxic effects were reported and undesirable side

effects were minimal and unimportant [7].

In two double-blind, crossover studies of irritable bowel syndrome with 16 and 29 patients respectively [25,26], enteric-coated peppermint oil (0.2 ml) capsules were compared with placebo. Three times daily the patients took 1 or 2 capsules depending on the severity of symptoms. Overall assessment of each treatment period showed that, compared to placebo, patients felt significantly better (p<0.01) while taking peppermint oil capsules and considered peppermint oil superior in relieving abdominal symptoms (p<0.005) [25].

In a double-blind, crossover study, 40 patients with irritable bowel syndrome were treated orally for 2 weeks with enteric-coated peppermint oil (0.2 ml) capsules or hyoscyamine (0.2 mg) or placebo. Treatment with peppermint oil tended to have a more pronounced effect on symptoms than hyoscyamine or placebo, but this was not statistically significant. These findings favour the short-term use of enteric-coated peppermint oil capsules as an antispasmodic in the treatment of irritable bowel syndrome [27].

In a double-blind clinical study 34 patients with irritable bowel syndrome, in whom pain was a prominent symptom, took 3 × 2 enteric-coated peppermint oil (0.2 ml) capsules or placebo daily. The patients' assessments at the end of 2 and 4 weeks of treatment showed no significant difference between peppermint oil and placebo in terms of overall symptoms [28].

In a randomized, double blind, placebo-controlled clinical study 110 outpatients (66 men and 44 women; 18-70 years of age) with symptoms of irritable bowel syndrome were assigned to oral treatment with 1 enteric-coated peppermint oil (0.2 ml) capsule or placebo 3-4 times daily, 15-30 minutes before meals, for a period of 1 month. The study was completed by 52 patients in the peppermint oil group and 49 in the placebo group. In the verum group, 79% of patients experienced a decrease in severity of abdominal pain (placebo group: 43%), 83% reported less abdominal distension (placebo group: 29%), 83% had reduced stool frequency (placebo group: 32%), 73% had fewer borborygmi (placebo group: 31%), and 79% less flatulence (placebo group: 22%). Improvements in all these symptoms were significantly better after peppermint oil than after placebo (p<0.05) [75].

In a randomized, double-blind, crossover study 18 patients with irritable bowel syndrome were treated orally with 3 enteric-coated peppermint oil (0.2 ml) capsules daily for 4 weeks and then changed to placebo for a further 4 weeks, or vice versa. Compared to placebo, peppermint oil produced a small but significant increase in frequency of defecation (p<0.05) but no significant change in scores for global severity of symptoms or scores for the specific symptoms of pain, bloating, urgent defecation and the sensation of incomplete evacuation [29].

A literature search revealed 8 randomized, controlled studies involving the use of enteric-coated peppermint oil capsules in irritable bowel syndrome and meeting pre-defined criteria for inclusion in a critical review; collectively they indicated that peppermint oil could be efficacious for symptomatic relief in irritable bowel syndrome. A meta-analysis of 5 of these studies (all double-blind, placebo-controlled) appeared to support this conclusion, showing a significant global improvement (p<0.001) in the symptoms of irritable bowel syndrome in patients treated with peppermint oil compared to placebo. However, in view of methodological flaws associated with most studies, no definitive judgement on efficacy could be given. The authors noted that well designed and carefully executed studies are needed to fully clarify the issue [76].

Tension-type headache
In a randomized, double-blind, placebo-controlled, crossover study involving 41 patients suffering from tension-type headaches, a total of 164 headache attacks were treated by oral medication (paracetamol 1000 mg or placebo) and simultaneously by cutaneous application of oil (a 10% solution of peppermint oil in ethanol, or a placebo with peppermint flavour). The oil was spread across the forehead and temples, and this was repeated after 15 and 30 minutes. Patients rated their pain intensities on a standardized category rating scale, making assessments after 15, 30, 45 and 60 minutes. The greatest effect was achieved with combined paracetamol/peppermint oil therapy (p≤0.001 compared to placebo). Both peppermint oil and paracetamol also significantly reduced the intensity of clinical headache (p<0.01 compared to placebo) over the 1-hour observation period with no significant difference between these groups [18].

Pharmacokinetic properties

Pharmacokinetics in animals
After oral administration of menthol to rats in the high dosage range of 0.1-1.0 g/kg, menthol glucuronide was the main conjugate in urine, whereas the sulphate was predominant in bile [63].

Pharmacokinetics in humans
Menthol and other terpene constituents of peppermint oil are fat-soluble and therefore rapidly absorbed from the proximal small intestine when taken orally [30,77].

Urinary excretion of menthol (as the glucuronide) was studied in 13 healthy subjects after oral administration of a single dose of 0.6 ml of peppermint oil, in the form of 3 enteric-coated peppermint oil (0.2 ml) capsules of one or the other of two different delayed-release preparations. With one of these formulations peak urinary excretion of menthol occurred 3 hours after administration; thereafter the levels rapidly decreased. The second preparation gave a peak urinary concentration of only about one-quarter of the first, but menthol excretion at this level was sustained over the period from 3 to 9 hours after administration [77].

In an earlier study, the pharmacokinetic profile of the second of the delayed-release preparations described above was compared with that of peppermint oil contained in soft gelatine capsules (which dissolve readily in the stomach). After oral administration to 6 healthy volunteers of a single dose providing 0.4 ml of peppermint oil, the total urinary excretion of menthol (as the glucuronide metabolite) was similar for both preparations, but peak menthol excretion levels were lower and excretion delayed with the delayed-release formulation [30].

Preclinical safety data
Peppermint oil was given orally (by gavage, diluted with soybean oil) to groups of 10 male and 10 female rats at 0, 10, 40 or 100 mg/kg body weight daily for 28 days. Histopathological changes, consisting of cyst-like spaces scattered in the white matter of the cerebellum, were seen at the higher dose levels of 40 and 100 mg/kg/day. There were no obvious signs of clinical symptoms due to the encephalopathy [78]. In a similar study in rats, but of longer duration, the same histopathological changes in the cerebellum were observed after oral administration of peppermint oil at 100 mg/kg/day for 90 days; in this study nephropathy was also observed in male rats at 100 mg/kg/day [79]. From these two studies the estimated no-effect-level of peppermint oil in rats was 10-40 mg/kg/day [78,79].

Oral administration of menthofuran to rats at a high dose level of 250 mg/kg/day for 3 days caused hepato-toxicity as indicated by a significant increase in serum glutamate pyruvate transaminase and decreases in glucose-6-phosphatase and aminopyrine N-demethyl-ase activities. A decrease was also observed in the levels of liver microsomal cytochrome P-450, whereas cytochrome b_5 and NAD(P)H-cytochrome c reductase activities were unaffected [80].

Clinical safety data
A total of 323 patients and healthy volunteers have been included in 9 studies where efficacy and safety in the use of peppermint oil were investigated. Oral administration in capsules or direct injection into the colon varied from a single dose to 2 or 4 weeks of treatment with daily doses of 3-6 × 0.2 ml of the oil. In these studies there were no reports of toxicity and

undesirable effects were minimal and unimportant; 1 patient developed a mild transient skin rash, and 1 experienced heartburn due to chewing the capsules [7,25-29,68,69,75].

REFERENCES

1. Peppermint Oil - Menthae piperitae aetheroleum. European Pharmacopoeia, Council of Europe.

2. Hänsel R, Sticher O, Steinegger E. Pfefferminzblätter, Pfefferminzöl. In: Pharmakognosie-Phytopharmazie, 6th ed. Berlin: Springer-Verlag, 1999:689-92 and 735-8.

3. Wichtl M. Menthae piperitae folium - Pfefferminzblätter. In: Wichtl M, editor. Teedrogen und Phytopharmaka. Ein Handbuch für die Praxis auf wissenschaftlicher Grundlage, 4th ed. Stuttgart: Wissenschaftliche Verlagsgesellschaft, 2002:390-3.

4. Wichtl M, Henke D. Pfefferminzöl - Menthae piperitae aetheroleum. In: Hartke K, Hartke H, Mutschler E, Rücker G, Wichtl M, editors. Kommentar zum Europäischen Arzneibuch. Stuttgart: Wissenschaftliche Verlagsgesellschaft, 1998(9. Lfg):P 29.

5. Stahl-Biskup E. Mentha. In: Hänsel R, Keller K, Rimpler H, Schneider G, editors. Hagers Handbuch der Pharmazeutischen Praxis, 5th ed. Volume 5: Drogen E-O. Berlin: Springer-Verlag, 1993:821-48.

6. Reynolds JEF, editor. Peppermint oil. In: Martindale. The Extra Pharmacopoeia. London: Pharmaceutical Press, 1993:899.

7. Fernández F. Menta piperita en el tratamiento de síndrome de colon irritable. Invest Med Inter 1990; 17:42-6.

8. Rhodes J, Evans BK. Carminative preparations for treating irritable colon syndrome. Brit UK Pat Appl 2,006,011 through Chem Abstr 1979;91:198934.

9. Rhodes J, Evans BK. Method of treating functional bowel disorders by the administration of peppermint oil to the intestine. U.S. US 4,687,667 through Chem Abstr 1987;107:183611.

10. Krag E. Irritable bowel syndrome: current concept and future trends. Scand J Gastroenterol 1985;20(Suppl 109):107-15.

11. Hänsel R, Haas H. Therapie mit Phytopharmaka. Berlin: Springer-Verlag, 1984:113,116,133,143,180 and 269.

12. Reiter M, Brandt W. Relaxant effects on tracheal and ileal smooth muscles of the guinea pig. Arzneim-Forsch/Drug Res 1985;35:408-14.

13. Eccles R, Jawad MS, Morris S. The effects of oral administration of (−)-menthol on nasal resistance to airflow and nasal sensation of airflow in subjects suffering from nasal congestion associated with common cold. J Pharm Pharmacol 1990;42:652-4.

14. Eccles R, Lancashire B, Tolley NS. The effect of L-

menthol on electromyographic activity of the alae nasi muscle in man. J Physiol 1989;412:34P.

15. Haen E. Expektoranzien, Antitussiva, Broncho-spasmolytika. Med Monatsschr Pharmazeuten 1989; 12:344-55.

16. Schilcher H. Pharmakologie und Toxikologie ätherischer Öle. Therapiewoche 1986;36:1100-12.

17. Seitz G, Schäfer-Korting M. Menthol. In: Hartke K, Hartke H, Mutschler E, Rücker G, Wichtl M, editors. DAB-Kommentar. Stuttgart: Wissenschaftliche Verlagsgesellschaft, 1993 (1. Lfg):M 41.

18. Göbel H, Fresenius J, Heinze A, Dworschak M, Soyka D. Effektivität von Oleum menthae piperitae und von Paracetamol in der Therapie des Kopfschmerzes vom Spannungstyp. Nervenarzt 1996;67:672-81

19. Gilchrest BA. Pruritus. Pathogenesis, therapy, and significance in systemic disease states. Arch Intern Med 1982;142:101-5.

20. Rajka G. Moderne Behandlung des atopischen Ekzems (Neurodermitis diffusia). Hautarzt 1977;28:348-52.

21. Osterler HB. The management of ocular Herpes virus infections. Surv Ophthalmol 1976;21:136-47.

22. Brown D. Herpes zoster of the vulva. Clin Obstet Gynecol 1972;15:1010-4.

23. Mentha piperita. In: British Herbal Pharmacopoeia 1983. Bournemouth: British Herbal Medicine Assoc-iation, 1983:141-2.

24. Fintelmann V, Menßen HG, Siegers C-P. Pfefferminzöl, Menthae piperitae aetheroleum. In: Phytotherapie Manual - Pharmazeutischer, pharmakologischer und therapeutischer Standard, 2nd ed. Stuttgart: Hippokrates Verlag, 1993:172-3.

25. Rees WDW, Evans BK, Rhodes J. Treating irritable bowel syndrome with peppermint oil. BMJ 1979:835-6.

26. Dew MJ, Evans BK, Rhodes J. Peppermint oil for the irritable bowel syndrome: A multicentre trial. Br J Clin Pract 1984;38:394-8.

27. Carling L, Svedberg LE, Hulten S. Short term treatment of the irritable bowel syndrome: a placebo-controlled trial of peppermint oil against hyoscyamine. Opuscula Medica 1989;34:55-7.

28. Nash P, Gould SR, Barnardo DE. Peppermint oil does not relieve the pain of irritable bowel syndrome. Br J Clin Pract 1986;40:292-3.

29. Lawson MJ, Knight RE, Tran K, Walker G, Robers-Thomson I. Failure of enteric-coated peppermint oil in the irritable bowel syndrome: A randomized double-blind crossover study. J Gastroent Hepatol 1988;3:235-8.

30. Somerville KW, Richmond CR, Bell GD. Delayed release peppermint oil capsules (Colpermin) for the spastic colon syndrome: a pharmacokinetic study. Br J Clin Pharmacol 1984;18:638-40.

31. Hänsel R, Sticher O, Steinegger E. Menthol. In: Pharmakognosie-Phytopharmazie, 6th ed. Berlin: Springer-Verlag, 1999:756-8.

32. Dorsch W, Loew D, Meyer-Buchtela E, Schilcher H. Menthae piperitae aetheroleum (Pfefferminzöl). In: Kooperation Phytopharmaka, editor. Kinderdosierung von Phytopharmaka, 3rd ed. Teil 1 - Empfehlungen zur Anwendung und Dosierung von Phytopharmaka, mono-graphierten Arzneidrogen und ihren Zubereitungen in der Pädiatrie. Bonn: Kooperation Phytopharmaka, 2002: 99-101.

33. Dooms-Goossens A, Degreef H, Holvoet C, Maertens M. Turpentine-induced hypersensitivity to peppermint oil. Contact Derm 1977;3:304-8.

34. Saito F, Oka K. Allergic contact dermatitis due to peppermint oil. Skin Res 1990;32(Suppl 9):161-7 [Japanese; English summary].

35. Fisher AA. Reactions to menthol. Cutis 1986;38:17-8.

36. Morton CA, Garioch J, Todd P, Lamey PJ, Forsyth A. Contact sensitivity to menthol and peppermint in patients with intra-oral symptoms. Contact Derm 1995;32:281-4.

37. Melis K, Janssens G, Bochner A. Accidentele nasale instillatie van eucalyptol en menthol bij kinderen. Tijdschr voor Geneeskunde 1990;46:1453-5. *Also published as*: Accidental nasal eucalyptol and menthol instillation. Acta Clin Belg 1990:45(Suppl.13):101-2.

38. Konietzko N. Mukolytika-Sekretolytika-Sekreto-motorika. Atemswegs- und Lungenkrankheiten 1983; 9;151-6.

39. Dupeyron J-P, Quattrocchi F, Castaing H, Fabiani P. Intoxication aiguë du nourisson par application cutanée d'une pommade révulsive locale et antiseptique pulmonaire. Eur J Toxicol 1976;9:313-20.

40. Lässig W, Graupner I, Leonhardt H, Pommerenke C. Bronchiale Obstruktion nach Inhalation ätherischer Öle. Z Klin Med 1990;45:969-71.

41. Tange RA. Gebruik menthol bij verkoudheden is niet aan te bevelen [Use of menthol in cases of cold is not to be recommended]. Apotheek in praktijk 1990; (January):9.

42. Javorka K, Tomori Z, Zavarska L. Protective and defensive airway reflexes in premature infants. Physiol Bohemoslov 1980;29:29-35.

43. Anon. Die gastroösophageale Refluxkrankheit. Dtsch Apoth Ztg 1990;130:2684.

44. Parys BT. Chemical burns resulting from contact with peppermint oil mar: a case report. Burns Incl Therm Inj 1983;9:374-5.

45. Weston CFM. Anal burning and peppermint oil. Postgrad Med J 1987;63:717.

46. Olowe SA, Ransome-Kuti O. The risk of jaundice in glucose-6-phosphate dehydrogenase deficient babies exposed to menthol. Acta Paediatr Scand 1980;69:341-5.

47. Familusi JB, Dawodu AH. A survey of neonatal jaundice in association with household drugs and chemicals in Nigeria. Ann Trop Paediatr 1985;5:219-22.

48. Owa JA. Relationship between exposure to icterogenic agents, glucose-6-phosphate dehydrogenase deficiency and neonatal jaundice in Nigeria. Acta Paediatr Scand 1989;78:848-52.

49. Luke E. Addiction to mentholated cigarettes. Lancet 1962:110-1.

50. O'Mullana NM, Joyce P, Kamath SV, Tham MK, Knass D. Adverse CNS effects of menthol-containing Olbas oil. Lancet 1982;I:1121.

51. Thomas JG. Peppermint fibrillation. Lancet 1962:222.

52. Brandt W. Spasmolytische Wirkung ätherischer Öle. Z Phytotherapie 1988;9:33-9.

53. Taddei I, Giachetti D, Taddei E, Mantovani P, Bianchi E. Spasmolytic activity of peppermint, sage and rosemary essences and their major constituents. Fitoterapia 1988;59:463-8.

54. Taylor BA, Luscombe DK, Duthie DL. Inhibitory effect of peppermint oil on gastrointestinal smooth muscle [Abstract]. Gut 1983;24:A992.

55. Hills JM, Aaronson PI. The mechanism of action of peppermint oil on gastrointestinal smooth muscle. An analysis using patch clamp electrophysiology and isolated tissue pharmacology in rabbit and guinea pig. Gastroenterology 1991;101:55-65.

56. Lis-Balchin M, Hart S. Studies on the mode of action of peppermint oil Mentha × piperita L. in the guinea-pig ileum in vitro. Med Sci Res 1999;27:307-9.

57. Teuscher E, Melzig M, Villmann E, Möritz KU. Untersuchungen zum Wirkungsmechanismus ätherischer Öle. Z Phytotherapie 1990;11:87-92.

58. Futami T. Actions of counterirritants on the muscle contractile mechanism and nervous system. Folia pharmacol Japon 1984;83:207-18. [Japanese; English summary].

59. Janssen AM, Chin NLJ, Scheffer JJC, Baerheim Svendsen A. Screening for antimicrobial activity of some essential oils by the agar overlay technique. Pharm Weekbl (Sci) 1986;8:289-92.

60. Osawa K, Saeki T, Yasuda H, Hamashima H, Sasatsu M, Arai T. The antibacterial activities of peppermint oil and green tea polyphenols, alone and in combination against enterohemorrhagic coli. Biocontrol Sci 1999; 4:1-7

61. Giachetti D, Taddei E, Taddei T. Pharmacological activity of Mentha piperita, Salvia officinalis and Rosmarinus officinalis essences on Oddi's sphincter. Planta Med 1986;52:543-4.

62. Steinmetzer K. Experimentelle Untersuchungen über Cholagoga. Wiener Klin Wochenschr 1926;39:1418-22 and 1455-7.

63. Mans M, Pentz R. Pharmacokinetics of menthol in the rat. Naunyn-Schmiedeberg's Arch Pharmacol 1987; 335(Suppl):R6.

64. Sant'Ambrogio FB, Anderson JW, Sant'Ambrogio G. Effect of l-menthol on laryngeal receptors. J Appl Physiol 1991;70:788-93.

65. Schäfer K, Braun HA, Isenberg C. Effect of menthol on cold-receptor activity. J Gen Physiol 1986;88:757-76.

66. Clegg RJ, Middleton B, Bell GD, White DA. Inhibition of hepatic cholesterol synthesis and S-3-hydroxy-3-methylglutaryl-CoA reductase by mono- and bicyclic monoterpenes administered in vivo. Biochem Pharmacol 1980;29:2125-7.

67. Clegg RJ, Middleton B, Bell GD, White DA. The mechanism of cyclic monoterpene inhibition of hepatic 3-hydroxy-3-methylglutaryl coenzyme A reductase in vivo in the rat. J Biol Chem 1982;257:2294-9.

68. Leicester RJ, Hunt RH. Peppermint oil to reduce colonic spasm during endoscopy. Lancet 1982;II:989.

69. Duthie HL. The effect of peppermint oil on colonic motility in man. Br J Surg 1981;68:820.

70. Eccles R, Jones AS. The effect of menthol on nasal resistance to airflow. J Laryngol Otol 1983;97:705-9.

71. Burrow A, Eccles R, Jones AS. The effects of camphor, eucalyptus and menthol vapour on nasal resistance to airflow and nasal sensation. Acta Otolaryngol (Stockh) 1983;96:157-61.

72. Eccles R. Menthol and related cooling compounds. J Pharm Pharmacol 1994;46:618-30.

73. Göbel H, Schmidt G, Soyka D. Effect of peppermint and eucalyptus oil preparations on neurophysiological and experimental algesimetric headache parameters. Cephalalgia 1994;14:228-34.
Reprinted with revisions and additions as: Göbel H, Schmidt G, Dworschak M, Stolze H, Heuss D. Essential plant oils and headache mechanisms. Phytomedicine 1995;2:93-102.
Also published with modifications as:
Göbel H, Schmidt G. Effekt von Pfefferminz- und Eukalyptusölpräparationen in experimentellen Kopfschmerzmodellen. Z Phytotherapie 1995;16:23-33.

74. Green BG. Menthol modulates oral sensations of warmth and cold. Physiol Behav 1985;35:427-34.

75. Lui JH, Chen GH, Yeh HZ, Huang CK, Poon SK. Enteric-coated peppermint-oil capsules in the treatment of irritable bowel syndrome: A prospective, randomized trial. J Gastroenterol 1997;32:765-8.

76. Pittler MH, Ernst E. Peppermint oil for irritable bowel syndrome: A critical review and metaanalysis. Am J Gastroenterol 1998;93:1131-5.

77. White DA, Thompson SP, Wilson CG, Bell GD. A pharmacokinetic comparison of two delayed-release peppermint oil preparations, Colpermin and Mintec, for treatment of the irritable bowel syndrome. Int J Pharmaceut 1987;40:151-5.

78. Thorup I, Würtzen G, Carstensen J, Olsen P. Short term toxicity study in rats dosed with peppermint oil. Toxicol Lett 1983;19:211-5.

79. Spindler P, Madsen C. Subchronic toxicity study of peppermint oil in rats. Toxicol Lett 1992;62:215-20.

80. Madyastha KM, Raj CP. Effects of menthofuran, a monoterpene furan on rat liver microsomal enzymes, in vivo. Toxicol 1994;89:119-25.

MENTHAE PIPERITAE FOLIUM

Peppermint Leaf

E/S/C/O/P
MONOGRAPHS
Second Edition

DEFINITION

Peppermint leaf consists of the whole or cut dried leaves of Mentha × piperita L. The whole drug contains not less than 12 ml/kg of essential oil. The cut drug contains not less than 9 ml/kg of essential oil.

The material complies with the monograph of the European Pharmacopoeia [1].

Fresh material may also be used, provided that when dried it complies with the monograph of the European Pharmacopoeia.

CONSTITUENTS

The main active component is essential oil (1-3%), of which the principal constituent is usually menthol, in the form of (-)-menthol (usually 35-55 %) with smaller amounts of stereoisomers such as (+)-neomenthol (ca. 3%) and (+)-isomenthol (ca. 3%), together with menthone (10-35%), menthyl acetate, menthofuran, cineole, limonene and other monoterpenes [2,3]. Small amounts of sesquiterpenes occur in the oil, notably viridoflorol [3].

Various flavonoids are present including luteolin and its 7-glycoside [4], rutin, hesperidin [5], eriocitrin [6-8] and highly oxygenated flavones [4,9]. Other constituents include phenolic acids [8,10] and small amounts of triterpenes [11].

CLINICAL PARTICULARS

Therapeutic indications
Used in the symptomatic treatment of digestive disorders such as dyspepsia [5,12-16], flatulence [16,17] and gastritis [15], although no clinical data are available in support of these indications.

Posology and method of administration

Dosage

Adults: As an infusion, 1.5-3 g of the drug to 150 ml of water, three times daily [15,16]. Tincture (1:5, 45% ethanol), 2-3 ml, three times daily [16].
Elderly: Dose as for adults.
Children from 4 years of age, daily dose as infusions only: *4-10 years, 3-5 g; 10-16 years, 3-6 g* [18].

Method of administration
For oral administration.

Duration of administration
If symptoms persist or worsen, medical advice should be sought.

Contra-indications
None known.

Special warnings and special precautions for use
None required.

Interaction with other medicaments and other forms of interaction
None reported.

Pregnancy and lactation
No harmful effects have been reported.

Effects on ability to drive and use machines
None known.

Undesirable effects
None reported.

Overdose
No toxic effects reported.

PHARMACOLOGICAL PROPERTIES

Pharmacodynamic properties
The pharmacological actions of peppermint leaf are largely, but not exclusively, attributable to the essential oil; other components such as flavonoids also appear to play a role [15,16]. Pharmacodynamic data relating to the essential oil are given in the monograph on Peppermint oil.

In vitro experiments
A 30%-ethanolic extract from peppermint leaf exhibited antispasmodic activity at concentrations of 2.5 and 10.0 ml/litre, causing significant and dose-dependent increases in ED_{50} values for acetylcholine- and histamine-induced contractions of isolated guinea pig ileum ($p<0.01$ and $p<0.0005$ respectively for histamine-induced contractions), and a significant decrease in the maximum possible contractility ($p<0.05$ and $p<0.001$ respectively for histamine-induced contractions). The effect of the extract at 10.0 ml/litre corresponded to that of 1.6 µg of atropine per litre [13]. A similar peppermint leaf extract inhibited carbachol-induced contractions of isolated guinea pig ileum [14].

A total flavonoid fraction from peppermint leaf, dissolved in water so that 1 ml corresponded to about 0.5 g of dried leaf, inhibited barium chloride-induced contractions of isolated guinea pig ileum [19].

In vivo experiments

Choleretic effects
In experiments with cannulated dogs, peppermint tea (0.4 g/kg body weight) increased the secretion of bile [20]. Flavonoids, as well as the essential oil, contribute to this action [5,21,22].

Mixed flavonoids from peppermint leaf (optimum dose 2 mg/kg) showed choleretic activity in dogs [21]. Flavomentin, a flavonoid preparation from peppermint leaf, stimulated bile secretion and the synthesis of bile acids in dogs at doses of 0.5-6 mg/kg (optimum 2 mg/kg) [22].

In experiments with cannulated rats, intravenous injection of a peppermint tea at 0.5 ml/rat or a flavonoid preparation (corresponding to a dose of 3.3 g of peppermint leaf per kg body weight) proved effective in increasing the amount of bile acids [19].

Anti-ulcerogenic effect
Oral pre-treatment of rats with an ethanolic liquid extract from peppermint leaf at 2.5-10 ml/kg body weight gave dose-dependent protection against oral indometacin-induced gastric ulcers (80% protection at 10 ml/kg); this was confirmed histologically. The extract also had gastric antisecretory and cyto-protective effects; compared to rats treated intraperitoneally with indometacin (10 mg/kg), analysis of the gastric contents of animals pre-treated orally with the extract indicated reduced acid output, an increase in prostaglandin E_2 release and a decrease in leukotrienes (all $p<0.05$ at 2.5 ml/kg) [23].

Other effects
A dry 80%-ethanolic extract from peppermint leaf showed antinociceptive effects in mice. When administered orally at 200 mg/kg or 400 mg/kg, the extract significantly reduced acetic acid-induced writhing ($p<0.01$ and $p<0.001$ respectively). The response time of mice to thermal stimulation in the hot-plate test also increased significantly 45 and 60 minutes after intraperitoneal administration of the extract at 400 mg/kg ($p<0.01$ and $p<0.001$ respectively) [24].

The same extract showed anti-inflammatory activity against acute and chronic inflammation in rodents. After oral administration it reduced xylene-induced ear oedema in mice (acute model) by 49% at 200 mg/kg and 50% at 400 mg/kg (both $p<0.05$). After intraperitoneal administration in the cotton pellet granuloma test in rats (chronic model), only the higher dose of 400 mg/kg had a significant inhibitory effect ($p<0.01$) [24].

A dry aqueous extract of peppermint leaf, administered orally to mice as single doses of 300 or 1000 mg/kg body weight, caused weak sedative effects in several tests: hexobarbital-induced sleep, exploratory behaviour, spontaneous motility and motor co-ordination. The same extract had a significant diuretic effect in mice at 100 and 300 mg/kg (p<0.05), but not at 1000 mg/kg [25].

Pharmacological studies in humans
The carminative action of peppermint leaf extracts is due to a reduction in tonus of the oesophageal sphincter, enabling release of entrapped air [17].

Pharmacokinetic properties
Pharmacokinetic data relating to the essential oil are given in the monograph on Peppermint oil.

Preclinical safety data
After oral administration of a dry peppermint leaf extract to 12 mice as a single dose at 4000 mg/kg body weight, none of the animals died and none showed macroscopic signs of toxicity over a 7-day period of observation [25].

REFERENCES

1. Peppermint Leaf - Menthae piperitae folium. European Pharmacopoeia, Council of Europe.

2. Lawrence BM. Progress in Essential Oils: Peppermint oil. Perfumer & Flavorist 1993;18(July/August):59-72.

3. Wichtl M, Egerer HP. Pfefferminzblätter - Menthae piperitae folium. In: Hartke K, Hartke H, Mutschler E, Rücker G, Wichtl M, editors. Kommentar zum Europäischen Arzneibuch. Stuttgart: Wissenschaftliche Verlagsgesellschaft, 1999(11. Lfg):P 28.

4. Barberan FAT. The flavonoid compounds from the Labiatae. Fitoterapia 1986;57:67-95.

5. Steinegger E, Hänsel R. Pfefferminzblätter und Pfefferminzöl. In: Pharmakognosie, 5th ed. Berlin: Springer-Verlag, 1992:302-4.

6. Hoffmann BG, Lunder LT. Flavonoids from Mentha piperita leaves. Planta Med 1984;51:361.

7. Duband F, Carnat AP, Carnat A, Petitjean-Freytet C, Clair G, Lamaison JL. Composition aromatique et polyphénolique de l'infusé de Menthe, Mentha × piperita L. Ann Pharm Fr 1992;50:146-55.

8. Guédon DJ, Pasquier BP. Analysis and distribution of flavonoid glycosides and rosmarinic acid in 40 Mentha × piperita clones. J Agric Food Chem 1994; 42:679-84.

9. Jullien F, Voirin B, Bernillon J, Favre-Bonvin J. Highly oxygenated flavones from Mentha piperita. Phyto-chemistry 1984;23:2972-3.

10. Litvinenko VI, Popova TP, Simonjan AV, Zoz IG, Sokolov VS. "Gerbstoffe" und Oxyzimtsäureab-kömmlinge in Labiaten. Planta Med 1975;27:372-80.

11. Croteau R, Loomis WD. Biosynthesis of squalene and other triterpenes in Mentha piperita from mevalonate-2-^{14}C. Phytochemistry 1973;12:1957-65.

12. Dinckler K. Über die biologische Wirkung verschiedener Reinstoffe im äetherischen Öl von Mentha-Arten. Pharm Zentrh 1936;77:281-90.

13. Forster HB, Niklas H, Lutz S. Antispasmodic effects of some medicinal plants. Planta Med 1980;40:309-19.

14. Forster H. Spasmolytische Wirkung pflanzlicher Carminativa. Z Allg Med 1983;59:1327-33.

15. Wichtl M. Menthae piperitae folium - Pfefferminz-blätter. In: Wichtl M, editor. Teedrogen und Phytopharmaka. Ein Handbuch für die Praxis auf wissenschaftlicher Grundlage, 4th ed. Stuttgart: Wissenschaftliche Verlagsgesellschaft, 2002:390-3.

16. Bradley PR, editor. Peppermint leaf. In: British Herbal Compendium, Volume 1. Bournemouth: British Herbal Medicine Association; 1992:174-6.

17. Demling L, Steger W. Zur Rechtfertigung der Volksmedizin: Pfefferminze und Zwiebel. Fortschr Med 1969;37:1305-6.

18. Dorsch W, Loew D, Meyer-Buchtela E, Schilcher H. Menthae piperitae folium (Pfefferminzblätter). In: Kooperation Phytopharmaka, editor. Kinderdosierung von Phytopharmaka, 3rd ed. Teil 1 - Empfehlungen zur Anwendung und Dosierung von Phytopharmaka, monographierten Arzneidrogen und ihren Zubereitungen in der Pädiatrie. Bonn: Kooperation Phytopharmaka, 2002:102-3.

19. Lallement-Guilbert N, Bézanger-Beauquesne L. Recherches sur les flavonoïdes de quelques Labiées médicinales (romarin, menthe poivrée, sauge officinale). Plantes Méd Phytothér 1970;4:92-107.

20. Steinmetzer K. Experimentelle Untersuchungen über Cholagoga. Wiener Klin Wschr 1926;39:1418-22;1455-7.

21. Pasechnik IK. Study of choleretic properties specific to flavonoids from Mentha piperita leaves. Farmakol Toksikol 1966;29:735-7, through Chem Abstr 1967; 66:54111.

22. Pasechnik IK, Gella EV. Choleretic preparation from peppermint. Farm Zh (Kiev) 1966;21:49-53, through Chem Abstr 1967;66:36450.

23. Khayyal MT, El-Ghazaly MA, Kenawy SA, Seif-El-Nasr M, Mahran LG, Kafafi YAH, Okpanyi SN. Anti-ulcerogenic effect of some gastrointestinally acting plant extracts and their combination. Arzneim-Forsch/Drug Res 2001;51:545-53.

24. Atta AH, Alkofahi A. Anti-nociceptive and anti-inflammatory effects of some Jordanian medicinal plant extracts. J Ethnopharmacol 1998;60:117-24.

25. Della Loggia R, Tubaro A, Lunder TL. Evaluation of some pharmacological activities of a peppermint extract. Fitoterapia 1990;61:215-21.

MYRRHA

Myrrh

E/S/C/O/P
MONOGRAPHS
Second Edition

DEFINITION

Myrrh consists of a gum-resin, hardened in air, obtained by incision or produced by spontaneous exudation from the stem and branches of *Commiphora molmol* Engler and/or other species of *Commiphora*.

The material complies with the monograph of the European Pharmacopoeia [1].

Species other than *Commiphora molmol* Engler [synonym: *C. myrrha* (Nees) Engler var. *molmol*] which may be acceptable sources of medicinal myrrh include *Commiphora abyssinica* (Berg) Engler and *C. schimperi* (Berg) Engler [2].

CONSTITUENTS

Myrrh can be separated into three components: volatile oil (2-10%), resin (25-40%) and gum (30-60%) [3].

The main constituents of the volatile oil are furano-sesquiterpenes of various structural types including furanoeudesma-1,3-diene (principal component), furanoeudesma-1,4-diene-6-one, lindestrene, curzerenone, furanodiene, 2-methoxyfuranodiene and 4,5-dihydrofuranodiene-6-one, together with sesquiterpenes such as α-copaene, elemene and bourbonene [4-8].

Characteristic constituents of the resin are α-, β- and γ-commiphoric acids, α- and β-heerabomyrrhols, heeraboresene and burseracin [7,8]; also various terpenes [9] and a sesquiterpene lactone, commiferin [10].

The gum consists mainly of a proteoglycan in which chains of alternating galactose and 4-*O*-methyl-glucuronic acid, and separate chains of arabinose, are attached to the protein through hydroxyproline links [3,11,12].

CLINICAL PARTICULARS

Therapeutic indications
Topical treatment of gingivitis, stomatitis (aphthous ulcers), minor skin inflammations, minor wounds and abrasions; supportive treatment for pharyngitis, tonsillitis [8,13-17].

Posology and method of administration

Dosage

Adults: As a gargle or mouthwash, 1-5 ml of tincture (1:5, ethanol 90% V/V) in a glass of water several times daily [8,13,17]. For use on skin, dab 2-3 times daily with diluted or undiluted tincture (1:5, ethanol 90% V/V) [8,13-16].

Elderly: as for adults.

Children: as for adults except using only diluted tincture on skin.

Method of administration
For topical application.

Duration of administration
No restriction.

Contra-indications
None known.

Special warnings and special precautions for use
None required.
Because of the alcohol content, a transient burning sensation on the skin may be experienced depending on the level of dilution of the tincture.

Interaction with other medicaments and other forms of interaction
None reported.

Pregnancy and lactation
No data available. In accordance with general medical practice the product should not be used during pregnancy or lactation without medical advice.

Effects on ability to drive and use machines
None known.

Undesirable effects
Very rare cases of allergic contact dermatitis have been reported [18,19].

Overdose
No toxic effects reported.

PHARMACOLOGICAL PROPERTIES

Pharmacodynamic properties

In vitro experiments

Antibacterial and antifungal effects
Various sesquiterpene-containing fractions from myrrh inhibited *Pseudomonas aeruginosa, Staphylococcus aureus, Escherichia coli* and *Candida albicans* with minimum inhibitory concentrations of 0.18-2.8 µg/ml [20].

In vivo experiments

Anti-inflammatory effects
In carrageenan-induced paw oedema and cotton pellet granuloma tests in rats a petroleum ether extract of myrrh (25:1), at an oral dose of 500 mg/kg body weight, exerted significant anti-inflammatory effects (Table 1) [21].

An ethanolic dry extract of myrrh (approximately 6:1), administered intraperitoneally to mice, exerted a significant anti-inflammatory effect (p<0.05) at 400 mg/kg body weight in the xylene-induced ear swelling model. The same extract significantly inhibited cotton pellet granuloma (p<0.05) in rats at an oral dose of 400 mg/kg [22].

Antipyretic effect
After oral administration to hyperpyretic mice of either an ethanolic or a petroleum ether extract of

TABLE 1

Treatment	Dose (mg/kg body weight)	Carrageenan-induced rat paw oedema		Cotton pellet-induced exudation	
		Mean increase in paw volume (ml ± SE)*	Per cent inhibition	Mean increase in weight of pellet (ml ± SE)*	Per cent inhibition
Control	Saline	0.86 ± 0.025	-	45.22 ± 2.18	-
Myrrh extract	500	0.33 ± 0.026	62.16	33.24 ± 3.65	26.49
Oxyphenbutazone	100	0.38 ± 0.017	55.32	Not tested	Not tested

*SE = Standard error of the mean

myrrh (25:1) at a dose of 500 mg/kg body weight a significant antipyretic effect (p<0.001) was demonstrated [21,23].

Stimulation of phagocytosis
Mice inoculated with *Escherichia coli* were treated intraperitoneally with either a dried ethanolic extract or the unsaponifiable fraction of myrrh, as solutions in aqueous ethanol (10% V/V) at 50 mg/kg (1 mg per 20 g animal). Both treatments stimulated phagocytosis in over 80% of the mice compared to controls [24].

Cytoprotective effect
Oral administration of myrrh to rats at 250, 500 and 1000 mg/kg body weight provided significant and dose-dependent protection to the gastric mucosa against the ulcerogenic effects of various necrotizing agents: 80% ethanol, 25% sodium chloride, 0.2 M sodium hydroxide, indometacin 30 mg/kg and combined ethanol 80%-indometacin 2.5 mg/kg (p<0.05 to p<0.001, depending on the dose). The same suspension significantly and dose-dependently protected against ethanol-induced depletion of gastric wall mucus (p<0.05 at 500 mg/kg; p<0.001 at 1000 mg/kg) [25].

Analgesic effects
In the hot plate test in mice a significant analgesic effect (p<0.01) was demonstrated after oral administration of myrrh at 1 mg/kg body weight [26].

Furanoeudesma-1,3-diene isolated from myrrh showed significant analgesic properties in mice when administered by intracerebroventricular injection at 1.25 mg/kg body weight (p<0.01) or orally at 50 mg/kg in the hot plate test, and also at 50 mg/kg in the writing test. The analgesic effects were reversed by naloxone at 1 mg/kg, indicating an interaction with brain opioid receptors. This interaction was subsequently demonstrated *in vitro*; furanoeudesma-1,3-diene concentration-dependently displaced the specific binding of [³H]diprenorphine to rat brain membrane [26,27].

An ethanolic dry extract of myrrh (approximately 6:1), administered orally to mice, exerted a significant and dose-dependent analgesic effect in the acetic acid-induced writhing test at 200 mg/kg (p< 0.05) and 400 mg/kg (p<0.01) [22].

Antitumour and cytotoxic effects
After oral treatment of Ehrlich solid tumour (EST)-bearing mice with an aqueous suspension of myrrh at daily doses of 250 or 500 mg/kg body weight, the higher dose produced significant decreases (p<0.05) after 25 days and 50 days in tumour weight, in the viability of EST cells and in levels of DNA, RNA and protein in EST cells. The antitumour potential of myrrh was found to be comparable to that of the cytotoxic drug cyclophosphamide [28].

The antitumour activity of an aqueous suspension of myrrh, equivalent to that of cyclophosphamide, has also been demonstrated in Ehrlich ascites carcinoma (EAC) cell-bearing mice. At 500 mg/kg, significant reductions in the DNA (p<0.05), RNA (p<0.01) and protein (p<0.01) contents of EAC cells, and in their viability (p<0.05), were observed together with an increased survival rate of the animals [29].

Hypoglycaemic effects
Intragastric treatment of normal and diabetic rats with a 5% m/V aqueous extract of myrrh (extracted with boiling water then filtered) daily for one week at 10 ml/kg body weight lowered fasting blood glucose levels in both groups and, in the oral glucose tolerance test, significantly increased glucose tolerance in both normal (p<0.02) and diabetic animals (p<0.05) [30].

Oral administration of two fractions (200-250 mg/kg body weight) and two pure furanosesquiterpenes (150-175 mg/kg) from myrrh (*C. myrrha*) to obese diabetic mice produced significant reductions in blood glucose at 27 hours post-dose (p<0.005 in all cases). One active fraction at 200 mg/kg reduced blood glucose by 50% (p<0.0001), compared to a 41% reduction with the oral antidiabetic metformin at 250 mg/kg [31].

Antithrombotic activity
Powdered myrrh (*C. molmol*), administered orally at 100 mg/kg body weight, provided 86% protection against experimental thrombosis in mice (p<0.05), comparable to the effect of acetylsalicylic acid at 20 mg/kg [32].

Local anaesthetic activity
A fraction from myrrh (*C. molmol*) composed of furanodiene-6-one and methoxyfuranoguaia-9-ene-8-one, administered as eye drops at a concentration of 280 µg/ml into the conjunctival sac of rabbits, had a strong local anaesthetic effect (p<0.01 compared to the vehicle as control) of about half that of procaine at 100 µg/ml [20].

Clinical studies

Anthelmintic effects
Oral treatment of 204 patients suffering from schistosomiasis with myrrh at 10 mg/kg body weight/day for 3 days in an open study produced a cure rate of 91.7%. Non-responding patients treated for 6 further days with the same dose gave a cure rate of 76.5%, increasing the overall rate to 98%. 20 patients provided biopsy specimens 6 months after treatment and none of them showed living ova [33].

In a preliminary open study 7 patients with fascioliasis (infection with parasitic liver flukes) were treated orally with a preparation consisting of 8 parts of myrrh resin and 3.5 parts of myrrh volatile oil at 12 mg/kg body weight/day for 6 days. The therapy proved to be effective, with pronounced improvement in the general condition of the patients and amelioration of all symptoms and signs. By the end of treatment a dramatic drop in the egg count was observed and eggs were no longer detectable in the faeces after 3 weeks or after a follow-up period of 3 months. High eosinophilic counts, elevated liver enzymes and *Fasciola* antibody titres returned to nearly normal [34].

Pharmacokinetic properties
No data available.

Preclinical safety data
The acute oral LD_{50} of myrrh oil has been determined as 1.65 g/kg [35].

Myrrh and the volatile oil of myrrh are reported to be non-irritating, non-sensitizing and non-phototoxic when applied to animal or human skin [16,35].

Oral toxicity studies of myrrh (*C. molmol*) were carried out in mice using acute doses of 0.5, 1.0 and 3.0 g/kg body weight and chronic doses of 100 mg/kg/day for 90 days. Compared to controls, no significant differences in mortality, weight gain or biochemical parameters were observed after acute or chronic treatment. After chronic treatment there were significant increases in weight of testes and seminal vesicles (p<0.05) and of caudae epididymis (p<0.01), and a significant increase in red blood cell count and haemoglobin (p<0.05). The toxicity studies supported the safe medicinal use of myrrh [36]

Genotoxicity and cytotoxicity
Myrrh administered orally to normal mice for 7 days at 125-500 mg/kg body weight/day as an aqueous suspension showed no mutagenicity in the micronucleus test. It caused a significant, dose-dependent reduction in the RNA content of hepatic cells (p<0.01 at 250 mg/kg), but not the DNA or protein content, and a highly significant, dose-dependent, mitosis-depressant effect in femoral cells (p<0.001) [29,37].

Clinical safety data
Myrrh was well tolerated with only mild and transient side effects when administered orally to 204 patients with schistosomiasis at 10 mg/kg body weight/day for 3-9 days [33]. No signs of toxicity or adverse effects were observed from treatment of 7 patients with fascioliasis with myrrh resin/volatile oil at 12 mg/kg body weight for 6 days [34].

Ethnopharmacological evidence [16] suggests that myrrh has been extensively used both internally and externally without serious adverse effects.

REFERENCES

1. Myrrh - Myrrha. European Pharmacopoeia, Council of Europe.

2. Wichtl M, Neubeck M. Myrrhe. In: Hartke K, Hartke H, Mutschler E, Rücker G, Wichtl M, editors. Kommentar zur Europäischen Arzneibuch. Stuttgart: Wissenschaftliche Verlagsgesellschaft, 1999 (12. Lfg.):M 87.

3. Wiendl RM, Franz G. Myrrhe - Neue Chemie einer alten Droge. Dtsch Apoth Ztg 1994;134:25-30.

4. Brieskorn CH, Noble P. Two furanoeudesmanes from the essential oil of myrrh. Phytochemistry 1983;22:187-9.

5. Brieskorn CH, Noble P. Furanosesquiterpenes from the essential oil of myrrh. Phytochemistry 1983;22:1207-11.

6. Brieskorn CH, Noble P. Inhaltsstoffe des etherischen Öls der Myrrhe. II: Sesquiterpene und Furanosesquiterpene. Planta Med 1982;44:87-90.

7. Martinetz D, Lohs K, Janzen J. Zur Chemie der Myrrhe. In: Weihrauch und Myrrhe. Kulturgeschichte und wirtschaftliche Bedeutung: Botanik, Chemie, Medizin. Stuttgart: Wissenschaftliche Verlagsgesellschaft, 1988: 169-80.

8. Hänsel R, Keller K, Rimpler H, Schneider G, editors. Commiphora. In: Hagers Handbuch der Pharmazeutischen Praxis, 5th ed. Volume 4: Drogen A-D. Berlin: Springer-Verlag, 1992:961-9.

9. Mincione E, Iavarone C. Terpeni dalla Commifera mirra arabica. Nota I. Chim Ind 1972;54:424-5.

10. Mincione E, Iavarone C. Terpeni dalla Commifera mirra arabica. Nota II. Chim Ind 1972;54:525-7.

11. Hough L, Jones JKN, Wadman WH. Some observations on the constitution of gum myrrh. J Chem Soc 1952:796-800.

12. Jones JKN, Nunn JR. The constitution of gum myrrh. Part II. J Chem Soc 1955:3001-4.

13. Bradley PR, editor. Myrrh. In: British Herbal Compendium, Volume 1. Bournemouth: British Herbal Medicine Association, 1992:163-5.

14. Czygan F-C, Hiller K. Myrrha - Myrrhe. In: Wichtl M, editor. Teedrogen und Phytopharmaka. Ein Handbuch für die Praxis auf wissenschaftlicher Grundlage, 4th ed. Stuttgart: Wissenschaftliche Verlagsgesellschaft, 2002:404-6.

15. Reynolds JEF, editor. Myrrh. In: Martindale - The Extra Pharmacopoeia, 31st ed. London: Royal Pharmaceutical Society, 1996:1730.

16. Martinetz D, Lohs K, Janzen J. Myrrhe als Arzneimittel. In: Weihrauch und Myrrhe. Kulturgeschichte und

wirtschaftliche Bedeutung: Botanik, Chemie, Medizin. Stuttgart: Wissenschaftliche Verlagsgesellschaft, 1989: 141-51.

17. Barnes J, Anderson LA and Phillipson JD. Myrrh. In: Herbal Medicines - A guide for healthcare professionals, 2nd ed. London-Chicago: Pharmaceutical Press, 2002: 357-9.

18. Gallo R, Rivara G, Cattarini G, Cozzani E, Guarrera M. Allergic contact dermatitis from myrrh. Contact Dermatitis 1999;41:230-1.

19. Al-Suwaidan SN, Gad el Rab MO, Al-Fakhiry S, Al Hoqail IA, Al-Maziad A, Sherif A-B. Allergic contact dermatitis from myrrh, a topical herbal medicine used to promote healing. Contact Dermatitis 1997;39:137.

20. Dolara P, Corte B, Ghelardini C, Pugliese AM, Cerbai E, Menichetti S, Lo Nostro A. Local anaesthetic, antibacterial and antifungal properties of sesquiterpenes from myrrh. Planta Med 2000;66:356-8.

21. Tariq M, Ageel AM, Al-Yahya MA, Mossa JS, Al-Said MS, Parmar NS. Anti-inflammatory activity of *Commiphora molmol*. Agents Actions 1985;17:381-2.

22. Atta AH, Alkofahi A. Anti-nociceptive and anti-inflammatory effect of some Jordanian medicinal plant extracts. J Ethnopharmacol 1998;60:117-24.

23. Mohsin A, Shah AH, Al-Yahya MA, Tariq M, Tanira MOM, Ageel AM. Analgesic, antipyretic activity and phytochemical screening of some plants used in traditional Arab system of medicine. Fitoterapia 1989; 60:174-7.

24. Delaveau P, Lallouette P, Tessier AM. Drogues végétales stimulant l'activité phagocytaire du système réticulo-endothélial. Planta Med 1980;40:49-54.

25. Al-Harbi MM, Qureshi S, Raza M, Ahmed MM, Afzal M, Shah AH. Gastric antiulcer and cytoprotective effect of *Commiphora molmol* in rats. J Ethnopharmacol 1997;55:141-50.

26. Dolara P, Luceri C, Ghelardini C, Monserrat C, Aiolli S, Luceri F et al. Analgesic effects of myrrh. Nature 1996; 379:29.

27. Dolara P, Moneti G, Pieraccini G, Romanelli N. Characterization of the action on central opioid receptors of furanoeudesma-1,3-diene, a sesquiterpene extracted from myrrh. Phytotherapy Res 1996; 10(Suppl.1):S81-3.

28. Al-Harbi MM, Qureshi S, Raza M, Ahmed MM, Giangreco AB, Shah AH. Anticarcinogenic effect of *Commiphora molmol* on solid tumors induced by Ehrlich carcinoma cells in mice. Chemotherapy 1994; 40:337-47.

29. Qureshi S, Al-Harbi MM, Ahmed MM, Raza M, Giangreco AB, Shah AH. Evaluation of the genotoxic, cytotoxic and antitumor properties of *Commiphora molmol* using normal and Ehrlich ascites carcinoma cell-bearing Swiss albino mice. Cancer Chemother Pharmacol 1993:33:130-8.

30. Al-Awadi FM, Gumaa KA. Studies on the activity of individual plants of an antidiabetic plant mixture. Acta Diabetol 1987;24:37-41.

31. Ubillas RP, Mendez CD, Jolad SD, Luo J, King SR, Carlson TJ, Fort DM. Antihyperglycemic furano-sesquiterpenes from *Commiphora myrrha*. Planta Med 1999;65:778-9.

32. Olajide OA. Investigation of the effects of selected medicinal plants on experimental thrombosis. Phytotherapy Res 1999;13:231-2.

33. Sheir Z, Nasr AA, Massoud A, Salama O, Badra GA, El-Shennawy H et al. A safe, effective, herbal antischistosomal therapy derived from myrrh. Am J Trop Med Hyg 2001;65:700-4.

34. Massoud A, El Sisi S, Salama O, Massoud A. Preliminary study of therapeutic efficacy of a new fasciolicidal drug derived from *Commiphora molmol* (myrrh). Am J Trop Med Hyg 2001;65:96-9.

35. Opdyke DLJ. Monographs on fragrance raw materials: Myrrh oil. Food Cosmet Toxicol 1976;14:621.

36. Rao RM, Khan ZA, Shah AH. Toxicity studies in mice of *Commiphora molmol* oleo-gum-resin. J Ethnopharmacol. 2001;76:151-4.

37. Al-Harbi MM, Qureshi S, Ahmed MM, Rafatullah S, Shah AH. Effect of *Commiphora molmol* (oleo-gum-resin) on the cytological and biochemical changes induced by cyclophosphamide in mice. Am J Chin Med 1994;22:77-82.

MYRTILLI FRUCTUS

Bilberry Fruit

DEFINITIONS

Dried bilberry fruit consists of the dried ripe fruit of *Vaccinium myrtillus* L. It contains not less than 1.0 percent of tannins, expressed as pyrogallol ($C_6H_6O_3$; M_r 126.1) and calculated with reference to the dried drug.

Fresh bilberry fruit consists of the fresh or frozen ripe fruit of *Vaccinium myrtillus* L. It contains not less than 0.30 per cent of anthocyanins, expressed as cyanidin-3-glucoside chloride (chrysanthemin $C_{21}H_{21}ClO_{11}$; M_r 485.5) and calculated with reference to the dried drug.

The materials comply with the respective monographs of the European Pharmacopoeia [1,2].

CONSTITUENTS

The main characteristic constituents are anthocyanins (anthocyanosides; 0.5% in dried bilberry fruit) [3]. Other constituents include tannins, hydroxycinnamic and hydroxy-benzoic acids, flavonol glycosides, flavan-3-ols, iridoids, terpenes, pectins and organic plant acids [3-7].

CLINICAL PARTICULARS

Therapeutic indications

Internal use
Extracts of bilberry fruit enriched in anthocyanins: symptomatic treatment of problems related to varicose veins, such as painful and heavy legs [8-17].
Dried bilberry fruit: supportive treatment of acute, non-specific diarrhoea [18,19].

External use
Topical treatment of mild inflammation of the mucous membranes of the mouth and throat [18].

Posology and method of administration

Dosage

Internal use
Standardized extracts of bilberry fruit containing 36% of anthocyanins: 320-480 mg/day [20-29]; equivalent preparations.
Dried bilberry fruit: 20-60 g daily [18,19].

External use
A 10% decoction of dried bilberry fruit [18].

E/S/C/O/P
MONOGRAPHS
Second Edition

Method of administration
For oral administration or local application.

Duration of administration
No restriction.
If diarrhoea persists for more than 3-4 days medical advice should be sought.

Contra-indications
None known.

Special warnings and special precautions for use
None required.

Interaction with other medicaments and other forms of interaction
None reported.

Pregnancy and lactation
Anthocyanins are well tolerated in pregnancy; they do not induce side-effects in the mother or offspring [17].

Effects on ability to drive and use machines
None known.

Undesirable effects
None reported.

Overdose
No toxic effects reported.

PHARMACOLOGICAL PROPERTIES

In the following text, unless stated otherwise, "standardized extract" of bilberry fruit refers to an extract containing 36% of anthocyanins.

Pharmacodynamic properties

In vitro experiments

Antioxidant activity
Anthocyanin-rich extract of bilberry fruit is reported to be a potent scavenger of free radicals, behaving both as a scavenger against superoxide anion [30-33] and as an inhibitor of lipid peroxidation induced by adenosine diphosphate (ADP)/Fe^{2+} and ascorbate in rat liver microsomes [31-33]. The radical scavenging properties have also been verified for individual anthocyanins [34]. Furthermore, an anthocyanin-rich extract inhibited the K^+ loss induced by free radicals in human erythrocytes as well as the cellular damage caused by oxidant compounds such as daunomycin and paraquat [35,36].

More recently an aqueous extract of bilberry fruit was shown to have a potent protective action on human low density lipoprotein (LDL) during copper-mediated oxidation [37], and a standardized extract containing 37% of anthocyanins prevented photo-induced oxidation of human LDL and fragmentation of apoprotein [38].

Platelet aggregation
A standardized extract of bilberry fruit showed activity against aggregation induced by ADP, collagen and sodium arachidonate in rabbit platelet-rich plasma [39]. This was confirmed *ex vivo* on ADP- and collagen-induced aggregation of platelets obtained from the blood of 30 healthy volunteers given 480 mg/day of the standardized extract orally for 30-60 days [40]. An anthocyanin extract of bilberry fruit also inhibited *in vitro* platelet aggregation induced by ADP or adrenaline in human plasma [41].

Effect on vascular tissues
Anthocyanin-rich extract of bilberry fruit is able to inhibit proteolytic enzymes such as elastase [42] and to interact with collagen metabolism by cross-linking collagen fibres, making them more resistant to collagenase action [43] and reducing the biosynthesis of polymeric collagen [44].

An anthocyanin-rich standardized extract (corresponding to 25% of anthocyanidins) had a slightly relaxing effect on various isolated vascular smooth muscle preparations and reduced the response to contraction inducers such as serotonin and barium [45-48].

In vivo experiments

Antioxidant activity
Oral pre-treatment of mice with 250 or 500 mg/kg of an anthocyanin-rich extract from bilberry fruit inhibited liver lipid peroxidation stimulated by a mixture of $FeCl_2$, ascorbic acid and ADP. The malonaldeyde content in the liver was significantly reduced (p<0.05) [33].

Vasoprotective activity
Anthocyanin-rich extracts of bilberry fruit exert modulating effects on capillary resistance and permeability, as demonstrated in various experimental models [20-22,49,50]. For example, an extract administered orally to rabbits at 200-400 mg/kg protected against increased capillary permeability induced by topical application of chloroform [20]. When administered orally to rats at 100-200 mg/kg, or intraperitoneally or intramuscularly at 25-100 mg/kg, the extract gave protection from capillary lesions induced by intradermal injection of bradykinin [20]. In a more recent study, the same extract was found to antagonise damage induced by ischaemia-reperfusion in the hamster cheek-pouch microcirculation model after oral administration at 100 mg/kg for 4 weeks [23].

Ophthalmic activity

An anthocyanin-rich extract of bilberry fruit, administered intravenously to rabbits at 3.2 mg/kg, reduced the permeability of vessels of the ciliary body, which had been increased by paracentesis [24].

Furthermore, a mixture of anthocyanins administered intravenously to rabbits at 160 mg/kg promoted dark adaptation after dazzling [25]. It was suggested that this improvement in visual function was probably due to an increase in the regeneration rate of rhodopsin [26].

Anti-inflammatory activity

The vasoprotective effect could also be responsible for anti-inflammatory activity exhibited by anthocyanins (50-500 mg/kg, given orally) against rat paw oedema induced by irritant agents such as carrageenan, histamine or hyaluronidase [20,27].

Wound healing and antiulcer activity

Topical application of 5-10 mg of an anthocyanin-rich extract of bilberry fruit accelerated the healing of experimental wounds in rats [28]. In another experimental model, healing delayed by prednisone, the same extract applied topically at concentrations of 0.5-2% for 3 days to skin wounds in rats promoted healing activity in comparison with prednisone-treated controls [29].

A standardized extract (corresponding to 25% of anthocyanidins), administered orally to rats at doses ranging from 25 to 200 mg/kg, showed antiulcer activity against acute gastric ulcers induced by pyloric ligation, non-steroidal anti-inflammatory drugs (NSAIDs) and reserpine [29].

Antiatherogenic activity

An anthocyanin-rich extract of bilberry fruit, administered intraperitoneally at 100 mg/kg for 45 days to rabbits fed on a cholesterol-rich diet, reduced the proliferation of intima and calcium and lipid deposition on the aortic wall [51].

Clinical studies

Peripheral vascular diseases

In 47 patients with lower limb varicose syndrome, oral treatment with bilberry fruit extract at 480 mg/day for 30 days led to improvements in objective symptoms such as limb oedema and dyschromic skin phenomena, and subjective symptoms such as heaviness, paraesthesia and pain [8].

Improvements in vessel fragility and objective symptoms after administration of bilberry fruit extract at 480 mg/day for 30-180 days have been confirmed in trials performed on 22 diabetic and dyslipidaemic patients [9], on 97 patients with complaints induced by stasis of the lower extremities such as prevaricose

syndrome, essential varices and post-phlebitic syndrome [10], and on 42 patients with severe arteriosclerotic vascular disease of the lower limbs [11].

In a double-blind, placebo-controlled study performed on 47 patients with peripheral vascular disorders of various origins, a standardized extract of bilberry fruit (480 mg/day for 30 days) reduced subjective symptoms such as paraesthesia, pain and heaviness, and improved oedema and mobility of finger joints [12].

The efficacy of a standardized extract of bilberry fruit has been evaluated in two clinical studies, each in 15 patients with venous insufficiency who were treated orally with 480 mg/day for 2-4 months. Significant improvements in plethysmographic (p<0.05) and duoregional rheographic (p<0.001) observations were reported [13,14].

In 24 patients with chronic venous insufficiency, oral administration of 480 mg of an anthocyanin-rich extract of bilberry fruit daily for 60 days induced a decrease in the total time of drainage after reactive hyperaemia evaluated by the strain gauge technique [15].

The efficacy of the same extract (480 mg/day for 30 days) was further demonstrated in a single-blind, placebo-controlled study carried out in 60 patients with different stages of venous insufficiency; this study showed significant activity of the extract (p<0.01 to p<0.001) on subjective parameters, namely feeling of pressure in the lower limbs and muscle cramps as well as oedema and leg and ankle girth [16].

Significant improvements in subjective symptoms (p<0.01) and reductions in oedema and capillary fragility were observed in 54 cases of phlebopathies induced by stasis during pregnancy after oral administration of 320 mg of extract daily for 60-90 days [17].

Ophthalmic disorders

Daily treatment of 14 patients suffering from tapetoretinal degeneration with 3 × 150 mg of a bilberry fruit extract resulted in an improvement in light sensitivity of the retina starting from the second day of treatment and remaining almost constant during the 3-month treatment period [52].

The efficacy of a standardized extract (320 mg/day) has been evaluated in 40 patients with refractory defects. Accurate ocular and electrofunctional examinations showed a significant increase in the flash electroretinogram amplitude in medium (p = 0.002) and high myopia (p = 0.008), indicating an improvement in retinal sensitivity [53]. In another study, daily administration of 320 mg of the extract for 3 months to 26 myopic patients resulted in improvement of electrophysiological functions [54].

In a double-blind, placebo-controlled study involving 40 healthy subjects the activity of an anthocyanin-rich extract, administered orally at 240 mg daily for 3 months, was evaluated from pupillary movements through examination of the direct photomotor reflex. The study demonstrated a more efficient pupillary photomotor response after administration of the extract compared to placebo [55].

Oral administration of a standardized extract of bilberry fruit at 480 mg/day for 180 days to 10 patients with type II diabetes mellitus and non-proliferative retinopathy resulted in improvement of the diabetic retinopathy, with marked reduction or disappearance of retinal haemorrhages [56].

In a double blind, placebo-controlled study, 40 patients with diabetic or hypertensive retinopathy were treated with 320 mg of a standardized extract of bilberry fruit or placebo daily for 30 days. An improvement in ophthalmoscopic and angiographic patterns was observed in 77-90% of the verum patients [57].

In another placebo-controlled study, involving 40 patients with diabetic retinopathy at a relatively early phase, a standardized extract of bilberry fruit administered at 320 mg/day for 12 months promoted the regression of hard exudates, which is considered a reliable index of altered permeability [58].

Pharmacokinetic properties
After oral administration to rats of a single dose of 400 mg/kg, a standardized extract of bilberry fruit was rapidly absorbed from the gastrointestinal tract with a C_{max} of 2.47 µg/ml and at a T_{max} of 15 min [59].

After intravenous or intraperitoneal administration of an anthocyanin-rich extract (equivalent to 25% of anthocyanidins) to rats at doses of 20-40 mg/kg or 25 mg/kg, respectively, anthocyanins were rapidly distributed to the tissues. Elimination occurred mainly in the urine (25-30% of the dose within 24 hours after administration) and to a lesser extent (15-20%) in bile [60].

Preclinical safety data

Acute toxicity
Intraperitoneal and intravenous LD_{50} values of an anthocyanin-rich extract from bilberry fruit containing about 70% of anthocyanins were determined as 4.11 g/kg and 0.84 g/kg in the mouse, and 2.35 g/kg and 0.24 g/kg in the rat, respectively. No deaths were observed following oral doses of up to 25 g/kg in the mouse and 20 g/kg in the rat [50].

Chronic toxicity
Treatment of rats for 90 days with the same extract at a daily dose corresponding to approximatively five times the human clinical dose (i.e. 600 mg/day) did not produce any toxic effects [50].

Mutagenicity and carcinogenicity
No data are available.

REFERENCES

1. Bilberry Fruit, Dried - Myrtilli fructus siccus. European Pharmacopoeia, Council of Europe.

2. Bilberry Fruit, Fresh - Myrtilli fructus recens. European Pharmacopoeia, Council of Europe.

3. Vaccinium. In: Hänsel R, Keller K, Rimpler H, Schneider G, editors. Hagers Handbuch der Pharmazeutischen Praxis, 5th ed. Volume 6: Drogen P-Z. Berlin: Springer-Verlag, 1994:1051-67.

4. Kröger C. Die Heidelbeere, *Vaccinium myrtillus* L. Pharmazie 1951;6:211-7.

5. Friedrich H, Schönert J. Untersuchungen über einige Inhaltsstoffe der Blätter und Früchte von *Vaccinium myrtillus*. Planta Med 1973;24:90-100.

6. Brenneisen R, Steinegger E. Zur Analytik der Polyphenole der Früchte von *Vaccinium myrtillus* L. (Ericaceae). Pharm Acta Helv 1981;56:180-5.

7. Baj A, Bombardelli E, Gabetta B, Martinelli EM. Qualitative and quantitative evaluation of *Vaccinium myrtillus* anthocyanins by high-resolution gas chromatography and high-performance liquid chromatography. J Chromatogr 1983;279:365-72.

8. Ghiringhelli C, Gregoratti L, Marastoni F. Attività capillarotropa di antocianosidi ad alto dosaggio nella stasi da flebopatia. Minerva Cardioangiol 1977;26:255-76.

9. Passariello N, Bisesti V, Sganbato S. Influenza degli antocianosidi sul microcircolo e sull'assetto lipidico in soggetti diabetici e dislipidemici. Gazz Med Ital 1979; 138:563-6.

10. Tori A, D'Errico F. Gli antocianosidi da *Vaccinium myrtillus* nella cura delle flebopatie da stasi degli arti inferiori. Gazz Med Ital 1980;139:217-24.

11. Nuti A, Curri SB, Vittori C, Lampertico M. Significance of anthocyanins in the treatment of peripheral vascular diseases. In: Reinis Z, Pokorný J, Linhart J, Hild R, Schirger, editors. Adaptability of Vascular Wall. Prague: Springer-Verlag, 1980:572-3.

12. Allegra C, Pollari G, Criscuolo A, Bonifacio M. Antocianosidi e sistema microvasculotessutale. Minerva Angiol 1982;7:39-44.

13. Signorini GP, Salmistrano G, Deotto GP, Maraglino GM. Ruolo delle moderne tecnologie strumentali angiologiche nella diagnostica non invasiva delle agiolo-flebopatie periferiche. Parte I. Fitoterapia 1983; 54(Suppl 3):3-18.

14. Signorini GP, Salmistrano G, Deotto GP, Maraglino GM. Ruolo delle moderne tecnologie strumentali angiologiche nella diagnostica non invasiva delle agiolo-flebopatie periferiche. Parte II. Fitoterapia 1983;54(Suppl 3):19-30.

15. Corsi C, Pollastri M, Tesi C, Borgioli A, Boscarini A. Contributo allo studio dell'attività degli antocianosidi sul microcircolo: valutazioni flussimetriche nell'insufficienza venosa cronica. Fitoterapia 1985; 56(Suppl 1):23-31.

16. Gatta L. Gli antocianosidi del mirtillo nel trattamento della stasi venosa: studio clinico controllato su sesenta pazienti. Fitoterapia 1988;59(Suppl 1):19-26.

17. Grismondi G.L. Contributo al trattamento delle flebopatie da stasi in gravidanza. Minerva Ginecol 1980;32:1-10.

18. Frohne D. Myrtilli fructus siccus - Getrocknete Heidelbeeren. In: Wichtl M, editor. Teedrogen und Phytopharmaka. Ein Handbuch für die Praxis auf wissenschaftlicher Grundlage, 4th ed. Stuttgart: Wissenschaftliche Verlagsgesellschaft, 2002:411-3.

19. Schilcher H. Diarrhoea. In: Phytotherapy in Paediatrics - Handbook for Physicians and Pharmacists. Stuttgart: Medpharm Scientific, 1997:49-51.

20. Lietti A, Cristoni A, Picci M. Studies on *Vaccinium myrtillus* anthocyanosides. I. Vasoprotective and antiinflammatory activity. Arzneim-Forsch/Drug Res 1976;26:829-32.

21. Robert AM, Godeau G, Moati F, Miskulin M. Action of anthocyanosides of *Vaccinium myrtillus* on the permeability of the blood brain barrier. J Medicine 1977;8:321-32.

22. Detre Z, Jellinek H, Miskulin M, Robert AM. Studies on vascular permeability in hypertension: action of anthocyanosides. Clin Physiol Biochem 1986;4:143-9.

23. Bertuglia S, Malandrino S, Colantuoni A. Effect of *Vaccinium myrtillus* anthocyanosides on ischemia-reperfusion injury in microcirculation. Scripta Phlebologica 1994;2:44.

24. Virno M, Pecori Giraldi J, Auriemma L. Antocianosidi di mirtillo e permeabilità dei vasi del corpo ciliare. Boll Ocul 1986;65:789-95.

25. Alfieri R, Sole P. Influence des anthocyanosides administrés par voie parentérale sur l'adapto-électrorétinogramme du lapin. CR Soc Biol 1964; 158:2338-41.

26. Tronche P, Bastide P, Komor J. Effet des glycosides d'anthocyanes sur la cinétique de régénération du pourpre rétinien chez le lapin. CR Soc Biol 1967; 161:2473-5.

27. Bonacina F, Galliani G, Pacchiano F. Attività degli antocianosidi nei processi flogistici acuti. Il Farmaco Ed Pr 1973;28:428-34.

28. Curri BS, Lietti A, Bombardelli E. Modificazioni morfoistochimiche del tessuto di granulazione delle ferite sperimentali indotte dall'apporto locale di antocianosidi. Giorn min Derm 1976;111:509-15.

29. Cristoni A, Magistretti MJ. Antiulcer and healing activity of *Vaccinium myrtillus* anthocyanosides. Il Farmaco Ed Prat 1987;42:29-43.

30. Salvayre R, Braquet P, Perruchot T, Douste-Blazy L. Comparison of the scavenger effect of bilberry anthocyanosides with various flavonoids. In: Farkas L, Gábor M, Kállay F, Wagner H, editors. Flavonoids and Bioflavonoids, 1981. Amsterdam: Elsevier, 1982: 437-42.

31. Meunier MT, Duroux E, Bastide P. Activité anti-radicalaire d'oligomères procyanidoliques et d'antho-cyanosides vis-à-vis de l'anion superoxyde et vis-à-vis de la lipoperoxydation. Plantes Méd Phytothér 1989; 23:267-74.

32. Martín-Aragón S, Basabe B, Benedì JM, Villar AM. Antioxidant action of *Vaccinium myrtillus* L. Phytotherapy Res 1998;12:S104-6.

33. Martín-Aragón S, Basabe B, Bebedì JM, Villar AM. In vitro and in vivo antioxidant properties of *Vaccinium myrtillus*. Pharmaceut Biol 1999;37:109-13.

34. Morazzoni P, Malandrino S. Anthocyanins and their aglycons as scavengers of free radicals and anti-lipoperoxidant agents. Pharmacol Res Commun 1988;20(Suppl 2):254.

35. Maridonneau I, Braquet P, Garay RP. Bioflavonoids protect human erythrocytes against the K^+-loss induced by free radicals. In: Farkas L, Gábor M, Kállay F, Wagner H, editors. Flavonoids and Bioflavonoids, 1981. Amsterdam: Elsevier, 1982:427-36.

36. Mavelli I, Rossi L, Autuori F, Braquet P, Rotilio G. Anthocyanosides inhibit cellular reactions of drugs producing oxy radicals. In: Cohen G, Greenwald RA, editors. Oxy Radicals: Their Scavenger Syst., Proc. Int. Conf. Superoxide - Superoxide Dismutase, 3rd. New York: Elsevier, 1982(Pub 1983);2:326-9; through Chem. Abstr. 1984;100:150g.

37. Laplaud PM, Lelubre A, Chapman MJ. Antioxidant action of *Vaccinium myrtillus* extract on human low density lipoproteins in vitro: initial observations. Fundam Clin Pharmacol 1997;11:35-40.

38. Rasetti MF, Caruso D, Galli G, Bosisio E. Extracts of *Gingko biloba* L. leaves and *Vaccinium myrtillus* L. fruits prevent photo-induced oxidation of low density lipoprotein cholesterol. Phytomedicine 1996/1997; 3:335-8.

39. Morazzoni P, Magistretti MJ. Activity of Myrtocyan®, an anthocyanoside complex from *Vaccinium myrtillus* (VMA), on platelet aggregation and adhesiveness. Fitoterapia 1990;61:13-21.

40. Pulliero G, Montin S, Bettini V, Martino R, Mogno C, Lo Castro G. *Ex vivo* study of the inhibitory effects of *Vaccinium myrtillus* anthocyanosides on human platelet aggregation. Fitoterapia 1989;60:69-75.

41. Serranillos Fdez MG, Zaragoza F, Alvarez P. Efectos sobre la agregación plaquetaria "in vitro" de los antocianósidos del *Vaccinium myrtillus* L. An Real Acad Farm 1983;49:79-90.

42. Jonadet M, Meunier MT, Bastide P. Anthocyanosides extraits de *Vitis vinifera*, de *Vaccinium myrtillus* et de *Pinus maritimus*. I. Activités inhibitrices vis-à-vis de l'élastase *in vitro*. II. Activités angioprotectrices comparées *in vivo*. J Pharm Belg 1983;38:41-6.

43. Robert AM, Miskulin M, Godeau G, Tixier JM. Action of anthocyanosides on the permeability of the blood-brain barrier. In: Robert L (editor). Frontiers of Matrix Biology, Volume 7. Basel: Karger, 1979:336-49; through Chem Abstr 1979;91:190464d.

44. Boniface R, Miskulin M, Robert L, Robert AM. Pharmacological properties of *Myrtillus* anthocyanosides: correlation with results of treatment of diabetic microangiopathy. In: Farkas L, Gábor M, Kállay F, Wagner H, editors. Flavonoids and Bioflavonoids, 1981. Amsterdam: Elsevier, 1982:293-301.

45. Bettini V, Mayellaro F, Ton P, Zanella P. Effects of *Vaccinium myrtillus* anthocyanosides on vascular smooth muscle. Fitoterapia 1984;55:265-72.

46. Bettini V, Mayellaro F, Patron E, Ton P, Terribile Wiel Marin V. Inhibition by *Vaccinium myrtillus* anthocyanosides of barium-induced contractions in segments of internal thoracic vein. Fitoterapia 1984;55:323-7.

47. Bettini V, Mayellaro F, Ton P, Zogno M. Interactions between *Vaccinium myrtillus* anthocyanosides and serotonin on splenic artery smooth muscle. Fitoterapia 1984;55:201-8.

48. Bettini V, Mayellaro F, Pilla I, Ton P, Terribile Wiel Marin V. Mechanical responses of isolated coronary arteries to barium in the presence of *Vaccinium myrtillus* anthocyanosides. Fitoterapia 1985;56:3-10.

49. Terrasse J, Moinade S. Premiers résultats obtenus avec un nouveau facteur vitaminique P - "les anthocyanosides" extraits du *Vaccinium myrtillus*. La Presse Médicale 1964;72:397-400.

50. Pourrat H, Bastide P, Dorier P, Pourrat A, Tronche P. Préparation et activité thérapeutique de quelques glycosides d'anthocyanes. Chimie Thérapeutique 1967; 2:33-8.

51. Kadar A, Robert L, Miskulin M, Tixier JM, Brechemier D, Robert AM. Influence of anthocyanoside treatment on the cholesterol-induced atherosclerosis in the rabbit. Arterial Wall 1979;5:187-206.

52. Zavarise G. Sull'effetto del trattamento prolungato con antocianosidi sul senso luminoso. Ann Ottal Clin Ocul 1968;94:209-14.

53. Spadea L, Giagnoli B, D'Amico M, Dragani T, Balestrazzi E. Antocianosidi del mirtillo ad alto dosaggio: risposte elettrofisiologiche nel soggetto normale, modesto miope e grande miope. Clin Ocul 1991;3:122-5.

54. Contestabile MT, Appolloni R, Suppressa F, D'Alba E, Pecorelli B. Trattamento prolungato con antocianosidi del mirtillo ad alto dosaggio: risposte elettrofisiologiche nel paziente miope. Boll Ocul 1991;70: 1157-69.

55. Vannini L, Samuelly R, Coffano M, Tibaldi L. Studio del comportamento pupillare in seguito a somministrazione di antocianosidi. Boll Ocul 1986;65:569-77.

56. Orsucci PL, Rossi M, Sabbatini G, Menci S, Berni M. Trattamento della retinopatia diabetica con antocianosidi. Indagine preliminare. Clin Ocul 1983;4:377-81.

57. Perossini M, Guidi S, Chiellini S, Siravo D. Studio clinico sull'impiego degli antocianosidi del mirtillo (Tegens) nel trattamento delle microangiopatie retiniche di tipo diabetico ed ipertensivo. Ann Ottal Clin Ocul 1987;113:1173-90.

58. Repossi P, Malagola R, De Cadilhac C. Influenza degli antocianosidi sulle malattie vasali da alterata permeabilità. Ann Ottal Clin Ocul 1987;113:357-61.

59. Morazzoni P, Livio S, Scilingo A, Malandrino S. *Vaccinium myrtillus* anthocyanosides. Pharmacokinetics in rats. Arzneim-Forsch/Drug Res 1991;41:128-31.

60. Lietti A, Forni G. Studies on *Vaccinium myrtillus* anthocyanosides. II. Aspects of anthocyanins pharmacokinetics in the rat. Arzneim-Forsch/Drug Res 1976;26:832-5.

ONONIDIS RADIX

Restharrow Root

E/S/C/O/P
MONOGRAPHS
Second Edition

DEFINITION

Restharrow root consists of the dried roots of *Ononis spinosa* L.

The material complies with the monograph of the European Pharmacopoeia [1].

CONSTITUENTS

Isoflavones including trifolirhizin [2,3], formononetin [3-5] together with its 7-O-glucoside-6″-malonate [4] and 7-O-glucoside (= ononin) [3,4], biochanin A 7-O-glucoside [4,5], medicarpin [6] and related compounds [3-5]; triterpenes, notably α-onocerin [3,7-9]; phytosterols, especially β-sitosterol [3,7]; phenolic acids [10]; tannins [11]; minerals [12] and about 0.02% of essential oil [13-15] containing mainly *trans*-anethole, carvone, menthol [13] and aromatic hydrocarbons [15]. The presence of flavonols such as rutin and kaempferol [5] has not been confirmed [16,17].

CLINICAL PARTICULARS

Therapeutic indications

Irrigation of the urinary tract, especially in cases of inflammation and renal gravel, and as an adjuvant in treatment of bacterial infections of the urinary tract [12,18-21].

Posology and method of administration

Dosage

Adults: An infusion of 2-3 g of dried material two to three times per day; equivalent preparations [22].

Method of administration

For oral administration. To prepare an infusion, boiling water is poured over the material and the mixture strained after 20-30 minutes.

Duration of administration

No restriction.

Contra-indications

None known.

Special warnings and special precautions for use

None required.

Interaction with other medicaments and other forms of interaction
None reported.

Pregnancy and lactation
No data available. In accordance with general medical practice, the product should not be used during pregnancy and lactation without medical advice.

Effects on ability to drive and use machines
None known.

Undesirable effects
None reported.

Overdose
No toxic effects reported.

PHARMACOLOGICAL PROPERTIES

Pharmacodynamic properties

Diuretic activity

In vivo experiments
In studies on 250 g rats, four preparations of restharrow (presumed to be from the root) were administered intragastrically to different groups of 4 rats, each dose being equivalent to 0.3 g of root and including 20 ml of water. The controls were water or theophylline (5 mg/kg), administered to the same rats several days later. The volumes of urine collected from the rats over a 5-hour period following administration of the respective preparations were: dried methanolic extract (rich in flavonoids) 19.9 ml, ash (rich in minerals, especially potassium) 18.7 ml, a mixture of methanolic extract and ash 20.9 ml, and aqueous infusion 21.4 ml, compared to 15.1 ml for water and 17.9 ml for theophylline. Corresponding amounts of sodium, determined by atomic absorption spectrophotometry in the urine collected over 5 hours, were 20, 32, 21 and 24 mg, compared to 6 and 16 mg with water and theophylline respectively. The potassium figures were 95, 79, 66 and 62 mg, compared to 44 and 61 mg with water and theophylline. These results demonstrated moderate diuretic (p<0.001) and saluretic activity, particularly natriuretic, of the preparations, in all cases higher than that of theophylline at 5 mg/kg. It was concluded that the diuretic activity of restharrow root was caused by its content of potassium salts and flavonoid glycosides [23].

An ethanolic extract (not defined) at a dose corresponding to 2 g of drug per kg body weight significantly increased urinary volume by 103% (p<0.05) compared to saline. No influence was observed on sodium or potassium elimination. Intraperitoneal administration did not show any diuretic effect at doses of drug up to 500 mg/kg [24].

Older studies gave the following results: an infusion from restharrow root administered orally to rabbits increased the urinary output by approx. 26% [25]; in mice an increase of urinary output and chloride excretion was demonstrated [25], while in rats the excretion of urea and chloride increased after oral administration [26].

After oral administration to rats, infusions of the root caused slight diuresis (average of 12%) and decoctions an antidiuretic effect of 7-20%. In these studies the aqueous residue after steam distillation showed an antidiuretic effect of 7-16% depending on the duration of distillation, whereas 0.5-1.0 ml of the essential oil obtained by steam distillation (2-4 hours) produced a diuretic effect [27]. The author [27] concluded that only the essential oil of restharrow root exhibits diuretic activity, a point which has been hotly disputed in the past [28-30].

Other effects

In vitro experiments
A methanolic restharrow root extract (6:1) was found to inhibit 5-lipoxygenase selectively with an IC_{50} of 7.8 µg/ml. The pterocarpan medicarpin, isolated from the extract, inhibited leukotriene B_4 formation with an IC_{50} of 6.7 µM [6].

Extracts of restharrow root have been shown to have antifungal activity [31].

In vivo experiments
No analgesic effects were observed in the hot plate test in mice after oral or intraperitoneal administration of an ethanolic restharrow root extract (not further defined). In the phenylquinone writhing test in mice, the extract reduced reaction to pain by up to 80% at doses of 100 and 500 mg per kg body weight after intraperitoneal administration, while no effect was observed after oral administration [24].

In the carrageenan-induced rat paw oedema test, the same extract significantly reduced oedema by a maximum of 46% after 3 hours (p<0.05) at an intraperitoneal dose corresponding to 500 mg of restharrow root per kg body weight, while no significant effects were observed at 100 mg/kg. Information on the controls was not stated [24].

Pharmacokinetic properties
No data available.

Preclinical safety data
An ethanolic extract (not further defined), administered orally or intraperitoneally at a daily dose corresponding to 2 g of drug per kg body weight for 14 days, did not cause any visible toxic effects [24].

REFERENCES

1. Restharrow Root - Ononidis radix. European Pharmacopoeia, Council of Europe.

2. Fujise Y, Toda T, Itô S. Isolation of trifolirhizin from *Ononis spinosa* L. Chem Pharm Bull 1965;13:93-5.

3. Háznagy A, Tóth G, Tamás J. Über die Inhaltsstoffe des wäßrigen Extraktes von *Ononis spinosa* L. Arch Pharm (Weinheim) 1978;311:318-23.

4. Köster J, Strack D, Barz W. High-performance liquid chromatographic separation of isoflavones and structural elucidation of isoflavone 7-O-glucoside 6'-malonates from *Cicer arietinum*. Planta Med 1983; 48:131-5.

5. Pietta P, Calatroni A, Zio C. High-performance liquid chromatographic analysis of flavonoids from *Ononis spinosa* L. J Chromatogr 1983;280:172-5.

6. Dannhardt G, Schneider G, Schwell B. Identification and 5-lipoxygenase inhibiting potency of medicarpin isolated from roots of *Ononis spinosa* L. Pharm Pharmacol Lett 1992;2:161-2.

7. Rowan MG, Dean PDG. α-Onocerin and sterol content of twelve species of *Ononis*. Phytochemistry 1972; 11:3263-5.

8. Spilková J, Hubík J. Pharmacognostic study of the species *Ononis arvensis* L. II. Flavonoids and onocerin in the vegetable drug. Cesk Farm 1982;31:24-6 [Czech; English summary].

9. Pauli GF. Comprehensive spectroscopic investigation of α-onocerin. Planta Med 2000;66:299-301.

10. Luczak S, Swiatek L. GC-MS investigation of phenolic acids in *Ononis spinosa* roots. Fitoterapia 1991;62:455-6.

11. Dedio I, Kozlowski J. Comparative morphological and phytochemical studies of *Ononis spinosa* L. and *Ononis arvensis* L. I. Biometric and chromatographic investigation of methanolic extracts. Acta Polon Pharm 1977;34:97-102 [Polish; English summary].

12. Steinegger E, Hänsel R. Hauhechelwurzel. In: Pharmakognosie, 5th ed. Berlin-Heidelberg-New York-London: Springer-Verlag, 1992:565-6.

13. Hilp K, Kating H, Schaden G. Inhaltsstoffe aus *Ononis spinosa* L. 1. Mitt. Das ätherische Öl der Radix Ononidis. Arch Pharm (Weinheim) 1975;308:429-33.

14. Dedio I, Kozlowski J. Comparative morphological and phytochemical studies of *Ononis spinosa* L. and *Ononis arvensis* L. II. Investigation of the oil. Acta Polon Pharm 1977;34:103-8 [Polish; English summary].

15. Hesse C, Hilp K, Kating H, Schaden G. Inhaltsstoffe aus *Ononis spinosa* L. 2. Mitt. Aromatische Kohlenwasserstoffe aus den ätherischen Ölen der Radix und Herba Ononidis. Arch Pharm (Weinheim) 1977; 310:792-5.

16. Kartnig T, Gruber A, Preuss M. Flavonoid-O-glykoside in *Ononis spinosa* L. (Fabaceae). Pharm Acta Helv 1985;60:253-5.

17. Kartnig T. Ononis. In: Blaschek W, Hänsel R, Keller K, Reichling J, Rimpler H, Schneider G, editors. Hagers Handbuch der Pharmazeutischen Praxis, 5th ed. Supplement Volume (Folgeband) 3: Drogen L-Z. Berlin-Heidelberg-New York-London: Springer, 1998: 263-71.

18. Weiß RF, Fintelmann V. Lehrbuch der Phytotherapie, 8th ed. Stuttgart: Hippokrates,1997:467.

19. Schilcher H. Pflanzliche Diuretika. Urologe B 1987; 27:215-22.

20. Schilcher H. Hauhechelwurzel. In: Loew D, Heimoth V, Kuntz E, Schilcher H, editors. Diuretika: Chemie, Pharmakologie und Therapie einschließlich Phytotherapie, 2nd ed. Stuttgart-New York: Thieme, 1990:273-4.

21. Hoppe HA. Drogenkunde, 8th ed. Berlin-New York: Walter de Gruyter, 1975:764-5.

22. Wichtl M. Ononidis radix - Hauhechelwurzel. In: Wichtl M, editor. Teedrogen und Phytopharmaka, 3rd ed. Stuttgart: Wissenschaftliche Verlagsgesellschaft, 1997:410-2.

23. Rebuelta M, San Roman L, G.-Serra Nillos M. Étude de l'effet diurétique de différentes préparations de l'*Ononis spinosa* L. Plantes Méd Phytothér 1981;15:99-108.

24. Bolle P, Faccendini P, Bello U, Panzironi C, Tita B. *Ononis spinosa* L. Pharmacological effect of ethanol extract. Pharmacol Res 1993;27(Suppl 1):27-8.

25. Vollmer H. Untersuchungen über die diuretische Wirkung der Folia betulae an Kaninchen und Mäusen. Vergleich mit anderen Drogen. Naunyn-Schmiedebergs Arch exp Path Pharmakol 1937;186:584-91.

26. Vollmer H, Hübner K. Untersuchungen über die diuretische Wirkung der Fructus juniperi, Radix levistici, Radix ononidis, Folia betulae, Radix liquiritiae und Herba equiseti an Ratten. Naunyn-Schmiedebergs Arch exp Path Pharmakol 1937;186:592-605.

27. Hilp K. Phytochemische und pharmakologische Untersuchungen der ätherischen Öle aus Wurzel und Kraut von *Ononis spinosa* L. [Dissertation]. University of Marburg, 1976.

28. Vollmer H. Über die diuretische Wirkung der Radix Ononidis und der Herba Equiseti. Arch Pharm (Weinheim) 1940;278:42-4.

29. Jaretzky R. Entgegnung zu vorstehenden Ausführungen Vollmers "Über die diuretische Wirkung der Radix Ononidis und der Herba Equiseti". Arch Pharm (Weinheim) 1940;278:44-7.

30. Vollmer H. Über die diuretische Wirkung der Radix ononidis. (Schlußwort zu den Ausführungen Jaretzkys auf Seite 44 bis 47). Arch Pharm (Weinheim) 1940; 278:283-4.

31. Wolters B. Die Verbreitung antibiotischer Eigenschaften bei Saponindrogen. Dtsch Apoth Ztg 1966;47:1729-33.

ORTHOSIPHONIS FOLIUM

Java Tea

DEFINITION

Java tea consists of the fragmented, dried leaves and tops of stems of *Orthosiphon stamineus* Benth. (*O. aristatus* Miq.; *O. spicatus* Bak.).

The material complies with the monograph of the European Pharmacopoeia [1].

CONSTITUENTS

Up to 12% of minerals with a high proportion of potassium [2-10], approx. 0.2% of lipophilic flavones including sinensetin and isosinensetin [2,3,6,7,11-18], flavonol glycosides [15,16], rosmarinic acid (0.1-0.5%) [3,16,18-20] and other caffeic acid depsides [15,16], inositol [8], phytosterols such as β-sitosterol [2] and up to 0.7% of essential oil [2,4,6,7,9,10,21]; pimarane, isopimarane and staminane diterpenes [18,22-29], triterpenes [2,6,7,9,16,29,30] and chromenes such as methylripariochromene A [28,31,32].

CLINICAL PARTICULARS

Therapeutic indications
Irrigation of the urinary tract, especially in cases of inflammation and renal gravel, and as an adjuvant in the treatment of bacterial infections of the urinary tract [2,7,16,33-35].

Posology and method of administration

Dosage
Adults: An infusion of 2-3 g of dried material in 150 ml of water two to three times per day; equivalent preparations [3,5,7,36].

Method of administration
For oral administration.

Duration of administration
No restriction.

Contra-indications
None known.

Special warnings and special precautions for use
Java tea should not be used in patients with oedema due to impaired heart and kidney function.

E/S/C/O/P
MONOGRAPHS
Second Edition

Interaction with other medicaments and other forms of interaction
None reported.

Pregnancy and lactation
No data available. In accordance with general medical practice, the product should not be used during pregnancy and lactation without medical advice.

Effects on ability to drive and use machines
None known.

Undesirable effects
None reported.

Overdose
No toxic effects reported.

PHARMACOLOGICAL PROPERTIES

Pharmacodynamic properties

In vitro experiments

Antibacterial activity
Bacteriostatic [8, 37] and fungistatic [38] activity has been demonstrated, and the bacteriostatic activity has been attributed to caffeic acid derivatives, particularly rosmarinic acid [16].

Effects on lipoxygenase activity
Various isolated lipophilic flavones inhibited 15-lipoxygenase from soybeans (used as a model for mammalian 15-lipoxygenase) [39]. In another study, flavonoids isolated from Java tea prevented inactivation of soybean 15-lipoxygenase, caused by bubbling air through the enzyme solution. The compounds with the strongest enzyme-stabilizing effects, 5,7,4'-trimethylapigenin, eupatorin and 5,7,3',4'-tetramethylluteolin, gave 50% protection at concentrations of 2.0, 2.4 and 4.3 µM respectively. However, none of the flavonoids were efficient as scavengers of the diphenylpicrylhydrazyl (DPPH) radical [40].

In vivo experiments

Diuretic activity
A 5% infusion of Java tea administered intravenously to rabbits had a diuretic effect [9]. This was also observed after subcutaneous injection of an aqueous extract into rabbits and dogs [41]. The volume of urine and excretion of electrolytes (K+, Na+, Cl-) were increased by intravenous infusion into dogs of a 50% ethanolic extract at 18.8 mg/kg/min [42]. Oral administration to rats of a lyophilized aqueous extract at 750 mg/kg body weight enhanced ion excretion (K+, Na+, Cl-) to a level comparable to that obtained

with furosemide at 100 mg/kg, but no aquaretic effect was observed [43].

Although it is not yet clear which are the active compounds [16], the diuretic effect could be partially due to the potassium content of Java tea [8,43] as well as to the flavones sinensetin and 3'-hydroxy-5,6,7,4'-tetramethoxyflavone, which exhibited diuretic activity in rats after intravenous administration of 10 mg/kg body weight [44].

Aqueous (5:1) and ethanolic (7:1, ethanol 70°) spray-dried extracts of Java tea were administered intragastrically to male rats as single doses at two levels: the aqueous extract at 18.0 mg/kg and 180 mg/kg, the ethanolic extract at 13.5 mg/kg and 135 mg/kg. Each extract was given to 5 rats, a further 5 rats receiving water as controls, and urine was collected over a period of 6 hours. After all doses the urine volume was between 2.99 and 3.36 ml per 100 g of rat, significantly higher (p≤0.05) than that of controls (2.15 ml). With both doses of the aqueous extract, a significant increase (p = 0.009) in sodium elimination was observed (0.1-0.12 mEq per 100 g of rat) compared to controls (0.05 mEq). The higher doses of aqueous and ethanolic extracts significantly (p = 0.009 and p = 0.02 respectively) increased chloride elimination (0.11 and 0.09 mEq per 100 g of rat) compared to controls (0.07 mEq). No significant changes were observed in elimination of potassium or urea [45].

A hydroethanolic extract was administered intraperitoneally to 13 male rats as a single dose of 50 mg/kg body weight; a control group of 28 rats received hypotonic saline solution. Another group of 10 rats received hydrochlorothiazide at 10 mg/kg body weight. After 8 hours the urine volume from rats treated with the extract was significantly higher (p<0.001) than that of the controls and was comparable to the volume after hydrochlorothiazide treatment [46].

Methylripariochromene A isolated from Java tea was suspended in 0.5% Tween 80 and administered orally to 5 rats at three dose levels (25, 50 and 100 mg/kg body weight) followed by oral administration of saline at 20 ml/kg. The highest dose produced a significant increase (p<0.01) in urinary volume over a period of 3 hours, comparable to that of hydrochlorothiazide at 25 mg/kg. Excretion of K+, Na+ and Cl- increased significantly at 100 mg/kg body weight compared to controls (p<0.05, p<0.01 and p<0.01 respectively), but less than with hydrochlorothiazide [28,47].

Anti-inflammatory effects
Orthosiphols A and B, applied topically at 200 µg per ear, inhibited inflammation of mouse ears induced by 2 µg of 12-O-tetradecanoylphorbol-13-acetate by 42% and 50% respectively [23].

Effects on aortic contractile responses
Various substances isolated from the leaves of Java tea had a concentration-dependent suppressive effect on contractile responses in endothelium-denuded rat thoracic aorta strips. IC_{50} values were between 1.01×10^{-1} µmol/ml for acetovanillochromene and 8.08×10^{-3} µmol/ml for tetramethylscutellarein; nifedipine as a positive control gave a value of 1.79×10^{-5} µmol/ml [25,28]. Methylripariochromene A at doses of 1.1×10^{-5} M, 3.8×10^{-5} M and 1.1×10^{-4} M decreased the maximum contractions caused by Ca^{2+} at 30mM to 73.8%, 47.0% and 21.0% respectively [28,47].

Hypoglycaemic effects
A dried aqueous extract of Java tea (yield 3.3%) redissolved in saline was administered to rats by gavage at doses of 0.5 and 1.0 g/kg body weight. The control group received saline at 5 ml/kg body weight. In rats treated with an oral glucose load or streptozotocin, the extract produced a hypoglycaemic effect (no values given). The effect of the extract on streptozotocin-induced diabetes in rats was comparable to that of 10 mg/kg of glibenclamide [48].

Effects on blood pressure and heart rate
Methylripariochromene A at doses of 50 and 100 mg/kg body weight was administered subcutaneously to conscious, stroke-prone, spontaneously hypertensive male rats. A decrease of 15-30 mm Hg in mean systolic blood pressure was observed from 3.5 to 24 hours with the higher dose (p<0.05 and p<0.01 respectively), whereas no changes were observed in the control group. The lower dose caused a significant decrease (p<0.05) only at 8 hours. The substance also caused significant reductions (p<0.01) of 75 and 45 beats/min at 6.0 and 8.5 hours respectively after administration of the higher dose, initial values in the treatment groups being 334 (at 50 mg/kg) and 340 (at 100 mg/kg) beats/min, and in the control group 345 beats/min. A slight decrease in heart rate was observed 6 hours after administration of the lower dose; the heart rate returned to baseline after 24 hours [28,47].

Ex vivo experiments

Suppression of contractile force
After cumulative applications at 3.8×10^{-5} M and 1.2×10^{-4} M to spontaneously beating isolated guinea pig atria, methylripariochromene A significantly suppressed the contractile force by 18.8% (p<0.05) and 54.7% (p<0.01) respectively without significantly reducing the beating rate [28,47].

Pharmacological studies in humans

Diuretic activity
No influence on 12- or 24-hour urine output or sodium excretion was observed in 40 healthy volunteers after administration of 600 ml (3 × 200 ml at 4-hour intervals) of a decoction equivalent to 10 g of dried leaf in a placebo-controlled, double-blind crossover study [49].

A study carried out on 6 healthy male volunteers, who drank 4 × 250 ml of a decoction of Java tea at 6-hourly intervals during one day, for comparison with the same intake of water on a separate control day, acidity of the urine increased 6 hours after ingestion. There were no changes in urine volume or electrolytes [50].

From much earlier observations, however, increased diuresis was reported after oral administration of aqueous extracts of Java tea (400 ml/day of a 3.75% extract, 400 ml/day of a 15% extract, 500 ml/day of a 3.3% extract) to healthy volunteers [51-53].

Clinical studies

Diuretic activity
In an open study involving 14 patients, who received a 12% infusion of the leaves (500 ml/day for a period of 10 days), increased diuresis and elimination of chlorides and urea was reported [41].

A study in 67 patients suffering from uratic diathesis did not reveal any influence of Java tea on diuresis, glomerular filtration, osmotic concentration, urinary pH, plasma content or excretion of calcium, inorganic phosphorus and uric acid during 3 months of treatment [54].

Choleretic activity
Increased choleresis and cholekinesis, together with an antibacterial effect in cholecystitis and cholangitis, has been reported in patients after oral administration of a Java tea extract [55]. However, in vivo studies in rats with the isolated flavones sinensetin and 3'-hydroxy-5,6,7,4'-tetramethoxyflavone administered intravenously at 10 mg/kg body weight did not confirm these findings [44].

Pharmacokinetic properties
No data available.

Preclinical safety data

In vitro experiments
Isolated diterpenes and flavonoids showed weak cytotoxicity towards murine colon carcinoma 26-L5 cells [29].

In a somatic segregation assay using the diploid strain *Aspergillus nidulans* D-30, no genotoxic effects (mitotic crossover, chromosome malsegregation, clastogenic damage) were detected after plate incorporation of a ethanolic extract of Java tea (7.4% dry matter) at 1.4 mg/ml [56].

In vivo experiments

A dry aqueous extract of Java tea redissolved in saline was administered to rats by gavage at 0.5 and 1.0 g/kg body weight, while a control group received saline only (5 ml/kg). Treatment of 6 normoglycaemic rats with the extract at 0.5 mg/kg body weight had no significant effect on fasting blood glucose levels during a 7-hour period. At 1.0 mg/kg, however, a significant decrease (p<0.05) in blood glucose concentration was observed in comparison with the control group [48].

REFERENCES

1. Java Tea - Orthosiphonis folium. European Pharmacopoeia, Council of Europe.

2. Steinegger E, Hänsel R. Orthosiphonblätter. In: Pharmakognosie, 5th ed. Berlin-Heidelberg-New York: Springer-Verlag,1992:566.

3. Hänsel R. Orthosiphonblätter. In: Phytopharmaka: Grundlagen und Praxis, 2nd ed. Berlin-Heidelberg-New York: Springer-Verlag,1991:234-5.

4. Hoppe HA. Orthosiphon. In: Drogenkunde, 8th ed. Berlin-New York: Walter de Gruyter,1975:774-5.

5. Weiß RF, Fintelmann V. In: Lehrbuch der Phytotherapie. 8th ed. Stuttgart: Hippokrates,1997:249-50.

6. Wagner H. Orthosiphonis folium. In: Pharmazeutische Biologie. 2. Drogen und ihre Inhaltsstoffe, 4th ed. Stuttgart-New York: Gustav Fischer, 1988:64.

7. Braun H, Frohne D. Orthosiphon aristatus (Blume) Miquel - Koemis Koetjing, Katzenbart. In: Heilpflanzenlexikon für Ärzte und Apotheker, 5th ed. Stuttgart-New York: Gustav Fischer, 1987:171.

8. Van der Veen T, Malingré TM, Zwaving JH. Orthosiphon stamineus, een geneeskruid met een diuretische werking. Fytochemisch en farmacologisch onderzoek. Pharm Weekbl 1979;114:965-70.

9. Fevrier C. Beiträge zur Kenntnis der Inhaltsbestandteile von Orthosiphon Stamineus Benth. [Dissertation]. University of Basel, 1933.

10. Van Itallie L. Over Orthosiphon stamineus. Nieuw Tijdschrift voor de Pharmacie in Nederland 1886:232 (cited in [8]).

11. Bombardelli E, Bonati A, Gabetta B, Mustich G. Flavonoid constituents of Orthosiphon stamineus Benth. Fitoterapia 1972;43:35-40.

12. Schneider G, Tan HS. Die lipophilen Flavone von Folia Orthosiphonis. Dtsch Apoth Ztg 1973;113:201-2.

13. Wollenweber E, Mann K. Weitere Flavonoide aus Orthosiphon spicatus. Planta Med 1985;51:459-60.

14. Malterud KE, Hanche-Olsen IM, Smith-Kielland I. Flavonoids from Orthosiphon spicatus. Planta Med 1989;55:569-70.

15. Sumaryono W, Proksch P, Wray V, Witte L, Hartmann T. Qualitative and quantitative analysis of the phenolic constituents from Orthosiphon aristatus. Planta Med 1991;57:176-80.

16. Proksch P. Orthosiphon aristatus (Blume) Miquel - der Katzenbart. Pflanzeninhaltsstoffe und ihre potentielle diuretische Wirkung. Z Phytotherapie 1992;13:63-9.

17. Pietta PG, Mauri PL, Gardana C, Bruno A. High-performance liquid chromatography with diode-array ultraviolet detection of methoxylated flavones in Orthosiphon leaves. J Chromatogr 1991;547:439-42.

18. Takeda Y, Matsumoto T, Terao H, Shingu T, Futatsuishi Y, Nohara T, Kajimoto T. Orthosiphol D and E, minor diterpenes from Orthosiphon stamineus. Phytochemistry 1993;33:411-5.

19. Lamaison JL, Petitjean-Freytet C, Carnat A. Teneurs en acide rosmarinique, en dérivés hydroxycinnamiques totaux et activité antioxydante chez les Apiacées, les Borraginacées et les Lamiacées médicinales. Ann Pharm Fr 1990;48:103-8.

20. Gracza L, Ruff P. Über Vorkommen und Analytik von Phenylpropanderivaten, 5. Mitt. Rosmarinsäure in Arzneibuchdrogen und ihre HPLC-Bestimmung. Arch Pharm (Weinheim) 1984;317:339-45.

21. Schut GA, Zwaving JH. Content and composition of the essential oil of Orthosiphon aristatus. Planta Med 1986;52;240-1.

22. Masuda T, Masuda K, Nakatani N. Orthosiphol A, a highly oxygenated diterpene from the leaves of Orthosiphon stamineus. Tetrahedron Lett 1992;33:945-6.

23. Masuda T, Masuda K, Shiragami S, Jitoe A, Nakatani N. Orthosiphol A and B, novel diterpenoid inhibitors of TPA (12-O-tetradecanoylphorbol-13-acetate)-induced inflammation, from Orthosiphon stamineus. Tetrahedron 1992;48:6787-92.

24. Shibuya H, Bohgaki T, Ohashi K. Two novel migrated pimarane-type diterpenes, neoorthosiphols A and B, from the leaves of Orthosiphon aristatus (Lamiaceae). Chem Pharm Bull 1999;47:911-2.

25. Ohashi K, Bohgaki T, Matsubara T, Shibuya H. Indonesian medicinal plants. XXIII. Chemical structures of two new migrated pimarane-type diterpenes, neoorthosiphols A and B, and suppressive effects on rat thoracic aorta of chemical constituents isolated from the leaves of Orthosiphon aristatus (Lamiaceae). Chem Pharm Bull 2000;48:433-5.

26. Stampoulis P, Tezuka Y, Banskota AH, Tran KQ, Saiki I, Kadota S. Staminolactones A and B and norstaminol A: three highly oxygenated staminane-type diterpenes from Orthosiphon stamineus. Org Lett 1999;1:1367-70.

27. Stampoulis P, Tezuka Y, Banskota AH, Tran KQ, Saiki

I, Kadota S. Staminol A, a novel diterpene from *Orthosiphon stamineus*. Tetrahedron Lett 1999; 40:4239-42.

28. Ohashi K, Bohgaki T, Shibuya H. Antihypertensive substance in the leaves of Kumis Kucing (*Orthosiphon aristatus*) in Java island. Yakugaku Zasshi 2000;120:474-82.

29. Tezuka Y, Stampoulis P, Banskota AH, Awale S, Tran KQ, Saiki I, Kadota S. Constituents of the Vietnamese medicinal plant *Orthosiphon stamineus*. Chem Pharm Bull 2000;48:1711-9.

30. Efimova FV, Inaishvili AD. Java tea (*Orthosiphon stamineus*) saponins. Aktual Vop Farm 1968;17-8, through Chem Abstr 1972;76:56594h.

31. Guérin J-C, Reveillère HP, Ducrey P, Toupet L. *Orthosiphon stamineus* as a potent source of methylripariochromene A. J Nat Prod 1989;52:171-3.

32. Shibuya H, Bohgaki T, Matsubara T, Watarai M, Ohashi K, Kitagawa I. Indonesian medicinal plants. XXII. Chemical structures of two new isopimarane-type diterpenes, orthosiphonones A and B, and a new benzochromene, orthochromene A, from the leaves of *Orthosiphon aristatus* (Lamiaceae). Chem Pharm Bull 1999;47:695-8.

33. Harnischfeger G, Stolze H. Orthosiphon stamineus – Katzenbart. In: Bewährte Pflanzendrogen in Wissenschaft und Medizin. Melsungen: notamed, 1983:172-80.

34. Schilcher H. Orthosiphonblätter. In: Loew D, Heimsoth V, Kuntz E, Schilcher H, editors. Diuretika: Chemie, Pharmakologie und Therapie einschließlich Phytotherapie. 2nd ed. Stuttgart-New York: Thieme, 1990: 275-6.

35. Schilcher H. Pflanzliche Diuretika. Urologe B 1987; 27:215-22.

36. Van Hellemont J. In: Fytotherapeutisch Compendium. Utrecht/Antwerpen: Bohn, Scheltema & Holkema, 1988:410-1.

37. Chen C-P, Lin C-C, Namba T. Screening of Taiwanese crude drugs for antibacterial activity against *Streptococcus mutans*. J Ethnopharmacol 1989;27:285-95.

38. Wolters B. Die Verbreitung antibiotischer Eigenschaften bei Saponindrogen. Dtsch Apoth Ztg 1966;47:1729-33.

39. Lyckander IM, Malterud KE. Lipophilic flavonoids from *Orthosiphon spicatus* as inhibitors of 15-lipoxygenase. Acta Pharm Nord 1992;4:159-66.

40. Lyckander IM, Malterud KE. Lipophilic flavonoids from *Orthosiphon spicatus* prevent oxidative inactivation of 15-lipoxygenase. Prostagland Leukotr Essent Fatty Acids 1996;54:239-46.

41. Mercier F, Mercier L-J. L'*Orthosiphon stamineus*, Médicament hépatorénal. Stimulant de la dépuration urinaire. Le Bulletin Médical 1936:523-31.

42. Chow S-Y, Liao J-F, Yang H-Y, Chen C-F. Pharmacological effects of Orthosiphonis Herba. J Formosan Med Assoc 1979;78:953-60.

43. Englert J, Harnischfeger G. Diuretic action of aqueous *Orthosiphon* extract in rats. Planta Med 1992;58:237-8.

44. Schut GA, Zwaving JH. Pharmacological investigation of some lipophilic flavonoids from *Orthosiphon aristatus*. Fitoterapia 1993;64:99-102.

45. Casadebaig-Lafon J, Jacob M, Cassanas G, Marion C, Puech A. Elaboration d'extraits végétaux adsorbés, réalisation d'extraits secs d'*Orthosiphon stamineus* Benth. Pharm Acta Helv 1989;64:220-4.

46. Beaux D, Fleurentin J, Mortier F. Effect of extracts of *Orthosiphon stamineus* Benth., *Hieracium pilosella* L., *Sambucus nigra* L. and *Arctostaphylos uva-ursi* (L.) Spreng. in rats. Phytotherapy Res 1998;12:498-501 and 1999;13:222-5.

47. Matsubara T, Bohgaki T, Watarai M, Suzuki H, Ohashi K, Shibuya H. Antihypertensive actions of methylripariochromene A from *Orthosiphon aristatus*, an Indonesian traditional medicinal plant. Biol Pharm Bull 1999;22:1083-8.

48. Mariam A, Asmawi MZ, Sadikun A. Hypoglycaemic activity of the aqueous extract of *Orthosiphon stamineus*. Fitoterapia 1996;67:465-8.

49. Doan DD, Nguyen NH, Doan HK, Nguyen TL, Phan TS, van Dau N et al. Studies on the individual and combined diuretic effects of four Vietnamese traditional herbal remedies (*Zea mays, Imperata cylindrica, Plantago major* and *Orthosiphon stamineus*). J Ethnopharmacol 1992;36:225-31.

50. Nirdnoy M, Muangman V. Effects of Folia Orthosiphonis on urinary stone promotors and inhibitors. J Med Assoc Thai 1991;74:318-21.

51. Schumann R. Über die diuretische Wirkung von Koemis Koetjing [Dissertation]. University of Marburg 1927:1-38.

52. Gürber A. Der indische Nierentee Koemis Koetjing. Dtsch Med Wochenschr 1927;(31):1299-1301.

53. Westing J. Weitere Untersuchungen über die Wirkung der Herba Orthosiphonis auf den menschlichen Harn [Dissertation]. University of Marburg 1928:1-23.

54. Tiktinsky OL, Bablumyan YA. The therapeutic effect of Java tea and *Equisetum arvense* in patients with uratic diathesis. Urol Nefrol 1983;(1):47-50.

55. Rutenbeck H. Klinische Untersuchungen über ein neues Präparat aus Koemis Koetjing, dem indischen Nierentee. Dtsch Med Wochenschr 1935;(10):377-8.

56. Ramos Ruiz A, De la Torre RA, Alonso N, Villaescusa A, Betancourt J, Vizoso A. Screening of medicinal plants for induction of somatic segregation activity in *Aspergillus nidulans*. J Ethnopharmacol 1996; 52:123-7.

PASSIFLORAE HERBA

Passion Flower

E/S/C/O/P
MONOGRAPHS
Second Edition

DEFINITION

Passion flower consists of the fragmented or cut, dried aerial parts of *Passiflora incarnata* L. It may also contain flowers and/or fruits. It contains not less than 1.5 per cent of total flavonoids expressed as vitexin ($C_{21}H_{20}O_{10}$; M_r 432.4), calculated with reference to the dried drug [1].

The material complies with the monograph of the European Pharmacopoeia [1].

Fresh material may also be used provided that when dried it complies with the monograph of the European Pharmacopoeia.

CONSTITUENTS

Flavonoids, mainly C-glycosides of apigenin and luteolin [2-11], e.g. isovitexin, isoorientin and their $2''$-β-D-glucosides, schaftoside, isoschaftoside, vicenin-2 [2,3,8-11] and swertisin [5, 8-11], with considerable variation in qualitative and quantitative composition according to source [7,12]; a small amount of maltol [13], possibly an artefact [12]; traces of essential oil containing more than 150 components [14]; a cyanogenic glycoside, gynocardin [15].

Traces of β-carboline alkaloids (e.g. harmol, harmalol, harman) may be present, depending on the source and maturity of the plant [16-21]. However, these alkaloids are undetectable in most commercial material [22].

CLINICAL PARTICULARS

Therapeutic indications
Tenseness, restlessness and irritability with difficulty in falling asleep [19,23,24].

Posology and method of administration

Dosage

Adult single dose, three to four times daily: 0.5-2 g of the drug; 2.5 g of drug as infusion; 1-4 ml of tincture (1:8); other equivalent preparations [19,23-25].
Elderly: dose as for adults.
Children from 3 to 12 years under medical supervision only: proportion of adult dose according to body weight.

Method of administration
For oral administration.

Duration of administration
No restriction; neither dependence nor withdrawal symptoms have been reported.

Contra-indications
None known.

Special warnings and special precautions for use
None required.

Interaction with other medicaments and other forms of interaction
None reported.

Pregnancy and lactation
No data available.
In accordance with general medical practice, the product should not be used during pregnancy and lactation without medical advice.

Effects on ability to drive and use machines
None known.
May cause drowsiness. The ability to drive a car or to operate machinery may be reduced. If affected do not drive or operate machinery.

Undesirable effects
Hypersensitivity possible in very rare cases [26,27]. One case of nausea, bradycardia and ventricular arrythmia has been reported [28].

Overdose
No toxic effects reported.

PHARMACOLOGICAL PROPERTIES

Pharmacodynamic properties

In vitro experiments
Two dry extracts of passion flower, containing 3.0% and 9.1% of total flavonoids respectively, were studied for their binding affinity to three receptors. In concentrations from 10 to 1000 µg/ml they did not interact with the binding sites, including benzodiazepine, dopaminergic and histaminergic subtypes. The two main flavonoids isovitexin-2″-glucoside and isoorientin-2″-glucoside did not inhibit the benzodiazepine binding site in concentrations up to 30 µM [29].

In vitro competition binding studies to various CNS receptors expressed in Chinese hamster ovary cells were performed with an ethanolic extract of passion flower. Neither opioid (μ, κ, δ, OFQ) nor serotonin (5-$HT_{1D\beta}$, 5-HT_6, 5-HT_7), oestrogen-α, histamine (H-1, H-2), neurokinin-1 and metabotropic glutamate

receptors were inhibited by the extract. Only binding of ^{3}H-GABA to the $GABA_A$ receptor was potently inhibited at 1 µg/ml [30].

In vivo experiments

Sedative effects
Passion flower has a sedative effect in rodents [31-38]. After intraperitoneal administration to rats at 160 mg/kg body weight an alcohol-free hydroethanolic extract significantly prolonged sleeping time induced by pentobarbital (p<0.01) and, at 50-400 mg/kg body weight, reduced spontaneous locomotor activity in a dose-dependent manner [31]. The same extract, administered orally or intraperitoneally at 160 mg/kg body weight, significantly raised the threshold to nociceptive stimuli in the tail flick and hot plate tests (p<0.05 to p<0.01) [31]. The activity of rats in a one-arm radial maze was reduced after one week of daily oral administration with an alcohol-free hydro-ethanolic extract of passion flower (10 ml/kg body weight, corresponding to 5 g/kg of the drug) [32].

Sedative effects of an extract of passion flower (drug to extract ratio 4.5:1, extracted with ethanol 70% and then inspissated) were investigated in male Swiss mice. To assess its effect on barbiturate-induced sleeping time, the extract (100 mg/kg body weight) was administered intraperitoneally 10 minutes before subcutaneous injection of sodium pentobarbital (40 mg/kg body weight). A distinct prolongation of mean sleeping time by 40% was observed in comparison with the control group. When administered by gastric tube one hour before subcutaneous injection of amphetamine sulphate (5 mg/kg body weight) the passion flower extract (50 mg/kg body weight) caused a significant reduction (p<0.05) in hypermotility, recorded using an activity cage. In comparison with the control group an average reduction in motility of 17% was observed 120 minutes after administration of amphetamine sulphate [33].

The activity of an alcohol-free hydroethanolic extract prepared from cryoground fresh plant was determined in mice [34]. The results indicated that oral treatment of mice with doses of 25 and 50 ml/kg body weight (corresponding to 1.25 and 2.5 g/kg of dried drug respectively [39]) reduced exploratory and spontaneous motor activities, prolonged sleeping time induced by pentobarbital, and inhibited aggressiveness and restlessness caused by amphetamine tartrate. The sedation index was comparable to that of meprobamate (250 mg/kg body weight) and higher than that of diazepam (10 mg/kg body weight) and chlordiazepoxide (10 mg/kg body weight) [34].

An aqueous extract of passion flower (drug to extract ratio 79:1), administered intraperitoneally to male Swiss mice, showed sedative activity at doses of 25, 50 and 100 mg/kg body weight. A dose-dependent reduction in locomotor activity, measured using an activity cage, was observed and motor coordination, evaluated 20, 40, 80 and 120 minutes after treatment using a rotarod apparatus, decreased significantly ($p<0.05$ to $p<0.01$). The pentobarbital-induced sleeping time was dose-dependently prolonged, significantly ($p<0.01$) at 50 and 100 mg/kg [35].

The sedative effect of a hydroethanolic dry extract of passion flower containing 2% of flavonoids was evaluated in Swiss mice. After intraperitoneal administration of 60, 125 and 250 mg/kg body weight a dose-dependent reduction in spontaneous locomotor activity was recorded using an activity cage, significant ($p<0.05$ and $p<0.01$ respectively) with the two higher doses. Oral (intragastric) administration of the extract at the same dose levels resulted in a less distinct decrease in activity. Oral treatment with 30, 60 and 125 mg/kg body weight of a more hydrophilic extract (lyophilized from a mixture obtained by two-step hydroethanolic and aqueous extraction, containing 7.4% of flavonoids) induced a dose-dependent reduction in locomotor activity, significant ($p<0.01$) at 60 and 125 mg/kg body weight; sodium pentobarbital-induced sleeping time increased significantly ($p<0.01$) at these doses. Furthermore, a significant ($p<0.01$) delay in the onset of convulsive episodes induced by intraperitoneal administration of pentylenetetrazole at 50 mg/kg body weight and an increase in the number of survivals were observed after oral pretreatment of the animals with 60 and 125 mg/kg body weight of the more hydrophilic extract [36].

Locomotor activity of male Swiss mice, recorded using an activity cage, declined significantly ($p<0.01$) after intraperitoneal administration of a hydroethanolic dry extract of passion flower at 65, 125 and 250 mg/kg body weight. The administration of 300, 400 and 600 mg/kg body weight of an extract prepared in a similar way from callus cultures of passion flower led to a less distinct decrease in locomotor activity, significant ($p<0.05$ to $p<0.01$) only for the higher concentrations [37].

The sedative and anxiolytic properties of two lyophilized extracts (hydroalcoholic, dry plant drug to extract ratio 7.2:1, and aqueous, dry plant drug to extract ratio 7.6:1) from cryoground fresh aerial parts of passion flower, as well as mixtures of harman and related alkaloids combined with maltol and of flavonoids combined with maltol, were assessed after intraperitoneal administration to male Swiss albino mice. The aqueous extract reduced activity in the staircase and free exploratory tests, and prolonged pentobarbital-induced sleeping time at 400 and 800 mg/kg body weight expressed in terms of dry plant material. Pretreatment with the benzodiazepine receptor antagonist flumazenil (10 mg/kg body weight) did not influence activity in the staircase test. The

hydroalcoholic extract significantly ($p<0.05$) enhanced activity in the staircase and light/dark avoidance tests at 400mg/kg body weight, thus suggesting an anxiolytic effect. Neither the alkaloid mixtures with maltol nor the flavonoid mixtures with maltol at doses corresponding to 0.5, 2, 8 and 18 g of dry plant material per kg body weight modified any behavioural parameters in the staircase test [38].

The sedative effect of passion flower was not confirmed in two different experimental procedures in mice, hexobarbital-induced sleeping time and exploratory activity, after oral administration of an alcohol-free 30% hydroethanolic extract at 1.75 and 3.5 ml/kg body weight [40].

In one study in mice, after oral administration of a dry extract of passion flower (800 mg/kg body weight) containing 2.6% of flavonoids, a significant ($p<0.01$) anxiolytic effect was observed with prolongation of hexobarbital-induced sleeping time, whereas locomotor activity remained unaffected [41].

The anxiolytic effects of extracts obtained by successive extraction of passion flower with petroleum ether, chloroform, methanol and water (in that order) were evaluated in the elevated plus-maze model in mice. After oral administration of 75 to 200 mg/kg body weight the petroleum ether, chloroform and water extracts did not modify behavioural parameters. In contrast, the methanolic extract produced significant effects ($p<0.001$) at doses of 75, 100, 125 and 200 mg/ kg body weight; at 125 and 200 mg/kg the effect was comparable to that of diazepam at 2 mg/kg body weight [42]. These findings were confirmed in another study using the same test model, in which similar extracts but from different plant parts (leaves, stems, flowers) were compared. The methanolic extracts from each plant part were the most effective ($p<0.001$ at 75-200 mg/kg body weight) [43].

Maltol isolated from passion flower inhibited spontaneous motor activity in mice (50% inhibition [13] and 66% inhibition [44] after subcutaneous injection of 75 and 135 mg/kg body weight respectively) and prolonged hexobarbital-induced sleeping time in a dose-dependent manner after oral administration at 300 and 500 mg/kg body weight [13]. The effective doses of maltol were, however, far beyond the amounts present in passion flower preparations [13,44].

In conclusion, the available pharmacodynamic studies generally support, with some conflicting results, the empirically acknowledged sedative and anxiolytic effects of passion flower but it is not yet clear which constituents are responsible for these effects [45].

Anti-inflammatory effects
In carrageenan-induced paw oedema, dextran pleurisy

and cotton pellet granuloma tests in rats, a dry extract of passion flower (lyophilized from a mixture obtained by two-step hydroethanolic and aqueous extraction) exerted a dose-dependent anti-inflammatory effect after oral administration. Significant inhibition of carrageenan-induced oedema at 125 (19.5%, p<0.05), 250 and 500 mg/kg body weight (48.1% and 55.7%, p<0.01) and of cotton pellet granuloma at 250 (15.7%, p<0.05) and 500 mg/kg body weight (20.2%, p<0.01) were observed [46].

Pharmacological studies in humans

In a randomized, placebo-controlled, double-blind study performed in a cross-over design, 12 healthy female volunteers received 1.2 g of a passion flower extract (drug to extract ratio 5.9:1) or 10 mg of diazepam or placebo and 140 minutes later 100 mg of caffeine. The current state of alertness was rated by the subjects on a visual analogue scale (VAS) from "wide awake" to "almost asleep". In the VAS results 120 minutes after treatment, compared to placebo those treated with passion flower extract reached about one third of the diazepam value. Quantitative EEG signals, for 5 minutes under vigilance-controlled reaction time conditions followed by 5 minutes under resting conditions, were measured before administration and 120 and 180 minutes after intake. The effects after administration of passion flower extract were difficult to distinguish from placebo [47].

Clinical studies

In a randomized, double-blind, controlled study in 36 patients with general anxiety disorder diagnosed in accordance with the Diagnostic and Statistical Manual of Mental Disorders (DSM IV) and a score of 14 or more on the Hamilton anxiety rating scale (HAM-A), 18 were treated with 45 drops/day of a hydroethanolic passion flower extract and a placebo tablet. Another 18 as the control group received 45 drops/day of placebo drops and 30 mg/day of oxazepam. HAM-A scores were assessed on days 0, 4, 7, 14, 21 and 28. There were no differences between groups in HAM-A scores on days 0, 21 and 28. On day 4 the score in the passion flower group was significantly higher (p<0.008) than in the oxazepam group; on days 7 and 14 the difference was not significant. These findings pointed to a slower onset of the effect of passion flower. At all stages the effect of both treatments was significant compared to baseline (p<0.001) [48].

A total of 65 opiate addicts undergoing withdrawal were treated in a randomized, double-blind, controlled study with 60 drops of a hydroethanolic passion flower extract and 0.8 mg of clonidine or placebo drops and clonidine. The severity of the withdrawal syndrome was measured on days 0, 1, 2, 3, 4, 7 and 14 using the Short Opiate Withdrawal Score (SOWS). Both protocols were equally effective with regard to the physical symptoms of withdrawal. However, the passion flower/clonidine treatment was superior to clonidine alone with respect to psychological symptoms [49].

Pharmacokinetic properties

No data available.

Preclinical safety data

Single dose toxicity

No acute toxicity was observed after intraperitoneal administration to mice of passion flower extracts in doses up to 500 mg/kg body weight [13] and 900 mg/kg body weight [31].

Repeated dose toxicity

Compared to control animals no change was observed in weight, rectal temperature and motor coordination of male Sprague-Dawley rats following 21 days of subacute oral treatment with a hydroethanolic extract of passion flower at 10 ml/kg body weight, equivalent to the dried herb at 5 g/kg body weight [32].

Mutagenicity

In the somatic segregation assay in the diploid strain *Aspergillus nidulans* D-30 no genotoxic effects (neither chromosomal damage caused by aneuploidy and clastogenic effects nor mitotic crossover) were detected after plate incorporation of 1.30 mg/ml of a fluid extract of passion flower (16.2% dry matter, 0.32% ethanol) [50].

REFERENCES

1. Passion Flower - Passiflorae herba. European Pharmacopoeia, Council of Europe.

2. Geiger H, Markham KR. The C-glycosylflavone pattern of *Passiflora incarnata* L. Z Naturforsch 1986;41c:949-50.

3. Qimin L, van den Heuvel H, Delorenzo O, Corthout J, Pieters LAC, Vlietinck AJ, Claeys M. Mass spectral characterization of C-glycosidic flavonoids isolated from a medicinal plant (*Passiflora incarnata*). J Chromatogr 1991;562:435-46.

4. Schmidt PC, Ortega GG. Passionsblumenkraut. Bestimmung des Gesamtflavonoidgehaltes von Passiflorae herba. Dtsch Apoth Ztg 1993;133:4457-66.

5. Rehwald A, Meier B, Sticher O. Qualitative and quantitative reversed-phase high-performance liquid chromatography of flavonoids in *Passiflora incarnata* L. Pharm Acta Helv 1994;69:153-8.

6. Glotzbach B, Rimpler H. Die Flavonoide von *Passiflora incarnata* L., *Passiflora quadrangularis* L. und *Passiflora pulchella* H.B.K. Planta Med 1968;16:1-7.

7. Schilcher H. Zur Kenntnis der Flavon-C-Glykoside in

Passiflora incarnata L. Z Naturforsch 1968;23b:1393.

8. Chimichi S, Mercati V, Moneti G, Raffaelli A, Toja E. Isolation and characterization of an unknown flavonoid in dry extracts from *Passiflora incarnata*. Nat Prod Lett 1998;11:225-32.

9. Rahman K, Krenn L, Kopp B, Schubert-Zsilavecz M, Mayer KK, Kubelka W. Isoscoparin-2$''$-O-glucoside from *Passiflora incarnata*. Phytochemistry 1997; 45:1093-4.

10. Voirin B, Sportouch M, Raymond O, Jay M, Bayet C, Dangles O, El Hajji H. Separation of flavone *C*-glycosides and qualitative analysis of *Passiflora incarnata* L. by capillary zone electrophoresis. Phytochem Anal 2000;11:90-8.

11. Raffaelli A, Moneti G, Mercati V, Toja E. Mass spectrometric characterization of flavonoids in extracts from *Passiflora incarnata*. J Chromatogr A 1997;777:223-31.

12. Meier B. Passiflorae herba - pharmazeutische Qualität. Z Phytother 1995;16:90-9.

13. Aoyagi N, Kimura R, Murata T. Studies on *Passiflora incarnata* dry extract. I. Isolation of maltol and pharmacological action of maltol and ethyl maltol. Chem Pharm Bull 1974;22:1008-13.

14. Buchbauer G, Jirovetz L. Volatile constituents of the essential oil of *Passiflora incarnata* L. J Essent Oil Res 1992;4:329-34.

15. Spencer KC, Seigler DS. Gynocardin from *Passiflora*. Planta Med 1984;50:356-7.

16. Löhdefink J, Kating H. Zur Frage des Vorkommens von Harmanalkaloiden in *Passiflora*-Arten. Planta Med 1974;25:101-4.

17. Brasseur T, Angenot L. Contribution à l'étude pharmacognostique de la Passiflore. J Pharm Belg 1984;39:15-22.

18. Lutomski J, Segiet E, Szpunar K, Grisse K. Die Bedeutung der Passionsblume in der Heilkunde. Pharm unserer Zeit 1981;10:45-9.

19. Hänsel R, Keller K, Rimpler H, Schneider G, editors. *Passiflora*. In: Hagers Handbuch der Pharmazeutischen Praxis, 5th ed. Volume 6: Drogen P-Z. Berlin:Springer-Verlag, 1994:34-49.

20. Tsuchiya H, Shimizu H, Iinuma M. Beta-carboline alkaloids in crude drugs. Chem Pharm Bull 1999;47:440-3.

21. Tsuchiya H, Hayashi H, Sato M, Shimizu H, Iinuma M. Quantitative analysis of all types of β-carboline alkaloids in medicinal plants and dried edible plants by high performance liquid chromatography with selective fluorometric detection. Phytochem Anal 1999;10:247-53.

22. Rehwald A, Sticher O, Meier B. Trace analysis of harman alkaloids in *Passiflora incarnata* by reversed-phase high performance liquid chromatography. Phytochem Anal 1995;6:96-100.

23. Bradley PR, editor. Passiflora. In: British Herbal Compendium, Volume 1. Bournemouth: British Herbal Medicine Association 1992:171-3.

24. Bisset NG, editor (translated from Wichtl M, editor. Teedrogen). Passiflorae herba. In: Herbal drugs and phytopharmaceuticals: a handbook for practice on a scientific basis. Stuttgart: Medpharm, Boca Raton-London: CRC Press, 1994:363-5.

25. Schilcher H. Pflanzliche Phytopharmaka. Eine neue Klassifizierung nach Indikationsgruppen. Dtsch Apoth Ztg 1995;135:1811-22.

26. Smith GW, Chalmers TM, Nuki G. Vasculitis associated with herbal preparation containing *Passiflora* extract. Br J Rheumatol 1993;32:87-8.

27. Echechipia S, Garcia BE, Alvarez MJ, Lizaso MT, Olaguibel JM, Rodriguez A, Tabar AI. Passiflora hyper-sensitivity in a latex allergic patient: cross reactivity study. Allergy 1996;51:49.

28. Fisher AA, Purcell P, Le Couteur DG. Toxicity of *Passiflora incarnata* L. Clin Toxicol 2000;38:63-6.

29. Burkard W, Kopp B, Krenn L, Berger D, Engesser A, Baureithel K, Schaffner W. Receptor binding studies in the CNS with extracts of *Passiflora incarnata*. Pharm Pharmacol Lett 1997;7:25-6.

30. Simmen U, Burkard W, Berger K, Schaffner W, Lundstrom K. Extracts and constituents of *Hypericum perforatum* inhibit the binding of various ligands to recombinant receptors expressed with the Semliki Forest virus system. J Receptor Signal Trandsduct Res 1999; 19:59-74.

31. Speroni E, Minghetti A. Neuropharmacological activity of extracts from *Passiflora incarnata*. Planta Med 1988; 54:488-91.

32. Sopranzi N, De Feo G, Mazzanti G, Tolu L. Parametri biologici ed elettroencefalografici nel ratto correlati a *Passiflora incarnata* L. Clin Ter 1990;132:329-33.

33. Capasso A, Pinto A Experimental investigations of the synergistic-sedative effect of Passiflora and Kava. Acta Ther 1995;21:127-40.

34. Galliano G, Foussard-Blanpin O, Bretaudeau J. Etude expérimentale du rôle du maltol dans les propriétés psycho-pharmacologiques de *Passiflora incarnata* L. (Passifloracées). Phytotherapy 1994;(40/41):18-22.

35. Capasso A, De Feo V, De Simone F, Sorrentino L. Pharmacological effects of aqueous extract from *Valeriana adscendens*. Phytother Res 1996;10:309-12.

36. Speroni E, Billi R, Mercati V, Boncompagni E, Toja E. Sedative effects of crude extract of *Passiflora incarnata* after oral administration. Phytother Res 1996;10:S92-4.

37. Speroni E, Billi R, Crespi Perellino N, Minghetti A. Role

of chrysin in the sedative effects of *Passiflora incarnata* L. Phytother Res 1996;10:S98-100.

38. Soulimani R, Younos C, Jarmouni S, Bousta D, Misslin R, Mortier F. Behavioural effects of *Passiflora incarnata* L.and its indole alkaloid and flavonoid derivatives and maltol in the mouse. J Ethnopharmacol 1997;57:11-20.

39. Chefaro-Ardeval, France: personal communication.

40. Weischer ML, Okpanyi SN. Pharmakologie eines pflanzlichen Schlafmittels. Z Phytother 1994;15:257-62.

41. Della Loggia R, Tubaro A, Redaelli C. Valutazione dell'attività sul S.N.C. del topo di alcuni estratti vegetali e di una loro associazione. Riv Neurol 1981;51:297-310.

42. Dhawan K, Kumar S, Sharma A. Comparative biological activity study on *Passiflora incarnata* and *P. edulis*. Fitoterapia 2001;72:698-702.

43. Dhawan K, Kumar S, Sharma A. Anxiolytic activity of aerial and underground parts of *Passiflora incarnata*. Fitoterapia 2001;72:922-6.

44. Kimura R, Matsui S, Ito S, Aimoto T, Murata T. Central depressant effects of maltol analogs in mice. Chem Pharm Bull 1980;28:2570-9.

45. Meier B. *Passiflora incarnata* L. - Passionsblume. Z Phytother 1995;16:115-26.

46. Borelli F, Pinto L, Izzo AA, Mascolo N, Capasso F, Mercati V et al. Anti-inflammatory activity of *Passiflora incarnata* L. in rats. Phytother Res 1996;10:S104-6.

47. Schulz H, Jobert M, Hübner WD. The quantitative EEG as a screening instrument to identify sedative effects of single doses of plant extracts in comparison with diazepam. Phytomedicine 1998;5:449-58.

48. Akhondzadeh S, Naghavi HR, Vazirian M, Shayegan-pour A, Rashidi H, Khani M. Passionflower in the treatment of generalized anxiety: a pilot double-blind randomized controlled trial with oxazepam. J Clin Pharm Therap 2001;26:363-7.

49. Akhondzadeh S, Kashani L, Mobaseri M, Hosseini SH, Nikzad S, Khani M. Passionflower in the treatment of opiates withdrawal: a double-blind randomized controlled trial. J Clin Pharm Therap 2001;26:369-73.

50. Ramos Ruiz A, De la Torre RA, Alonso N, Villaescusa A, Betancourt J, Vizoso A. Screening of medicinal plants for induction of somatic segregation activity in *Aspergillus nidulans*. J Ethnopharmacol 1996;52:123-7.

PIPERIS METHYSTICI RHIZOMA

Kava-Kava

DEFINITION

Kava-kava consists of the dried rhizome, usually free from roots and sometimes scraped, of *Piper methysticum* G. Forst. It contains not less than 3.5% of kavalactones calculated as kavain ($C_{14}H_{14}O_3$; M_r 230.2).

The material complies with the monograph of the Deutscher Arzneimittel Codex [1] or of the British Herbal Pharmacopoeia [2].

CONSTITUENTS

The characteristic constituents of kava-kava are α-pyrones, known as kavalactones or kavapyrones, of which at least 18 have been identified [3]; the major ones are (+)-kavain, (+)-dihydrokavain, (+)-methysticin, (+)-dihydromethysticin, yangonin and demethoxy-yangonin [3-8]. Proportions of individual kavalactones vary but the total amount is often over 5% [5,9].

Other constituents include three chalcone pigments, flavokavins A-C [3,5,10], bornyl cinnamate, stigmasterol and small amounts of two N-cinnamoyl pyrrolidine alkaloids [6].

CLINICAL PARTICULARS

Therapeutic indications
Anxiety, tension and restlessness arising from various causes of non-psychotic origin [11-21].

Posology and method of administration

Dosage

Adult daily dose: dried rhizome or extracts corresponding to 60-120 mg of kavalactones [15,19-25].

Elderly: dose as for adults.

No data available for children

Method of administration
For oral administration.

Duration of administration
Usually 1 month; at most 2 months [25].

Contra-indications
Existing liver diseases; alcohol abuse.

E/S/C/O/P
MONOGRAPHS
Second Edition

Special warnings and special precautions for use
Unusual fatigue, weakness or loss of appetite and unintended weight loss, yellow discolouration of the conjunctiva or of the skin, dark urine or colourless stool can be signs of damage to the liver. If such symptoms occur, the medication should be discontinued and a doctor should be consulted immediately.

Avoid concomitant medication with beta-blockers, antidepressants and anti-migraine preparations. Be cautious with alcohol [25].

Major depression should not be treated with kava-kava without medical advice [5].

Interaction with other medicaments and other forms of interaction
None confirmed.

A single, unsubstantiated case of possible interaction has been reported between an unspecified kava-kava product and the benzodiazepine drug alprazolam, resulting in a semicomatose state. However, the patient had also taken cimetidine (a histamine H_2-receptor antagonist) and terazosin (an antihypertensive); no dosages were reported for any of the four medications [26]. The semicomatose state could have been caused by alprazolam alone, but a combination of cimetidine and terazosin can also lead to somnolence. Furthermore, interaction between cimetidine and alprazolam can result in delayed elimination of alprazolam and thus an increased blood level of the benzodiazepine [27]. No additive effects were observed in a study in which kava-kava extract and bromazepam (another benzodiazepine) were taken concurrently for 14 days [28] or, in another study, when one of several benzodiazepines (including alprazolam) were taken concurrently for up to 14 days [11]. In this complicated situation, therefore, the contributing role of kava-kava to the semicomatose state appears highly questionable.

Pregnancy and lactation
No data available. In accordance with general medical practice the product should not be used during pregnancy or lactation without medical advice.

Effects on ability to drive and use machines
No negative influence on ability to drive or use machines [28,29].

Undesirable effects

Hepatotoxicity
The health status of 39 users of kava-kava (dried rhizome, prepared as an infusion in cold water) in an Australian aboriginal community was assessed in 1988; 20 were classified as very heavy users (mean consumption, 440 g/week), 15 as heavy users (310 g/week) and 4 as occasional users (100 g/week). Various adverse effects were observed from these extra-

ordinarily high intakes, but with respect to plasma biochemistry only γ-glutamyl transferase (γ-GT) levels (U/litre) were clearly outside the normal range of variation: very heavy users 251, heavy users 312 and occasional users 77, compared to 58 for non-users (values below 60 considered to be normal). Bilirubin levels (μmol/litre) were within the normal range (less than 20), slightly lower in heavy and very heavy users (4.2-4.3) than in non-users (6.7). The authors com-mented that "the markedly-elevated plasma levels of γ-glutamyl transferase provide strong circumstantial evidence for a hepatotoxic effect of kava, although it has not yet been possible to confirm this by examin-ation of liver biopsies. Such an effect on the liver has not been described in the literature previously" [30].

No reports of hepatotoxicity associated with the use of kava-kava extracts at therapeutic dose levels appear to have been published until the late 1990s, when cases of severe liver damage linked to the use of kava-kava preparations, although rare, began to emerge and were increasingly reported in the literature and to regulatory authorities. Some examples follow.

Necrotizing hepatitis in a 39-year-old woman was attributed to the daily intake of 60 mg of kavalactones. Commencement and discontinuation of the kava-lactones preparation coincided, on two occasions separated by an interval of 6 months, with sharp increases and subsequent normalization of serum transaminase levels [31].

After taking 300 mg of kava-kava extract (containing 210 mg of kavalactones) daily for at least 2 months, a 33-year-old woman became ill with fatigue and anorexia; 6 weeks later she developed jaundice. Liver parameters worsened even 10 days after discontinuing the preparation, bilirubin reaching almost 400 μmol/litre and transaminase 2500 U/litre with only slightly elevated alkaline phosphatase. The levels eventually recovered within 1 month of discontinuation of the drug. Histology and serological parameters ruled out hepatitis due to Epstein-Barr virus. Two further cases of jaundice reported to the Swiss authorities were possibly due to kava-kava extract but complicated by the use of additional medication(s) [32].

Jaundice was diagnosed in a 50-year-old man, who took no other drugs and did not consume alcohol, after he had taken 3-4 capsules of kava-kava extract (equivalent to 210-280 mg of kavalactones) daily for 2 months; he had developed a 'tanned' skin and dark urine. Liver function tests revealed 60-fold and 70-fold increases in aspartate aminotransferase and alanine aminotransferase concentrations respectively. Levels of alkaline phosphatase, γ-glutamyltransferase, lactase dehydrogenase, and total and conjugated bilirubin were also very much higher than normal ranges, and the prothrombin time was 25%. Ultrasonography showed a slight increase in liver size but no ascites or portal vein thrombosis. Blood tests for hepatitis A, B, C and E, HIV, cytomegalovirus and Epstein-Barr virus gave negative results. Following rapid deterioration of his condition, including stage IV encephalopathy and a prothrombin time of 10%, the patient received a liver transplant and recovered uneventfully. The removed liver was atrophic, and subhepatic and portal veins were free; histology showed extensive and severe hepatocellular necrosis, and extensive lobular and portal infiltration of lymphocytes and numerous eosinophils. The physicians concluded that the chronology of the case, together with histological findings and exclusion of other causes of hepatitis, supported a relationship between ingestion of kava-kava and fulminant hepatic failure; causality was assessed as probable [33].

A 60-year-old woman, admitted to hospital due to fatigue, weight loss over several months and jaundice with icteric skin and dark urine, had taken kava-kava extract in varying doses in the past year, and also occasional doses of etilefrine hydrochloride and piretanide. She was subsequently transferred to intensive care because of progressive liver failure, concomitant renal failure and progressive encephalopathy. Biochemical tests revealed high levels of aspartate aminotransferase and alanine aminotransferase, and total and conjugated bilirubin; prothrombin time was less than 10%. Viral hepatitis and metabolic or autoimmune causes of liver failure were ruled out by serological tests. No pathological changes were detected by tomography or ultrasonography. Due to her deteriorating physical condition, with progressive liver failure, respiratory insufficiency and stage IV encephalopathy, the patient received a liver transplant 11 days after admission. From histological evidence and exclusion of other causes, the physicians considered kava-kava to be the most likely cause of acute liver failure [34].

A 50-year-old woman who had taken a kava-kava preparation equivalent to 60 mg of kavalactones daily for 7 months, and concomitantly a sulfonylurea derivative (for diabetes mellitus) and an oestrogen preparation, was admitted to hospital with jaundice. Her bilirubin level was ca. 400 µmol/litre, various other serological parameters were abnormal and a liver biopsy revealed ca. 45% liver cell necrosis. Following continued clinical deterioration leading to hepatic coma, the patient received a liver transplant and recovered without complication [35].

A female patient who had taken a kava-kava preparation providing 240 mg of kavalactones daily for 4 months was admitted to hospital with jaundice; she had fatigue and elevated bilirubin (10.5 mg/dl) and transaminases (GPT 519 U/dl). Toxicological screening, including for hepatitis A, B and C, gave negative results. Within 3 days fulminant liver damage developed, and also lung and cardiac-circulatory problems and stage III encephalopathy; a liver transplant was performed as soon as possible. Histological examination of the removed organ revealed a liver much reduced in weight (780 g) with marked necrosis and complete destruction of the parenchyma. The physicians attributed the liver damage to kava-kava [36].

By July 2002, 68 cases of suspected hepatotoxicity associated with the use of products containing kava-kava extracts or isolated kavalactones had been reported worldwide, including cases of liver failure resulting in 6 liver transplants and 3 deaths [37]. After assessment of the implications, health authorities in some countries took action to ban the use of kava-kava preparations, at least until the position becomes clearer.

Following such regulatory action in Germany, Loew and Gaus reviewed the available data from 37 case reports of hepatotoxicity involving kava-kava extracts. They pointed out that, from the often rather inadequate data in these reports, an adverse effect from kava-kava extracts could be assumed (i.e. probable or definite) in only 15 cases and was definite in only 2 cases. Taking dosage and duration of intake into account, serious liver failure had been reported only after daily doses of extracts corresponding to over 210 mg of kavalactones or when the duration of administration was longer than 8 weeks [25]. Members of the German Commission E expressed unease at the decision of their regulatory authority, stating that they remained convinced by scientific data of the efficacy of kava-kava, and considered the risk/benefit ratio and the therapeutic benefit for the patient to be positive under correct and stipulated use of kava-kava preparations; they considered the following recommendations necessary and sufficient [25,38]:

- Medical prescription only for preparations containing kava-kava.
- Clear indications: mild to moderately severe generalized anxiety disorders; depression is not an indication.
- Maximum daily dose corresponding to 120 mg of kavalactones.
- Package size limited to 30 daily doses.
- Usual duration of therapy: 1 month; maximum 2 months.
- Determination of liver parameters (GPT and γ-GT) before treatment and once a week thereafter.
- Avoidance of concomitant medication with potentially hepatotoxic medications, especially beta-blockers, antidepressants and anti-migraine preparations. Caution in the consumption of alcohol.

Correlation of data from the MEDIPLUS database for a recent 12-month period, September 1999 to August 2000, on the relative incidence of hepatotoxicity reported for benzodiazepine drugs and kava-kava extracts indicated a comparably low potential for hepatotoxic adverse effects. For bromazepam, diazepam, oxazepam and kava-kava extracts (ethanolic and acetone-water), the incidence of hepatotoxicity including toxic hepatosis was 0.90, 2.12, 1.23 and 0.89 cases per million daily doses of the respective drugs [39]. The incidence of reported hepatoxicity for ethanolic kava-kava extracts has been estimated as 0.008 cases per million daily doses and compared to estimates of the incidence of elevated transaminase values of 2.1 per 100,000 doses of omeprazole and the incidence of acute hepatic adverse effects of 3.6 cases per 100,000 doses of diclofenac [40].

Other effects

On the basis of case studies on four patients who developed involuntary dyskinesia and other symptoms suggesting central dopaminergic antagonism after taking kava-kava preparations (in two cases within hours of the first dose), a potential for extrapyramidal side effects (EPS) was noted by the physicians [41]. One of the kava-kava extracts in question, and a number of kavalactones and flavokavins, were therefore tested in rats using the 'bar test' as a rodent model of catalepsy. After single oral doses of 100 or 200 mg/kg of the extract, or 100 mg/kg of individual kavalactones or flavokavins, no cataleptogenic effects could be detected, whereas under similar conditions a 0.2 mg/kg subcutaneous dose of haloperidol always induced catalepsy. Subsequent experiments using the same test demonstrated that cataleptogenic effects of 0.2 mg/kg s.c. of haloperidol were actually inhibited by pre-treatment with kava-kava extract at 100 mg/kg and 200 mg/kg (p<0.01) and, to a lesser extent, by dihydrokavain at 100 mg (p<0.01) but not by other kavalactones or flavokavins (p<0.01). It was concluded that the kava-kava extract is devoid of haloperidol-like cataleptogenic properties. Extrapyramidal side effects reported in the above case studies remain unclarified but central dopaminergic antagonism from kava-kava appears unlikely [42].

A delayed-type hypersensitivity reaction, resulting in a generalized rash and severe itching, was reported in a 36-year-old woman 4 days after the termination of a 3-week course of daily treatment with 120 mg of kava-kava extract [43].

Overdose

Kava-kava beverages
The traditional ceremonial drinking of kava beverages in South Pacific islands may be considered as overdosage in relation to medicinal doses of kava-kava. Since the early 1980s, the drinking of kava beverages, often in considerably greater amounts than in the South Pacific, has been adopted by some aboriginal communities in Australia [30]. Various effects of heavy kava drinking have been noted in ethnomedicinal literature including a local anaesthetic

effect in the mouth and yellowing of the skin and finger/toe nails. The yellow colouration, which is reversible on cessation of kava drinking, has been attributed to accumulation of some as yet unidentified constituent(s) of kava-kava in skin and nails; it has not been observed from medicinal use of kava-kava at therapeutic dose levels [44] and is presumably unrelated to yellowing of the skin in cases of jaundice.

Heavy users of kava-kava beverages in Australia and Pacific islands have been reported to develop a typical scaly rash due to pellagroid dermatopathy [30,45-47], attributed to niacin deficiency [46] or interference with cholesterol metabolism [47]; it is reversible on cessation of kava-kava ingestion [47]. Loss of body weight (up to 20%) is also common, although it is not clear whether this is a clinical effect or simply due to malnutrition (since heavy use of kava-kava causes loss of appetite and nausea) or detached feelings and less interest in (or less to spend on) food [30,45].

A detailed study in an Australian aboriginal community, involving clinical, physiological and biochemical assessments, showed that chronic heavy consumption of kava-kava (up to 440 g of dried rhizome per week) led to various detrimental effects: reduced plasma levels of albumin, protein, urea and bilirubin, increased HDL cholesterol, haematuria, changes in haematological parameters, shortness of breath and other symptoms [30].

Case reports
An acute neurological syndrome involving generalized choreoathetosis was reported three times in the same patient as a symptom of acute intoxication from excessive drinking of a kava beverage; it was settled by intravenous diazepam and the patient was asymptomatic within 12 hours [48].

Visual effects such as reduced near-point accommodation, increased pupil diameter and disturbed oculomotor balance were observed in an experiment when a male subject (with no previous experience of kava-kava) drank 600 ml of a kava-kava beverage within 15 minutes [49].

A man aged 29 years who admitted to drinking kava-kava tea 5-6 times daily for 6 months had a range of overdose symptoms: a feeling of chronic intoxication, loss of appetite, diarrhoea, emaciation, yellow skin and finger/toe nails, marked dermatoses, difficulty in focusing his eyes, poor hearing and moderate ataxia. The symptoms gradually disappeared after discontinuing the tea [50].

In another case report, a man aged 44 years, who had experienced generalized erythema from taking kava-kava 3 months previously, drank more than 4 cups of kava-kava tea in one evening. He awoke with a confluent non-pruritic extreme erythema involving his entire head and neck, and the upper parts of his back and chest [51].

PHARMACOLOGICAL PROPERTIES

Pharmacodynamic properties

In vitro experiments

Interaction with GABA and benzodiazepine receptors
A hydroethanolic extract of kava-kava concentration-dependently enhanced the binding of [³H] muscimol (a GABA$_A$ receptor agonist) to GABA$_A$ binding sites in membrane fractions from different regions of the rat brain: hippocampus (HIP), amygdala (AMY), medulla oblongata (MED), frontal cortex (FC) and cerebellum (CER). Except for CER, the EC$_{50}$ values ranged between 200 and 300 μM of kavalactones, and maximum potentiation was obtained in the HIP (358% compared to the control) followed by AMY and MED, the three main target brain centres of kava-lactone action. The effects of the kavalactones were attributed to an increase in the number of receptor binding sites (B$_{max}$) rather than a change in affinity. At a kavalactone concentration of 500 μM the order of enhancement in B$_{max}$ was HIP = AMY > MED > FC > CER (p<0.001 vs. control in each region) [52].

In another investigation, isolated kavalactones (including kavain, dihydrokavain, methysticin, yangonin and tetrahydroyangonin) were tested at concentrations ranging from 100 μM to 1 mM for their ability to compete with [³H]-diazepam binding to GABA$_A$ and benzodiazepine receptors in rat forebrain membranes [53,54]. Weak binding of kavalactones to GABA$_A$ and benzodiazepine receptors was observed, whereas no binding to GABA$_B$ was evident.

The influence of kavalactones on the GABA$_A$ receptor in rat brain cortex was demonstrated using radio-receptor assays. Maximal enhancements of 18-28% in specific binding of [³H]bicuculline methochloride were exhibited by (+)-kavain, (+)-methysticin and (+)-dihydromethysticin at 0.1 μM, by yangonin at 1 μM and by (+)-dihydrokavain at 10 μM, while demethoxy-yangonin had no effect. No inhibition of specific binding of [³H]flunitrazepam was observed, indicating that the influence of the kavalactones on the GABA$_A$ receptor was not based on interaction with the benzo-diazepine receptor [55].

Inhibition of monoamine uptake
(+)-Methysticin, (+)-kavain and the synthetic racemate (±)-kavain were tested at concentrations ranging from 10 to 400 μM for their ability to block the uptake of [³H]-noradrenaline and [³H]-serotonin in synaptosomes prepared from the cerebral cortex and hippocampus of rats. (+)-Kavain and (±)-kavain potently and concentration-dependently inhibited the uptake of [³H]-noradrenaline, by 70-80% of the control at 400 μM; (+)-methysticin was less potent, with 45% inhibition at 400 μM. None of the kavalactones efficiently blocked the uptake of [³H]-serotonin [56].

Modulation of 5-HT$_{1A}$ receptor activity
(+)-Kavain and (+)-dihydromethysticin at 20, 50 and 100 μM concentration-dependently reduced field potential changes induced on hippocampal slices from guinea-pig brain by the serotonin (5-HT$_{1A}$) agonist ipsapirone, suggesting that these kavalactones modulate 5-HT$_{1A}$ activity [57].

In a related experiment on guinea pig hippocampal slices, kavain and dihydromethysticin at 5-40 μM and 10-40 μM respectively reversibly reduced the frequency of occurrence of field potential changes induced by the omission of extracellular Mg^{2+}. The kavalactones showed additive actions [58].

Anticonvulsive activity
Isolated methysticin at concentrations of 10-100 μM reversibly blocked epileptiform activity in various types of *in vitro* seizure models using rat temporal cortex slices containing the hippocampus and ento-rhinal cortex [59]. (+)-Kavain and its synthetic race-mate (±)-kavain rapidly and non-stereospecifically inhibited veratridine-activated voltage-dependent Na$^+$-channels [60-63]. Other data suggested that (±)-kavain, at concentrations sufficient to completely block Na$^+$-channels, only moderately inhibits the non-activated Ca^{2+}-channels in mammalian pre-synaptic nerve endings [62,63].

In a radiological binding assay using rat cerebro-cortical synaptosomes, (+)-kavain, (±)-kavain, (+)-dihydrokavain, (±)-dihydrokavain and (+)-dihydro-methysticin significantly decreased the apparent total number of binding sites (B$_{max}$) for [³H]-batrachotoxin-A 20α-benzoate (control: 0.5 pmol/mg protein, kava-lactones: 0.2-0.27 pmol/mg protein) with little change in the equilibrium constants for [³H]-batrachotoxin-A 20α-benzoate. The results indicated that kavalactones non-competitively and non-stereospecifically inhibit [³H]-batrachotoxin-A 20α-benzoate binding to receptor site 2 of voltage-gated Na$^+$-channels [64].

Spasmolytic activity
Dihydromethysticin from kava-kava inhibited hista-mine-, acetylcholine-, 5-HT- and barium chloride-induced spasms in isolated guinea-pig ileum with ED$_{50}$ values (2.6-7.2 × 10^{-6} g/ml) of the same order as those of papaverine [65].

Synthetic (±)-kavain and (+)-methysticin at concen-trations of 1-400 μM inhibited voltage-dependent Na$^+$ channels in rat CA1 hippocampal neurons [66].

Synthetic (±)-kavain (1 μM to 1 mM) dose-dependently reduced contractions of guinea pig ileum evoked by carbachol (10 µM), BAY K 8644 (0.3 µM) or substance P (0.05 µM). While nifedipine also inhibited contractions evoked by BAY K 8644 and substance P, it failed, even at a high concentration (1µM), to completely block the contraction evoked by carbachol (10 µM); the nifedipine-resistant contraction was completely suppressed by (±)-kavain (400 µM). Pretreatment of longitudinal ileum strips with pertussis toxin markedly reduced carbachol-induced contractions; remaining contractions were eliminated by (±)-kavain (400 µM). However, (±)-kavain had no effect on caffeine-induced (20 mM) contractions of ileum strips and failed to affect Ca^{2+}-evoked contractions of skinned muscles. These results suggested that (±)-kavain may act in a non-specific musculotropic way on the smooth muscle membrane [67].

Neuromodulatory activity in abdominal ganglia
The potential of kava-kava to block action currents in nerve tissue (abdominal ganglia) isolated from crayfish was demonstrated using biomagnetic sensors. The time required to completely block the action currents correlated with the kavalactone concentrations in extracts passed through a flow cell containing the nerve tissue [68].

Inhibition of cyclooxygenase
Pre-treatment of human platelets with (+)-kavain 5 minutes before application of arachidonic acid dose-dependently diminished platelet aggregation (IC_{50}: 78 µmol/litre), ATP release (IC_{50}: 115 µmol/litre) and the synthesis of thromboxane A_2 (IC_{50}: 71 µmol/litre) and prostaglandin E_2 (IC_{50}: 86 µmol/litre). The similarity of IC_{50} values suggested inhibition of cyclooxygenase by (+)-kavain as the primary target, thus suppressing the generation of thromboxane A_2 which induces aggregation of platelets and exocytosis of ATP by its binding to thromboxane A2 receptors [69].

In vivo experiments
Studies with lipophilic and aqueous extracts of kava-kava, and isolated constituents, have revealed the most important pharmacological actions of kavalactones: tranquillization, sedation, centrally-induced muscle relaxation and also anticonvulsive and neuroprotective effects [5,57,70-80]. In some experiments the dichloromethane extract (6% yield) and the aqueous extract (6% yield), obtained by successive extraction of the same plant material, were used to compare their activity. The lipid-soluble fraction decreased spontaneous motility and reduced motor control; hypnosis, analgesia and a local anaesthetic effect were also evident. The aqueous extract caused a loss of spontaneous activity, without loss of muscle tone; no hypnotic effect was observed and the anticonvulsant effect against strychnine was only slight, while a certain analgesic effect could be demonstrated [70,72,73]. The pharmacological effects of kava-kava therefore appear to be due to central activity of compounds present in the lipid-soluble fraction, which contains mainly kavalactones. Synergistic actions between kavalactones have been reported [78] and could partly be explained by the synergism of uptake of these compounds into brain tissue [81].

Sedative/tranquillizing/muscle relaxing effects
Dichloromethane and aqueous extracts of kava-kava reduced amphetamine-induced hypermotility in mice. In rats, the aqueous extract administered intraperitoneally at doses of 30-500 mg/kg body weight had no effect on conditioned avoidance responses in a "shelf-jump" apparatus. However, 125 mg/kg of dichloromethane extract reduced the number of conditioned avoidance responses by 18%, while 150 mg/kg caused ataxia and sedation [70].

The steam distillate from kava-kava was separated in two fractions, F1 and F2, the latter containing kavalactones. Both fractions decreased spontaneous motor activity at dose levels that did not alter forced motor activity of mice. The estimated intraperitoneal ED_{50} was 31.6 mg/kg for F1 and 5.4 mg/kg for F2. Brain levels of endogenous serotonin did not change within 1 hour after intraperitoneal administration of F1, F2 or isolated dihydromethysticin [71].

Intraperitoneal administration of dichloromethane or aqueous extracts of kava-kava in rats at 120 mg/kg body weight suppressed apomorphine-induced hyperactivity. In mice, intraperitoneal administration of aqueous extract at 62.5 mg/kg decreased spontaneous activity for 2 hours without loss of muscle tone. However, at doses of 500 mg/kg to 2.5 g/kg, orally administered aqueous extract was not active in rats or mice. A dichloromethane extract administered intraperitoneally at 150 mg/kg decreased spontaneous motility by 46%, markedly reduced motor control and produced hypnosis and analgesia in mice [72].

The hypnotic-sedative properties of a dichloromethane extract from kava-kava administered intraperitoneally to mice at 300 mg/kg were prolonged significantly (p<0.001) by concurrent administration of ethanol at 2 g/kg. Intraperitoneal or intragastric administration of aqueous or dichloromethane extracts in mice at 150-250 mg/kg produced analgesia, as measured in the tail-flick test and acetic acid writhing test [73].

(±)-Kavain at 10-50 mg/kg and a kava-kava extract in arachis oil (corresponding to kavalactones at 50-100 mg/kg body weight), administered intraperitoneally to cats, reduced muscle tone by about 50%. The extract also produced marked effects on the electroencephalogram, inducing high amplitude delta waves, spindle-like formations and continuous alpha- or beta-synchronization in amygdaloid nucleus recordings (p<0.001). Hippocampal responses following stimulation of the amygdaloid nucleus increased in amplitude in cats treated intraperitoneally with (±)-kavain at 50 mg/kg (p<0.05) or the extract equivalent to kavalactones at 100 mg/kg (p<0.001) [74].

Central nervous system depression was observed in rats after intraperitoneal administration of aqueous extracts of kava-kava [75].

Kavain, methysticin, dihydromethysticin and yangonin isolated from kava-kava showed strong centrally-mediated muscle relaxing activity after intravenous administration in rabbits. Yangonin proved to be the most potent kavalactone, almost completely suppressing electromyographically measured impulses at 5-10 mg/kg; the other kavalactones required doses 2-3 times larger to produce the same effect. From simultaneously obtained cortical EEGs, high voltage synchronised waves developed with relaxing doses of the kavalactones. The results indicated that the sedative effect of kava-kava is probably a result of both depression of muscle tone and depression of the cortical activation system and limbic areas by kava-lactones [82].

The effects of a single oral dose of (+)-dihydromethysticin at 100 mg/kg body weight on striatal and cortical tissue concentrations of dopamine, serotonin, 3,4-dihydroxyphenylacetic acid and 5-hydroxyindolacetic acid, as well as on dopamine and serotonin turnover, were evaluated in rats. Other rats were fed for 78 days with a diet containing 0.48 g of (±)-kavain per kg, leading to an intake of ca. 10.8 mg of (±)-kavain per day, to evaluate the influence of chronic treatment with kavalactones on neurotransmitters. The results clearly demonstrated that neither (+)-dihydromethysticin in a high single dose nor (±)-kavain administered chronically significantly altered the dopaminergic or serotonergic tissue levels in rats [83].

Anticonvulsant effects
The effects of intraperitoneally administered kavain, dihydrokavain, methysticin and dihydromethysticin were evaluated in mice poisoned with varying doses of strychnine (of which the LD_{50} is 1.45 mg/kg). All the kavalactones showed a marked antagonistic effect on the convulsant and lethal action of strychnine. Kavain or dihydrokavain at 200 mg/kg and methysticin or dihydromethysticin at 150 mg/kg completely prevented convulsions due to strychnine at up to 4-5 mg/kg. ED_{50} values which antagonized the lethal effects of strychnine at 2 mg/kg were: kavain 76 mg/kg, dihydrokavain 122 mg/kg, methysticin 16 mg/kg and dihydromethysticin 18 mg/kg, compared to mephenesin 215 mg/kg and phenobarbital 34 mg/kg [84]. Similar results from other experiments indicate that the chloroform extract of kava-kava, and methysticin and dihydromethysticin, have particularly marked anticonvulsant activity [78,85].

Both dihydromethysticin and dihydrokavain inhibited electroshock-induced seizures in rats and mice at intraperitoneal doses of 25 and 60 mg/kg [86].

Neuroprotective effects
The neuroprotective effects of an acetone-water extract of kava-kava (70% kavalactones) and isolated kavalactones were evaluated in rodent models of focal cerebral ischaemia. The kava-kava extract, administered orally at 150 mg/kg one hour before induction of ischaemia, diminished the infarct area in mouse brain (p<0.05) and the infarct volume in rat brain (p<0.05). Intraperitoneally administered methysticin and dihydromethysticin at 10 and 30 mg/kg, and memantine (a typical anticonvulsant) at 20 mg/kg, significantly reduced the infarct area in mouse brain, while kavain, dihydrokavain and yangonin had no beneficial effect. The neuroprotective effect of kava-kava extract was therefore probably mediated by methysticin and dihydromethysticin [87,88].

The effects of kava-kava extract and individual kava-lactones on neurotransmitter levels were investigated in the nucleus accumbens of rats. A low intraperitoneal dose of kava-kava extract (20 mg/kg body weight) caused changes in rat behaviour and concentrations of dopamine in the nucleus accumbens; a higher dose (120 mg/kg) raised the levels of dopamine. Low doses of (±)-kavain (30 mg/kg) diminished dopamine levels, while higher amounts either increased or did not change dopamine concentrations. Yangonin (120 mg/kg) decreased dopamine levels to below the detection limit and demethoxyyangonin (120 mg/kg) increased dopamine levels. Dihydrokavain (120 mg/kg), methysticin (120 mg/kg) and dihydromethysticin (120 mg/kg) produced no significant changes in dopamine levels. (±)-Kavain caused a decrease in 5-HT concentrations and some other kavalactones also affected 5-HT levels. The results suggested that the relaxing and slightly euphoric actions of kavalactones may be caused by activation of mesolimbic dopaminergic neurones. Changes in the activity of 5-HT neurones could explain the sleep-inducing action [89].

The effect on dopamine release under ischaemic conditions was evaluated in animals using two kava-kava extracts: a dry extract with 30% kavalactones (I) and a viscous (spissum) extract with 60% kavalactones (II). The animals were treated with amounts of the extracts equivalent to 25, 50 or 100 mg of kavalactones/kg/day for 5 days. 4 hours after administration of the last dose, the animals were subjected to mild hypoxia for 18 hours; dopamine release was then monitored for 24 hours using a radioactive marker. Pre-treatment of animals with extract I had no effect on dopamine release at the 25 mg/kg dose; higher doses were effective. However pre-treatment with extract II showed a marked effect on dopamine release at 25 mg/kg; at 100 mg/kg the diminution of dopamine release under hypoxic conditions was totally eliminated. The stronger effect of extract II compared to I was attributed to its higher proportion of methysticin and dihydromethysticin, which have been shown to have neuroprotective activity [90].

Pharmacological studies in humans

Cognitive performance

In a randomized, double-blind crossover study, 12 healthy young volunteers were assessed by a recognition memory task. Three types of medication, packaged to appear identical, were used: placebo; 3 × 200 mg of an acetone-water kava-kava extract containing 70% of kavalactones daily for 5 days; oxazepam, 15 mg the day before testing and 75 mg on the morning of the test day. The task was to distinguish between words being visually presented for the first time (new words) and words being repeated (old words). Highly significant medication effects were observed after oxazepam, reflected in greatly reduced performance, while kava-kava extract did not alter performance compared to placebo [91,92].

The effects of kava-kava on alertness and speed of access to information from long-term memory were investigated in a single-blind study using a letter-match task; 9 healthy undergraduates took no kava-kava while 9 others drank 250 ml of an aqueous preparation from 30 g of kava-kava thirty minutes prior to the test. As a separate experiment, a further 9 undergraduates drank 500 ml of an aqueous preparation, individually prepared to contain the equivalent of kava-kava at 1 g/kg body weight, one hour prior to the test. Kava-kava was found to have no discernible effect on cognitive performance [93].

Vigilance

In a single-blind study, 6 healthy volunteers were given 300 or 600 mg of an acetone-water kava-kava extract containing 70% of kavalactones, or placebo, daily for one week. The quantitative EEGs obtained in the kava-kava group showed an increase in the beta/alpha index typical of the EEG profile of anxiolytics. No sedative-hypnotic effects were evident, even after 600 mg. The results of evoked potential studies indicated that information processing may be improved in the cortical areas studied, i.e. vigilance is increased. These findings correlated with results from psychometric tests, which indicated increased activation and improvement in emotional stability [94].

In a double-blind, 3-fold crossover study 12 healthy volunteers received as a single dose, on test days separated by a 7-day interval, an ethanolic kava-kava extract containing 120 mg of kavalactones or 10 mg of diazepam or placebo. All tests were done immediately before, 2 hours after and 6 hours after administration of the preparations. After kava-kava extract or diazepam the EEGs showed an increase in the relative intensity of slow waves and a decrease in relative intensity of alpha-waves. The specific increase in beta activity with diazepam was not observed with kava-kava extract. In psycho-physiological tests the critical flicker frequency was reduced more by kava-kava extract or diazepam than by placebo. In tests of mental performance (Pauli test, simple reaction time test and complex multiple choice reaction time test) subjects taking kava-kava produced significantly better results than those on placebo. No significant improvement over placebo was observed in those taking diazepam [95].

Sleeping pattern

In a single-blind study with 12 healthy volunteers the effects on sleeping-pattern of either 150 or 300 mg of an acetone-water kava-kava extract in comparison with placebo were tested by EEG recordings during sleep. The results showed a tendency towards a shorter time before onset of sleep and shorter duration of periods of light sleep in the kava-kava group, while phases of deep sleep (III and IV) and periods of REM sleep were clearly prolonged. All the results indicated improved quality of sleep during treatment with kava-kava extract [96].

Sedative effects

Two multiple crossover studies were performed with 12 healthy female volunteers (mean age 53.7 years) to screen for acute sedative effects by quantitative EEG analysis after a single oral dose of 600 mg of a kava-kava extract (drug to extract ratio 12.5:1). An increase in power of both the theta and slow alpha bands was noted 2 hours after administration. The increase in theta power was still present 3 hours after administration, while fronto-centrally a decrease in power was evident in the high frequency beta 3 band. Although the quantitative EEG can indicate drug-induced CNS changes, it is not easy to conclude whether such changes are valid predictors of sedation or anxiolysis [97].

ABBREVIATIONS used in the summaries of clinical studies

Bf-S	von Zerssen's Health Status Scale (Befindlichkeits-Skala)
CGI	Clinical Global Impressions Scale [98]
DSM-III-R	Diagnostic and Statistical Manual of Mental Disorders, 3rd ed., revised [99]
DSM-IV	Diagnostic and Statistical Manual of Mental Disorders, 4th ed. [100]
HAMA	Hamilton Anxiety Scale [101]
ICD-10	International Statistical Classification of Diseases and Related Health Problems, Tenth Revision [102]

Clinical studies

General anxiety, nervousness and restlessness

Controlled studies
Patients with nervous anxiety, tension and restlessness of non-psychotic origin, diagnosed in accordance with DSM-III-R criteria for generalized anxiety disorder (300.02; 12 cases), social (300.23; 14 cases) or simple (300.29; 11 cases) phobia, agoraphobia (300.22; 2 cases) or adaptation disturbances (309.24; 1 case), and with a minimum history of 4.5 weeks (mean duration 21 months) of uninterrupted treatment with benzodiazepines (lorazepam, bromazepam, alprazolam or oxazepam), were included in a 5-week randomized, placebo-controlled double-blind study; all had a medical indication for discontinuation of benzodiazepine treatment and change to an alternative anxiolytic. To exclude severe disorders, a total score not exceeding 14 on the Hamilton anxiety scale (HAMA) and a score of at least 12 in an intelligence test based on vocabulary were required. With the patients' knowledge, pre-existing medication with benzodiazepines was tapered off to zero at a steady rate over the first 2 weeks of the study. Simultaneously, the patients received daily either kava-kava extract (70% kavalactones), gradually increasing from 50 mg to 300 mg over the first week (n = 20), or placebo (n = 20). Thus in the final 3 weeks of the study, patients received daily monotherapy with 300 mg of kava-kava extract or placebo. Kava-kava extract was superior to placebo with respect to the primary outcome measures, reductions from baseline in HAMA (p = 0.01) and a subjective well-being scale (Bf-S, p = 0.002) scores and in the secondary efficacy measures, CGI and Erlanger anxiety, tension and aggression scales. Over the 5-week period, the median HAMA score in the kava-kava group decreased by 7.5, whereas in the placebo group it increased by 1 point. During a 3-week follow-up phase, 14 patients whose HAMA scores had improved while taking kava-kava in the 5-week study received placebo; 9 of these patients showed a recurrence of the basic symptoms of anxiety disorder [11].

In a randomized, double-blind study, 101 outpatients suffering from anxiety of non-psychotic origin (DSM-III-R diagnostic criteria: agoraphobia, specific phobia, generalized anxiety disorder or adjustment disorder with anxiety) were treated daily for 25 weeks with either 3 × 100 mg of an acetone-water extract of kava-kava containing 70% of kavalactones (n = 52) or placebo (n = 49). By week 8 the patients taking kava-kava extract had significantly better HAMA total scores (p = 0.02) than those on placebo and the difference increased during subsequent weeks (p<0.001 at weeks 16, 20 and 24). Verum patients also showed significantly greater improvements in HAMA sub-scores for somatic and mental anxiety (p = 0.02 by week 8), CGI (p = 0.001 after 12 weeks; p = 0.015

after 24 weeks) and a Self-report Symptom Inventory (p<0.05 from week 12). Adverse events were rare and distributed evenly in both groups [12].

In a double-blind multicentre study 172 patients with non-psychotic anxiety conditions were randomized into three groups and treated daily for 6 weeks with 3 × 100 mg of an acetone-water extract of kava-kava containing 70% of kavalactones (n = 57) or 3 × 5 mg of oxazepam (n = 59) or 3 × 3 mg of bromazepam (n = 56). Therapeutically relevant improvements in HAMA and CGI scales were observed in all groups with no significant differences between groups [13].

In a further randomized, double-blind study, two groups of 29 patients with non-psychotic anxiety syndromes were treated daily for 4 weeks with either 3 × 100 mg of an acetone-water extract of kava-kava containing 70% of kavalactones or placebo. Therapeutic efficacy was assessed by HAMA, CGI and an Adjectives Checklist after 1, 2 and 4 weeks of treatment. After 1 week of treatment the HAMA total score for anxiety symptoms had decreased significantly in the kava-kava group compared to the placebo group and this difference widened during the course of the study (p = 0.0035 after 4 weeks). Results from secondary target variables (HAMA sub-scores for somatic and mental anxiety, CGI and Adjectives Checklist) were in agreement with the HAMA total score, demonstrating the efficacy of kava-kava extract in patients with anxiety disorders. No adverse events were noted during the medication period [14].

In a randomized, double-blind, reference-controlled, three-armed, multicentre study, 129 outpatients (aged from 18 to 65) with generalized anxiety disorder diagnosed in accordance with ICD-10 (F 41.1) were assigned to one of the following treatments daily for 8 weeks: 400 mg of a 96%-ethanolic kava-kava extract (containing 120 mg of kavalactones) or 10 mg of buspirone (an anxiolytic) or 100 mg of opipramol (a tricyclic antidepressant). The average duration of existing illness was 40 months and 62% of the patients had not previously been treated. After 8 weeks, in comparison with initial levels the proportion of patients classified as responders (defined by a reduction in HAMA score of 50% or to less than 9 points) was 76.7% in the kava-kava group, 76.2% in the opipramol group and 73.8% in the buspirone group. Seven secondary efficacy parameters including Clinical Global Impressions also showed no differentiation between the three treatments, each of which led to significant and clinically relevant effects [15].

In a randomized, double-blind, placebo-controlled study, 38 patients (31 female, 7 male; aged 31-75 years, mean 52 years) meeting DSM-IV criteria for general anxiety disorder and having a Hamilton Anxiety Scale (HAMA) score ≥ 16 were assigned, following a 1-week placebo run-in, to 4 weeks of treatment with a kava-kava extract corresponding to 2 × 70 mg of kavalactones daily in the first week and 2 × 140 mg of kavalactones for the last three weeks, or placebo. Data were evaluable on 35 patients (17 verum, 18 placebo). Assessments were carried out using the HAMA, the Hospital Anxiety and Depression Scale (HADS) and the Self-Assessment of Resilience and Anxiety (SARA). Improvements were noted in both the verum and placebo groups, with response rates (≥ 50% reduction in baseline HAMA score) of 35% and 50% respectively, but no significant differences between groups were evident in any of the efficacy assessments. However, analysis of SARA scores in a subgroup with relatively low baseline anxiety revealed greater improvement after kava-kava treatment (p<0.01) than after placebo [103].

Although not yet published in full, limited data are available in the literature on three randomized, controlled studies in which daily doses of kava-kava extracts, equivalent to 105 or 140 mg of kavalactones, were used:

- 141 patients with anxiety, stress and restlessness diagnosed in accordance with DSM-III-R were assigned to treatment with 150 mg of an acetone-water extract of kava-kava (corresponding to 105 mg of kavalactones) or placebo daily for 28 days. Compared to the placebo group, significant improvements were observed in the kava-kava group using four efficacy parameters: the Anxiety Status Inventory, the Erlanger Scale for Anxiety, Aggression and Stress, the Bf-S and CGI [22, 104].

- 50 patients with non-psychotic anxiety diagnosed in accordance with DSM-IV-R were treated with 150 mg of an acetone-water extract of kava-kava (corresponding to 105 mg of kavalactones) or placebo daily for 28 days. Compared to the placebo group, the kava group showed significant improvement with respect to HAMA scores [23,104].

- 61 patients with sleep disorders, anxiety, stress and/or restlessness diagnosed in accordance with DSM-III-R, were treated with 200 mg of an acetone-water extract of kava-kava (corresponding to 140 mg of kavalactones) or placebo daily for 28 days. Compared to the placebo group, patients in the kava-kava group showed significant improvements with respect to HAMA, Bf-S and CGI results and a sleep questionnaire subscore for quality of sleep [104,105].

In a randomized, double-blind study, hospital patients (aged 25-81 years) undergoing surgery under epidural (regional) anaesthesia were premedicated at 9.00 pm on the evening before the operation and again 1 hour before the operation with 300 mg of a kava-kava ext-

ract corresponding to 60 mg of kavalactones (n = 28) or placebo (n = 28). Based on a 10-point anxiety questionnaire, completed by each patient and compared as 'matched pairs' within four subgroups according to the duration of surgery (< 40 to > 120 minutes), the verum group experienced significantly (p<0.05) less anxiety than the placebo group. Sleep quality (p<0.05), psychostatus (p<0.01) and post-operative assessment (p<0.01) were also superior in the verum group [16].

A randomized study compared the acute sedative and anxiolytic effects of a viscous (spissum) kava-kava extract (group K; n = 26) with those of benzo-diazepines (group B; n = 27) as pre-medication in women (average age, 68.3 years) waiting to undergo hysterectomy under regional anaesthesia. On the evening before the operation, both groups received 25 mg of promethazine orally; group K also received kava-kava extract equivalent to 100 mg of kava-lactones orally, while group B received 1-2 mg of flunitrazepam orally. On the morning of the operation, 45 minutes before transfer to the operating room, both groups received 0.5-1 mg of atropine intramuscularly (dose adjusted for body weight); group K also received kava-kava extract equivalent to 100 mg of kavalactones orally, while group B received 10 mg of diazepam intramuscularly. Physician and patient assessments of extent of anxiety and quality of medication-induced sedation (3-step scale), together with blood pressure, pulse frequency and blood oxygen saturation values, showed comparable efficacy of the kava-kava extract and benzodiazepines. Significantly higher systolic blood pressures (p = 0.029) were recorded in the benzodiazepines group. Adverse events of nausea and vomiting were at the same level (5 cases) in both groups but could not be attributed to the medication. The study also demonstrated the rapid onset of effect of the kava-kava extract [17].

Open studies
766 patients with anxiety syndrome were treated daily for 4 weeks with 3 × 100 mg of kava-kava extract (70% kavalactones) in an open multicentric study and assessed by the modified HAMA. Overall HAMA scores decreased by 70% from 30 to 9 (p<0.0001) and efficacy was considered excellent or good by 93.7% of physicians and 86.9% of patients. Tolerability of the preparation was considered good or very good in 95.8% of patients [106].

In an open, multicentre observational study, 52 out-patients suffering from non-psychotic anxiety, with (n = 26) or without (n = 26) concomitant depression, were treated with capsules of unit dose 100 mg of an ethanolic kava-kava extract (50 mg of kavalactones). The dosage varied from 2 to 6 capsules and the mean treatment duration was 51 days. On a global five-point improvement scale 42 patients (81%) rated the treatment as very good or good and all three symptoms showed a marked decrease from the baseline. Before treatment 42%, 50% and 40% of patients rated as "severe" the three target symptoms: anxiety, tension and restlessness respectively. By the end of the study no patients had "severe" ratings and 38%, 29% and 35% reported absence of the respective symptoms [107].

1673 patients aged from 8 to 90 years (average 48.8 years) and suffering from anxiety (n = 1421) and/or nervousness and restlessness (n = 1631) participated in a post-marketing surveillance study and were treated daily with 400 mg of a ethanolic kava-kava extract (120 mg of kavalactones) for a minimum of 4 weeks with final evaluation after 34.5 days on average. Based on questionnaires, 75% of patients rated the efficacy, and 93% the tolerability, of the treatment as good or very good. Anxiety symptoms decreased in average intensity from 2.33 to 0.74 and nervousness symptoms from 2.7 to 0.99 [108].

In a very large, open, multicentre surveillance study, the 4049 participating patients were diagnosed as suffering from states of nervous anxiety, tension and restlessness arising from various causes, the most frequent being over-stretched or over-demanding situations, but also including anxious moods, bereavements or climacteric complaints. They were treated with an acetone extract of kava-kava, usually at a daily dose level of 150 mg of extract (containing 105 mg of kavalactones) for 6 weeks. By the end of treatment, based on the HAMA the total score for "psychic symptoms" had dropped from 2.54 to 0.79 and the total score for "vegetative symptoms" from 2.13 to 0.62. The efficacy of the treatment was assessed by the physicians as good to very good in 74% of cases, and 87% of the patients rated their general quality of life as improved [109].

Anxiety in the climacteric phase

Controlled studies
In a randomized, double-blind study 40 women, aged 45-60 years and in the peri- or post-menopausal phase with psychovegetative symptoms (anxiety, restlessness and sleep disorders) and psychosomatic symptoms correlating with gynaecological dysfunction, were treated for 8 weeks with either 3 × 100 mg of an acetone-water extract of kava-kava containing 70% of kavalactones (n = 20) or placebo (n = 20), with assessment after 0, 1, 4 and 8 weeks. After 1 week of treatment the average HAMA score in the verum group had decreased by more than 50% (from 31.10 to 14.65), significantly more (p<0.001) than in the placebo group (decrease from 30.15 to 27.50). The difference widened by the end of weeks 4 and 8 (p<0.0005). Other parameters such as the Depressive Status Inventory (DSI) scale, the CGI and the Kuppermann Menopause Index (severity of climacteric

symptoms) also demonstrated a high level of efficacy of the kava-kava extract over the treatment period, together with good tolerance of the preparation [18].

In another randomized, double-blind study, 40 women with climacteric syndrome (primarily anxiety and vegetative dysregulation in peri- and post-menopausal phases) were treated daily for 12 weeks with either 2 × 150 mg of a kava-kava extract corresponding to 2 × 30 mg of kavalactones (n = 20) or a placebo preparation (n = 20). At the end of 4 and 8 weeks, assessment using the Kuppermann Menopause Index (severity of climacteric symptoms) and ASI scale (rating of anxiety disorders) showed significant improvements (p<0.001) in the verum group, in which 11 patients reduced their daily dose to 1 × 150 mg of extract in the final weeks of the study (mainly from week 9). Due to a high drop-out rate during weeks 6-10, primarily because of lack of efficacy (2 in the verum group, 14 in the placebo group), statistical comparisons were not reliable after 12 weeks. In the verum group 5 patients reported minor adverse effects such as lowering of vigilance or tiredness in the morning; 2 verum and 3 placebo patients reported gastrointestinal complaints [19].

Perimenopausal women with climacteric symptoms participating in a randomized, open study to evaluate the effects of calcium supplementation and a kava-kava extract (containing 55% of kavain) were randomized into three groups and assigned to one of the following oral treatments daily for 3 months: 100 mg of kava-kava extract + 1 g of calcium (n = 20) or 2 × 100 mg of kava-kava extract + 1 g of calcium (n = 20) or 1 g of calcium only as a control (n = 40); data on 68 patients (n = 15, n = 19 and n = 34 respectively) were available for evaluation. Anxiety was evaluated using the State Trait Anxiety Inventory (STAI, 20 items), while depression was evaluated by Zung's Self-Evaluation Scale and climacteric symptoms by Greene's Scale. In the calcium-only control group, anxiety, depression and climacteric symptoms declined slightly, but not significantly. Compared to the control group, scores for anxiety in both kava-kava groups declined significantly (p<0.009; two-factors ANOVA for the combined kava-kava groups, n = 34). Compared to baseline, scores for anxiety in the combined kava-kava groups (n = 34) declined significantly (p<0.0001), in the 100 mg group from 47.3 to 43.2 after 1 month and 42.7 after 3 months (p<0.025), and in the 200 mg group from 46.6 to 43.1 after 1 month and 41.3 after 3 months (p<0.0003). Although scores for depression and climacteric symptoms declined more in the kava-kava groups than in the control group and were significant compared to baseline after 3 months, the differences were not statistically significant compared to the control group [20].

To evaluate the efficacy of a kava-kava extract

(containing 55% of kavain) in combination with hormone replacement therapy and to compare it with hormone replacement therapy alone in the treatment of menopausal anxiety, 40 women patients in physiological or surgical menopause with generalized anxiety in accordance with DSM III criteria were assigned to one of four treatments for 6 months in a randomized study. Patients in physiological menopause received either natural oestrogens with progestin + 100 mg/day of kava-kava extract (HRT + K; n = 13) or natural oestrogens with progestin + placebo (HRT; n = 9). Those in surgical menopause received daily either natural oestrogens + 100 mg of kava-kava extract (ERT + K; n = 11) or natural oestrogens + placebo (ERT; n = 7). Initial HAMA scores of all patients were at least 19 (mean initial scores in all groups were ≥ 26). Significant reductions in HAMA scores compared to baseline were observed after 3 and 6 months of treatment in all four groups, but greater reductions were achieved in groups using combination therapy (HRT + K, 55.5%; ERT + K, 53.3%) than in groups treated with hormones only (HRT, 23.0%; ERT, 25.8%). Furthermore, in both groups given combination treatments (HRT + K or ERT + K), reductions in the HAMA subscores for both somatic anxiety and psychic anxiety were significantly greater (p<0.05) than in corresponding groups treated with hormones only [21].

Open studies
In an open study 15 women with psychosomatic and psychovegetative complaints leading to anxiety syndrome during the climacteric period were treated daily for 12 weeks with 2 × 150 mg of a kava-kava extract providing 2 × 30 mg of kavalactones. The patients were evaluated by a Self-Assessment Scale (SAS) and the Kuppermann Menopause Index. After 8 weeks the SAS score had decreased from 37 to 18 and the Kuppermann Index from 38 to 22. Four patients dropped out between weeks 8 and 12, one due to neurotic psychosis and three on account of insufficient effectiveness. After week 8 a reduction to half of the initial daily dose was considered adequate for 9 of the 11 patients who completed the study. At the end of 12 weeks the SAS score had decreased further to 5.5 and the Kuppermann Index to 7 [110].

Clinical reviews
A systematic review of 7 double-blind, randomized, placebo-controlled studies of oral kava-kava extract in the treatment of anxiety [12,14,16,18,19 and two others], involving a total of 377 patients, suggested superiority of kava extract in all the studies assessed. A meta-analysis of 3 of these studies [12,14,18] which assessed a common outcome measure, involving a total of 198 patients, suggested a significant difference in favour of kava-kava extract in reduction of the total HAMA score. The reviewed data implied that kava extract is superior to placebo as a symptomatic treatment for anxiety [111].

Pharmacokinetic properties

Pharmacokinetics in animals
Kavain, dihydrokavain, yangonin and demethoxy-yangonin were administered intraperitoneally to mice at 100 mg/kg. At specific time intervals after administration (5, 15, 30 and 45 minutes) animals were sacrificed and brain concentrations of these kavalactones determined. Kavain and dihydrokavain attained maximum concentrations in the brain within 5 minutes and were then rapidly eliminated. In contrast, yangonin and demethoxyyangonin had poorly defined maxima and were more slowly eliminated. When crude kava resin (120 mg/kg containing 44 mg of kavain, 23 mg of dihydrokavain, 18 mg of yangonin and 16 mg of demethoxyyangonin) was administered intraperitoneally, brain concentrations of kavain and yangonin markedly increased (2 and 20 times respectively) relative to values measured after their individual injection, whereas dihydrokavain and demethoxyyangonin remained at the percentage incorporation into brain tissue established for their individual injection [81].

After oral administration of a kava-kava extract to mice at 100 mg/kg, maximum plasma levels of individual kavalactones (kavain, dihydrokavain, methysticin and dihydromethysticin, but not yangonin), ranging between 300 and 900 ng/ml, were attained within 5 minutes; the elimination half-life was approx. 30 minutes. When mice and rats were treated orally with 100 mg/kg of a kava-kava extract formulation, bioavailability clearly increased, with maximum plasma levels of kavalactones in mice reaching 1.7-2.5 µg/ml (except yangonin, 0.3 µg/ml) 0.5 hours after administration; in rats, however, two absorption peaks of the lactones were observed, at 15 min. and approx. 2 hours. Surprisingly, kavalactone levels in the brain showed peak concentrations (1.1-2 µg/g of brain) at the same time as in plasma. Elimination half-lives in mouse plasma and brain were approx. 1 hour, and even longer in the rat. In contrast to results from rodents, dogs showed quite wide variations in t_{max} (0.7-4 hours) and elimination half-lives varied from 90 minutes to several hours after administration of an extract formulation or a blend of individual kavalactones [112].

In metabolic studies in rats, approx. half the oral dose of dihydrokavain (400 mg/kg) was found in the urine within 48 hours; about two-thirds consisted of hydroxylated metabolites, p-hydroxydihydrokavain being the most abundant, while the remaining third consisted of metabolites formed by scission of the 5,6-dihydro-α-pyrone ring and included hippuric acid (9-13% of the dose). Lower amounts of urinary metabolites were excreted when kavain was given, but both hydroxylated and open-ring metabolites were formed. Methysticin gave rise to only small amounts of two urinary metabolites formed by demethylation of the methylenedioxyphenyl moiety. Urinary metabolites of yangonin and 7,8-dihydroxyyangonin were formed via *ortho*-demethylation; no open-ring metabolites were detected [113].

Synergistic pharmacological effects from combinations of kavalactones have been suggested on the basis of results from various experiments [78,81].

Pharmacokinetics in humans

After ingestion by healthy male subjects of a kava-kava beverage prepared by the traditional method of aqueous extraction, all 7 major and several minor kavalactones were identified in the urine. Metabolic transformations included reduction of the 3,4-double bond and/or demethylation of the 4-methoxyl group of the α-pyrone system. In contrast to metabolism in rats, no dihydroxylated metabolites of kavalactones or products from ring opening of the 2-pyrone ring system were identified in human urine [114].

After a single oral dose of 200 mg of kavain in humans, approx. 80% is absorbed, of which up to 98% is metabolized, mainly to more hydrophilic *p*-hydroxykavain, on first pass through the liver. Maximum plasma levels of *p*-hydroxykavain sulphate conjugate (50 ng/ml) and kavain (18 ng/ml) are attained within 1.7-1.8 hours. The elimination half-life of *p*-hydroxykavain sulphate is about 29 hours, while elimination of kavain shows a biphasic pattern with half-lives of 50 min for the first phase and approx. 9 hours for the second [44].

Preclinical safety data

Acute toxicity
The LD_{50} values in mice and rats of an acetone-water extract of kava-kava (11-20:1, 70% kavalactones) have been determined as > 1500 mg/kg (oral) and > 360 mg/kg body weight (intraperitoneal). Acute reactions were dose-dependent and manifested by reduced spontaneous motility, ataxia, sedation, lying on their sides with reduced reflex excitability, unconsciousness and death from respiratory paralysis [5,25,104].

For individual kavalactones the oral, intraperitoneal and intravenous LD_{50} values respectively in mice were found to be (in mg/kg body weight): kavain, 1130, 420 and 69; dihydrokavain, 980, 490 and 53; methysticin, > 800, 530 and 49; dihydromethysticin, 1050, 420 and 67; demethoxyyangonin, > 800, > 800 and 55; yangonin, > 1500, >1500 and 41 [85].

Chronic toxicity
An acetone-water extract of kava-kava (11-20:1, 70% kavalactones) administered orally to 40 rats (20 male, 20 female) at 20, 80 and 320 mg/kg bodyweight, and to 8 beagle dogs (4 male, 4 female) at 8, 24 and 60 mg/

kg bodyweight, daily for 26 weeks caused no extract-related deaths. Low-degree histopathological changes in liver tissues (centrilobular hypertrophy) and kidney tissues of the rats (hyaline drops and epithelial pigmentation of the proximal tubuli) observed at the higher doses were interpreted as adaptation of the organs to the large amounts of the test substance reported. No effects were observed, and no pathological changes in tissues were evident, from doses of 20 mg/kg/day in the rats or 24 mg/kg/day in the dogs [5,25,104].

An ethanolic kava-kava extract was incorporated into the diet of rats at two levels, 0.01% and 0.1%, for periods of 3 and 6 months. In the 3-month study, no deaths occurred and no changes occurred in (body) weight or in haematological and blood chemistry parameters, in particular with respect to liver enzymes. Macroscopically the investigated organs were normal with respect to weight; in individual liver lobes slight oedematous swelling and lymphocyte infiltration of the portal and biliary tissues, and in glomerular and kidney tissues a leukocyte and lymphocyte infiltration was recorded in both controls and treated cases. Blood chemistry, laboratory chemistry, macroscopic and histological findings were similarly normal after 6-month feeding with the same extract [25].

Reproductive toxicity
No teratogenic effects were evident in the F_1 or F_2 generations after intraperitoneal administration of dihydromethysticin to rats at 50 mg/kg body weight 3 times per week for 3 months [5]. No other data appears to be available.

Cytotoxicity
The cytotoxicity of ethanolic and acetone-water extracts, as well as 6 kavalactones, was evaluated in the MTT test [3-(4,5-dimethylthiazole-2-yl)-2,4-diphenyltetrazolium bromide] in rat hepatocytes and human HepG2 cells. The extracts used gave no signs of hepatotoxicity in either system. The EC_{50} in rat hepatocytes was well over 500 μg/ml and could not be determined in human HepG2 cells. On the other hand, the 6 kavalactones showed dose-dependent cytotoxicity in rat hepatocytes, which was less marked in human HepG2 cells. Kavain was the most toxic in rat hepatocytes with an EC_{50} value of 45 μg/ml. With about 20% of kavain in the total extract and complete absorption, a plasma concentration of 3.33 μg/ml would be achieved from a daily dose of 20 mg of kavain, which means a 13-fold safety margin from the EC_{50}. The safety margin for the other kavalactones is even more marked [25].

Mutagenicity
In the Ames test, using *Salmonella typhimurium* strains TA98, TA100, TA1535, TA1537 and TA1538 with and without metabolic S9 activation, an acetone-water extract of kava-kava (11-20:1, 70% kava-

lactones) did not increase the number of revertants and showed no evidence of mutagenicity at levels of up to 2.5 mg/plate (the highest dose being toxic to the test organisms). In the micronucleus test in mice, after oral doses of 150, 300 and 600 mg/kg bodyweight on two successive days, no evidence of genotoxic potential was detected [5,25,104].

Clinical safety data

Over 500 patients have been treated with kava-kava extracts in controlled clinical studies [11-23,103,105] and a further 6500 in open studies [106-110]. Adverse effects were reported in about 2.3% of patients; none were of a serious nature, mild gastrointestinal complaints being the most prevalent. In placebo-controlled studies, the level of adverse effects was generally no higher in patients treated with kava-kava than in patients receiving placebo.

In a recent systematic review of the safety of kava-kava extracts, data from clinical studies (including short-term post-marketing surveillance studies) and spontaneous reporting schemes (World Health Organization and national drug regulatory bodies) suggested that, in general, adverse events are rare, mild and reversible. However, serious adverse events have been reported, most notably liver damage. Controlled studies suggest that kava-kava extracts do not impair cognitive performance and vigilance or potentiate the effects of central nervous system depressants. It was concluded that, when taken as a short-term monotherapy at recommended dose levels, kava-kava extracts appear to be well tolerated by most users. The serious adverse events require further research to determine their nature and frequency [115].

REFERENCES

1. Kavakavawurzelstock - Kava-Kava rhizoma. Deutscher Arzneimittel-Codex.

2. Kava-Kava. In: British Herbal Pharmacopoeia 1996. Bournemouth: British Herbal Medicine Association, 1996:118-9.

3. He X-g, Lin L-z, Lian L-z. Electrospray high performance liquid chromatography-mass spectrometry in phytochemical analysis of Kava (Piper methysticum) extract. Planta Med 1997;63:70-4.

4. Hänsel R, Lazar J. Kawapyrone - Inhaltsstoffe des Rauschpfeffers in pflanzlichen Sedativa. Dtsch Apoth Ztg 1985;125:2056-8.

5. Hänsel R, Keller K, Rimpler H, Schneider G, editors. Piper. In: Hagers Handbuch der Pharmazeutischen Praxis. 5th ed. Volume 6: Drogen P-Z. Berlin-Heidelberg-New York-London: Springer-Verlag 1992: 191-221.

6. Cheng D, Lidgard RO, Duffield PH, Duffield AM, Brophy JJ. Identification by methane chemical ionization gas chromatography/mass spectrometry of the products obtained by steam distillation and aqueous acid extraction of commercial Piper methysticum. Biomed Environ Mass Spectrom 1988;17:371-6.

7. Lechtenberg M, Quandt B, Kohlenberg F-J, Nahrstedt A. Qualitative and quantitative micellar electrokinetic chromatography of kavalactones from dry extracts of Piper methysticum Forst. and commercial drugs. J Chromatogr A 1999;848:457-64.

8. Shao Y, He K, Zheng B, Zheng Q. Reversed-phase high-performance liquid chromatographic method for quantitative analysis of the six major kavalactones in Piper methysticum. J Chromatogr A 1998;825:1-8.

9. Lebot V, Levesque J. Genetic control of kavalactone chemotypes in Piper methysticum cultivars. Phytochemistry 1996;43:397-403.

10. Hänsel R, Ranft G, Bähr P. Zwei Chalkonpigmente aus Piper methysticum Forst. 4. Mitt. Zur Frage der Biosythese der Kawalaktone. Z Naturforsch 1963;18b:370-3.

11. Malsch U, Kieser M. Efficacy of kava-kava in the treatment of non-psychotic anxiety, following pre-treatment with benzodiazepines. Psychopharmacology 2001;157:277-83.

12. Volz H-P, Kieser M. Kava-kava extract WS 1490 versus placebo in anxiety disorders - a randomised placebo-controlled 25-week outpatient trial. Pharmacopsychiatry 1997;30:1-5.

13. Woelk H, Kapoula O, Lehrl S, Schröter K, Weinholz P. Behandlung von Angst-Patienten. Doppelblindstudie: Kava-Spezialextrakt WS 1490 versus Benzodiazepine. Z Allg Med 1993;69:271-7.

14. Lehmann E, Kinzler E, Friedemann J. Efficacy of a special kava extract (Piper methysticum) in patients with states of anxiety, tension and excitedness of non-mental origin - a double-blind placebo-controlled study of four weeks treatment. Phytomedicine 1996; 3:113-9.
    Previously published in German as:
    Kinzler E, Krömer J, Lehmann E. Wirksamkeit eines Kava-Spezial-Extraktes bei Patienten mit Angst-, Spannungs- und Erregungszuständen nicht-psychotischer Genese. Arzneim-Forsch/Drug Res 1991;41:584-8.

15. Boerner RJ, Sommer H, Berger W, Kuhn U, Schmidt U, Mannel M. Kava-kava extract LI 150 is as effective as opipramol and buspirone in generalised anxiety disorder - an 8-week randomized, double-blind multi-centre clinical trial in 129 outpatients. Phytomedicine 2003;10 (Suppl 4):38-49.
    Summary previously published as:
    Boerner RJ, Berger W, Mannel N. Kava-Kava in der Therapie der generalisierten Angststörung. Nervenarzt 2000;71 (Suppl 1):Abstract P533.

16. Bhate H, Gerster G, Gracza E. Orale Prämedikation mit Zubereitungen aus Piper methysticum bei operativen

Eingriffen in Epiduralanästhesie. Erfahrungsheilkunde 1989;6:339-45.

17. Mittman U, Schmidt M, Vrastyakova J. Akut-anxiolytische Wirksamkeit von Kava-Spissum-Spezialextrakt und Benzodiazepinen als Prämedikation bei chirurgischen Eingriffen - Ergebnisse einer randomisierten, referenzkontrollierten Studie. J Pharmakol Ther 2000;9:99-108.

18. Warnecke G. Psychosomatische Dysfunktionen im weiblichen Klimakterium. Klinische Wirksamkeit und Verträglichkeit von Kava-Extrakt WS 1490. Fortschr Med 1991;109:119-22.

19. Warnecke G, Pfaender H, Gerster G, Gracza E. Wirksamkeit von Kawa-Kawa-Extrakt beim Klimakterischen Syndrom. Eine Doppelblindstudie mit einem neuen Monopräparat. Z Phytotherapie 1990;11:81-6.

20. Cagnacci A, Arangino S, Renzi A, Zanni AL, Malmusi S, Volpe A. Kava-kava administration reduces anxiety in perimenopausal women. Maturitas 2003;44:103-9.

21. De Leo V, La Marca A, Lanzetta D, Palazzi S, Torricelli M, Facchini C, Morgante G. Valutazione dell'associazione di estratto di kava-kava e terapia ormonale sostitutiva nel trattamento d'ansia in postmenopausa. Minerva Ginecol 2000;52:263-7.

22. Gastpar M, Klimm HD. Treatment of anxiety, tension and restlessness states with kava special extract WS 1490 in general practice. A randomized placebo-controlled double-blind multicenter trial (submitted for publication); cited by Loew in references 25 and 104.

23. Geier FP, Konstantinowicz T. Kava treatment in patients with anxiety. Phytotherapy Res (in press); cited by Loew in references 25 and 104.

24. Czygan F-C, Hiller K. Kava-Kava rhizoma - Kavakavawurzelstock. In: Wichtl M, editor. Teedrogen und Phytopharmaka. Ein Handbuch für die Praxis auf wissenschaftlicher Grundlage, 4th ed. Stuttgart: Wissenschaftliche Verlagsgesellschaft, 2002:324-6.

25. Loew D, Gaus W. Kava-Kava. Tragödie einer Fehlbeurteilung. Z Phytotherapie 2002;23:267-81.

26. Almeida JC, Grimsley EW. Coma from the health food store: interaction between kava and alprazolam. Ann Intern Med 1996;125:940-1.

27. Xanax (alprazolam tablets, USP). In: Physicians' Desk Reference, 50th edition. Montvale, NJ: Medical Economics Company, 1996.

28. Herberg K-W. Alltagssicherheit unter Kava-Kava-Extrakt, Bromazepam und deren Kombination. Z Allg Med 1996;72:973-7.

29. Herberg K-W. Fahrtüchtigkeit nach Einnahme von Kava-Spezial-Extrakt WS 1490. Doppelblinde, placebokontrollierte Probandenstudie. Z Allg Med 1991;67:842-6.

30. Mathews JD, Riley MD, Fejo L, Munoz E, Milns NR, Gardner ID et al. Effects of the heavy usage of kava on physical health: summary of a pilot survey in an Aboriginal community. Med J Aust 1988;148:548-55.

31. Strahl S, Ehret V, Dahm HH, Maier KP. Nekrotisierende Hepatitis nach Einnahme pflanzlicher Heilmittel. Dtsch med Wschr 1998;123:1410-4.

32. Stoller R. Leberschädigungen unter Kava-Extrakten. Schweiz Ärztezeitung 2000;81:1335-6.

33. Escher M, Desmeules J. Hepatitis associated with Kava, a herbal remedy for anxiety. Brit Med J 2001;322:139.

34. Kraft M, Spahn TW, Menzel J, Senninger N, Dietl K-H, Herbst H et al. Fulminantes Leberversagen nach Einnahme des pflanzlichen Antidepressivums Kava-Kava. Dtsch Med Wschr 2001;126:970-2.

35. Saß M, Schnabel S, Kröger J, Liebe S, Schareck WD. Akutes Leberversagen durch Kava-Kava - eine seltene Indikation zur Lebertransplantation. Z Gastroentrol 2001;39:491 (Abstract P29).

36. Brauer RB, Pfab R, Becker K, Berger H, Stangl M. Fulminantes Leberversagen nach Einnahme des pflanzlichen Heilmittels Kava-Kava. Z Gastroenterol 2001;39:491 (P30).

37. UK Medicines Control Agency. Consultation letter MLX 286 (25 July 2002): Proposals to prohibit the herbal ingredient kava-kava (Piper methysticum) in unlicensed medicines.

38. Commission E of the German Health Authority (BfArM). Declaration of Commission E on kava-kava. July 2002.

39. Schulze J, Meng G, Siegers C-P. Safety assessment of kavalactone-containing herbal drugs in comparison to other psychotropics. Naunyn-Schmiederberg's Arch Pharmacol 2001;364 (3, Suppl.):R22 (Abstract 27) and associated poster from The Swiss Society of Pharmacology and Toxicology meeting in Berne, Switzerland, on 1-2 October 2001.

40. Schmidt M, Nahrstedt A, Lüpke NP. Piper methysticum (Kava) in der Diskussion: Betrachtungen zu Qualität, Wirksamkeit und Unbedenklichkeit. Wien Med Wschr 2002;152:382-8.

41. Schelosky L, Raffauf C, Jendroska K, Poewe W. Kava and dopamine antagonism. J Neurol Neurosurg Psychiat 1995;58:639-40.

42. Nöldner M, Chatterjee SS. Inhibition of haloperidol-induced catalepsy in rats by root extracts from Piper methysticum F. Phytomedicine 1999;6:285-6.

43. Schmidt P, Boehncke W-H. Delayed-type hypersensitivity reaction to kava-kava extract. Contact Dermatitis 2000;42:363-4.

44. Hänsel R, Woelk H, editors. Unerwünschte Wirkungen des Kavatrinkens/Toxikologie. In: Spektrum Kava-Kava, 2nd ed. Basel: Aesopus Verlag 1995:19-20 and 41-2.

45. Cawte J. Parameters of kava used as a challenge to alcohol. Aust NZ J Psychiat 1986;20:70-6.

46. Ruze P. Kava-induced dermopathy: a niacin deficiency? Lancet 1990;335:1442-5.

47. Norton SA, Ruze P. Kava dermopathy. J Amer Acad Dermatol 1994;31:89-97.

48. Spillane PK, Fisher DA, Currie BJ. Neurological manifestations of kava intoxication Med J Austr 1997; 167:172-3.

49. Garner LF, Klinger JD. Some visual effects caused by the beverage Kava. J Ethnopharmacol 1985;13:307-11.

50. Siegel RK. Herbal Intoxication. Psychoactive effects from herbal cigarettes, tea and capsules. JAMA 1976; 236:473-6.

51. Levine R, Taylor WB. Take tea and see. Arch Dermatol 1986;122:856.

52. Jussofie A, Schmiz A, Hiemke C. Kavapyrone enriched extract from Piper methysticum as modulator of the GABA binding site in different regions of rat brain. Psychopharmacology 1994;116:469-74.

53. Davies LP, Drew CA, Duffield P, Johnston GAR, Jamieson DD. Kava pyrones and resin: studies on GABA_A, GABA_B and benzodiazepine binding sites in rodent brain. Pharmacol Toxicol 1992;71:120-6.

54. Davies L, Drew C, Duffield P, Jamieson D. Effects of kava on benzodiazepine and GABA receptor binding. Eur J Pharmacol 1990;183:558.

55. Boonen G, Häberlein H. Influence of genuine kava-pyrone enantiomers on the GABA_A binding site. Planta Med 1998;64:504-6.

56. Seitz U, Schüle A, Gleitz J. [³H]-Monoamine uptake inhibition properties of kava pyrones. Planta Med 1997;63:548-9.

57. Walden J, von Wegerer J, Winter U, Berger M. Actions of kavain and dihydromethysticin on ipsapirone-induced field potential changes in the hippocampus. Human Psychopharmacol 1997;12:265-70.

58. Walden J, von Wegerer J, Winter U, Berger M, Grunze H. Effects of kawain and dihydromethysticin on field potential changes in the hippocampus. Progress Neuropsychopharmacol Biol Psychiat 1997;21:697-706.

59. Schmitz D, Zhang CL, Chatterjee SS, Heinemann U. Effects of methysticin on three different models of seizure like events studied in rat hippocampal and entorhinal cortex slices. Naunyn-Schmiedeberg's Arch Pharmacol 1995;351:348-55.

60. Gleitz J, Gottner N, Ameri A, Peters T. Kavain inhibits non-stereospecifically veratridine-activated Na⁺ channels. Planta Med 1996;62:580-1.

61. Gleitz J, Beile A, Peters T. (±)-Kavain inhibits veratridine-activated voltage-dependent Na⁺ channels in synaptosomes prepared from rat cerebral cortex. Neuropharmacology 1995;34:1133-8.

62. Gleitz J, Beile A, Peters T. (±)-Kavain inhibits the veratridine- and KCl-induced increase in intracellular Ca²⁺ and glutamate-release of rat cerebrocortical synaptosomes. Neuropharmacology 1996;35:179-86.

63. Gleitz J, Friese J, Beile A, Ameri A, Peters T. Anticonvulsive action of (±)-kavain estimated from its properties on stimulated synaptosomes and Na⁺ channel receptor sites. Eur J Pharmacol 1996;315:89-97.

64. Friese J, Gleitz J. Kavain, dihydrokavain and dihydromethysticin non-competitively inhibit the specific binding of [³H]-batrachotoxinin-A 20-α-benzoate to receptor site 2 of voltage-gated Na⁺ channels. Planta Med 1998;64:458-9.

65. Meyer HJ. Spasmolytische Effekte von Dihydromethysticin, einem Wirkstoff aus Piper methysticum Forst. Arch Int Pharmacodyn 1965;154:449-67.

66. Magura EI, Kopanitsa MV, Gleitz J, Peters T, Krishtal OA. Kava extract ingredients, (+)-methysticin and (±)-kavain inhibit voltage-operated Na⁺-channels in rat CA1 hippocampal neurons. Neuroscience 1997;81: 345-51.

67. Seitz U, Ameri A, Pelzer H, Gleitz J, Peters T. Relaxation of evoked contractile activity of isolated guinea-pig ileum by (±)-kavain. Planta Med 1997;63:303-6.

68. Rechnitz GA, Coon D, Babb C, Ogunseitan A, Lee A. Sensing neuroactive agents in Hawaiian plants. Analyt Chim Acta 1997;337:297-303.

69. Gleitz J, Beile A, Wilkens P, Ameri A, Peters T. Antithrombotic action of the kava pyrone (+)-kavain prepared from Piper methysticum on human platelets. Planta Med 1997;63:27-30.

70. Duffield PH, Jamieson DD, Duffield AM. Effect of aqueous and lipid-soluble extracts of kava on the conditioned avoidance response in rats. Arch Int Pharmacodyn 1989;301:81-90.

71. O'Hara MJ, Kinnard WJ, Buckley JP. Preliminary characterization of aqueous extracts of Piper methysticum (kava, kawa kawa). J Pharm Sci 1965;54:1021-5.

72. Jamieson DD, Duffield PH, Cheng D, Duffield AM. Comparison of the central nervous system activity of the aqueous and lipid extract of kava (Piper methysticum). Arch Int Pharmacodyn 1989;301:66-80.

73. Jamieson DD, Duffield PH. The antinociceptive actions of kava components in mice. Clin Exptl Pharmacol Physiol 1990;17:495-507.

74. Holm E, Staedt U, Heep J, Kortsik C, Behne F, Kaske A, Mennicke I. Untersuchungen zum Wirkungsprofil von D,L-Kavain. Zerebrale Angriffsorte und Schlaf-Wach-Rhythmus im Tierexperiment. Arzneim-Forsch/Drug Res 1991;41:673-83.

75. Furgiuele AR, Kinnard WJ, Aceto MD, Buckley JP. Central activity of aqueous extracts of Piper methysticum (kava). J Pharm Sci 1965;54:247-52.

76. Kretzschmar R, Meyer HJ, Teschendorf HJ, Zöllner B. Spasmolytische Wirksamkeit von aryl-substituierten

α-Pyronen und wässrigen Extrakten aus *Piper methysticum* Forst. Arch Int Pharmacodyn 1969;180:475-91.

77. Kretzschmar R, Teschendorf HJ. Pharmakologische Untersuchungen zur sedativ-tranquilisierenden Wirkung des Rauschpfeffers (*Piper methysticum* Forst). Chem-Ztg 1974;98:24-8.

78. Klohs MW, Keller F, Williams RE, Toekes MI, Cronheim GE. A chemical and pharmacological investigation of *Piper methysticum* Forst. J Med Pharm Chem 1959;1:95-103.

79. Edwards J, Wang M, Pecore N, La Granoe L. The LD$_{50}$ of kavalactones extracted from *Piper methysticum* in rats. FASEB J 1998;12(4):A464 (Abstract 2698).

80. Klimke A, Klieser E, Lehmann E, Strauss WH. Effectivity of cavain in tranquillizer indication. Psychopharmacology 1988;96(Suppl):354 (Abstract 33.03.19).

81. Keledjian J, Duffield PH, Jamieson DD, Lidgard RO, Duffield AM. Uptake into mouse brain of four compounds present in the psychoactive beverage kava. J Pharm Sci 1988;77:1003-6.

82. Kretzschmar R, Teschendorf HJ, Ladous A, Ettehadieh D. On the sedative action of the kava rhizome. Acta Pharmacol Toxicol 1971;29 (Suppl 4):26.

83. Boonen G, Ferger B, Kuschinsky K, Häberlein H. *In vivo* effects of the kavapyrones (+)-dihydromethysticin and (±)-kavain on dopamine, 3,4-dihydroxyphenylacetic acid, serotonin and 5-hydroxyindoleacetic acid levels in striatal and cortical brain regions. Planta Med 1998;64:507-10.

84. Kretzschmar R, Meyer HJ, Teschendorf HJ. Strychnine antagonistic potency of pyrone compounds of the kava root (*Piper methysticum* Forst). Experientia 1970;26:283-4.

85. Kretzschmar R, Meyer HJ. Vergleichende Untersuchungen über die antikonvulsive Wirksamkeit der Pyronverbindungen aus *Piper methysticum* Forst. Arch Int Pharmacodyn 1969;177:261-77.

86. Meyer HJ, Meyer-Burg J. Hemmung des Elektrokrampfes durch die Kawa-Pyrone Dihydromethysticin und Dihydrokawain. Arch Int Pharmacodyn 1964;148:97-110.

87. Backhauß C, Krieglstein J. Extract of kava (*Piper methysticum*) and its methysticin constituents protect brain tissue against ischemic damage in rodents. Eur J Pharmacol 1992;215:265-9.

88. Backhauß C, Krieglstein J. Neuroprotective activity of kava extract (*Piper methysticum*) and its methysticin constituents *in vivo* and *in vitro*. In: Krieglstein J and Oberpichler-Schwenk H, editors. Pharmacology of Cerebral Ischemia 1992. Stuttgart: Wissenschaftliche Verlagsgesellschaft, 1992:501-7.

89. Baum SS, Hill R, Rommelspacher H. Effect of kava extract and individual kavapyrones on neurotransmitter levels in the nucleus accumbens of rats. Progress Neuropsychopharmacol Biol Psychiat 1998;22:1105-20.

90. Bergsträßer E. Kava-Kava beeinflußt die Dopaminfreisetzung nach Hypoxie. Z Phytother 1997;18:224-6.

91. Heinze HJ, Münte TF, Steitz J, Matzke M. Pharmacopsychological effects of oxazepam and kava-extract in a visual search paradigm assessed with event-related potentials. Pharmacopsychiatry 1994;27:224-30.

92. Münte TF, Heinze HJ, Matzke M, Steitz J. Effects of oxazepam and an extract of kava roots (*Piper methysticum*) on event-related potentials in a word recognition task. Neuropsychobiology 1993;27:46-53.

93. Russell PN, Bakker D, Singh NN. The effects of kava on alerting and speed of access of information from long-term memory. Bull Psychonomic Soc 1987;25:236-7.

94. Johnson D, Frauendorf A, Stecker K, Stein U. Neurophysiologisches Wirkprofil und Verträglichkeit von Kava-Extrakt WS 1490. TW Neurol Psychiat 1991;5:349-54.

95. Gessner B, Cnota P. Untersuchung der Vigilanz nach Applikation von Kava-Kava-Extrakt, Diazepam oder Placebo. Z Phytotherapie 1994;15:30-7.

96. Emser W, Bartylla K. Verbesserung der Schlafqualität. Zur Wirkung von Kava-Extrakt WS 1490 auf das Schlafmuster bei Gesunden. TW Neurol Psychiat 1991;5:636-42.

97. Schulz H, Jobert M, Hübner WD. The quantitative EEG as a screening instrument to identify sedative effects of single doses of plant extracts in comparison with diazepam. Phytomedicine 1998;5:449-58.

98. Guy W. Clinical global impressions. In: ECDEU assessment manual for psychopharmacology, revised. Rockville MD: US Department of Health, Education and Welfare, National Institute of Mental Health, 1967:217-22.

99. American Psychiatric Association. Diagnostic and statistical manual of mental disorders, 3rd ed. revised. Washington DC: American Psychiatric Association Press, 1987.

100. American Psychiatric Association. Diagnostic and statistical manual of mental disorders, 4th ed. Washington DC: American Psychiatric Association Press, 1994.

101. Hamilton M. The assessment of anxiety states by rating. Brit J Med Psychol 1959;32:50-5.

102. World Health Organisation. ICD-10: International Statistical Classification of Diseases and Related Health Problems. Tenth Revision. Geneva: WHO, 1992.

103. Connor KM, Davidson JRT. A placebo-controlled study of kava kava in generalized anxiety disorder. Int Clin Psychopharmacol 2002;17:185-8.

104. Loew D. Kava-Kava-Extrakt. Dtsch Apoth Ztg 2002;142:1012-20.

105. Lehrl S. Clinical efficacy of kava extract WS 1490 in sleep disturbances associated with anxiety disorders. J Affective Disord (in press); cited by Loew in references 25 and 104.

106. Neto JT. Eficácia e tolerabilidade do extrato de kava-kava WS 1490 em estados de ansiedade. Estudo multicêntrico brasileiro. Rev Bras Med 1999;56:280-4.

107. Scherer J. Kava-kava extract in anxiety disorders: an outpatient observational study. Advances Ther 1998; 15:261-9.

108. Spree MH, Croy HH. Antares®- ein standardisiertes Kava-Kava-Präparat mit dem Spezialextrakt KW 1491. Der Kassenarzt 1992;(17):44-51.

109. Siegers C-P, Honold E, Krall B, Meng G, Habs M. Ergebnisse der Anwendungsbeobachtung L 1090 mit Laitan® Kapseln. Verträglichkeit in 96% der Fälle sehr gut oder gut. Ärztl Forsch 1992;39:7-11.

110. Warnecke G. Langzeittherapie psychischer und vegetativer Dysregulationen mit Zubereitungen aus Piper methysticum. Erfahrungsheilkunde 1989:6:333-8.

111. Pittler MH, Ernst E. Efficacy of kava extract for treating anxiety: systematic review and meta-analysis. J Clin Psychopharmacol 2000;20:84-9.

112. Biber A, Nöldner M, Schlegelmilch R. Development of a formulation of kava-kava extract through pharmacokinetic experiments in animals. Naunyn-Schmiedebergs Arch Pharmacol 1992:R24 (Abstract 93).

113. Rasmussen AK, Scheline RR, Solheim E. Metabolism of some kava pyrones in the rat. Xenobiotica 1979;9:1-16.

114. Duffield AM, Jamieson DD, Lidgard RO, Duffield PH, Bourne DJ. Identification of some human urinary metabolites of the intoxicating beverage kava. J Chromatogr 1989;475:273-81.

115. Stevinson C, Huntley A, Ernst E. A systematic review of the safety of kava extract in the treatment of anxiety. Drug Safety 2002;25:251-61.

PLANTAGINIS LANCEOLATAE FOLIUM/HERBA

Ribwort Plantain Leaf/Herb

E/S/C/O/P
MONOGRAPHS
Second Edition

DEFINITIONS

Ribwort plantain leaf consists of the dried leaves of *Plantago lanceolata* L. It contains not less than 1.5 per cent of total *ortho*-dihydroxycinnamic acid derivatives, expressed as acteoside ($C_{29}H_{36}O_{15}$; M_r 624.6) and calculated with respect to the dried drug.

Ribwort plantain herb consists of the dried flowering aerial parts of *Plantago lanceolata* L.

Ribwort plantain leaf complies with the monograph of the European Pharmacopoeia for ribwort plantain [1]. Until recently, a monograph for ribwort plantain herb appeared in the Deutsches Arzneibuch [2].

Fresh material may also be used, provided that when dried it complies with the monograph of the respective pharmacopoeia.

CONSTITUENTS

The characteristic constitue... polysaccharides, iridoid glyc... aucubin and catalpol) and pher... side, isoacteoside and plantama, ...

CLINICAL PARTICULARS

Therapeutic indications
Catarrhs of the respiratory tract [3,13-17].
Temporary, mild inflammations of the oral and pharyngeal mucosa [3,16,17].

Posology and method of administration

Dosage

Adults: average daily dose, 3-6 g of the drug or equivalent preparations [13,14,17].
Elderly: dose as for adults.
Children, average daily dose: *>1-4 years of age*, 1-2 g; *4-10 years*, 2-4 g; *10-16 years*, 3-6 g [15,18].

Mode of administration
For oral administration.

Duration of administration
If symptoms persist or worsen, medical advice should be sought.

Contra-indications
None known.

Special warnings and special precautions for use
None required.

Interaction with other medicaments and other forms of interaction
None reported.

Pregnancy and lactation
No data available. In accordance with general medical practice, the product should not be used during pregnancy and lactation without medical advice.

Effects on ability to drive and use machines
None known.

Undesirable effects
None known.

Overdose
No toxic effects reported.

PHARMACOLOGICAL PROPERTIES

Pharmacodynamic properties
Ribwort plantain herb and its characteristic constituents exert anti-inflammatory, antibacterial, spasmolytic and immunostimulatory effects. The pharmacologically active constituents are considered to be mucilage polysaccharides, iridoid glycosides and phenylethanoids [10,12,19].

In vitro experiments

Anti-inflammatory activity
Four different freeze-dried extracts (ethanol 28%) from ribwort plantain herb were evaluated for anti-inflammatory activity in a modified hen's egg chorio-allantoic membrane (HET-CAM) test using sodium dodecyl sulphate as the membrane irritant. At concentrations of 500 µg/pellet all the extracts inhibited the formation of blood vessels around the granuloma and the total blood vessel net appeared normal. Two extracts inhibited membrane irritation by 100%, the other two by 67 and 93% respectively. The activity of the extracts was comparable to that of hydrocortisone, phenylbutazone and diclofenac, each at 50 µg/pellet [10,19].

Acteoside and plantamajoside inhibited 5-lipoxygenase with IC_{50} values of 13.6 and 3.75×10^{-7} M respectively [20].

In human polymorphonuclear leukocytes acteoside inhibited the production of 5-HETE with an IC_{50} of 4.85 µM and leukotriene B_4 with an IC_{50} of 2.93 µM. In peritoneal leukocytes from mice, 5-HETE production was inhibited with an IC_{50} of 5.27 µM [21].

Antibacterial and antiviral activity
Expressed juice and aqueous, methanolic and ethan-olic extracts of ribwort plantain leaf have shown inhibitory activity against various microorganisms such as *Bacillus subtilis*, *B. cereus*, *Klebsiella pneumoniae*, *Micrococcus flavus*, *Mycobacterium phlei*, *Pseudomonas aeruginosa*, *Proteus vulgare*, *Staphylococcus aureus*, *Streptococcus aureus*, *S. β-haemolyticus* and *S. pyocyaneus*, and against several strains of *Salmonella* and *Shigella* in the plate diffusion test [3,22-26].

Aucubigenin, the aglycone of aucubin, has been shown to be mainly responsible for antibacterial activity of the drug and extracts [8,23,25,27,28]. Extracts without aucubin exerted no antibacterial effects [27].

Aucubin preincubated with β-glucosidase suppressed hepatitis B virus DNA replication in HepG2 cell cultures in a dose-dependent manner [29].

Spasmolytic activity
A fluid extract (1:1) from ribwort plantain herb inhibited contractions of isolated guinea pig ileum induced by acetylcholine, histamine, K^+ and Ba^{2+} by 50% at 10 mg/ml and 100% at higher concentrations. The effects were comparable to those of atropine, diphenhydramine and papaverine. With preparations of isolated guinea pig trachea, only Ba^{2+}-induced contractions were inhibited, by 30% at 10 mg/ml [30].

Aucubin and catalpol peracetates dose-dependently inhibited acetylcholine- and calcium-induced contractions of rat uterine strips in a similar way to papaverine. The antagonism was non-competitive against acetylcholine (pD_2' values: peracetylated aucubin 5.74, peracetylated catalpol 5.59, papaverine 5.32) and competitive against calcium (pA_2 values: peracetylated aucubin 6.34, peracetylated catalpol 6.48, papaverine 6.23) [31].

Acteoside inhibited histamine- and bradykinin-induced contractions of isolated guinea-pig ileum with pA values of 6.31 and 6.51 respectively [32].

Immunostimulant activity
At a concentration of 0.0002% the polysaccharides of ribwort plantain leaf increased phagocytosis of granulocytes by 20.5%. Chemiluminescence was increased by 36% at a concentration of 0.001% [22].

Coagulant activity
A diluted infusion of ribwort plantain herb [33] and an aqueous extract of ribwort plantain leaf [34] accelerated clotting of canine or rabbit blood *in vitro*.

Other effects
The mucociliary transport velocity in isolated ciliated epithelium from the frog oesophagus was not influenced by application of 200 µl of an infusion from

ribwort plantain herb (4.6 g per 100 ml of water) [35].

In vivo experiments

Anti-inflammatory effects

Oral pre-treatment of rats with a dry 80%-ethanolic extract from ribwort plantain leaf at 100 mg/kg body weight inhibited carrageenan-induced paw oedema by 11% (not significant) compared to 45% inhibition by indometacin at 5 mg/kg [36].

A freeze-dried extract from ribwort plantain leaf, administered intraperitoneally to rats, reduced the inflammatory effect and leukocyte infiltration induced by simultaneous subplantar injection of carrageenan and prostaglandin E_1 [37].

Aucubin administered orally at 100 mg/kg body weight inhibited carrageenan-induced mouse paw oedema by 33.0% after 3 hours (p<0.01), compared to 44% inhibition by oral indometacin at 7 mg/kg (p<0.01). In the 12-O-tetradecanoylphorbol acetate (TPA)-induced mouse ear oedema test, aucubin applied topically at 1 mg/ear inhibited oedema by 80% (p<0.01), compared to 87% inhibition by indometacin at 0.5 mg/ear (p<0.01) [38].

Oral pretreatment of rats with acteoside at 150 mg/kg body weight significantly inhibited carrageenan-induced rat paw oedema by 96 and 94% after 2 and 4 hours respectively compared to vehicle controls; oral indometacin at 10 mg/kg caused 25 and 40% inhibition after 2 and 4 hours respectively [32].

Topical pretreatment with acteoside or plantamajoside at 3 mg/ear inhibited arachidonic acid-induced mouse ear oedema by 14% (p<0.05) and 25% (p<0.01) respectively, compared to 38% inhibition by phenidone at 0.1 mg/ear (p<0.01) [39].

Immunostimulant effects

Interferon production in mice increased by 15-fold and 3-fold respectively 24 and 48 hours after intravenous administration of 0.2 ml of a decoction from ribwort plantain leaf (2 g in 100 ml of water) [40].

An aqueous extract from ribwort plantain leaf increased SRBC-antibody production and the liberation of angiogenesis factor in mice [41].

Pharmacological studies in humans

No data available.

Clinical studies

In an open study 593 patients with acute respiratory complaints such as acute bronchitis and post-infectious dry cough were treated, for 10 days on average, with a mean daily dose of 31.3 ml of a syrup, equivalent to about 6.3 g of ribwort plantain herb (100 ml of the syrup contained 20 g of fluid extract 1:1 of the herb).

Symptoms declined significantly (p<0.001), the overall symptom score declining by about 65%. Compared to initial values, the subjective score reductions were: cough frequency, 65.5%; cough intensity, 66.9%; cough-related chest pain, 79.9%; dry cough, 68.5%; dyspnoea, 69.6%; rales, 69.9%; and obstructive "whistling", 74.6%. Expectoration improved by 73.3% and purulent sputum decreased by 66.4%. Global efficacy evaluated by the physicians was excellent in 25.9% of patients, good in 61.8%, moderate in 7.8% and minimal in 2% [13,14].

Similar results were reported in a subgroup of the 91 patients under 18 years of age (58 of them under 13 years) in the above study. In this subgroup the mean daily dose was 22.4 ml of the syrup, equivalent to about 4.5 g of ribwort plantain herb, and the mean duration of treatment was 8.8 days. The overall symptom score declined by about 58.3%. The physicians evaluated global efficacy as excellent in 22%, good in 63.7%, moderate in 9.9% and minimal in 1.1% of patients [15].

Pharmacokinetic properties

No data available.

Preclinical safety data

No acute, repeated-dose or reproductive toxicity data are available.

A tincture of ribwort plantain herb (1:5, 70 % ethanol) showed no mutagenicity in the Ames Test using *Salmonella typhimurium* strains TA98 and TA100, with or without metabolic activation [42].

In a somatic segregation assay in the diploid strain *Aspergillus nidulans* D-30 no genotoxic effects (neither chromosomal damage caused by aneuploidy and clastogenic effects nor mitotic crossover) were detected after plate incorporation of 4.76 mg/ml of a fluid extract of ribwort plantain leaf [43].

Clinical safety data

In the open study involving 593 patients there were only 7 minor adverse events, mainly diarrhoea (n = 5) [13-15].

REFERENCES

1. Ribwort Plantain - Plantago lanceolatae folium. European Pharmacopoeia, Council of Europe.

2. Spitzwegerichkraut - Plantaginis lanceolatae herba. Deutsches Arzneibuch.

3. Bräutigam M. Plantago. In: Hänsel R, Keller K, Rimpler H, Schneider G, editors. Hagers Handbuch der

Pharmazeutischen Praxis, 5th ed. Volume 6: Drogen P-Z. Berlin-Heidelberg-New York-London: Springer-Verlag, 1994:221-39.

4. Bräutigam M, Franz G. Schleimpolysaccharide aus Spitzwegerichblättern. Dtsch Apoth Ztg 1985;125:58-62.

5. Bräutigam M, Franz G. Structural features of *Plantago lanceolata* mucilage. Planta Med 1985;51:293-7.

6. Darrow K, Bowers MD. Phenological and population variation in iridoid glycosides of *Plantago lanceolata* (Plantaginaceae). Biochem Syst Ecol 1997;25:1-11.

7. Handjieva N, Saadi H. Iridoid glycosides from *Plantago altissima* L., *Plantago lanceolata* L., *Plantago atrata* Hoppe and *Plantago argentea* Chaix. Z Naturforsch 1991;46c:963-5.

8. Háznagy A, Tóth G, Bula E. Apigenin-7-O-monoglucosid im Kraut von *Plantago lanceolata*. Pharmazie 1976;31:482-3.

9. Kardosova A. Polysaccharides from the leaves of *Plantago lanceolata* L., var. LIBOR: an alpha-D-glucan. Chem Papers 1992;46:127-30.

10. Marchesan M, Hose S, Paper DH, Franz G. Spitzwegerich. Neue Untersuchungen zur antiinflammatorischen Wirkung. Dtsch Apoth Ztg 1998;138:2987-92.

11. Murai M, Tamayama Y, Nishibe S. Phenylethanoids in the herb of *Plantago lanceolata* and inhibitory effect on arachidonic acid-induced mouse ear edema. Planta Med 1995;61:479-80.

12. Paper DH, Marchesan M. Spitzwegerich (*Plantago lanceolata* L.). Inhaltsstoffe - Analytik - Pharmakologie - Standardisierung. Z Phytotherapie 1999;20:231-8.

13. Kraft K. Efficacy of a *Plantago lanceolata* fluid extract (PLFE) in acute respiratory diseases (ARD). In: Abstracts of 2nd International Congress on Phytomedicine. Munich, 11-14 September 1996. *Published as*: Phytomedicine 1996;3(Suppl 1):150 (Abstract SL-121).

14. Kraft K. Therapeutisches Profil eines Spitzwegerichkraut-Fluidextraktes bei akuten respiratorischen Erkrankungen im Kindes- und Erwachsenenalter. In: Loew D, Rietbrock N, editors. Phytopharmaka III. Forschung und klinische Anwendung. Darmstadt: Steinkopff, 1997:199-209.

15. Kraft K. Spitzwegerich-Fluidextrakt als Antitussivum. Anwendung bei unspezifischen respiratorischen Erkrankungen im Kindes- und Jugendalter. Z Phytother 1998;19:219.

16. Schilcher H, Kammerer S. In: Leitfaden Phytotherapie. München: Urban & Fischer, 2000.

17. Willuhn G. Plantaginis lanceolatae folium/herba (Spitzwegerichblätter/kraut). In: Wichtl M, editor. Teedrogen und Phytopharmaka - Ein Handbuch für die Praxis auf wissenschaftliche Grundlage, 4th ed. Stuttgart: Wissenschaftliche Verlagsgesellschaft, 2002:456-60.

18. Dorsch W, Loew D, Meyer-Buchtela E, Schilcher H.

Plantaginis lanceolatae herba (Spitzwegerichkraut). In: Kooperation Phytopharmaka, editor. Kinderdosierung von Phytopharmaka, 3rd ed. Teil 1 - Empfehlungen zur Anwendung und Dosierung von Phytopharmaka, monographierten Arzneidrogen und ihren Zubereitungen in der Pädiatrie. Bonn: Kooperation Phytopharmaka, 2002: 118-9.

19. Marchesan M, Paper DH, Hose S, Franz G. Investigation of the antiinflammatory activity of liquid extracts of *Plantago lanceolata* L. Phytother Res 1998;12:S33-S34.

20. Ravn H, Nishibe S, Sasahara M, Xuebo L. Phenolic compounds from *Plantago asiatica*. Phytochemistry 1990;29:3627-31.

21. Kimura Y, Okuda H, Nishibe S, Arichi S. Effects of caffeoylglycosides on arachidonate metabolism in leukocytes. Planta Med 1987;53:148-53.

22. Bräutigam M. Untersuchungen über die Schleimpolysaccharide aus Plantaginis lanceolatae folium und Versuche zur Gewebekultur von schleimbildenden pflanzlichen Geweben [Dissertation]. Universität Regensburg, 1985.

23. Elich J. Die antibakterielle Aktivität einiger einheimischer Plantago-Arten. Dtsch Apoth Ztg 1966;106: 428.

24. Felklová M. Antibakterielle Eigenschaften der Extrakte aus *Plantago lanceolata* L. Pharm Zentralh 1958;97:61-5.

25. Hänsel R. Glykosidische Bitterstoffe der Monoterpenreihe. Dtsch Apoth Ztg 1966;106:1761-7.

26. Tarle D, Petricic J, Kupinic M. Antibiotic effect of aucubin, saponins and extract of plantain leaf - herba or folium Plantaginis lanceolatae. Farm Glas 1981; 37:351-4.

27. Elich J. Das antibakterielle Prinzip unserer einheimischen Plantagoarten. Pharmazie 1962;17:639-40.

28. Háznagy A. Neuere Untersuchungsergebnisse über Plantaginis folium. Herba Hung 1970;9:57-63.

29. Chang IM. Antiviral activity of aucubin against hepatitis B virus replication. Phytother Res 1997;11:189-92.

30. Fleer H, Verspohl EJ, Nahrstedt A. In-vitro spasmolytische Aktivität von Extrakten aus *Cynara scolymus* und *Plantago lanceolata*. In: Proceedings of 8th Congress on Phytotherapy. Würzburg, 27-28 November 1997.

31. Ortiz de Urbina AV, Martín ML, Fernández B, San Román L, Cubillo L. *In vitro* antispasmodic activity of peracetylated penstemonoside, aucubin and catalpol. Planta Med 1994;60:512-5.

32. Schapoval EES, Vargas MRW, Chaves CG, Bridi R, Zuanazzi JA, Henriques AT. Antiinflammatory and antinociceptive activities of extracts and isolated compounds from *Stachytarpheta cayennensis*. J Ethnopharmacol 1998;60:53-9.

33. Keeser ED. Untersuchung einiger Blutstillungsmittel. Dtsch Med Wschr 1939;65:375-6.

34. Monastyrskaya BI, Petropavlovskaya AA. Hemostatic and wound-healing effects of plantain. Farmakol Toksikol 1953;16:30-2.

35. Müller-Limmroth W, Fröhlich H-H. Wirkungsnachweis einiger phytotherapeutischer Expektorantien auf den mukoziliaren Transport. Fortschr Med 1980;98:95-101.

36. Mascolo N, Autore G, Capasso F, Menghini A, Fasulo MP. Biological screening of Italian medicinal plants for anti-inflammatory activity. Phytother Res 1987;1:28-31.

37. Shipochliev T, Dimitrov A, Aleksandrova E. Study on the antiinflammatory effect of a group of plant extracts. Vet-Med Nauk (Vet Sci Sofia) 1981;18(6):87-94.

38. Recio MC, Giner RM, Mañez S, Ríos JL. Structural considerations on the iridoids as anti-inflammatory agents. Planta Med 1994;60:232-4.

39. Murai M, Tamayama Y, Nishibe S. Phenylethanoids in the herb of *Plantago lanceolata* and inhibitory effect on arachidonic acid-induced mouse ear edema. Planta Med 1995;61:479-80.

40. Plachcinska J, Matacz D, Krzysztofik R, Dabrowa A, Brzosko WJ, Ozarowski A. Influence of medicinal herbs on the immune system. I. Induction of endogenous interferon. Fitoterapia 1984;55:346-8.

41. Strzelecka H, Glinkowska G, Skopínska-Rózewska E, Malkowska-Zwierz W, Sikorska E, Sokolnicka I. Immunotropic activity of plant extracts, I. Influence of water extracts of chosen crude drugs on humoral and cellular immune response. Herba Pol 1995;41:23-32.

42. Schimmer O, Krüger A, Paulini H, Haefele F. An evaluation of 55 commercial plant extracts in the Ames mutagenicity test. Pharmazie 1994;49:448-51.

43. Ramos Ruiz A, De la Torre RA, Alonso N, Villaescusa A, Betancourt J, Vizoso A. Screening of medicinal plants for induction of somatic segregation activity in *Aspergillus nidulans*. J Ethnopharmacol 1996;52:123-7.

PLANTAGINIS OVATAE SEMEN

Ispaghula Seed

E/S/C/O/P
MONOGRAPHS
Second Edition

DEFINITION

Ispaghula seed consists of the dried ripe seeds of *Plantago ovata* Forssk. (*Plantago ispaghula* Roxb.).

The material complies with the monograph of the European Pharmacopoeia [1].

CONSTITUENTS

About 80% [2] of total dietary fibre when determined by the AOAC method [3], consisting predominantly of insoluble fibre (ratio of soluble to insoluble fibre, 47:53) [2]. Soluble fibre occurs in the epidermis as a mucilage polysaccharide consisting mainly of a highly-branched arabinoxylan with a xylan backbone and branches of arabinose, xylose and 2-*O*-(galactosyl-uronic acid)-rhamnose residues [4,5].

The seeds also contain proteins, fixed oil, sterols and the trisaccharide planteose [6-8].

CLINICAL PARTICULARS

Therapeutic indications
Treatment of occasional constipation [9-13].
Conditions in which easy defecation with soft stools is desirable, e.g. in cases of anal fissures or haemorrhoids [14], after rectal or anal surgery, and during pregnancy.
Conditions which need an increased daily intake of fibre, e.g. irritable bowel syndrome [15,16].
Adjuvant symptomatic therapy in cases of diarrhoea from various causes [17-19].

Posology and method of administration

Dosage

Adults and children over 12 years of age: as a laxative, 7-30 g of the seeds [9,13,15] or equivalent preparations daily; in cases of diarrhoea, up to 40 g daily, divided into 2-3 doses.
Children 6-12 years: half the adult dose.

Method of administration
For oral administration.

It is very important to take the seeds with a large amount of liquid, e.g. mix approx. 5 g with 150 ml of cool water, stir briskly and swallow as quickly as possible, then maintain adequate fluid intake.

Ispaghula seed should preferably be taken at meal-times; it should not be taken immediately prior to going to bed. Any other medications should be taken at least 30-60 minutes before ispaghula seed in order to avoid delayed absorption.

Duration of administration
In cases of diarrhoea, medical advice should be sought if the symptoms persist for more than 3 days in order to ensure definitive diagnosis of the cause.

Contra-indications
Children under 6 years of age.
Known hypersensitivity to ispaghula seed [9,20-22].

Ispaghula seed should not be used by patients with the following conditions unless advised by a physician: faecal impaction; undiagnosed abdominal symptoms; a sudden change in bowel habit that persists for more than 2 weeks; rectal bleeding; failure to defecate following the use of a laxative; abnormal constrictions in the gastrointestinal tract; potential or existing intestinal obstruction (ileus); diseases of the oesophagus and cardia; megacolon [9,10]; diabetes mellitus which is difficult to regulate [10,11,23].

Special warnings and special precautions for use
A sufficient amount of liquid should always be taken: at least 150 ml of water per 5 g of seed [9].

Taking ispaghula seed without adequate fluid may cause it to swell and block the throat or oesophagus and may cause choking. Intestinal obstruction may occur should adequate fluid intake not be maintained. Do not take ispaghula seed if you have ever had difficulty in swallowing or have any throat problems. If you experience chest pain, vomiting, or difficulty in swallowing or breathing after taking it, seek immediate medical attention. Treatment of the elderly and debilitated patients requires medical supervision. Administration to the elderly should be supervised.

In cases of diarrhoea sufficient intake of water and electrolytes is important.

Interactions with other medicaments and other forms of interaction
Enteral absorption of concomitantly administered minerals (e.g. calcium, iron, lithium, zinc), vitamins (B12), cardiac glycosides and coumarin derivatives may be delayed [10,11,23]. For this reason, other medications should be taken at least 30-60 minutes before ispaghula seed. In the case of insulin-dependent diabetics it may be necessary to reduce the insulin dose [11,23-25].

Pregnancy and lactation
No restriction [26].
A risk is not to be expected since the constituents of ispaghula seed are not absorbed and have no systemic effects.

Effects on ability to drive and use machines
None known.

Undesirable effects
Flatulence may occur, but generally disappears during the course of treatment. Abdominal distension and risk of oesophageal or intestinal obstruction and faecal impaction may occur, particularly if ispaghula seed is ingested without sufficient fluid.

There is a risk of allergic reaction from inhalation of the powder during occupational exposure [27]. Due to the allergic potential of ispaghula seed, patients must be aware of reactions of hypersensitivity including anaphylactic reactions in single cases [9,20-22].

Overdose
Overdosage may cause abdominal discomfort and flatulence, or even intestinal obstruction. Adequate fluid intake should be maintained and management should be symptomatic.

PHARMACOLOGICAL PROPERTIES

Pharmacodynamic properties

Bulk-forming laxative effect
Ispaghula seed increases the volume of intestinal contents by the binding of fluid, which leads to physical stimulation of the gut [6,28,29]. The intra-luminal pressure is decreased and colon transit is accelerated [15].

Ispaghula seed increases stool weight and water content due to the fibre residue, the water bound to that residue, and the increased faecal bacterial mass [6,12,13].

Antidiarrhoeal effect
In cases of diarrhoea, ispaghula seed increases the viscosity of intestinal contents by the binding of fluid [30], thereby normalizing transit time and frequency of defecation [18,19,31].

Metabolic effects
Ispaghula seed lowers blood cholesterol levels by binding bile acids and increasing their faecal excretion which, in turn, results in further bile salt synthesis from cholesterol [2,32-38].

It reduces peak levels of blood glucose by delaying intestinal absorption of sugar [20,39-41].

Mucosa-protective effects
It has been shown in animal studies that ispaghula seed decreases the β-glucuronidase activity of colonic

bacteria, thus inhibiting the cleavage of toxic compounds from their liver conjugates [2,42-45]. Reduced bacterial conversion of primary bile acids to the more toxic secondary ones has been observed in rats [35].

Short-chain fatty acids (acetate, propionate, butyrate) released from the digestible part of the fibre by bacterial fermentation have a trophic and differentiating effect on the mucosal cells, as could be demonstrated *in vitro* and *in vivo* in experiments on rats [2,46,47].

Pharmacokinetic properties
The vegetable fibre of ispaghula seed is resistant to digestion in the upper intestinal tract; thus it is not absorbed. Part of the fibre is degraded by colonic bacteria [11].

Preclinical safety data
Not relevant.

REFERENCES

1. Ispaghula seed - Plantaginis ovatae semen. European Pharmacopoeia, Council of Europe.

2. Leng-Peschlow E. *Plantago ovata* seeds as dietary fibre supplement: physiological and metabolic effects in rats. Br J Nutr 1991;66:331-49.

3. Prosky L, Asp N-G, Furda I, DeVries JW, Schweizer TF, Harland BF. Determination of total dietary fiber in foods and food products: collaborative study. J Assoc Off Anal Chem 1985;68:677-9.

4. Kennedy JF, Sandhu JS, Southgate DAT. Structural data for the carbohydrate of ispaghula husk ex *Plantago ovata* Forsk. Carbohydr Res 1979;75:265-74.

5. Sandhu JS, Hudson GJ, Kennedy JF. The gel nature and structure of the carbohydrate of ispaghula husk ex *Plantago ovata* Forsk. Carbohydr Res 1981;93:247-59.

6. Sharma PK, Koul AK. Mucilage in seeds of *Plantago ovata* and its wild allies. J Ethnopharmacol 1986; 17:289-95.

7. Heckers H, Zielinsky D. Fecal composition and colonic function due to dietary variables. Results of a long-term study in healthy young men consuming 10 different diets. Motility (Lisbon) 1984:24-9.

8. Wichtl M. Indische Flohsamen - Plantaginis ovatae semen. In: Hartke K, Hartke H, Mutschler E, Rücker G, Wichtl M, editors. Kommentar zum Europäischen Arzneibuch. Stuttgart: Wissenschaftliche Verlagsgesellschaft, 1999(12. Lfg):F 12.

9. Sweetman SC, editor. Ispaghula. In: Martindale - The complete drug reference. 33rd ed. London: Royal Pharmaceutical Society, 2002:1229.

10. Brunton LL. Agents affecting gastrointestinal water flux and motility, digestants and bile acids. In: Gilman AG, Rall TW, Nies AS, Taylor P, editors. The Pharmacological Basis of Therapeutics, 8th ed. New York: Pergamon Press, 1990:914-24.

11. Kay RM, Strasberg SM. Origin, chemistry, physiological effects and clinical importance of dietary fibre. Clin Invest Med 1978;1:9-24.

12. Sölter H, Lorenz D. Summary of clinical results with Prodiem Plain, a bowel-regulating agent. Today's Therapeutic Trends 1983;1:45-59.

13. Marlett JA, Li BUK, Patrow CJ, Bass P. Comparative laxation of psyllium with and without senna in an ambulatory constipated population. Am J Gastroenterol 1987;82:333-7.

14. Webster DJT, Gough DCS, Craven JL. The use of bulk evacuant in patients with haemorrhoids. Br J Surg 1978;65:291-2.

15. Ligny G. Therapie des Colon irritabile. Kontrollierte Doppelblindstudie zur Prüfung der Wirksamkeit einer hemizellulosehaltigen Arzneizubereitung. Therapeutikon 1988;7:449-53.

16. Koch H. Adjuvante Therapie bei Morbus Crohn mit Agiocur®. Therapiewoche 1984;34:4545-8.

17. Bradshaw MJ, Harvey RF. Antidiarrhoeal agents: clinical pharmacology and therapeutic use. Curr Ther 1983:65-73.

18. Kovar F. Was tun bei akuter, nicht bakteriell bedingter Diarrhö? Ärztl Praxis 1983;35:1498.

19. Hamouz W. Die Behandlung der akuten und chronischen Diarrhö mit Agiocur®. Med Klin 1984; 79:32-3.

20. Zaloga GP, Hierlwimmer UR, Engler RJ. Anaphylaxis following psyllium ingestion. J Allergy Clin Immunol 1984;74:79-80.

21. Suhonen R, Kantola I, Björksten F. Anaphylactic shock due to ingestion of psyllium laxative. Allergy 1983; 38:363-5.

22. Lantner RR, Espiritu BR, Zumerchik P, Tobin MC. Anaphylaxis following ingestion of a psyllium-containing cereal. JAMA 1990; 264:2534-6.

23. Cummings JH. Nutritional implications of dietary fiber. Am J Clin Nutr 1978;31:S21-9.

24. Capani F, Consoli A, Del Ponte A, Lalli G, Sensi S. A new dietary fibre for use in diabetes. IRCS J Med Sci 1980;8:661.

25. Frati-Munari AC, Flores-Garduño MA, Ariza-Andraca R, Islas-Andrade S, Chavez NA. Efecto de diferentes dosis de mucilago de Plantago psyllium en la prueba de tolerancia a la glucosa. Archivos Invest Méd (Mexico) 1989;20:147-52.

26. Lewis JH, Weingold AB. The use of gastrointestinal

drugs during pregnancy and lactation. Am J Gastroenterol 1985;80:912-23.

27. Busse WW, Schoenwetter WF. Asthma from psyllium in laxative manufacture. Ann Intern Med 1975;83:361-2.

28. Read NW. Dietary fiber and bowel transit. In: Vahouny GV, Kritchevsky D, editors. Dietary fiber. Basic and clinical aspects. New York-London: Plenum Press, 1986:81-100.

29. Stevens J, VanSoest PJ, Robertson JB, Levitsky DA. Comparison of the effects of psyllium and wheat bran on gastrointestinal transit time and stool characteristics. J Am Dietetic Assoc 1988;88:323-6.

30. Russell J, Bass P. Effects of laxative and nonlaxative hydrophilic polymers on canine small intestinal motor activity. Digest Dis Sci 1986;31:281-8.

31. Qvitzau S, Matzen P, Madsen P. Treatment of chronic diarrhoea: loperamide versus ispaghula husk and calcium. Scand J Gastroenterol 1988;23:1237-40.

32. Leng-Peschlow E. Cholesterol-lowering effect of *Plantago ovata* seeds. In: Abstracts of 10th International Symposium on drugs affecting lipid metabolism. Houston, 8-11 November 1989:101.

33. Burton R, Manninen V. Influence of a psyllium-based fibre preparation on faecal and serum parameters. Acta Med Scand (Suppl) 1982;668:91-4.

34. Anderson JW, Zettwoch N, Feldman T, Tietyen-Clark J, Oeltgen P, Bishop CW. Cholesterol-lowering effects of psyllium hydrophilic mucilloid for hypercholesterolemic men. Arch Intern Med 1988;148:292-6.

35. Vahouny GV, Khalafi R, Satchithanandam S, Watkins DW, Story JA, Cassidy MM, Kritchevsky D. Dietary fiber supplementation and fecal bile acids, neutral steroids and divalent cations in rats. J Nutr 1987; 117:2009-15.

36. Forman DT, Garvin JE, Forestner JE, Taylor CB. Increased excretion of fecal bile acids by an oral hydrophilic colloid. Proc Soc Exp Biol Med 1968; 127:1060-3.

37. Kritchevsky D, Tepper SA, Klurfeld DM. Influence of psyllium preparations on plasma and liver lipids of cholesterol-fed rats. Artery 1995;21:303-11.

38. Segawa K, Kataoka T, Fukuo Y. Cholesterol-lowering effects of psyllium seed associated with urea metabolism. Biol Pharm Bull 1998;21:184-7.

39. Mahapatra SC, Bijlani RL, Nayar U. Effect of cellulose and ispaghula on intestinal function of hamsters maintained on diets of varying fibre content. Indian J Med Res 1988;88:175-80.

40. Welsh JD, Manion CV, Griffiths WJ, Bird PC. Effect of psyllium hydrophilic mucilloid on oral glucose tolerance and breath hydrogen in postgastrectomy patients. Digest Dis Sci 1982;27:7-12.

41. Fagerberg S-E. The effects of a bulk laxative (Metamucil®) on fasting blood glucose, serum lipids and other variables in constipated patients with non-insulin dependent adult diabetes. Curr Ther Res 1982; 31:166-72.

42. Costa MA, Mehta T, Males JR. Effects of dietary cellulose, psyllium husk and cholesterol level on fecal and colonic microbial metabolism in monkeys. J Nutr 1989;119:986-92.

43. Bauer HG, Asp N-G, Öste R, Dahlqvist A, Fredlund PE. Effect of dietary fiber on the induction of colorectal tumors and fecal β-glucuronidase activity in the rat. Cancer Res 1979;39:3752-6.

44. Sun Y, Li Y. Induction of beta-glucuronidase activity during dimethylhydrazine carcinogenesis and additive effects of cholic acid and indole. Cancer Lett 1988; 39:69-76.

45. Takada H, Hirooka T, Hiramatsu Y, Yamamoto M. Effect of β-glucuronidase inhibitor on azoxymethane-induced colonic carcinogenesis in rats. Cancer Res 1982;42:331-4.

46. Sakata T. Depression of intestinal epithelial cell production rate by hindgut bypass in rats. Scand J Gastroenterol 1988;23:1200-2.

47. Muller DE, Laeng H, Schindler R. Butyrate-induced cell differentiation of cell-cycle mutants and 'wild-type' mastocytoma cells: histamine, 5-hydroxy-tryptamine and metachromatic granules as independently regulated differentiation markers. Differentiation 1986;32:82-8.

PLANTAGINIS OVATAE TESTA

Ispaghula Husk
Blond Psyllium Husk

DEFINITION

Ispaghula husk consists of the episperm and collapsed adjacent layers removed from the seeds of *Plantago ovata* Forssk. (*P. ispaghula* Roxb.).

The material complies with the monograph of the European Pharmacopoeia [1].

CONSTITUENTS

Dietary fibre, principally as mucilage polysaccharide consisting of a highly-branched arabinoxylan with a xylan backbone and branches of arabinose, xylose and 2-*O*-(galactosyluronic acid)-rhamnose residues [2-4].

CLINICAL PARTICULARS

Therapeutic indications
Treatment of occasional constipation [5-12].
Conditions in which easy defecation with soft stools is desirable, e.g. in cases of anal fissures or haemorrhoids [13], after rectal or anal surgery, and during pregnancy.
Conditions which need an increased daily intake of fibre, e.g. irritable bowel syndrome [14-16].
Adjuvant symptomatic therapy in cases of diarrhoea from various causes [17-23].
As an adjunct to a low fat diet in the treatment of mild to moderate hypercholesterolaemia [24-54].

Posology and method of administration

Dosage

Adults and children over 12 years of age: 4-20 g daily, divided into 2-3 doses.
Children 6-12 years: half the adult dose.

Special Dosage Instructions
For the treatment of hypercholesterolaemia approx. 10 g of ispaghula husk should be given daily in 2 or 3 doses [24-37,39-42,44-47,50,54].

Method of administration
For oral administration.

It is very important to take the material with a large amount of liquid, e.g. mix approx. 5 g with 150 ml of cool water, stir briskly and swallow as quickly as possible, then maintain adequate fluid intake.

Ispaghula husk should preferably be taken at meal-

E/S/C/O/P
MONOGRAPHS
Second Edition

times; it should not be taken immediately prior to going to bed. Any other medications should be taken at least 30-60 minutes before ispaghula husk in order to avoid delayed absorption.

Duration of administration
In cases of diarrhoea, medical advice should be sought if the symptoms persist for more than 3 days in order to ensure definitive diagnosis of the cause.

Contra-indications
Children under 6 years of age.
Known hypersensitivity to ispaghula husk [5,6,55-57].

Ispaghula husk should not be used by patients with the following conditions unless advised by a physician: faecal impaction; undiagnosed abdominal symptoms; a sudden change in bowel habit that persists for more than 2 weeks; rectal bleeding; failure to defecate following the use of a laxative; abnormal constrictions in the gastrointestinal tract; potential or existing intestinal obstruction (ileus); diseases of the oesophagus and cardia; megacolon [5,6]; diabetes mellitus which is difficult to regulate [6,7,58].

Special warnings and special precautions for use
A sufficient amount of liquid should always be taken: at least 150 ml of water per 5 g of material [11].

If you experience chest pain, vomiting, or difficulty in swallowing or breathing after taking ispaghula husk, seek immediate medical attention. Administration to the elderly should be supervised.

In cases of diarrhoea sufficient intake of water and electrolytes is important.

Interactions with other medicaments and other forms of interaction
Enteral absorption of concomitantly administered minerals (e.g. calcium, iron, lithium, zinc), vitamins (B12), cardiac glycosides and coumarin derivatives may be delayed [6,7,58,59]. For this reason, other medications should be taken at least 30-60 minutes before ispaghula husk. In the case of insulin-dependent diabetics it may be necessary to reduce the insulin dose [7,54,60-63].

Pregnancy and lactation
No restriction.
A risk is not to be expected since the components of ispaghula husk are not absorbed and have no systemic effects [64].

Effects on ability to drive and use machines
None known.

Undesirable effects
Flatulence may occur, but generally disappears dur-

ing the course of treatment. Abdominal distension and risk of oesophageal or intestinal obstruction and faecal impaction may occur, particularly if ispaghula husk is ingested without sufficient fluid.

There is a risk of allergic reaction from inhalation of the powder during occupational exposure. Due to the allergic potential of ispaghula husk, patients must be aware of reactions of hypersensitivity including anaphylactic reactions in single cases [55-57].

Overdose
Overdosage may cause abdominal discomfort and flatulence, or even intestinal obstruction. Adequate fluid intake should be maintained and management should be symptomatic.

PHARMACOLOGICAL PROPERTIES

Pharmacodynamic properties
Dietary fibre such as ispaghula husk binds water and swells to form a demulcent gel or viscous solution in the intestine. By virtue of binding water in the colon, the faeces are softened and their bulk increased, thus promoting peristalsis and reducing transit time [5,6,9,10]. Degradation products of dietary fibre resulting from bacterial action in the colon may also contribute to the laxative effect [6,7].

The ability to absorb abundant water and to convert fluid in the intestine into a more viscous mass also makes ispaghula husk useful for the symptomatic relief of acute diarrhoea, enabling the patient to pass a formed stool [6,17,21].

In vivo experiments
Ispaghula husk reduces experimentally-induced hyperlipidaemia and atherosclerosis in animals [65-74]. Beneficial changes in serum lipid and lipoprotein profiles were greater in rats fed a mixture of ispaghula husk and margarine (rich in *trans*, as well as *cis*, fatty acids) than in rats fed a mixture of ispaghula husk and corn oil/olive oil (rich in *cis*, but free from *trans*, fatty acids) [75].

Ispaghula husk had little or no effect on the faecal excretion of neutral steroids or on cholesterol absorption [65-67] but apparently enhanced bile acid loss, due to its gel-forming ability and its viscosity [68,69].

Ispaghula husk was shown to increase the activity of hepatic 7α-hydroxylase, the initial and rate-limiting enzyme in the conversion of cholesterol to bile acids [69-71]. The conversion of hepatic cholesterol into bile acids has been established as a mechanism for reducing serum cholesterol [69,72,73] with a net negative sterol balance across the liver [65].

Guinea pigs were fed diets containing two levels of ispaghula husk (none or 7.5%) and two levels of cholesterol (0.04% and 0.25%) to determine the mechanisms by which ispaghula husk lowers plasma low-density lipoprotein (LDL) concentrations. Intake of ispaghula husk as 7.5% of the diet reduced plasma LDL by 30% and 54% respectively (p<0.001) in the 0.04% and the 0.25% cholesterol groups. Ispaghula husk altered hepatic cholesterol homeostasis by increasing the activity of HMG-CoA reductase (p<0.001) and reducing hepatic acyl-CoA:cholesterol acyltransferase activity (p<0.001). It increased hepatic membrane apoB/E receptor number (p<0.005) and modified LDL composition and size compared to LDL from control animals. The LDL from treated animals had a lower proportion of cholesteryl ester, a higher proportion of triacylglycerol, a lower molecular weight, a smaller diameter and a higher peak density (p<0.001) [71].

Pharmacological studies in humans

In 10 healthy subjects, 20 g of ispaghula husk per day significantly decreased fat digestibility (p<0.05) and increased faecal fat excretion (p<0.05) [76]. However it did not affect faecal steroid excretion (neutral steroids and bile acids) [63,77]. 16 healthy volunteers consumed 7 g of ispaghula husk per day for 8 weeks; faecal lithocholic and isolithocholic acids and the weighted ratio of lithocholic to deoxycholic acid were significantly lower after treatment. These changes in faecal bile acid profiles indicate a reduction in the hydrophobicity of bile acids in the enterohepatic circulation [78].

Using radiotelemetry in patients with left sided diverticular disease, it was shown that ispaghula husk stimulates colonic motility and thus reduces mouth to rectum transit time, predominantly by decreasing the duration of right colonic transit [11].

Clinical studies

Laxative effect
In a 2-week randomized study, the effects of ispaghula husk (2 × 5.1 g per day) were compared with those of docusate sodium (200 mg per day) in 170 patients suffering from chronic idiopathic constipation. Ispaghula husk was significantly superior to docusate sodium for softening stools by increasing stool water content and had greater overall laxative efficacy [12].

Antidiarrhoeal effect
In a crossover study 9 volunteers with diarrhoea induced by phenolphthalein were consecutively treated in a random sequence with 18 g of ispaghula husk, 6 g of calcium polycarbophil, 42 g of unprocessed wheat bran or placebo daily for 4 days. Only ispaghula husk treatment made stools firmer (p<0.01) and increased faecal viscosity (p<0.001). In a dose-response study in 6 subjects, doses of 9, 18 and 30 g

of ispaghula husk per day caused a near linear increase in faecal viscosity [23].

Cholesterol-lowering effects
A meta-analysis has been conducted on 5 published studies [24-28] and 3 unpublished studies involving a total of 656 subjects with mild to moderate hyper-cholesterolaemia (384 in ispaghula husk groups and 272 in placebo groups); 7 studies used a randomized, double-blind, placebo-controlled design, while one study [28] used a crossover design. All the studies met the following criteria: ispaghula husk was used as an adjunct to an American Heart Association (AHA) Step 1 diet (i.e. a diet with no more than 30% of calories from total fat, less than 10% of calories from saturated fat, and less than 300 mg of cholesterol daily) with a pretreatment dietary lead-in period of 8-12 weeks; the subjects consumed 10.2 g of ispaghula husk daily in 2 or 3 divided doses for 8 weeks (4 studies), or 12-26 weeks (4 studies). The conclusions were that ispaghula husk significantly lowered serum total cholesterol concentrations by an additional 3.9% (p<0.0001) and serum LDL-cholesterol concentrations by an additional 6.7% (p<0.0001) relative to placebo in subjects already consuming a low fat diet. Ispaghula husk also significantly lowered serum ratios of apo-lipoprotein B to apolipoprotein A-I by an additional 6% (p<0.05) relative to placebo, but had little effect on serum HDL-cholesterol or triglyceride concentrations [29].

340 patients with mild to moderate hyper-cholesterolaemia entered an initial 8-week diet-only period followed by a 12-week randomized, double-blind comparison of ispaghula husk and placebo groups. Ispaghula husk at daily doses of 7.0 g (p = 0.009) and 10.5 g (p<0.001) produced significantly greater reductions in serum LDL-cholesterol levels (8.7% and 9.7% respectively) than did placebo (4.3%). At both dose levels ispaghula husk also produced significantly greater reductions in total cholesterol levels than did placebo (7.0 g/day versus placebo, p = 0.040; 10.5 g/day versus placebo, p = 0.010) [30].

The long-term cholesterol-lowering effect of ispaghula husk as an adjunct to diet therapy (AHA Step 1) was evaluated in a randomized, double-blind, placebo-controlled study involving 248 subjects with primary hypercholesterolaemia. After 24-26 weeks, daily treatment with 10.2 g of ispaghula husk had significantly reduced (p<0.001) serum total cholesterol (4.7%) and LDL-cholesterol (6.7%) compared to placebo [31].

In a randomized, double-blind study in patients with mild to moderate hypercholesterolaemia, 2 × 5.1 g of ispaghula husk daily for 16 weeks as an adjunct to a low fat diet (AHA Step 1) significantly reduced total cholesterol (p<0.02), LDL-cholesterol (p<0.01) and apolipoprotein B (p<0.04) in comparison with placebo or diet alone [32-34]. An open, 28-week extension of this study confirmed the reductions in total cholesterol and LDL-cholesterol after taking 2 × 5.1 g of ispaghula husk daily in conjunction with a low fat diet [35-37].

These results [24-28,30-37] and another study [38] showed that, where a good reduction of blood lipids has already been achieved by use of a low fat diet, a further reduction is possible by taking ispaghula husk as an adjunct to the diet.

Another meta-analysis was performed to determine the effects of ispaghula husk-enriched cereal products on blood total cholesterol, and LDL- and HDL-cholesterol levels, in mild to moderate hypercholesterolaemic adults who consumed a low fat diet. The 8 published [39-45] and 4 unpublished studies included, involving a total of 404 patients, met the criteria of randomized, controlled studies in adults using either a crossover design (7 studies) or a design with parallel arms (5 studies) to compare treatment and control conditions for determining the effects of ispaghula husk-enriched cereals on blood lipids, with control groups that ate cereals providing ≤ 3 g of soluble fibre per day. Three studies [41,44 and one other] had no dietary lead-in period whereas the others had a 3- to 6-week dietary lead-in period, during which time the subjects were instructed to adhere to a low fat diet. The daily dose of ispaghula husk was 9.4-12 g in 9 studies, but lower (3.0, 6.7 and 7.6 g) in the other 3 studies. The conclusions from this meta-analysis were that treatment with ispaghula husk-enriched cereals significantly lowered total cholesterol (by 5%; p<0.0002) and LDL-cholesterol (by 9%; p<0.0001) but had no effect on HDL-cholesterol. The results confirmed that consuming an ispaghula husk-enriched cereal as part of a low fat diet improves the blood lipid profile of hypercholesterolaemic adults beyond that which can be achieved with a low fat diet alone [46].

The results of a randomized, double-blind, controlled study in patients with mild to moderate hypercholesterolaemia suggested that consumption of foods containing 10.2 g of ispaghula husk daily in conjunction with a low fat diet (AHA Step 1) results in the maintenance of reduced LDL-cholesterol concentrations without affecting HDL-cholesterol or triacylglycerol concentrations. At the conclusion of the 24-week treatment period, the mean LDL-cholesterol concentration was 5.3% lower in the verum group than in the control group (p<0.05) [47].

After 8 weeks of diet stabilisation, the effects of an ispaghula husk-enriched cereal (providing 6.4 g of ispaghula husk per day) or a matched control cereal, administered during 6-week phases (separated by a 6-week washout period) of a randomized, double-blind, crossover study, were compared in 25 hypercholesterolaemic children aged 6-18 years. Reductions in serum total cholesterol and LDL-

cholesterol concentrations were highly significant in favour of the ispaghula husk-enriched cereal (p = 0.03 and 0.01 respectively); the reduction in LDL-cholesterol was 7% in the ispaghula husk group compared to nil in the control group [48]. In contrast, in a study involving 20 children aged 5-17 years with elevated serum LDL-cholesterol, who had already been on a low total fat, low saturated fat, low cholesterol diet for at least 3 months, treatment with an ispaghula husk-enriched cereal (providing 6 g of ispaghula husk per day) for 4-5 weeks had no additional lowering effect on total cholesterol or LDL-cholesterol levels [79].

In a randomized, double-blind, placebo-controlled study, after a low fat diet for 1 year (AHA Step 2, i.e. a diet with no more than 30% of calories from total fat, less than 7% of calories from saturated fat and less than 200 mg of cholesterol daily), 105 moderately hypercholesterolaemic patients received either 5 g of colestipol (a bile acid sequestrant resin), 2.5 g of colestipol + 2.5 g of ispaghula husk, 5 g of ispaghula husk or 5 g of cellulose (as placebo) three times daily before meals for 10 weeks. The combination of colestipol + ispaghula husk reduced the ratio of total cholesterol to HDL-cholesterol significantly more than did colestipol alone or ispaghula husk alone (p<0.05). These findings suggested that adding ispaghula husk to half the usual dose of bile acid sequestrant resin maintains the efficacy and improves the tolerability of the resin [49]. In another controlled study, ispaghula husk treatment significantly reduced the frequency and severity of constipation (p<0.05), abdominal discomfort (p<0.01) and heart-burn (p<0.05) induced by cholestyramine therapy [80].

In a randomized, placebo-controlled, double-blind study, significant reductions (p<0.01) in serum total cholesterol (by 14.8%), LDL-cholesterol (by 20.2%) and the ratio of LDL- to HDL-cholesterol (by 14.8%) relative to baseline values were shown after 8 weeks of daily treatment with 10.2 g of ispaghula husk in 12 men with mild to moderate hypercholesterolaemia who maintained their usual diets. No significant reductions from baseline in these parameters were observed in 12 other volunteers after placebo treatment [50].

In a randomized, double-blind, placebo-controlled, crossover study involving 20 men with moderate hypercholesterolaemia who took 15 g of ispaghula husk daily for 40 days, a significant increase in bile acid synthesis was observed in those subjects whose LDL-cholesterol was lowered by more than 10% (p<0.0002), suggesting that ispaghula husk acts by stimulating bile acid synthesis [51]. These findings are consistent with those of another randomized, double-blind, placebo-controlled, crossover study in which, besides significantly decreased serum LDL-cholesterol levels, significantly increased levels of the serum cholesterol precursors lathosterol and Δ8-cholestanol were observed after daily treatment with 10.2 g of ispaghula husk for 8 weeks (p = 0.02 vs. placebo), indicating increased endogenous cholesterol synthesis caused by elimination of bile acids. A trend towards decreased LDL production in response to ispaghula husk treatment was observed, suggesting that the reduction in serum LDL-cholesterol may be due to decreased LDL production [28].

The requirement that ispaghula husk should be consumed together with food for the treatment of hypercholesterolaemia has been shown in a study in which serum total cholesterol and LDL-cholesterol levels remained unchanged when ispaghula husk was taken between meals, whereas they fell significantly when ispaghula husk was incorporated into a breakfast cereal. This suggests that the effect could be dependent on an interaction of ispaghula husk with other components of the meal [81].

In a 6-week randomized, double-blind, placebo-controlled study, significant reductions in serum total cholesterol (p = 0.03), LDL-cholesterol (p = 0.01) and triglycerides (p = 0.005), and a significant increase in HDL-cholesterol (p<0.0001), were observed in 125 patients with type II diabetes after 6 weeks of daily treatment with 3 × 5 g of ispaghula husk [52]. The hypolipidaemic effect of ispaghula husk in patients with type II diabetes has also been shown in other studies [53,62].

Hypoglycaemic effects
A randomized, double-blind, crossover study was conducted in 18 non-insulin-dependent, type II diabetes patients, to whom 6.8 g of ispaghula husk or placebo was administered twice, immediately before breakfast and dinner (but none before lunch), during each 15-hour phase. Relative to placebo, for meals eaten immediately after ispaghula husk ingestion, postprandial maximum serum glucose elevations were reduced by 14% after breakfast and 20% after dinner; second meal effects after lunch showed a 31% reduction. Postprandial insulin concentrations measured after breakfast were reduced by 12% [82].

A number of studies have shown that ispaghula husk lowers peak blood glucose levels due to delayed intestinal absorption [7,58,60-63,81,83].

Other effects
Consistency of the faeces, ease of defecation and general bowel habit were significantly improved (p<0.01) in 53 patients with haemorrhoids after a 6-week course of 2 × 3.5 g of ispaghula husk daily when compared to results from the 6-week placebo phase in a double-blind, crossover study [13].

In a 4-month randomized, double-blind, placebo-controlled, crossover study, ispaghula husk (2 × 3.5 g

daily) was found to be superior to placebo (p<0.001) in relieving gastrointestinal symptoms, with a lower score on all of the eight scales (e.g. abdominal pain, diarrhoea, loose stools, bloating) in 36 colitis patients in remission. Less symptoms were reported in 69% of the patients while taking ispaghula husk, compared to 7% who felt better with placebo (p<0.001) [84].

In another controlled crossover study a significant improvement (p<0.05) was observed from overall assessment after patients with irritable bowel syndrome had taken ispaghula husk for 3 weeks, the best results being obtained in spastic colitis (p<0.01) and relief in severity of abdominal pain (p<0.05) [15]. Ispaghula husk was also shown to alleviate the symptoms of left-sided diverticular disease [11].

Pharmacokinetic properties
The vegetable fibre of ispaghula husk is resistant to digestion in the upper intestinal tract and thus is not absorbed. Subsequent degradation of the fibre by colonic bacteria results in the production of gas and short chain fatty acids. Studies in animals have demonstrated at least partial absorption of short chain fatty acids [6,7,85].

Preclinical safety data
Not relevant.

REFERENCES

1. Ispaghula Husk - Plantaginis ovatae testa. European Pharmacopoeia, Council of Europe.

2. Kennedy JF, Sandhu JS, Southgate DAT. Structural data for the carbohydrate of ispaghula husk ex *Plantago ovata* Forsk. Carbohydr Res 1979;75:265-74

3. Sandhu JS, Hudson GJ, Kennedy JF. The gel nature and structure of the carbohydrate of ispaghula husk ex *Plantago ovata* Forsk. Carbohydr Res 1981;93:247-59.

4. Hänsel R, Sticher O, Steinegger E. Flohsamen. In: Pharmakognosie - Phytopharmazie, 6th ed. Berlin: Springer-Verlag, 1999:366-7.

5. Sweetman SC, editor. Ispaghula. In: Martindale - The complete drug reference, 33rd ed. London: Royal Pharmaceutical Society, 2002:1229.

6. Brunton LL. Agents affecting gastrointestinal water flux and motility, digestants, and bile acids. In: Gilman AG, Rall TW, Nies AS, Taylor P, editors. The Pharmacological Basis of Therapeutics, 8th ed. New York: Pergamon Press, 1990:914-24.

7. Kay RM, Strasberg SM. Origin, chemistry, physiological effects and clinical importance of dietary fibre. Clin Invest Med 1978;1:9-24.

8. Borgia M, Sepe N, Brancato V, Costa G, Simone P,

Borgia R, Lugli R. Treatment of chronic constipation by a bulk-forming laxative (Fibrolax®). J Int Med Res 1983; 11:124-7.

9. Stephen AM, Cummings JH. Mechanism of action of dietary fibre in the human colon. Nature 1980;284:283-4.

10. Marlett JA, Li BUK, Patrow CJ, Bass P. Comparative laxation of psyllium with and without senna in an ambulatory constipated population. Am J Gastroenterol 1987;82:333-7.

11. Thorburn HA, Carter KB, Goldberg JA, Finlay IG. Does ispaghula husk stimulate the entire colon in diverticular disease? Gut 1992;33:352-6.

12. McRorie JW, Daggy BP, Morel JG, Diersing PS, Miner PB, Robinson M. Psyllium is superior to docusate sodium for treatment of chronic constipation. Aliment Pharmacol Ther 1998;12:491-7.

13. Webster DJT, Gough DCS, Craven JL. The use of bulk evacuant in patients with haemorrhoids. Br J Surg 1978;65:291-2.

14. Prior A, Whorwell PJ. Double blind study of ispaghula in irritable bowel syndrome. Gut 1987;28:1510-3.

15. Golecha AC, Chadda VS, Chadda S, Sharma SK, Mishra SN. Role of ispaghula husk in the management of irritable bowel syndrome (a randomized double-blind crossover study). J Assoc Physicians India 1982;30:353-5.

16. Kumar A, Kumar N, Vij JC, Sarin SK, Anand BS. Optimum dosage of ispaghula husk in patients with irritable bowel syndrome: correlation of symptom relief with whole gut transit time and stool weight. Gut 1987;28:150-5.

17. Bradshaw MJ, Harvey RF. Antidiarrhoeal agents: clinical pharmacology and therapeutic use. Curr Ther 1983:65-73.

18. Qvitzau S, Matzen P, Madsen P. Treatment of chronic diarrhoea: loperamide versus ispaghula husk and calcium. Scand J Gastroenterol 1988;23:1237-40.

19. Hamouz W. Die Behandlung der akuten und chronischen Diarrhö mit Agiocur®. Med Klin 1984; 79:32-3.

20. Bobrove AM. Misoprostol, diarrhea and psyllium mucilloid. Ann Intern Med 1990;112:386.

21. Smalley JR, Klish WJ, Campbell MA, Brown MR. Use of psyllium in the management of chronic nonspecific diarrhea of childhood. J Pediatr Gastroenterol Nutr 1982;1:361-3.

22. Frank HA, Green LC. Successful use of a bulk laxative to control the diarrhea of tube feeding. Scand J Plast Reconstr Surg 1979;13:193-4.

23. Eherer AJ, Santa Ana CA, Porter J, Fordtran JS. Effect of psyllium, calcium polycarbophil and wheat bran on secretory diarrhea induced by phenolphthalein.

Gastroenterology 1993;104:1007-12.

24. Bell LP, Hectorne K, Reynolds H, Balm TK, Hunninghake DB. Cholesterol-lowering effects of psyllium hydrophilic mucilloid. JAMA 1989;261:3419-23.

25. Levin EG, Miller VT, Muesing RA, Stoy DB, Balm TK, LaRosa JC. Comparison of psyllium hydrophilic mucilloid and cellulose as adjuncts to a prudent diet in the treatment of mild to moderate hypercholesterolemia. Arch Intern Med 1990;150:1822-7.

26. Anderson JW, Floore TL, Geil PB, O'Neal DS, Balm TK. Hypocholesterolemic effects of different bulk-forming hydrophilic fibers as adjuncts to dietary therapy in mild to moderate hypercholesterolemia. Arch Intern Med 1991;151:1597-1602.

27. Sprecher DL, Harris BV, Goldberg AC, Anderson EC, Bayuk LM, Russell BS et al. Efficacy of psyllium in reducing serum cholesterol levels in hypercholesterolemic patients on high- or low-fat diets. Ann Intern Med 1993;119:545-54.

28. Weingand KW, Le N-A, Kuzmak BR, Brown WV, Daggy BP, Miettinen TA et al. Effects of psyllium on cholesterol and low-density lipoprotein metabolism in subjects with hypercholesterolemia. Endocrinol Metab 1997;4:141-50.

29. Anderson JW, Allgood LD, Lawrence A, Altringer LA, Jerdack GR, Hengehold DA, Morel JG. Cholesterol-lowering effects of psyllium intake adjunctive to diet therapy in men and women with hypercholesterolemia: meta-analysis of 8 controlled trials. Am J Clin Nutr 2000;71:472-9.

30. MacMahon M, Carless J. Ispaghula husk in the treatment of hypercholesterolemia: a double-blind controlled study. J Cardiovasc Risk 1998;5:167-72.

31. Anderson JW, Davidson MH, Blonde L, Brown WV, Howard WJ, Ginsberg HH et al. Long-term cholesterol-lowering effects of psyllium as an adjunct to diet therapy in the treatment of hypercholesterolemia. Am J Clin Nutr 2000;71:1433-8.

32. Clinical Study Report CCP #89-004A. A randomized, double-blind, parallel study comparing psyllium to placebo used as adjunct therapy in patients with mild to moderate hypercholesteremia who are placed on an AHA step 1 diet. Unpublished Report: Ciba Consumer Pharmaceuticals, New Jersey. October 1992.

33. Clinical Study Report CCP #89-004B. A randomized, double-blind, parallel study comparing psyllium to placebo in patients with mild to moderate hypercholesteremia who maintain their usual diet. Unpublished Report: Ciba Consumer Pharmaceuticals, New Jersey. September 1992.

34. Clinical Study Report CCP #89-004A and CCP #89-004B. An overall summary of efficacy. Unpublished Report: Ciba Consumer Pharmaceuticals, New Jersey. December 1992.

35. Clinical Study Report CCP #89-004AE. An open-label extension in patients with mild to moderate

hypercholesteremia who have completed protocol CCP #89-004A (AHA Step 1 Diet). Unpublished Report: Ciba Consumer Pharmaceuticals, New Jersey. April 1993.

36. Clinical Study Report CCP #89-004BE. An open-label extension in patients with mild to moderate hypercholesteremia who have completed protocol CCP #89-004B (Usual Diet). Unpublished Report: Ciba Consumer Pharmaceuticals, New Jersey. April 1993.

37. Clinical Study Report CCP #89-004AE and CCP #89-004BE. An overall summary of safety and efficacy. Unpublished Report: Ciba Consumer Pharmaceuticals, New Jersey. April 1993.

38. Neal GW, Balm TK. Synergistic effects of psyllium in the dietary treatment of hypercholesterolemia. Southern Med J 1990;83:1131-7.

39. Bell LP, Hectorn KJ, Reynolds H, Hunninghake DB. Cholesterol-lowering effects of soluble-fiber cereals as part of a prudent diet for patients with mild to moderate hypercholesterolemia. Am J Clin Nutr 1990;52:1020-6.

40. Anderson JW, Riddell-Mason S, Gustafson NJ, Smith SF, Mackey M. Cholesterol-lowering effects of psyllium-enriched cereal as an adjunct to a prudent diet in the treatment of mild to moderate hypercholesterolemia. Am J Clin Nutr 1992;56:93-8.

41. Roberts DCK, Truswell AS, Benke A, Dewar HM, Farmakalidis E. The cholesterol-lowering effect of a breakfast cereal containing psyllium fibre. Med J Aust 1994;161:660-4.

42. Stoy DB, LaRosa JC, Brewer BK, Mackey M, Meusing RA. Cholesterol-lowering effects of ready-to-eat cereal containing psyllium. J Am Dietetic Assoc 1993;93:910-2.

43. Wolever TMS, Jenkins DJA, Mueller S, Patten R, Relle LK, Boctor D et al. Psyllium reduces blood lipids in men and women with hyperlipidemia. Am J Med Sci 1994; 307:269-73.

44. Summerbell CD, Manley P, Barnes D, Leeds A. The effects of psyllium on blood lipids in hypercholesterolaemic subjects. J Hum Nutr Diet 1994;7:147-51.

45. Jenkins DJA, Wolever TMS, Vidgen E, Kendall CWC, Ransom TPP, Mehling CC et al. Effect of psyllium in hypercholesterolemia at two monounsaturated fatty acid intakes. Am J Clin Nutr 1997;65:1524-33.

46. Olson BH, Anderson SM, Becker MP, Anderson JW, Hunninghake DB, Jenkins DJA et al. Psyllium-enriched cereals lower blood total cholesterol and LDL cholesterol, but not HDL cholesterol, in hypercholesterolemic adults: results of a meta-analysis. J Nutr 1997;127:1973-80.

47. Davidson MH, Maki KC, Kong JC, Dugan LD, Torri SA, Hall HA et al. Long-term effects of consuming foods containing psyllium seed husk on serum lipids in subjects with hypercholesterolemia. Am J Clin Nutr 1998;67:367-76.

48. Davidson MH, Dugan LD, Burns JH, Sugimoto D, Story K, Drennan K. A psyllium-enriched cereal for the treatment of hypercholesterolemia in children: a controlled, double-blind, crossover study. Am J Clin Nutr 1996;63:96-102.

49. Spence JD, Huff MW, Heidenheim P, Viswanatha A, Munoz C, Lindsay R et al. Combination therapy with colestipol and psyllium mucilloid in patients with hyperlipidemia. Ann Intern Med 1995;123:493-9.

50. Anderson JW, Zettwoch N, Feldman T, Tietyen-Clark J, Oeltgen P, Bishop CW. Cholesterol-lowering effects of psyllium hydrophilic mucilloid for hypercholesterolemic men. Arch Intern Med 1988;148:292-6.

51. Everson GT, Daggy BP, McKinley C, Story JA. Effects of psyllium hydrophilic mucilloid on LDL-cholesterol and bile acid synthesis in hypercholesterolemic men. J Lipid Res 1992;33:1183-92.

52. Rodríguez-Morán M, Guerrero-Romero F, Lazcano-Burciaga G. Lipid- and glucose-lowering efficacy of Plantago psyllium in type II diabetes. J Diabet Complic 1998;12:273-8.

53. Gupta RR, Agrawal CG, Singh GP, Ghatak A. Lipid-lowering efficacy of psyllium hydrophilic mucilloid in non insulin dependent diabetes mellitus with hyperlipidaemia. Indian J Med Res 1994;100:237-41.

54. USA Department of Health and Human Services: Food and Drug Administration. 21 CFR, Part 101. Food labelling: health claims; soluble fiber from certain foods and coronary heart disease. Federal Register 1998;63(32):8103-21 (February 18,1998).

55. Zaloga GP, Hierlwimmer UR, Engler RJ. Anaphylaxis following psyllium ingestion. J Allergy Clin Immunol 1984;74:79-80.

56. Suhonen R, Kantola I, Björksten F. Anaphylactic shock due to ingestion of psyllium laxative. Allergy 1983; 38:363-5.

57. Lantner RR, Espiritu BR, Zumerchik P, Tobin MC. Anaphylaxis following ingestion of a psyllium-containing cereal. JAMA 1990;264:2534-6.

58. Cummings JH. Nutritional implications of dietary fiber. Am J Clin Nutr 1978;31:S21-9.

59. Perlmann BB. Interaction between lithium salts and ispaghula husk. Lancet 1990:416.

60. Fagerberg S-E. The effects of a bulk laxative (Metamucil®) on fasting blood glucose, serum lipids and other variables in constipated patients with non-insulin dependent adult diabetes. Curr Ther Res 1982;31:166-72.

61. Capani F, Consoli A, Del Ponte A, Lalli G, Sensi S. A new dietary fibre for use in diabetes. IRCS J Med Sci 1980;8:661.

62. Frati-Munari AC, Flores-Garduño MA, Ariza-Andraca R, Islas-Andrade S, Chavez NA. Efecto de diferentes

dosis de mucilago de Plantago psyllium en la prueba de tolerancia a la glucosa. Archivos Invest Méd (Mexico) 1989;20:147-52.

63. Abraham ZD, Mehta T. Three-week psyllium-husk supplementation: effect on plasma cholesterol concentrations, fecal steroid excretion, and carbohydrate absorption in men. Am J Clin Nutr 1988;47:67-74.

64. Lewis JH, Weingold AB. The use of gastrointestinal drugs during pregnancy and lactation. Am J Gastroenterology 1985;80:912-23.

65. Turley SD, Daggy BP, Dietschy JM. Psyllium augments the cholesterol-lowering action of cholestyramine in hamsters by enhancing sterol loss from the liver. Gastroenterology 1994;107:444-52.

66. Turley SD, Daggy BP, Dietschy JM. Cholesterol-lowering action of psyllium mucilloid in the hamster: sites and possible mechanisms of action. Metabolism 1991; 40:1063-73.

67. McCall MR, Mehta T, Leathers CW, Foster DM. Psyllium husk I: effect on plasma lipoproteins, cholesterol metabolism and atherosclerosis in African green monkeys. Am J Clin Nutr 1992;56:376-84.

68. Gallaher DD, Hassel CA, Lee K-J, Gallaher CM. Viscosity and fermentability as attributes of dietary fiber responsible for the hypocholesterolemic effect in hamsters. J Nutr 1993;123:244-52.

69. Matheson HB, Colón IS, Story JA. Cholesterol 7α-hydroxylase activity is increased by dietary modification with psyllium hydrocolloid, pectin, cholesterol and cholestyramine in rats. J Nutr 1995;125:454-8.

70. Horton JD, Cuthbert JA, Spady DK. Regulation of hepatic 7α-hydroxylase expression by dietary psyllium in the hamster. J Clin Invest 1994;93:2084-92.

71. Fernandez ML, Ruiz LR, Conde AK, Sun D-M, Erickson SK, McNamara DJ. Psyllium reduces plasma LDL in guinea pigs by altering hepatic cholesterol homeostasis. J Lipid Res 1995;36:1128-38.

72. Arjmandi BH, Ahn J, Nathani S, Reeves RD. Dietary soluble fiber and cholesterol affect serum cholesterol concentration, hepatic portal venous short-chain fatty acid concentration and fecal sterol excretion in rats. J Nutr 1992;122:246-53.

73. Matheson HB, Story JA. Dietary psyllium hydrocolloid and pectin increase bile acid pool size and change bile acid composition in rats. J Nutr 1994;124:1161-5.

74. McCall MR, Mehta T, Leathers CW, Foster DM. Psyllium husk II: effect on the metabolism of apolipoprotein B in African green monkeys. Am J Clin Nutr 1992;56:385-93.

75. Fang C. Dietary psyllium reverses hypercholesterolemic effect of trans fatty acids in rats. Nutr Res 2000;20:695-705.

76. Ganji V, Kies CV. Psyllium husk fibre supplementation to soybean and coconut oil diets of humans: effect on fat digestibility and faecal fatty acid excretion. Eur J Clin Nutr 1994;48:595-7.

77. Gelissen IC, Brodie B, Eastwood MA. Effect of Plantago ovata (psyllium) husk and seeds on sterol metabolism: studies in normal and ileostomy subjects. Am J Clin Nutr 1994;59:395-400.

78. Chaplin MF, Chaudhury S, Dettmar PW, Sykes J, Shaw AD, Davies GJ. Effect of ispaghula husk on the faecal output of bile acids in healthy volunteers. J Steroid Biochem Mol Biol 2000;72:283-92.

79. Dennison BA, Levine DM. Randomized, double-blind, placebo-controlled, two-period crossover clinical trial of psyllium fiber in children with hypercholesterolemia. J Pediatr 1993;123:24-9.

80. Maciejko JJ, Brazg R, Shah A, Patil S, Rubenfire M. Psyllium for the reduction of cholestyramine-associated gastrointestinal symptoms in the treatment of primary hypercholesterolemia. Arch Fam Med 1994;3:955-60.

81. Wolever TMS, Jenkins DJA, Mueller S, Boctor DL, Ransom TPP, Patten R et al. Method of administration influences the serum cholesterol-lowering effect of psyllium. Am J Clin Nutr 1994;59:1055-9.

82. Pastors JG, Blaisdell PW, Balm TK, Asplin CM, Pohl SL. Psyllium fiber reduces rise in postprandial glucose and insulin concentrations in patients with non-insulin-dependent diabetes. Am J Clin Nutr 1991;53:1431-5.

83. Florholmen J, Arvidsson-Lenner R, Jorde R, Burhol PG. The effect of metamucil on postprandial blood glucose and plasma gastric inhibitory peptide in insulin-dependent diabetics. Acta Med Scand 1982;212:237-9.

84. Hallert C, Kaldma M, Petersson B-G. Ispaghula husk may relieve gastrointestinal symptoms in ulcerative colitis in remission. Scand J Gastroenterol 1991;26:747-50.

85. Cummings JH. Dietary fibre. Br Med Bull 1981;37:65-70.

POLYGALAE RADIX

Senega Root

E/S/C/O/P
MONOGRAPHS
Second Edition

DEFINITION

Senega root consists of the dried and usually fragmented root and root-crown of *Polygala senega* L. or of certain other closely related species or of a mixture of these *Polygala* species.

The material complies with the monograph of the European Pharmacopoeia [1].

Polygala senega L. var. *latifolia* Torr. et Gray and *Polygala tenuifolia* Willd. are generally accepted as sources of senega root closely related to *Polygala senega* L. [2-5]. In the Japanese Pharmacopoeia [6] and in Japanese scientific literature the names Senega (Senegae radix) and Polygala Root (Polygalae radix) refer to the roots of *Polygala senega* var. *latifolia* and *Polygala tenuifolia* respectively.

CONSTITUENTS

The characteristic constituents of *Polygala senega* [7,8], *P. senega* var. *latifolia* [9-15] and *Polygala tenuifolia* [16,17] are bidesmosidic triterpene saponins, 6-12% [5], based on one aglycone, presenegenin.

The structures of saponins in the root of *P. senega* var. *latifolia* have been elucidated [9-15]. All are 3-glucosides of presenegenin with tetra-, penta- or hexaglycosyl groups attached through an ester linkage at C-28, including a 4″-methoxycinnamoyl or 3″,4″-dimethoxycinnamoyl fucosyl moiety which gives rise to *E*-and *Z*-cinnamoyl isomers of each saponin [13-15]. The first saponins to be characterized, senegins II, III, and IV [9-12], were *E*-isomers but more recently *Z*-isomers of these, together with *E*- and *Z*-isomers of senegasaponins a, b and c, have also been isolated and characterized [13-15].

Other constituents of *P. senega* var. *latifolia* include a variety of mono- and oligosaccharides [18], a series of oligosaccharide multi-esters called senegoses A-O [19-21], and up to 0.2% of essential oil containing 25-45% of methyl salicylate, which imparts an aromatic odour to the drug [22].

From the root of *P. tenuifolia* 7 saponins, named onjisaponins A-G, have been isolated; they are similar, in one case identical (onjisaponin B = senegin III), to the saponins of *P. senega* var. *latifolia* [16,17]. Other constituents identified are various xanthones [23-26]; a series of phenylpropanoid sugar esters including tenuifolisides A-E [26,27]; a series of oligosaccharide multi-esters named tenuifolioses A-P, which are similar to the senegoses in *P. senega* var. *latifolia* [28-30]; and traces of β-carboline alkaloids [31].

P. senega is less investigated but the root saponins are chromatographically almost identical to those of *P. tenuifolia* [8].

CLINICAL PARTICULARS

Therapeutic indications
Productive cough [32]; catarrh of the respiratory tract [33,34]; chronic bronchitis [5,32,34].

Posology and method of administration

Dosage

Adult daily dose, taken in small amounts as necessary: 1.5-3 g of the drug in hydroethanolic preparations (liquid extracts, tinctures) or solid dosage forms [3,33,34]; 2.5-5 g of the drug in aqueous preparations (e.g. decoctions) [35]; other equivalent preparations.
Elderly: Dose as for adults.
Children: Proportion of adult dose according to age and bodyweight, in alcohol-free preparations.

Method of administration
For oral administration in liquid or solid dosage forms.

Duration of administration
No restriction.

Contra-indications
Gastritis, gastric ulcer [34].

Special warnings and special precautions for use
None required.

Interaction with other medicaments and other forms of interaction
None reported.

Pregnancy and lactation
No data available. In view of this, and its potentially irritant properties, senega root should not be taken during pregnancy or lactation [36].

Effects on ability to drive and use machines
None known.

Undesirable effects
Normally none at the recommended dosage [33]. In sensitive individuals gastrointestinal disturbance may occur [37,38].

Overdose
Overdosage may lead to stomach upset, vomiting or diarrhoea [36-38].

PHARMACOLOGICAL PROPERTIES

Pharmacodynamic properties
Senega root has an expectorant action arising primarily from local irritation of the gastric mucosa by saponins; this provokes a reflex increase in bronchial secretion [2,5,37,39,40] which dilutes the mucus, reducing its viscosity and facilitating its removal by ciliary action and coughing [41,42].

Few pharmacodynamic studies have been carried out on the expectorant action of senega root because, as with other expectorants, precise measurement of the effects is difficult. However, two animal studies [39,40] and one human study [43] of its effect on respiratory tract secretions are described below.

Other pharmacological effects of senega root have been investigated in a variety of *in vitro* [44-49] and *in vivo* [13-15,46,50-58] studies.

In vitro experiments
A hexane extract (50 µg/ml) of *Polygala senega* root inhibited COX (cyclooxygenase)-1 and COX-2 by 54% and 71% respectively [44].

A methanolic extract of *Polygala tenuifolia* inhibited the activity of prolyl endopeptidase (PEP) with an IC_{50} of 58 µg/ml. PEP is thought to hydrolyze proline-containing neuropeptides which participate in learning and memory processes, and its inhibition may have anti-amnesic effects [45].

The butanol-soluble fraction (containing onji-saponins) from a methanolic extract of *Polygala tenuifolia* showed 73% inhibition of cyclic adenosine monophosphate (cAMP) phosphodiesterase at a concentration of 100 µl/ml. Isolated onjisaponins E, F and G also showed high inhibitory effects with IC_{50} values ($\times 10^{-5}$ M) of 3.1, 2.9 and 3.7 respectively, similar in potency to papaverine with a value of 3.0 [46].

Serum from the blood of guinea pigs taken 2 hours after abdominal administration of a solution containing 600 mg of a lyophilized aqueous extract of *Polygala tenuifolia* inhibited the growth of herpes simplex virus type 1 (HSV-1) in Vero cells at a therapeutically meaningful level. The mean virus yield (100% for water) was 8.3%, the second lowest value obtained in comparative antiviral assays of 32 herbal extracts previously selected for potential anti-HSV-1 activity [47].

An unspecified senegin from *Polygala senega* exhibited activity against influenza (A2/Japan 305) virus, producing 34% inhibition at a concentration of 12.5 µl/ml [48].

A hydromethanolic extract from the root of *Polygala senega* inhibited the growth of a range of fungi [49].

In vivo experiments

Expectorant effects

Respiratory tract fluid (RTF) was collected from the trachea of decerebrate or urethanized animals for 3 hours before and 4 hours after administration by stomach tube of fluid extract of senega root in doses from 0.1 to 10 ml. In the third or fourth hour after administration the output of RTF increased by up to 173% in cats and 186% in guinea pigs, but no effect was observed in rabbits. Control animals showed increases or decreases in RTF output of less than 30% over the 4 hours. It was concluded that senega root acts as an expectorant by way of a reflex from the stomach [39].

A more sensitive method of recording RTF output involved determining electrical resistance between electrodes inserted into the trachea of anaesthetized dogs and calibrated *in situ* with saline before each experiment. Oral administration of senega syrup (3 ml/kg, equivalent to 90 mg/kg of senega root) produced an increase in RTF volume within 5 minutes and a rapid increase within 30 minutes. The total RTF in 2 hours was 0.114 ml (n = 5; p<0.001) compared to 0.010 ml per hour with saline. Intravenous administration of senega syrup had no effect, suggesting that the secretagogic activity was a reflex action following stimulation of the gastric mucosa [40].

Diuretic effects

Dry, 50%-methanolic extracts from roots of *Polygala tenuifolia* and *P. senega* var. *latifolia*, administered orally to rats in aqueous suspension as single doses of 2000 mg/kg bodyweight, produced 100% and 62% inhibition of congestive oedema respectively and also significantly increased 24-hour urine volume (p<0.01 for *P. tenuifolia*; p<0.05 for *P. senega* var. *latifolia*) compared to control animals. Under the same conditions furosemide at 100 mg/kg produced 100% inhibition of congestive oedema and significantly increased 24-hour urine volume (p<0.001) [50].

Effects on alcohol absorption

E,Z-senegin II and *E,Z*-senegasaponins a and b from *Polygala senega* var. *latifolia* exhibit potent inhibitory effects on alcohol absorption in rats. After single oral administrations of 100 mg of *E,Z*-senegasaponins a or b per kg bodyweight, the ethanol concentration in blood was 0.06-0.07 mg/ml after 1 hour and 0.02-0.07 mg/ml after 2 hours compared to 0.50 mg/ml after 1 hour and 0.19 mg/ml after 2 hours in control animals (p<0.01) [14]. Under similar conditions, 100 mg/kg of *E,Z*-senegin II produced an ethanol concentration of 0.09 mg/ml after 1 hour compared to 0.54 mg/ml in control animals [13]. The 28-oligoglycosyl moiety with a 4''-methoxycinnamoyl group was found to be important for the inhibition of ethanol absorption [13,14].

Hypoglycaemic effects

Four hours after intraperitoneal administration at 5 mg/kg body weight, the n-butanol fraction from senega root (*P. senega* var. *latifolia*) had reduced blood glucose levels from 191 to 120 mg/dl (p<0.001) in normal mice and from 469 to 244 mg/dl (p<0.001) in KK-Ay mice (a model of non-insulin dependent diabetes mellitus), but had no effect on streptozotocin-induced diabetic mice (a model of insulin-dependent diabetes mellitus). The results suggested that the butanol fraction, of which senegin II was shown to be an active component, produced hypoglycaemic effects without altering the insulin concentration, but required the presence of insulin in order to act [51]. It was subsequently demonstrated that intraperitoneally administered senegins II [52,53] and III [53] significantly reduced blood glucose levels in both normal and KK-Ay mice.

In the oral glucose tolerance test in rats, following oral administration of 100 mg/kg of *E,Z*-senegasaponins a or b, plasma glucose levels after 0.5 hour were 107.5-122.9 mg/ml compared to 150 mg/ml in control animals (p<0.01) [14]. *E,Z*-senegins II, III and IV and *E,Z*-senegasaponin c similarly inhibited the elevation of plasma glucose levels and it was shown that the methoxycinnamoyl group of senegins and senegasaponins is required for hypoglycaemic activity [15]. The conclusion from other experiments in glucose-loaded rats was that orally administered *E,Z*-senegin II had neither insulin-like nor insulin-releasing activity, but inhibited glucose absorption by suppressing the transfer of glucose from the stomach to the small intestine and by inhibiting glucose transport at the small intestinal brush border [54].

Effects on blood lipids

The n-butanol fraction, containing senegin II, of a methanolic extract of senega root (from *Polygala senega* var. *latifolia*), administered intraperitoneally at 5 mg/kg, reduced the blood triglyceride level in normal mice after 7 hours to 65 mg/100ml compared to 152 mg/100ml in control animals (p<0.05); pure senegin II at 5 mg/kg also significantly lowered blood triglycerides (p<0.01). Under the same conditions, the n-butanol fraction lowered blood cholesterol in hypercholesterolaemic (cholesterol-fed) mice and blood triglyceride levels in Triton-induced hyperlipidaemic mice (p<0.05 in both cases). Repeated daily administration of the n-butanol fraction for 5 days to hypercholesterolaemic mice produced significant decreases in blood cholesterol to 193 mg/dl (p<0.01) and blood triglyceride levels to 74 mg/dl (p<0.05) compared to 276 and 117 mg/dl respectively in control animals [55].

Sedative effects

A methanolic extract of *Polygala tenuifolia*, various fractions from it and pure onjisaponins B, F and G prolonged hexobarbital sleeping time in mice. The butanol-soluble fraction produced sleeping times of 52, 61, 84 and 62 minutes after intraperitoneal administration of 6.25, 12.5, 25 and 50 mg/kg respectively (p<0.01), compared to 61 minutes for chlorpromazine hydrochloride at 3 mg/kg and 26 minutes for control animals. Onjisaponin F produced sleeping times of 33 and 35 minutes at 5 and 20 mg/kg respectively (p<0.05) compared to 42 minutes for chlorpromazine hydrochloride at 2 mg/kg and 24 minutes for control animals. These results were considered to provide support for the traditional use of *Polygala tenuifolia* as a sedative in oriental medicine [46].

Other effects
When applied to the bald backs of mice, four compounds isolated from *Polygala senega* var. *latifolia* stimulated hair regrowth, particularly senegose A (p<0.001 compared to the control, 13 days after a single application of 1 mg) but also senegins II and III and senegasaponin b [56].

An aqueous extract of *Polygala tenuifolia*, administered intragastrically at 100-500 mg/kg for 7 days, induced choline acetyltransferase activity (p<0.01) in the cerebral cortex of basal forebrain lesioned rats (an animal dementia model); the effect appeared to be due to cinnamoyl metabolites from the extract. Significant *in vitro* activity of the extract on choline acetyltransferase activity in rat basal forebrain cell cultures was also demonstrated (p<0.01) [57].

A total saponin preparation (denoted as 'senegin') extracted from *Polygala senega* var. *latifolia* produced increased plasma levels of adreno-corticotropic hormone (ACTH), corticosterone and glucose 30 minutes after intraperitoneal administration to rats. At a dose of 25 mg/kg of 'senegin', plasma ACTH determined by the radio-immunoassay method was 1128 pg/ml compared to 95 pg/ml for control animals (p<0.01). The ED_{50} for corticosterone secretion-inducing activity, determined by the competitive protein binding method, was 2.3 mg/kg. The haemolytic concentration of the saponin extract was 27.2 µg/ml and haemolytic index 36700 [58].

Pharmacological studies in humans
Physical and chemical evaluation of sputum collected by postural drainage and bronchoscopic suction from patients with brochiectasis before and after administration of expectorant showed that fluid extract of senega root markedly reduced the viscosity [43].

Pharmacokinetic properties
Triterpene saponins are poorly absorbed in animals after oral administration. They are either excreted unchanged or metabolized in the gut, but few data are available [2].

After oral administration of an aqueous extract of the root of *Polygala tenuifolia* the compounds 3,4,5-trimethoxycinnamic acid (TMCA), methyl-3,4,5-trimethoxycinnamate (M-TMCA) and p-methoxycinnamic acid (PMCA) were detected in the blood and bile of rats [59]. Following oral administration of the extract at 5 g/kg bodyweight (equivalent to crude drug 20 g/kg), TMCA and M-TMCA were detected in the blood plasma of rats, both at concentrations of approximately 1 µg/ml after 15 minutes; plasma levels then remained fairly constant for about 3 hours [60].

From related experiments in which pure compounds were administered intravenously to rats it was shown that:
- part of the TCMA could be metabolized in the rat liver and excreted into the small intestine with bile in the form of M-TMCA, which could then be reabsorbed into blood.
- M-TCMA in the blood can be converted rapidly to TCMA.
- TMCA and PMCA were rapidly cleared from rat plasma with half-lives of 14.0 and 17.4 minutes respectively.
It was suggested that the TMCA and M-TCMA found in rat plasma at fairly constant levels for 3 hours after oral administration of the extract are metabolites derived, by hydrolysis at differing rates, from constituents which have a 3,4,5-trimethoxy-cinnamoyl (TMC) moiety in their structures [60]. The TMC moiety occurs in onjisaponins E, F and G [16,17] and in certain tenuifolisides [27].

Preclinical safety data
Aqueous and methanolic extracts from the roots of *Polygala senega* and *P. tenuifolia* gave negative results from mutagenicity screening by the rec-assay with *Bacillus subtilis* and also by the reversion assay with Ames strains TA98 and TA100 of *Salmonella typhimurium*, with or without metabolic activation [61].

The LD_{50} of *Polygala tenuifolia* root after intragastric administration in mice was found to be approximately 17 g/kg whereas the root bark gave a lower LD_{50} of 10 g/kg and the root core was not lethal in doses up to 75 g/kg. The root core is reported to have a much lower saponin content than the root bark [38].

Generally, the oral toxicity of saponins in mammals is relatively low due to their poor absorption [2]; LD_{50} values between 50 and 960 mg/kg have been reported for various saponins [62]. In contrast, a mixture of senegins administered parenterally to rats gave an LD_{50} of 3 mg/kg; it also inhibited the growth of Walker carcinoma in rats with an ED_{50} of 1.5 mg/kg, too close to the LD_{50} to be of practical significance [63].

REFERENCES

1. Senega Root - Polygalae radix. European Pharmacopoeia, Council of Europe.

2. Hostettmann K, Marston A. Senegae radix (senega root). In: Saponins. Cambridge: Cambridge University Press, 1995:323.

3. Pharmaceutical Society of Great Britain. Senega. In: British Pharmaceutical Codex 1973. London: Pharmaceutical Press, 1973:436.

4. Evans WC. Senega root. In: Trease and Evans' Pharmacognosy, 14th ed. London-Philadelphia: WB Saunders, 1996:308-9.

5. Wichtl M, Schäfer-Korting M. Senegawurzel - Polygalae radix. In: Hartke K, Hartke H, Mutschler E, Rücker G and Wichtl M, editors. Arzneibuch-Kommentar. Wissenschaftliche Erläuterungen zum Europäischen Arzneibuch und zum Deutschen Arzneibuch. Stuttgart: Wissenschaftliche Verlagsgesellschaft, 1999 (11 Lfg.):S 30.

6. Senega - Senegae Radix, Polygala Root - Polygalae Radix. In: The Japanese Pharmacopoeia (English version). Tokyo: Society of Japanese Pharmacopoeia.

7. Brieskorn CH, Renke F. Chemischer Aufbau, physikalische Eigenschaften und Unterscheidungsmerkmale einiger Polygala-Saponine. Dtsch Apoth Ztg 1968;108:1601-5.

8. Pelletier SW, Nakamura S, Soman R. Constituents of Polygala species. The structure of tenuifolin, a prosapogenin from P. senega and P. tenuifolia. Tetrahedron 1971;27:4417-27.

9. Shoji J, Kawanishi S, Tsukitani Y. Studies on the constituents of Senegae radix I. Isolation and quantitative analysis of the glycosides. Yakugaku Zasshi 1971; 91:198-202.

10. Shoji J, Kawanishi S, Tsukitani Y. On the structure of senegin-II of Senegae radix. Chem Pharm Bull 1971; 19:1740-2.

11. Tsukitani Y, Kawanishi S, Shoji J. Studies on the constituents of Senegae radix. II. The structure of senegin-II, a saponin from Polygala senega Linné var. latifolia Torry et Gray. Chem Pharm Bull 1973;21:791-9.

12. Tsukitani Y, Shoji J. Studies on the constituents of Senegae radix. III. The structures of senegin-III and -IV, saponins from Polygala senega Linné var. latifolia Torry et Gray. Chem Pharm Bull 1973;21:1564-74.

13. Yoshikawa M, Murakami T, Ueno T, Kadoya M, Matsuda H, Yamahara J, Murakami N. E-Senegasaponins A and B, Z-senegasaponins A and B, Z-senegins II and III, new type inhibitors of ethanol absorption in rats from Senegae radix, the roots of Polygala senega L. var. latifolia Torrey et Gray. Chem Pharm Bull 1995;43:350-2.

14. Yoshikawa M, Murakami T, Ueno T, Kadoya M, Matsuda H, Yamahara J, Murakami N. Bioactive saponins and glycosides. I. Senega radix (1): E-Senegasaponins a and b and Z-senegasaponins a and b, their inhibitory effect on alcohol absorption and hypoglycemic activity. Chem Pharm Bull 1995;43:2115-22.

15. Yoshikawa M, Murakami T, Matsuda H, Ueno T, Kadoya M, Yamahara J, Murakami N. Bioactive saponins and glycosides. II. Senegae radix (2): Chemical structures, hypoglycemic activity and ethanol absorption-inhibitory effect of E-senegasaponin c, Z-senegasaponin c and Z-senegins II, III and IV. Chem Pharm Bull 1996;44:1305-13.

16. Sakuma S, Shoji J. Studies on the constituents of the root of Polygala tenuifolia Willdenow. I. Isolation of saponins and the structures of onjisaponins G and F. Chem Pharm Bull 1981;29:2431-41.

17. Sakuma S, Shoji J. Studies on the constituents of the root of Polygala tenuifolia Willdenow. II. On the structures of onjisaponins A, B and E. Chem Pharm Bull 1982; 30:810-21.

18. Takiura K, Yamamoto M, Murata H, Takai H, Honda S, Yuki H. Studies on oligosaccharides XIII. Oligosaccharides in Polygala senega and structures of glycosyl-1,5-anhydro-D-glucitols. Yakugaku Zasshi 1974;94:998-1003.

19. Saitoh H, Miyase T, Ueno A. Senegoses A-E, oligosaccharide multi-esters from Polygala senega var. latifolia Torr. et Gray. Chem Pharm Bull 1993;41:1127-31.

20. Saitoh H, Miyase T, Ueno A. Senegoses F-I, oligosaccharide multi-esters from the roots of Polygala senega var. latifolia Torr. et Gray. Chem Pharm Bull 1993;41:2125-8.

21. Saitoh H, Miyase T, Ueno A, Atarashi K, Saiki Y. Senegoses J-O, oligosaccharide multi-esters from the roots of Polygala senega L. Chem Pharm Bull 1994; 42:641-5.

22. Hayashi S, Kameoka H. Volatile compounds of Polygala senega L. var. latifolia Torrey et Gray roots. Flavour Fragrance J 1995;10:273-80.

23. Ito H, Taniguchi H, Kita T, Matsuki Y, Tachikawa E, Fujita T. Xanthones and a cinnamic acid derivative from Polygala tenuifolia. Phytochemistry 1977; 16:1614-6.

24. Ikeya Y, Sugama K, Okada M, Mitsuhashi H. Two xanthones from Polygala tenuifolia. Phytochemistry 1991;30:2061-5.

25. Fujita T, Liu D-Y, Ueda S, Takeda Y. Xanthones from Polygala tenuifolia. Phytochemistry 1992;31:3997-4000.

26. Ikeya Y, Sugama K, Maruno M. Xanthone C-glycoside and acylated sugar from Polygala tenuifolia. Chem Pharm Bull 1994;42:2305-8.

27. Ikeya Y, Sugama K, Okada M, Mitsuhashi H. Four new phenolic glycosides from Polygala tenuifolia. Chem

Pharm Bull 1991;39:2600-5.

28. Miyase T, Iwata Y, Ueno A. Tenuifolioses A-F, oligosaccharide multi-esters from the roots of *Polygala tenuifolia* Willd. Chem Pharm Bull 1991;39:3082-4.

29. Miyase T, Iwata Y, Ueno A. Tenuifolioses G-P, oligosaccharide multi-esters from the roots of *Polygala tenuifolia* Willd. Chem Pharm Bull 1992;40:2741-8.

30. Miyase T, Ueno A. Sucrose derivatives from the roots of *Polygala tenuifolia*. Shoyakugaku Zasshi 1993; 47:267-78.

31. Tsuchiya H, Hayashi H, Sato M, Shimizu H, Iinuma M. Quantitative analysis of all types of β-carboline alkaloids in medicinal plants and dried edible plants by high performance liquid chromatography with selective fluorimetric detection. Phytochem Analysis 1999; 10:247-53.

32. Steinegger E, Hänsel R. Senegine und Senegawurzel. In: Pharmakognosie, 5th ed. Berlin: Springer-Verlag, 1992:212-3.

33. Bisset NG (translated from Wichtl M, Teedrogen). Polygalae radix. In: Herbal Drugs and Phyto-pharmaceuticals: a handbook for practice on a scientific basis. Stuttgart: Medpharm, 1994:384-5.

34. Bradley PR, editor. Senega. In: British Herbal Compendium, Volume 1. Bournemouth: British Herbal Medicine Association, 1992:196-8.

35. Tisanes: Polygala (racine). In: Pharmacopée Française Xe.

36. Newall CA, Anderson LA, Phillipson JD. Senega. In: Herbal Medicines. A guide for health-care professionals. London: Pharmaceutical Press, 1996:241-2.

37. Briggs CJ. Senega Snakeroot. A traditional Canadian herbal medicine. Can Pharm J 1988;121:199-201.

38. De Smet PAGM. *Polygala* Species. In: De Smet PAGM, Keller K, Hänsel R, Chandler RF. Adverse Effects of Herbal Drugs, Volume 2. Berlin-Heidelberg: Springer-Verlag, 1993:275-82.

39. Boyd EM, Palmer ME. The effect of Quillaia, Senega, Squill, Grindelia, Sanguinaria, Chionanthus and Dioscorea upon the output of respiratory tract fluid. Acta Pharmacol 1946;2:235-46.

40. Misawa M, Yanaura S. Continuous determination of tracheobronchial secretory activity in dogs. Japan J Pharmacol 1980;30:221-9.

41. Boyd EM. Expectorants and respiratory tract fluid. J Pharm Pharmacol 1954;6:521-42.

42. Reynolds JEF, editor. Cough suppressants, expectorants and mucolytics. In: Martindale - The Extra Pharmacopoeia, 31st ed. London: Royal Pharmaceutical Society, 1996:1059-60,1074.

43. Basch FP, Holinger P, Poncher HG. Physical and chemical properties of sputum. II. Influence of drugs, steam, carbon dioxide and oxygen. Am J Dis Child 1941;62:1149-71.

44. Lohmann K, Reininger E, Bauer R. Screening of European anti-inflammatory herbal drugs for inhibition of cyclooxygenase-1 and -2 [Poster]. In: Abstracts of 3rd International Congress on Phytomedicine. Munich, 11-13 October 2000. *Published as*: Phytomedicine 2000;7(Suppl. 2):99 (P-91).

45. Tezuka Y, Fan W, Kasimu R, Kadota S. Screening of crude drug extracts for prolyl endopeptidase inhibitory activity. Phytomedicine 1999;6:197-203.

46. Nikaido T, Ohmoto T, Saitoh H, Sankawa U, Sakuma S, Shoji J. Inhibitors of cyclic adenosine monophosphate phosphodiesterase in *Polygala tenuifolia*. Chem Pharm Bull 1982;30:2020-4.

47. Kurokawa M, Ohyama H, Hozumi T, Namba T, Nakano M, Shiraki K. Assay for antiviral activity of herbal extracts using their absorbed sera. Chem Pharm Bull 1996;44:1270-2.

48. Rao GS, Sinsheimer JE, Cochran KW. Antiviral activity of triterpenoid saponins containing acylated β-amyrin aglycones. J Pharm Sci 1974;63:471-3.

49. Wolters B. Die Verbreitung antibiotischer Eigenschaften bei Saponindrogen. Dtsch Apoth Ztg 1966;106:1729-33.

50. Yamahara J, Takagi Y, Sawada T, Fujimura H, Shirakawa K, Yoshikawa M, Kitagawa I. Effects of crude drugs on congestive edema. Chem Pharm Bull 1979;27:1464-8.

51. Kako M, Miura T, Nishiyama Y, Ichimaru M, Moriyasu M, Kato A. Hypoglycemic effect of the rhizomes of *Polygala senega* in normal and diabetic mice and its main component, the triterpenoid glycoside senegin II. Planta Med 1996;62:440-3.

52. Kako M, Miura T, Usami M, Nishiyama Y, Ichimaru M, Moriyasu M, Kato A. Effect of senegin-II on blood glucose in normal and NIDDM mice. Biol Pharm Bull 1995;18;1159-61.

53. Kako M, Miura T, Nishiyama Y, Ichimaru M, Moriyasu M, Kato A. Hypoglycemic activity of some triterpenoid glycosides. J Nat Prod 1997;60:604-5.

54. Matsuda H, Murakami T, Li Y, Yamahara J, Yoshikawa M. Mode of action of escins Ia and IIa and *E,Z*-senegin II on glucose absorption in gastrointestinal tract. Bioorg Med Chem 1998;6:1019-23.

55. Masuda H, Ohsumi K, Kako M, Miura T, Nishiyama Y, Ichimaru M et al. Intraperitoneal administration of Senegae radix extract and its main component, senegin II, affects lipid metabolism in normal and hyperlipidemic mice. Biol Pharm Bull 1996;19:315-7.

56. Ishida H, Inaoka Y, Okada M, Fukushima M, Fukazawa H and Tsuji K. Studies of the active substances in herbs used for hair treatment. III. Isolation of hair-regrowth substances from *Polygala senega* var. *latifolia* Torr. et Gray. Biol Pharm Bull 1999;22:1249-50.

57. Yabe T, Iizuka S, Komatsu Y, Yamada H. Enhancements of choline acetyltransferase activity and nerve growth factor secretion by Polygalae radix extract containing active ingredients in Kami-untan-to. Phytomedicine 1997;4:199-205.

58. Yokoyama H, Hiai S, Oura H, Hayashi T. Effects of total saponins extracted from several crude drugs on rat adrenocortical hormone secretion. Yakugaku Zasshi 1982;102:555-9.

59. Wang S, Kozuka K, Saito K, Kano Y. Pharmacological properties of galenical preparations (XVII): Active compounds in blood and bile of rats after oral administration of extracts of Polygalae radix. J Traditional Med 1994;11;44-9.

60. Wang S, Kozuka K, Saito K, Komatsu K, Kano Y. Pharmacological properties of galenical preparations (XVIII): Pharmacokinetics of active compounds of Polygalae radix. J Traditional Med 1994;11;168-75.

61. Morimoto I, Watanabe F, Osawa T, Okitsu T, Kada T. Mutagenicity screening of crude drugs with *Bacillus subtilis* rec-assay and *Salmonella*/microsome reversion assay. Mutation Res 1982;97:81-102.

62. George AJ. Legal status and toxicity of saponins. Food Cosmet Toxicol 1965;3:85-91.

63. Tschesche R, Wulff G. Chemie und Biologie der Saponine. In: Herz W, Grisebach H, Kirby GW, editors. Fortschritte der Chemie organischer Naturstoffe - Progress in the Chemistry of Organic Natural Products, Volume 30. Vienna-New York: Springer-Verlag, 1973: 461-606.

PRIMULAE RADIX

Primula Root

E/S/C/O/P
MONOGRAPHS
Second Edition

DEFINITION

Primula root consists of the whole or cut, dried rhizome and root of *Primula veris* L. or *P. elatior* (L.) Hill.

The material complies with the monograph of the European Pharmacopoeia [1].

CONSTITUENTS

The characteristic constituents are triterpene saponins [2-9], usually in the range of 3-10 % [7,10-12], and phenolic glycosides [7,13].

The principal saponins of *Primula veris* and *P. elatior* are closely related and have a branched chain of at least four sugars (glucuronic acid, glucose, galactose and rhamnose) at C-3 [7-9]; an additional xylose residue is present in one saponin [9]. It remains debatable whether the saponins of the two species are identical [7] or different [8]. Two main saponins appear to be present [9,14], those of *P. elatior* being derived from protoprimulagenin A [8,12]. The most recent study of *P. veris* (as subsp. *macrocalyx*) [8] indicated saponins derived from the aglycones priverogenin B and its 22-acetate, and also anagalligenin A [8,12].

The phenolic glycosides primverin and primulaverin occur in both species, in very variable amounts up to 2.3 %; they are the 2-primeverosides of 4-methoxy- and 5-methoxysalicylic acid methyl esters respectively [7,13]. These two esters as aglycones have been identified as the main components of essential oil (0.1-0.2%) obtained from the roots of *P. veris* (= *P. officinalis*) [15] and *P. elatior* [16].

CLINICAL PARTICULARS

Therapeutic indications
Productive cough [17,18]; catarrh of the respiratory tract [17,19]; chronic bronchitis [12,17,18].

Posology and method of administration

Dosage

Adult daily dose: 0.5-1.5 g of the drug as a decoction or equivalent preparation, taken in small amounts as necessary [12,17-19]; higher daily doses of 5-10 g of the drug have also been recommended [20,21]. *Elderly*: dose as for adults.

Children: 4-10 years, 0.5-1.0 g daily; 10-16 years, 0.5-1.5 g daily [22].

Method of administration
For oral administration.

Duration of administration
No restriction.

Contra-indications
Gastritis, gastric ulcer.

Special warnings and special precautions for use
None required.

Interaction with other medicaments and other forms of interaction
None reported.

Pregnancy and lactation
No data available. In accordance with general medical practice, the product should not be used during pregnancy or lactation without medical advice.

Effects on ability to drive and use machines
None known.

Undesirable effects
Normally none at the recommended dosage. In rare cases gastrointestinal disturbance may occur [19].

Overdose
Overdosage may lead to stomach upset, vomiting or diarrhoea [12,17,19].

PHARMACOLOGICAL PROPERTIES

Pharmacodynamic properties

Primula root has an expectorant action arising primarily from local irritation of the gastric mucosa by saponins; this provokes a reflex increase in bronchial secretion, which dilutes the mucus and reduces its viscosity [19,23]. Irritation of mucous membranes in the throat and respiratory tract by saponins may also cause an increase in bronchial secretions and the surface tension-lowering action of saponins might help to reduce the viscosity of sputum, making it easier to eject [24].

In vitro experiments
A hexane extract (50 μg/ml) of *Primula veris* root inhibited COX (cyclooxygenase)-1 and COX-2 by 54% and 66% respectively [25].

Primula root saponins inhibit the growth of a variety of bacteria and fungi [26,27]. An unspecified saponin mixture from *Primula veris* exhibited activity against influenza (A_2/Japan 305) virus, producing 89%

inhibition at a concentration of 6.2 μg/ml [28,29].

In vivo experiments
An undefined mixture of saponins from primula root at a concentration of 1:10,000 increased the ciliary activity of throat epithelium of curarized frog. This effect was assumed to be due to a decrease in surface tension of the mucus. The ciliary activity was less at a concentration of 1:6,000 and ceased at 1:3,000 due to toxic effects [30].

An unspecified primula saponin, administered parenterally, inhibited the growth of Walker carcinoma in rats with an ED_{50} of 40 mg/kg, although this dose was too toxic in relation to the LD_{50} of 70 mg/kg to be of practical significance [31].

Clinical studies
None reported.

Pharmacokinetic properties
No specific data are available on the pharmacokinetics of primula root saponins. In general, saponins are poorly absorbed by the body [24].

Preclinical safety data
The oral toxicity of saponins in mammals is relatively low due to their poor absorption from the gastrointestinal tract [24]; oral LD_{50} values determined in rodents for various saponins ranged from 50 to 960 mg/kg [32]. Although their oral LD_{50} values have not been reported, primula saponins are considered to have a favourable risk-benefit ratio [24].

The dietary intake of saponins has been estimated as 15 mg per person per day in an average UK family; for vegetarians the figure is substantially higher at 110 mg, and sometimes over 200 mg, per person per day. With a few exceptions (such as liquorice), no negative effects are apparent from prolonged intake of edible plants containing saponins [24].

REFERENCES

1. Primula Root - Primulae radix. European Pharmacopoeia, Council of Europe.

2. Tschesche R, Tjoa BT, Wulff G. Über Triterpene XXIII. Über Struktur und Chemie der Priverogenine. Tetrahedron Lett 1968:183-8.

3. Grecu L, Cucu V. Saponine aus *Primula officinalis* und *Primula elatior*. Planta Med 1975;27:247-53.

4. Tschesche R, Ballhorn L. Protoprimulagenin A als Aglykon des Hauptsaponins von *Primula elatior*. Phytochemistry 1975;14:305-6.

5. Tschesche R, Wiemann W. Über Triterpene XXXII.

Über die Zuckerkette des Hauptsaponins aus den Wurzeln von *Primula elatior* L. Schreber. Chem Ber 1977;110:2407-15.

6. Tschesche R, Wagner R, Widera W. Saponine aus den Wurzeln von *P. elatior* (L.) Schreber. Konstitution eines Nebensaponins und Revision der Zuckerkette des Hauptsaponins. Liebigs Ann Chem 1983:993-1000.

7. Wagner H, Reger H. Radix Primulae-Extrakte. HPLC-Analyse. Dtsch Apoth Ztg 1986;126:1489-93.

8. Çalis I, Yürüker A, Rüegger H, Wright AD, Sticher O. Triterpene saponins from *Primula veris* subsp. *macrocalyx* and *Primula elatior* subsp. *meyeri*. J Nat Prod. 1992;55:1299-1306.

9. Siems K, Jaensch M, Jakupovic J. Structures of the two saponins isolated from commercially available root extract of *Primula* sp. Planta Med 1998;64:272-4.

10. Jentzsch K, Kubelka W, Kvarda B. Untersuchungen über den Saponingehalt von Radix Primulae veris L. im Verlauf mehrjähriger Kultur. Sci Pharm 1973;41:162-5.

11. Glasl H, Ihrig M. Quantitative Bestimmung von Triterpensaponinen in Drogen. Pharm Ztg 1984;129:2619-22.

12. Wichtl M, Neubeck M. Primelwurzel - Primulae radix. In: Hartke K, Hartke H, Mutschler E, Rücker G and Wichtl M, editors. Kommentar zum Europäischen Arzneibuch. Stuttgart: Wissenschaftliche Verlagsgesellschaft, Eschborn: Govi-Verlag, 1999 (12. Lfg.):P 92.

13. Thieme H, Winkler H-J. Über Vorkommen und Akkumulation von Phenolglykosiden in der Familie der Primulaceen. Pharmazie 1971;26:434-6.

14. Hahn-Deinstrop E, Koch A, Müller M. HPTLC measured values of primula saponins in extracts of Primulae radix: a comparison after derivatization between handspraying, dipping and autospraying. Chromatographia 2000;51(Suppl.):S302-4.

15. Frigot P, Goris A. Nouvelles recherches sur la composition des essences des organes souterrains de quelques Primevères. Ann Pharm Fr 1968;26:287-90.

16. Goris A, Frigot P. Sur la composition de l'essence retirée des organes souterrains de *Primula elatior* Jacq. Ann Pharm Fr 1974;32:233-6.

17. Bisset NG (translated from Wichtl M, editor. Teedrogen, 2nd ed.). Primulae radix. In: Herbal Drugs and Phytopharmaceuticals: a handbook for practice on a scientific basis. Boca Raton-London: CRC Press, Stuttgart: Medpharm, 1994:390-2.

18. Steinegger E, Hänsel R. Primulasaponine und Primel-wurzel. In: Pharmakognosie, 5th ed. Berlin: Springer-Verlag, 1992:210-1.

19. Hänsel R, Keller K, Rimpler H, Schneider G, editors. Primula. In: Hagers Handbuch der Pharmazeutischen Praxis, 5th ed. Volume 6: Drogen P-Z. Berlin: Springer-Verlag, 1994:269-87.

20. Tisanes: Primevère racine. In: Pharmacopée Française, Xe.

21. Garnier G, Bézanger-Beauquesne L, Debraux G. Primulacées. In: Ressources Médicinales de la Flore Française, Volume II. Paris: Vigot Frères, 1961:972-6.

22. Dorsch W, Loew D, Meyer E, Schilcher H. Primulae radix. In: Empfehlungen zu Kinderdosierungen von monographierten Arzneidrogen und ihren Zubereitungen. Bonn: Kooperation Phytopharmaka, 1993: Table 75.

23. Boyd EM. Expectorants and respiratory tract fluid. J Pharm Pharmacol 1954;6:521-42.

24. Hostettman K, Marston A. In: Saponins. Cambridge: Cambridge University Press, 1995:266-7 and 284-6.

25. Lohmann K, Reininger E, Bauer R. Screening of European anti-inflammatory herbal drugs for inhibition of cyclooxygenase-1 and -2 [Poster]. In: Abstracts of 3rd International Congress on Phytomedicine. Munich, Germany, 11-13 October 2000. *Published as*: Phytomedicine 2000;7(Suppl 2):99 (Poster P-91).

26. Wolters B. Die Verbreitung antibiotischer Eigenschaften bei Saponindrogen. Dtsch Apoth Ztg 1966;106:1729-33.

27. Tschesche R, Wulff G. Über die antimikrobielle Wirksamkeit von Saponinen. Z Naturforsch 1965; 20b:543-6.

28. Rao GS, Sinsheimer JE, Cochran KW. Antiviral activity of triterpenoid saponins containing acylated β-amyrin aglycones. J Pharm Sci 1974;63:471-3.

29. Büechi S. Antivirale Saponine. Pharmakologische und klinische Untersuchungen. Dtsch Apoth Ztg 1996; 136:89-98.

30. Vogel G. Zur Pharmakologie von Saponinen. Planta Med 1963;11:362-76.

31. Tschesche R, Wulff G. Chemie und Biologie der Saponine. In: Herz W, Grisebach H, Kirby GW, editors. Fortschritte der Chemie organischer Naturstoffe/Progress in the Chemistry of Organic Natural Products, Volume 30. Vienna-New York: Springer-Verlag, 1973:461-606.

32. Oakenfull D. Saponins in food - a review. Food Chemistry 1981;7:19-40.

PSYLLII SEMEN

Psyllium Seed

DEFINITION

Psyllium seed consists of the ripe, whole, dry seeds of *Plantago afra* L. (*Plantago psyllium* L.) or *Plantago indica* L. (*Plantago arenaria* Waldstein and Kitaibel).

The material complies with the monograph of the European Pharmacopoeia [1].

CONSTITUENTS

Mucilage polysaccharide (10-15%) [2,3] in the epidermis, consisting of xylose, galacturonic acid, arabinose and rhamnose residues [2]. The seeds also contain protein (15-20%), fixed oil (5-13%) [4], the trisaccharide planteose [4,5] and small amounts of phytosterols, triterpenes [4,5], the iridoid glucoside aucubin and alkaloids (plantagonine, indicaine and indicamine) [4-6], but no starch [2,3].

CLINICAL PARTICULARS

Therapeutic indications
Treatment of occasional constipation.
Conditions in which easy defecation with soft stools is desirable, e.g. in cases of anal fissures or haemorrhoids, after rectal or anal surgery, and during pregnancy [3,7,8].
Adjuvant symptomatic therapy in cases of diarrhoea from various causes [9].

Posology and method of administration

Dosage

Adults and children over 12 years of age: as a laxative, 10-30 g daily of the seeds [3,7] or equivalent preparations; in cases of diarrhoea, up to 40 g daily [3] divided into 2-3 doses.
Children 6-12 years: as a laxative, half the adult dose [10].

Method of administration
For oral administration.

It is very important to take the seeds with a large amount of liquid, e.g. mix approx. 5 g with 150 ml of cool water, stir briskly and swallow as quickly as possible, then maintain adequate fluid intake.

Psyllium seed should preferably be taken at mealtimes; it should not be taken immediately prior to going to bed. Any other medications should be taken at least

30-60 minutes before psyllium seed in order to avoid delayed absorption.

Duration of administration
In cases of diarrhoea, medical advice should be sought if the symptoms persist for more than 3 days in order to ensure definitive diagnosis of the cause.

Contra-indications
Children under 6 years of age.
Known hypersensitivity to psyllium seed [11].

Psyllium seed should not be used by patients with the following conditions unless advised by a physician: faecal impaction; undiagnosed abdominal symptoms; a sudden change in bowel habit that persists for more than 2 weeks; rectal bleeding; failure to defecate following the use of a laxative; abnormal constrictions in the gastrointestinal tract; potential or existing intestinal obstruction (ileus); diseases of the oesophagus and cardia; megacolon [3]; diabetes mellitus which is difficult to regulate [3].

Special warnings and special precautions for use
A sufficient amount of liquid should always be taken: at least 150 ml of water per 5 g of seed [11].

Taking psyllium seed without adequate fluid may cause it to swell and block the throat or oesophagus and may cause choking. Intestinal obstruction may occur should adequate fluid intake not be maintained. Do not take psyllium seed if you have ever had difficulty in swallowing or have any throat problems. If you experience chest pain, vomiting, or difficulty in swallowing or breathing after taking it, seek immediate medical attention. Treatment of the elderly and debilitated patients requires medical supervision. Administration to the elderly should be supervised.

In cases of diarrhoea sufficient intake of water and electrolytes is important.

Interaction with other medicaments and other forms of interaction
Enteral absorption of concomitantly administered minerals (e.g. calcium, iron, lithium, zinc), vitamins (B12), cardiac glycosides and coumarin derivatives may be delayed [3,8,9,12-14]. For this reason, other medications should be taken at least 30-60 minutes before psyllium seed. In the case of insulin-dependent diabetics it may be necessary to reduce the insulin dose [14-16].

Pregnancy and lactation
No restriction [17].
A risk is not to be expected since the constituents of psyllium seed are not absorbed and have no systemic effects.

Effects on ability to drive and use machines
None known.

Undesirable effects
Flatulence may occur, but generally disappears during the course of treatment.
Abdominal distension and risk of oesophageal or intestinal obstruction and faecal impaction may occur, particularly if psyllium seed is ingested with insufficient fluid.

There is a risk of allergic reaction from inhalation of the powder during occupational exposure. Due to the allergic potential of psyllium seed, patients must be aware of reactions of hypersensitivity including anaphylactic reactions in single cases [11].

Overdose
Overdosage may cause abdominal discomfort and flatulence, or even intestinal obstruction. Adequate fluid intake should be maintained and management should be symptomatic.

PHARMACOLOGICAL PROPERTIES

Pharmacodynamic properties

Laxative effects
Psyllium seed increases the volume of intestinal contents by the binding of fluid, resulting in increased faecal weights. This leads to physical stimulation of the gut [3,9,12]. The intraluminal pressure is decreased and colonic transit is accelerated [12].

Psyllium seed increases stool weight and water content due to the fibre residue, the water bound to that residue [3,9,12] and the increased faecal bacterial mass [9,18].

Antidiarrhoeal effects
In cases of diarrhoea, psyllium seed binds fluids and thus increases the viscosity of intestinal contents [9], thereby normalizing transit time and frequency of defecation [3,12].

Metabolic effects
Psyllium seed significantly lowers serum cholesterol (5-15%) [2,12] and LDL-cholesterol levels (8-20%) in hypercholesterolaemic subjects without significant changes in HDL-cholesterol or triglycerides [3,19]. The mechanism for this effect is still under discussion, one possible explanation being the increased faecal excretion of bile acids which, in turn, results in further bile salt synthesis from cholesterol [3,9,15].

Psyllium seed reduces peak levels of blood glucose by delaying intestinal absorption of sugar [3,12,20].

Pharmacokinetic properties

The vegetable fibre of psyllium seed is resistant to digestion in the upper intestinal tract; thus it is not absorbed. Part of the fibre is degraded by colonic bacteria [3,15].

Preclinical safety data

After 125 days on a diet containing 25% of psyllium seed, albino rats showed a dark pigmentation of the suprarenal gland, the kidney marrow and the liver. Dogs showed a grey colour of the kidneys after being fed a diet containing 25% of psyllium seed for 30 days. Similar effects have not been observed in humans. The pigment probably originates from the black pericarp of *Plantago afra*. When the seeds were extracted with hot water prior to feeding and then fed to the animals as whole seeds no pigmentation was observed [3].

REFERENCES

1. Psyllium seed - Psyllii semen. European Pharmacopoeia, Council of Europe.

2. Karawya MS, Balbaa SI, Afifi MSA. Investigation of the carbohydrate contents of certain mucilaginous plants. Planta Med 1971;20:14-23

3. Hänsel R, Keller K, Rimpler H, Schneider G, editors. Plantago. In: Hagers Handbuch der Pharmazeutischen Praxis, 5th ed. Volume 6: Drogen P-Z. Berlin: Springer-Verlag, 1994:221-39.

4. Hänsel R, Sticher O, Steinegger E. Flohsamen. In: Pharmakognosie - Phytopharmazie. 6th ed. Berlin: Springer-Verlag, 1999:366-7.

5. Balbaa SI, Karawya MS, Afifi MS. Pharmacognostical study of the seeds of certain *Plantago* species growing in Egypt. UAR J Pharm Sci 1971;12:35-52, through Chem Abstr 1972;77:156311.

6. Karawya MS, Balbaa SI, Afifi MS. Alkaloids and glycosides in *Plantago psyllium* growing in Egypt. UAR J Pharm Sci 1971;12:53-61, through Chem Abstr 1973; 78:13729.

7. Wichtl M. Flohsamen. In: Wichtl M, editor. Teedrogen und Phytopharmaka, 4th ed. Stuttgart: Wissenschaftliche Verlagsgesellschaft, 2002:478-9.

8. Laxatives (Local). In: USP Dispensing Information, 14th ed. Volume I: Drug information for the health care professional. Rockville MD: The United States Pharmacopoeial Convention, 1994:1703-9.

9. Brunton LL. Agents affecting gastrointestinal water flux and motility; emesis and antiemetics; bile acids and pancreatic enzymes. In: Hardman JG, Limbird LE, Molinoff PB, Ruddon RW, Gilman AG, editors. Goodman & Gilman's The Pharmacological Basis of Therapeutics, 9th ed. New York: McGraw-Hill, 1996: 917-36.

10. Dorsch W, Loew D, Meyer E, Schilcher H. Psyllii semen. In: Empfehlungen zu Kinderdosierungen von monographierten Arzneidrogen und ihren Zubereitungen. Bonn: Kooperation Phytopharmaka, 1993:89.

11. Sweetman SC, editor. Ispaghula. In: Martindale - The complete drug reference, 33rd ed. London: Royal Pharmaceutical Society, 2002:1229.

12. Kies C. Purified psyllium seed fiber, human gastrointestinal tract function and nutritional status of humans. In: Furda I, editor. Unconventional sources of dietary fiber. Physiological and *in vitro* functional properties. ACS Symposium Series 214. Washington DC: American Chemical Society, 1983:61-70.

13. Drews LM, Kies C, Fox HM. Effect of dietary fiber on copper, zinc and magnesium utilization by adolescent boys. Am J Clin Nutr 1979;32:1893-7.

14. Cummings JH. Nutritional implications of dietary fiber. Am J Clin Nutr 1978;31:S21-9.

15. Kay RM, Strasberg SM. Origin, chemistry, physiological effects and clinical importance of dietary fibre. Clin Invest Med 1978;1:9-24.

16. Uribe M, Dibildox M, Malpica S, Guillermo E, Villallobos A, Nieto L et al. Beneficial effect of vegetable protein diet supplemented with Psyllium Plantago in patients with hepatic encephalopathy and diabetes mellitus. Gastroenterology 1985;88:901-7.

17. Lewis JH, Weingold AB. The use of gastrointestinal drugs during pregnancy and lactation. Am J Gastroenterol 1985;80:912-23.

18. de Lourdes Rossano Garcia M, Mirabent M. Estudio comparativo de policarbófilo cálcico y *Psyllium plantago* en el tratamiento de la constipación. Investigación Médica Internacional 1992;19:75-82.

19. Lerman GI, Lagunas M, Sienra PJC, Ahumada AM, Saldaña A, Cardoso SG, Posadas RC. Efecto del Psyllium Plantago en pacientes con hipercolesterolemia leve a moderada. Arch Inst Cardiol Méx 1990;60:535-9.

20. Frati-Munari AC, Flores-Garduño MA, Ariza-Andraca R, Islas-Andrade S, Chavez NA. Efecto de diferentes dosis de mucilago de Plantago psyllium en la prueba de tolerancia a la glucosa. Archivos Invest Méd (Mexico) 1989;20:147-52.

RHAMNI PURSHIANI CORTEX

Cascara

E/S/C/O/P
MONOGRAPHS
Second Edition

DEFINITION

Cascara consists of the dried, whole or fragmented bark of *Rhamnus purshianus* D.C. [*Frangula purshiana* (D.C.) A. Gray ex J.C. Cooper]. It contains not less than 8.0 per cent of hydroxyanthracene glycosides of which not less than 60 per cent consists of cascarosides, both expressed as cascaroside A ($C_{27}H_{32}O_{14}$; M_r 580.5) and calculated with reference to the dried drug.

The material complies with the monograph of the European Pharmacopoeia [1].

CONSTITUENTS

The main active constituents are cascarosides A, B, C, D, E and F [2,3]. Cascarosides A and B are mixed anthrone-C- and O-glycosides, being the 8-O-β-D-glucosides of 10-(S)-deoxyglucosyl aloe-emodin anthrone and of 10-(R)-deoxyglucosyl aloe-emodin anthrone (aloins A and B) respectively. Cascarosides C and D are the 8-O-β-D-glucosides of 10-(R)(S)-deoxyglucosyl chrysophanol anthrone (chrysaloins A and B) [2]. Cascarosides E and F are 8-O-β-D-glucosides of 10-deoxyglucosyl emodin anthrone [3]. The cascarosides comprise between 60 and 70% of the total hydroxyanthracene complex. Aloins A and B together with chrysaloins A and B account for 10-30% of the total hydroxyanthracene content. The remaining 10-20% consists of a mixture of hydroxyanthracene O-glycosides including the mono-glucosides of aloe-emodin, chrysophanol, emodin and physcion together with the corresponding aglycones [2].

CLINICAL PARTICULARS

Therapeutic indications
For short term use in cases of occasional constipation [4].

Posology and method of administration

Dosage

The correct individual dosage is the smallest required to produce a comfortable soft-formed motion.

Adults and children over 10 years
Dried bark: 0.3-1 g in a single daily dose [4].
Infusion: 1.5-2 g of dried bark in 150 ml of hot water [2].

Preparations equivalent to 20-30 mg of hydroxy-anthracene derivatives (calculated as cascaroside A) daily [2].

Elderly: dose as for adults.
Not recommended for use in children under 10 years of age.

The pharmaceutical form must allow lower dosages.

Method of administration
For oral administration.

Duration of administration
Stimulant laxatives should not be used for periods of more than 2 weeks without medical advice.

Contra-indications
Intestinal obstruction and stenosis, atony, inflammatory diseases of the colon (e.g. Crohn's disease, ulcerative colitis), appendicitis; abdominal pain of unknown origin; severe dehydration states with water and electrolyte depletion [5,6].
Children under 10 years.

Special warnings and special precautions for use
As for all laxatives, cascara should not be given when any undiagnosed acute or persistent abdominal symptoms are present.

If laxatives are needed every day the cause of the constipation should be investigated. Long term use of laxatives should be avoided. Use for more than 2 weeks requires medical supervision. Chronic use may cause pigmentation of the colon (pseudo-melanosis coli) which is harmless and reversible after drug discontinuation. Abuse, with diarrhoea and consequent fluid and electrolyte losses, may cause: dependence with possible need for increased dosages; disturbance of the water and electrolyte (mainly hypokalaemia) balance; an atonic colon with impaired function. Intake of anthranoid-containing laxatives for more than a short period of time may result in aggravation of constipation. Hypokalaemia can result in cardiac and neuromuscular dysfunction, especially if cardiac glycosides, diuretics or corticosteroids are taken. Chronic use may result in albuminuria and haematuria.

In chronic constipation, stimulant laxatives are not an acceptable alternative to a change in diet [5-8].

Note: A detailed text with advice concerning changes in dietary habits, physical activities and training for normal bowel evacuation should be included on the package leaflet. An example is given in the booklet "Médicaments á base de plantes", published by the French health authority (Paris: Agence du Médicament, 1998).

Interaction with other medicaments and other forms of interaction
Hypokalaemia (resulting from long term laxative abuse) potentiates the action of cardiac glycosides and interacts with antiarrhythmic drugs or with drugs which induce reversion to sinus rhythm (e.g. quinidine). Concomitant use with other drugs inducing hypokalaemia (e.g. thiazide diuretics, adreno-corticosteroids and liquorice root) may aggravate electrolyte imbalance [6].

Pregnancy and lactation

Pregnancy
Experimental studies, as well as many years of experience, do not indicate undesirable or damaging effects from anthranoid laxatives during pregnancy or on the foetus when used at the recommended dosage [9,10]. However, in view of experimental data concerning a genotoxic risk from several anthranoids (e.g. aloe-emodin), avoid during the first trimester or take only under medical supervision.

Lactation
Breastfeeding is not recommended as there are insufficient data on the excretion of metabolites in breast milk. Small amounts of active metabolites (rhein) may appear in breast milk. However, a laxative effect in breast-fed babies has not been reported [5,11].

Effects on ability to drive and use machines
None.

Undesirable effects
Abdominal spasms and pain, in particular with irritable colon; yellowish-brown or red (pH dependent) dis-colouration of urine by metabolites, which is not clinically significant [5,6,12,13].

Overdose
The major symptoms are griping and severe diarrhoea with consequent losses of fluid and electrolytes, which should be replaced [6]. Treatment should be supportive with generous amounts of fluid. Electrolytes, especially potassium, should be monitored; this is particularly important in the elderly and the young.

PHARMACOLOGICAL PROPERTIES

Pharmacodynamic properties

Laxative effects
1,8-dihydroxyanthracene derivatives possess a laxative effect [14,15]. The cascarosides, and aloins A and B and chrysaloins A and B, are precursors which are not absorbed in the upper gut. Studies have established that glycosidases from the intestinal flora

are responsible for metabolism of the glycosides [16]. Caecal incubates from rats hydrolysed cascarosides into the corresponding aloins and chrysaloins. Subsequently these were reductively cleaved to the corresponding aloe-emodin anthrone or chrysophanol anthrone [16]. Various bacterial isolates from human faeces have given similar results [16-18,19].

In male rats positive to aloin A, the cathartic activity of aloins A and B was found to be dose-dependent and nearly equivalent (ED$_{50}$ of approx. 20 mg/kg) [20].

In rats, cascara increased the constitutive, Ca^{2+}-dependent NO synthase activity and also induced the Ca^{2+}-independent isoform of NO synthase. NO is a possible mediator for the laxative effect of 1,8-dihydroxyanthracene derivatives [21].

The main active metabolite is aloe-emodin-9-anthrone which acts specifically on the colon [22].

There are two different mechanisms of action [23]:

(i) an influence on the motility of the large intestine (inhibition of the Na$^+$/K$^+$ pump and of Cl$^-$ channels at the colonic membrane) resulting in accelerated colonic transit [22,24,25] and

(ii) an influence on secretion processes (stimulation of mucus and chloride secretion) resulting in enhanced fluid secretion [22,26,27].

The motility effects are mediated by direct stimulation of colonic neurons [22] and possibly by prostaglandins [28].

Defecation takes place after a delay of 6-12 hours due to the time taken for transport to the colon and transformation into the active compound.

Other effects
Aloe-emodin inhibited the growth of human neuro-ectodermal tumours in tissue cultures and in mice (50 mg/kg body weight/day; p<0.05) with severe combined immunodeficiency [29].

Aloe-emodin pretreatment (2 × 50 mg/kg body weight intraperitoneally) significantly reduced acute liver injury induced by carbon tetrachloride (p<0.05), and changes in hepatic albumin and tumour necrosis factor-α mRNA were normalized (p<0.05) [30].

Pharmacokinetic properties
No pharmacokinetic data have been directly obtained with cascara or its extracts. However, a human pharmacokinetic study using a mixture of aloins and their corresponding 3-rhamnosides (aloinosides A and B) has been reported. In this study, the equivalent of 16.4 mg of hydroxyanthracene derivatives was administered orally for 7 days during which aloe-emodin was detected only sporadically as a metabolite in the plasma, with maximum concentrations of less than 2 ng/ml. In the same study, rhein was detected in the plasma in concentrations ranging from 6 to 28 ng/ml (median c_{max} 13.5 ng/ml at median t_{max} 16 hours) after single dose administration. In the 7-day administration there was no evidence of accumulation of rhein [31].

From another study it was concluded that free anthranoids absorbed systemically in humans are partly excreted in the urine as rhein or as conjugates, even when rhein is not present in the administered drug (as in cascara) [32]. It is not known to what extent aloe-emodin anthrone is absorbed. However, in the case of senna, animal experiments with radio-labelled rheinanthrone administered directly into the caecum have shown that only a very small proportion (less than 10%) of rheinanthrone is absorbed [33].

Systemic metabolism of free anthranoids depends upon their ring constituents [34,35]. In the case of aloe-emodin, it has been shown in animal experiments that at least 20-25% of an oral dose will be absorbed. The bioavailability of aloe-emodin is much lower than the absorption, because it is quickly oxidized to rhein and an unknown metabolite, or conjugated. Maximum plasma values of aloe-emodin were reached 1.5-3 hours after administration. Maximum concentrations in plasma were about 3 times higher than those in ovaries and 10 times higher than those in testes [36].

Oral administration of emodin to rabbits at 10 mg/kg body weight resulted in a very low serum concentration (approximately 2.5 μg/ml). Emodin was found to be highly bound (99.6%) to serum protein [37].

Preclinical safety data

Repeated dose toxicity
No specific data are available for cascara or the cascarosides. Studies with aloin showed low acute and subchronic toxicity in rats and mice [9,38,39]. Aloin at doses of up to 60 mg/kg daily for 20 weeks showed no specific toxic effects in mice [40,41].

Reproductive toxicity
Aloin A at doses of up to 200 mg/kg body weight showed no evidence of any embryolethal, teratogenic or foetotoxic effects in rats [38,42].

Mutagenicity
No specific data are available for cascara or the cascarosides. Data for aloin derived from aloes indicate no genotoxic risk [36,43-48]. Aloe-emodin showed positive and negative results *in vitro* but was clearly negative *in vivo* [49,50]. Emodin was mutagenic in

the Ames test [51,52] but gave inconsistent results in gene mutation assays (V79 HGPRT) [53-55], positive results in the UDS test with primary rat hepatocytes [53] but negative results in the SCE assay [54].

Carcinogenicity
Data on the carcinogenicity of cascara or the cascarosides are not available.

Aloin fed to male NMRI mice in the diet at a level of 100 mg/kg/day for 140 days did not lead to the promotion of colorectal tumours [41].

In a 2-year study, male and female F344/N rats were exposed to 280, 830 or 2500 ppm of emodin in the diet, corresponding to an average daily dose of emodin of 110, 320 or 1000 mg/kg body weight in male rats and 120, 370 or 1100 mg/kg in female rats. No evidence of carcinogenic activity of emodin was observed in male rats. A marginal increase in the incidence of Zymbal's gland carcinoma occurred in female rats treated with the high dosage but was interpreted as questionable [56].

In a further 2-year study, on B6C3F$_1$ mice, males were exposed to 160, 312 or 625 ppm of emodin (corresponding to an average daily dose of 15, 35 or 70 mg/kg body weight) and females to 312, 625 or 1250 ppm of emodin (corresponding to an average daily dose of 30, 60 or 120 mg/kg). There was no evidence of carcinogenic activity in female mice. A low incidence of renal tubule neoplasms in exposed males was not considered relevant [56].

In a case control study with retrospective and prospective evaluation, no causal relationship between anthranoid laxative use and colorectal cancer could be detected [57,58].

Hepatotoxicity
In one case report, cascara was reported to be associated with the development of cholestatic hepatitis, complicated by portal hypertension after intake of 3 × 425 mg of cascara (containing 5% cascarosides) daily for 3 days, but a causal relationship could not be demonstrated [59].

REFERENCES

1. Cascara - Rhamni purshianae cortex. European Pharmacopoeia, Council of Europe.

2. Hänsel R, Keller K, Rimpler H, Schneider G, editors. Rhamnus. In: Hagers Handbuch der Pharmazeutischen Praxis, 5th ed. Volume 6: Drogen P-Z. Berlin: Springer, 1994:392-410.

3. Manitto P, Monti D, Speranza G, Mulinacci N, Vincieri F, Griffini A, Pifferi G. Studies on cascara, Part 2. Structure of cascarosides E and F. J Nat Prod 1995; 58:419-23.

4. USA Department of Health and Human Services: Food and Drug Administration. 21 CFR Part 334. Laxative drug products for over-the-counter human use; Tentative final monograph. Federal Register 1985;50:2124-58.

5. Reynolds JEF, editor. Cascara. In: Martindale - The Extra Pharmacopoeia 31st ed. London: Royal Pharmaceutical Society, 1996:1209,1240-1.

6. Brunton LL. Agents affecting gastrointestinal water flux and motility; emesis and antiemetics; bile acids and pancreatic enzymes. In: Hardman JG, Limbird LE, Molinoff PB, Ruddon RW, Gilman AG, editors. Goodman & Gilman's The Pharmacological Basis of Therapeutics, 9th ed. New York: McGraw-Hill, 1996: 917-36.

7. Steinegger E, Hänsel R. Cascararinde. In: Pharmakognosie, 5th ed. Berlin: Springer, 1992:431-3.

8. Müller-Lissner S. Adverse effects of laxatives: fact and fiction. Pharmacology 1993;47(Suppl 1):138-45.

9. Schmidt L. Vergleichende Pharmakologie und Toxikologie der Laxantien. Arch Exper Path Pharmakol 1955;226:207-18.

10. Westendorf J. Anthranoid derivatives - general discussion. In: De Smet PAGM, Keller K, Hänsel R, Chandler RF, editors. Adverse effects of herbal drugs. Volume 2. Berlin: Springer, 1993:105-18.

11. Faber P, Strenge-Hesse A. Relevance of rhein excretion into breast milk. Pharmacology 1988;36(Suppl 1):212-20.

12. Tedesco FJ. Laxative use in constipation. Am J Gastroenterol 1985;80:303-9.

13. Ewe K, Karbach U. Factitious diarrhoea. Clin Gastroenterol 1986;15:723-40.

14. Fairbairn JW. Chemical structure, mode of action and therapeutical activity of anthraquinone glycosides. Pharm Weekbl Sci Ed 1965;100:1493-9.

15. Fairbairn JW, Moss MJR. The relative purgative activities of 1,8-dihydroxyanthracene derivatives. J Pharm Pharmacol 1970;22:584-93.

16. Dreessen M, Lemli J. Studies in the field of drugs containing anthraquinone derivatives. XXXVI. The metabolism of cascarosides by intestinal bacteria. Pharm Acta Helv 1988;63:287-9.

17. Hattori M, Kanda T, Shu Y-Z, Akao T, Kobashi K, Namba T. Metabolism of barbaloin by intestinal bacteria. Chem Pharm Bull 1988;36:4462-6.

18. Che Q-M, Akao T, Hattori M, Kobashi K, Namba T. Isolation of a human intestinal bacterium capable of transforming barbaloin to aloe-emodin anthrone. Planta Med 1991;57:15-9.

19. Ishii Y, Tanizawa H, Takino Y. Studies on Aloe. III. Mechanism of cathartic effect. Chem Pharm Bull 1990; 38:197-200.

20. Akao T, Che Q-M, Kobashi K, Hattori M, Nama T. A

purgative action of barbaloin is induced by *Eubacterium* sp. strain BAR, a human intestinal anaerobe, capable of transforming barbaloin to aloe-emodin anthrone. Biol Pharm Bull 1996;19:136-8.

21. Ishii Y, Takino Y, Toyooka T, Tanizawa H. Studies of Aloe. VI. Cathartic effect of isobarbaloin. Biol Pharm Bull 1998;21:1226-7.

22. Izzo AA, Sautebin L, Rombolà L, Capasso F. The role of constitutive and inducible nitric oxide synthase in senna- and cascara-induced diarrhoea in the rat. Eur J Pharmacol 1997; 323:93-7.

23. Ewe K. Therapie der Obstipation. Dtsch Med Wschr 1989;114:1924-6.

24. Hönig J, Geck P, Rauwald HW. Inhibition of Cl⁻ channels as a possible base of laxative action of certain anthraquinones and anthrones. Planta Med 1992: 58(Suppl 1):586-7.

25. Rauwald HW, Hönig J, Flindt S, Geck P. Different influence of certain anthraquinones/anthrones on energy metabolism: An approach for interpretation of known synergistic effects in laxative action? Planta Med 1992: 58(Suppl 1):587-8.

26. Ishii Y, Tanizawa H, Takino Y. Studies of Aloe. IV. Mechanism of cathartic effects. (3). Biol Pharm Bull 1994;17:495-7.

27. Ishii Y, Tanizawa H, Takino Y. Studies of Aloe. V. Mechanisms of cathartic effect. Biol Pharm Bull 1994; 17:651-3.

28. Capasso F, Mascolo N, Autore G, Duraccio MR. Effect of indomethacin on aloin and 1,8-dioxianthraquinone-induced production of prostaglandins in rat isolated colon. Prostaglandins 1993;26:557-62.

29. Pecere T, Gazzola MV, Mucignat C, Parolin C, Dalla Vecchia F, Cavaggioni A et al. Aloe-emodin is a new type of anticancer agent with selective activity against neuroectodermal tumors. Cancer Res 2000;60:2800-4.

30. Arosio B, Gagliano N, Fusaro LMP, Parmeggiani L, Taglabue J, Galetti P et al. Aloe-emodin quinone pretreatment reduces acute liver injury induced by carbon tetrachloride. Pharmacol Toxicol (Copenhagen) 2000;87:229-33.

31. Schulz HU. Investigation into the pharmacokinetics of anthranoids after single and multiple oral administration of Laxatan® Dragees (Study in 6 healthy volunteers). Research Report, LAFAA, March 1993.

32. Vyth A, Kamp PE. Detection of anthraquinone laxatives in the urine. Pharm Weekbl Sci Ed 1979;114:456-9.

33. De Witte P, Lemli J. Excretion and distribution of [¹⁴C]rhein and [¹⁴C]rhein anthrone in rat. J Pharm Pharmacol 1988:40:652-5.

34. de Witte P, Lemli J. Metabolism of ¹⁴C-rhein and ¹⁴C-rhein anthrone in rats. Pharmacology 1988;36(Suppl 1): 152-7.

35. Sendelbach LE. A review of the toxicity and carcinogenicity of anthraquinone derivatives. Toxicology 1989;57:227-40.

36. Lang W. Pharmacokinetic-metabolic studies with ¹⁴C-aloe emodin after oral administration to male and female rats. Pharmacology 1993;47(Suppl 1):110-9.

37. Liang JW, Hsiu SL, Wu PP and Chao PDL. Emodin pharmacokinetics in rabbits. Planta Med 1995;61:406-8.

38. Bangel E, Pospisil M, Roetz R, Falk W. Tierexperimentelle pharmakologische Untersuchungen zur Frage der abortiven und teratogenen Wirkung sowie zur Hyperämie von Aloe. Steiner-Informationsdienst 1975; 4:1-25.

39. Nelemans FA. Clinical and toxicological aspects of anthraquinone laxatives. Pharmacology 1976;14(Suppl 1):73-7.

40. Siegers CP, Younes M, Herbst EW. Toxikologische Bewertung anthrachinonhaltiger Laxantien. Z Phytotherapie 1986;7:157-9.

41. Siegers C-P, Siemers J, Baretton G. Sennosides and aloin do not promote dimethylhydrazine-induced colorectal tumors in mice. Pharmacology 1993; 47(Suppl 1): 205-8.

42. Schmähl D. Henk-Pharma; Internal Report, 1975.

43. Bootman J, Hodson-Walker G, Dance C. U.-No. 9482: Assessment of clastogenic action on bone marrow erythrocytes in the micronucleus test. Eye, LSR, Internal Report 1987:87/SIR 004/386.

44. Bootman J, Hodson-Walker G, Dance C. Reinsubstanz 104/5 AA (Barbaloin): Assessment of clastogenic action on bone marrow erythrocytes in the micronucleus test. Eye, LSR, Internal Report 1987: 87/SIR 006/538.

45. CCR, *Salmonella typhimurium* reverse mutation assay with EX AL 15. Rossdorf 1992: Project No. 280416.

46. CCR, Chromosome aberration assay in Chinese hamster ovary (CHO) cells in vitro with EX AL 15. Rossdorf 1992: Project No. 280438.

47. CCR, Gene mutation assay in Chinese hamster V79 cells in vitro with EX AL 15. Rossdorf 1992: Project No. 280427.

48. Marquardt H, Westendorf J, Piasecki A, Ruge A, Westendorf B. Untersuchungen zur Genotoxizität von Bisacodyl, Sennosid A, Sennosid B, Aloin, Aloe-Extrakt. Steiner Internal Report; Hamburg 1987.

49. Heidemann A, Miltenburger HG, Mengs U. The genotoxicity status of senna. Pharmacology 1993; 47(Suppl 1):178-86.

50. Nitz D, Krumbiegel G. Bestimmung von Aloeemodin und Rhein im Serum von Ratte und Maus nach oraler Gabe von Fructus sennae und Aloeemodin. Madaus Report 18.05.1992, unpublished.

51. Brown JP, Brown RJ. Mutagenesis by 9,10-anthra-

quinone derivatives and related compounds in *Salmonella typhimurium*. Mutat Res 1976;40:203-24.

52. Tikkanen L, Matsushima T, Natori S. Mutagenicity of anthraquinones in the *Salmonella* preincubation test. Mutat Res 1983;116:297-304.

53. Westendorf J, Marquardt H, Poginsky B, Dominiak M, Schmidt J, Marquardt H. Genotoxicity of naturally occurring hydroxyanthraquinones. Mutat Res 1990; 240;1-12.

54. Bruggeman IM, van der Hoeven JCM. Lack of activity of the bacterial mutagen emodin in HGPRT and SCE assay with V79 Chinese hamster cells. Mutat Res 1984; 138:219-24.

55. Müllerschön H. Gene mutation assay in Chinese hamster V79 cells in vitro with EX FR10. CCR Report 10.09.1992, unpublished.

56. NTP Technical Report 493. Toxicology and carcinogenesis studies of emodin (CAS No. 518-82-1) in F344/N rats and B6C3F$_1$ mice. NIH Publication No. 99-3952, 1999.

57. Loew D, Bergmann U, Schmidt M, Überla KH. Anthranoidlaxantien. Ursache für Kolonkarzinom? Dtsch Apoth Ztg 1994;134:3180-3.

58. Loew D. Pseudomelanosis coli durch Anthranoide. Z Phytotherapie 1994;16:312-8.

59. Nadir A, Reddy D, Van Thiel DH. Cascara sagrada-induced intrahepatic cholestasis causing portal hypertension: case report and review of herbal hepatotoxicity. Am J Gastroenterol 2000;95:3634-7.

RHEI RADIX

Rhubarb

DEFINITION

Rhubarb consists of the whole or cut, dried underground parts of *Rheum palmatum* L. or of *Rheum officinale* Baillon or of hybrids of these two species or of a mixture. The underground parts are often divided; the stem and most of the bark with the rootlets are removed. It contains not less than 2.2 per cent of hydroxyanthracene derivatives, expressed as rhein ($C_{15}H_8O_6$; M_r 284.2), calculated with reference to the dried drug.

The material complies with the monograph of the European Pharmacopoeia [1].

CONSTITUENTS

The main active constituents are hydroxyanthracene derivatives (3-12%, depending on the method of determination) consisting mainly (60-80%) of mono- and diglucosides of rhein, chrysophanol, aloe-emodin, physcion and emodin, and only small amounts of the respective aglycones. Dianthrone glycosides (sennosides) are also present and small amounts of anthrone glycosides depending on the time of harvesting and the conditions of drying [2-6].

Other constituents include gallotannins (ca. 5%) [4-7], chromones, phenylbutanones and traces of volatile oil [5,6,8].

CLINICAL PARTICULARS

Therapeutic indications
For short-term use in cases of occasional constipation [7,9-11].

Posology and method of administration

Dosage

The correct individual dose is the smallest required to produce a comfortable soft-formed motion.

Adults and children over 10 years: drug or preparations equivalent to 15-50 mg of hydroxyanthracene derivatives (calculated as rhein) daily, preferably taken in one dose at night [6,10,11].

Not recommended for use in children under 10 years of age.

The pharmaceutical form must allow lower dosages.

E/S/C/O/P
MONOGRAPHS
Second Edition

419

Method of administration
For oral administration.

Duration of administration
Stimulant laxatives should not be used for periods of more than 2 weeks without medical advice.

Contra-indications
Pregnancy and lactation; children under 10 years of age [6].

Not to be used in cases of intestinal obstruction and stenosis, atony, inflammatory colon diseases (e.g. Crohn's disease, ulcerative colitis), appendicitis, abdominal pain of unknown origin [6]; severe dehydration states with electrolyte depletion.

Special warnings and special precautions for use
As for all laxatives, rhubarb should not be given when any undiagnosed acute or persistent abdominal symptoms are present.

If laxatives are needed every day the cause of the constipation should be investigated. Long term use of laxatives should be avoided. Use for more than 2 weeks requires medical supervision. Chronic use may cause pigmentation of the colon (pseudo-melanosis coli) which is harmless and reversible after drug discontinuation. Abuse, resulting in loss of fluid and electrolytes, may cause [12]: dependence with possible need for increased dosages; disturbance of the water and electrolyte (mainly hypokalaemia) balance; an atonic colon with impaired function. Intake of anthranoid-containing laxatives for more than a short period of time may result in aggravation of constipation. Hypokalaemia can result in cardiac and neuromuscular dysfunction, especially if cardiac glycosides, diuretics or corticosteroids are taken. Chronic use may result in albuminuria and haematuria.

In chronic constipation, stimulant laxatives are not an acceptable alternative to a change in diet.

Note: A detailed text with advice concerning changes in dietary habits, physical activities and training for normal bowel evacuation should be included on the package leaflet. An example is given in the booklet "Médicaments á base de plantes" published by the French health authority (Paris: Agence du Médicament).

Interaction with other medicaments and other forms of interaction
Hypokalaemia (resulting from long term laxative abuse) potentiates the action of cardiac glycosides and interacts with anti-arrhythmic drugs or with drugs which induce reversion to sinus rhythm (e.g. quinidine). Concomitant use with other drugs inducing hypokalaemia (e.g. thiazide diuretics, adreno-corticosteroids and liquorice root) may aggravate electrolyte imbalance.

Pregnancy and lactation

Pregnancy
Not recommended during pregnancy.
There are no reports of undesirable or damaging effects during pregnancy or on the foetus when used in accordance with the recommended dosage schedule. However, experimental data concerning a genotoxic risk from several anthranoids (e.g. emodin) are not counterbalanced by sufficient studies to eliminate a possible risk.

Lactation
Breast-feeding is not recommended as there are insufficient data on the excretion of metabolites in breast milk. Excretion of active principles in breast milk has not been investigated. However, small amounts of active metabolites (e.g. rhein) from other anthranoids are known to be excreted in breast milk. A laxative effect in breast-fed babies has not been reported [13].

Effects on ability to drive and use machines
None known.

Undesirable effects
Abdominal spasms and pain, in particular in patients with irritable colon; yellow or red-brown (pH dependent) discoloration of urine by metabolites, which is not clinically significant [14-16].

Overdose
The major symptoms are griping and severe diarrhoea with consequent losses of fluid and electrolyte, which should be replaced.

Treatment should be supportive with generous amounts of fluid. Electrolytes, especially potassium, should be monitored; this is particularly important in the elderly and the young.

PHARMACOLOGICAL PROPERTIES

Pharmacodynamic properties

1,8-dihydroxyanthracene derivatives possess a laxative effect [12,17]. The β-linked glucosides in rhubarb are not absorbed in the upper gut; they are converted by the bacteria of the large intestine into active metabolites (anthrones).

Based on experimental studies and studies in humans with Tinnevelly senna pods and isolated sennosides, two distinct mechanisms of action are assumed [18]:

(i) an influence on the motility of the large intestine (stimulation of peristaltic contractions and inhibition of local contractions) resulting in accelerated colonic transit, thus reducing fluid absorption [19,20], and

(ii) an influence on secretion processes (stimulation of mucus and active chloride secretion) resulting in enhanced fluid secretion [18,21].

Defecation takes place after a delay of 8-12 hours due to the time taken for transport to the colon and metabolic conversion of hydroxyanthracene glycosides to the active compounds.

In vitro experiments
Methanolic extracts from *Rheum palmatum* and *Rheum officinale* showed radical scavenging activity, reducing 40 µM α,α-diphenyl-β-picrylhydrazyl (DPPH) radical by 50% at concentrations of 5.2 and 3.3 µg/ml respectively. IC_{50} values on superoxide anion radical in the xanthine/xanthine oxidase system were 5.0 and 3.8 µg/ml [22]. Pyrogallol autoxidation and hydroxyl radicals generated via the Fenton reaction were inhibited by anthraquinones from rhubarb [23].

A hot water extract of rhubarb inhibited rat squalene epoxidase, an enzyme that catalyzes a rate-limiting step of cholesterol biosynthesis, by 70% at a concentration of 50 µg/ml; several galloyl compounds isolated from rhubarb were found to be potent inhibitors of the enzyme [24].

Bioassay-guided fractionation of an ethyl acetate extract from rhubarb showed emodin to be a selective inhibitor of casein kinase II with an IC_{50} of 2 µM [25].

In an agar plate assay, strong inhibition of *Helicobacter pylori* was observed with a water extract of rhubarb (MIC < 1 mg) [26]. An ethanolic extract of rhubarb inhibited *Helicobacter pylori* growth with a MIC of 17.24 µg/ml; in this test the MICs of anthraquinone compounds isolated from rhubarb were 0.40 µg/ml (emodin), 0.60 µg/ml (rhein), 0.78 µg/ml (chrysophanol) and 0.85 µg/ml (aloe-emodin) [27].

An ethanolic extract of rhubarb exhibited antiviral activity against *Herpes simplex* by preventing virus attachment and penetration [28].

The antimycotic activity of an aqueous extract of rhubarb against *Aspergillus fumigatus* and *Candida albicans* was comparable to that of nystatin. The growth of *Geotrichum candidum* and *Rhodotorula rubra* was inhibited to a lesser extent [29].

Rhein isolated from rhubarb showed strong antibacterial properties against *Candida albicans* and *Bacteroides fragilis* [30].

Methanolic extracts from *Rheum palmatum* and *Rheum officinalis* rhizomes significantly (p<0.01)

enhanced proliferation of the oestrogen-sensitive MCF-7 cell line at concentrations of 100 and 30 µg/ml, respectively. This effect was mainly attributed to emodin and emodin-8-O-β-D-glucoside, which bound to human oestrogen receptors α and β [31].

Several phenolic compounds from rhubarb showed cytotoxicity against human oral squamous cell carcinoma and salivary gland tumor cell lines as well as human gingival fibroblasts [32]. Aloe-emodin induced apoptotic cell death in human lung squamous cell carcinoma [33].

In vivo experiments
In rats with adenine-induced chronic renal failure a hot water extract from rhubarb decreased levels of urea nitrogen and creatinine in serum, as well as the hepatic urea concentration, in a dose-dependent manner. The effects were significant at doses of 15 and 35 mg/rat/day (p<0.01 to p<0.05) and 55 mg/rat/day (p<0.001). Hypocalcaemia and hyperphosphataemia and the concentrations of guanidino compounds in the serum, liver and kidney were improved. Proanthocyanidin oligomers were shown to be the active substances [34,35].

Rats with streptozotocin-induced diabetic nephropathy were treated orally with 125 mg/kg body weight/day of a hot water extract of rhubarb (drug to extract ratio 4:1) over a period of 80 days. At the end of the experimental period treated animals showed decreases in blood glucose levels, serum triglycerides and total cholesterol, and increases in urinary excretion of urea nitrogen and creatinine. All the changes were significant (p<0.01) compared to untreated controls [36].

A hot water extract from rhubarb was administered orally to rats after subtotal nephrectomy (SN) at a dose of 150 mg/day from day 30 to day 120. The treated animals had significantly less proteinuria (p<0.05) compared to untreated SN controls on days 90 and 120 after SN. Renal function was similar in the two groups, but the severity of glomerulosclerosis was significantly reduced by the treatment (p<0.5) [37].

Anti-inflammatory activity of rhubarb was demonstrated in 12-O-tetradecanoylphorbol-13-acetate (TPA)-induced mouse ear oedema. After single or multiple topical application of TPA, an extract (50% ethanol, drug to extract ratio 3:1) applied topically at 0.5 mg/ear led to significant inhibition of oedema (p<0.01). Increased myeloperoxidase activity in the tissue after multiple application of TPA was significantly reduced by the extract (p<0.01) [38].

Pharmacokinetic properties
No systematic data are available on rhubarb. It is assumed that aglycones present in the drug are

absorbed in the upper gut, but that (by analogy with sennosides from senna) the β-linked glucosides are neither absorbed in the upper gut nor split by human digestive enzymes. They are converted by the bacteria of the large intestine into aglycones and subsequently to the active compounds, the anthrones [39].

In rat liver microsomes emodin was metabolized to 6-hydroxyaloe-emodin and 2-hydroxyemodin, and chrysophanol was converted to aloe-emodin [40].

Preclinical safety data

There are no studies on single dose toxicity, repeated dose toxicity, reproductive toxicity or *in vivo* tests on carcinogenicity of rhubarb or preparations from it. In the *Salmonella* microsome assay an ethanolic extract of rhubarb showed mutagenic effects against *S. typhimurium* strain TA 1537 [41]. Some isolated anthraquinones (aloe-emodin, emodin, physcion and chrysophanol) gave positive results in *in vitro* genotoxicity studies [42-45]. All *in vivo* genotoxicity studies were negative [44-46]. Sennosides A and B and rhein gave negative results in *in vitro* and *in vivo* mutagenicity tests [45,47].

In a 2-year study, male and female F344/N rats were exposed to 280, 830 or 2500 ppm of emodin in the diet, corresponding to an average daily dose of emodin of 110, 320 or 1000 mg/kg body weight in male rats and 120, 370 or 1100 mg/kg body weight in female rats. No evidence of carcinogenic activity of emodin was observed in male rats. A marginal increase in the incidence of Zymbal's gland carcinoma occurred in female rats treated with the high dosage but was interpreted as questionable [48].

In a further 2-year study, on B6C3F$_1$ mice, males were exposed to 160, 312 or 625 ppm of emodin (corresponding to an average daily dose of 15, 35 or 70 mg/kg body weight) and females to 312, 625 or 1250 ppm of emodin (corresponding to an average daily dose of 30, 60 or 120 mg/kg body weight). There was no evidence of carcinogenic activity in female mice. A low incidence of renal tubule neoplasms in exposed males was not considered relevant [48].

Clinical safety data

Despite a lack of formal preclinical data on rhubarb, epidemiological studies suggest that there is no carcinogenic risk to humans from the use of anthranoid laxatives [49-55].

REFERENCES

1. Rhubarb - Rhei radix. European Pharmacopoeia, Council of Europe.

2. van Os FHL. Anthraquinone derivatives in vegetable laxatives. Pharmacology 1976;14 (Suppl. 1):7-17.

3. Chirikdjian JJ, Kopp B, Beran H. Über die laxative Wirkung eines neuen Anthrachinonglykosides aus Radix Rhei. Planta Med 1983;48:34-7.

4. Engelshowe R. Rhabarber: eine alte Droge - noch immer aktuell. Pharm unserer Zeit 1985;14:40-9.

5. Hänsel R, Sticher O, Steinegger E. Rhabarberwurzel. In: Pharmakognosie-Phytopharmazie, 6th ed. Berlin-Heidelberg: Springer-Verlag, 1999: 921-3.

6. Hänsel R, Keller K, Rimpler H, Schneider G, editors. Rheum. In: Hagers Handbuch der Pharmazeutischen Praxis, 5th ed. Volume 6: Drogen P-Z. Berlin-Heidelberg: Springer-Verlag, 1994:411-39.

7. Weiß RF. Rheum, Rhabarber. In: Lehrbuch der Phytotherapie. 6th ed. Stuttgart: Hippokrates Verlag, 1990:142-4.

8. Miyazawa M, Minamino Y, Kameoka H. Volatile components of the rhizomes of *Rheum palmatum* L. Flavour Fragr J 1996;11:57-60.

9. Reynolds JEF, editor. Rhubarb. In: Martindale - The Extra Pharmacopoeia, 31st ed. London: Royal Pharmaceutical Society, 1996:1239-40.

10. Wichtl M, editor. Rhabarber. In: Teedrogen und Phytopharmaka, 3rd ed. Stuttgart: Wissenschaftliche Verlagsgesellschaft, 1997:492-6.

11. Schilcher H, Kammerer S. Rhabarberwurzel. In: Leitfaden Phytotherapie. München-Jena: Fischer Verlag, 2000:188-9.

12. Leng-Peschlow E. Senna and its rational use. Pharmacology 1992;44(Suppl 1):1-52.

13. Faber P, Strenge-Hesse A. Relevance of rhein excretion into breast milk. Pharmacology 1988; 36(Suppl 1):212-20.

14. Cooke WT. Laxative abuse. Clin Gastroenterol 1977; 6:659-73.

15. Tedesco FJ. Laxative use in constipation. Am J Gastroenterol 1985;80:303-9.

16. Ewe K, Karbach U. Factitious diarrhoea. Clin Gastroenterol 1986;15:723-40.

17. Fairbairn JW, Moss MJR. The relative purgative activities of 1,8-dihydroxyanthracene derivatives. J Pharm Pharmacol 1970;22:584-93.

18. Leng-Peschlow E. Dual effect of orally administered sennosides on large intestine transit and fluid absorption in the rat. J Pharm Pharmacol 1986;38:606-10.

19. Garcia-Villar R, Leng-Peschlow E, Ruckebusch Y. Effect of anthraquinone derivatives on canine and rat intestinal motility. J Pharm Pharmacol 1980;32:323-9.

20. Bueno L, Fioramonti J, Frexinos J, Ruckebusch Y. Colonic myoelectrical activity in diarrhea and

constipation. Hepato-Gastroenterology 1980; 27:381-9.

21. Leng-Peschlow E. Effects of sennosides A + B and bisacodyl on rat large intestine. Pharmacology 1989; 38:310-8.

22. Matsuda H, Morikawa T, Toguchida I, Park J-Y, Harima S, Yoshikawa M. Antioxidant constituents from rhubarb: structural requirements of stilbenes for the activity and structures of two new anthraquinone glucosides. Bioorg Med Chem 2001;9:41-50

23. Yuan Z, Gao R. Anti-oxidant actions of anthraquinolines contained in *Rheum*. Pharm Pharmacol Lett 1997;7:9-12.

24. Abe I, Seki T, Noguchi H, Kashiwada Y. Galloyl esters from rhubarb are potent inhibitors of squalene epoxidase, a key enzyme in cholesterol biosynthesis. Planta Med 2000;66:753-6.

25. Yim H, Lee YH, Lee CH, Lee SK. Emodin, an anthraquinone derivative isolated from the rhizomes of *Rheum palmatum*, selectively inhibits the activity of casein kinase II as a competitive inhibitor. Planta Med 1999; 65:9-13.

26. Bae EA, Han MJ, Kim NJ, Kim DH. Anti-*Helicobacter pylori* activity of herbal medicines. Biol Pharm Bull 1998;21:990-2.

27. Gou K, Sun L, Lou W, Ling C, Wang Y. Four compounds of anthraquinone in *Rheum officinale* on *Helicobacter pylori* inhibition. Zhongguo Yaoxue Zazhi (Beijing) 1997;32:278-80.

28. Hsiang CY, Hsieh CL, Wu SL, Lai IL, Ho TY. Inhibitory effect of anti-pyretic and anti-inflammatory herbs on *Herpes simplex* virus replication. Am J Chin Med 2001; 29:459-67.

29. Blaszczyk T, Krzyzanowska J, Lamer-Zarawska E. Screening for antimycotic properties of 56 traditional Chinese drugs. Phytother Res 2000;14:210-2.

30. Cyong J-C, Matsumoto T, Arakawa K, Kiyohara H, Yamada H, Otsuka Y. Anti-*Bacteroides fragilis* substance from rhubarb. J Ethnopharmacol 1987;19:279-83.

31. Matsuda H, Shimoda H, Morikawa T, Yoshikawa M. Phytoestrogens from the roots of *Polygonum cuspidatum* (Polygonaceae): structure-requirement of hydroxy-anthraquinones for estrogenic activity. Bioorg Med Chem Lett 2001;11:1839-42.

32. Shi Y-Q, Fukai T, Sakagami H, Kuroda J, Miyaoka R, Tamura M et al. Cytotoxic and DNA damage-inducing activities of low molecular weight phenols from rhubarb. Anticancer Res 2001;21:2847-54.

33. Lee H-Z, Hsu S-L, Liu M-C, Wu C-H. Effects and mechanisms of aloe-emodin on cell death in human lung squamous cell carcinoma. Eur J Pharmacol 2001; 431:287-95.

34. Yokozawa T, Suzuki N, Oura H, Nonaka G-I, Nishioka I. Effect of extracts obtained from rhubarb in rats with

chronic renal failure. Chem Pharm Bull 1986;34:4718-23.

35. Yokozawa T, Suzuki N, Zheng PD, Oura H, Nishioka I. Effect of orally administered rhubarb extract in rats with chronic renal failure. Chem Pharm Bull 1984; 32:4506-13.

36. Yokozawa T, He L-Q, Muto Y, Nagasaki R, Hattori M, Oura H. Effects of rhubarb extract in rats with diabetic nephropathy. Phytother Res 1997;11:73-5.

37. Zhang G, El Nahas AM. The effect of rhubarb extract on experimental renal fibrosis. Nephrol Dial Transplant 1996;11:186-90.

38. Cuéllar MJ, Giner RM, Recio MC, Mánez S, Ríos JL. Topical anti-inflammatory activity of some Asian medicinal plants used in dermatological disorders. Fitoterapia 2001;72:221-9.

39. Kobashi K, Nishimura T, Kusaka M, Hattori M, Namba T. Metabolism of sennosides by human intestinal bacteria. Planta Med 1980;40:225-36.

40. Mueller SO, Stopper H, Dekant W. Biotransformation of the anthraquinones emodin and chrysophanol by cytochrome P450 enzymes. Bioactivation to genotoxic metabolites. Drug Metab Dispos 1998;26:540-6.

41. Paneitz A, Westendorf J. Anthranoid contents of rhubarb (*Rheum undulatum* L.) and other *Rheum* species and their toxicological relevance. Eur Food Res Technol 1999;210:97-101.

42. Westendorf J, Marquardt H, Poginsky B, Dominiak M, Schmidt J, Marquardt H. Genotoxicity of naturally occurring hydroxyanthraquinones. Mutat Res 1990; 240:1-12.

43. Bruggeman IM, van der Hoeven JCM. Lack of activity of the bacterial mutagen emodin in HGPRT and SCE assay with V79 Chinese hamster cells. Mutat Res 1984;138:219-24.

44. Heidemann A, Völkner W, Mengs U. Genotoxicity of aloeemodin in vitro and in vivo. Mutat Res 1996; 367:123-33.

45. Heidemann A, Miltenburger HG, Mengs U. The genotoxicity status of senna. Pharmacology 1993;47 (Suppl 1):178-86.

46. Mengs U, Krumbiegel G, Völkner W. Lack of emodin genotoxicity in the mouse micronucleus assay. Mutat Res 1997;393:289-93.

47. Mengs U, Heidemann A. Genotoxicity of sennosides and rhein in vitro and in vivo. Med Sci Res 1993;21:749-50.

48. NTP Technical Report 493. Toxicology and carcinogenesis studies of emodin (CAS No. 518-82-1) in F344/N rats and B6C3F$_1$ mice. NIH Publication No. 99-3952, 1999.

49. Siegers C-P, von Hertzberg-Lottin E, Otte M, Schneider B. Anthranoid laxative abuse - a risk for colorectal

cancer? Gut 1993;34:1099-101.

50. Nusko G, Schneider B, Müller G, Kusche J, Hahn EG. Retrospective study on laxative use and melanosis coli as risk factors for colorectal neoplasma. Pharmacology 1993;47 (Suppl 1):234-41.

51. Sonnenberg A, Müller AD. Constipation and cathartics as risk factors of colorectal cancer: A meta-analysis. Pharmacology 1993;47 (Suppl 1):224-33.

52. Kune GA. Laxative use not a risk for colorectal cancer: data from the Melbourne colorectal cancer study. Z Gastroenterol 1993;31:140-3.

53. Kune GA. Causes and control of colorectal cancer. Boston-Dordrecht-London: Kluwer Academic, 1996: 179-90.

54. Loew D, Bergmann U, Dirschedl P, Schmidt M, Melching K, Hues B, Überla K. Retro- und prospektive Fall-Kontroll-Studien zu Anthranoidlaxanzien. In: Loew D, Rietbrock N, editors. Phytopharmaka II. Forschung und klinische Anwendung. Darmstadt: Steinkopff, 1996:175-84.

55. Loew D, Bergmann U, Dirschedl P, Schmidt M, Überla KH. Anthranoidlaxanzien. Dtsch Apoth Ztg 1997; 137:2088-92.

RIBIS NIGRI FOLIUM

Blackcurrant Leaf

E/S/C/O/P
MONOGRAPHS
Second Edition

DEFINITION

Blackcurrant leaf consists of the dried leaves of *Ribes nigrum* L. It contains not less than 1.5 per cent of flavonoids, expressed as rutin ($C_{27}H_{30}O_{16} \cdot 3H_2O$; M_r 665) and calculated with reference to the dried drug.

The material complies with the monograph of the Pharmacopée Française [1].

Fresh material may also be used, provided that when dried it complies with the monograph of the Pharmacopée Française.

CONSTITUENTS

Characteristic constituents are: mono- and di-glycosides of quercetin and kaempferol, mainly isoquercitrin and rutin [2-4]; a flavanone, sakuranetin [5]; monomeric flavanols (mainly gallocatechin and epigallocatechin) [6-8]; proanthocyanidins [6-9], especially di- and trimeric prodelphinidins [7-9]; hydroxycinnamic acid derivatives including chlorogenic, caffeic and *p*-coumaric acids [4]; and traces of essential oil [10,11].

CLINICAL PARTICULARS

Therapeutic indications
Adjuvant in the treatment of rheumatic conditions [11-16].

Posology and method of administration

Dosage

Adults: Dried leaf as an infusion (20-50 g/litre, infused for 15 minutes), 250-500 ml daily [12-14]; fluid extract (1:1), 5 ml twice daily, taken before meals [12-15].

Method of administration
For oral administration.

Duration of administration
No restriction.

Contra-indications
None known.

Special warnings and special precautions for use
None required.

Interaction with other medicaments and other forms of interaction

None reported.
Blackcurrant leaf has a diuretic action [11,12,14], therefore it should not be taken concurrently with diuretics indicated for cardiac or renal insufficiency except on medical advice.

Pregnancy and lactation

No data available.
In accordance with general medical practice, the product should not be used during pregnancy or lactation without medical advice.

Effects on ability to drive and use machines

None known.

Undesirable effects

None reported.

Overdose

No toxic effects reported.

PHARMACOLOGICAL PROPERTIES

Pharmacodynamic properties

In vitro experiments

Effects on biosynthesis and release of prostaglandins
A purified flavonoid extract obtained from blackcurrant leaf inhibited the biosynthesis and release of prostaglandins (IC_{30}: 1.03 mg/ml flavonoids) in isolated perfused rabbit heart. The flavonoid extract was 2.2 and 3.6 times more effective than isoquercitrin and rutin respectively [17].

Antioxidant effects
Antioxidant properties of methanolic crude extracts from fresh blackcurrant leaf (2.4 g in 50 ml) of three different varieties were demonstrated by measuring the inhibition of lipid oxidation induced in rat liver microsomes by ferrous sulfate-ADP-ascorbic acid (IC_{50}: 6.44-7.29 µl of methanolic extract per ml) or by t-butyl hydroperoxide (IC_{50}: 8.63-9.31 µl of methanolic extract per ml) [18].

In vivo experiments

Anti-inflammatory effects
A 14%-ethanolic extract from blackcurrant leaf (60 g per litre), administered orally at 1 and 10 ml/kg body weight, produced dose-dependent anti-inflammatory effects corresponding respectively to 30% and 54% reductions in carrageenan-induced rat paw oedema compared to controls. Comparable activities were observed with reference substances: indometacin produced 63% reduction at 2.5 mg/kg and 66% at 5 mg/kg; niflumic acid produced 19% reduction at 25

mg/kg and 70% at 50 mg/kg. 21-day oral treatment with the extract reduced oedema compared to control animals by 30% at 0.33 ml/kg, 42.5% at 1 ml/kg and 46% at 10 ml/kg, the last being statistically identical with the activities of indometacin at 1.66 mg/kg (49% reduction) and niflumic acid at 12.5 mg/kg (53% reduction). 21-day oral treatment with a lyophilizate of the 14%-ethanolic extract (1 g of lyophilizate equivalent to 30 ml of extract or 1.8 g of leaf) gave an ED_{50} of 0.67 g/kg for the lyophilizate compared to 0.43 mg/kg for indometacin. The efficacy of the blackcurrant leaf extract was apparent in both the proliferative and exudative phases of inflammation [19].

A lyophilizate prepared after maceration of blackcurrant leaf (100 g/litre) in 15% ethanol for 10 days at 20°C and administered intraperitoneally to rats exhibited potent anti-inflammatory activity in comparison with controls [20]. In the carrageenan-induced rat paw oedema test at 50 and 100 mg/kg body weight, the lyophilizate produced dose-dependent inhibition of inflammation (p<0.01), its effect at 100 mg/kg (70% inhibition) being similar to that of indometacin at 5 mg/kg (77% inhibition). In the cotton pellet-induced granuloma test, the lyophilizate at 150 mg/kg reduced inflammation by 18.6%, comparable to the 24% reduction with indometacin at 3 mg/kg. In the Freund adjuvant-induced arthritis test, the lyophilizate produced a dose-dependent reduction in inflammation of 18.7% at 150 mg/kg and 34.6% at 300 mg/kg, the latter being statistically identical to the 37.7% reduction obtained with indometacin at 3 mg/kg [20].

Prodelphinidins isolated from blackcurrant leaf, administered intraperitoneally, had a dose-dependent anti-inflammatory effect in the carrageenan-induced rat paw oedema model: 18%, 40% and 55% reductions in inflammation with 5, 10 and 40 mg/kg respectively. In a similar experiment, a crude aqueous extract from blackcurrant leaf produced 57% inhibition at 60 mg/kg, comparable to 44% with indometacin at 4 mg/kg and 47% with aspirin at 200 mg/kg [8].

Analgesic effects
A lyophilizate prepared after maceration of blackcurrant leaf (100 g/litre) in 15% ethanol for 10 days exhibited potent analgesic activity, which may be of peripheral origin, in the acetic acid-induced writhing test after single dose intraperitoneal administration to mice. The lyophilizate had an ED_{50} of 61.5 mg/kg and a therapeutic index (LD_{50}/ED_{50}) of 17.7. Paracetamol (acetaminophen) administered to the control group gave a higher ED_{50} of 132 mg/kg and a lower therapeutic index of 3.8 [20].

Diuretic activity
A fluid extract (1:1) of blackcurrant leaf showed a salidiuretic action (diuretic quotient 1.56) in rats

when administered orally at a dose equivalent to 1500 mg dried leaf/kg; this was similar to the effect of furosemide at 50 mg/kg (diuretic quotient 1.52) [21].

The potassium-sodium ratios in blackcurrant leaf and blackcurrant leaf decoction were found to be 128:1 and 242:1 respectively, which may contribute to a diuretic effect [22].

Antihypertensive effects
A fluid extract (1:1) of blackcurrant leaf had an anti-hypertensive effect on cats, with an antihypertensive quotient of 1.82 at an oral dose equivalent to 400 mg dried leaf/kg, the effect lasting for 15-20 minutes; tolazoline had comparable antihypertensive quotients, 1.69 at 0.75 mg/kg and 2.12 at 1.0 mg/kg, but the effect lasted for only 5 minutes [21].

An infusion of blackcurrant leaf (20 g/litre), administered intravenously to normotensive rats at a dose equivalent to 360 mg dried leaf/kg body weight, produced a rapid fall of 45% in arterial blood pressure and the decrease was still 30% after 30 minutes [23].

Pharmacokinetic properties
No data available.

Preclinical safety data
A lyophilized 14%-ethanolic extract (1 g of lyophilizate equivalent to 1.8 g of blackcurrant leaf), administered orally to rats at 2 g/kg/day for 21 days or 1.34 g/kg/day for 28 days, revealed no signs of toxicity and no gastric ulceration was observed [19].

Rats treated orally for 28 days with a lyophilizate prepared after maceration of blackcurrant leaf (100 g/litre) in 15% ethanol for 10 days had no gastric ulceration. Compared to control animals no changes were apparent in food and fluid consumption or body weight, nor in results from blood analysis and histopathological evaluation of 14 different organs. In an acute toxicity study of the same lyophilizate in mice, the intraperitoneal LD_{50} was 1.09 g/kg; oral doses up to 3 g/kg showed no overt toxicity [20].

The intraperitoneal LD_0 and LD_{50} values of a blackcurrant leaf fluid extract (1:1) in mice were 22 and 49 g/kg respectively [21].

REFERENCES

1. Cassis (feuille de) - Ribis nigri folium. Pharmacopée Française.

2. Calamita O, Malinowski J, Strzelecka H. Flavonoid compounds of black currant leaves (*Ribes nigrum* L.). Acta Polon Pharm 1983;40:383-7.

3. Trajkovski V. Resistance to *Sphaerotheca mors-uvae* (Schw.) Berk. in *Ribes nigrum* L. 3. Identification by thin-layer chromatography of flavonoids in varieties of *Ribes nigrum*. Swedish J Agric Res 1974;4:99-108.

4. Trajkovski V. Resistance to *Sphaerotheca mors-uvae* (Schw.) Berk. in *Ribes nigrum* L. 4. Developmental changes in phenolic compounds in leaves of *Ribes nigrum*. Swedish J Agric Res 1974;4:143-50.

5. Atkinson P, Blakeman JP. Seasonal occurrence of an antimicrobial flavanone, sakuranetin, associated with glands on leaves of *Ribes nigrum*. New Phytol 1982; 92:63-74.

6. Buzun GA, Dzhemukhadze KM, Mileshko LF. *Ortho*-diphenoloxidases and catechins of plants. Fiziologiya Rastenii 1978;25:1185-90, as English translation in Russian Plant Physiol 1978;25:937-41.

7. Tits M, Angenot L, Poukens P, Warin R, Dierckxsens Y. Prodelphinidins from *Ribes nigrum*. Phytochemistry 1992;31:971-3.

8. Tits M, Poukens P, Angenot L, Dierckxsens Y. Thin-layer chromatographic analysis of proanthocyanidins from *Ribes nigrum* leaves. J Pharmaceut Biomed Anal 1992;10:1097-100.

9. Tits M, Angenot L, Damas J, Dierckxsens Y, Poukens P. Anti-inflammatory prodelphinidins from black currant (*Ribes nigrum*) leaves. Planta Med 1991;57(Suppl. 2):A 134.

10. Andersson J, Bosvik R, von Sydow E. The composition of the essential oil of black currant leaves (*Ribes nigrum* L.). J Sci Food Agric 1963;14:834-40.

11. Hänsel R, Keller K, Rimpler H, Schneider G, editors. Ribes. In: Hagers Handbuch der Pharmazeutischen Praxis, 5th ed. Volume 6: Drogen P-Z. Berlin: Springer-Verlag, 1994:466-74.

12. Fiches de documentation de pratique officinale: Cassis, *Ribes nigrum* L. Pharmacopée Française, 9th ed. 1978.

13. Leclerc H. Cassis (*Ribes nigrum* L.). Synonyme: Gros-eillier noir (Ribésiacées). In: Précis de phytothérapie, 5th ed. Paris: Masson, 1983:75-6.

14. Wichtl M. Ribis nigri folium - Schwarze Johannis-beerblätter. In: Wichtl M, editor. Teedrogen und Phytopharmaka, 4th ed. Stuttgart: Wissenschaftliche Verlagsgesellschaft, 2002:516-8.

15. Decaux F. La feuille de cassis dans le traitement des manifestations de l'arthritisme. Le Courrier Médical 1930:77-9.

16. Garnier G, Bezanger-Beauquesne L, Debraux G. Ribésiacées. *Ribes nigrum* L. - Cassis. In : Ressources médicinales de la flore Française. Paris: Vigot Frères 1961:707-8.

17. Pham Huu Chanh, Ifansyah N, Chahine R, Mounayar-Chalfoun A, Gleye J, Moulis C. Comparative effects of total flavonoids extracted from *Ribes nigrum* leaves,

rutin and isoquercitrin on biosynthesis and release of prostaglandins in the ex-vivo rabbit heart. Prostagland Leukotr Med 1986;22:295-300.

18. Costantino L, Rastelli G, Rossi T, Bertoldi M, Albasini A. Activité antilipoperoxydante d'extraits poly-phénoliques de Ribes nigrum L. Plantes Méd Phytothér 1993;26:207-14.

19. Declume C. Anti-inflammatory evaluation of a hydro-alcoholic extract of black currant leaves (Ribes nigrum). J Ethnopharmacol 1989;27:91-8.

20. Mongold JJ, Susplugas P, Taillade C, Serrano JJ. Anti-inflammatory activity of Ribes nigrum leaf extract in rats. Plantes Méd Phytothér 1993;26:109-16.

21. Rácz-Kotilla E, Rácz G. Salidiuretische und hypotensive Wirkung der Auszüge von Ribes Blättern. Planta Med 1977;32:110-4.

22. Szentmihályi K, Kéry A, Then M, Lakatos B, Sándor Z, Vinkler P. Potassium-sodium ratio for the character-ization of medicinal plant extracts with diuretic activity. Phytother Res 1998;12:163-6.

23. Lasserre B, Kaiser R, Pham Huu Chanh, Ifansyah N, Gleye J, Moulis C. Effects on rats of aqueous extracts of plants used in folk medicine as antihypertensive agents. Naturwissenschaften 1983;70:95-6.

ROSMARINI FOLIUM

Rosemary Leaf

DEFINITION

Rosemary leaf consists of the whole, dried leaves of *Rosmarinus officinalis* L. It contains not less than 12 ml/kg of essential oil and not less than 3 per cent of total hydroxycinnamic derivatives expressed as rosmarinic acid ($C_{18}H_{16}O_8$; M_r 360), both calculated with respect to the anhydrous drug.

The material complies with the monograph of the European Pharmacopoeia [1].

CONSTITUENTS

1-2.5% V/m of essential oil [2,3], the composition of which may vary according to the chemotype or other factors [2,4-7]. Characteristic components of the oil are: 1,8-cineole (20-50%), α-pinene (15-26%), camphor (10-25%), bornyl acetate (1-5%), borneol (1-6%), camphene (5-10%) and α-terpineol (12-24%) [1-5,8-16]. Limonene, β-pinene, β-caryophyllene and myrcene are also present in the oil [5,8,11-13,15,16].

Other characteristic constituents are phenolic diterpenes such as carnosol (up to 4.6%), carnos(ol)ic acid, rosmanol, isorosmanol, epirosmanol and rosmaridiphenol [2,3,17-25]; rosmariquinone [17,24]; hydroxycinnamic derivatives, e.g. rosmarinic acid (2-3%) [3,20,26]; flavonoids such as nepetin and nepitrin [3,19,20,27,28] and triterpenoids such as oleanolic acid, ursolic acid, α- and β-amyrin, and rofficerone [2,3,17,20,29,30].

CLINICAL PARTICULARS

Therapeutic indications

Internal use
Improvement of hepatic and biliary function and in dyspeptic complaints [2,3,20,31,32].

External use
Adjuvant therapy in rheumatic conditions and peripheral circulatory disorders [2,3,31-35].
Promotion of wound healing and as a mild antiseptic [20,33,34].

Posology and method of administration

Dosage

Adults:
Internal use
Infusion: 2-4 g of rosemary leaf daily [2,34].

E/S/C/O/P
MONOGRAPHS
Second Edition

Fluid extract (1:1, 45% ethanol V/V): 1.5-3 ml daily [2].

Tincture (1:5, 70% ethanol): 3-8.5 ml daily [2].

External use
Ethanolic extract (1:20) [33].
Essential oil (2% V/V) in ethanol, as an antiseptic [34].
1 litre of a decoction (1:20) added to bath water (twice weekly) [2,3,35].

Method of administration
For oral administration and topical application.

Duration of administration
If symptoms persist or worsen, medical advice should be sought.

Contra-indications
Hypersensitivity to rosemary leaf and its preparations, especially those containing carnosol [36].

Special warnings and special precautions for use
Hot baths containing rosemary preparations should be avoided by patients with large open wounds, large skin lesions, feverish conditions or acute inflammation, severe circulatory disorders or hypertension.

Interaction with other medicaments and other forms of interaction
None reported.

Pregnancy and lactation
No data available. In accordance with general medical practice, rosemary leaf should not be used medicinally during pregnancy and lactation without medical advice.

Effects on ability to drive and use machines
None known.

Undesirable effects
Contact dermatitis of the hands, forearms and face was reported in a man working with an extract made from rosemary leaf. The diterpene carnosol was identified as the irritant by patch testing [36].

Overdose
No toxic effects reported.

PHARMACOLOGICAL PROPERTIES

Pharmacodynamic properties

Cholagogic, choleretic and antihepatotoxic effects

In vitro experiments
A lyophilised aqueous extract of rosemary shoots (16.2% w/v) significantly reduced the hepatotoxicity of *tert*-butyl hydroperoxide to rat hepatocytes, causing a dose-dependent decrease in malonaldehyde formation and significantly decreasing the release of lactate dehydrogenase and aspartate aminotransferase ($p<0.01$ to $p<0.05$) [37,38].

In vivo experiments
A lyophilisate of an ethanolic tincture of rosemary, dissolved in perfusate, was injected in doses corresponding to the crude drug at 0.5 g, 1 g or 2 g/kg body weight into the jugular vein of bile duct-cannulated rats under constant infusion with sodium taurocholate solution. A significant and rapid increase in bile flow was observed ($p<0.001$ compared to perfusate only); it reached a maximum in 30 minutes then returned to baseline within 2 hours after 1 g or 2 g/kg, and within 1 hour after 0.5 g/kg [39].

Intravenous administration of a lyophilised 15%-alcoholic extract of rosemary flowering tops to bile duct cannulated guinea pigs at 100 mg/kg body weight caused a 138% increase in bile flow within 30 minutes, followed by a period of slower activity but reaching a second peak of 218% after 105-120 minutes. The results indicated both cholagogic and choleretic activity of the extract [40].

Intraperitoneal pretreatment of rats with a lyophilised aqueous extract from fresh rosemary shoots, corresponding to the crude drug at 1 g/kg body weight, 30 minutes before intraperitoneal injection of carbon tetrachloride (CCl_4) resulted in a 78% decrease in plasma glutamic-pyruvic transaminase ($p<0.001$), indicating hepatoprotective activity. This effect was not seen in rats given the aqueous extract 30 minutes after exposure to CCl_4 [39].

In another experiment, intragastric administration of an ethanolic rosemary extract to rats at 1500 mg/kg for 3 weeks produced a pronounced hepatoprotective effect (CCl_4 model) comparable to that of silymarin. The effects were evaluated from serum and liver parameters, and were confirmed by histopathological examination of the liver tissue [41].

Supplementation of the diet of rats with rosemary extract at a level as low as 0.25% enhanced the activity of the important liver enzymes GSH-transferase and NAD(P)H-quinone reductase [42].

Antispasmodic and anticonvulsant effects

In vitro experiments
Rosemary essential oil inhibited acetylcholine-induced contractions of rabbit tracheal smooth muscle (IC_{50}: 0.40 mg/ml) and histamine-induced contractions of guinea pig tracheal smooth muscle (IC_{50}: 0.19 mg/ml) [43].

Half-maximal inhibition of contractility of isolated, non-stimulated guinea pig atria was observed with rosemary essential oil at a concentration of 250 nl/ml, or 1,8-cineole at 100 nl/ml (6×10^{-4} M) or bornyl acetate at 400 nl/ml (2×10^{-3} M). Similarly, half-maximal inhibition of acetylcholine-induced contractions of guinea pig ileum was achieved with rosemary essential oil at 465 nl/ml, or 1,8-cineole at 414 nl/ml (2.5×10^{-3} M) or bornyl acetate at 112 nl/ml (5.7×10^{-4} M) [44].

A 30%-ethanolic rosemary extract at a concentration of 10 ml/litre exhibited antispasmodic activity on histamine-induced contractions of isolated guinea pig ileum, increasing the median ED_{50} for histamine by 38.7 µg/litre (p<0.005); no significant effect was observed on ED_{50} values for acetylcholine, but the maximal contractility of both histamine- and acetylcholine-induced contractions was reduced (p<0.001 and p<0.005 respectively) [45].

Noradrenaline- and potassium-induced contractions of rabbit vascular smooth muscle (as isolated aortic rings) were significantly and dose-dependently reduced by rosemary leaf essential oil with ID_{50} values of 0.68 mg/ml and 0.24 mg/ml respectively [46].

Rosemary essential oil at concentrations of 0.25-2.5 µl/ml dose-dependently inhibited acetylcholine-induced contractions of isolated guinea pig ileum; similar effects were observed with 1,8-cineole at 0.25-2.5 µl/ml and bornyl acetate at 0.025-2.5 µl/ml [47].

In vivo experiments
Rosemary leaf essential oil, administered intra-venously (in an emulsion) to male guinea pigs at a dose of 25 mg/kg body weight, completely reversed morphine-induced blockage of Oddi's sphincter [48].

Intraperitoneal pretreatment of female mice with an aqueous extract of dried rosemary leaf at 6 mg/kg delayed the onset of picrotoxin-induced convulsions from 10.73 to 12.44 minutes compared to a saline control, while a similar extract from fresh rosemary leaf had a stronger effect, delaying the onset of convulsions from 10.73 to 15.82 minutes (p<0.001) and reducing the mortality rate from 84% to 36% [49].

Antioxidant effects

In vitro experiments
The antioxidant activity of various extracts and certain constituents of rosemary has been demonstrated by a variety of test methods [6,24,50-54]. Both lipophilic and hydrophilic fractions showed activity, which has been attributed to diterpenes, e.g. carnosol, rosmanol and carnos(ol)ic acid [17,24,55]; 90% of the activity is believed to be due to carnosol and carnosic acid [17,56].

Antimicrobial effects

In vitro experiments
Rosemary essential oil has exhibited antibacterial and antifungal activity against a range of test organisms [5,8,11,57]. Aqueous extract from rosemary showed activity against *Salmonella typhi* [58] while the evidence for activity against *Candida albicans* is contradictory [59,60].

Antiviral activity

In vitro experiments
A dry rosemary leaf extract (obtained by extraction with 95% ethanol of the solid residue after removal of essential oil by steam distillation) dose-dependently inhibited *Herpes simplex* virus type 2 plaque formation, 10 µg/ml producing 50% inhibition [61].

Carnosic acid exhibited strong inhibitory activity against HIV-1 protease (IC_{90}: 0.08 µg/ml) and against HIV-1 virus replication (IC_{90}: 0.32 µg/ml). However, the cytotoxic EC_{90} on cultured H9 lymphocytes was only 0.36 µg/ml, which was very close to the effective antiviral dose [18,62].

Anti-inflammatory effects

In vitro experiments
Rosmarinic acid has been shown to inhibit complement-dependent mechanisms of inflammatory reactions [63-65].

In vivo experiments
Rosmarinic acid administered intravenously to rats inhibited cobra venom factor-induced paw oedema at 0.1-1.0 mg/kg and inhibited passive cutaneous anaphylaxis (ID_{50}: ca. 1 mg/kg) [64]. When applied topically (5% in vehicle) to rhesus monkeys, rosmarinic acid reduced both gingival and plaque indices over a 3-week period compared to placebo treatment (p<0.001) [66].

Topical application of 3.6 mg of a dry methanolic extract from rosemary leaf to the backs of mice twice daily for 4 days inhibited skin inflammation and hyperplasia induced by 12-O-tetradecanoylphorbol-13-acetate (TPA) [56]. A similar extract, applied topically at 0.02-0.24 mg/ear, inhibited arachidonic acid-induced mouse ear oedema by 16-54% [17].

Anti-ulcerogenic effects

In vivo experiments
A 70%-ethanolic extract from rosemary herb was tested for anti-ulcerogenic activity in several rat models. At 1000 mg/kg body weight the extract significantly reduced the index of indometacin-induced ulcerative lesions (by 44%, p<0.05 compared to saline), as did cimetidine at 100 mg/kg

(p<0.001) as positive control. In the ethanol-induced ulcer model, the extract at 500 and 1000 mg/kg reduced the index (by 70% and 74.6% respectively, p<0.01), as did carbenoxolone at 200 mg/kg as positive control (p<0.01). In the reserpine-induced ulcer model, the extract at 1000 mg/kg reduced the index by 51.8% (p<0.01), as did atropine at 10 mg/kg as positive control (p<0.01). Further experiments indicated that the mechanism of action had no relationship with nitric oxide or prostaglandins. The results suggested that the hydroethanolic extract may increase the mucosal content of non-protein sulfhydryl groups (a class of endogen cytoprotective substances believed to reduce free radicals in gastric mucosa), possibly linked with general antioxidant activity [67].

Tumour inhibition and cytotoxicity

In vitro experiments
The precipitate from the aqueous phase (after partition with hexane) of a 70%-ethanolic extract of rosemary leaf inhibited KB-cells (an assay for anti-cancer agents) by 87% at 50 μg/ml [68].

In vivo experiments
Topical pre-treatment of the backs of mice with a dry methanolic extract from rosemary leaf reduced the initiation and promotion of tumours by carcinogens; application of 1.2 mg or 3.6 mg of the extract 5 minutes before [^{3}H]benzo[*a*]pyrene (BP) reduced the formation of BP metabolite-DNA adducts by 30% and 54% respectively [17,56].

Supplementation of the diet of rats with 1% of a rosemary extract for 21 weeks reduced the frequency of 7,12-dimethylbenz[*a*]anthracene (DMBA)-induced mammary carcinoma from 76% in the control group to 40% in the treated group [2,69].

Rosemary essential oil at concentrations from 1.2 to 300 mg/ml had cytotoxic effects on leukaemia cells [70].

Hyperglycaemic activity

In vivo experiments
In a glucose tolerance test, rosemary leaf essential oil administered intramuscularly (in a solution) to normal adult rabbits at 25 mg/kg body weight 5 minutes before intraperitoneal glucose loading had a hyperglycaemic effect, increasing plasma glucose levels by 20% (p<0.05), 27% (p<0.01) and 55% (p<0.001) at 60, 90 and 120 min respectively compared to the vehicle control group; a 30% decrease in serum insulin (p<0.002) was observed after 30 minutes. When alloxan diabetic rabbits were given the same intramuscular dose of rosemary leaf essential oil, fasting glucose levels 6 hours after treatment increased by 17% (p<0.005) compared to the control group [71].

Diuretic activity

In vivo experiments
Daily oral administration of an aqueous rosemary leaf extract to rats in an amount corresponding to 0.8 g of crude drug for 7 days significantly enhanced urine volume on days 5-7 compared to controls (p<0.01 on day 5); twice this dosage had no significant effect. Urinary excretion of sodium, potassium and chloride also increased, with the most significant effects on day 6 (p<0.001 in all cases), while creatinine clearance had decreased by day 7 (p<0.01) [72].

Aldose reductase inhibition

In vitro experiments
Two highly oxygenated flavonoids isolated from rosemary have shown potential anti-cataract activity by inhibiting aldose reductase in homogenized rat eye lenses: at concentrations of 10^{-5} M, 10^{-6} M and 10^{-7} M, nepitrin (a flavone glycoside) caused inhibition of 72.2%, 69% and 30.9%, and nepetin (a flavone) caused inhibition of 62.0%, 59.5% and 30.9%, respectively [28].

Effects on metabolism of oestrogens

In vivo experiments
Enhanced liver microsomal metabolism of endogenous oestrogens by a methanolic extract from rosemary leaf have been demonstrated in female CD-1 mice. Incorporation of 2% of the extract in the diet for 3 weeks increased liver microsomal 2-hydroxylation by ca. 150% and 6-hydroxylation by ca. 30% of both oestradiol and oestrone, and inhibited the 16α-hydroxylation of oestradiol by ca. 50%. Liver microsomal glucuronidation of oestradiol and oestrone were stimulated by 54-67% and 37-56% respectively. When ovariectomized CD-1 mice were fed on a diet supplemented with 2% of the extract for 3 weeks the uterotropic action of oestradiol and oestrone was inhibited by 35-50% compared with animals fed a control diet. The authors concluded that the anti-oestrogenic effect of the dietary rosemary leaf extract may contribute to its inhibitory effect on DMBA-induced mammary tumours in experimental animals [73].

CNS stimulation

In vivo experiments
Inhalation of the vapour of rosemary oil (0.5 ml of oil per cage) resulted in a 4-fold increase in locomotor activity in mice over a period of 30 minutes (p<0.001). A similar effect was observed after oral administration of 20 μl of the oil to mice [74].

Pharmacokinetic properties
After oral administration of rosmarinic acid to rats at

200 mg/kg six metabolites were detected in the urine, principally *m*-hydroxyphenylpropionic acid and *trans-m*-coumaric acid 3-*O*-sulphate with smaller amounts of *trans*-ferulic acid 4-*O*-sulphate, *trans-m*-coumaric acid, *trans*-caffeic acid and *trans*-caffeic acid 4-*O*-sulphate, and a small amount of unchanged rosmarinic acid; the first five compounds were also detected in the plasma. Cumulative amounts of these compounds excreted in the urine over 48 hours represented about 32% of the administered dose; none were found in the bile [75].

Inhalation by mice of rosemary oil vapour (0.5 ml of oil per cage) resulted in detectable levels of 1,8-cineole in the blood. Elimination of 1,8-cineole from the blood was biphasic: a rapid phase with a half-life of 6 minutes followed by a slower rate during a second phase with a half-life of 45 minutes, indicating a two-compartment model [74].

Preclinical safety data

Acute toxicity
No mortality was seen in rats or mice given a single intraperitoneal dose of 2 g/kg of a 15%-alcoholic extract of rosemary herb and no change was observed in their behaviour over a period of 15 days. Macroscopic examination during autopsy revealed no visible abnormalities [40].

Mutagenicity and carcinogenicity
A rosemary extract high in antioxidants, as well as isolated carnosic acid (but not carnosol), markedly and dose-dependently reduced *tert*-butyl hydroperoxide-induced mutagenicity in *Salmonella typhimurium* strain TA102 at a concentration approximately 10 times lower than that of ascorbic acid. The antimutagenic effect was attributed principally to carnosic acid [76].

Skin tumours were initiated on the backs of mice with 7,12-dimethylbenz[*a*]anthracene then the test animals were simultaneously treated topically with either acetone alone or with 3.6 mg of rosemary leaf extract in acetone twice a week for 19 weeks; none of these animals developed tumours, indicating that rosemary is not a tumour promoter. Other mice were treated topically with 3.6 mg of rosemary leaf extract and then tumours were promoted with 5 nmol of 12-*O*-tetradecanoylphorbol-13-acetate twice a week for 19 weeks; none of these animals developed tumours, indicating that rosemary is not a tumour initiator on mouse skin [56].

REFERENCES

1. Rosemary Leaf - Rosmarini folium. European Pharmacopoeia, Council of Europe.

2. Stahl-Biskup E. Rosmarinus. In: Hänsel R, Keller K, Rimpler H, Schneider G, editors. Hagers Handbuch der Pharmazeutischen Praxis, 5th ed. Volume 6: Drogen P-Z. Berlin-Heidelberg-New York: Springer-Verlag, 1994:490-503.

3. Czygan F-C, Hiller K. Rosmarini folium - Rosmarinblätter. In: Wichtl M, editor. Teedrogen und Phytopharmaka. Ein Handbuch für die Praxis auf wissenschaftlicher Grundlage, 4th ed. Stuttgart: Wissenschaftliche Verlagsgesellschaft, 2002:523-5.

4. Maffei M, Mucciarelli M, Scannerini S. Environmental factors affecting the lipid metabolism in *Rosmarinus officinalis* L. Biochem Syst Ecol 1993;21:765-84.

5. Panizzi L, Flamini G, Cioni PL, Morelli I. Composition and antimicrobial properties of essential oils of four Mediterranean Lamiaceae. J Ethnopharmacol 1993; 39:167-70.

6. Svoboda KP, Deans SG. A study of the variability of rosemary and sage and their volatile oils on the British market: their antioxidative properties. Flavour Fragrance J 1992;7:81-7.

7. Vokou D, Margaris NS. Variation of volatile oil concentration of Mediterranean aromatic shrubs *Thymus capitatus* Hoffmag et Link, *Satureja thymbra* L., *Teucrium polium* L. and *Rosmarinus officinalis*. Int J Biometeorol 1986;30:147-55.

8. Héthelyi E, Koczka I, Tétényi P. Phytochemical and antimicrobial analysis of essential oils. Herba Hung 1989;28:99-115.

9. Konstantopoulou I, Vassilopoulou L, Mavragani-Tsipidou P, Scouras ZG. Insecticidal effects of essential oils. A study of the effects of essential oils extracted from eleven Greek aromatic plants on *Drosophila auraria*. Experientia 1992;48:616-9.

10. Jain M, Banerji R, Nigam SK, Scheffer JJC, Chaturvedi HC. *In vitro* production of essential oil from proliferating shoots of *Rosmarinus officinalis*. Planta Med 1991;57: 122-4.

11. Montes MA, Wilkomirsky T, Valenzuela L, Bello H, Osses F. Esencias de algunas Labiadas aclimatadas en la región del Bío-Bío, Chile. *Rosmarinus officinalis* L., *Mentha pulegium* L., *Mentha spicata*. Constituyentes y propiedades antimicrobianas. An Real Acad Farm 1991; 57:425-38.

12. Pérez-Alonso MJ, Velasco-Negueruela A, Duru ME, Harmandar M, Esteban JL. Composition of the essential oils of *Ocimum basilicum* var. *glabratum* and *Rosmarinus officinalis* from Turkey. J Essent Oil Res 1995;7:73-5.

13. Reglero G, Herraiz M, Herraiz T. Capillary gas chromatographic determination of volatiles in solid matrices by direct introduction using a programmable-temperature vaporizer. J Chromatogr 1989;483:43-50.

14. Regnault-Roger C, Hamraoui A, Holeman M, Theron E, Pinel R. Insecticidal effect of essential oils from Mediterranean aromatic plants upon *Acanthoscelides obtectus*

SAY (Coleoptera, Bruchidae), a pest of kidney bean (*Phaseolus vulgaris* L.). J Chem Ecol 1993;19:1233-44.

15. Tateo F, Fellin M. Produzione HPE di oleoresina da *Rosmarinus officinalis* L. Mitt Gebiete Lebensm Hyg 1987;78:325-35.

16. Tateo F, Fellin M. Production of rosemary oleoresin using supercritical carbon dioxide. Perfumer & Flavorist 1988;13(Oct-Nov):27-34.

17. Huang M-T, Ho C-T, Wang ZY, Ferraro T, Lou Y-R, Stauber K et al. Inhibition of skin tumorigenesis by rosemary and its constituents carnosol and ursolic acid. Cancer Res 1994;54:701-8.

18. Paris A, Strukelj B, Renko M, Turk V, Pukl M, Umek A, Korant BD. Inhibitory effect of carnosolic acid on HIV-1 protease in cell-free assays. J Nat Prod 1993;56:1426-30.

19. Venturella P, Venturella G, Marino ML, Mericli AH, Cubukcu B. Phytochemical investigation of the Labiatae *Dorystoechas hastata*. Giorn Bot Ital 1988;122:291-4.

20. Paris RR, Moyse H. Romarin (*Rosmarinus officinalis* L.). In: Matière Medicale, Volume 3. Paris: Masson, 1971:277-9.

21. Schwarz K, Ternes W. Antioxidative constituents of *Rosmarinus officinalis* and *Salvia officinalis*. I. Determination of phenolic diterpenes with antioxidative activity amongst tocochromanols using HPLC. Z Lebensm Unters Forsch 1992;195:95-8.

22. Schwarz K, Ternes W. Antioxidative constituents of *Rosmarinus officinalis* and *Salvia officinalis*. II. Isolation of carnosic acid and formation of other phenolic diterpenes. Z Lebensm Unters Forsch 1992;195:99-103.

23. Fraga BM, Gonzalez AG, Herrera JR, Luis JG, Perales A, Ravelo AG. A revised structure for the diterpene rosmanol. Phytochemistry 1985;24:1853-4.

24. Houlihan CM, Ho C-T, Chang SS. The structure of rosmariquinone - a new antioxidant isolated from *Rosmarinus officinalis* L. JAOCS 1985;62:96-8.

25. Schwarz K, Ternes W, Schmauderer E. Antioxidative constituents of *Rosmarinus officinalis* and *Salvia officinalis*. III. Stability of phenolic diterpenes of rosemary extracts under thermal stress as required for technological processes. Z Lebensm Unters Forsch 1992;195:104-7.

26. Verotta L. Isolation and HPLC determination of the active principles of *Rosmarinus officinalis* and *Gentiana lutea*. Fitoterapia 1985;56:25-9.

27. Okamura N, Haraguchi H, Hashimoto K, Yagi A. Flavonoids in *Rosmarinus officinalis* leaves. Phytochemistry 1994;37:1463-6.

28. Tomás-Barberán FA, López-Gómez C, Villar A, Tomás-Lorente F. Inhibition of lens aldose reductase by Labiatae flavonoids. Planta Med 1986;52:239-40.

29. Evans WC. Rosemary oil. In: Trease and Evans'

Pharmacognosy, 14th ed. London-Philadelphia: WB Saunders, 1996:262-3.

30. Ganeva Y, Tsankova E, Simova S, Apostolova B, Zaharieva E. Rofficerone: a new triterpenoid from *Rosmarinus officinalis*. Planta Med 1993;59:276-7.

31. Hänsel R. Rosmarinöl; Einreibemittel. In: Phytopharmaka, 2nd ed. Berlin-Heidelberg: Springer-Verlag, 1991:134 and 214.

32. Weiß RF. Rosmarinus officinalis, echter Rosmarin. In: Lehrbuch der Phytotherapie. Stuttgart: Hippokrates Verlag, 1991;246-7.

33. Velasco Negueruela A, Perez Alonso MJ, Bonet Carrasquilla C, Marcos Samaniego N. Datos sobre la composición quimica (terpenoides) de plantas aromaticas de la provincia de Toledo. In: Instituto Nacional de Investigación y Tecnologia Agraria y Alimentaria, editor. I. Jornadas Ibericas de Plantas Medicinales, Aromaticas y Aceites Esenciales. Madrid: Ministerio de Agricultura, Pesca y Alimentación, 1992: 291-301.

34. del Río Hijas ME. El uso de las plantas medicinales en los distintos metodos terapeuticos. First Iberian Symposium on medicinal, aromatic plants and essential oils. Madrid, 1992; 399-407.

35. Rulffs W. Rosmarinöl-Badezusatz. Wirksamkeitsnachweis. Münch med Wschr 1984;126:207-8.

36. Hjorther AB, Christophersen C, Hausen BM, Menné T. Occupational allergic contact dermatitis from carnosol, a naturally-occuring compound present in rosemary. Contact Derm 1997;37:99-100.

37. Joyeux M, Rolland A, Fleurentin J, Mortier F, Dorfman P. *Tert*-butyl hydroperoxide-induced injury in isolated rat hepatocytes: a model for studying antihepatotoxic crude drugs. Planta Med 1990;56:171-4.

38. Joyeux M, Mortier F, Fleurentin J. Screening of antiradical, antilipoperoxidant and hepatoprotective effects of nine plant extracts used in Caribbean folk medicine. Phytotherapy Res 1995;9:228-30.

39. Hoefler C, Fleurentin J, Mortier F, Pelt JM, Guillemain J. Comparative choleretic and hepatoprotective properties of young sprouts and total plant extracts of *Rosmarinus officinalis* in rats. J Ethnopharmacol 1987;19:133-43.

40. Mongold JJ, Camillieri S, Susplugas P, Taillade C, Masse JP, Serrano JJ. Activité cholagogue/cholérétique d'un extrait lyophilisé de *Rosmarinus officinalis* L. Plantes Méd Phytothér 1991;25:6-11.

41. Fahim FA, Esmat AY, Fadel HM, Hassan KFS. Allied studies on the effect of *Rosmarinus officinalis* L. on experimental hepatotoxicity and mutagenesis. Int J Food Sci Nutr 1990;50:413-27.

42. Singletary K, Gutierrez E. Rosemary extract increases liver GSH-transferase and quinone reductase activities. Faseb Journal 1993;7:A866.

43. Aqel MB. Relaxant effect of the volatile oil of *Rosmarinus*

officinalis on tracheal smooth muscle. J Ethnopharmacol 1991;33:57-62.

44. Hof S, Ammon HPT. Negative inotropic action of rosemary oil, 1,8-cineole and bornyl acetate. Planta Med 1989;55:106-7.

45. Forster HB, Niklas H, Lutz S. Antispasmodic effects of some medicinal plants. Planta Med 1980;40:309-19.

46. Aqel MB. A vascular smooth muscle relaxant effect of *Rosmarinus officinalis*. Int J Pharmacog 1992;30:281-8.

47. Hof S, Gropper B, Ammon HPT. Different sensitivities of the CNS and smooth musculature of the guinea-pig ileum to the effects of rosemary oil and its individual components. Arch Pharm (Weinheim) 1988;321:702.

48. Giachetti D, Taddei E, Taddei I. Pharmacological activity of essential oils on Oddi's sphincter. Planta Med 1988; 54:389-92.

49. Abdul-Ghani A-S, El-Lati SG, Sacaan AI, Suleiman MS, Amin RM. Anticonvulsant effects of some Arab medicinal plants. Int J Crude Drug Res 1987;25:39-43.

50. Fang X, Wada S. Enhancing the antioxidant effect of α-tocopherol with rosemary in inhibiting catalyzed oxidation caused by Fe^{2+} and hemoprotein. Food Res Int 1993;26:405-11.

51. Guerreiro M, Cunha A. Hydroxyl scavenger activity of *Rosmarinus officinalis* L. XXI Congrès International de la Societé de Pharmacie de la Mediterranée Latine, Messina-Lipari (Italy), 7-9 October 1994.

52. Guerreiro M, Amaral MT, Proença da Cunha A. Effects of rosemary extracts on lipid oxidation. In: Abstracts of XVII International Conference, Palma de Maiorca, May 1994.

53. Guerreiro M, Dinis TC, Almeida LM, Proença da Cunha A. Free radical scavenger activity of some extracts from *Rosmarinus officinalis* L. In: Abstracts of World Congress of Pharmacy 1994 - 54th International Congress of FIP. Lisbon, Portugal, 4-9 September 1994 (Abstract P101).

54. Tateo F, Fellin M, Santamaria L, Bianchi A, Bianchi L. *Rosmarinus officinalis* L. extract. Production, antioxidant and antimutagenic activity. Perfumer & Flavorist 1988; 13(Dec):48-54.

55. Haraguchi H, Saito T, Okamura N, Yagi A. Inhibition of lipid peroxidation and superoxide generation by diterpenoids from *Rosmarinus officinalis*. Planta Med 1995;61:333-6.

56. Ho C-T, Ferraro T, Chen Q, Rosen RT, Huang M-T. Phytochemicals in teas and rosemary and their cancer-preventive properties. In: Ho C-T, Osawa T, Huang M-T, Rosen RT, editors. Food Phytochemicals for Cancer Prevention II: Teas, Spices and Herbs. ACS Symposium Series 547. Washington DC: American Chemical Society, 1994:2-19.

57. Benjilali B, Tantaoui-El-Araki A, Ismaili-Alaoui M, Ayadi A. Méthode d'étude des propriétés antiseptiques des huîles essentielles par contact direct en milieu gélosé. Plantes Méd Phytothér 1986;20:155-67.

58. Perez C, Anesini C. In vitro antibacterial activity of Argentine folk medicinal plants against *Salmonella typhi*. J Ethnopharmacol 1994;44:41-6.

59. Larrondo JV, Calvo MA. Effect of essential oils on *Candida albicans*: a scanning electron microscope study. Biomed Lett 1991;46:269-72.

60. Soliman FM, El-Kashoury EA, Fathy MM, Gonaid MH. Analysis and biological activity of the essential oil of *Rosmarinus officinalis* L. from Egypt. Flavour Fragrance J 1994;9:29-33.

61. Romero E, Tateo F, Debiaggi M. Antiviral activity of a *Rosmarinus officinalis* L. extract. Mitt Gebiete Lebensm Hyg 1989;80:113-9.

62. Pukl M, Umek A, Paris A, Strukelj B, Renko M, Korant BD, Turk V. Inhibitory effect of carnosolic acid on HIV-1 protease. Planta Med 1992;58(Suppl 1):A632.

63. Rampart M, Beetens JR, Bult H, Herman AG, Parnham MJ, Winkelmann J. Complement-dependent stimulation of prostacyclin biosynthesis; inhibition by rosmarinic acid. Biochem Pharmacol 1986;35:1397-1400.

64. Parnham MJ, Kesselring K. Rosmarinic acid. Drugs of the Future 1985;10:756-7.

65. Gracza L, Koch H, Löffler E. Isolierung von Rosmarin-säure aus *Symphytum officinale* und ihre anti-inflammatorische Wirksamkeit in einem In-vitro-Modell. Arch Pharm (Weinheim) 1985;318:1090-5.

66. Van Dyke TE, Braswell L, Offenbacher S. Inhibition of gingivitis by topical application of ebselen and rosmarinic acid. Agents Actions 1986;19:376-7.

67. Dias PC, Foglio MA, Possenti A, de Carvalho JE. Antiulcerogenic activity of crude hydroalcoholic extract of *Rosmarius officinalis* L. J Ethnopharmacol 2000; 69:57-62.

68. Hayashi T, Arisawa M, Bandome T, Namose Y, Shimizu M, Suzuki S et al. Studies on medicinal plants in Paraguay; studies on "Romero"; Part I. Planta Med 1987;53:394.

69. Singletary K. Inhibition of DMBA-induced mammary tumorigenesis by rosemary extract. Faseb Journal 1991; 5:A927.

70. Ilarionova M, Todorov D, Burov P, Dimitrova N, Parvanova V. Cytotoxic effect on leukemic cells of the essential oils from rosemary, wild geranium and nettle and concrete of royal Bulgarian rose. Anticancer Res 1992;12:1915.

71. Al-Hader AA, Hasan ZA, Aqel MB. Hyperglycemic and insulin release inhibitory effects of *Rosmarinus officinalis*. J Ethnopharmacol 1994;43:217-21.

72. Haloui M, Louedec L, Michel J-B, Lyoussi B. Experimental diuretic effects of *Rosmarinus officinalis*

and *Centaurium erythraea*. J Ethnopharmacol 2000; 71:465-72.

73. Zhu BT, Loder DP, Cai MX, Ho C-T, Huang M-T, Conney AH. Dietary administration of an extract from rosemary leaves enhances the liver microsomal metabolism of endogenous estrogens and decreases their uterotropic action in CD-1 mice. Carcinogenesis 1998;19:1821-7.

74. Kovar KA, Gropper B, Friess D, Ammon HPT. Blood levels of 1,8-cineole and locomotor activity of mice after inhalation and oral administration of rosemary oil. Planta Med 1987;53:315-8.

75. Nakazawa T, Ohsawa K. Metabolism of rosmarinic acid in rats. J Nat Prod 1998;61:993-6.

76. Minnunni M, Wolleb U, Mueller O, Pfeifer A, Aeschbacher HU. Natural antioxidants as inhibitors of oxygen species induced mutagenicity. Mutation Res 1992;269: 193-200.

RUSCI RHIZOMA

Butcher's Broom

E/S/C/O/P
MONOGRAPHS
Second Edition

DEFINITION

Butcher's Broom consists of the dried, whole or fragmented underground parts of *Ruscus aculeatus* L. It contains not less than 1.0 per cent of total sapogenins, expressed as ruscogenins [a mixture of neoruscogenin ($C_{27}H_{40}O_4$; M_r 428.6) and ruscogenin ($C_{27}M_{42}O_4$; M_r 430.6)] and calculated with reference to the dried drug.

The material complies with the monograph of the European Pharmacopoeia [1].

CONSTITUENTS

The characteristic constituents are steroidal saponins based upon (25R)-spirost-5-ene-1β,3β-diol (ruscogenin) and spirosta-5,25(27)-diene-10,3β-diol (neoruscogenin), such as ruscoside, ruscin, deglucoruscoside and deglucoruscin. Minor constituents include flavonoids, anthraquinones, benzofurans, essential oil (mainly monoterpenes) and sterols [2-6].

CLINICAL PARTICULARS

Therapeutic indications

Supportive therapy for symptoms of chronic venous insufficiency, such as painful, tired and heavy legs, tingling and swelling [7]. Supportive therapy for symptoms of haemorrhoids, such as itching and burning [8,9].

Posology and method of administration

Dosage

Adult daily dose: Solid or liquid extracts in amounts corresponding to 7-11 mg of total ruscogenins [8].

Method of administration
For oral administration.

Duration of administration
No restriction; long-term administration may be advisable. If symptoms persist or worsen, medical advice should be sought.

Contra-indications
None known.

Special warnings and special precautions for use
None required.

Interaction with other medicaments and other forms of interaction
None reported.

Pregnancy and lactation
In accordance with general medical practice, the product should not be used during pregnancy and lactation without medical advice.

No adverse effects have been reported in mothers or newborn babies when used in late pregnancy [9,10].

Effects on ability to drive and use machines
None known.

Undesirable effects
None reported.

Overdose
No toxic effects reported.

PHARMACOLOGICAL PROPERTIES

Pharmacodynamic properties

In vitro experiments

Vasoconstriction
In rings of saphenous vein from ovarectomized female rabbits, a butcher's broom extract (0.001-1 mg/ml) induced dose-dependent contractions. This effect was insensitive to blockade by either prazosin or rauwolscine, but was partially inhibited by both substances in rings isolated from oestradiol-treated animals [11].

Butcher's broom extract enhanced the response to noradrenaline in isolated normal or stenosed canine saphenous veins. In a second model, butcher's broom extract ensured valvular closure when the veins were perfused inverse to the normal blood stream [12].

A hydroalcoholic butcher's broom extract caused dose-dependent contraction in segments of isolated canine saphenous veins (effective dose: 30 μg/ml and higher). The maximal contraction caused by the extract averaged $80 \pm 12\%$ of the response to 10^{-4} M noradrenaline. Prazosin and rauwolscine given alone decreased, and the presence of both substances eliminated, the response to butcher's broom extract (0.1-1 mg/ml, n = 5 each concentration). Cocaine reduced the contraction evoked by butcher's broom extract suggesting also an indirect sympathomimetic effect of the extract. The contractile response to the butcher's broom extract was also depressed by phentolamine, adenosine, verapamil and by chemical sympathectomy with 6-hydroxydopamine. Tetrodotoxin, atropine, methysergide and indometacin did not significantly influence the effect of butcher's broom extract; acetylcholine enhanced the increase in tension. Warming augmented the contractile response to butcher's broom extract (0.2 mg/ml), while cooling inhibited it [13-16].

Femoral vein rings and coronary arterial rings were isolated from adult female mongrel dogs. Butcher's broom extract (0.001 mg/ml) induced dose-dependent contractions of the vein preparations. The effect was modulated by the integrity of the endothelial cells and the hormonal status of the animals. Treatment with prazosin plus rauwolscine reduced the contractions evoked by butcher's broom extract following progesterone treatment; inhibition of α-adrenergic receptors in veins from oestrogen-treated animals augmented the contractions evoked by the extract [17,18].

In both the venous and arterial rings with endothelium, butcher's broom extract (4-6 g/ml) relaxed contractions induced by noradrenaline (veins) or prostaglandin F_{2a} (PGF_{2a}; arteries) in a dose-dependent manner. The relaxing effect was inhibited by atropine and by inactivation of the endothelial relaxing factors. The authors concluded that butcher's broom can initiate the release of vasoactive factors from the endothelium [17].

Saponin mixtures and ruscogenin provoked remarkable vasoconstrictive effects in the isolated rabbit ear. The ED_{50} of ruscogenin was 20-25 fold lower than for the saponins [19].

Butcher's broom extract (0.001-1 mg/ml) induced dose-dependent contractions in rings from greater saphenous veins and varicose tributaries of patients (3 male, 17 female) who underwent vein stripping for primary varicosity (n = 5-7 for each experiment). Blocking of α- and β-adrenergic receptors with phentolamine and propranolol reduced the maximal tonus induced by butcher's broom extract in each type of vein [20].

Butcher's broom extract caused comparable and moderate contraction of human saphenous veins with and without endothelium isolated from healthy volunteers (n = 8; 3 female, 5 male) and patients with primary varicosity (n = 14; 11 female, 3 male). The threshold dose ranged between 0.01 and 0.1 mg/ml. Contractions of the varicose tributaries were about two-fold greater than those of saphenous veins from the same patients. In veins from varicose patients, α_2-blockade with rauwolscine was more effective than α_1-blockade with prazosin in reducing contractions induced by butcher's broom in rings with and without endothelium [21].

Maximal contractions induced by butcher's broom extract (1 mg/ml) in human veins taken from women undergoing varicectomy were independent from the oestrogen level during the menstrual cycle. Comparable effects were seen in veins from menopausal women [22].

A water-soluble butcher's broom extract (0.01, 0.1 and 1 mg/ml) caused dose-dependent reduction of noradrenaline accumulation in isolated normal and varicose human saphenous veins. The highest concentration caused a reduction of about 50% in the normal vein and reduced the formation of all metabolites of noradrenaline [23].

Effects on permeability
Damage to isolated pig ear vein induced by ethacrynic acid was diminished by pre-incubation with butcher's broom extract (0.005%). This effect was related to reduced permeability to both water and protein [24].

Vasoprotection
In the presence of butcher's broom extract the viability of human umbilical vein endothelial cells exposed to hypoxia increased by up to 60%. A pronounced effect was observed when cells under hypoxia were incubated for 48 hours with concentrations higher than 330 µg/ml [25]. Butcher's broom extract at 0.05 µg/ml provided only slight protection from the hypoxia-induced decrease in ATP, while 50 µg/ml totally prevented the effect of hypoxia (n = 9 for each concentration). Inhibition of phospholipase A_2 activation by 50%, observed with butcher's broom extract at 0.05 µg/ml, increased slightly with higher extract concentrations (0.5 µg/ml, 5 µg/ml and 50 µg/ml). The extract also dose-dependently inhibited hypoxia-induced adherence of neutrophils to the endothelial cells: 0% at 0.05 µg/ml and 88% at 50 µg/ml [26].

Effects on lymphatic vessels
Noradrenaline (10^{-8} to 10^{-4} M) and butcher's broom extract (0.01-1 mg/ml) caused dose-dependent contractions in isolated canine lymphatic thoracic duct. The activity of butcher's broom extract was partially inhibited by prazosin and rauwolscine, whereas phentolamine completely eliminated the contractile response [27].

Addition of butcher's broom extract (30 µg/ml) increased the contraction frequency caused by electrical field stimulation in isolated bovine mesenteric lymphatic vessels (n = 8) by about 50%. Noradrenaline blocked the response to the field stimulation (n = 6) [28].

Elastase activity
Ruscogenins from butcher's broom inhibited the activity of porcine pancreatic elastase (IC_{50}: 119µM; competitive inhibition) [29].

In vivo experiments

Vasoconstriction, vasoprotection
Butcher's broom extract increased the rise in, and the final level of, venous pressure in the extracorporal (carotid-femoral arteries) circulation of anaesthetized

dogs; this effect was reversible [12].

Butcher's broom extract was added to the superfusion solution applied to cheek pouch preparations of male hamsters. The venules constricted with doses above 0.05 mg/ml/min, while arterioles remained unchanged. Venular constriction evoked by the extract at 0.2 mg/ml/min was blocked by prazosin (10^{-9} M), by diltiazem (10^{-9} M) and by high concentrations of rauwolscine (10^{-6} M) [30].

The vasoconstrictive effects of butcher's broom extract applied topically to hamster cheek pouch preparations were found to be temperature-dependent. At 25°C venules and arterioles dilated. At 36.5°C venules constricted, whereas arterioles either dilated with extract concentrations of up to 0.05 mg/ml or remained unchanged even with higher concentrations of the extract. At 40°C constriction of venules was more pronounced than at the lower temperatures, whereas arterioles only constricted with higher concentrations of the extract (above 0.01 mg/ml) [31].

Intravenous administration of butcher's broom extract at 5 mg/kg body weight caused venular constriction in the cheek pouch of male hamsters, but did not affect the arteriolar diameter. Mean arterial pressure was not affected at this dose level [31].

Oral administration of a solution of butcher's broom extract at 150 mg/kg body weight for 28 days resulted in constriction of the venules by 30% and dilatation of the arterioles by 37% in the hamster cheek pouch (n = 6) compared to water-treated controls (n = 6). Arteriolar and venular side branches were not affected [31].

The vasoconstrictive effects of butcher's broom extract were investigated in lower leg muscle preparations of 12 anaesthetized young adult cats. Following intra-arterial administration of 0.4 mg/min/kg body weight, arterial, arteriolar and venular resistance increased by 30-35% within 90 seconds, while higher doses (0.8 mg/min/kg and 3 mg/min/kg) produced sustained dilator effects. This pattern of response was consistent in all experiments (n = 24). Intravenous administration of the extract at 1-9 mg/min/kg resulted in a dose-dependent venoconstrictive response (n = 10) [32].

In dogs (n = 4), constant infusion of butcher's broom extract at 50 µg/hour/kg body weight for 5 days (total doses: 60-84 mg) had beneficial effects on alterations caused by denervation of the lateral saphenous vein segments. The increase in smooth muscle cell diameter was completely prevented by this treatment. Butcher's broom extract increased the O-methylating capacity of the denervated and the non-denervated tissues [33].

Effects on permeability; oedema-protective and anti-inflammatory effects
Topical application of butcher's broom extract (0.002-

2.0 mg/ml/min) to male hamster cheek pouch preparations dose-dependently inhibited the increase in macromolecular permeability caused by histamine. A concentration of 0.2 mg/ml/min elicited 50% inhibition of the histamine-induced permeability. This effect was blocked by prazosin and by diltiazem, but not by rauwolscine (all applied topically) [34].

Intravenously administered butcher's broom extract (5 mg/kg body weight) showed protective effects against leakage of dextran in the hamster cheek pouch after topical administration of various permeability-increasing substances such as bradykinin, leukotriene B_4 or histamine [35].

The oedema-protective effects of a butcher's broom extract (containing 2.5% of ruscogenin) and ruscogenin were demonstrated in a perfusion model of the hindleg of anaesthetized cats. Oedema was induced by perfusion with 0.1% of ethacrynic acid for 10 minutes. Butcher's broom extract (200 or 400 mg/kg body weight) or ruscogenin (20 or 80 mg/kg body weight) were administered orally 4 hours before induction of oedema. Alternatively, the extract at 10 or 20 mg/kg or ruscogenin at 4 mg/kg were administered intravenously 1 hour prior to oedema induction. Each treatment group comprised 5 or 6 animals and 16 animals served as controls. After an additional 45-minute perfusion with sodium chloride solution, the blood, protein and water contents in the oedema of the skin and muscle were measured. The optimal protective dose of butcher's broom extract was 20 mg/kg body weight when administered intravenously, whereas an oral dose 10- to 20-fold higher was necessary. An intravenous dose of ruscogenin at 4 mg/kg body weight was as effective as an oral dose of 20 mg/kg [36].

Butcher's broom extract showed anti-inflammatory activity in rats when administered by the intraperitoneal route (100, 200 or 300 mg/kg body weight) or the rectal route (suppositories, 275 mg/kg body weight). The effect of 300 mg/kg of butcher's broom extract (i.p.) was equivalent to 72% of the activity of phenylbutazone (165 mg/kg i.p). Two other purified extracts with higher concentrations of ruscogenins were effective at lower doses [37].

Purified sapogenins isolated from butcher's broom were evaluated for antiphlogistic and anti-inflammatory activity in the rat. Oedema was induced by injection of dextran, histamine, serotonin or hyaluronidase. Intraperitoneal administration of the sapogenins at 20, 40 or 80 mg/kg body weight reduced limb oedema; this antiphlogistic activity was suppressed by adrenalectomy. Slight anti-inflammatory activity was observed against granulomas induced by subcutaneous implantation of cotton pellets. When the purified sapogenins were administered orally neither antiphlogistic nor anti-inflammatory activity

was observed [38].

Saponins and ruscogenins isolated from butcher's broom showed anti-inflammatory activity in carrageenan- and brewer's yeast-induced rat paw oedema when administered intraperitoneally or intravenously. In the rabbit, only the ruscogenins (80 mg/kg body weight i.p.) decreased capillary permeability significantly (p = 0.05). These substances were not active against capillary fragility [19].

Effects on lymph vessels
Intravenous administration of a water-soluble butcher's broom extract at 1, 2 or 5 mg/kg body weight dose-dependently enhanced flow duration and intensity in isolated lymph vessels of anaesthetized dogs. A similar effect was seen in the veins. The activity of the extract was not influenced by injection of nifedipine [39].

Pharmacological studies in humans
In a randomized, double-blind, crossover, 4-armed study 20 healthy volunteers (11 men and 9 women aged between 20 and 43 years) took a single oral dose of four different treatments, separated by 1-week wash-out periods: 450 mg of butcher's broom extract, 450 mg of trimethylhesperidin chalcone (TMHC), a combination of both substances, or a placebo. Venous function, capillary filtration rate, tissue and blood volume were monitored before intake and after 50, 70, 90, 120 and 150 minutes. Compared to placebo, butcher's broom extract significantly decreased venous capacity (p<0.01), reduced the blood pool in the lower leg (p< 0.05) and reduced tissue volumes in the foot and ankle (p<0.01). TMHC did not influence venous capacity and its influence on tissue volume was about 3 times weaker than that of butcher's broom extract [40].

In a double-blind, placebo-controlled study the influence of venous stasis on several microrheological factors and the effects of taking butcher's broom extract for 30 days were investigated in 25 patients suffering from chronic venous insufficiency (13 verum, 12 placebo). All parameters were also measured in 20 untreated healthy controls. In patients treated with butcher's broom extract there was no increase in haematocrit after stasis, while haematocrit values rose in the placebo group. Butcher's broom extract prevented an increase in plasma viscosity after stasis and improved red cell deformability. The red blood cell aggregation index after stasis was similar to that of control subjects, while it increased after stasis in the placebo group [41].

Clinical studies

Chronic venous insufficiency, varicoses
The efficacy of a dry extract from butcher's broom (15-20:1; methanol 60%) was evaluated in a

randomized, double-blind, placebo-controlled study involving 166 women suffering from chronic venous insufficiency (Widmer grades I and II; CEAP[1] 3-4). After a placebo run-in period of 2 weeks, the patients were randomly assigned to either 72-75 mg of the butcher's broom extract or placebo daily for 12 weeks. Data relating to 148 patients (30-89 years, 150-182 cm height, 49-97 kg weight), with mean disease durations of 14.6 years in the butcher's broom extract group (n = 77) and 15.1 years in the placebo group (n = 71), were eligible for efficacy analysis. Significant differences in favour of the verum treatment were found for reductions in lower leg volume and ankle circumference after 8 and 12 weeks (p<0.001), and in leg circumference (p<0.001) and the main subjective symptoms (p<0.05) after 12 weeks. There was a clear relationship between the changes in lower leg volume and the subjective symptoms "tired, heavy legs", "sensation of tension" and "tingling sensation" (p<0.05). Global assessment by the investigators also confirmed the superiority of the butcher's broom extract treatment (p<0.05) compared to placebo [7].

Haemorrhoids
In observational studies more than 1800 patients (including 26 pregnant women) suffering from haemorrhoids and anorectal complaints have been treated topically with isolated ruscogenins in suppositories (each containing 8 mg) and/or creams (0.8%) for 2 days to 13 weeks. Improvements were reported with respect to symptoms and objective evaluation by the physicians. The efficacy of treatment was estimated as very good or good in 85-93% of cases [9,42,43].

Pharmacokinetic properties

Pharmacokinetics in animals
The pharmacokinetic characteristics of a radiolabelled extract from butcher's broom were investigated in two male Wistar rats. The activity of the extract was 2.8 mCi/mg, with 94% of the total radioactivity bound to saponins. Each animal received 1 ml of extract orally. Radioactivity was detected in the blood 15 minutes after administration. After 2 hours, 39% of the radioactivity was found in the blood samples. After 3.5 hours, in 10 ml samples of blood a maximum radioactivity of 0.41% and 0.45% was observed and was maintained until the end of the 24-hour observation period. The extract was eliminated mainly in the faeces but also renally in a ratio of 2:1, 46% of the administered radioactivity being excreted within 96 hours. Biliary excretion within 24 hours was 8.5 and 10.8% [44].

The bioavailability of a ^{3}H-labelled butcher's broom extract after oral, topical and intravenous administration was studied in rats. Male Wistar rats were

treated orally with 1 ml of an aqueous solution containing 0.1 ml of a fluid extract (2% saponins, 70 µCi). Male Atrichi rats were treated topically with 250 mg of a combination of labelled butcher's broom extract, melilotus extract and dextran sulphate, corresponding to 25µCi. By the intravenous route male Wistar rats received 0.5 ml of an aqueous solution containing 50 mg of the butcher's broom extract (56 µCi). Based on radioactivity in the blood and urine, absorption by the oral route was estimated at 65% and by the local route at 25%. After intravenous administration the existence of an enterohepatic cycle was demonstrated and one-third of the radioactivity was eliminated via the faeces. Following oral administration maximum radioactivity was found in the blood after 2 hours and was maintained for 24 hours. In similar experiments with orally-treated Atrichi rats 80% of the radioactivity was eliminated within 72 hours, 35% of the dose being found in the urine [45].

Macaca monkeys (3 females, 3 males) were treated with a tritiated butcher's broom extract (1.5 mCi/kg body weight) by the oral (n = 4) or intravenous (n = 1) routes, or topically in a fixed combination (n = 1). Thin layer chromatography showed that 80-83% of the labelling was fixed in the sapogenin fraction of the extract. Most of the radioactivity was found in the bile, the digestive tract and the urinary tract 2 hours after oral administration, while liver and kidneys were moderately radioactive. After 7 hours, radioactivity had further increased only in the urinary tract, the bile and the faeces. Radioactivity after 24 hours was markedly lower in all measured tissues. Percutaneous absorption was about 20% compared to absorption after oral administration. Maximum urinary excretion occurred after about 7.5 hours and sapogenins were identified as the major urinary metabolites. A considerable proportion of the radioactivity was excreted in urine and faeces within 24 hours [46]:

Administration	Excretion within 24 hours	
	Urine	Faeces
Intravenous	26%	6.5%
Oral	20%	23%
Topical	4%	9%

Pharmacokinetics in humans
The presence of butcher's broom saponins in the blood was clearly demonstrated after oral administration of 1 g of butcher's broom extract to three volunteers. Plasma levels of the spirostanol glycosides deglucneoruscin and deglucoruscin were measured

[1] **C**linical signs, **E**tiological classification, **A**natomic distribution, **P**athophysiology

by HPLC for 4 hours at 30-minute intervals. The T_{max} for degluconeoruscin was 90-120 minutes after dosing, with a C_{max} of 2.5 µg/ml [47].

Preclinical safety data

Acute toxicity

The acute toxicity of an ethanolic extract from butcher's broom was investigated in dogs and guinea pigs. In 6 male and female dogs death occurred within 1 hour following intravenous infusion of the extract at doses between 0.83 and 1.8 g/kg body weight. By the intraperitoneal route no toxic signs were found in guinea pigs at doses lower than 1.5 g/kg body weight; animals receiving doses of 2 g/kg body weight and above died. Toxic and subtoxic doses affected the respiratory function, and lethal doses resulted in hyperventilation followed by fatal apnoea [48,49].

Estimation of the oral and intraperitoneal LD_{50} values of a butcher's broom fluid extract (ethanol 50% V/V) in rats and mice revealed differences depending on the harvest time of the plant, the route of administration and the use of roots or rhizomes. The oral LD_{50} of the rhizome extracts was 2.07-2.39 ml/kg body weight in rats and 24.69-33.73 ml/kg in mice; after intraperitoneal administration the toxicity was 10-20 fold higher. Root extract was found to be more toxic than rhizome extract (1.4-1.8 fold in rats and 4-5 fold in mice). The observed symptoms of intoxication were convulsion, paralysis and gastro-intestinal inflammation with dysentery. Animals died following respiratory failure. Autopsies revealed pronounced irritation of the mucosa and strong visceral congestion [50].

Oral LD_{50} values of ruscogenin and *Ruscus* saponins were estimated to be greater than 3g/kg body weight in mice and rats [19].

Repeated dose toxicity

Butcher's broom extract was given to male rabbits in their diet for 26 weeks, 17 animals receiving 2 g/kg body weight and 19 receiving 5 g/kg while 16 animals served as controls. Body weights and blood counts did not reveal any differences between treated animals and controls [51].

Rats were treated with 300 mg/kg of ruscogenin or *Ruscus* saponins by gavage daily for 8 weeks (10 animals per group, with 10 untreated rats as controls). No toxic signs or differences in body and organ weight were observed. Histological examination did not reveal any pathological changes in any group. Blood glucose and liver function did not reveal any significant differences between groups. An increase in diuresis and excretion of electrolytes was observed in the ruscogenin group but not in animals treated with saponins [19].

Reproductive toxicity

Reproductive toxicity was studied with a preparation containing an ethanolic butcher's broom extract (10%), TMHC, citric acid, methyl-4-esculetol and ascorbic acid; 5 ml of the ethanolic fluid contained 0.5 ml of the butcher's broom extract. Twenty female Wistar rats received a daily dose of 2.4 ml of the preparation, equivalent to 25 times the recommended dose for humans; 20 untreated animals served as controls. Treatment started one week before conception and continued until delivery. The animals tolerated the drug without any signs of intoxication. The fertility of females in the treatment group was comparable to that in the control group and the offspring did not show any teratogenic signs [52].

Clinical safety data

A butcher's broom dry extract (15-20:1, methanol 60%) taken orally by 77 women at a dosage of 72-75 mg daily for 12 weeks was well tolerated. Overall tolerability was assessed as very good by 76.8% and good by 23.2% of subjects and was comparable to that of placebo treatment. Laboratory data, comparison of vital signs and physical examination before and after treatment did not reveal any treatment-related changes [7].

Combination preparations

Placebo-controlled and open studies with combination preparations containing butcher's broom extracts have not revealed any specific side effects. Moderate gastric complaints were observed [53,54].

Single cases of diarrhoea and lymphocytic colitis have been reported following the use of combinations containing butcher's broom extract [55-57].

Reproductive toxicity

Ruscogenin-containing suppositories were well tolerated by 30 pregnant women without any apparent effects on the newborn babies [9].

REFERENCES

1. Butcher's Broom - Rusci rhizoma. European Pharmacopoeia, Council of Europe.

2. Sticher O. Mäusedornwurzelstock. In: Hänsel R, Sticher O, Steinegger E. Pharmakognosie - Phytopharmazie, 6th ed. Berlin-Heidelberg-New York: Springer-Verlag, 1999:568-70.

3. Schneider G. Saponine. In: Arzneidrogen. Mannheim-Wien-Zürich: BI-Wiss.-Verlag, 1990:153-62.

4. Mimaki Y, Kuroda M, Kameyama A, Yokosuka A, Sashida Y. New steroidal constituents of the underground parts of *Ruscus aculeatus* and their cytostatic activity on HL-60 cells. Chem Pharm Bull 1998;46:298-303.

5. Mimaki Y, Kuroda M, Kameyama A, Yokosuka A, Sashida Y. Steroidal saponins from the underground parts of *Ruscus aculeatus* and their cytostatic activity on HL-60 cells. Phytochemistry 1998;48:485-93.

6. Rauwald HW, Janßen B. Desglucoruscin und Desglucoruscosid als Leitstoffe des *Ruscus aculeatus*-Wurzelstock. Pharm Ztg Wiss 1988;133/1:61-8.

7. Vanscheidt W, Jost V, Wolna P, Lücker PW, Müller M, Theurer C, Patz B, Grützner KI. Efficacy and safety of a butcher's broom preparation (*Ruscus aculeatus* L. extract) compared to placebo in patients suffering from chronic venous insufficiency. Arzneim-Forsch/Drug Res 2002;52:243-50.

8. Willuhn G. Rusci rhizoma - Mäusedornwurzelstock. In: Wichtl M, editor. Teedrogen und Phytopharmaka. Ein Handbuch für die Praxis auf wissenschaftlicher Grundlage, 4th ed. Stuttgart: Wissenschaftliche Verlagsgesellschaft, 2002:531-3.

9. Anger H, Nietsch P. Ruscorectal bei Analerkrankungen. Med Welt 1981;33:1450-2.

10. Baudet JH, Collet D, Aubard Y, Renaudie P. Therapeutic test of *Ruscus* extract in pregnant women: evaluation of the fetal tolerance applying the pulse Doppler's method of the cord. In: Vanhoutte PM, editor. Return circulation and norepinephrine: an update. Paris: John Libbey Eurotext 1991:63-71.

11. Harker CT, Marcelon G, Vanhoutte PM. Temperature, oestrogens and contractions of venous smooth muscle of the rabbit. Phlebology 1988;3(Suppl 1):77-82.

12. Lauressergues H, Vilain P. Pharmacological activities of *Ruscus* extract on venous smooth muscle. Int Angiol 1984;3:70-3.

13. Marcelon G, Verbeuren TJ, Lauressergues H, Vanhoutte PM. Effect of *Ruscus aculeatus* on isolated canine cutaneous veins. Gen Pharmacol 1983;14:103-6.

14. Marcelon G, Vanhoutte PM. Venotonic effect of *Ruscus* under variable temperature conditions in vitro. Phlebology 1988;3(Suppl 1):51-4.

15. Marcelon G, Vanhoutte PM. Mechanism of action of *Ruscus* extract. Int Angiol 1984;3:74-6.

16. Rubanyi, F, Marcelon G, Vanhoutte PM. Effect of temperature on the responsiveness of cutaneous veins to the extract of *Ruscus aculeatus*. Gen Pharmacol 1994;15:431-4.

17. Miller VM, Marcelon G, Vanhoutte PM. *Ruscus* extract releases endothelium-derived relaxing factor in arteries and veins. In: Vanhoutte PM, editor. Return circulation and norepinephrine: an update. Paris: John Libbey Eurotext 1991:31-42.

18. Miller VM, Marcelon G, Vanhoutte PM. Progesterone augments the venoconstrictor effect of *Ruscus* without altering adrenergic reactivity. Phlebology 1991;6:261-8.

19. Capra C. Studio farmacologico e tossicologico di componenti del *Ruscus aculeatus* L. Fitoterapia 1972;43:99-113.

20. Miller VM, Rud K, Gloviczki P. Interactions of *Ruscus* extract with endothelin-receptors in human varicose veins. Clin Hemorheol 1994;14:S37-S45.

21. Miller VM, Rud KS, Gloviczki. Pharmacological assessment of adrenergic receptors in human varicose veins. Int Angiol 2000;19:176-183.

22. Marcelon G, Vieu S, Pouget G, Tisne-Versailles J. Oestrogenous impregnation and *Ruscus* action on the human vein in vitro, depending on preliminary results. Phlebology 1988;3(Suppl 1):83-5.

23. Branco D, Osswald W. The influence of *Ruscus* extract on the uptake and metabolism of noradrenaline in the normal and varicose human saphenous vein. Phlebology 1988;3 (Suppl 1):33-9.

24. Hönig I, Felix W. Effect on the permeability of the isolated ear vein of the pig; a comparison between flavonoid and saponins. In: Davy A, Stemmer R, editors. Phlébologie. Paris: John Libbey Eurotext, 1989:680-2.

25. Baurain R, Dom G, Trouet A. Protecting effect of Cyclo 3 Fort and its constituents for human endothelial cells under hypoxia. Clin Hemorheol 1994;14:S15-S21.

26. Bouaziz N, Michiels C, Janssens D, Berna N, Eliaers F, Panconi E, Remacle J. Effect of *Ruscus* extract and hesperidin methylchalcone on hypoxia-induced activation of endothelial cells. Int Angiol 1999;18:306-12.

27. Marcelon G, Pouget G, Tisne-Versailles J. Effect of *Ruscus* on the adrenoceptors of the canine lymphatic thoracic duct. Phlebology 1988;3(Suppl 1):109-112.

28. McHale NG. Mechanism of noradrenaline action in lymphatic vessels. In: Vanhoutte PM, editor. Return circulation and norepinephrine: an update. Paris: John Libbey Eurotext 1991:73-88.

29. Maffei Facino R, Carini M, Stefani R, Aldini G, Saibene L. Anti-elastase and anti-hyaluronidase activities of saponins and sapogenins from *Hedera helix*, *Aesculus hippocastanum* and *Ruscus aculeatus*: factors contributing to their efficacy in the treatment of venous insufficiency. Arch Pharm (Weinheim) 1995;328:720-4.

30. Bouskela E, Cyrino FZGA, Marcelon G. Possible mechanism for the venular constriction elicited by *Ruscus* extract on hamster cheek pouch. J Cardiovasc Pharmacol 1994;24:165-70.

31. Bouskela E. Microcirculatory responses to *Ruscus* extract in the hamster cheek pouch. In : Vanhoutte PM, editor. Return circulation and norepinephrine: an update. Paris: John Libbey Eurotext, 1991:207-18.

32. Mellander S, Maspers M, Ekelund U. Sympathetic nervous control of tonus in large bore arterial vessels, arterioles and veins, and of capillary pressure and fluid exchange in cat skeletal muscle (comparative effects evoked by *Ruscus aculeatus* extract). In: Vanhoutte

PM, editor. Return circulation and norepinephrine: an update. Paris: John Libbey Eurotext, 1991:181-96.

33. Teixeira AA, Oswald W. Effects of *Ruscus aculeatus* extract on the structural and functional alterations caused by sympathetic denervation of the saphenous vein. Phlebology 1988;3(Suppl 1):27-31.

34. Bouskela E, Cyrino FZGA. Possible mechanisms for the effects of *Ruscus* extract on microvascular permeability and diameter. Clin Hemorheol 1994;14:S23-S36.

35. Bouskela E, Cyrino FZGA, Marcelon G. Inhibitory effect of the *Ruscus* extract and of the flavonoid hesperidine methylchalcone on increased microvascular permeability induced by various agents in the hamster cheek pouch. J Cardiovasc Pharmacol 1993; 22:225-30.

36. Felix W, Nieberle J, Schmidt G. Protektive Wirkung von Trimethylhesperidinchalkon und *Ruscus aculeatus* gegenüber dem Etacrynsäureödem am Hinterlauf der narkotisierten Katze. Phlebol Proktol 1983;12:209-18.

37. Chevillard L, Ranson M, Senault B. Activité anti-inflammatoire d'extraits de fragon épineux (*Ruscus aculeatus* L.). Med Pharmacol 1965;12:109-14.

38. Cahn J, Herold M, Senault B. Antiphlogistic and anti-inflammatory activity of F191 (purified sapogenins of *Ruscus aculeatus*). Proc Int Symposium on non-steroidal anti-inflammatory drugs. Mailand, 8-10 Sept 1964. Amsterdam 1965:293-8.

39. Pouget G, Ducros L, Marcelon G. Effect of *Ruscus* extract on peripheral lymphatic vessel pressure and flow. In: Vanhoutte PM, editor. Return circulation and norepinephrine: an update. Paris: John Libbey Eurotext, 1991:89-95.

40. Rudofsky G. Venentonisierung und Kapillarabdichtung. Fortschr Med 1989;107:430-4.

41. Le Devehat C, Khodabandehlou T, Vimeux M, Bondoux G. Hemorheological concepts in venous insufficiency and implications for treatment with *Ruscus* extract. In: Vanhoutte PM, editor. Return circulation and norepinephrine: an update. Paris: John Libbey Eurotext, 1991:225-36.

42. Salzmann P, Ehresmann U, Adler U. *Ruscus aculeatus* L. - der Mäusedorn: ein Therapeutikum in der Proktologie. Fortschr Med 1977;95:1419-22.

43. Bärmig H. Ruscorectal - ein neues anorektales Therapeutikum. Therapiewoche 1978;28:7279-80.

44. Chanal JL, Cousse H, Sicart MT, Derocq JM. Étude cinétique de l'absorption d'un extrait de *Ruscus*

radiomarqué. Travaux Soc Pharm Montpellier 1978; 38:43-8.

45. Chanal JL, MBatchi B, Sicart MT, Cousse H, Fauran F. Comparaison de la biodisponibilité d'extrait de *Ruscus* tritié chez le rat en fonction de la voie d'administration. Travaux Soc Pharm Montpellier 1981;41:263-72.

46. Bernard P, Cousse H, Rico AG, Fauran F. Etude autoradiographique de la distribution du tritium chez des singes macaques traité par un extrait de *Ruscus* tritié. Ann Pharm Fr 1985;43:573-84.

47. Rauwald HW, Grünwidl J. *Ruscus aculeatus* extract: unambiguous proof of the absorption of spirostanol glycosides in human plasma after oral administration. Planta Med 1991;57(Suppl 2):A75-A76.

48. Moscarella C. Contribution a l'étude pharmaco-dynamique du *Ruscus aculeatus* L. [Thesis]. Université de Toulouse, 1953.

49. Caujolle F, Mériel P, Stanislas E. Sur les propriétés pharmacologiques de l'extrait de *Ruscus aculeatus*. Ann Pharm Fr 1953;11:109-20.

50. Boucard M, Beaulaton IS, Reboul C. Étude de la toxicité aiguë de divers extraits fluides de fragon épineux (*Ruscus aculeatus* L.). Travaux Soc Pharm Montpellier 1967;27:187-91.

51. Roux G. Toxikologisches Gutachten für *Ruscus aculeatus*. Faculté Med Pharm, Université de Toulouse, 1969 (Unpublished).

52. Labie C. Gutachten über die teratogene Wirkung des Präparates "Cyclo 3" (Unpublished).

53. Monteil-Seurin J, Ladure P. Efficacy of *Ruscus* extract in the treatment of the premenstrual syndrome. In: Vanhoutte PM, editor. Return circulation and norepinephrine: an update. Paris: John Libbey Eurotext, 1991:43-53.

54. Parrodo F, Buzzi A. A study of the efficacy and tolerability of a preparation containing *Ruscus aculeatus* in the treatment of chronic venous insufficiency of the lower limbs. Clin Drug Invest 1999;18:255-61.

55. Beaugerie L, Luboinski J, Brousse N, Cosnes J, Chatelet FP, Gendre JP, Quintrec YL. Drug induced lymphocytic colitis. Gut 1994;35:426-8.

56. Maechel H. Diarrhée chronique secondaire au Cirkan®. Gastroenterol Clin Biol 1992;16:373.

57. Rassiat E, Michiels C, Piard F, Faivre J. Colite lympho-cytaire chez une femme ayant une maladie de Biermer et traitée par Cirkan®. La Presse Medicale 2001;30:970.

SALICIS CORTEX

Willow Bark

E/S/C/O/P
MONOGRAPHS
Second Edition

DEFINITION

Willow bark consists of the whole or fragmented dried bark of young branches or whole dried pieces of current year twigs of various species of the genus *Salix* including *S. purpurea* L., *S. daphnoides* Vill. and *S. fragilis* L. The drug contains not less than 1.5 per cent of total salicylic derivatives, expressed as salicin ($C_{13}H_{18}O_7$; M_r 286.3) and calculated with reference to the dried drug.

The material complies with the monograph of the European Pharmacopoeia [1].

CONSTITUENTS

The characteristic constituents are derivatives of salicin, mainly salicortin, 2'-*O*-acetylsalicortin and/or tremulacin [2-7].

The bark of *Salix purpurea* L. contains 4-8% of total salicin (determined after hydrolysis) [2]. Phenol glucosides present include salicortin (up to 9%), tremulacin (rarely more than 1%) and salireposide (0.1-1.2%), with small amounts of syringin and purpurein (up to 0.4%) [4,5,8]. Other constituents include the yellow chalcone isosalipurposide (0.15-2.2%), the flavanones eriodictyol-7-glucoside (0.18-0.4%) and (+)- and (–)-naringenin-5-glucoside (0.4-1.5% each) [5,7,8], approximately 0.5% of (+)-catechin [5] and 5% of polyphenols [3]. Young twigs (bark and wood) contain the same constituents in lower concentrations than the bark alone.

The bark of *Salix daphnoides* Villars contains more than 4% of total salicin [2]. Phenol glucosides present include salicortin (3-11%), tremulacin (up to 1.5%) and salicin (up to 1%) [3-5,8]; a small amount of syringin (up to 0.2%) also occurs [8]. Other constituents include the yellow chalcone isosalipurposide (0.2-1.5%), the flavanones (+)- and (–)-naringenin-5-glucoside (0.3-1.0% each) and naringenin-7-glucoside (0.3-1.5%) [7,8], approximately 0.5% of (+)-catechin [5] and 5% of polyphenols [3]. Young twigs (bark and wood) contain the same constituents in lower concentrations than the bark alone.

CLINICAL PARTICULARS

Therapeutic indications
Relief of low back pain [9-12,17,18]; symptomatic relief of mild osteoarthritic and rheumatic complaints [9-11,13-16].

Posology and method of administration

Dosage
Adult daily dose: dried hydroalcoholic or aqueous extracts, tinctures or fluid extracts, equivalent to 120-240 mg of total salicin [9,11,12,16-18].
Elderly: dose as for adults.
Children: not recommended for children.

Method of administration
For oral administration.

Duration of administration
No restriction.

Contra-indications
None known.

Special warnings and special precautions for use
The treatment of children with willow bark extracts is not recommended because of the structural similarity of salicylic derivatives in willow bark to acetylsalicylic acid. The use of synthetic acetylsalicylic acid (aspirin) in children is still associated with the so-called Reye's syndrome, although the number of reported cases appears to be declining with the availability of better diagnostic tools [19,20].

Interaction with other medicaments and other forms of interaction
None reported.
The irreversible inhibition of platelet aggregation by acetylsalicylic acid is less likely to be induced by the structurally different salicin [7,21].

Pregnancy and lactation
No data available. In accordance with general medical practice, the product should not be used during pregnancy and lactation without medical advice.

Effects on ability to drive and use machines
None known.

Undesirable effects
None reported.
In cases of sensitivity to salicylates, the use of willow bark preparations should be avoided.

Overdose
No toxic effects reported.

PHARMACOLOGICAL PROPERTIES

Pharmacodynamic properties

In vitro experiments

Anti-inflammatory effects
The hen's egg chorioallantoic membrane test system [22,23] has been used to study the anti-inflammatory effect of the willow bark constituents salicin and tremulacin [24]. Onset of this anti-inflammatory effect is delayed in comparison with saligenin (salicyl alcohol), sodium salicylate and acetylsalicylic acid, indicating that the active principles may be metabolites of salicin and tremulacin [24].

In vivo experiments

Anti-inflammatory effects
Isolated tremulacin, subcutanously injected at 100 mg/kg body weight, significantly inhibited carrageenan-induced paw oedema ($p<0.001$ in hours 3-6 after carrageenan injection) and peritoneal leucocyte migration (by 50%, $p<0.01$) in rats, and croton oil-induced ear oedema (by 43%, $p<0.001$) and acetic-acid induced writhing ($p<0.01$ to $p<0.001$) in mice. Inhibition of leukotriene B_4 biosynthesis in pleural leucocytes (obtained from rats 4 hours after intrapleural injection of carrageenan) also supported its anti-inflammatory activity in acute inflammatory animal models [25].

Antipyretic effects
Salicin administered orally to rats at 5 mmol/kg body weight significantly reduced yeast-induced fever, producing a normal temperature, and completely prevented fever when administered simultaneously with yeast. However, salicin at this dose level did not affect the rectal body temperature of afebrile rats. On the other hand, both sodium salicylate and saligenin at 5 mmol/kg lowered body temperature significantly in afebrile rats [26].

Pharmacological studies in humans
None reported.

Clinical studies
A standardized willow bark extract in coated tablets was evaluated in osteoarthritis patients in a randomized, double-blind, placebo-controlled study at an oral dosage corresponding to 240 mg of salicin (n = 39) or placebo (n = 39) daily for 2 weeks following a washout phase with placebo only for 4-6 days. Efficacy was assessed by means of the WOMAC Osteoarthritis Index [27]. The WOMAC pain score in the willow bark group decreased significantly (–14%, p = 0.047) compared to that of the placebo group (+ 2%). The final overall assessments showed significant superiority of the willow bark extract over placebo (physicians' assessment, p = 0.0073; patients' assessment, p = 0.0002) and demonstrated a moderate analgesic effect in osteoarthritis. The authors suggested that 2 weeks may not have been long enough to reach the maximum treatment effect [16].

In a randomized, double-blind, placebo-controlled, three-arm study, patients with an exacerbation of chronic low back pain were assigned to one of three treatments: a standardized willow bark extract in coated tablets corresponding to either 2 × 120 mg of salicin (n = 70) or 2 × 60 mg of salicin (n = 70), or placebo (n = 70), daily for 4 weeks. Efficacy was assessed using the Arhus Low Back Pain Index, and tramadol (an opoid analgesic) was the sole rescue medication. From intention-to-treat analysis, the number of pain-free patients without rescue medication (responders) in the last week of the study was significantly higher (p<0.001) in the verum groups and also dose-dependent: 27 out of 70 (39%) in the high-dose group and 15 out of 70 (21%) in the low-dose group, compared to 4 out of 70 (6%) in the placebo group. Significantly more patients in the placebo group required tramadol (p<0.001) during each week of the study. Willow bark extract thus appeared to be a useful and safe treatment for low back pain [17].

In an open, randomized, controlled, post-marketing study, patients with acute exacerbations of low back pain were assigned to treatment with a willow bark extract (corresponding to 240 mg of salicin, n = 114) or the synthetic anti-rheumatic rofecoxib, a selective COX-2 inhibitor (12.5 mg, n = 114) daily for 4 weeks. All patients were free to use whatever additional conventional treatments were thought necessary. About 20 patients were pain-free (visual analogue scale score < 2) in each group after 4 weeks of treatment. About 60% of patients in each group responded well to treatment, as judged by improvement of ≥ 30% in the Total Pain Index. Only a few patients resorted to additional conventional treatment options. The incidence of adverse events was similar in the two groups and there was no significant difference in efficacy between willow bark extract and the COX-2 inhibitor [12].

In an open, non-randomized, post-marketing study, groups of patients with acute exacerbations of low back pain received willow bark extract corresponding to 120 mg (n = 115) or 240 mg (n = 112) of salicin daily or, as controls, no treatment with willow bark (n = 224). All patients had access to conventional treatments according to the budget of the general practitioner. Better pain relief and less reliance on supplementary conventional treatments was evident in the group treated with 240 mg of salicin than in the group treated with 120 mg of salicin. The average cost incurred in the group not using willow bark was reduced by 14-40% in the willow bark groups [18].

Pharmacokinetic properties

Pharmacokinetics in vitro

Hydrolysis of salicin
Salicin is stable under acidic conditions (0.5% hydrochloric acid, with or without pepsin) [28,29]

and produces no saligenin (salicyl alcohol), even after incubation with human saliva at pH 7.2 [28].

Hydrolysis of salicortin
Salicortin was unchanged after 1 hour of incubation in artificial gastric juice (pH 1.0). After 6 hours of incubation with artificial intestinal juice (pH 7.4-7.6 at 37°C) salicortin was degraded to salicin with $t_{0.5}$ = 4.02 hours [7,21].

Enzymatic hydrolysis and esterification
β-Glucosidase extracted from almonds (EC 3.2.1.21) and β-glucosidase derived from guinea pig liver converted salicin and salicortin to saligenin [30,31]; however, salicin derivatives acetylated on the sugar moiety (2'-O-acetylsalicin and 2'-O-acetylsalicortin) and tremulacin were not decomposed by β-glucosidase. Non-specific esterases (EC 3.1.1.1) from rabbit and porcine liver transformed salicortin to salicin (98.1%), acetylsalicortin to acetylsalicin (75.5%) and tremulacin to tremuloidin (63.9%) [30]. Pancreatic proteases degraded salicortin to salicin and tremulacin to tremuloidin [32].

Erythrocyte membrane permeability
Transport of salicin and saligenin into erythrocytes was rapid for saligenin (1 minute to saturation) and delayed for salicin (4 hours to saturation). The process was reversible, release being rapid for saligenin and slower for salicin [33].

Protein binding
Saligenin and salicin both bind to human serum albumin but saligenin has a significantly higher affinity [33].

Metabolic transformation by homogenised kidney, liver and lung
Saligenin was transformed into salicylic acid by homogenised liver, kidney and lung. Gentisic acid was qualitatively detectable in homogenised liver after incubation with saligenin [34]. Salicin was partially metabolised to saligenin and salicylic acid after incubation with homogenised kidney from rats [35].

Intestinal metabolism
Salicin injected into an isolated, closed-off section of the male rat intestine, appendix and colon was hydrolysed by intestinal bacteria to its main metabolite saligenin [34].

Transport through intestinal wall
Transport of salicin and saligenin through the isolated intestinal wall was confirmed using the closed-off posterior section of the male rat intestine. When salicin and saligenin were injected into the closed intestine both passed the ileal wall unchanged. Saligenin appeared to penetrate the intestinal wall faster than salicin [35].

Pharmacokinetics in animals

Serum concentration-time curve
and metabolism in rats
The concentration of the metabolite salicylic acid was determined in the serum of rats after oral administration of salicin (400 mg/kg) or sodium salicylate (29 mg/kg). With salicin, no salicylic acid appeared during the first 2 hours but then it appeared in the serum, gradually increased and peaked at 5 hours with C_{max} = 82.4 µg/ml. After administration of sodium salicylate, salicylic acid appeared rapidly and reached a maximum concentration at 1.5 hours with C_{max} = 104.2 µg/ml. Elimination was slower after administration of sodium salicylate than after salicin. The relative bioavailability of salicylic acid from salicin was only 3.25% of that from sodium salicylate [36]; a discrepancy exists between this result and an earlier report [29] postulating good absorption of salicin in rats.

After oral administration of salicin to 4 male Wistar rats at 1 mmol/kg (0.268 g/kg) the urinary metabolites were: unchanged salicin (ca. 15% of the dose), saligenin (ca. 0.1%), salicylic acid (ca. 30%), conjugated salicylic acid (ca. 5%) and gentisic acid (ca. 2%). After oral administration of a total of 2.5 g of salicin in successive daily doses of 1 mmol/kg, only unchanged salicin was identified in the faeces [29].

Plasma levels of salicin, saligenin and salicylic acid were measured and compared to sodium salicylate after oral administration of each compound to rats at 1, 2.5 and 5 mmol/kg body weight. Salicin appears to be a prodrug, which is gradually transported to the lower part of the intestine, hydrolysed to saligenin by intestinal bacteria and converted to salicylic acid after absorption. Salicin absorption is slow compared to that of saligenin or salicylic acid [26].

Metabolism of radioactively-labelled salicin in mice
^{14}C-labelled salicin (8.9 mg/mouse) was rapidly and completely metabolised after oral administration to mice. Free salicylic acid was detected in the blood. Elimination was mainly by the renal route. Salicortin (4 mg/mouse) and tremulacin (11 mg/mouse) were partially metabolised. The metabolite gentisic acid was transiently detected in the small intestine [32].

Pharmacokinetics in humans

Absorption of salicin in humans
Salicin (4.0 g, corresponding to 1730 mg of saligenin) and, as a separate experiment, 2.0 g of sodium salicylate were taken as self-medication by the investigator to study and compare the kinetics. The maximum plasma concentration of free salicylates was reached about 2 hours after administration of salicin with C_{max} = 100 µg/ml. Sodium salicylate yielded C_{max} = 150 µg/ml, also after about 2 hours.

Metabolites equivalent to more than 86% of the administered salicin were recovered in 24-hour urine: salicyluric acid (51%), salicyl glucuronide (14%), salicylic acid (12%), gentisic acid (5%) and saligenin (4%), together with a small amount of unchanged salicin [28].

The urinary metabolite spectrum of oral acetylsalicylic acid in man [37] is very similar to that of salicin taken orally [21]. Populin (6'-*O*-benzoyl salicin) is not metabolised after oral administration in man [28].

Absorption and metabolism
of willow bark extract in humans
A standardized willow bark extract preparation corresponding to 240 mg of salicin was administered to 10 healthy volunteers in two equal doses at 0 and 3 hours. Urine and serum collected over a 24-hour period showed that salicylic acid was the major metabolite in serum (86% of total salicylates). Peak levels of salicylic acid were reached after 2 hours (1.2 mg/litre) and the area under the curve (AUC) was equivalent to that expected from an intake of 87 mg of acetylsalicylic acid. From this study it was concluded that willow bark extract leads to much lower serum salicylate levels than observed after analgesic doses of synthetic salicylates. The formation of salicylic acid alone does not therefore explain the analgesic or antirheumatic effects of willow bark [38].

12 male volunteers took 3 tablets containing willow bark extract (standardized to provide a total dose of 55 mg salicin) and cola nut extract. The plasma C_{max} of salicylic acid was 130 ng/ml, reached 3 hours after administration, and the plasma half-life was calculated as 2.5 hours. An exceptional increase in the plasma level of salicylic acid observed in one volunteer 4-6 hours after administration was attributed to the effects of eating lunch during this period. Administration of a second dose of 3 tablets four hours after the first dose produced a C_{max} of 311 ng/ml six hours after the first dose. This level was not increased further by a third dose of 3 tablets eight hours after the first dose [39].

Peak levels of salicylic acid in the serum of 10 healthy volunteers who received a willow bark extract corresponding to 240 mg of salicin per day were approximately 1.4 mg/litre. In contrast, peak levels of 35-50 mg/litre have been reported after the intake of 500 mg of acetylsalicylic acid. The observed analgesic effect of willow bark may not, therefore, be attributed to salicylic acid alone. It can be speculated that other constituents (e.g. tannins, flavonoids, salicin, salicin esters or others) may contribute to the overall effect of willow bark [16].

Other authors have suggested that the serum salicylate levels achieved by daily intake of willow bark corresponding to 240 mg of salicin are bioequivalent to an intake of about 50 mg of acetylsalicylate, which is a cardioprotective rather than an analgesic dose. Salicylate metabolites cannot be responsible for all the effects of willow bark extract, therefore other components of the extract may contribute to the overall analgesic effects [17].

Preclinical safety data

Inhibition of human platelet aggregation
Two randomized, double-blinded groups of patients with chronic low back pain were treated with willow bark extract corresponding to 240 mg of salicin (n = 19) or placebo (n = 16) daily for 28 days; a third group of patients suffering from chronic ischaemic heart disease (n = 16) received 100 mg of acetylsalicylate daily during the study period. Arachidonic acid-induced platelet aggregation, measured *ex vivo* in blood samples taken from the patients after 28 days of treatment, was minimally inhibited by the willow bark extract, but to a far lesser degree than by acetyl-salicylic acid. The mean percentages of maximal arachidonic acid-induced platelet aggregation were 61%, 78% and 13% in the willow bark extract, placebo and acetylsalicylate groups respectively [40].

Induction of gastric lesions
Salicin did not induce gastric lesions in rats even at a dose of 5 mmol/kg body weight. On the other hand, saligenin and sodium salicylate induced severe gastric lesions in a dose-dependent manner in the range of 1-5 mmol/kg [26].

Clinical safety data

From a total of 1149 patients and healthy volunteers treated with various preparations containing willow bark adverse events, predominantly mild, were reported in only 58 cases (5%) [15-18,39-42].

During 2 weeks of treatment with tablets each containing willow bark extract (360 mg, standardized to 11% of total salicin) and passiflora extract (40 mg), at a dosage of 6 tablets daily in the first week and 3 tablets daily in the second week, minor adverse events were reported in 10 patients (2.3%) out of 441. There were 5 reports of stomach ache, 2 of nausea, 1 of dizziness, 1 of sweating and 1 of a reversible skin rash, which were correlated with taking the preparation [41].

From daily treatment of 11 patients for 14 days with 6 tablets of the same combination product (extracts of willow bark and passiflora), no significant adverse reactions were reported in 10 patients; 1 patient dropped out due to stomach ache, which appeared unrelated to taking the preparation [15].

In a 2-week randomized study involving osteoarthritis patients, the number of patients experiencing adverse

events was the same in the placebo group (16 out of 39) as in those treated with willow bark extract corresponding to 240 mg of salicin per day (16 out of 39). However, more adverse events were reported in the placebo group (28) than in the verum group (17), the most frequent being allergic skin reactions and gastrointestinal upsets. The most important adverse event in the verum group was a skin rash starting on day 10, but the patient had a medical history of frequent allergic reactions [16].

In a 4-week randomized, three-arm study in patients with low back pain (three groups of 70), an allergic reaction (skin rash, swollen eyes, pruritus) reported by 1 patient receiving low-dose willow bark extract (2 × 60 mg of salicin per day) was attributed to the extract; dizziness reported by 2 patients taking the extract at the higher dose (2 × 120 mg of salicin per day) was attributed to tramadol rescue medication. In the placebo group, 3 patients reported dizziness and other symptoms attributed to tramadol, and 3 reported mild gastrointestinal ailments [17].

In 227 patients treated with willow bark extract (corresponding to 120 or 240 mg of salicin daily), occasional mild adverse events occurred and 3 cases of allergy appeared to be specific to willow bark [18].

Reversible gastrointestinal complaints were reported in 13 patients (5.7%) out of 228 treated for one day (one tablet, repeated if necessary every two hours) with a combination product containing willow bark extract (340 mg, standardized to 11% total salicin) and dry extract of cola nut (80 mg, standardized to 22.5 % caffeine) [42].

During treatment of 12 male volunteers for 2 days with tablets each containing willow bark extract (166.6 mg, standardized to 11% total salicin) and dry extract of cola nut (38 mg, standardized to 25% caffeine), at a dosage of 3 tablets on the first day and 9 tablets on the second day, no adverse events were reported [39].

From 41 patients with chronic arthritic pain, treated with a combination product containing 200 mg of willow bark per dose in a 2-month double-blind study, 3 adverse events were reported: one of dyspeptic symptoms, one of diarrhoea and one of headache [43].

A review of the safety of willow bark extract preparations treatments concluded that the incidence of adverse effects is low [44].

An extensive review of *Salix* studies supported the hypothesis that willow bark extract is less prone to cause adverse reactions in the stomach, as are known to be caused by acetylsalicylic acid. This appears to be because willow bark does not inhibit cyclooxygenase in the stomach wall, since its active metabolites are generated in the intestine after passing through the stomach as intact glycosides; the development of stomach lesions is therefore unlikely [45].

REFERENCES

1.   Willow Bark - Salicis cortex. European Pharmacopoeia, Council of Europe.

2.   Meier B, Sticher O, Bettschart A. Weidenrinden-Qualität. Gesamtsalicinbestimmung in Weidenrinden und Weidenpräparaten mit HPLC. Dtsch Apoth Ztg 1985;125:341-7.

3.   Julkunen-Tiitto R. Distribution of certain phenolics in *Salix* species (Salicaceae) [Dissertation]. University of Joensuu, Finland: Publications in Sciences No. 15, 1989.

4.   Egloff CP. Phenolglykoside einheimischer *Salix*-Arten [Dissertation]. Eidg Techn Hochschule (ETH) Zürich, Switzerland. Nr. 7138, 1982.

5.   Shao Y. Phytochemischer Atlas der Schweizer Weiden [Dissertation]. Eidg Techn Hochschule (ETH) Zürich, Switzerland. Nr. 9532, 1991.

6.   Meier B, Julkunen-Tiitto R, Tahvanainen J, Sticher O. Comparative high-performance liquid and gas-liquid chromatographic determination of phenolic glucosides in Salicaceae species. J Chromatogr 1988;442:175-86.

7.   Meier B. Analytik, chromatographisches Verhalten und potentielle Wirksamkeit der Inhaltsstoffe salicylat-haltiger Arzneipflanzen Mitteleuropas [Habilitations-schrift]. Eidg Techn Hochschule (ETH) Zürich, Switzer-land, 1987.

8.   Meier B, Lehmann D, Sticher O, Bettschart A. Identifikation und Bestimmung von je acht Phenol-glycosiden in *Salix purpurea* und *Salix daphnoides* mit moderner HPLC. Pharm Acta Helv 1985;60:269-75.

9.   Willuhn G. Salicis cortex - Weidenrinde. In: Wichtl M, editor. Teedrogen und Phytopharmaka. Ein Handbuch für die Praxis auf wissenschaftlicher Grundlage, 4th ed. Stuttgart: Wissenschaftliche Verlagsgesellschaft, 2002: 534-7.

10.   Hänsel R. Weidenrinde, Salicis cortex. In: Phyto-pharmaka, 2nd ed. Berlin-Heidelberg-New York: Springer-Verlag, 1991:96-7.

11.   Meier B, Meier-Liebi M. Salix. In: Blaschek W, Hänsel R, Keller K, Reichling J, Rimpler H and Schneider G, editors. Hagers Handbuch der Pharmazeutischen Praxis, 5th ed. Supplement Volume (Folgeband) 3: Drogen L-Z. Berlin-Heidelberg-New York-London: Springer, 1998:469-96.

12.   Chrubasik S, Künzel O, Model A, Conradt C, Black A. Treatment of low back pain with a herbal or synthetic anti-rheumatic: a randomized controlled study. Willow bark extract for low back pain. Rheumatology 2001;

40:1388-93.

13.   Wagner H, Wiesenauer M. Salicylathaltige Drogen zur internen und externen Anwendung. In: Phytotherapie - Phytopharmaka und pflanzliche Homöopathika. Stuttgart-Jena-New York: Gustav Fischer, 1995:232-4.

14.   Meier B. Pflanzliche versus synthetische Arzneimittel. Schweiz Apoth Ztg 1989;127:472-7.
Also published as:
Meier B. Pflanzliche versus synthetische Arzneimittel. Z Phytotherapie 1989;10:182-9.

15.   Schaffner W. Weidenrinde - Ein Antirheumatikum der modernen Phytotherapie? In: Chrubasik S, Wink M, editors. Rheumatherapie mit Phytopharmaka. Stuttgart: Hippokrates, 1997:125-7.

16.   Schmid B, Lüdtke R, Selbmann H-K, Kötter I, Tschirdewahn B, Schaffner W, Heide L. Wirksamkeit und Verträglichkeit eines standardisierten Weiden-rindenextraktes bei Arthrose-Patienten: Randomisierte, Placebo-kontrollierte Doppelblindstudie. Z Rheumatol 2000;59:314-20.
English translation published as:
Schmid B, Lüdtke R, Selbmann H-K, Kötter I, Tschirdewahn B, Schaffner W, Heide L. Efficacy and tolerability of a standardized willow bark extract in patients with osteoarthritis: randomized placebo-controlled, double blind clinical trial. Phytother Res 2001;15:344-50.

17.   Chrubasik S, Eisenberg E, Balan E, Weinberger T, Luzzati R, Conradt C. Treatment of low back pain exacerbations with willow bark extract: a randomized double-blind study. Am J Med 2000;109:9-14.

18.   Chrubasik S, Künzel O, Black A, Conradt C, Kerschbaumer F. Potential economic impact of using a proprietary willow bark extract in outpatient treatment of low back pain: An open non-randomized study. Phytomedicine 2001;8:241-51.

19.   McGovern MC, Glasgow JFT, Stewart MC. Reye's syndrome and aspirin: lest we forget. BMJ 2001; 322:1591-2.

20.   Clark I, Whitten R, Molyneux M, Taylor T. Salicylates, nitric oxide, malaria and Reye's syndrome. Lancet 2001;357:625-7. *Subsequent correspondence*: Casteels-Van Daele M, Van Geet C, Wouters C, Eggermont E. Reye's syndrome *and authors' reply*: Clark I, Whitten R, Molyneux M, Taylor T. Reye's syndrome. ibid. 2001;358:334.

21.   Meier B, Liebi M. Salicinhaltige pflanzliche Arzneimittel. Überlegungen zur Wirksamkeit und Unbedenklichkeit. Z Phytotherapie 1990;11:50-8.

22.   Luepke NP. Hen's egg chorioallantoic membrane test for irritation potential. Food Chem Toxicol 1985;23:287-91.

23.   Luepke NP, Kemper FH. The HET-CAM test: an alternative to the Draize eye test. Food Chem Toxicol 1986;24:495-6.

24.   Steinegger E, Hövel H. Analytische und biologische

Untersuchungen an Salicaceen-Wirkstoffen, insbesondere an Salicin. I. Identifizierungs-, Isolierungs- und Bestimmungsmethoden. Pharm Acta Helv 1972; 47:133-41.

25. Cheng GF, Liu DP, Yang DX, He KQ, Bai JY, Zhu XY. Antiinflammatory effects of tremulacin, a salicin-related substance isolated from *Populus tomentosa* Carr. leaves. Phytomedicine 1994;1:209-11.

26. Akao T, Yoshino T, Kobashi K, Hattori M. Evaluation of salicin as an antipyretic prodrug that does not cause gastric injury. Planta Med 2002;68:714-8.

27. Bellamy N, Buchanan WW, Goldsmith CH, Campbell J, Stitt LW. Validation study of WOMAC: a health status instrument for measuring clinically important patient relevant outcomes to antirheumatic drug therapy in patients with osteoarthritis of the hip or knee. J Rheumatol 1988;15:1833-40.

28. Steinegger E, Hövel H. Analytische und biologische Untersuchungen an Salicaceen-Wirkstoffen, insbesondere an Salicin. II. Biologische Untersuchungen. Pharm Acta Helv 1972;47:222-34.

29. Fötsch G, Pfeifer S, Bartoszek M, Franke P, Hiller K. Biotransformation der Phenolglycoside Leiocarposid und Salicin. Pharmazie 1989;44:555-8.

30. Julkunen-Tiitto R, Meier B. The enzymatic decomposition of salicin and its derivatives obtained from Salicaceae species. J Nat Prod 1992;55:1204-12.

31. Gopalan V, Pastuszyn A, Galey WR, Glew RH. Exolytic hydrolysis of toxic plant glucosides by guinea pig liver cytosolic β-glucosidase. J Biol Chem 1992;267:14027-32.

32. Wutzke A. Radioisotopenmarkierung und Pharmakokinetik von Phenolglycosiden aus *Populus* spec., insbesondere aus *P. trichocarpa* Hook. sowie Untersuchungen zur Analytik und Wirkung [Dissertation]. Philipps-Universität Marburg, Germany, 1991.

33. Matsumoto Y, Ohsako M, Takadate A, Goto S. Reduction of erythrocyte membrane permeability and protein binding of low-molecular-weight drugs following glycoside derivatization. J Pharm Sci 1993;82:399-403.

34. Fötsch G, Pfeifer S. Die Biotransformation der Phenolglycoside Leiocarposid und Salicin - Beispiele für Besonderheiten von Absorption und Metabolismus glycosidischer Verbindungen. Pharmazie 1989;44:710-2.

35. Adamkiewicz VW, Fortier AA. Passage of salicin and saligenin across the wall of the rat ileum. Can J Biochem Physiol 1961;39:1097-9.

36. Fötsch G, Pfeifer S. Vergleichende Serumspiegeluntersuchung von Salicylsäure nach oraler Applikation von Salicin bzw. Natriumsalicylat in Ratten. Pharmazie 1990;45:535-6.

37. Dinnendahl V, Fricke U, editors. Acetylsalicylsäure. In: Arzneistoff-profile. Basisinformation über arzneiliche Wirkstoffe. 1. Ergänzungs-Lieferung. Arbeitsgemeinschaft für Pharmazeutische Information (API). Frankfurt: Govi-Verlag, 1982.

38. Schmid B, Kötter I, Heide L. Pharmacokinetics of salicin after oral administration of a standardised willow bark extract. Eur J Clin Pharmacol 2001;57:387-91.

39. Pentz R, Busse HG, König R, Siegers C-P. Bioverfügbarkeit von Salicylsäure und Coffein aus einem phytoanalgetischen Kombinationspräparat. Dtsch Apoth Ztg 1989;129:277-9.

40. Krivoy N, Pavlotzky E, Chrubasik S, Eisenberg E, Brook G. Effect of Salicis cortex extract on human platelet aggregation. Planta Med 2001;67:209-12.
Also published as:
Krivoy N, Brook G. Effect of a Salicis cortex extract on platelet aggregation. In: Chrubasik S, Roufogalis BD, editors. Herbal Medicinal Products for the Treatment of Pain. Lismore, Australia: Southern Cross University Press, 2000:79-84.

41. Feldstudie mit Zeller Rheuma-Dragées forte. Max Zeller Söhne AG, CH-8590 Romanshorn. Unpublished report 1990.

42. Erfolgschancen eines pflanzlichen Heilmittels bei Kopfschmerzen. Max Zeller Söhne AG, CH-8590 Romanshorn. Unpublished report 1992.

43. Mills SY, Jakoby RK, Chacksfield M, Willoughby M. Effect of a proprietary herbal medicine on the relief of chronic arthritic pain: a double-blind study. Brit J Rheumatol 1996;35:874-8.

44. Chrubasik S, Eisenberg E. Efficacy and safety of *Salix* extract preparations. In: Chrubasik S, Roufogalis BD editors. Herbal Medicinal Products for the Treatment of Pain. Lismore, Australia: Southern Cross University Press, 2000:74-8.

45. Kaul R, Lagoni N. Weidenrinde. Renaissance eines Phytoanalgetikums. Dtsch Apoth Ztg 1999;139:3439-46.

451

SALVIAE OFFICINALIS FOLIUM

Sage Leaf

DEFINITION

Sage leaf consists of the whole or cut dried leaves of *Salvia officinalis* L. The whole drug contains not less than 15 ml/kg of essential oil and the cut drug not less than 10 ml/kg of essential oil, both calculated with reference to the anhydrous drug.

The material complies with the monograph of the European Pharmacopoeia [1].

Fresh material may also be used, provided that when dried it complies with the monograph of the European Pharmacopoeia.

CONSTITUENTS

Essential oil, up to 2.5% [2], containing monoterpenes such as α- and β-thujone (up to 63% and 13% respectively), camphor and 1,8-cineole [3,4]. Monoterpene glycosides [5,6]. Diterpenoids such as carnosic acid and its derivatives, e.g. carnosol [7,8], and a quinone methide [9]. Triterpenoids including ursolic acid, oleanolic acid and their derivatives [10,11]. Flavonoids, e.g. 5-methoxysalvigenin [12,13]. Phenolic compounds, e.g. rosmarinic acid and derivatives [14,15], a caffeic acid trimer [16], and flavonoid and phenolic glycosides [17-19].

CLINICAL PARTICULARS

Therapeutic indications
Inflammations and infections of the mouth and throat such as stomatitis, gingivitis and pharyngitis [10,20]; hyperhidrosis [10,20-22].

Posology and method of administration

Dosage

Topical use
An infusion of 3 g of the drug in 150 ml of water as a mouthwash or gargle [21,23].

Oral use (in hyperhidrosis)
Tincture: (1:10) in 55% ethanol, 75 drops daily [23].
Infusion: 1-1.5 g of dried herb in 150 ml of water, once or several times daily [21,23].
Dry extract: 160 mg of dry aqueous extract corresponding to 880 mg of drug three times daily [22].

Method of administration
For oral administration or topical application.

Duration of administration

In hyperhidrosis, treatment for 2-4 weeks is recommended, using an aqueous preparation [22].

Contra-indications

None known.

Special warnings and special precautions for use

Caution is required with the use of alcoholic preparations because of the presence of thujone.

Interaction with other medicaments and other forms of interaction

None reported.

Pregnancy and lactation

Given the potential toxicity of some constituents of the essential oil [24-27], the use of sage leaf is not recommended during pregnancy or lactation.

Effects on ability to drive and use machines

None known.

Undesirable effects

None reported.

Overdose

No toxic effects reported.

PHARMACOLOGICAL PROPERTIES

Pharmacodynamic properties

In vitro experiments

Sage oil exhibited bactericidal and fungicidal properties when tested on Gram-positive and Gram-negative bacteria, filamentous fungi and yeasts, e.g. *Candida albicans* [28,29]. An aqueous and a 50%-ethanolic extract of sage leaf exhibited strong inhibitory effects on the collagenolytic activity of *Porphyromonas gingivalis* [30]. Aerial parts of sage contain diterpenes with antiviral activity against vesicular stomatitis virus [31-33].

A 50%-methanolic extract from aerial parts of sage considerably inhibited lipid peroxidation in both enzyme-dependent and enzyme-independent test systems [34,35]. Two phenolic glycosides isolated from sage leaf, 6-*O*-caffeoyl-β-D-fructofuranosyl-(2→1)-α-D-glucopyranoside and 1-*O*-caffeoyl-β-D-apiofuranosyl-(1→6)-β-D-glucopyranoside, were found to have moderate antioxidant activity in the DPPH and metmyoglobin tests [19].

Rosmarinic acid has been shown to have anti-inflammatory activity [36,37].

In vivo experiments

Chloroform and *n*-hexane dry extracts from sage leaf dose-dependently inhibited croton oil-induced ear oedema in mice, chloroform extracts being the more potent with ID_{50} values of 106-140 µg/cm^2. The main component of the chloroform extract and the major contributor to its anti-inflammatory activity was found to be ursolic acid (ID_{50}: 0.14 µM/cm^2), which had twice the potency of indometacin (ID_{50}: 0.26 µM/cm^2) in this test. Oleanolic acid also showed anti-inflammatory activity but was less effective (ID_{50}: 0.36 µM/cm^2) [38].

When applied topically (5% in vehicle) to rhesus monkeys, rosmarinic acid significantly lowered both gingival and plaque indices in comparison with placebo [39].

Clinical studies

A dialysate of an aqueous extract from fresh sage leaf showed antihyperhidrotic activity in humans [40-42]. Excessive sweat production induced by pilocarpine was inhibited [42,43].

In an open study, patients with idiopathic hyperhidrosis were treated daily for 4 weeks with either 440 mg of a dry aqueous extract corresponding to 2.6 g of sage leaf (n = 40) or an infusion from 4.5 g of sage leaf (n = 40). The achieved reduction in sweat secretion (less than 50%) was comparable in the two groups, although slightly greater in the group treated with extract [22,44].

Pharmacokinetic properties

α-Thujone incubated with rabbit (but not mouse) liver cytosol in the presence of NADPH gave thujol and neothujol in low yield. On incubation with mouse liver cytosol alone, α-thujone was stable, but in the presence of NADPH it was rapidly metabolized, the major product being 7-hydroxy-α-thujone together with 4-hydroxy-α-thujone, 4-hydroxy-β-thujone and other minor metabolites [45].

In mice treated intraperitoneally with α-thujone, the brain levels of α-thujone and 7-hydroxy-α-thujone were dose- and time-dependent, but α-thujone appeared at much lower levels and was less persistent than 7-hydroxy-α-thujone. The latter compound is less toxic to mice; at 50 mg/kg administered intraperitoneally, α-thujone was lethal but 7-hydroxy-α-thujone and other metabolites were not lethal [45].

Preclinical safety data

The oral LD_{50} of the essential oil in rats was determined as 2.6 g/kg [26]. After intraperitoneal administration of sage oil to rats, cortical phenomena remained subclinical below 0.3 g/kg whereas convulsions appeared above 0.5 g/kg and became lethal above 3.2 g/kg [25].

The oral LD_{50} of thujone ($\alpha + \beta$) in rats was found to be 192 mg/kg. In subchronic toxicity tests in rats, thujone ($\alpha + \beta$) given orally to rats at 10 mg/kg daily produced convulsions in only 1 out of 20 animals by the 38th day [27].

Subcutaneous LD_{50} values in mice were determined as 87.5 mg/kg body weight for α-thujone and 442.4 mg/kg for β-thujone [46]; thus α-thujone, which is present as a higher proportion of the essential oil, is more toxic than β-thujone [3,45,46]. α-Thujone is a convulsant, the intraperitoneal LD_{50} in mice being about 45 mg/kg; at 60 mg/kg it is lethal to mice within 1 minute whereas at 30-45 mg/kg the mice either die or recover. The mechanism of α-thujone neurotoxicity has recently been elucidated; it is a reversible modulator of the γ-aminobutyric acid (GABA) type A receptor, but it is rapidly metabolized and detoxified [45].

A sage leaf tincture at doses up to 200 µl/plate showed no mutagenic activity in the Ames test using *Salmonella typhimurium* strains TA98 and TA100 with or without S9 metabolic activation [47]. Sage oil showed no mutagenic or DNA-damaging potential in the Ames test or *Bacillus subtilis* rec-assay [48].

REFERENCES

1. Sage Leaf (Salvia officinalis) - Salviae officinalis folium. European Pharmacopoeia, Council of Europe.

2. Steinegger E, Hänsel R. Salbei und Salbeiöle. In: Pharmakognosie, 5th ed. Berlin-Heidelberg: Springer-Verlag, 1992:343-5.

3. Lawrence BM. Progress in essential oils. Perfumer & Flavorist. 1998;23(March/April):47-57.

4. Müller J, Köll-Weber M, Kraus W. Effect of drying on the essential oil of *Salvia officinalis*. Planta Med 1992;58(Suppl 1):A678.

5. Croteau R, El-Bialy H, El-Hindawi S. Metabolism of monoterpenes: lactonization of (+)-camphor and conversion of the corresponding hydroxy acid to the glucoside-glucose ester in sage (*Salvia officinalis*). Arch Biochem Biophys 1984;228:667-80.

6. van den Dries JMA, Baerheim Svendsen A. A simple method for detection of glycosidic bound monoterpenes and other volatile compounds occurring in fresh plant material. Flavour Fragrance J 1989;4:59-61.

7. Rutherford DM, Nielsen MPC, Hansen SK, Witt M-R, Bergendorff O, Sterner O. Isolation and identification from *Salvia officinalis* of two diterpenes which inhibit *t*-butylbicyclophosphoro[^{35}S]thionate binding to chloride channel of rat cerebrocortical membranes in vitro. Neurosci Lett 1992;135:224-6.

8. Brieskorn CH, Dömling HJ. Natürliche und synthetische Derivate der Carnosolsäure. Arch Pharm 1969;302:641-5.

9. Tada M, Hara T, Hara C, Chiba K. A quinone methide from *Salvia officinalis*. Phytochemistry 1997;45:1475-7.

10. Brieskorn CH. Salbei - seine Inhaltsstoffe und sein therapeutischer Wert. Z Phytotherapie 1991;12:61-9.

11. Brieskorn CH, Kapadia Z. Bestandteile von *Salvia officinalis* XXIV: Triterpenalkohole, Triterpensäuren und Pristan im Blatt von *Salvia officinalis* L. Planta Med 1980;38:86-90.

12. Brieskorn CH, Biechele W. Flavone aus *Salvia officinalis* L. Arch Pharm 1971;304:557-61.

13. Brieskorn CH, Kapadia Z. Constituents of *Salvia officinalis* XXIII: 5-methoxysalvigenin in leaves of *Salvia officinalis*. Planta Med 1979;35:376-8.

14. Gracza L, Ruff P. Rosmarinsäure in Arzneibuchdrogen und ihre HPLC-Bestimmung. Arch Pharm (Weinheim) 1984;317:339-45.

15. Lu Y, Foo LY. Rosmarinic acid derivatives from *Salvia officinalis*. Phytochemistry 1999;51:91-4.

16. Lu Y, Foo LY, Wong H. Sagecoumarin, a novel caffeic acid trimer from *Salvia officinalis*. Phytochemistry 1999;52:1149-52.

17. Lu Y, Foo LY. Flavonoid and phenolic glycosides from *Salvia officinalis*. Phytochemistry 2000;55:263-7.

18. Wang M, Kikuzaki H, Zhu N, Sang S, Nakatani N, Ho C-T. Isolation and structure elucidation of two new glycosides from sage (*Salvia officinalis* L.). J Agric Food Chem 2000;48:235-8.

19. Wang M, Shao Y, Li J, Zhu N, Rangarajan M, LaVoie EJ, Ho C-T. Antioxidative phenolic glycosides from sage (*Salvia officinalis*). J Nat Prod 1999;62:454-6.

20. Weiss RF, Fintelmann V. Sage leaves (Salviae folium). In: Herbal Medicine, 2nd ed. (translated from Lehrbuch der Phytotherapie, 9th ed.). Stuttgart-New York: Thieme, 2000:36 and 422.

21. Wichtl M. Salviae officinalis folium - Salbeiblätter. In: Wichtl M, editor. Teedrogen und Phytopharmaka. Ein Handbuch für die Praxis auf wissenschaftlicher Grundlage. Stuttgart: Wissenschaftliche Verlags-gesellschaft, 2002:538-42.

22. Rösing S. Sweatosan-Studie; Untersuchungsbericht. Äquivalenz der Wirksamkeit und Vergleich der Verträglichkeit von Sweatosan und Salbeitee bei Patienten mit idiopathischer Hyperhidrosis in der dermatologischen Poliklinik. Zyma 1989; unpublished.

23. Van Hellemont J. In: Fytotherapeutisch compendium, 2nd ed. Utrecht: Bohn, Scheltema & Holkema, 1988: 539-41.

24. Gessner O. *Salvia officinalis* L., Salbei (Labiatae). In: Gift- und Arzneipflanzen in Mitteleuropa, 3rd ed. 1974:255-7.

25. Millet Y, Tognetti P, Lavaire-Pierlovisi M, Steinmetz M-

D, Arditti J, Jouglard J. Étude expérimentale des propriétés toxiques convulsivantes des essences de sauge et d'hysope du commerce. Rev EEG Neurophysiol 1979;9:12-8.

26. von Skramlik E. Über die Giftigkeit und Verträglichkeit von ätherischen Ölen. Pharmazie 1959;14:435-45.

27. Pinto-Scognamiglio W. Connaissances actuelles sur l'activité pharmacodynamique de la thuyone, aromatisant naturel d'un emploi étendu. Boll Chim Farm 1967;106:292-300.

28. Jalsenjak V, Peljnjak S, Kustrak D. Microcapsules of sage oil: essential oils content and antimicrobial activity. Pharmazie 1987;42:419-20.

29. Janssen AM. Antimicrobial activities of essential oils - a pharmacognostical study [Dissertation]. Leiden: Rijksuniversiteit te Leiden, 1989:91-108.

30. Osawa K, Matsumoto T, Yasuda H, Kato T, Naito Y, Okuda K. The inhibitory effect of plant extracts on the collagenolytic activity and cytotoxicity of human gingival fibroblasts by *Porphyromonas gingivalis* crude enzyme. Bull Tokyo Dent Coll 1991;32:1-7.

31. Tada M, Takakuwa T, Nagai M, Yoshii T. Antiviral and antimicrobial activity of 2,4-diacylphloroglucinols, 2-acylcyclohexane-1,3-diones and 2-carboxamidocyclo-hexane-1,3-diones. Agric Biol Chem 1990;54:3061-3.

32. Chiba K, Takakuwa T, Tada M, Yoshii T. Inhibitory effect of acylphloroglucinol derivatives on the replication of vesicular stomatitis virus. Biosci Biotech Biochem 1992;56:1769-72.

33. Tada M, Okuno K, Chiba K, Ohnishi E, Yoshii T. Antiviral diterpenes from *Salvia officinalis*. Phytochemistry 1994;35:539-41.

34. Hohmann J, Zupkó I, Rédei D, Csányi M, Falkay G, Máthé I, Janicsák G. Protective effects of the aerial parts of *Salvia officinalis*, *Melissa officinalis* and *Lavandula angustifolia* and their constituents against enzyme-dependent and enzyme-independent lipid peroxidation. Planta Med 1999;65:576-8.

35. Zupkó I, Hohmann J, Rédei D, Falkay G, Janicsák G, Máthé I. Antioxidant activity of leaves of *Salvia* species in enzyme-dependent and enzyme-independent systems of lipid peroxidation and their phenolic constituents. Planta Med 2001;67:366-8.

36. Verweij-van Vught AMJJ, Appelmelk BJ, Groeneveld ABJ, Sparrius M, Thijs LG, MacLaren DM. Influence of rosmarinic acid on opsonization and intracellular killing of *Escherichia coli* and *Staphylococcus aureus* by porcine and human polymorphonuclear leucocytes. Agents Actions 1987;22:288-94.

37. Rampart M, Beetens JR, Bult H, Herman AG, Parnham MJ, Winkelmann J. Complement-dependent stimulation of prostacyclin biosynthesis: inhibition by rosmarinic acid. Biochem Pharmacol 1986;35:1397-400.

38. Baricevic D, Sosa S, Della Loggia R, Tubaro A, Simonovska B, Krasna A, Zupancic A. Topical anti-inflammatory activity of *Salvia officinalis* L. leaves: the relevance of ursolic acid. J Ethnopharmacol 2001; 75:125-32.

39. Van Dyke TE, Braswell L, Offenbacher S. Inhibition of gingivitis by topical application of ebselen and rosmarinic acid. Agents Actions 1986;19:376-7.

40. Jost A. Über den Nachweis der schweißhemmenden Wirkung der Salbeidroge [Dissertation]. Bayerischen Ludwig-Maximilians-Universität zu München, 1934:1-25.

41. Schlegel B, Böttner H. Über den Einfluß der Salbeidroge auf den unmerklichen Gewichtsverlust des Gesunden. Z Ges exp Med 1940;107:267-74.

42. Mayr JK. Der Wasser- und Kochsalzstoffwechsel bei Dermatosen. Arch Dermatol Syph 1930;162:146-9.

43. Mayr JK. Studien zur Hautwasserabgabe. II. Mitteilung. Über die Wirkung allgemeiner Antihidrotica. Virchows Arch Pathol Anat Physiol 1933;287:297-308.

44. Council of Europe. Plant preparations used as ingredients of cosmetic products, 1st ed. Strasbourg, 1989.

45. Höld KM, Sirisoma NS, Ikeda T, Narahashi T, Casida JE. α-Thujone (the active component of absinthe): γ-aminobutyric acid type A receptor modulation and metabolic detoxification. Proc Natl Acad Sci USA 2000;97:3826-31.

46. Rice KC, Wilson RS. (–)-3-Isothujone, a small non-nitrogenous molecule with antinociceptive activity in mice. J Med Chem 1976;19:1054-7

47. Schimmer O, Krüger A, Paulini H, Haefele F. An evaluation of 55 commercial plant extracts in the Ames mutagenicity test. Pharmazie 1994;49:448-51.

48. Zani F, Massimo G, Benvenuti S, Bianchi A, Albasini A, Melegari M et al. Studies on the genotoxic properties of essential oils with *Bacillus subtilis* rec-assay and *Salmonella*/microsome reversion assay. Planta Med 1991;57:237-41.

SENNAE FOLIUM

Senna Leaf

DEFINITION

Senna leaf consists of the dried leaflets of *Cassia senna* L. (*C. acutifolia* Delile), known as Alexandrian or Khartoum senna, or *Cassia angustifolia* Vahl, known as Tinnevelly senna, or a mixture of the two species. It contains not less than 2.5 per cent of hydroxyanthracene glycosides, calculated as sennoside B ($C_{42}H_{38}O_{20}$; M_r 863) with reference to the dried drug.

The material complies with the monograph of the European Pharmacopoeia [1].

CONSTITUENTS

The main active constituents are sennosides A and B (ca. 2.5%), which are rhein-dianthrone diglucosides. Smaller amounts of other dianthrone diglucosides, monoanthraquinone glucosides and aglycones are also present [2-6].

CLINICAL PARTICULARS

Therapeutic indications
For short-term use in cases of occasional constipation [7-21].

Posology and method of administration

Dosage

The correct individual dose is the smallest required to produce a comfortable soft formed motion.

Adults and children over 10 years: preparations equivalent to 15-30 mg of hydroxyanthracene derivatives, calculated as sennoside B, to be taken once daily at night [11,14,15,20-24].
Elderly: dose as for adults [25,26].

Not recommended for use in children under 10 years of age [27-32].

The pharmaceutical form must allow lower dosages.

Method of administration
For oral administration.

Contra-indications
Not to be used in cases of: intestinal obstruction and stenosis, atony, inflammatory colon diseases (e.g. Crohn's disease, ulcerative colitis), appendicitis; abdominal pain of unknown origin; severe dehydration

E/S/C/O/P
MONOGRAPHS
Second Edition

states with water and electrolyte depletion. Children under 10 years.

Special warnings and special precautions for use

As for all laxatives, senna leaf should not be given when any undiagnosed acute or persistent abdominal symptoms are present.

If laxatives are needed every day the cause of the constipation should be investigated. Long term use of laxatives should be avoided. Use for more than 2 weeks requires medical supervision. Chronic use may cause pigmentation of the colon (pseudo-melanosis coli) which is harmless and reversible after drug discontinuation. Abuse, with diarrhoea and consequent fluid and electrolyte losses, may cause: dependence with possible need for increased dosages; disturbance of the water and electrolyte (mainly hypokalaemia) balance; an atonic colon with impaired function. Intake of anthranoid-containing laxatives for more than a short period of time may result in aggravation of constipation. Hypokalaemia can result in cardiac and neuromuscular dysfunction, especially if cardiac glycosides, diuretics or corticosteroids are taken. Chronic use may result in albuminuria and haematuria.

In chronic constipation stimulant laxatives are not an acceptable alternative to a change in diet [33-42].

Note: A detailed text with advice concerning changes in dietary habits, physical activities and training for normal bowel evacuation should be included on the package leaflet. An example is given in the booklet "Médicaments á base de plantes" published by the French health authority (Paris: Agence du Médicament).

Interaction with other medicaments and other forms of interaction

Hypokalaemia (resulting from long term laxative abuse) potentiates the action of cardiac glycosides and interacts with antiarrhythmic drugs or with drugs which induce reversion to sinus rhythm (e.g. quinidine). Concomitant use with other drugs inducing hypokalaemia (e.g. thiazide diuretics, adreno-corticosteroids and liquorice root) may aggravate electrolyte imbalance.

Pregnancy and lactation

Pregnancy

There are no reports of undesirable or damaging effects during pregnancy or on the foetus when used in accordance with the recommended dosage schedule. However, in view of experimental data concerning a genotoxic risk from several anthranoids (e.g. emodin and aloe-emodin), avoid during the first trimester or take only under medical supervision [33,43-54].

Lactation

Breastfeeding is not recommended as there are insufficient data on the excretion of metabolites in breast milk. Small amounts of active metabolites (e.g. rhein) are excreted in breast milk. A laxative effect in breast-fed babies has not been reported [18,33,46, 52,55-61].

Effects on ability to drive and use machines

None known.

Undesirable effects

Abdominal spasms and pain, particularly in patients with irritable colon; yellow or red-brown (pH dependent) discoloration of urine by metabolites, which is not clinically significant [61-64].

Overdose

The major symptoms are griping and severe diarrhoea with consequent losses of fluid and electrolyte, which should be replaced.

Treatment should be supportive with generous amounts of fluid. Electrolytes, especially potassium, should be monitored; this is particularly important in the elderly and the young.

PHARMACOLOGICAL PROPERTIES

Pharmacodynamic properties

1,8-dihydroxyanthracene derivatives possess a laxative effect [65-68]. The β-linked glucosides (sennosides) are not absorbed in the upper gut; they are converted by the bacteria of the large intestine into the active metabolite (rhein anthrone) [69-73]. There are two different mechanisms of action [68]:

(i) an influence on the motility of the large intestine (stimulation of peristaltic contractions and inhibition of local contractions) resulting in accelerated colonic transit, thus reducing fluid absorption [74-82], and

(ii) an influence on secretion processes (stimulation of mucus and active chloride secretion) [81,83,84] resulting in enhanced fluid secretion [68,81,85-91].

Defecation takes place after a delay of 8-12 hours due to the time taken for transport to the colon and metabolization into the active compound.

Aloe-emodin stimulated a release of platelet activating factor (PAF) in experiments with human gastro-intestinal mucosal cells, while rhein had no effect [92].

Pharmacokinetic properties

The β-linked glucosides (sennosides) are neither absorbed in the upper gut nor split by human digestive enzymes. They are converted by the bacteria of the large intestine into the active metabolite (rhein anthrone). Aglycones are absorbed in the upper gut. Animal experiments with radio-isotope-labelled rhein anthrone administered directly into the caecum demonstrated less than 10% absorption.

In contact with oxygen, rhein anthrone is oxidized into rhein and sennidins which can be found in the blood, mainly in the form of glucuronides and sulphates. After oral administration of sennosides, 3-6% of the metabolites are excreted in the urine; some are excreted in bile. Most of the sennosides (ca. 90%) are excreted in the faeces as polymers (polyquinones) together with 2-6% of unchanged sennosides, sennidins, rhein anthrone and rhein. In human pharmacokinetic studies, with senna pod powder (20 mg of sennosides) administered orally for 7 days, a maximum rhein concentration of 100 ng/ml was found in the blood. No accumulation of rhein was observed.

Active metabolites, e.g. rhein, pass into breast milk in small amounts. Animal experiments demonstrated that passage of rhein through the placenta is low [69-73,93-100].

Preclinical safety data
No new systematic preclinical studies are available for senna leaf or preparations from it.

Most data refer to extracts from senna pods containing 1.4 to 3.5% of anthranoids, corresponding to 0.9 to 2.3% of potential rhein, 0.05 to 0.15% of potential aloe-emodin and 0.001 to 0.006% of potential emodin, or to isolated active constituents, e.g. rhein or sennosides A and B. The acute oral toxicity in rats and mice of senna pods, of specified extracts from them and of sennosides and rhein was found to be low. From the results of investigations involving parenteral administration in mice, extracts are thought to possess higher toxicity than purified glucosides, possibly due to their content of aglycones [101-106].

Sennosides displayed no specific toxicity when tested at doses of up to 500 mg/kg in dogs for 4 weeks and up to 100 mg/kg in rats for 6 months. No data are available for crude drug preparations [103,107,108].

There was no evidence of any embryolethal, teratogenic or fetotoxic effects in rats or rabbits after oral treatment with sennosides. Furthermore, there was no effect on the postnatal development of young rats, on rearing behaviour of dams or on male and female fertility in rats. No data are available for crude drug preparations [43].

In the Ames test a senna extract, emodin and aloe-emodin were mutagenic. Sennosides A and B and rhein gave negative results. Comprehensive *in vivo*

testing of a defined extract of senna pods and its anthranoid constituents revealed no genotoxicity [109-118]. An ethanolic extract has been reported to be antimutagenic [119].

A senna extract given orally at doses of 5, 15 or 25 mg/kg for 2 years was not carcinogenic in male or female Sprague-Dawley rats. The extract investigated contained approx. 40.8% of anthranoids of which 35% were sennosides, corresponding to about 25.2% of potential rhein, 2.3% of potential aloe-emodin and 0.007% of potential emodin, and 142 ppm of free aloe-emodin and 9 ppm of free emodin [120].

In a 2-year study, male and female F344/N rats were exposed to 280, 830 or 2500 ppm of emodin in the diet, corresponding to an average daily dose of emodin of 110, 320 or 1000 mg/kg body weight in male rats and 120, 370 or 1100 mg/kg body weight in female rats. No evidence of carcinogenic activity of emodin was observed in male rats. A marginal increase in the incidence of Zymbal's gland carcinoma occurred in female rats treated with the high dosage but was interpreted as questionable [121].

In a further 2-year study, on B6C3F$_1$ mice, males were exposed to 160, 312 or 625 ppm of emodin (corresponding to an average daily dose of 15, 35 or 70 mg/kg body weight) and females to 312, 625 or 1250 ppm of emodin (corresponding to an average daily dose of 30, 60 or 120 mg/kg body weight). There was no evidence of carcinogenic activity in female mice. A low incidence of renal tubule neoplasms in exposed males was not considered relevant [121].

REFERENCES

1. Senna Leaf - Sennae folium. European Pharmacopoeia, Council of Europe.

2. Hänsel R, Keller K, Rimpler H, Schneider G, editors. Cassia. In: Hagers Handbuch der pharmazeutischen Praxis, 5th ed. Volume 4: Drogen A-D. Berlin: Springer-Verlag, 1992:701-25.

3. Hänsel R, Sticher O, Steinegger E. Sennesblätter und Sennesfrüchte. In: Pharmakognosie, 6th ed. Berlin: Springer-Verlag, 1999:910-4.

4. Nakajima K, Yamauchi K, Kuwano S. Isolation of a new aloe-emodin dianthrone diglucoside from senna and its potentiating effect on the purgative activity of sennoside A in mice. J Pharm Pharmacol 1985;37:703-6.

5. Lemli J. The chemistry of senna. Fitoterapia 1986;57:33-40.

6. van Os FHL. Anthraquinone derivatives in vegetable laxatives. Pharmacology 1976;14(Suppl 1):7-17.

7. Slanger A. Comparative study of a standardized senna

liquid and castor oil in preparing patients for radiographic examination of the colon. Dis Colon Rectum 1979;22:356-9.

8. Georgia EH. Management of drug-induced constipation in psychiatric outpatients. Curr Ther Res 1983;33:1018-22.

9. Izard MW, Ellison FS. Treatment of drug-induced constipation with a purified senna derivative. Conn Med 1962;26:589-92.

10. Pers M, Pers B. A crossover comparative study with two bulk laxatives. J Int Med Res 1983;11:51-3.

11. Gould SR, Williams CB. Castor oil or senna preparation before colonoscopy for inactive chronic ulcerative colitis. Gastrointest Endosc 1982;28:6-8.

12. Marlett JA, Li BUK, Patrow CJ, Bass P. Comparative laxation of psyllium with and without senna in an ambulatory constipated population. Am J Gastroenterol 1987;82:333-7.

13. Maguire LC, Yon JL, Miller E. Prevention of narcotic-induced constipation [Letter]. New Engl J Med 1981; 305:1651.

14. Slanger A. Cleansing of the sigmoid flexure and rectum preparatory to sigmoidoscopy: Report of a controlled study. Dis Colon Rectum 1966;9:109-12.

15. Dickie J, James WB, Hume R, Robertson D. A comparison of three substances used for bowel preparation prior to radiological examination. Clin Radiol 1970;21:201-2.

16. Reis Neto JA, Quilici FA, Oliveira LAR, Faria PC, Cordeiro F, Reis JA Jr. Eficácia e segurança de uma associação laxativa no pós-operatório imediato de cirurgias colo-proctológicas. Rev Bras Clín Terap 1986; 15:26-30.

17. Maddi VI. Regulation of bowel function by a laxative/stool softener preparation in aged nursing home patients. J Am Geriatr Soc 1979;27:464-8.

18. Duncan AS. Standardized senna as a laxative in the puerperium. A clinical assessment. Br Med J 1957;1:439-41.

19. Godding EW. Laxatives and the special role of senna. Pharmacology 1988;36(Suppl 1):230-6.

20. USA Department of Health and Human Services: Food and Drug Administration. 21 CFR Part 334. Laxative Drug Products for Over-the-Counter Human Use; Tentative Final Monograph. Federal Register 1985; 50(10):2124, 2151-8 (January 15, 1985).

21. Binder HJ. Use of laxatives in clinical medicine. Pharmacology 1988;36(Suppl 1):226-9.

22. Kovar F. Sennatin® tabl. - Dosage, efficacy and tolerance in bedridden patients with constipation. Köln: Madaus Report 14.11.1984, unpublished.

23. Brusis O. Sennatin® in acute constipation. Köln: Madaus Report 25.07.1986. Double-blind study, unpublished.

24. Jähnig L. Offene, monozentrische, randomisierte klinische Prüfung zur Bestimmung des Wirkungseintritts und der Wirkqualität unterschiedlicher Dosen von AX14E0 bei chronischer Obstipation (AX14E0.53). Köln: Madaus Report 27.04.1993, unpublished.

25. McClure Browne JC, Edmunds V, Fairbairn JW, Reid DD. Clinical and laboratory assessments of senna preparations. Br Med J 1957:436-9.

26. Smith CW, Evans PR. Bowel motility. A problem in institutionalized geriatric care. Geriatrics 1961;16:189-92.

27. Berg I, Jones KV. Functional faecal incontinence in children. Arch Dis Childh 1964;39:465-72.

28. Campbell-Mackie M. The re-educative treatment of bowel dysfunction in infants and children. S Afr Med J 1963;37:675-8.

29. Clayden GS. Constipation and soiling in childhood. Br Med J 1976;1:515-7.

30. Campbell-Mackie M. The treatment of bowel dysfunction in infants and young children. Practitioner 1959;183:732-6.

31. Wherry CA. Treating chronic constipation in children. Nursing Times 1977:1829-31.

32. Braid F. The treatment of constipation in children. Medical Press 1954;231:521-4.

33. Leng-Peschlow E. Senna and its rational use. Pharmacology 1992;44(Suppl 1):1-52.

34. Sonnenberg A, Sonnenberg GS. Epidemiologie der Obstipation. In: Müller-Lissner SA, Ackermans LMA, editors. Chronische Obstipation und Stuhlinkontinenz. Berlin: Springer-Verlag, 1989:141-56.

35. Preston DM, Lennard-Jones JE. Severe chronic constipation of young women: 'Idiopathic slow transit constipation'. Gut 1986;27:41-8.

36. Klauser A, Peyerl C, Schindlbeck N, Müller-Lissner S. Obstipierte unterscheiden sich nicht von Gesunden hinsichtlich Ernährung und körperlicher Aktivität [Abstract]. Z Gastroenterol 1990;28:494.

37. Müller-Lissner SA. Effect of wheat bran on weight of stool and gastrointestinal transit time: a meta-analysis. Br Med J 1988;296:615-7.

38. Klauser A, Beck A, Schindlbeck N, Müller-Lissner S. Dursten beeinflußt die Colonfunktion bei Probanden [Abstract]. Z Gastroenterol 1990;28:493.

39. Coenen C, Schmidt G, Wegener M, Hoffmann S, Wedmann B. Beeinflußt körperliche Aktivität den oro-analen Transit? - Eine prospektive, kontrollierte Studie [Abstract]. Z Gastroenterol 1990;28:469.

40. Bingham SA, Cummings JH. Effect of exercise and physical fitness on large intestinal function. Gastro-

enterology 1989;97:1389-99.

41. Bingham S. Does exercise affect large gut function? J Hum Nutr Diet 1991;4:281-5.

42. Klauser AG, Flaschenträger J, Gehrke A, Müller-Lissner SA. Abdominal wall massage: effect on colonic function in healthy volunteers and in patients with chronic constipation. Z Gastroenterol 1992;30:247-51.

43. Mengs U. Reproductive toxicological investigations with sennosides. Arzneim-Forsch/Drug Res 1986;36:1355-8.

44. Garcia-Villar R. Evaluation of the effects of sennosides on uterine motility in the pregnant ewe. Pharmacology 1988; 36(Suppl 1):203-11.

45. Herland AL, Lowenstein A. Physiologic rehabilitation of the constipated colon in pregnant women. Use of a standardized senna derivative. Q Rev Surg 1957;14:196-202.

46. Greenhalf JO, Leonard HSD. Laxatives in the treatment of constipation in pregnant and breast-feeding mothers. Practitioner 1973;210:259-63.

47. Wager HP, Melosh WD. The management of constipation in pregnancy. Q Rev Surg 1958;15:30-4.

48. Scott RS. Management of constipation in obstetrics: A clinical report on 592 cases. West Med 1965;6:342-4.

49. Girotti M, Hauser GA. Therapie der Obstipation in der Schwangerschaft und bei gynäkologischen Patientinnen. Ther Umsch 1971;28:490-3.

50. Mahon R, Palmade J. Traitement de la constipation chez la femme enceinte. Gaz Med Fr 1974;81:3259-60.

51. Gram U. Bedeutung der normalen Darmtätigkeit während der Schwangerschaft. Med Welt 1969; 20:2613-5.

52. Kaltstein A. Zur Behandlung der Schwangerschafts- und Wochenbettobstipation. Fortschr Med 1969; 87:723-5.

53. Roth OA. Therapeutische Beobachtungen bei Obstipation. Med Welt 1969;20:536-7.

54. Bauer H. Behandlung der Obstipation mit Laxariston® in der gynäkologischen Praxis. Ther Gegenwart 1977; 116:2305-12.

55. Baldwin WF. Clinical study of senna administration to nursing mothers: Assessment of effects on infant bowel habits. Can Med Assoc J 1963;89:566-8.

56. Dubecq JP, Palmade J. Étude clinique de l'administration de tamarine chez la mère qui allaite. Gaz Med Fr 1974; 81:5173-5.

57. Shelton MG. Standardized senna in the management of constipation in the puerperium. A clinical trial. S Afr Med J 1980;57:78-80.

58. Suarez J, Castillo AG, Shepard J. The use of a new standardized senna derivative in the management of puerperal constipation. Int Rec Med 1960;173:639-42.

59. Faber P, Strenge-Hesse A. Relevance of rhein excretion into breast milk. Pharmacology 1988;36(Suppl 1):212-20.

60. Cameron BD, Phillips MWA, Fenerty CA. Milk transfer of rhein in the rhesus monkey. Pharmacology 1988; 36(Suppl 1):221-5.

61. Reynolds JEF, editor. Senna. In: Martindale - The Extra Pharmacopoeia, 31st ed. London: Royal Pharmaceutical Society, 1996:1240-1.

62. Cooke WT. Laxative abuse. Clin Gastroenterol 1977; 6:659-73.

63. Tedesco FJ. Laxative use in constipation. Am J Gastroenterol 1985;80:303-9.

64. Ewe K, Karbach U. Factitious diarrhoea. Clin Gastroenterol 1986;15:723-40.

65. Brittain RT, D'Arcy PF, Grimshaw JJ. Observations on the use of a mouse bioassay method for investigating purgative activity. J Pharm Pharmacol 1962;14:715-21.

66. Fairbairn JW. Chemical structure, mode of action and therapeutical activity of anthraquinone glycosides. Pharm Weekbl (Sci) 1965;100:1493-9.

67. Fairbairn JW, Moss MJR. The relative purgative activities of 1,8-dihydroxyanthracene derivatives. J Pharm Pharmacol 1970;22:584-93.

68. Leng-Peschlow E. Dual effect of orally administered sennosides on large intestine transit and fluid absorption in the rat. J Pharm Pharmacol 1986;38:606-10.

69. Lemmens L. The laxative action of anthracene derivatives. 2. Absorption, metabolism and excretion of sennoside A and B in the rat. Pharm Weekbl (Sci) 1979;114:178-85.

70. Lemli J, Lemmens L. Metabolism of sennosides and rhein in the rat. Pharmacology 1980;20(Suppl 1):50-7.

71. Kobashi K, Nishimura T, Kusaka M, Hattori M, Namba T. Metabolism of sennosides by human intestinal bacteria. Planta Med 1980;40:225-36.

72. Dreessen M, Eyssen H, Lemli J. The metabolism of sennosides A and B by the intestinal microflora: in vitro and in vivo studies on the rat and the mouse. J Pharm Pharmacol 1981;33:679-81.

73. Hattori M, Kim G, Motoike S, Kobashi K, Namba T. Metabolism of sennosides by intestinal flora. Chem Pharm Bull 1982;30:1338-46.

74. Hardcastle JD, Wilkins JL. The action of sennosides and related compounds on human colon and rectum. Gut 1970;11:1038-42.

75. Garcia-Villar R, Leng-Peschlow E, Ruckebusch Y. Effect of anthraquinone derivatives on canine and rat intestinal

motility. J Pharm Pharmacol 1980;32:323-9.

76. Bueno L, Fioramonti J, Frexinos J, Ruckebusch Y. Colonic myoelectrical activity in diarrhea and constipation. Hepatogastroenterology 1980;27:381-9.

77. Leng-Peschlow E. Acceleration of large intestine transit time in rats by sennosides and related compounds. J Pharm Pharmacol 1986;38:369-73.

78. Fioramonti J, Staumont G, Garcia-Villar R, Buéno L. Effect of sennosides on colon motility in dogs. Pharmacology 1988;36(Suppl 1):23-30.

79. Staumont G, Frexinos J, Fioramonti J, Buéno L. Sennosides and human colonic motility. Pharmacology 1988;36(Suppl 1):49-56.

80. Staumont G, Fioramonti J, Frexinos J, Buéno L. Changes in colonic motility induced by sennosides in dogs: evidence of a prostaglandin mediation. Gut 1988; 29:1180-7.

81. Leng-Peschlow E. Effects of sennosides A + B and bisacodyl on rat large intestine. Pharmacology 1989; 38:310-8.

82. Frexinos J, Staumont G, Fioramonti J, Buéno L. Effects of sennosides on colonic myoelectrical activity in man. Dig Dis Sci 1989;34:214-9.

83. Clauss W, Domokos G, Leng-Peschlow E. Effect of rhein on electrogenic chloride secretion in rabbit distal colon. Pharmacology 1988;36(Suppl 1):104-10.

84. Goerg KJ, Wanitschke R, Schwarz M, Meyer z. Büschenfelde KH. Rhein stimulates active chloride secretion in the short-circuited rat colonic mucosa. Pharmacology 1988;36(Suppl 1):111-9.

85. Lemmens L, Borja E. The influence of dihydroxy-anthracene derivatives on water and electrolyte movement in rat colon. J Pharm Pharmacol 1976; 28:498-501.

86. Ewe K. Effect of rhein on the transport of electrolytes, water and carbohydrates in the human jejunum and colon. Pharmacology 1980;20(Suppl 1):27-35.

87. Ewe K, Wanitschke R. The effect of cathartic agents on transmucosal electrical potential difference in the human rectum. Klin Wochenschr 1980;58:299-306.

88. Leng-Peschlow E. Inhibition of intestinal water and electrolyte absorption by senna derivatives in rats. J Pharm Pharmacol 1980;32:330-5.

89. Donowitz M, Wicks J, Battisti L, Pike G, DeLellis R. Effect of Senokot on rat intestinal electrolyte transport. Evidence of Ca^{++} dependence. Gastroenterology 1984;87:503-12.

90. Beubler E, Kollar G. Stimulation of PGE_2 synthesis and water and electrolyte secretion by senna anthraquinones is inhibited by indomethacin. J Pharm Pharmacol 1985;37:248-51.

91. Beubler E, Kollar G. Prostaglandin-mediated action of sennosides. Pharmacology 1988;36(Suppl 1):85-91.

92. Tavares IA, Mascolo N, Izzo AA, Capasso F. Effects of anthraquinone derivatives on PAF release by human gastrointestinal mucosa in vitro. Phytother Res 1996; 10:20-1.

93. Krumbiegel G, Schulz HU. Rhein and aloe-emodin kinetics from senna laxatives in man. Pharmacology 1993;47(Suppl 1):120-4.

94. Lang W. Pharmacokinetic-metabolic studies with ^{14}C-aloe emodin after oral administration to male and female rats. Pharmacology 1993;47(Suppl 1):110-9.

95. de Witte P, Lemli J. Metabolism of ^{14}C-rhein and ^{14}C-rhein anthrone in rats. Pharmacology 1988;36(Suppl 1):152-7.

96. de Witte P, Lemli J. Excretion and distribution of ^{14}C-rhein and ^{14}C-rhein anthrone in rat. J Pharm Pharmacol 1988;40:652-5.

97. de Witte P, Cuveele J, Lemli J. In vitro deterioration of rhein anthraquinone in cecal content of rats. Pharm Acta Helv 1992;67:198-203.

98. Hattori M, Namba T, Akao T, Kobashi K. Metabolism of sennosides by human intestinal bacteria. Pharmacology 1988;36(Suppl 1):172-9.

99. Hietala P, Lainonen H, Marvola M. New aspects on the metabolism of the sennosides. Pharmacology 1988; 36(Suppl.1):138-43.

100. Lemli J. Metabolismus der Anthranoide. Z Phytother 1986;7:127-9.

101. Mengs U. SF48-WI006: Acute oral toxicity study in rats. Köln: Madaus Report 23.04.1993, unpublished.

102. Mengs U. AX14-WI025: Acute oral toxicity study in mice. Köln: Madaus Report 22.04.1993, unpublished.

103. Mengs U. Toxic effects of sennosides in laboratory animals and in vitro. Pharmacology 1988;36(Suppl. 1):180-7.

104. Marvola M, Koponen A, Hiltunen R, Hietala P. The effect of raw material purity on the acute toxicity and laxative effect of sennosides. J Pharm Pharmacol 1981;33:108-9.

105. Mengs U. Akute Toxizität von Rhein an weiblichen Ratten nach intragastraler Applikation. Köln: Madaus Report 04.11.1985, unpublished.

106. Mengs U. Akute Toxizität von Rhein an männlichen und weiblichen Mäusen nach intragastraler Applikation. Köln: Madaus Report 04.07.1983, unpublished.

107. Rudolph RL, Mengs U. Electron microscopical studies on rat intestine after long-term treatment with sennosides. Pharmacology 1988;36(Suppl. 1):188-93.

108. Dufour P, Gendre P. Ultrastructure of mouse intestinal mucosa and changes observed after long-term anthraquinone administration. Gut 1984;25:1358-63.

461

109. Mengs U, Heidemann A. Genotoxicity of sennosides and rhein in vitro and in vivo. Med Sci Res 1993;21:749-50.

110. Westendorf J, Marquardt H, Poginsky B, Dominiak M, Schmidt J, Marquardt H. Genotoxicity of naturally occurring hydroxyanthraquinones. Mutat Res 1990; 240:1-12.

111. Heidemann A, Miltenburger HG, Mengs U. The genotoxicity status of senna. Pharmacology 1993;47(Suppl 1):178-86.

112. Nitz D, Krumbiegel G. Bestimmung von Aloeemodin und Rhein im Serum von Ratte und Maus nach oraler Gabe von Fructus sennae und Aloeemodin. Köln: Madaus Report 18.05.1992, unpublished.

113. Sandnes D, Johansen T, Teen G, Ulsaker G. Mutagenicity of crude senna and senna glycosides in Salmonella typhimurium. Pharmacol Toxicol 1992;71:165-72.

114. Müller SO, Eckert I, Lutz WK, Stopper H. Genotoxicity of the laxative drug components emodin, aloe-emodin and danthron in mammalian cells: topoisomerase II mediated? Mut Res 1996;165-73.

115. Mengs U, Krumbiegel G, Völkner W. Lack of emodin genotoxicity in the mouse micronucleus assay. Mut Res 1997;393:289-93.

116. Mukhopadhyay MJ, Saha A, Dutta A, De B, Mukherjee A. Genotoxicity of sennosides on the bone marrow cells of mice. Food Chem Toxicol 1998;36:937-40.

117. Mueller SO, Lutz WK, Stopper H. Factors affecting the genotoxic potency ranking of natural anthraquinones in mammalian cell culture systems. Mut Res 1998;125-9.

118. Mengs U, Grimminger W, Krumbiegel G, Schuler D, Silber W, Völkner W. No clastogenic activity of a senna extract in mouse micronucleus assay. Mut Res 1999; 444:421-6.

119. Al-Dakan AA, Al-Tuffail M, Hannan MA. Cassia senna inhibits mutagenic activities of benzo[a]pyrene, aflatoxine B_1, shamma and methyl methanesulfonate. Pharmacol Toxicol 1995;77:288-92.

120. Sokolowski AL, Montin G, Nilsson A, Olofsson IM, Sjöberg P. Two-year carcinogenicity study with senna in the rat. VI. Int. Congress of Toxicology, Rome 1992.

121. NTP Technical Report 493. Toxicology and carcinogenesis studies of emodin (CAS No. 518-82-1) in F344/N rats and B6C3F$_1$ mice. NIH Publication No. 99-3952, 1999.

SENNAE FRUCTUS ACUTIFOLIAE

Alexandrian Senna Pods

E/S/C/O/P
MONOGRAPHS
Second Edition

DEFINITION

Alexandrian senna pods consist of the dried fruit of *Cassia senna* L. *(C. acutifolia* Delile*)*. They contain not less than 3.4 per cent of hydroxyanthracene glycosides, calculated as sennoside B ($C_{42}H_{38}O_{20}$; M_r 863) with reference to the dried drug.

The material complies with the monograph of the European Pharmacopoeia [1].

CONSTITUENTS

The main active constituents are sennosides A and B (ca. 4%), which are rhein-dianthrone diglucosides. Smaller amounts of other dianthrone diglucosides, monoanthraquinone glucosides and aglycones are also present [2-6].

CLINICAL PARTICULARS

Therapeutic indications
For short-term use in cases of occasional constipation [7-21].

Posology and method of administration

Dosage

The correct individual dose is the smallest required to produce a comfortable soft-formed motion.

Adults and children over 10 years: preparations equivalent to 15-30 mg of hydroxyanthracene derivatives, calculated as sennoside B, to be taken once daily at night [11,14,15,20-24].
Elderly: dose as for adults [25,26].

Not recommended for use in children under 10 years of age [27-32].

The pharmaceutical form must allow lower dosages.

Method of administration
For oral administration.

Contra-indications
Not to be used in cases of: intestinal obstruction and stenosis, atony, inflammatory colon diseases (e.g. Crohn's disease, ulcerative colitis), appendicitis; abdominal pain of unknown origin; severe dehydration states with water and electrolyte depletion.
Children under 10 years.

Special warnings and special precautions for use

As for all laxatives, senna pods should not be given when any undiagnosed acute or persistent abdominal symptoms are present.

If laxatives are needed every day the cause of the constipation should be investigated. Long term use of laxatives should be avoided. Use for more than 2 weeks requires medical supervision. Chronic use may cause pigmentation of the colon (pseudo-melanosis coli) which is harmless and reversible after drug discontinuation. Abuse, with diarrhoea and consequent fluid and electrolyte losses, may cause: dependence with possible need for increased dosages; disturbance of the water and electrolyte (mainly hypokalaemia) balance; an atonic colon with impaired function. Intake of anthranoid-containing laxatives for more than a short period of time may result in aggravation of constipation. Hypokalaemia can result in cardiac and neuromuscular dysfunction, especially if cardiac glycosides, diuretics or corticosteroids are taken. Chronic use may result in albuminuria and haematuria.

In chronic constipation, stimulant laxatives are not an acceptable alternative to a change in diet [33-42].

Note: A detailed text with advice concerning changes in dietary habits, physical activities and training for normal bowel evacuation should be included on the package leaflet. An example is given in the booklet "Médicaments á base de plantes" published by the French health authority (Paris: Agence du Médicament).

Interaction with other medicaments and other forms of interaction

Hypokalaemia (resulting from long term laxative abuse) potentiates the action of cardiac glycosides and interacts with antiarrhythmic drugs or with drugs which induce reversion to sinus rhythm (e.g. quinidine). Concomitant use with other drugs inducing hypokalaemia (e.g. thiazide diuretics, adreno-corticosteroids and liquorice root) may aggravate electrolyte imbalance.

Pregnancy and lactation

Pregnancy

Wording for extracts identical to those investigated (see Preclinical safety data)
There are no reports of undesirable or damaging effects during pregnancy or on the foetus when used in accordance with the recommended dosage schedule. However, the usual precautionary measures for the use of medicinal products should be observed, especially in the first 3 months of pregnancy.

Wording for all other preparations
There are no reports of undesirable or damaging effects during pregnancy or on the foetus when used in accordance with the recommended dosage schedule. However, in view of experimental data concerning a genotoxic risk from several anthranoids (e.g. emodin and aloe emodin), avoid during the first trimester or take only under medical supervision [33,43-54].

Lactation
Breastfeeding is not recommended as there are insufficient data on the excretion of metabolites in breast milk. Small amounts of active metabolites (e.g. rhein) are excreted in breast milk. A laxative effect in breast-fed babies has not been reported [18,33, 46,52,55-61].

Effects on ability to drive and use machines
None known.

Undesirable effects
Abdominal spasms and pain, particularly in patients with irritable colon; yellow or red-brown (pH dependent) discoloration of urine by metabolites, which is not clinically significant [61-64].

Overdose
The major symptoms are griping and severe diarrhoea with consequent losses of fluid and electrolyte, which should be replaced.

Treatment should be supportive with generous amounts of fluid. Electrolytes, especially potassium, should be monitored; this is particularly important in the elderly and the young.

PHARMACOLOGICAL PROPERTIES

Pharmacodynamic properties
1,8-dihydroxyanthracene derivatives possess a laxative effect [65-68]. The β-linked glucosides (sennosides) are not absorbed in the upper gut; they are converted by the bacteria of the large intestine into the active metabolite (rhein anthrone) [69-73]. There are two different mechanisms of action [68]:

(i) an influence on the motility of the large intestine (stimulation of peristaltic contractions and inhibition of local contractions) resulting in accelerated colonic transit, thus reducing fluid absorption [74-82], and

(ii) an influence on secretion processes (stimulation of mucus and active chloride secretion) [81,83,84] resulting in enhanced fluid secretion [68,81,85-91].

Defecation takes place after a delay of 8-12 hours due to the time taken for transport to the colon and metabolization into the active compound.

Aloe-emodin stimulated a release of platelet activating factor (PAF) in experiments with human gastrointestinal mucosal cells, while rhein had no effect [92].

Pharmacokinetic properties

The β-linked glucosides (sennosides) are neither absorbed in the upper gut nor split by human digestive enzymes. They are converted by the bacteria of the large intestine into the active metabolite (rhein anthrone). Aglycones are absorbed in the upper gut. Animal experiments with radio-isotope-labelled rhein anthrone administered directly into the caecum demonstrated less than 10% absorption.

In contact with oxygen, rhein anthrone is oxidized into rhein and sennidins which can be found in the blood, mainly in the form of glucuronides and sulphates. After oral administration of sennosides, 3-6% of the metabolites are excreted in the urine; some are excreted in bile. Most of the sennosides (ca. 90%) are excreted in the faeces as polymers (polyquinones) together with 2-6% of unchanged sennosides, sennidins, rhein anthrone and rhein. In human pharmacokinetic studies with senna pod powder (20 mg of sennosides), administered orally for 7 days, a maximum rhein concentration of 100 ng/ml was found in the blood. No accumulation of rhein was observed.

Active metabolites, e.g. rhein, pass in small amounts into breast milk. Animal experiments demonstrated that passage of rhein through the placenta is low [69-73,93-100].

Preclinical safety data

Most data refer to extracts containing 1.4 to 3.5% of anthranoids, corresponding to 0.9 to 2.3% of potential rhein, 0.05 to 0.15% of potential aloe emodin and 0.001 to 0.006% of potential emodin, or to isolated active constituents, e.g. rhein or sennosides A and B. The acute oral toxicity in rats and mice of senna pods, of specified extracts from them and of sennosides was found to be low. From the results of investigations involving parenteral administration in mice, extracts are thought to possess higher toxicity than purified glucosides, possibly due to their content of aglycones [101-106].

Sennosides displayed no specific toxicity when tested at doses of up to 500 mg/kg in dogs for 4 weeks and up to 100 mg/kg in rats for 6 months. No data are available for crude drug preparations [103,107,108].

There was no evidence of any embryolethal, terato-genic or fetotoxic effects in rats or rabbits after oral treatment with sennosides. Furthermore, there was no effect on the postnatal development of young rats, on rearing behaviour of dams or on male and female fertility in rats. No data are available for crude drug preparations [43].

In the Ames test a senna extract, emodin and aloe-emodin were mutagenic. Sennosides A and B and rhein gave negative results. Comprehensive in vivo testing of a defined extract of senna pods and its anthranoid constituents revealed no genotoxicity (109-118). An ethanolic extract has been reported to be antimutagenic [119].

A senna extract given orally at doses of 5, 15 or 25 mg/kg for 2 years was not carcinogenic in male or female Sprague-Dawley rats. The extract investigated contained approx. 40.8% of anthranoids of which 35% were sennosides, corresponding to about 25.2% of potential rhein, 2.3% of potential aloe-emodin and 0.007% of potential emodin, and 142 ppm of free aloe-emodin and 9 ppm of free emodin [120].

In a 2-year study, male and female F344/N rats were exposed to 280, 830 or 2500 ppm of emodin in the diet, corresponding to an average daily dose of emodin of 110, 320 or 1000 mg/kg body weight in male rats and 120, 370 or 1100 mg/kg body weight in female rats. No evidence of carcinogenic activity of emodin was observed in male rats. A marginal increase in the incidence of Zymbal's gland carcinoma occurred in female rats treated with the high dosage but was interpreted as questionable [121].

In a further 2-year study, on B6C3F$_1$ mice, males were exposed to 160, 312 or 625 ppm of emodin (corresponding to an average daily dose of 15, 35 or 70 mg/kg body weight) and females to 312, 625 or 1250 ppm of emodin (corresponding to an average daily dose of 30, 60 or 120 mg/kg body weight). There was no evidence of carcinogenic activity in female mice. A low incidence of renal tubule neoplasms in exposed males was not considered relevant [121].

REFERENCES

1. Senna Pods, Alexandrian - Sennae fructus acutifoliae. European Pharmacopoeia, Council of Europe.

2. Hänsel R, Keller K, Rimpler H, Schneider G, editors. Cassia. In: Hagers Handbuch der pharmazeutischen Praxis, 5th ed. Volume 4: Drogen A-D. Berlin: Springer-Verlag, 1992:701-25.

3. Hänsel R, Sticher O, Steinegger E. Sennesblätter und Sennesfrüchte. In: Pharmakognosie, 6th ed. Berlin: Springer-Verlag, 1999:910-4.

4. Nakajima K, Yamauchi K, Kuwano S. Isolation of a new aloe-emodin dianthrone diglucoside from senna and its potentiating effect on the purgative activity of sennoside A in mice. J Pharm Pharmacol 1985;37:703-6.

5. Lemli J. The chemistry of senna. Fitoterapia 1986;57:33-40.

6. van Os FHL. Anthraquinone derivatives in vegetable laxatives. Pharmacology 1976;14(Suppl 1):7-17.

7. Slanger A. Comparative study of a standardized senna liquid and castor oil in preparing patients for radiographic examination of the colon. Dis Colon Rectum 1979;22:356-9.

8. Georgia EH. Management of drug-induced constipation in psychiatric outpatients. Curr Ther Res 1983;33:1018-22.

9. Izard MW, Ellison FS. Treatment of drug-induced constipation with a purified senna derivative. Conn Med 1962;26:589-92.

10. Pers M, Pers B. A crossover comparative study with two bulk laxatives. J Int Med Res 1983;11:51-3.

11. Gould SR, Williams CB. Castor oil or senna preparation before colonoscopy for inactive chronic ulcerative colitis. Gastrointest Endosc 1982;28:6-8.

12. Marlett JA, Li BUK, Patrow CJ, Bass P. Comparative laxation of psyllium with and without senna in an ambulatory constipated population. Am J Gastroenterol 1987;82:333-7.

13. Maguire LC, Yon JL, Miller E. Prevention of narcotic-induced constipation [Letter]. New Engl J Med 1981; 305:1651.

14. Slanger A. Cleansing of the sigmoid flexure and rectum preparatory to sigmoidoscopy: Report of a controlled study. Dis Colon Rectum 1966;9:109-12.

15. Dickie J, James WB, Hume R, Robertson D. A comparison of three substances used for bowel preparation prior to radiological examination. Clin Radiol 1970;21:201-2.

16. Reis Neto JA, Quilici FA, Oliveira LAR, Faria PC, Cordeiro F, Reis JA Jr. Eficácia e segurança de uma associação laxativa no pós-operatório imediato de cirurgias colo-proctológicas. Rev Bras Clín Terap 1986;15:26-30.

17. Maddi VI. Regulation of bowel function by a laxative/stool softener preparation in aged nursing home patients. J Am Geriatr Soc 1979;27:464-8.

18. Duncan AS. Standardized senna as a laxative in the puerperium. A clinical assessment. Br Med J 1957;1:439-41.

19. Godding EW. Laxatives and the special role of senna. Pharmacology 1988;36(Suppl 1):230-6.

20. USA Department of Health and Human Services: Food and Drug Administration. 21 CFR Part 334. Laxative Drug Products for Over-the-Counter Human Use; Tentative Final Monograph. Federal Register 1985;50(10):2124, 2151-8 (January 15, 1985).

21. Binder HJ. Use of laxatives in clinical medicine. Pharmacology 1988;36(Suppl 1):226-9.

22. Kovar F. Sennatin® tabl. - Dosage, efficacy and tolerance in bedridden patients with constipation. Köln: Madaus Report 14.11.1984, unpublished.

23. Brusis O. Sennatin® in acute constipation. Köln: Madaus Report 25.07.1986. Double-blind study, unpublished.

24. Jähnig L. Offene, monozentrische, randomisierte klinische Prüfung zur Bestimmung des Wirkungseintritts und der Wirkqualität unterschiedlicher Dosen von AX14E0 bei chronischer Obstipation (AX14E0.53). Köln: Madaus Report 27.04.1993, unpublished.

25. McClure Browne JC, Edmunds V, Fairbairn JW, Reid DD. Clinical and laboratory assessments of senna preparations. Br Med J 1957:436-9.

26. Smith CW, Evans PR. Bowel motility. A problem in institutionalized geriatric care. Geriatrics 1961:189-92.

27. Berg I, Jones KV. Functional faecal incontinence in children. Arch Dis Child 1964;39:465-72.

28. Campbell-Mackie M. The re-educative treatment of bowel dysfunction in infants and children. S Afr Med J 1963;37:675-8.

29. Clayden GS. Constipation and soiling in childhood. Br Med J 1976;1:515-7.

30. Campbell-Mackie M. The treatment of bowel dysfunction in infants and young children. Practitioner 1959;183:732-6.

31. Wherry CA. Treating chronic constipation in children. Nursing Times 1977:1829-31.

32. Braid F. The treatment of constipation in children. Medical Press 1954;231:521-4.

33. Leng-Peschlow E. Senna and its rational use. Pharmacology 1992;44(Suppl 1):1-52.

34. Sonnenberg A, Sonnenberg GS. Epidemiologie der Obstipation. In: Müller-Lissner SA, Ackermans LMA, editors. Chronische Obstipation und Stuhlinkontinenz. Berlin: Springer-Verlag, 1989:141-56.

35. Preston DM, Lennard-Jones JE. Severe chronic constipation of young women: 'Idiopathic slow transit constipation'. Gut 1986;27:41-8.

36. Klauser A, Peyerl C, Schindlbeck N, Müller-Lissner S. Obstipierte unterscheiden sich nicht von Gesunden hinsichtlich Ernährung und körperlicher Aktivität [Abstract]. Z Gastroenterol 1990;28:494.

37. Müller-Lissner SA. Effect of wheat bran on weight of stool and gastrointestinal transit time: a meta analysis. Br Med J 1988;296:615-7.

38. Klauser A, Beck A, Schindlbeck N, Müller-Lissner S. Dursten beeinflußt die Colonfunktion bei Probanden [Abstract]. Z Gastroenterol 1990;28:493.

39. Coenen C, Schmidt G, Wegener M, Hoffmann S, Wedmann B. Beeinflußt körperliche Aktivität den oro-analen Transit? - Eine prospektive, kontrollierte Studie

[Abstract]. Z Gastroenterol 1990;28:469.

40. Bingham SA, Cummings JH. Effect of exercise and physical fitness on large intestinal function. Gastroenterology 1989;97:1389-99.

41. Bingham S. Does exercise affect large gut function? J Hum Nutr Diet 1991;4:281-5.

42. Klauser AG, Flaschenträger J, Gehrke A, Müller-Lissner SA. Abdominal wall massage: effect on colonic function in healthy volunteers and in patients with chronic constipation. Z Gastroenterol 1992;30:247-51.

43. Mengs U. Reproductive toxicological investigations with sennosides. Arzneim-Forsch/Drug Res 1986;36: 1355-8.

44. Garcia-Villar R. Evaluation of the effects of sennosides on uterine motility in the pregnant ewe. Pharmacology 1988; 36(Suppl 1):203-11.

45. Herland AL, Lowenstein A. Physiologic rehabilitation of the constipated colon in pregnant women. Use of a standardized s enna derivative. Q Rev Surg 1957;14: 196-202.

46. Greenhalf JO, Leonard HSD. Laxatives in the treatment of constipation in pregnant and breast-feeding mothers. Practitioner 1973;210:259-63.

47. Wager HP, Melosh WD. The management of constipation in pregnancy. Q Rev Surg 1958;15:30-4.

48. Scott RS. Management of constipation in obstetrics: A clinical report on 592 cases. West Med 1965;6:342-4.

49. Girotti M, Hauser GA. Therapie der Obstipation in der Schwangerschaft und bei gynäkologischen Patientinnen. Ther Umsch 1971;28:490-3.

50. Mahon R, Palmade J. Traitement de la constipation chez la femme enceinte. Gaz Med Fr 1974;81:3259-60.

51. Gram U. Bedeutung der normalen Darmtätigkeit während der Schwangerschaft. Med Welt 1969; 20:2613-5.

52. Kaltstein A. Zur Behandlung der Schwangerschafts- und Wochenbettobstipation. Fortschr Med 1969;87: 723-5.

53. Roth OA. Therapeutische Beobachtungen bei Obstipation. Med Welt 1969;20:536-7.

54. Bauer H. Behandlung der Obstipation mit Laxariston® in der gynäkologischen Praxis. Ther Gegenwart 1977; 116:2305-12.

55. Baldwin WF. Clinical study of senna administration to nursing mothers: Assessment of effects on infant bowel habits. Can Med Assoc J 1963;89:566-8.

56. Dubecq JP, Palmade J. Étude clinique de l'administration de tamarine chez la mère qui allaite. Gaz Med Fr 1974;81:5173-5.

57. Shelton MG. Standardized senna in the management of constipation in the puerperium. A clinical trial. S Afr Med J 1980;57:78-80.

58. Suarez J, Castillo AG, Shepard J. The use of a new standardized senna derivative in the management of puerperal constipation. Int Rec Med 1960;173:639-42.

59. Faber P, Strenge-Hesse A. Relevance of rhein excretion into breast milk. Pharmacology 1988;36(Suppl 1):212-20.

60. Cameron BD, Phillips MWA, Fenerty CA. Milk transfer of rhein in the rhesus monkey. Pharmacology 1988; 36(Suppl 1):221-5.

61. Reynolds JEF, editor. Senna. In: Martindale - The Extra Pharmacopoeia, 31st ed. London: Royal Pharmaceutical Society, 1996:1240-1.

62. Cooke WT. Laxative abuse. Clin Gastroenterol 1977; 6:659-73.

63. Tedesco FJ. Laxative use in constipation. Am J Gastroenterol 1985;80:303-9.

64. Ewe K, Karbach U. Factitious diarrhoea. Clin Gastroenterol 1986;15:723-40.

65. Brittain RT, D'Arcy PF, Grimshaw JJ. Observations on the use of a mouse bioassay method for investigating purgative activity. J Pharm Pharmacol 1962;14:715-21.

66. Fairbairn JW. Chemical structure, mode of action and therapeutical activity of anthraquinone glycosides. Pharm Weekbl (Sci) 1965;100:1493-9.

67. Fairbairn JW, Moss MJR. The relative purgative activities of 1,8-dihydroxyanthracene derivatives. J Pharm Pharmacol 1970;22:584-93.

68. Leng-Peschlow E. Dual effect of orally administered sennosides on large intestine transit and fluid absorption in the rat. J Pharm Pharmacol 1986;38:606-10.

69. Lemmens L. The laxative action of anthracene derivatives. 2. Absorption, metabolism and excretion of sennoside A and B in the rat. Pharm Weekbl (Sci) 1979;114:178-85.

70. Lemli J, Lemmens L. Metabolism of sennosides and rhein in the rat. Pharmacology 1980;20(Suppl 1):50-7.

71. Kobashi K, Nishimura T, Kusaka M, Hattori M, Namba T. Metabolism of sennosides by human intestinal bacteria. Planta Med 1980;40:225-36.

72. Dreessen M, Eyssen H, Lemli J. The metabolism of sennosides A and B by the intestinal microflora: in vitro and in vivo studies on the rat and the mouse. J Pharm Pharmacol 1981;33:679-81.

73. Hattori M, Kim G, Motoike S, Kobashi K, Namba T. Metabolism of sennosides by intestinal flora. Chem Pharm Bull 1982;30:1338-46.

74. Hardcastle JD, Wilkins JL. The action of sennosides and related compounds on human colon and rectum. Gut 1970;11:1038-42.

75. Garcia-Villar R, Leng-Peschlow E, Ruckebusch Y. Effect of anthraquinone derivatives on canine and rat intestinal motility. J Pharm Pharmacol 1980;32:323-9.

76. Bueno L, Fioramonti J, Frexinos J, Ruckebusch Y. Colonic myoelectrical activity in diarrhea and constipation. Hepatogastroenterology 1980;27:381-9.

77. Leng-Peschlow E. Acceleration of large intestine transit time in rats by sennosides and related compounds. J Pharm Pharmacol 1986;38:369-73.

78. Fioramonti J, Staumont G, Garcia-Villar R, Buéno L. Effect of sennosides on colon motility in dogs. Pharmacology 1988;36(Suppl 1):23-30.

79. Staumont G, Frexinos J, Fioramonti J, Buéno L. Sennosides and human colonic motility. Pharmacology 1988;36(Suppl 1):49-56.

80. Staumont G, Fioramonti J, Frexinos J, Buéno L. Changes in colonic motility induced by sennosides in dogs: evidence of a prostaglandin mediation. Gut 1988; 29:1180-7.

81. Leng-Peschlow E. Effects of sennosides A + B and bisacodyl on rat large intestine. Pharmacology 1989; 38:310-8.

82. Frexinos J, Staumont G, Fioramonti J, Buéno L. Effects of sennosides on colonic myoelectrical activity in man. Dig Dis Sci 1989;34:214-9.

83. Clauss W, Domokos G, Leng-Peschlow E. Effect of rhein on electrogenic chloride secretion in rabbit distal colon. Pharmacology 1988;36(Suppl 1):104-10.

84. Goerg KJ, Wanitschke R, Schwarz M, Meyer z. Büschenfelde KH. Rhein stimulates active chloride secretion in the short-circuited rat colonic mucosa. Pharmacology 1988;36(Suppl 1):111-9.

85. Lemmens L, Borja E. The influence of dihydroxy-anthracene derivatives on water and electrolyte movement in rat colon. J Pharm Pharmacol 1976; 28:498-501.

86. Ewe K. Effect of rhein on the transport of electrolytes, water and carbohydrates in the human jejunum and colon. Pharmacology 1980;20(Suppl 1):27-35.

87. Ewe K, Wanitschke R. The effect of cathartic agents on transmucosal electrical potential difference in the human rectum. Klin Wochenschr 1980;58:299-306.

88. Leng-Peschlow E. Inhibition of intestinal water and electrolyte absorption by senna derivatives in rats. J Pharm Pharmacol 1980;32:330-5.

89. Donowitz M, Wicks J, Battisti L, Pike G, DeLellis R. Effect of Senokot on rat intestinal electrolyte transport. Evidence of Ca^{++} dependence. Gastroenterology 1984;87:503-12.

90. Beubler E, Kollar G. Stimulation of PGE_2 synthesis and water and electrolyte secretion by senna anthraquinones is inhibited by indomethacin. J Pharm Pharmacol 1985; 37:248-51.

91. Beubler E, Kollar G. Prostaglandin-mediated action of sennosides. Pharmacology 1988;36(Suppl 1):85-91.

92. Tavares IA, Mascolo N, Izzo AA, Capasso F. Effects of anthraquinone derivatives on PAF release by human gastrointestinal mucosa in vitro. Phytother Res 1996; 10:20-1.

93. Krumbiegel G, Schulz HU. Rhein and aloe-emodin kinetics from senna laxatives in man. Pharmacology 1993;47(Suppl 1):120-4.

94. Lang W. Pharmacokinetic-metabolic studies with ^{14}C-aloe emodin after oral administration to male and female rats. Pharmacology 1993;47(Suppl 1):110-9.

95. de Witte P, Lemli J. Metabolism of ^{14}C-rhein and ^{14}C-rhein anthrone in rats. Pharmacology 1988;36(Suppl 1):152-7.

96. de Witte P, Lemli J. Excretion and distribution of ^{14}C-rhein and ^{14}C-rhein anthrone in rat. J Pharm Pharmacol 1988;40:652-5.

97. de Witte P, Cuveele J, Lemli J. In vitro deterioration of rhein anthraquinone in cecal content of rats. Pharm Acta Helv 1992;67:198-203.

98. Hattori M, Namba T, Akao T, Kobashi K. Metabolism of sennosides by human intestinal bacteria. Pharmacology 1988;36(Suppl 1):172-9.

99. Hietala P, Lainonen H, Marvola M. New aspects on the metabolism of the sennosides. Pharmacology 1988; 36(Suppl.1):138-43.

100. Lemli J. Metabolismus der Anthranoide. Z Phytother 1986;7:127-9.

101. Mengs U. SF48-WI006: Acute oral toxicity study in rats. Köln: Madaus Report 23.04.1993, unpublished.

102. Mengs U. AX14-WI025: Acute oral toxicity study in mice. Köln: Madaus Report 22.04.1993, unpublished.

103. Mengs U. Toxic effects of sennosides in laboratory animals and in vitro. Pharmacology 1988;36(Suppl. 1):180-7.

104. Marvola M, Koponen A, Hiltunen R, Hietala P. The effect of raw material purity on the acute toxicity and laxative effect of sennosides. J Pharm Pharmacol 1981;33:108-9.

105. Mengs U. Akute Toxizität von Rhein an weiblichen Ratten nach intragastraler Applikation. Köln: Madaus Report 04.11.1985, unpublished.

106. Mengs U. Akute Toxizität von Rhein an männlichen und weiblichen Mäusen nach intragastraler Applikation. Köln: Madaus Report 04.07.1983, unpublished.

107. Rudolph RL, Mengs U. Electron microscopical studies on rat intestine after long-term treatment with sennosides. Pharmacology 1988;36(Suppl. 1):188-93.

108. Dufour P, Gendre P. Ultrastructure of mouse intestinal mucosa and changes observed after long-term

anthraquinone administration. Gut 1984;25:1358-63.

109. Mengs U, Heidemann A. Genotoxicity of sennosides and rhein in vitro and in vivo. Med Sci Res 1993;21:749-50.

110. Westendorf J, Marquardt H, Poginsky B, Dominiak M, Schmidt J, Marquardt H. Genotoxicity of naturally occurring hydroxyanthraquinones. Mutat Res 1990; 240:1-12.

111. Heidemann A, Miltenburger HG, Mengs U. The genotoxicity status of senna. Pharmacology 1993; 47(Suppl 1):178-86.

112. Nitz D, Krumbiegel G. Bestimmung von Aloeemodin und Rhein im Serum von Ratte und Maus nach oraler Gabe von Fructus sennae und Aloeemodin. Köln: Madaus Report 18.05.1992, unpublished.

113. Sandnes D, Johansen T, Teen G, Ulsaker G. Mutagenicity of crude senna and senna glycosides in *Salmonella typhimurium*. Pharmacol Toxicol 1992;71:165-72.

114. Müller SO, Eckert I, Lutz WK, Stopper H. Genotoxicity of the laxative drug components emodin, aloe-emodin and danthron in mammalian cells: topoisomerase II mediated? Mut Res 1996;165-73.

115. Mengs U, Krumbiegel G, Völkner W. Lack of emodin genotoxicity in the mouse micronucleus assay. Mut Res 1997;393:289-93.

116. Mukhopadhyay MJ, Saha A, Dutta A, De B, Mukherjee A. Genotoxicity of sennosides on the bone marrow cells of mice. Food Chem Toxicol 1998;36:937-40.

117. Mueller SO, Lutz WK, Stopper H. Factors affecting the genotoxic potency ranking of natural anthraquinones in mammalian cell culture systems. Mut Res 1998;125-9.

118. Mengs U, Grimminger W, Krumbiegel G, Schuler D, Silber W, Völkner W. No clastogenic activity of a senna extract in mouse micronucleus assay. Mut Res 1999; 444:421-6.

119. Al-Dakan AA, Al-Tuffail M, Hannan MA. Cassia senna inhibits mutagenic activities of benzo[a]pyrene, aflatoxine B_1, shamma and methyl methanesulfonate. Pharmacol Toxicol 1995;77:288-92.

120. Sokolowski AL, Montin G, Nilsson A, Olofsson IM, Sjöberg P. Two-year carcinogenicity study with senna in the rat. VI. Int. Congress of Toxicology, Rome 1992.

121. NTP Technical Report 493. Toxicology and carcinogenesis studies of emodin (CAS No. 518-82-1) in F344/N rats and B6C3F$_1$ mice. NIH Publication No. 99-3952, 1999.

SENNAE FRUCTUS ANGUSTIFOLIAE

Tinnevelly Senna Pods

DEFINITION

Tinnevelly senna pods consist of the dried fruit of *Cassia angustifolia* Vahl. They contain not less than 2.2 per cent of hydroxyanthracene glycosides, calculated as sennoside B ($C_{42}H_{38}O_{20}$; M_r 863) with reference to the dried drug.

The material complies with the monograph of the European Pharmacopoeia [1].

CONSTITUENTS

The main active constituents are sennosides A and B (ca. 2.5%), which are rhein-dianthrone diglucosides. Smaller amounts of other dianthrone diglucosides, monoanthraquinone glucosides and aglycones are also present [2-6].

CLINICAL PARTICULARS

Therapeutic indications
For short-term use in cases of occasional constipation [7-21].

Posology and method of administration

Dosage

The correct individual dose is the smallest required to produce a comfortable soft-formed motion.

Adults and children over 10 years: preparations equivalent to 15-30 mg of hydroxyanthracene derivatives, calculated as sennoside B, to be taken once daily at night [11,14,15,20-24].
Elderly: dose as for adults [25,26].

Not recommended for use in children under 10 years of age [27-32].

The pharmaceutical form must allow lower dosages.

Method of administration
For oral administration.

Contra-indications
Not to be used in cases of: intestinal obstruction and stenosis, atony, inflammatory colon diseases (e.g. Crohn's disease, ulcerative colitis), appendicitis; abdominal pain of unknown origin; severe dehydration states with water and electrolyte depletion.
Children under 10 years.

Special warnings and special precautions for use
As for all laxatives, senna pods should not be given when any undiagnosed acute or persistent abdominal symptoms are present.

If laxatives are needed every day the cause of the constipation should be investigated. Long term use of laxatives should be avoided. Use for more than 2 weeks requires medical supervision. Chronic use may cause pigmentation of the colon (pseudo-melanosis coli) which is harmless and reversible after drug discontinuation. Abuse, with diarrhoea and consequent fluid and electrolyte losses, may cause: dependence with possible need for increased dosages; disturbance of the water and electrolyte (mainly hypokalaemia) balance; an atonic colon with impaired function. Intake of anthranoid-containing laxatives for more than a short period of time may result in an aggravation of constipation. Hypokalaemia can result in cardiac and neuromuscular dysfunction, especially if cardiac glycosides, diuretics or corticosteroids are taken. Chronic use may result in albuminuria and haematuria.

In chronic constipation, stimulant laxatives are not an acceptable alternative to a change in diet [33-42].

Note: A detailed text with advice concerning changes in dietary habits, physical activities and training for normal bowel evacuation should be included on the package leaflet. An example is given in the booklet "Médicaments á base de plantes" published by the French health authority (Paris: Agence du Médicament).

Interaction with other medicaments and other forms of interaction
Hypokalaemia (resulting from long term laxative abuse) potentiates the action of cardiac glycosides and interacts with antiarrhythmic drugs or with drugs which induce reversion to sinus rhythm (e.g. quinidine). Concomitant use with other drugs inducing hypokalaemia (e.g. thiazide diuretics, adreno-corticosteroids and liquorice root) may aggravate electrolyte imbalance.

Pregnancy and lactation

Pregnancy

Wording for extracts identical to those investigated (see Preclinical safety data)
There are no reports of undesirable or damaging effects during pregnancy or on the foetus when used in accordance with the recommended dosage schedule. However, the usual precautionary measures for the use of medicinal products should be observed, especially in the first 3 months of pregnancy.

Wording for all other preparations
There are no reports of undesirable or damaging

effects during pregnancy or on the foetus when used in accordance with the recommended dosage schedule. However, in view of experimental data concerning a genotoxic risk from several anthranoids (e.g. emodin and aloe emodin), avoid during the first trimester or take only under medical supervision [33,43-54].

Lactation
Breastfeeding is not recommended as there are insufficient data on the excretion of metabolites in breast milk. Small amounts of active metabolites (e.g. rhein) are excreted in breast milk. A laxative effect in breast-fed babies has not been reported [18,33,46, 52,55-61].

Effects on ability to drive and use machines
None known.

Undesirable effects
Abdominal spasms and pain, particularly in patients with irritable colon; yellow or red-brown (pH dependent) discoloration of urine by metabolites, which is not clinically significant [61-64].

Overdose
The major symptoms are griping and severe diarrhoea with consequent losses of fluid and electrolyte, which should be replaced.

Treatment should be supportive with generous amounts of fluid. Electrolytes, especially potassium, should be monitored; this is particularly important in the elderly and the young.

PHARMACOLOGICAL PROPERTIES

Pharmacodynamic properties
1,8-dihydroxyanthracene derivatives possess a laxative effect [65-68]. The β-linked glucosides (sennosides) are not absorbed in the upper gut; they are converted by the bacteria of the large intestine into the active metabolite (rhein anthrone) [69-73]. There are two different mechanisms of action [68]:

(i) an influence on the motility of the large intestine (stimulation of peristaltic contractions and inhibition of local contractions) resulting in accelerated colonic transit, thus reducing fluid absorption [74-82], and

(ii) an influence on secretion processes (stimulation of mucus and active chloride secretion) [81,83,84] resulting in enhanced fluid secretion [68,81,85-91].

Defecation takes place after a delay of 8-12 hours due to the time taken for transport to the colon and metabolization into the active compound.

Aloe-emodin stimulated a release of platelet activating factor (PAF) in experiments with human gastrointestinal mucosal cells, while rhein had no effect [92].

Pharmacokinetic properties

The β-linked glucosides (sennosides) are neither absorbed in the upper gut nor split by human digestive enzymes. They are converted by the bacteria of the large intestine into the active metabolite (rhein anthrone). Aglycones are absorbed in the upper gut. Animal experiments with radio-isotope-labelled rhein anthrone administered directly into the caecum demonstrated less than 10% absorption.

In contact with oxygen, rhein anthrone is oxidized into rhein and sennidins which can be found in the blood, mainly in the form of glucuronides and sulphates. After oral administration of sennosides, 3-6% of the metabolites are excreted in the urine; some are excreted in bile. Most of the sennosides (ca. 90%) are excreted in the faeces as polymers (polyquinones) together with 2-6% of unchanged sennosides, sennidins, rhein anthrone and rhein. In human pharmacokinetic studies with senna pod powder (20 mg of sennosides), administered orally for 7 days, a maximum rhein concentration of 100 ng/ml was found in the blood. No accumulation of rhein was observed.

Active metabolites, e.g. rhein, pass in small amounts into breast milk. Animal experiments demonstrated that passage of rhein through the placenta is low [70-74,93-100].

Preclinical safety data

Most data refer to extracts containing 1.4 to 3.5% of anthranoids, corresponding to 0.9 to 2.3% of potential rhein, 0.05 to 0.15% of potential aloe emodin and 0.001 to 0.006% of potential emodin or to isolated active constituents, e.g. rhein or sennosides A and B. The acute oral toxicity in rats and mice of senna pods, of specified extracts from them and of sennosides was found to be low. From the results of investigations involving parenteral administration in mice, extracts are thought to possess higher toxicity than purified glucosides, possibly due to their content of aglycones [100-106].

Sennosides displayed no specific toxicity when tested at doses of up to 500 mg/kg in dogs for 4 weeks and up to 100 mg/kg in rats for 6 months. No data are available for crude drug preparations [103,107,108].

There was no evidence of any embryolethal, terato-genic or fetotoxic effects in rats or rabbits after oral treatment with sennosides. Furthermore, there was no effect on the postnatal development of young rats, on rearing behaviour of dams or on male and female fertility in rats. No data are available for crude drug preparations [43].

In the Ames test a senna extract, emodin and aloe-emodin were mutagenic. Sennosides A and B and rhein gave negative results. Comprehensive in vivo testing of a defined extract of senna pods and its anthranoid constituents revealed no genotoxicity (109-118). An ethanolic extract has been reported to be antimutagenic [119].

A senna extract given orally at doses of 5, 15 or 25 mg/kg for 2 years was not carcinogenic in male or female Sprague-Dawley rats. The extract investigated contained approx. 40.8% of anthranoids of which 35% were sennosides, corresponding to about 25.2% of potential rhein, 2.3% of potential aloe-emodin and 0.007% of potential emodin, and 142 ppm of free aloe-emodin and 9 ppm of free emodin [120].

In a 2-year study, male and female F344/N rats were exposed to 280, 830 or 2500 ppm of emodin in the diet, corresponding to an average daily dose of emodin of 110, 320 or 1000 mg/kg body weight in male rats and 120, 370 or 1100 mg/kg body weight in female rats. No evidence of carcinogenic activity of emodin was observed in male rats. A marginal increase in the incidence of Zymbal's gland carcinoma occurred in female rats treated with the high dosage but was interpreted as questionable [121].

In a further 2-year study, on B6C3F$_1$ mice, males were exposed to 160, 312 or 625 ppm of emodin (corresponding to an average daily dose of 15, 35 or 70 mg/kg body weight) and females to 312, 625 or 1250 ppm of emodin (corresponding to an average daily dose of 30, 60 or 120 mg/kg body weight). There was no evidence of carcinogenic activity in female mice. A low incidence of renal tubule neoplasms in exposed males was not considered relevant [121].

REFERENCES

1. Senna Pods, Tinnevelly - Sennae fructus angustifoliae. European Pharmacopoeia, Council of Europe.

2. Hänsel R, Keller K, Rimpler H, Schneider G, editors. Cassia. In: Hagers Handbuch der pharmazeutischen Praxis, 5th ed. Volume 4: Drogen A-D. Berlin: Springer-Verlag, 1992:701-25.

3. Hänsel R, Sticher O, Steinegger E. Sennesblätter und Sennesfrüchte. In: Pharmakognosie, 6th ed. Berlin: Springer-Verlag, 1999:910-4.

4. Nakajima K, Yamauchi K, Kuwano S. Isolation of a new aloe-emodin dianthrone diglucoside from senna and its potentiating effect on the purgative activity of sennoside A in mice. J Pharm Pharmacol 1985;37:703-6.

5. Lemli J. The chemistry of senna. Fitoterapia 1986;57:33-40.

6. van Os FHL. Anthraquinone derivatives in vegetable laxatives. Pharmacology 1976;14(Suppl 1):7-17.

7. Slanger A. Comparative study of a standardized senna liquid and castor oil in preparing patients for radiographic examination of the colon. Dis Colon Rectum 1979;22:356-9.

8. Georgia EH. Management of drug-induced constipation in psychiatric outpatients. Curr Ther Res 1983;33:1018-22.

9. Izard MW, Ellison FS. Treatment of drug-induced constipation with a purified senna derivative. Conn Med 1962;26:589-92.

10. Pers M, Pers B. A crossover comparative study with two bulk laxatives. J Int Med Res 1983;11:51-3.

11. Gould SR, Williams CB. Castor oil or senna preparation before colonoscopy for inactive chronic ulcerative colitis. Gastrointest Endosc 1982;28:6-8.

12. Marlett JA, Li BUK, Patrow CJ, Bass P. Comparative laxation of psyllium with and without senna in an ambulatory constipated population. Am J Gastroenterol 1987;82:333-7.

13. Maguire LC, Yon JL, Miller E. Prevention of narcotic-induced constipation [Letter]. New Engl J Med 1981; 305:1651.

14. Slanger A. Cleansing of the sigmoid flexure and rectum preparatory to sigmoidoscopy: Report of a controlled study. Dis Colon Rectum 1966;9:109-12.

15. Dickie J, James WB, Hume R, Robertson D. A comparison of three substances used for bowel preparation prior to radiological examination. Clin Radiol 1970;21:201-2.

16. Reis Neto JA, Quilici FA, Oliveira LAR, Faria PC, Cordeiro F, Reis JA Jr. Eficácia e segurança de uma associação laxativa no pós-operatório imediato de cirurgias colo-proctológicas. Rev Bras Clín Terap 1986; 15:26-30.

17. Maddi VI. Regulation of bowel function by a laxative/stool softener preparation in aged nursing home patients. J Am Geriatr Soc 1979;27:464-8.

18. Duncan AS. Standardized senna as a laxative in the puerperium. A clinical assessment. Br Med J 1957;1:439-41.

19. Godding EW. Laxatives and the special role of senna. Pharmacology 1988;36(Suppl 1):230-6.

20. USA Department of Health and Human Services: Food and Drug Administration. 21 CFR Part 334. Laxative Drug Products for Over-the-Counter Human Use; Tentative Final Monograph. Federal Register 1985; 50(10):2124, 2151-8 (January 15, 1985).

21. Binder HJ. Use of laxatives in clinical medicine. Pharmacology 1988;36(Suppl 1):226-9.

22. Kovar F. Sennatin® tabl. - Dosage, efficacy and tolerance

in bedridden patients with constipation. Köln: Madaus Report 14.11.1984, unpublished.

23. Brusis O. Sennatin® in acute constipation. Köln: Madaus Report 25.07.1986. Double-blind study, unpublished.

24. Jähnig L. Offene, monozentrische, randomisierte klinische Prüfung zur Bestimmung des Wirkungseintritts und der Wirkqualität unterschiedlicher Dosen von AX14E0 bei chronischer Obstipation (AX14E0.53). Köln: Madaus Report 27.04.1993, unpublished.

25. McClure Browne JC, Edmunds V, Fairbairn JW, Reid DD. Clinical and laboratory assessments of senna preparations. Br Med J 1957:436-9.

26. Smith CW, Evans PR. Bowel motility. A problem in institutionalized geriatric care. Geriatrics 1961:189-92.

27. Berg I, Jones KV. Functional faecal incontinence in children. Arch Dis Child 1964;39:465-72.

28. Campbell-Mackie M. The re-educative treatment of bowel dysfunction in infants and children. S Afr Med J 1963;37:675-8.

29. Clayden GS. Constipation and soiling in childhood. Br Med J 1976;1:515-7.

30. Campbell-Mackie M. The treatment of bowel dysfunction in infants and young children. Practitioner 1959;183:732-6.

31. Wherry CA. Treating chronic constipation in children. Nursing Times 1977:1829-31.

32. Braid F. The treatment of constipation in children. Medical Press 1954;231:521-4.

33. Leng-Peschlow E. Senna and its rational use. Pharmacology 1992;44(Suppl 1):1-52.

34. Sonnenberg A, Sonnenberg GS. Epidemiologie der Obstipation. In: Müller-Lissner SA, Ackermans LMA, editors. Chronische Obstipation und Stuhlinkontinenz. Berlin: Springer-Verlag, 1989:141-56.

35. Preston DM, Lennard-Jones JE. Severe chronic constipation of young women: 'Idiopathic slow transit constipation'. Gut 1986;27:41-8.

36. Klauser A, Peyerl C, Schindlbeck N, Müller-Lissner S. Obstipierte unterscheiden sich nicht von Gesunden hinsichtlich Ernährung und körperlicher Aktivität [Abstract]. Z Gastroenterol 1990;28:494.

37. Müller-Lissner SA. Effect of wheat bran on weight of stool and gastrointestinal transit time: a meta analysis. Br Med J 1988;296:615-7.

38. Klauser A, Beck A, Schindlbeck N, Müller-Lissner S. Dursten beeinflußt die Colonfunktion bei Probanden [Abstract]. Z Gastroenterol 1990;28:493.

39. Coenen C, Schmidt G, Wegener M, Hoffmann S, Wedmann B. Beeinflußt körperliche Aktivität den oro-analen Transit? - Eine prospektive, kontrollierte Studie

[Abstract]. Z Gastroenterol 1990;28:469.

40. Bingham SA, Cummings JH. Effect of exercise and physical fitness on large intestinal function. Gastroenterology 1989;97:1389-99.

41. Bingham S. Does exercise affect large gut function? J Hum Nutr Diet 1991;4:281-5.

42. Klauser AG, Flaschenträger J, Gehrke A, Müller-Lissner SA. Abdominal wall massage: effect on colonic function in healthy volunteers and in patients with chronic constipation. Z Gastroenterol 1992;30:247-51.

43. Mengs U. Reproductive toxicological investigations with sennosides. Arzneim-Forsch/Drug Res 1986;36: 1355-8.

44. Garcia-Villar R. Evaluation of the effects of sennosides on uterine motility in the pregnant ewe. Pharmacology 1988; 36(Suppl 1):203-11.

45. Herland AL, Lowenstein A. Physiologic rehabilitation of the constipated colon in pregnant women. Use of a standardized senna derivative. Q Rev Surg 1957; 14:196-202.

46. Greenhalf JO, Leonard HSD. Laxatives in the treatment of constipation in pregnant and breast-feeding mothers. Practitioner 1973;210:259-63.

47. Wager HP, Melosh WD. The management of constipation in pregnancy. Q Rev Surg 1958;15:30-4.

48. Scott RS. Management of constipation in obstetrics: A clinical report on 592 cases. West Med 1965;6:342-4.

49. Girotti M, Hauser GA. Therapie der Obstipation in der Schwangerschaft und bei gynäkologischen Patientinnen. Ther Umsch 1971;28:490-3.

50. Mahon R, Palmade J. Traitement de la constipation chez la femme enceinte. Gaz Med Fr 1974;81:3259-60.

51. Gram U. Bedeutung der normalen Darmtätigkeit während der Schwangerschaft. Med Welt 1969; 20:2613-5.

52. Kaltstein A. Zur Behandlung der Schwangerschafts- und Wochenbettobstipation. Fortschr Med 1969; 87:723-5.

53. Roth OA. Therapeutische Beobachtungen bei Obstipation. Med Welt 1969;20:536-7.

54. Bauer H. Behandlung der Obstipation mit Laxariston® in der gynäkologischen Praxis. Ther Gegenwart 1977; 116:2305-12.

55. Baldwin WF. Clinical study of senna administration to nursing mothers: Assessment of effects on infant bowel habits. Can Med Assoc J 1963;89:566-8.

56. Dubecq JP, Palmade J. Étude clinique de l'administration de tamarine chez la mère qui allaite. Gaz Med Fr 1974; 81:5173-5.

57. Shelton MG. Standardized senna in the management of constipation in the puerperium. A clinical trial. S Afr Med J 1980;57:78-80.

58. Suarez J, Castillo AG, Shepard J. The use of a new standardized senna derivative in the management of puerperal constipation. Int Rec Med 1960;173:639-42.

59. Faber P, Strenge-Hesse A. Relevance of rhein excretion into breast milk. Pharmacology 1988;36(Suppl 1):212-20.

60. Cameron BD, Phillips MWA, Fenerty CA. Milk transfer of rhein in the rhesus monkey. Pharmacology 1988; 36(Suppl 1):221-5.

61. Reynolds JEF, editor. Senna. In: Martindale - The Extra Pharmacopoeia, 31st ed. London: Royal Pharmaceutical Society, 1996:1240-1.

62. Cooke WT. Laxative abuse. Clin Gastroenterol 1977; 6:659-73.

63. Tedesco FJ. Laxative use in constipation. Am J Gastroenterol 1985;80:303-9.

64. Ewe K, Karbach U. Factitious diarrhoea. Clin Gastroenterol 1986;15:723-40.

65. Brittain RT, D'Arcy PF, Grimshaw JJ. Observations on the use of a mouse bioassay method for investigating purgative activity. J Pharm Pharmacol 1962;14:715-21.

66. Fairbairn JW. Chemical structure, mode of action and therapeutical activity of anthraquinone glycosides. Pharm Weekbl (Sci) 1965;100:1493-9.

67. Fairbairn JW, Moss MJR. The relative purgative activities of 1,8-dihydroxyanthracene derivatives. J Pharm Pharmacol 1970;22:584-93.

68. Leng-Peschlow E. Dual effect of orally administered sennosides on large intestine transit and fluid absorption in the rat. J Pharm Pharmacol 1986;38:606-10.

69. Lemmens L. The laxative action of anthracene derivatives. 2. Absorption, metabolism and excretion of sennoside A and B in the rat. Pharm Weekbl (Sci) 1979;114:178-85.

70. Lemli J, Lemmens L. Metabolism of sennosides and rhein in the rat. Pharmacology 1980;20(Suppl 1):50-7.

71. Kobashi K, Nishimura T, Kusaka M, Hattori M, Namba T. Metabolism of sennosides by human intestinal bacteria. Planta Med 1980;40:225-36.

72. Dreessen M, Eyssen H, Lemli J. The metabolism of sennosides A and B by the intestinal microflora: in vitro and in vivo studies on the rat and the mouse. J Pharm Pharmacol 1981;33:679-81.

73. Hattori M, Kim G, Motoike S, Kobashi K, Namba T. Metabolism of sennosides by intestinal flora. Chem Pharm Bull 1982;30:1338-46.

74. Hardcastle JD, Wilkins JL. The action of sennosides and related compounds on human colon and rectum. Gut 1970;11:1038-42.

75. Garcia-Villar R, Leng-Peschlow E, Ruckebusch Y. Effect of anthraquinone derivatives on canine and rat intestinal motility. J Pharm Pharmacol 1980;32:323-9.

76. Bueno L, Fioramonti J, Frexinos J, Ruckebusch Y. Colonic myoelectrical activity in diarrhea and constipation. Hepatogastroenterology 1980;27:381-9.

77. Leng-Peschlow E. Acceleration of large intestine transit time in rats by sennosides and related compounds. J Pharm Pharmacol 1986;38:369-73.

78. Fioramonti J, Staumont G, Garcia-Villar R, Buéno L. Effect of sennosides on colon motility in dogs. Pharmacology 1988;36(Suppl 1):23-30.

79. Staumont G, Frexinos J, Fioramonti J, Buéno L. Sennosides and human colonic motility. Pharmacology 1988;36(Suppl 1):49-56.

80. Staumont G, Fioramonti J, Frexinos J, Buéno L. Changes in colonic motility induced by sennosides in dogs: evidence of a prostaglandin mediation. Gut 1988; 29:1180-7.

81. Leng-Peschlow E. Effects of sennosides A + B and bisacodyl on rat large intestine. Pharmacology 1989; 38:310-8.

82. Frexinos J, Staumont G, Fioramonti J, Buéno L. Effects of sennosides on colonic myoelectrical activity in man. Dig Dis Sci 1989;34:214-9.

83. Clauss W, Domokos G, Leng-Peschlow E. Effect of rhein on electrogenic chloride secretion in rabbit distal colon. Pharmacology 1988;36(Suppl 1):104-10.

84. Goerg KJ, Wanitschke R, Schwarz M, Meyer z. Büschenfelde KH. Rhein stimulates active chloride secretion in the short-circuited rat colonic mucosa. Pharmacology 1988;36(Suppl 1):111-9.

85. Lemmens L, Borja E. The influence of dihydroxy-anthracene derivatives on water and electrolyte movement in rat colon. J Pharm Pharmacol 1976; 28:498-501.

86. Ewe K. Effect of rhein on the transport of electrolytes, water and carbohydrates in the human jejunum and colon. Pharmacology 1980;20(Suppl 1):27-35.

87. Ewe K, Wanitschke R. The effect of cathartic agents on transmucosal electrical potential difference in the human rectum. Klin Wochenschr 1980;58:299-306.

88. Leng-Peschlow E. Inhibition of intestinal water and electrolyte absorption by senna derivatives in rats. J Pharm Pharmacol 1980;32:330-5.

89. Donowitz M, Wicks J, Battisti L, Pike G, DeLellis R. Effect of Senokot on rat intestinal electrolyte transport. Evidence of Ca^{++} dependence. Gastroenterology 1984; 87:503-12.

90. Beubler E, Kollar G. Stimulation of PGE_2 synthesis and water and electrolyte secretion by senna anthraquinones is inhibited by indomethacin. J Pharm Pharmacol 1985;37:248-51.

91. Beubler E, Kollar G. Prostaglandin-mediated action of sennosides. Pharmacology 1988;36(Suppl 1):85-91.

92. Tavares IA, Mascolo N, Izzo AA, Capasso F. Effects of anthraquinone derivatives on PAF release by human gastrointestinal mucosa in vitro. Phytother Res 1996; 10:20-1.

93. Krumbiegel G, Schulz HU. Rhein and aloe-emodin kinetics from senna laxatives in man. Pharmacology 1993;47(Suppl 1):120-4.

94. Lang W. Pharmacokinetic-metabolic studies with ^{14}C-aloe emodin after oral administration to male and female rats. Pharmacology 1993;47(Suppl 1):110-9.

95. de Witte P, Lemli J. Metabolism of ^{14}C-rhein and ^{14}C-rhein anthrone in rats. Pharmacology 1988;36(Suppl 1):152-7.

96. de Witte P, Lemli J. Excretion and distribution of ^{14}C-rhein and ^{14}C-rhein anthrone in rat. J Pharm Pharmacol 1988;40:652-5.

97. de Witte P, Cuveele J, Lemli J. In vitro deterioration of rhein anthraquinone in cecal content of rats. Pharm Acta Helv 1992;67:198-203.

98. Hattori M, Namba T, Akao T, Kobashi K. Metabolism of sennosides by human intestinal bacteria. Pharmacology 1988;36(Suppl 1):172-9.

99. Hietala P, Lainonen H, Marvola M. New aspects on the metabolism of the sennosides. Pharmacology 1988; 36(Suppl.1):138-43.

100. Lemli J. Metabolismus der Anthranoide. Z Phytother 1986;7:127-9.

101. Mengs U. SF48-WI006: Acute oral toxicity study in rats. Köln: Madaus Report 23.04.1993, unpublished.

102. Mengs U. AX14-WI025: Acute oral toxicity study in mice. Köln: Madaus Report 22.04.1993, unpublished.

103. Mengs U. Toxic effects of sennosides in laboratory animals and in vitro. Pharmacology 1988;36(Suppl. 1):180-7.

104. Marvola M, Koponen A, Hiltunen R, Hietala P. The effect of raw material purity on the acute toxicity and laxative effect of sennosides. J Pharm Pharmacol 1981;33:108-9.

105. Mengs U. Akute Toxizität von Rhein an weiblichen Ratten nach intragastraler Applikation. Köln: Madaus Report 04.11.1985, unpublished.

106. Mengs U. Akute Toxizität von Rhein an männlichen und weiblichen Mäusen nach intragastraler Applikation. Köln: Madaus Report 04.07.1983, unpublished.

107. Rudolph RL, Mengs U. Electron microscopical studies on rat intestine after long-term treatment with senno-sides. Pharmacology 1988;36(Suppl. 1):188-93.

108. Dufour P, Gendre P. Ultrastructure of mouse intestinal mucosa and changes observed after long-term

anthraquinone administration. Gut 1984;25:1358-63.

109. Mengs U, Heidemann A. Genotoxicity of sennosides and rhein in vitro and in vivo. Med Sci Res 1993;21:749-50.

110. Westendorf J, Marquardt H, Poginsky B, Dominiak M, Schmidt J, Marquardt H. Genotoxicity of naturally occurring hydroxyanthraquinones. Mutat Res 1990; 240:1-12.

111. Heidemann A, Miltenburger HG, Mengs U. The genotoxicity status of senna. Pharmacology 1993;47(Suppl 1):178-86.

112. Nitz D, Krumbiegel G. Bestimmung von Aloeemodin und Rhein im Serum von Ratte und Maus nach oraler Gabe von Fructus sennae und Aloeemodin. Köln: Madaus Report 18.05.1992, unpublished.

113. Sandnes D, Johansen T, Teen G, Ulsaker G. Mutagenicity of crude senna and senna glycosides in *Salmonella typhimurium*. Pharmacol Toxicol 1992;71:165-72.

114. Müller SO, Eckert I, Lutz WK, Stopper H. Genotoxicity of the laxative drug components emodin, aloe-emodin and danthron in mammalian cells: topoisomerase II mediated? Mut Res 1996;165-73.

115. Mengs U, Krumbiegel G, Völkner W. Lack of emodin genotoxicity in the mouse micronucleus assay. Mut Res 1997;393:289-93.

116. Mukhopadhyay MJ, Saha A, Dutta A, De B, Mukherjee A. Genotoxicity of sennosides on the bone marrow cells of mice. Food Chem Toxicol 1998;36:937-40.

117. Mueller SO, Lutz WK, Stopper H. Factors affecting the genotoxic potency ranking of natural anthraquinones in mammalian cell culture systems. Mut Res 1998;125-9.

118. Mengs U, Grimminger W, Krumbiegel G, Schuler D, Silber W, Völkner W. No clastogenic activity of a senna extract in mouse micronucleus assay. Mut Res 1999;444:421-6.

119. Al-Dakan AA, Al-Tuffail M, Hannan MA. Cassia senna inhibits mutagenic activities of benzo[a]pyrene, aflatoxine B_1, shamma and methyl methanesulfonate. Pharmacol Toxicol 1995;77:288-92.

120. Sokolowski AL, Montin G, Nilsson A, Olofsson IM, Sjöberg P. Two-year carcinogenicity study with senna in the rat. VI. Int. Congress of Toxicology, Rome 1992.

121. NTP Technical Report 493. Toxicology and carcinogenesis studies of emodin (CAS No. 518-82-1) in F344/N rats and B6C3F$_1$ mice. NIH Publication No. 99-3952, 1999.

SERENOAE REPENTIS FRUCTUS (SABAL FRUCTUS)

Saw Palmetto Fruit

DEFINITION

Saw palmetto fruit consists of the dried, ripe fruit of *Serenoa repens* (Bartram) Small [*Sabal serrulata* (Michaux) Nichols].

The material complies with the monograph of the United States Pharmacopeia [1].

A draft monograph on Sabal, intended for inclusion in the European Pharmacopoeia, has been published [2].

CONSTITUENTS

Free fatty acids, especially capric, caproic, caprylic, lauric, myristic, oleic, linoleic, linolenic, stearic and palmitic acids. Sterols, principally β-sitosterol and its 3-glucoside (and fatty acid derivatives of these), campesterol and stigmasterol. Triglycerides, triterpenes, alkanols, polysaccharides, flavonoids, essential oil and anthranilic acid [3-12].

Esters of the above fatty acids may be present in extracts prepared using an alcohol; due to the presence of an esterase, esterification can easily occur during the extraction process [6].

CLINICAL PARTICULARS

Therapeutic indications
Symptomatic treatment of micturition disorders (dysuria, pollakisuria, nocturia, urine retention) in mild to moderate benign prostatic hyperplasia (BPH) [3,12-49], i.e. stages I and II as defined by Alken [50], stages II and III as defined by Vahlensieck [51] or a comparable severity of symptoms as evaluated by the International Prostate Symptom Score and associated diagnostic tests [52].

Note: *The stages of BPH defined by Alken [50] and Vahlensieck [51] are tabulated in the monograph on Urticae radix.*

Posology and method of administration

Dosage

Daily dose: 1-2 g of the drug or 320 mg of lipophilic extract [3,12-49]; other equivalent preparations.

Method of administration
For oral administration.

E/S/C/O/P
MONOGRAPHS
Second Edition

Duration of administration
No restriction.

Contra-indications
None known.

Special warnings and special precautions for use
Difficulties in micturition require clarification by a physician in every case and regular medical checks to exclude the need for other treatment, e.g. surgical intervention. Consultation with a physician is especially necessary in cases of blood in the urine or acute retention of urine.

Interaction with other medicaments and other forms of interaction
None reported.

Pregnancy and lactation
Not applicable.

Effects on ability to drive and use machines
None known.

Undesirable effects
Minor gastrointestinal complaints [3,13,22,36,37, 40,42,44,46,48].

Overdose
No toxic effects reported.

PHARMACOLOGICAL PROPERTIES

Pharmacodynamic properties

In vitro experiments

Inhibition of 5α-reductase and other enzymes
Lipophilic extracts from saw palmetto fruit inhibit the activity of 5α-reductase, an enzyme catalysing the conversion of testosterone into dihydrotestosterone (DHT) [8,53-60]. Various extracts (hexane, ethanol, hypercritical CO_2) gave IC_{50} values between 25 µg/ml and 2200 µg/ml depending on the assay [8,57-59]. Dose-dependent and non-competitive inhibition of 5α-reductase was observed in both the prostatic epithelium and the stroma: the mean inhibitory effect of an ethanolic extract at a concentration of 500 µg/ml was about 29% in the epithelium and 45% in the stroma [57]. The inhibition is mainly due to free fatty acids in the saponifiable fraction [8,57,59]. The non-saponifiable fraction, containing phytosterols, triterpenes and fatty alcohols, and the hydrophilic components proved to be inactive [8]. In a comparative study with finasteride, IC_{50} values of between 5.6 µg/ml and 40 µg/ml were obtained with the various lipophilic extracts (hexane, ethanol, hypercritical CO_2), compared to an IC_{50} of 1 ng/ml for finasteride [61]. The hexanic extract non-competitively inhibited

both isoforms of 5α-reductase with IC_{50} values of 4 µg/ml for type 1 and 7 µg/ml for type 2, whereas finasteride was a competitive inhibitor of both isozymes, with a more selective inhibition of type 2 (IC_{50}: 400 nM for type 1; 10.7 nM for type 2) [62].

A hexanic extract from saw palmetto fruit inhibited the formation not only of dihydrotestosterone but also of the testosterone metabolites androstenedione and 5α-androstane-3,17-dione in primary cultures of human stromal and epithelial cells derived from benign prostatic hyperplasia tissues, suggesting that it inhibits the activity of both 5α-reductase and 17β-hydroxysteroid dehydrogenase [63]. An ethanolic extract (IC_{50}: 132 µg/ml) and a hexanic extract (IC_{50}: 91 µg/ml) inhibited the enzyme aromatase, which catalyses the conversion of androgens into oestrogens [59].

Influence on androgen-receptor binding
A hexanic extract from saw palmetto fruit inhibited the receptor binding of androgens [53,64-66]; in contrast, no inhibition of androgen receptor binding by this extract was observed in another investigation [61]. In the human prostatic cell lines LNCaP (lymph node carcinoma of the prostate) and PC3 (bone metastasis of prostatic carcinoma), which are respectively responsive and unresponsive to androgen stimulation, a hexanic extract at 100 µg/ml induced a double proliferative-differentiative effect in the LNCaP cell line, indicating a role of the androgen receptor in mediating the effects of the extract in these cells. In PC3 cells cotransfected with wild-type androgen receptors and CAT (chloramphenicol acetyl coenzyme A transferase) receptor genes under the control of an androgen responsive element, the extract inhibited androgen-induced CAT transcription by 70% at 25 µg/ml [67]. Ethanolic and CO_2 extracts had no, or only very weak, inhibitory activity on the receptor binding of androgens [53-55,59,61,64,65].

Inhibition of α₁-receptor binding
Six extracts from saw palmetto fruit (two powders, four oils) inhibited [³H]-tamsulosin binding to human prostatic α₁-adrenoceptors (IC_{50}: 0.005-0.01%), [³H]-prazosin binding to cloned human α₁-adrenoceptors (IC_{50}: 0.001-0.002%) and agonist-induced [³H]-inositol phosphate formation by cloned α₁-adrenoceptors (63-69% inhibition by 400 µg/ml of extract powders, 33-46% inhibition by 0.08% of extracted oils). The inhibition was non-competitive [68,69].

Inhibition of eicosanoid synthesis
A hexanic extract inhibited the calcium ionophore A23187-stimulated production of 5-lipoxygenase metabolites in human polymorphonuclear neutrophils at concentrations ≥ 5 µg/ml; the IC_{50} for inhibition of leukotriene B_4 (LTB_4) was approximately 13 µg/ml [70]. A hypercritical CO_2 extract was found to be a dual inhibitor of the cyclooxygenase (IC_{50}: 28.1 µg/ml)

and 5-lipoxygenase pathways (IC$_{50}$: 18.0 μg/ml); a fraction containing acidic lipophilic compounds inhibited the biosynthesis of cyclooxygenase and 5-lipoxygenase metabolites with the same intensity as the native extract, while β-sitosterol and fractions containing sterols and fatty alcohols as main components did not show inhibitory effects on either of the enzymes [55,71]. An ethanolic extract inhibited formation of the cyclooxygenase product thromboxane B$_2$ (TXB$_2$) (IC$_{50}$: 15.3 μg/ml) and synthesis of the 5-lipoxygenase product LTB$_4$ (IC$_{50}$: 8.3 μg/ml) [59]. An alcoholic extract inhibited synthesis of the prostaglandins prostacyclin (PGI$_2$) and prostaglandin E$_2$ (PGE$_2$) [7].

Spasmolytic effects
A total lipidic extract and a saponifiable fraction from saw palmetto fruit relaxed tonic contractions induced in various smooth muscle preparations by vanadate (EC$_{50}$: extract, 43.9 μg/ml; fraction, 11.4 μg/ml) [72], noradrenaline (EC$_{50}$: extract, 530 μg/ml; fraction, 560 μg/ml) [73], KCl (EC$_{50}$: extract, 350 μg/ml; fraction, 430 μg/ml) [73] and acetylcholine (EC$_{50}$: acetylcholine, 4.41 μM; extract at 1 mg/ml, 23.66 μM; fraction at 1 mg/ml, 35.42 μM) [73] or by electrical stimulation [74], and inhibited calmodulin-dependent cAMP phosphodiesterase activity (IC$_{50}$: extract, 25.1 μg/ml; fraction, 28.6 μg/ml) [72-75].

Other effects
A hexanic extract (1-30 μg/ml) inhibited Ca^{2+}-dependent K$^+$ channels, prolactin-stimulated Ca^{2+} mobilization from intracellular stores and Ca^{2+} influx and protein kinase C, suggesting possible blocking effects on prolactin-induced prostate growth by inhibiting several steps of prolactin receptor signal transduction [76].

A hexanic extract inhibited basic fibroblast growth factor (b-FGF)-induced proliferation of human prostate cell cultures, this effect was significant at 30 μg extract/ml (p<0.01) [77].

In vivo experiments

Antiandrogenic effects
In castrated or prepubescent mice and rats treated with testosterone or gonadotrophin, oral administration of a hexanic extract from saw palmetto fruit (300 mg/animal per day for 4-12 days) resulted in a loss of weight of the accessory sex glands; the extract did not show oestrogenic or progestogenic properties and had no adverse effect on the neuroendocrine feedback mechanism [64]. In castrated rats treated with testosterone, oestradiol and the hexanic extract (50 mg/kg/day orally for 30, 60 or 90 days), the weight of the dorsal prostate lobe was significantly lower at days 30, 60 and 90 and the weight of the lateral prostate lobe was significantly reduced at day 60, whereas the effect on the ventral lobe was very weak

[78]. In another study, the hexanic extract (180 or 1800 mg/day orally over 7 days) did not show any effect on prostate growth in either testosterone- or dihydrotestosterone-stimulated castrated rats [61]. An ethanolic extract administered orally (0.15 ml/ 25 g body weight once weekly for 2 months), caused inhibition of prostatic growth in athymic nude mice, into which human benign hyperplastic prostatic tissue had been transplanted and which was stimulated with dihydrotestosterone and oestradiol [79]. In castrated rats treated with testosterone, the same ethanolic extract (100, 300 or 1000 mg/kg orally for 6 days) reduced the weight of the ventral prostate and the seminal vesicles including the coagulation glands [59].

A fraction from a methanolic extract of saw palmetto fruit (2.5 and 5 mg/animal, administered subcutaneously for 3 days) and β-sitosterol isolated from it (2-50 μg/animal subcutaneously) showed oestrogenic activity (increase in uterine weight) in immature female mice [80].

Anti-inflammatory, anti-oedematous effects
Capillary permeability was reduced by oral administration of a hexanic extract from saw palmetto fruit (5-10 ml extract/kg body weight) in various models of inflammation in rats, mice and guinea pigs [64,81]. An ethanolic extract (10 mg/kg orally) inhibited carrageenan-induced rat paw oedema [7]. In the croton oil-induced mouse ear oedema test, local application of an ethanolic extract (500 μg) inhibited the oedema by 42% [59]. An acidic polysaccharide (0.1-1 mg/kg, administered intravenously) isolated from an aqueous extract of saw palmetto fruit showed anti-inflammatory activity against carrageenan-induced rat paw oedema and in the pellet test in rats [82,83].

Pharmacological studies in humans
In a double-blind, placebo-controlled study, 35 patients with BPH were treated orally for 3 months with a hexanic extract from saw palmetto fruit (320 mg daily) or placebo up to the day before transvesical adenectomy. At the end of treatment, both nuclear oestrogen and progesterone receptors in prostatic tissue were significantly lower (p<0.01 each) in the verum group than in the placebo group, while cytosolic oestrogen and progesterone receptors remained almost unchanged [84].

In a double-blind, placebo-controlled trial 18 patients with BPH received an extract (1920 mg) or placebo daily for 3 months [85,86]. The activity of 5α-reductase, 3α- and 3β-hydroxysteroid oxidoreductases, and creatine kinase was determined in mechanically separated epithelium and stroma from BPH patients, obtained by suprapubic prostatectomy. The extract slightly decreased the substrate affinity of 5α-reductase in the epithelium; in the stroma, the

V_{max} value of creatine kinase increased to a greater extent than that of the 3α- and 3β-hydroxysteroid oxidoreductases [85]. A reduction in periglandular stromal oedema, mucoid degeneration, intraglandular congestion and congestive prostatitis was observed in patients treated with the extract [86].

A total of 32 healthy male volunteers were enrolled in a one-week, randomized, open study comparing the effects of the 5α-reductase inhibitor finasteride (5 mg daily) with a hexanic extract of saw palmetto (320 mg daily) or placebo. 5α-Reductase activity was assessed by determination of serum levels of dihydro-testosterone (DHT). As in the placebo group, the extract had no effect on serum DHT levels, whereas finasteride significantly reduced serum DHT levels (p<0.01 vs baseline) by 65% (first single dose) and 52-60% (multiple doses). No significant difference was detected between groups with respect to serum testosterone [87].

In another study 25 patients with BPH were randomly assigned to treatment with a hexanic extract from saw palmetto fruit (320 mg daily for 3 months; n = 10) or to an untreated control group (n = 15). After suprapubic prostatectomy, concentrations of testosterone (T), dihydrotestosterone (DHT) and epidermal growth factor (EGF) were determined in prostatic tissue. In the group treated with the extract significant reductions were observed in DHT levels (p<0.001) and EGF levels (p<0.01), whereas T levels were increased (p<0.001) [88].

In an open study 20 patients with BPH received a liposterolic extract (320 mg daily for 30 days). No changes were detected in plasma levels of test-osterone, follicle-stimulating hormone or luteinizing hormone [89].

Clinical studies
In a 6-month randomized, double-blind study the effects of a hexanic extract (320 mg daily) were compared with those of the 5α-reductase inhibitor finasteride (5 mg daily) in 1098 men with moderate BPH using the International Prostate Symptom Score (IPSS) as the primary criterion. At the end of treatment, mean total IPSS had decreased from baseline by 37% among men receiving the extract and by 39% among finasteride recipients, the difference between treatment groups not being statistically significant. Quality of life improved in both the extract and finasteride groups, by 38% and 41% respectively, again with no significant difference between groups. Peak urinary flow rate increased in both groups, by 25% and 30% respectively (p = 0.035 in favour of finasteride), with no statistical difference in the percentage of responders with a 3 ml/sec improvement. The reduction in prostate volume due to finasteride (18%) was significantly greater than that due to the extract (6%) (p<0.001). Serum levels of prostate specific antigen (PSA) dropped

markedly after finasteride (41%), but remained unchanged after the extract (p<0.001). The extract showed an advantage over finasteride in a sexual function questionnaire (p<0.001), giving rise to fewer complaints of decreased libido and impotence [14].

The following double-blind, placebo-controlled studies were performed in BPH patients using a hexanic extract from saw palmetto fruit (320 mg daily). Symptoms such as nocturnal and daytime urinary frequency and dysuria were evaluated together with objective measurements such as urinary flow rate and residual volume

In a 30-day study involving 176 patients (who had previously been unresponsive to the placebo effect), greater improvement in dysuria was seen in the verum group (31.3%) than in the placebo group (16.1%) (p = 0.02). Daytime urinary frequency decreased by 11.3% in the verum group, but was unchanged in the placebo group (p = 0.012). Nocturnal urinary frequency decreased to a greater extent in the verum group (32.5%) than in the placebo group (17.7%) (p = 0.03). The mean peak urinary flow rate increased by 28.9% in the verum group compared to 8.9% in the placebo group (p = 0.04). The global efficacy of the extract was judged to be satisfactory or better in 71.3% of cases by the patients and 56.6% of cases by the physicians; corresponding values for placebo were 67.5% and 47.2%, and the difference between groups was not significant [15].

In a study involving 146 patients, nocturnal urinary frequency had decreased by 33.3% after 30 days of treatment with the extract compared to 14.7% after placebo (p<0.001); corresponding daytime reductions were 19.5% after the extract and 1.3% after placebo (p<0.001). Residual urine volume decreased by 14.7% in the verum group and increased by 53.2% in the placebo group (p<0.05) [16].

Nocturnal urinary frequency decreased by 45.8% after the extract and by 15.0% after placebo (p<0.001) in a 30-day study with 110 patients. Urinary flow rate increased by 50.5% after the extract and by 5.0% after placebo (p<0.001), while residual urine volume decreased by 41.9% after the extract and increased by 9.3% after placebo (p<0.001). Global efficacy for the extract was rated higher than for placebo by both the patients and the physicians (p<0.001) [17].

In another study, 30 patients received the extract or placebo for 30 days. There were greater reductions in nocturnal and daytime urinary frequencies, and a greater increase in peak urinary flow, with the extract than with placebo. The extract diminished dysuria in 92.3% of the patients compared to 33.3% with placebo [18].

Night-time and daytime urinary frequencies decreased

more, and peak urinary flow rate increased more (p<0.05), in the extract group than in the placebo group in a study over 58-69 days involving 27 patients [19].

Treatment of 22 patients for 60 days resulted in increased voiding volume and peak and mean urinary flow rates, and reduced nocturnal urinary frequency and dysuria in the verum group. Other disturbances including duration of voiding, residual urine volume and daytime urinary frequency generally showed improvements but were similar for both groups [20].

When 80 patients were treated for a 12-week period, improvements in urinary flow rate and subjective assessment of symptoms were found in both groups [21].

Open and uncontrolled studies [22-32] conducted in patients with BPH have shown improvements in symptoms such as nocturnal and daytime urinary frequency and dysuria as well as in objective measurements such as urinary flow rate and residual urine volume. A 24-week study, in which 24 patients were treated with 320 mg and 25 patients with 960 mg of extract daily, demonstrated similar efficacy from the two dosage levels with respect to urinary frequency, dysuria, peak urinary flow rate and voiding volume [24].

The following studies were performed in BPH patients using an extract prepared by extraction of saw palmetto fruit with supercritical carbon dioxide

In a double-blind study, 238 patients received the extract (320 mg daily) or placebo for 3 months. Pollakisuria and nocturia decreased by 51% and 67% respectively after the extract and by 32% and 47% after placebo (p<0.05 each); urgency and dysuria improved by 57% and 44% respectively after the extract and by 21% and 19% after placebo (p<0.01 each). Significant improvements were observed in the verum group for urinary volume (p<0.05), total symptom score (day 60, p<0.05; day 90, p<0.01) and quality of life as evaluated by both the patients (p = 0.015 after 1 month; p<0.001 after 2 and 3 months) and the physicians (p = 0.002 after 1 month; p<0.001 after 3 months). Differences between verum and placebo groups were not significant for mean and maximal urinary flow rates or residual urinary volume [90].

In a double-blind, placebo-controlled study, 40 patients with BPH received the extract (320 mg daily) or placebo for 3 months. In the verum group nocturnal and daytime urinary frequencies and residual urine volume, and subjective symptoms such as dysuria, significantly improved (p<0.01 to p<0.05 vs. baseline). No significant changes were observed in prostate size [37].

In a 3-month open study, the efficacy of a saw palmetto fruit extract (320 mg daily) was evaluated in 305 patients. Compared to initial values, the IPSS decreased from 19.0 to 12.4 points and the quality of life score improved in 78% of the patients. The peak urinary flow rate increased, residual urine volume decreased and prostate volume decreased. The treatment did not significantly alter concentrations of serum prostate specific antigen [40].

Two dosage regimens (320 mg once daily or 160 mg twice daily) were compared in an open trial over a 1-year treatment period in 132 patients. Both regimens gave rise to improvements in efficacy parameters: IPSS (60%), quality of life score (85% of patients were satisfied), prostatic volume (12% after 1 year), peak urinary flow rate (22%), mean urinary flow rate (17%) and residual urinary volume (16%). No differences were observed between the two dosage regimens [33].

The following results were obtained in post-marketing surveillance studies (daily dose: 320 mg of extract):

- After treatment of 1965 patients for 6 months IPSS and quality of life scores had improved by about 50%. Peak urinary flow rate increased by 37% and residual urine volume decreased by 48% [34].

- In 1334 patients who were treated for 12 weeks, pollakisuria decreased on average by 37%, nocturia by 54% and residual urine volume by 50%. The percentage of patients with dysuric pain decreased from 75% to 37% [35].

- In 578 patients treated for 12 weeks, urinary flow increased by 46%, residual urine volume decreased by 30% and reductions were observed in nocturnal and daytime urinary frequency [48].

- When 176 patients were treated for 6 months, nocturia decreased by 58%, diuria by 39% and residual urine volume by 61%. The proportion of patients with dysuric pain decreased from 81% to 29% [36].

The following studies were performed with other preparations

In a randomized, double-blind study lasting for 3 weeks, the efficacy of an undefined saw palmetto fruit extract (320 mg daily) was compared with the α_1-receptor antagonist alfuzosin (7.5 mg daily) in 63 patients with BPH. In terms of Boyarsky's total, obstructive and irritative scores, overall symptoms improved in both treatment groups. Alfuzosin produced a greater reduction in the total score (38.8% for alfuzosin and 26.9% for the saw palmetto fruit extract respectively; p = 0.01) and in the obstructive score (37.1% for alfuzosin and 23.1% for the saw palmetto fruit extract; p = 0.01). However, no significant difference was found with respect to irritative symptoms (decrease of 39.8% for alfuzosin and 30.3% for the saw palmetto fruit extract; p = 0.32). Increases in urinary flow rates in alfuzosin-treated patients were not significantly different from those found in patients who received the saw palmetto fruit extract (51.1% and 26.8% respectively for peak urinary flow rate, p = 0.276; 46.5% and 17.7% for mean urinary flow rate, p = 0.207). Both treatments reduced residual urine volume (54.2% for alfuzosin and 30.1% for the saw palmetto fruit extract) [38].

A long-term, open multicentre study was carried out in 435 BPH patients over a period of 3 years using 320 mg of a saw palmetto fruit extract daily. By the end of treatment nocturia had decreased in 73.3% and sensation of incomplete voiding in 75.9% of patients; daytime urinary frequency normalized in 41.6% of patients. An increase in peak flow rate of 45.5% was observed and residual urine volume decreased from 64 ml to 32 ml [39].

In two open studies, 42 patients [41] and 38 patients [91] with BPH were treated with a saw palmetto fruit extract (320 mg daily) for 1 year. In the first study, nocturia decreased in 68.4% of patients, peak urinary flow rate increased from 11.0 to 15.2 ml/s and residual urine volume decreased from 62.8 to 12.3 ml [41]. In the second study, subjective complaints improved by 74%, peak urinary flow rate increased from 10.36 ml to 14.44 ml/s and mean urinary flow rate from 6.02 ml/s to 7.45 ml/s, and the average residual urinary volume decreased by 47 ml [91].

In two further open studies [44,45] involving 109 and 60 patients respectively, 12 weeks of daily treatment with 320 mg of an ethanolic extract from saw palmetto fruit (10-14.3:1, ethanol 90%) led to an increase in peak urinary flow and a decrease in residual urine volume.

In an open study 50 men with previously untreated lower urinary tract symptoms, presumed secondary to BPH, were treated with a preparation of saw palmetto fruit (320 mg daily) for 6 months. The mean IPSS score improved from 19.5 to 12.5 points (p<0.001). No significant changes were observed in peak urinary flow rate, residual urine volume or detrusor pressure at peak flow [47].

The following results were obtained in post-marketing surveillance studies:

In 6967 patients with BPH a decrease in IPSS total score from 18 to 10 points and an improvement in quality of life score from 3.2 to 1.8 points were noted after daily treatment with 320 mg of a lipophilic extract for 6 months [42].

In 1533 patients with BPH, daily treatment with 320 mg of an ethanolic extract for 3 months reduced the IPSS total score from 18.3 points to 10.9 points, improved the quality of life score from 3.51 to 1.9 points, increased peak urinary flow from 12.0 ml/s to 15.7 ml/s and decreased residual urine volume from 60.7 to 36.2 ml [46].

In 630 patients with BPH who received 320 mg of an extract daily for 100 days, nocturia, diuria and sensation of incomplete voiding improved, and peak urinary flow rate and residual urine volume decreased [43].

Pharmacokinetic properties

After oral administration to rats of 10 mg of a hexanic extract from saw palmetto fruit supplemented with ^{14}C-labelled oleic acid, the ratios of radioactivity in tissues compared to plasma showed a greater uptake of radioactivity in the prostate than in other genital organs (i.e. the seminal vesicles) or other organs such as the liver [92].

Plasma concentrations of an unspecified component of a lipophilic extract (retention time 26.4 minutes in a high-performance liquid chromatography assay) were measured using plasma samples taken after single dose oral administration of 320 mg of the extract to 12 healthy young male volunteers in the fasting state. A mean peak plasma concentration of 2.6 µg/ml was achieved 1.5 hours after oral administration; the mean value of the AUC was 8.4 µg h/ml and of the elimination half-life 1.73 hours [93].

Preclinical safety data

The oral LD_{50} of a hexanic extract from saw palmetto fruit was determined as 54 ml/kg in male rats. Oral doses of 10 ml/kg caused no toxic effects in rats. No mortality occurred after oral administration of 50 ml/kg to male mice [81].

REFERENCES

1. Saw Palmetto. United States Pharmacopeia.

2. Sabal - Sabalis serrulatae fructus. Pharmeuropa 2001;13:208-12.

3. Hiermann A, Hübner W, Schulz V. Serenoa. In: Hänsel R, Keller K, Rimpler H, Schneider G, editors. Hagers Handbuch der Pharmazeutischen Praxis, 5th ed. Volume 6: Drogen P-Z. Berlin: Springer-Verlag, 1994:680-7.

4. Hatinguais P, Belle R, Basso Y, Ribet JP, Bauer M,

Pousset JL. Composition de l'extrait hexanique de fruits de *Serenoa repens* Bartram. Trav Soc Pharm Montpellier 1981;41:253-62.

5. Jommi G, Verotta L, Gariboldi P, Gabetta B. Constituents of the lipophilic extract of the fruits of *Serenoa repens* (Bart.) Small. Gazz Chim Ital 1988;118:823-6.

6. Harnischfeger G, Stolze H. *Serenoa repens* - Die Sägezahnpalme. Z Phytother 1989;10:71-6.

7. Hiermann A. Über Inhaltsstoffe von Sabalfrüchten und deren Prüfung auf entzündungshemmende Wirkung. Arch Pharm (Weinheim) 1989;322:111-4.

8. Niederprüm H-J, Schweikert H-U, Zänker KS. Testosterone 5α-reductase inhibition by free fatty acids from Sabal serrulata fruits. Phytomedicine 1994;1:127-33.

9. De Swaef SI, Vlietinck AJ. Simultaneous quantitation of lauric acid and ethyl laureate in *Sabal serrulata* by capillary gas chromatography and derivatisation with trimethyl sulphonium hydroxide. J Chromatogr A 1996; 719:479-82.

10. Schöpflin G, Rimpler H, Hänsel R. β-Sitosterin als möglicher Wirkstoff der Sabalfrüchte. Planta Med 1966;14:402-7.

11. Wajda-Dubos J-P, Farines M, Soulier J, Cousse H. Étude comparative de la fraction lipidique des pulpes et graines de *Serenoa repens* (Palmaceae). Ol Corps Gras Lipides 1996;3:136-9.

12. Bombardelli E, Morazzoni P. *Serenoa repens* (Bartram) J.K. Small. Fitoterapia 1997;68:99-113.

13. Plosker GL, Brogden RN. Serenoa repens (Permixon®). A review of its pharmacology and therapeutic efficacy in benign prostatic hyperplasia. Drugs Aging 1996; 9:379-95.

14. Carraro J-C, Raynaud J-P, Koch G, Chisholm GD, Di Silverio F, Teillac P et al. Comparison of phytotherapy (Permixon®) with finasteride in the treatment of benign prostate hyperplasia: a randomized international study of 1,098 patients. Prostate 1996;29:231-40.

15. Descotes JL, Rambeaud JJ, Deschaseaux P, Faure G. Placebo-controlled evaluation of the efficacy and tolerability of Permixon® in benign prostatic hyperplasia after exclusion of placebo responders. Clin Drug Invest 1995;9:291-7.

16. Cukier, Ducassou, Le Guillou, Leriche, Lobel, Toubol et al. Permixon versus placebo. Résultats d'une étude multicentrique. Comptes Rend Therap Pharmacol Clin 1985;4:15-21.

17. Champault G, Bonnard AM, Cauquil J, Patel JC. Traitement médical de l'adénome prostatique. Essai contrôlé: PA 109 vs placebo chez cent dix patients. Ann Urol 1984;18:407-10.
Also published as:
Champault G, Patel JC, Bonnard AM. A double-blind trial of an extract of the plant *Serenoa repens* in benign prostatic hyperplasia. Br J Clin Pharmacol 1984;18:461-2.

18. Emili E, Lo Cigno M, Petrone U. Risultati clinici su un nuovo farmaco nella terapia dell'ipertrofia della prostata (Permixon). Urologia 1983;50:1042-8.

19. Tasca A, Barulli M, Cavazzana A, Zattoni F, Artibani W, Pagano F. Trattamento della sintomatologia ostruttiva da adenoma prostatico con estratto di Serenoa repens. Studio clinico in doppio cieco vs. placebo. Minerva Urol Nefrol 1985;37:87-91.

20. Boccafoschi C, Annoscia S. Confronto fra estratto di Serenoa repens e placebo mediante prova clinica controllata in pazienti con adenomatosi prostatica. Urologia 1983;50:1257-68.

21. Reece Smith H, Memon A, Smart CJ, Dewbury K. The value of Permixon in benign prostatic hypertrophy. Br J Urol 1986;58:36-40.

22. Authie D, Cauquil J. Appréciation de l'efficacité de Permixon en pratique quotidienne. Étude multicentrique. Comptes Rend Thérapeut 1987;(56):4-13.

23. Cirillo-Marucco E, Pagliarulo A, Tritto G, Piccinno A, Di Rienzo U. L'estratto di Serenoa repens (Permixon®) nel trattamento precoce, dell'ipertrofia prostatica. Urologia 1983;50:1269-77.

24. Dathe G, Schmid H. Phytotherapie der benignen Prostatahyperplasie (BPH) mit Extractum Serenoa repens (Permixon®). Urologe [B] 1991;31:220-3.

25. Mancuso G, Guillot F, Migaleddu V, Satta U. La Serenoa repens nel trattamento medico dell'ipertrofia prostatica benigna. Nostra esperienza. Urologia 1986; 53:709-14.

26. Martorana G, Giberti C, Pizzorno R, Natta GD, Brancadoro MT, Barreca T et al. Studio a lungo termine con estratto di Serenoa repens nei pazienti affetti da adenoma prostatico. Urologia 1986;53:366-9.

27. Olle Carreras J. Nuestra experiencia con extracto hexánico de *Serenoa repens* en el tratamiento de la hipertrofia benigna de próstata. Arch Esp de Urol 1987; 40:310-3.

28. Orfei S, Grumelli B, Galetti G. Valutazione clinica e uroflussimetrica di Permixon® in geriatria. Urologia 1988;55:373-81.

29. Paoletti PP, Francalanci R, Tenti S, Paoletti G, Pedaccini P. Trattamento medico dell'ipertrofia prostatica. Esperienza con l'impiego terapeutico di Serenoa repens. Urologia 1986;53:182-7.

30. Pescatore D, Calvi P, Michelotti P. Valutazione urodinamica del trattamento nei pazienti affetti da adenoma prostatico con estratto di Serenoa repens. Urologia 1986;53:894-7.

31. Proietti G. Impiego dell'estratto lipido-sterolico di Serenoa repens in pazienti affetti da prostatite cronica e prostatite abatterica. Urologia 1986;53:361-5.

32. Vespasiani G, Cesaroni M, Parziani S, Rosi P, Valentini P, Porena M. La Serenoa repens nel trattamento dell'ipertrofia prostatica benigna. Urologia 1987;54:145-9.

33. Braeckman J, Bruhwyler J, Vandekerckhove K, Geczy J. Efficacy and safety of the extract of Serenoa repens in the treatment of benign prostatic hyperplasia: therapeutic equivalence between twice and once daily dosage forms. Phytother Res 1997;11:558-63.

34. Schneider HJ, Uysal A. Internationaler Prostata-Symptomenscore (IPSS) im klinischen Alltag. Urologe [B] 1994;34:443-7.

35. Vahlensieck W, Völp A, Lubos W, Kuntze M. Benigne Prostatahyperplasie - Behandlung mit Sabalfrucht-Extrakt. Eine Anwendungsbeobachtung an 1334 Patienten. Fortschr Med 1993;111:323-6.

36. Fabricius PG, Vahlensieck W. Therapie der benignen Prostatahyperplasie. Sabalfrucht-Extrakt: Einmalgabe reicht! Therapiewoche 1993;43:1616-20.

37. Mattei FM, Capone M, Acconcia A. Impiego dell'estratto di Serenoa repens nel trattamento medico della ipertrofia prostatica benigna. Urologia 1988;55:547-52.
   Also published as:
   Mattei FM, Capone M, Acconcia A. Medikamentöse Therapie der benignen Prostatahyperplasie mit einem Extrakt der Sägepalme. TW Urol Nephrol 1990;2:346-50.

38. Grasso M, Montesano A, Buonaguidi A, Castelli M, Lania C, Rigatti P et al. Comparative effects of alfuzosin versus Serenoa repens in the treatment of symptomatic benign prostatic hyperplasia. Arch Esp de Urol 1995; 48:97-103.

39. Bach D. Medikamentöse Langzeitbehandlung der BPH. Ergebnisse einer prospektiven 3-Jahres-Studie mit dem Sabalextrakt IDS 89. Urologe [B] 1995;35:178-83.

40. Braeckman J. The extract of Serenoa repens in the treatment of benign prostatic hyperplasia: a multicenter open study. Curr Ther Res 1994;55:776-85.

41. Romics I, Schmitz H, Frang D. Experience in treating benign prostatic hypertrophy with Sabal serrulata for one year. Int Urol Nephrol 1993;25:565-9.

42. Eickenberg HU. Behandlung der benignen Prostata-hyperplasie mit einem lipophilen Extrakt aus Sägepalmenfrüchten (Sita). Urologe [B] 1997;37:130-3.

43. Schneider HJ. Benigne Prostata-Hyperplasie. Zwergsägepalme 1 × täglich. Ärztl Prax 1993;45:11-4.

44. Ziegler J, Hölscher U. Wirksamkeit des Spezialextraktes WS 1473 aus Sägepalmenfrüchten bei Patienten mit benigner Prostatahyperplasie im Stadium I-II nach Alken - Offene Multicenterstudie. Jatros Uro 1998;14:34-43.

45. Redecker K-D, Funk P. Sabal-Extrakt WS 1473 bei benigner Prostatahyperplasie. Extracta Urologica 1998;21(3):23-5.

46. Derakhshani P, Geerke H, Böhnert KJ, Engelmann U. Beeinflussung des Internationalen Prostata-Symptomen-Score unter der Therapie mit Sägepalmenfrüchteextrakt bei täglicher Einmalgabe. Urologe [B] 1997;37:384-91.

47. Gerber GS, Zagaja GP, Bales GT, Chodak GW, Contreras BA. Saw Palmetto (Serenoa repens) in men with lower urinary tract symptoms: effects on urodynamic parameters and voiding symptoms. Urology 1998;51:1003-7.

48. Vahlensieck W Jr, Völp A, Kuntze M, Lubos W. Änderung der Miktion bei Patienten mit benigner Prostatahyperplasie unter Sabalfruchtbehandlung. Urologe [B] 1993;33:380-3.

49. Wilt TJ, Ishani A, Stark G, MacDonald R, Lau J, Mulrow C. Saw palmetto extracts for treatment of benign prostatic hyperplasia. A systematic review. JAMA 1998;280: 1604-9.

50. Alken CE. Konservative Behandlung des Prostata-Adenoms und Stadien-Einteilung. Urologe B 1973;13: 95-8.

51. Vahlensieck W, Fabricius PG. Benigne Prostata-hyperplasie (BPH). Therapeutische Möglichkeiten durch medikamentöse Therapie. Therapiewoche 1996;33: 1796-802.

52. Cockett AT, Aso Y, Denis L, Murphy G, Khoury S, Abrams P et al. 1994 Recommendations of the International Consensus Committee concerning: 1. Prostate Symptom Score (I-PSS) and Quality of Life Assessment. 2. Diagnostic work-up of patients presenting with symptoms suggestive of prostatism. 3. Standardization of the evaluation of treatment modalities. 4. BPH treatment recommendations. In: Cockett ATK, Khoury S, Aso Y, Chatelain C, Denis L, Griffiths K, Murphy G, editors. The 2nd International Consultation on Benign Prostatic Hyperplasia (BPH). Paris, June 27-30, 1993: Proceedings 2. Jersey, Channel Islands: Scientific Communication International, 1993:553-64.

53. Sultan C, Terraza A, Devillier C, Carilla E, Briley M, Loire C, Descomps B. Inhibition of androgen metabolism and binding by a liposterolic extract of "Serenoa repens B" in human foreskin fibroblasts. J Steroid Biochem 1984;20:515-9.

54. Düker E-M, Kopanski L, Schweikert H-U. Inhibition of 5α-reductase activity by extracts from Sabal serrulata. In: Abstracts of 37th Annual Congress on Medicinal Plant Research (Society for Medicinal Plant Research). Braunschweig, 5-9 September 1989:5 (Abstract L2-2). Published in: Planta Med 1989;55:587.

55. Breu W, Stadler F, Hagenlocher M, Wagner H. Der Sabalfrucht-Extrakt SG 291. Ein Phytotherapeutikum zur Behandlung der benignen Prostatahyperplasie. Z Phytother 1992;13:107-15.

56. Koch E, Biber A. Pharmakologische Wirkungen von Sabal- und Urtikaextrakten als Grundlage für eine rationale medikamentöse Therapie der benignen Prostatahyperplasie. Urologe [B] 1994;34:90-5.

57. Weisser H, Tunn S, Behnke B, Krieg M. Effects of the Sabal serrulata extract IDS 89 and its subfractions on 5α-reductase activity in human benign prostatic hyperplasia. Prostate 1996;28:300-6.

58. Hagenlocher M, Romalo G, Schweikert HU. Spezifische

Hemmung der 5α-Reduktase durch einen neuen Extrakt aus Sabal serrulata. Akt Urol 1993;24:147-50.

59. Koch E. Pharmakologie und Wirkmechanismen von Extrakten aus Sabalfrüchten (Sabal fructus), Brennesselwurzeln (Urticae radix) und Kürbissamen (Cucurbitae peponis semen) bei der Behandlung der benignen Prostatahyperplasie. In: Loew D, Rietbrock N, editors. Phytopharmaka in Forschung und klinischer Anwendung, Steinkopff, Darmstadt 1995:57-79.

60. Palin M-F, Faguy M, LeHoux J-G, Pelletier G. Inhibitory effects of *Serenoa repens* on the kinetic of pig prostatic microsomal 5α-reductase activity. Endocrine 1998; 9:65-9.

61. Rhodes L, Primka RL, Berman C, Vergult G, Gabriel M, Pierre-Malice M, Gibelin B. Comparison of finasteride (Proscar®), a 5α-reductase inhibitor, and various commercial plant extracts in *in vitro* and *in vivo* 5α-reductase inhibition. Prostate 1993;22:43-51.

62. Iehlé C, Délos S, Guirou O, Tate R, Raynaud J-P, Martin P-M. Human prostatic steroid 5α-reductase isoforms - a comparative study of selective inhibitors. J Steroid Biochem Molec Biol 1995;54:273-9.

63. Délos S, Carsol J-L, Ghazarossian E, Raynaud J-P, Martin P-M. Testosterone metabolism in primary cultures of human prostate epithelial cells and fibroblasts. J Steroid Biochem Molec Biol 1995;55:375-83.

64. Stenger A, Tarayre J-P, Carilla E, Delhon A, Charveron M, Morre M, Lauressergues H. Étude pharmacologique et biochimique de l'extrait hexanique de Serenoa repens B (PA 109). Gaz Méd France 1982;89:2041-8.

65. Carilla E, Briley M, Fauran F, Sultan C. Binding of Permixon, a new treatment for prostatic benign hyperplasia, to the cytosolic androgen receptor in the rat prostate. J Steroid Biochem 1984;20:521-3.

66. Magdy El-Sheikh M, Dakkak MR, Saddique A. The effect of Permixon on androgen receptors. Acta Obstet Gynecol Scand 1988;67:397-9.

67. Ravenna L, Di Silverio F, Russo MA, Salvatori L, Morgante E, Morrone S et al. Effects of the lipidosterolic extract of *Serenoa repens* (Permixon®) on human prostatic cell lines. Prostate 1996;29:219-30.

68. Goepel M, Hecker U, Krege S, Rubben H, Michel MC. Saw palmetto extracts potently and noncompetitively inhibit human α₁-adrenoceptors in vitro. Prostate 1999;38:208-15.

69. Goepel M, Hecker U, Rübben H, Michel MC. Sabalfruchtextrakte enthalten α₁-Adrenozeptor-hemmende Wirkstoffe. Urologe [A] 1998;37(Suppl 1):23 (Abstract P2.13).

70. Paubert-Braquet M, Mencia Huerta J-M, Cousse H, Braquet P. Effect of the lipidic lipidosterolic extract of *Serenoa repens* (Permixon®) on the ionophore A23187-stimulated production of leukotriene B₄ (LTB₄) from human polymorphonuclear neutrophils. Prostagland Leukotr Essent Fatty Acids 1997;57:299-304.

71. Breu W, Hagenlocher M, Redl K, Tittel G, Stadler F, Wagner H. Antiphlogistische Wirkung eines mit hyperkritischem Kohlendioxid gewonnenen Sabalfrucht-Extraktes. In-vitro-Hemmung des Cyclooxygenase- und 5-Lipoxygenase-Metabolismus. Arzneim-Forsch/Drug Res 1992;42:547-51.

72. Gutierrez M, Hidalgo A, Cantabrana B. Possible involvement of calmodulin in the spasmolytic effect of extracts from Sabal serrulata fruits. Pharm Sci 1995;1:403-5.

73. Gutierrez M, García de Boto MJ, Cantabrana B, Hidalgo A. Mechanisms involved in the spasmolytic effect of extracts from Sabal serrulata fruit on smooth muscle. Gen Pharmac 1996;27:171-6.

74. Odenthal KP, Rauwald HW. Kontraktionshemmende Eigenschaften von lipophilem Extrakt aus Sabal serrulata. Akt Urol 1996;27:152-8.

75. Gutiérrez M, Hidalgo A, Cantabrana B. Spasmolytic activity of a lipid extract from *Sabal serrulata* fruits: further study of the mechanisms underlying this activity. Planta Med 1996;62:507-11.

76. Vacher P, Prevarskaya N, Skryma R, Audy MC, Vacher AM, Odessa MF, Dufy B. The lipidosterolic extract from *Serenoa repens* interferes with prolactin receptor signal transduction. J Biomed Sci 1995;2:357-65.

77. Paubert-Braquet M, Cousse H, Raynaud J-P, Mencia-Huerta JM, Braquet P. Effect of the lipidosterolic extract of *Serenoa repens* (Permixon®) and its major components on basic fibroblast growth factor-induced proliferation of cultures of human prostate biopsies. Eur Urol 1998; 33:340-7.

78. Paubert-Braquet M, Richardson FO, Servent-Saez N, Gordon WC, Monge MC, Bazan NG et al. Effect of *Serenoa repens* extract (Permixon®) on estradiol/testosterone-induced experimental prostate enlargement in the rat. Pharmacol Res 1996;34:171-9.

79. Otto U, Wagner B, Becker H, Schröder S, Klosterhalfen H. Transplantation of human benign hyperplastic prostate tissue into nude mice: first results of systemic therapy. Urol Int 1992;48:167-70.

80. Elghamry MI, Hänsel R. Activity and isolated phytoestrogen of shrub palmetto fruits (*Serenoa repens* Small), a new estrogenic plant. Experientia 1969;25:828-9.

81. Tarayre JP, Delhon A, Lauressergues H, Stenger A. Action anti-oedémateuse d'un extrait hexanique de drupes de *Serenoa repens* Bartr. Ann Pharm Fr 1983; 41:559-70.

82. Wagner H, Flachsbarth H. Über ein neues antiphlogistisches Wirkprinzip aus Sabal serrulata I. Planta Med 1981;41:244-51.

83. Wagner H, Flachsbarth H, Vogel G. Über ein neues antiphlogistisches Wirkprinzip aus Sabal serrulata II. Planta Med 1981;41:252-8.

84. Di Silverio F, D'Eramo G, Lubrano C, Flammia GP, Sciarra A, Palma E et al. Evidence that *Serenoa repens* extract displays an antiestrogenic activity in prostatic

tissue of benign prostatic hypertrophy patients. Eur Urol 1992;21:309-14.

85. Weisser H, Behnke B, Helpap B, Bach D, Krieg M. Enzyme activities in tissue of human benign prostatic hyperplasia after three months' treatment with the Sabal serrulata extract IDS 89 (Strogen®) or placebo. Eur Urol 1997;31:97-101.

86. Helpap B, Oehler U, Weisser H, Bach D, Ebeling L. Morphology of benign prostatic hyperplasia after treatment with Sabal extract IDS 89 or placebo. Results of a prospective, randomized, double-blind trial. J Urologic Pathol 1995;3:175-82.

87. Strauch G, Perles P, Vergult G, Gabriel M, Gibelin B, Cummings S et al. Comparison of finasteride (Proscar®) and Serenoa repens (Permixon®) in the inhibition of 5-alpha reductase in healthy male volunteers. Eur Urol 1994;26:247-52.

88. Di Silverio F, Monti S, Sciarra A, Varasano PA, Martini C, Lanzara S et al. Effects of long-term treatment with Serenoa repens (Permixon®) on the concentrations and regional distribution of androgens and epidermal growth factor in benign prostatic hyperplasia. Prostate 1998; 37:77-83.

89. Casarosa C, Cosci o di Coscio M, Fratta M. Lack of effects of a liposterolic extract of Serenoa repens on plasma levels of testosterone, follicle-stimulating hormone and luteinizing hormone. Clin Ther 1988; 10:585-8.

90. Braeckman J, Denis L, de Leval J, Keuppens F, Cornet A, De Bruyne R et al. A double-blind, placebo-controlled study of the plant extract Serenoa repens in the treatment of benign hyperplasia of the prostate. Eur J Clin Res 1997;9:247-59.

91. Kondás J, Philipp V, Diószeghy G. Sabal serrulata extract (Strogen forte) in the treatment of symptomatic benign prostatic hyperplasia. Int Urol Nephrol 1996; 28:767-72.

92. Chevalier G, Benard P, Cousse H, Bengone T. Distribution study of radioactivity in rats after oral administration of the lipido/sterolic extract of Serenoa repens (Permixon®) supplemented with [1-^{14}C]-lauric acid, [1-^{14}C]-oleic acid or [4-^{14}C]-β-sitosterol. Eur J Drug Metab Pharmacokinet 1997;22:73-83.

93. De Bernardi di Valserra M, Tripodi AS, Contos S, Germogli R. Serenoa repens capsules: a bioequivalence study. Acta Toxicol Ther 1994;15:21-39.

SOLIDAGINIS VIRGAUREAE HERBA

European Golden Rod

DEFINITION

European golden rod consists of the dried, flowering aerial parts of *Solidago virgaurea* L.

The material complies with the monograph of the Pharmacopée Française [1] or of the Deutsches Arzneibuch [2].

Fresh material may also be used, provided that when dried it complies with the monograph of one of the above pharmacopoeias.

A draft monograph on European golden rod, intended for inclusion in the European Pharmacopoeia, has been published [3].

CONSTITUENTS

Flavonoids (minimum 1.5%) including astragalin, hyperoside, isoquercitrin, nicotiflorin, quercitrin and rutin [4-7]; triterpene saponins of the oleanane type (up to 2%) derived from virgaureagenin, polygalacic acid and other sapogenins [8-15]; the bisdesmosidic phenol glycosides leiocarposide and virgaureoside A [16-20]; diterpenoid lactones of the *cis*-clerodane type [5,21]; phenolic acids such as caffeic acid and chlorogenic acid [22-24] and small amounts of essential oil [5,25-27].

CLINICAL PARTICULARS

Therapeutic indications
Irrigation of the urinary tract, especially in cases of inflammation and renal gravel, and as an adjuvant in the treatment of bacterial infections of the urinary tract [28-34].

Posology and method of administration

Dosage

Adults: An infusion of 3-4 g of dried herb in 150 ml of water, 2-3 times daily; equivalent preparations [29,31]. *Children*: 1-4 years of age, 1-2 g of dried herb; 4-10 years of age, 2-5 g; 10-16 years of age: 4-8 g [35].

Method of administration
For oral administration.

Duration of administration
No restriction.

E/S/C/O/P
MONOGRAPHS
Second Edition

Contra-indications
European golden rod should not be used in patients with oedema due to impaired heart or kidney function [31].

Special warnings and special precautions for use
None required.

Interaction with other medicaments and other forms of interaction
None reported.

Pregnancy and lactation
No data available. In accordance with general medical practice, the product should not be used during pregnancy and lactation without medical advice.

Effects on ability to drive and use machines
None known.

Undesirable effects
None reported.

Overdose
No toxic effects reported.

PHARMACOLOGICAL PROPERTIES

Pharmacodynamic properties

In vitro experiments

Spasmolytic activity
A 60%-hydroethanolic extract from European golden rod inhibited acetylcholine-induced spasms in isolated guinea pig ileum with 15% of the activity of papaverine [36]. The extract also inhibited acetylcholine-induced spasms in isolated rat bladder [37].

Anti-inflammatory activity
In some *in vitro* models, European golden rod aqueous extracts have exhibited antioxidant characteristics in the sense of reduced production of reactive oxygen species (inhibition of lipid peroxidation, ability to donate hydrogen atoms and to scavenge OH radicals) [38]. A hydroethanolic extract from European golden rod (containing 0.52 mg/ml of rutin, 0.64 mg/ml of flavonoids and 45.6% V/V of ethanol) at concentrations from 0.01 to 5% inhibited biochemical model reactions (including xanthine oxidase, diaphorase in the presence of the auto-oxidizable quinone juglone, lipoxygenase, dihydrofolate reductase), and photodynamic reactions driven by riboflavin or rose bengal, representing inflammatory situations [39-41].

The anti-inflammatory activity is supported by results with 3,5-O-caffeoylquinic acid and the flavonoids from European golden rod, which inhibited the leucocyte elastase [42].

In vivo experiments

Diuretic effects
Significant increases (p<0.01) in diuresis and excretion of sodium, potassium and chloride were demonstrated in rats after oral administration of an aqueous infusion of European golden rod containing 0.3% of flavonoids at 4.64 and 10.0 ml/kg body weight, although the increases in sodium, potassium and chloride were considered due to the electrolyte content of the administered extracts. The increase in volume of urine was more pronounced at the lower dose level [43].

Isolated leiocarposide had a diuretic effect (20% weaker than that of furosemide at 6 mg/kg) after oral or intraperitoneal administration to rats at 25 mg/kg body weight, but did not influence urinary mineral excretion [44-47]. Furthermore, leiocarposide had an inhibitory effect on the growth of human urinary calculi implanted into the rat bladder [46].

Anti-inflammatory effects
Anti-inflammatory and analgesic effects of a hydro-alcoholic extract from European golden rod have been demonstrated in various models of inflammation [48].

A 46%-ethanolic extract from European golden rod, administered orally at 5 ml/kg on days 15-21 after injection of the adjuvant, significantly reduced the intensity of inflammation in Freund's adjuvant-induced arthritis of rat paw; the inhibition was nearly 40% of the control value on day 21 (p<0.05) [49].

Isolated leiocarposide showed anti-inflammatory and analgesic effects after subcutaneous administration to rodents. It inhibited carrageenan-induced rat paw oedema by 20% at 100 mg/kg and 27% at 200 mg/kg (p<0.05) after 5 hours, compared to 54% by phenylbutazone at 50 mg/kg. The analgesic effect of leiocarposide at 200 mg/kg in the hot plate test in mice was similar to that of aminophenazone at 50 mg/kg after 0.5 and 1 hour, but considerably weaker after 2 hours [50].

A mixture of saponins from European golden rod, administered intravenously at 1.25-2.5 mg/kg body weight, had an inhibitory effect on sodium nucleinate-induced rat paw oedema [51].

Other effects
Immunomodulatory and antitumoral effects of triterpenoid saponins from European golden rod have been investigated. Mitogeneic effects on murine spleen and thymus cells, and on human mononuclear cells, were demonstrated *in vitro*. The activity of murine bone marrow macrophages was stimulated in a chemoluminescence assay, and induction of cytotoxic macrophages and TNF-α release from murine

macrophages were observed [52]. The mitogeneic and TNF-α releasing virgaureasaponin E showed *in vivo* antitumoral effects in the allogeneic sarcoma 180 tumour model and in the syngeneic DBA/2-MC.SC-1 fibrosarcoma tumour model. In mice treated with virgaureasaponin E, phagocytosis of bone marrow cells and proliferation of spleen and bone marrow cells were stimulated in an *ex vivo* assay; the TNF-α concentration in blood increased considerably compared to the control group [52,53].

Hypotensive and sedative effects of European golden rod extracts have been demonstrated in rats (180 and 360 mg/kg of a 2% aqueous extract administered intravenously) [54] and in dogs (150 mg/kg of a non-specified extract of the leaves) [55].

Pharmacological studies in humans

In a double-blind, crossover study involving 22 healthy volunteers, a single oral dose of 100 drops of a tincture (65% ethanol) made from fresh plants (0.57 g per g of tincture) produced a 30% rise in the amount of urine compared to placebo [56].

Clinical studies

In an open study in 53 patients suffering from urinary tract inflammation, symptoms disappeared in 70-73% of cases after treatment with a daily dose of 5 ml of an ethanolic extract (HAB) made from fresh plants [56].

In an open, post-marketing study, 745 patients with irritable bladder were treated daily with 3 × 380 mg of a European golden rod dry extract (5.4:1). After 2 weeks of treatment, micturition frequency had decreased and symptom-related responder rates were between 69 and 85% [32].

The efficacy of a dry extract from European golden rod (5.0-7.1:1, ethanol 30% m/m; 3 × 424.8 mg of extract daily for 4 weeks on average) was investigated in another post-marketing study involving a total of 1487 patients, with subgroups for urinary tract infections, irritable bladder and urinary calculi/renal gravel. For patients with recurrent urinary tract infections (n = 555) the extract alone was as effective as when combined with initial antibiotic treatment [33,34]. In patients suffering from chronic or recurrent irritable bladder symptoms (n = 512), even incontinence could be improved or eliminated in 2 out of 3 cases. The subgroup with "urinary calculi/renal gravel" comprised 427 patients (32% of whom had additional urinary tract infections and 11% had additional symptoms of irritable bladder); for the typical symptoms, responder rates of 81% (feeling of pressure in the area of the bladder) to 98% (colics) were determined. Global improvement (CGI-scale) under treatment was evaluated by the physicians as "very much or much better" in 79% of the cases [34].

Case reports on 10 patients treated with the above

extract during ESWL therapy (extracorporeal shock wave lithotripsy) in hospital and during 4-week aftercare indicated a positive spasmolytic effect from treatment with the extract: no colics occurred and additional spasmolytic drugs were unnecessary [34].

Pharmacokinetic properties

Experiments in rats demonstrated that leiocarposide is excreted mostly unchanged in the urine after parenteral administration [57]. *In vitro* experiments showed that microbial breakdown of ester and glycosidic bonds of leiocarposide takes place predominantly in the caecum and the colon of rats [57].

Preclinical safety data

The oral LD_{50} of leiocarposide in rats was determined as 1.55g/kg body weight [44].

Clinical safety data

Two drug monitoring studies showed very good to good tolerability in 97-98% of patients (n = 745 and 1487) during 2-4 weeks of treatment One suspected case of a minor adverse drug reaction (heart burn) was reported [32,33].

A case of allergic contact dermatitis after oral treatment with a European golden rod fluid extract was reported [58].

REFERENCES

1. Solidage - Solidago virga-aurea. Pharmacopée Française.

2. Echtes Goldrutenkraut - Solidaginis virgaureae herba. Deutches Arzneibuch.

3. Golden Rod, European - Solidaginis virgaureae herba. Pharmeuropa 2001;13:104-6.

4. Budzianowski J, Skrzypczak L, Wesolowska M. Flavonoids and leiocarposide in four *Solidago* taxa. Sci Pharm 1990;58:15-23.

5. Hiller K, Bader G. Goldruten-Kraut. Die Gattung *Solidago* - eine pharmazeutische Bewertung. Portrait einer Arzneipflanze. Z Phytotherapie 1996;17:123-30.

6. Bader G. *Solidago*. In: Hänsel R, Keller K, Rimpler H, Schneider G, editors. Hagers Handbuch der Pharmazeutischen Praxis, 5th ed. Volume 6: Drogen P-Z. Berlin: Springer-Verlag, 1994:759-65.

7. Wittig J, Veit M. Analyse der Flavonolglycoside von *Solidago*-Spezies in einem zusammengesetzten Pflanzenextrakt. Drogenreport 1999;12:18-20.

8. Hiller K, Genzel S, Murach M, Franke P. Zur Kenntnis

der Saponine der Gattung *Solidago*. 1. Mitteilung: Über die Saponine von *Solidago virgaurea* L. Pharmazie 1975;30:188-90.

9. Bader G, Grimm A, Hiller K. Quantitative determination of triterpenoid saponins in *Solidago virgaurea*. Planta Med 1991;57 (Suppl. 2):A67-8.

10. Hiller K, Bader G, Reznicek G, Jurenitsch J, Kubelka W. Die Hauptsaponine der arzneilich genutzten Arten der Gattung *Solidago*. Pharmazie 1991;46:405-8.

11. Bader G, Wray V, Hiller K. Virgaureasaponin 3. A 3,28-bisdesmosidic triterpenoid saponin from *Solidago virgaurea*. Phytochemistry 1992;31:621-3.

12. Inose Y, Miyase T, Ueno A. Studies on the constituents of *Solidago virga-aurea* L. I. Structural elucidation of saponins in the herb. Chem Pharm Bull 1991;39:2037-42.

13. Inose Y, Miyase T, Ueno A. Studies on the constituents of *Solidago virga-aurea* L. II. Structures of Solidago-saponins X-XX. Chem Pharm Bull 1992;40:946-53.

14. Miyase T, Inose Y, Ueno A. Studies on the constituents of *Solidago virga-aurea* L. III. Structures of Solidago-saponins XXI-XXIX. Chem Pharm Bull 1994;42:617-24.

15. Bader G, Wray V, Hiller K. The main saponins from the aerial parts and the roots of *Solidago virgaurea* subsp. *virgaurea*. Planta Med 1995;61:158-61.

16. Hiller K, Gil-Rjong R, Franke P, Gründemann E. Über die Saponine der Gattung *Solidago virgaurea* L. *var. leiocarpa* (Benth.) A. Gray. 3. Mitteilung: Zur Kenntnis der Saponine der Gattung *Solidago*. Pharmazie 1979; 34:360-1.

17. Hiller K, Dube G, Zeigan D. Virgaureosid A - ein neues, bisdesmosidisches Phenolglycosid aus *Solidago virgaurea* L. Pharmazie 1985;40;795-6.

18. Hiller K, Fötsch G. Zur quantitativen Verteilung der Phenolglykoside Virgaureosid A und Leiocarposid in *Solidago virgaurea* L. Pharmazie 1986;41:415-6.

19. Bader G, Janka M, Hannig H-J, Hiller K. Zur quantitativen Bestimmung von Leiocarposid in *Solidago virgaurea* L. Pharmazie 1990;45:380-1.

20. Fötsch G, Gründemann E, Pfeifer S, Hiller K, Salzwedel D. Zur Struktur von Leiocarposid. Pharmazie 1988; 43:278-80.

21. Goswami A, Barua RN, Sharma RP, Baruah JN, Kulanthaivel P, Herz W. Clerodanes from *Solidago virgaurea*. Phytochemistry 1984;23:837-41.

22. Kalemba D. Phenolic acids in four *Solidago* species. Pharmazie 1992;47:471-2.

23. Poetsch F, Pauli GF, Nahrstedt A. Specific access to the structures of quinic acid diesters - an example from *Solidago* spec. In: Abstracts of 45th Ann Congr Soc Med Plant Res, 1997:C22.

24. Poetsch F. Kaffeesäure-Derivate in *Solidago*-Arten. Drogenreport 1999;12:15-8.

25. Bader G. Wirksamkeitsmitbestimmende Inhaltsstoffgruppen der Gattung Solidago. Drogenreport 1999; 12:13-5.

26. Fujita S. On the components of the essential oils of *Solidago virgaurea* Linn. ssp. (Miscellaneous contributions to the essential oils of plants from various territories. Part 52). Nippon Nogeikagaku Kaishi 64:1729-33; through Chem. Abstr. 1990;114:98252.

27. Bornschein U. Pharmakognostische, phytochemische und biosynthetische Untersuchungen über *Solidago virgaurea, Solidago gigantea* und *Solidago canadensis* [Dissertation]. University of Berlin, 1987.

28. Schilcher H. In: Loew D, Heimsoth V, Kuntz E, Schilcher H, editors. Diuretika: Chemie, Pharmakologie und Therapie einschließlich Phytotherapie, 2nd ed. Stuttgart-New York: Thieme, 1990:270-2.

29. Weiß RF, Fintelmann V. In: Lehrbuch der Phytotherapie. 9th ed. Stuttgart: Hippokrates, 1999.

30. Schilcher H. In: Phytotherapie in der Urologie. Stuttgart:Hippokrates, 1992:11-8,24-5,57-8,97-101.

31. Schilcher H, Kammerer S. In: Leitfaden Phytotherapie. München-Jena:Urban & Fischer, 2000:97-8,633-5,648-9,660-2,664-7.

32. Schmitt M. Echte Goldrute normalisiert die Reizblase. Effective und nebenwirkungsarme Behandlung abakterieller Cystitiden. TW Urol Nephrol 1996;8:133-5.

33. Laszig R. Goldrutenkraut bei chronischen/rezidivierenden Harnwegsinfekten. Jatros Uro 1999;15:39-43.

34. Laszig R, Smiszek R, Stammwitz U, Henneicke-von Zepelin H-H, Akçetin Z. Klinische Anwendungsbeobachtungen zur Wirksamkeit und Sicherheit bei Monographie-konformem Einsatz eines Goldrutenextrakt-Präparates. Drogenreport 1999;12:38-40.

35. Dorsch W, Loew D, Meyer-Buchtela E, Schilcher H. Solidaginis virgaureae herba (Goldrutenkraut). In: Kinderdosierungen von Phytopharmaka. Teil I: Empfehlungen zur Anwendung und Dosierung von Phytopharmaka, monographierten Arzneidrogen und ihren Zubereitungen in der Pädiatrie, 2nd ed. Bonn: Kooperation Phytopharmaka, 1998:129.

36. Westendorf J, Vahlensieck W. Spasmolytische und kontraktile Einflüsse eines pflanzlichen Kombinationspräparates auf die glatte Muskulatur des isolierten Meerschweinchendarms. Arzneim-Forsch/Drug Res 1981;31:40-3.

37. Westendorf J, Vahlensieck W. Spasmolytische Einflüsse des pflanzlichen Kombinationspräparates Urol® auf die isolierte Rattenharnblase. Therapiewoche 1983;33: 936-44.

38. Filípek J. Antioxidative properties of *Alchemilla xanthochlora, Salvia officinalis* and *Solidago virgaurea* water extracts. Biologia (Bratislava) 1994;49:359-64.

39. Meyer B, Elstner EF. Antioxidative properties of leaf extracts from *Populus*, *Fraxinus* and *Solidago* as components of the anti-inflammatory plant drug "Phytodolor®". Planta Med 1990;56:666.

40. Meyer B, Schneider W, Elstner EF. Antioxidative properties of alcoholic extracts from *Fraxinus excelsior*, *Populus tremula* and *Solidago virgaurea*. Arzneim-Forsch/Drug Res 1995;45:174-6.

41. Strehl E, Schneider W, Elstner EF. Inhibition of dihydrofolate reductase activity by alcoholic extracts from *Fraxinus excelsior*, *Populus tremula* and *Solidago virgaurea*. Arzneim-Forsch/Drug Res 1995;45:172-3.

42. Melzig MF, Löser B, Bader G, Papsdorf G. Echtes Goldrutenkraut als entzündungshemmende Droge. Molekularpharmakologische Untersuchungen zur entzündungshemmenden Wirksamkeit von *Solidago-virgaurea*-Zubereitungen. Z Phytotherapie 2000;21:67-70.

43. Schilcher H, Rau H. Nachweis der aquaretischen Wirkung von Birkenblätter- und Goldrutenkraut-auszügen im Tierversuch. Urologe B 1988;28:274-80.

44. Chodera A, Dabrowska K, Senczuk M, Wasik-Olejnik A, Skrzypczak L, Budzianowski J, Ellnain-Wojtaszek M. [Studies on the diuretic action of the glucoside ester from the *Solidago* L. genus]. Acta Polon Pharm 1985;42:199-204.

45. Chodera A, Dabrowska K, Skrzypczak L, Budzianowski J. [Further studies on diuretic activity of leiocarposide]. Acta Polon Pharm 1986;43:499-503.

46. Chodera A, Dabrowska K, Bobkiewicz-Kozlowska T, Tkaczyk J, Skrzypczak L, Budzianowski J. [Effect of leiocarposide on experimental urolithiasis in rats]. Acta Polon Pharm 1988;45:181-6.

47. Budzianowski J. Die urologische Wirkung des Leiocarposids. Drogenreport 1999;12:20-1.

48. Okpanyi SN, Schirpke-von Paczensky R, Dickson D. Antiphlogistische, analgetische und antipyretische Wirkung unterschiedlicher Pflanzenextrakte und deren Kombination im Tiermodell. Arzneim-Forsch/Drug Res 1989;39:698-703.

49. El-Ghazaly M, Khayyal MT, Okpanyi SN, Arens-Corell M. Study of the anti-inflammatory activity of *Populus tremula*, *Solidago virgaurea* and *Fraxinus excelsior*. Arzneim-Forsch/Drug Res 1992;42:333-6.

50. Metzner J, Hirschelmann R, Hiller K. Antiphlogistische und analgetische Wirkungen von Leiocarposid, einem phenolischen Bisglucosid aus *Solidago virgaurea* L. Pharmazie 1984;39:869-70.

51. Jacker H-J, Voigt G, Hiller K. Zum antiexsudativen Verhalten einiger Triterpensaponine. Pharmazie 1982;37:380-2.

52. Plohmann B, Bader G, Hiller K, Franz G. Immuno-modulatory and antitumoral effects of triterpenoid saponins. Pharmazie 1997;52:953-7.

53. Plohmann B, Franz G, Bader G, Hiller K. Immuno-modulatorische und antitumorale Aktivität von Triterpensaponinen aus *Solidago virgaurea* L. Drogenreport 1999;12:29-30.

54. Lasserre B, Kaiser R, Huu Chanh P, Ifansyah N, Gleye J, Moulis C. Effects on rats of aqueous extracts of plants used in folk medicine as antihypertensive agents. Naturwissenschaften 1983;70:95-6.

55. Racz-Kotilla E, Racz G. Hypotensive and sedative effect of extracts obtained from *Solidago virgaurea* L. (Abstract 1977). *Published as*: Racz-Kotilla E, Mayer M, Racz G. Actiunea hipotensiva si sedativa a extractelar de *Solidago virgaurea* L. Proc Acad Sc Bucuresti, Note Botanice 1977;13:1-5.

56. Brühwiler K, Frater-Schröder M, Kalbermatten R, Tobler M. Research project on *Solidago virgaurea* tincture. In: Abstracts of 4th and International Congress on Phytotherapy. Munich, 10-13 September 1992 (Abstract SL 20).

57. Fötsch G, Pfeifer S. Die Biotransformation der Phenolglycoside Leiocarposid und Salicin - Beispiele für Besonderheiten von Absorption und Metabolismus glycosidischer Verbindungen. Pharmazie 1989;44:710-2.

58. Schätzle M, Agathos M, Breit R. Allergic contact dermatitis from goldenrod (Herba Solidaginis) after systemic administration. Contact Dermatitis 1998;39:271-2.

TANACETI PARTHENII HERBA

Feverfew

E/S/C/O/P
MONOGRAPHS
Second Edition

DEFINITION

Feverfew consists of the dried, whole or fragmented aerial parts of *Tanacetum parthenium* (L.) Schultz Bip. It contains not less than 0.20 per cent of parthenolide ($C_{15}H_{20}O_3$; M_r 248.3), calculated with reference to the dried drug.

The material complies with the monograph of the European Pharmacopoeia [1].

Fresh material may also be used provided that, when dried, it complies with the monograph of the European Pharmacopoeia.

CONSTITUENTS

The characteristic constituents are sesquiterpene lactones with an α-methylenebutyrolactone structure [2-4] of which parthenolide [2-7], a germacranolide, is the major component [8-10]. The others, which occur in significantly smaller amounts, are mainly guaianolides including canin, 10-*epi*-canin, tanaparthin-α- and -β-peroxides, artecanin and 8-hydroxyestafiatin [2,3].

Other constituents include monoterpenes, principally camphor and trans-chrysanthenyl acetate; poly-acetylene compounds (spiroketal enol ethers) [2,11-13]; lipophilic flavonoids such as 6-hydroxy-kaempferol-3,6-dimethylether, 6-hydroxykaempferol-3,6,4′-trimethylether (=santin), quercetagenin-3,6,3′-trimethylether and quercetagenin-3,6,4′-trimethyl-ether; and hydrophilic flavonoids, principally apigenin-7-glucuronide and luteolin-7-glucuronide [14].

CLINICAL PARTICULARS

Therapeutic indications
Prophylaxis of migraine [15-23].

Posology and method of administration

Dosage
Adult daily dose: 50-120 mg of powdered feverfew [18,19,22,23]; equivalent preparations.

Method of administration
For oral administration.

Duration of administration
Treatment for at least a few months is recommended

[19]. From time to time a pause in treatment is advisable with gradual reduction of dosage during the preceding month.

Contra-indications
Hypersensitivity to feverfew or other members of the Compositae [24].

Special warnings and special precautions for use
None required.

Interactions with other medicaments and other forms of interaction
None reported.
No adverse side effects were noted in a large number of individuals taking feverfew together with other medications [15,16].

Pregnancy and lactation
No data available.
In accordance with general medical practice, the product should not be used during pregnancy and lactation without medical advice.

Effects on ability to drive and use machines
None known.

Undesirable effects
In rare cases, allergic contact dermatitis [24-31], mouth ulceration or tongue irritation and inflammation [15,16,22,24,32] may occur. Cases of abdominal pain and indigestion in patients who have taken feverfew for long periods have been reported [15,19,22,32,33]. Rare cases of diarrhoea, flatulence, nausea or vomiting have been noted [22,24].

In two clinical studies the incidence of adverse effects was higher in the placebo groups than in the verum groups [18,19].

Overdose
No toxic effects reported.

PHARMACOLOGICAL PROPERTIES

Pharmacodynamic properties

In vitro experiments
Much of the biological activity of parthenolide (and the other sesquiterpene lactones) can be explained by the presence of the α-methylenebutyrolactone functional group and its possible interaction with biologically active thiol (sulphydryl) groups [16,34-40].

There is no firmly established link between the constituents of feverfew and its migraine prophylactic properties. However, many experimental observations, mainly *in vitro*, suggest such a link. Most of these results have been obtained using crude plant extracts although some have been obtained using pure parthenolide or other sesquiterpene lactones from feverfew [37-39].

Anti-inflammatory effects
Feverfew extracts or pure parthenolide inhibit the production of prostaglandins, which are mediators of inflammation [16]. Sesquiterpene lactones having an α-methylenebutyrolactone group are known to have anti-inflammatory activity [41]. Feverfew extracts have been shown to inhibit prostaglandin biosynthesis in bovine seminal vesicular mitochondrial fraction, probably by interfering with the action of phospholipase A_2 at the beginning of the arachidonic acid cascade rather than at the cyclo-oxygenase step [36,42-44].

Feverfew extracts inhibited thromboxane B_2 and leukotriene B_4 production in leukocytes indicating that they are presumably inhibitors of both 5-lipoxygenase and cyclo-oxygenase [36,45].

An acetone extract of feverfew inhibited phorbol myristate acetate-induced chemiluminescence of human polymorphonuclear leucocytes with an IC_{50} of 0.79 mg of leaf dry weight per ml of whole blood [46].

Parthenolide dose-dependently suppressed inducible nitric oxide synthase (iNOS) promoter activity from 2.5 μM with an IC_{50} of 10μM, thus reducing the formation of NO radicals. The TPA-induced increase in iNOS promoter activity was also suppressed with an IC_{50} of 2 μM [47].

A 70% ethanolic extract of feverfew (1:80) and parthenolide (2 μg/ml) inhibited the expression of intercellular adhesion molecule-1 induced by cytokines IL-1 (up to 95% suppression), TNF-α (up to 93% suppression) and interferon-γ (up to 39% suppression) [48].

Parthenolide was shown to bind to IκB kinase β, the kinase subunit that plays an important role in cytokine-mediated signalling. A biotinylated parthenolide derivative directly inhibited IκB kinase β [40].

Pretreatment of A549 cells with parthenolide inhibited TNF-α mediated interleukin-8 (IL-8) gene expression (p<0.05), activation of the IL-8 promoter (p<0.05), translocation of NF-κB and degradation of the NF-κB inhibitory protein [49].

In rat peritoneal leucocytes, 6-hydroxykaempferol-3,6-dimethylether and santin inhibited cyclooxygenase (CO) (IC_{50} values of 182 and 27 μM respectively) and 5-lipoxygenase (5-LO) (IC_{50} values of 182 and 58 μM respectively) in the same way. In contrast, quercetagenin-3,6,3'-trimethylether showed preferential activity against CO with IC_{50} values of 22µM for CO and 167 µM for 5-LO [14].

Serotonergic effects

Feverfew extracts inhibit the secretion of serotonin (5-HT) from blood platelets and also prevent aggregation in response to external chemical stimuli [37,50,51]; it is unclear whether phospholipase A_2 inhibition is involved in these processes [16,38]. The effects on platelets are probably due to the Michael addition mechanism since prior addition of a thiol to the extracts or pure parthenolide removes this bioactivity [16,39].

Parthenolide displaced [³H] ketanserin from 5-HT_{2A} receptors from rat and rabbit brain and from cloned 5-HT_{2A} receptors [52].

Parthenolide did not show agonistic or antagonistic effects towards serotonin in isolated rat stomach fundus at concentrations from 1 to 10 µM. However, parthenolide non-competitively antagonised the effects of fenfluramine and dextroamphetamine, two indirect acting serotonergics, at a concentration of 10 µM [53].

Similar results were obtained in another study. Furthermore it was shown that in contrast to parthenolide, a dichloromethane extract of feverfew blocked 5-HT_{2A} and 5-HT_{2B} receptors and neuronally released serotonin at a concentration of 10 µM [54].

Other effects

Parthenolide also interferes markedly with both contractile and relaxant mechanisms in blood vessels, almost certainly due to the presence of the α-methylenebutyrolactone functional group; when this is blocked, these activities are lost [34,35].

Various sesquiterpene lactones with an α-methylene-butyrolactone group, including parthenolide, have been shown to be cytotoxic towards several human tumour cell lines [55,56]. Parthenolide inhibits the incorporation of thymidine into DNA and thus the cytotoxic activity may occur at the DNA replication level [57,58]. Parthenolide inhibited cell growth irreversibly after 24 hours of exposure time at concentrations above 5 µM in mouse fibrosarcoma and human lymphoma cell lines. However, at lower concentrations parthenolide had a cytostatic effect and approx. 85% of the cells were able to proliferate after removal of parthenolide [59].

The lactones and an ethanolic extract exhibited antimicrobial activity, inhibiting the growth of Gram-positive (but not Gram-negative) bacteria, yeasts and filamentous fungi [60,61]. The essential oil was bactericidal and fungicidal against mainly Gram-negative bacteria, yeasts and fungi [62].

In vivo experiments

Anti-inflammatory activity

Significant inhibition of collagen-induced broncho-constriction in guinea pigs (p<0.01), observed after intravenous administration of 1 ml of a feverfew extract (prepared by homogenising 1 g of chopped fresh leaf in 2.5 ml distilled water), was interpreted as inhibition of phospholipase A_2 activity [63]. Similarly, inhibition of prostanoid biosynthesis was suggested as the mechanism by which parthenolide inhibited experimentally-induced nephrocalcinosis in rats [16].

An extract of feverfew administered orally at 10-40 mg/kg body weight and parthenolide administered intraperitoneally at 1-2 mg/kg led to significant antinociceptive (p<0.05 to p<0.001) and anti-inflammatory (p<0.05) effects against acetic acid-induced writhing in mice and carrageenan-induced paw oedema in rats respectively. Naloxone failed to reverse the induced antinociception. Higher doses of the extract (up to 60 mg/kg orally) did not alter locomotor activity, potentiate pentobarbital-induced sleep time or change rectal temperature in rats [64].

Parthenolide decreased phorbol myristate acetate-induced contact sensitivity in the murine ear oedema model of inflammation (0.5 mg/ear). However, chemically reduced parthenolide (i.e. without the exocyclic methylene moiety) showed no activity in this test, demonstrating that the exocyclic methylene is required for anti-inflammatory activity [40].

Anti-ulcerogenic activity

Gastric ulcers induced by oral administration of absolute ethanol to rats were dose-dependently reduced after oral pre-treatment with a chloroform extract of feverfew (2.5-80 mg/kg) or parthenolide (5-40 mg/kg). The level of protection ranged between 34 and 100% with the extract and 27 and 100% with parthenolide. The mean ulcer index was reduced from 4.8 (control) to 1.4 (extract 40 mg/kg) and 0.5 (parthenolide 40 mg/kg) [65].

Pharmacological studies in humans

Platelet aggregation responses in 10 patients taking feverfew for from 3.5 to 8 years were indistinguishable from those of a control group of 4 patients who had stopped taking feverfew at least 6 months previously [16,66].

Clinical studies

A systematic review of six randomized, double-blind, placebo-controlled clinical studies [18,19,23,67-69] of feverfew mono-preparations in the prevention of migraine concluded that feverfew is likely to be effective in the prevention of migraine [22].

In a randomized, double-blind, placebo-controlled study, an oral dose of 2 × 25 mg of dried feverfew leaf was administered daily for 6 months to 8 migraine patients, while 9 other patients took placebo. All patients had previously treated themselves daily with raw feverfew leaf for 3-4 years, with substantial alleviation of symptoms. The mean frequency of headaches in the verum group was 1.69 per month during the 6 months and 1.5 per month during the final 3 months, compared with 3.13 and 3.43 respectively in the placebo group (p<0.02). Nausea or vomiting, or both, occurred on only 39 occasions in the verum group compared with 116 occasions in the placebo group (p<0.05) [18].

In a randomized, double-blind, placebo-controlled, crossover study in 59 migraine patients, after a 1-month run-in period on placebo (dried cabbage leaf) each patient received feverfew for 4 months then placebo for 4 months (or vice versa). The verum groups received one capsule daily containing 70-114 mg of dried feverfew leaf, equivalent to 0.545 mg of parthenolide. There was a 24% reduction in the number of migraine attacks (p<0.005) during feverfew treatment compared with the placebo phase and, although no significant change in the duration of individual attacks, a significant reduction (p<0.002) in nausea and vomiting during attacks. Global assessments also showed that feverfew was significantly superior to placebo (p<0.01) [19].

In another crossover study 57 migraine patients were treated in 3 phases. In the first phase (open) all patients received 100 mg of powdered feverfew leaf per day for 2 months. In the second and third phases, with a randomized, double-blind, crossover design, the patients received feverfew (same dosage) or placebo consecutively, each for an additional month. Compared to placebo treatment, feverfew caused a significant reduction in pain intensity (p<0.01) and in the severity of typical symptoms such as nausea, vomiting, sensitivity to light (all p<0.001) and sensitivity to noise (p<0.03) [23].

In a randomized, double-blind, placebo-controlled, crossover study, 50 migraine patients received placebo daily for 1 month. Over the following 4 months the patients received 1 capsule daily containing a 90% ethanolic extract of feverfew standardized to 0.5 mg of parthenolide and subsequently placebo for 4 months (or vice versa). No significant prophylactic effect could be demonstrated for the feverfew preparation, but the patients tended to use less of other medications [67].

Prophylactic effects of feverfew have also been claimed with regard to various forms of arthritis [15-17,21,24]. However, a double-blind, placebo-controlled, 6-week study, involving 40 female patients with rheumatoid arthritis receiving either 70-86 mg of dried leaf per day or placebo, showed no beneficial effects [70].

Pharmacokinetic properties
No data available.

Preclinical safety data
No data available.

Clinical safety data
A systematic review of 6 clinical studies using feverfew mono-preparations for the prevention of migraine led to the conclusion that there are no major safety problems [22].

Comparisons have been made between 30 female migraine patients who had taken feverfew daily (12.5-250 mg) for more than 11 consecutive months and a matched control group of 30 female migraine patients who had not used feverfew. No statistically significant difference in the mean frequency of chromosomal aberrations and sister chromatid exchanges in lymphocytes were observed over a period of several months. Urine from feverfew-using migraine patients did not induce a significant increase in the mean number of revertants in the Ames mutagenicity assay, with or without metabolic activation, in comparison with urine from matched non-user migraine patients [71,72].

REFERENCES

1. Feverfew - Tanaceti parthenii herba. European Pharmacopoeia, Council of Europe.

2. Bohlmann F, Zdero C. Sesquiterpene lactones and other constituents from *Tanacetum parthenium*. Phytochemistry 1982;21:2543-9.

3. Begley MJ, Hewlett MJ, Knight DW. Revised structures for guaianolide α-methylenebutyrolactones from feverfew. Phytochemistry 1989;28:940-3.

4. Fischer NH, Olivier EJ, Fischer HD. The biogenesis and chemistry of sesquiterpene lactones. Fortschr Chem Org Naturst 1979;38:47-390.

5. Soucek M, Herout V, Sorm F. Constitution of parthenolide. Collect Czech Chem Commun 1961;26:803-10.

6. Govindachari TR, Joshi BS, Kamat VN. Structure of parthenolide. Tetrahedron 1965;21:1509-19.

7. Quick A, Rogers D. Crystal and molecular structure of parthenolide [4,5-epoxygermacra-1(10),11(13)-dien-12,6-olactone]. J Chem Soc Perkin Trans 2 1976;465-9.

8. Groenewegen WA, Heptinstall S. Amounts of feverfew in commercial preparations of the herb. Lancet 1986;i:44-5.

9. Heptinstall S, Awang DVC, Dawson BA, Kindack D,

Knight DW, May J. Parthenolide content and bioactivity of feverfew (*Tanacetum parthenium* (L.) Schultz-Bip.). Estimation of commercial and authenticated feverfew products. J Pharm Pharmacol 1992;44:391-5.

10. Dolman DM, Knight DW, Salan U, Toplis D. A quantitative method for the estimation of parthenolide and other sesquiterpene lactones containing α-methylene-butyrolactone functions present in feverfew, *Tanacetum parthenium*. Phytochem Anal 1992;3:26-31.

11. Bohlmann F, Arndt C, Bornowski H, Kleine KM, Herbst P. Neue Acetylenverbindungen aus *Chrysanthemum*-Arten. Chem Ber 1964;97:1179-92.

12. Bohlmann F, von Kap-Herr W, Fanghänel L, Arndt C. Über einige neue Inhaltsstoffe aus dem Tribus *Anthemidae*. Chem Ber 1965;98:1411-5.

13. Knight DW. Feverfew: Chemistry and biological activity. Nat Prod Rep 1995;12:271-6.

14. Williams CA, Harborne JB, Geiger H, Hoult JRS. The flavonoids of *Tanacetum parthenium* and *T. vulgare* and their anti-inflammatory properties. Phytochemistry 1999;51:417-23.

15. Johnson S. Feverfew. A traditional herbal remedy for migraine and arthritis. London: Sheldon Press, 1984.

16. Groenewegen WA, Knight DW, Heptinstall, S. Progress in the medicinal chemistry of the herb feverfew. In: Ellis GP, Luscombe DK, editors. Progress in Medicinal Chemistry, Volume 29. Amsterdam: Elsevier, 1992:217-38.

17. Hancock K. Feverfew. Your headache may be over. New Canaan CT: Keats Publishing, 1986.

18. Johnson ES, Kadam NP, Hylands DM, Hylands PJ. Efficacy of feverfew as prophylactic treatment of migraine. Brit Med J 1985;291:569-73.

19. Murphy JJ, Heptinstall S, Mitchell JRA. Randomised double-blind placebo-controlled trial of feverfew in migraine prevention. Lancet 1988;ii:189-92.

20. Heptinstall S. Feverfew - an ancient remedy for modern times ? J Royal Soc Med 1988;81:373-4.

21. Berry MI. Feverfew faces the future. Pharm J 1984; 232:611-4.

22. Ernst E, Pittler MH. The efficacy and safety of feverfew (*Tanacetum parthenium* L.): an update of a systematic review. Public Health Nutr 2000;3(4A):509-14.

23. Palevitch D, Earon G, Carasso R. Feverfew (*Tanacetum parthenium*) as a prophylactic treatment for migraine: a double-blind placebo-controlled study. Phytotherapy Res 1997;11:508-11.

24. Hausen BM. Sesquiterpene lactones - *Tanacetum parthenium*. In: De Smet PAGM, Keller K, Hänsel R, Chandler RF, editors. Adverse Effects of Herbal Drugs, Volume 1. Berlin: Springer-Verlag, 1992:255-60.

25. Mitchell JC, Geissman TA, Dupuis G, Towers GHN.

Allergic contact dermatitis caused by *Artemisia* and *Chrysanthemum* species. J Invest Derm 1971;56:98-101.

26. Guin JD, Skidmore G. Compositae dermatitis in childhood. Arch Dermatol 1987;123:500-2.

27. Senff H, Kuhlwein A, Hausen BM. Aerogene Kontaktdermatitis. Akt Dermatol 1986;12:153-4.

28. Hausen BM, Osmundsen PE. Contact allergy to parthenolide in *Tanacetum parthenium* (L.) Schultz-Bip.(feverfew, Asteraceae) and cross-reactions to related sesquiterpene lactone containing Compositae species. Acta Derm Venereol (Stockh) 1983;63:308-14.

29. Fernandez de Corres L. Contact dermatitis from *Frullania*, Compositae and other plants. Contact Derm 1984;11:74-9.

30. Mattes H, Hamada K, Benezra C. Stereospecificity in allergic contact dermatitis to simple substituted methylenelactone derivatives. J Med Chem 1987; 30:1948-51.

31. Talaga P, Schaeffer M, Mattes H, Benezra C, Stampf J-L. Synthesis of Boc-Cys-Ala-OMe and its stereoselective addition to α-methylene-γ-butyrolactones. Tetrahedron 1989;45:5029-38.

32. Turner P. Adverse reactions to drugs in migraine: some recent reports. Hum Toxicol 1985;4:475-6.

33. Baldwin CA, Anderson LA, Phillipson JD. What pharmacists should know about feverfew. Pharm J 1987;239:237-8.

34. Barsby RWJ, Salan U, Knight DW, Hoult JRS. Feverfew extracts and parthenolide irreversibly inhibit vascular responses of the rabbit aorta. J Pharm Pharmacol 1992; 44:737-40.

35. Barsby RWJ, Salan U, Knight DW, Hoult JRS. Feverfew and vascular smooth muscle: extracts from fresh and dried plants show opposing pharmacological profiles, dependent upon sesquiterpene lactone content. Planta Med 1993;59:20-5.

36. Sumner H, Salan U, Knight DW, Hoult JRS. Inhibition of 5-lipoxygenase and cyclo-oxygenase in leukocytes by feverfew. Biochem Pharmacol 1992;43:2313-20.

37. Groenewegen WA, Knight DW, Heptinstall S. Compounds extracted from feverfew that have anti-secretory activity contain an α-methylene butyrolactone unit. J Pharm Pharmacol 1986;38:709-12.

38. Heptinstall S, Groenewegen WA, Knight DW, Spangenberg P, Loesche W. Studies on feverfew and its mode of action. In: Rose FC, editor. Advances in headache research. London: John Libbey, 1987:129-34.

39. Heptinstall S, Groenewegen WA, Spangenberg P, Loesche W. Extracts of feverfew may inhibit platelet behaviour via neutralization of sulphydryl groups. J Pharm Pharmacol 1987;39:459-65.

40. Kwok BHB, Koh B, Ndubuisi MI, Elofsson M, Crews

CM. The anti-inflammatory natural product parthenolide from the medicinal herb feverfew directly binds to and inhibits IκB kinase. Chemistry & Biology 2001;8:759-66.

41. Hall IH, Lee KH, Starnes CO, Sumida Y, Wu RY, Waddell TG et al. Anti-inflammatory activity of sesquiterpene lactones and related compounds. J Pharm Sci 1979;68:537-42.

42. Collier HOJ, Butt NM, McDonald-Gibson WJ, Saeed SA. Extract of feverfew inhibits prostaglandin biosynthesis. Lancet 1980;ii:922-3.

43. Pugh WJ, Sambo K. Prostaglandin synthetase inhibitors in feverfew. J Pharm Pharmacol 1988;40:743-5.

44. Thakkar JK, Sperelakis N, Pang D, Franson RC. Characterization of phospholipase A_2 activity in rat aorta smooth muscle cells. Biochim Biophys Acta 1983;750:134-40.

45. Capasso F. The effect of an aqueous extract of Tanacetum parthenium L. on arachidonic acid metabolism by rat peritoneal leucocytes. J Pharm Pharmacol 1986;38:71-2.

46. Brown AMG, Edwards CM, Davey MR, Power JB, Lowe KC. Effects of extracts of Tanacetum species on human polymorphonuclear leucocyte activity in vitro. Phytotherapy Res 1997;11:479-84.

47. Fukuda K, Hibiya Y, Mutoh M, Ohno Y, Yamashita K, Akao S, Fujiwara H. Inhibition by parthenolide of phorbol ester-induced transcriptional activation of inducible nitric oxide synthase gene in a human monocyte cell line THP-1. Biochem Pharmacol 2000; 60:595-600.

48. Piela-Smith TH, Liu X. Feverfew extracts and the sesquiterpene lactone parthenolide inhibit intercellular adhesion molecule-1 expression in human synovial fibroblasts. Cellular Immunol 2001;209:89-96.

49. Mazor RL, Menedez IY, Ryan MA, Fiedler MA, Wong HR. Sesquiterpene lactones are potent inhibitors of interleukine 8 gene expression in cultered human respiratory epithelium. Cytokine 2000;12:239-45.

50. Makheja AN, Bailey JM. The active principle in feverfew. Lancet 1981;ii:1054.

51. Makheja AN, Bailey JM. A platelet phospholipase inhibitor from the medicinal herb feverfew (Tanacetum parthenium). Prostagland Leukotr Med 1982;8:653-60.

52. Weber JT, O'Connor M-F, Hayataka K, Colson N, Medora R, Russo EB, Parker KK. Activity of parthenolide at $5HT_{2A}$ receptors. J Nat Prod 1997;60:651-3.

53. Béjar E. Parthenolide inhibits the contractile responses of rat stomach fundus to fenfluramine and dextroamphetamine but not serotonin. J Ethnopharmacol 1996;50:1-12.

54. Mittra S, Datta A, Singh SK, Singh A. 5-Hydroxytryptamine-inhibiting property of feverfew: role of

parthenolide content. Acta Pharmacol Sin 2000;21: 1106-14.

55. Lee K-H, Huang E-S, Piantadosi C, Pagano JS, Geissman TA. Cytotoxicity of sesquiterpene lactones. Cancer Res 1971;31:1649-54.

56. Hoffmann JJ, Torrance SJ, Wiedhopf RM, Cole JR. Cytotoxic agents from Michelia champaca and Talauma ovata: parthenolide and costunolide. J Pharm Sci 1977; 66:884-5.

57. Woynarowski JM, Konopa J. Inhibition of DNA biosynthesis in HeLa cells by cytotoxic and antitumor sesquiterpene lactones. Molec Pharmacol 1981;19:97-102.

58. Woynarowski JW, Beerman TA, Konopa J. Induction of deoxyribonucleic acid damage in HeLa S3 cells by cytotoxic and antitumor sesquiterpene lactones. Biochem Pharmacol 1981;30:3005-7.

59. Ross JJ, Arnason JT, Birnboim HC. Low concentrations of the feverfew component parthenolide inhibit in vitro growth of tumor lines in a cytostatic fashion. Planta Med 1999;65:126-9.

60. Blakeman JP, Atkinson P. Antimicrobial properties and possible rôle in host-pathogen interactions of parthenolide, a sesquiterpene lactone isolated from glands of Chrysanthemum parthenium. Physiol Plant Pathol 1979;15:183-92.

61. Kalodera Z, Pepeljnjak S, Petrak T. The antimicrobial activity of Tanacetum parthenium extract. Pharmazie 1996;51:995-6.

62. Kalodera Z, Pepljnjak S, Blazevic N, Petrak T. Chemical composition and antimicrobial activity of Tanacetum parthenium essential oil. Pharmazie 1997;52:885-6.

63. Keery RJ, Lumley P. Does feverfew extract exhibit phospholipase A_2 inhibitory activity in vivo? Br J Pharmacol 1986;89:834P.

64. Jain NK, Kulkarni SK. Antinociceptive and anti-inflammatory effects of Tanacetum parthenium L. extract in mice and rats. J Ethnopharmacol 1999;68:251-9.

65. Tournier H, Schinella G, De Balsa EM, Buschiazzo H, Manez S, De Buschiazzo PM. Effects of the chloroform extract of Tanacetum vulgare and one of its active principles, parthenolide, on experimental gastric ulcer in rats. J Pharm Pharmacol 1999;51:215-9.

66. Biggs MJ, Johnson ES, Persaud NP, Ratcliffe DM. Platelet aggregation in patients using feverfew for migraine. Lancet 1982;ii:776.

67. De Weerdt CJ, Bootsma HPR, Hendriks H. Herbal medicines in migraine prevention: randomized double-blind placebo-controlled crossover trial of a feverfew preparation. Phytomedicine 1996;3:225-30.

68. Kuritzky A, Elhacham Y, Yerushalmi Z, Hering R. Feverfew in the treatment of migraine: its effect on serotonin uptake and platelet activity. Neurology 1994;44(Suppl 2):293P (cited in 22).

69. Pfaffenrath V, Fischer M, Friede M, Heinneicke V, Zepelin HH. Clinical dose-response study for the investigation of efficacy and tolerability of *Tanacetum parthenium* in migraine prophylaxis. Proceedings of Deutscher Schmerzkongress, 1999 (cited in 22).

70. Pattrick M, Heptinstall S, Doherty M. Feverfew in rheumatoid arthritis: a double blind, placebo controlled study. Ann Rheum Dis 1989;48:547-9.

71. Johnson ES, Kadam NP, Anderson D, Jenkinson PC, Dewdney RS, Blowers SD. Investigation of possible genotoxic effects of feverfew in migraine patients. Hum Toxicol 1987;6:533-4.

72. Anderson D, Jenkinson PC, Dewdney RS, Blowers SD, Johnson ES, Kadam NP. Chromosomal aberrations and sister chromatid exchanges in lymphocytes and urine mutagenicity of migraine patients: a comparison of chronic feverfew users and matched non-users. Hum Toxicol 1988;7:145-52.

TARAXACI FOLIUM

Dandelion Leaf

DEFINITION

Dandelion leaf consists of the dried leaves of *Taraxacum officinale* Weber *s.l.,* collected before the flowering period.

The material complies with the monograph of the British Herbal Pharmacopoeia [1].

Fresh material may also be used provided that when dried it complies with the monograph of the British Herbal Pharmacopoeia [1].

CONSTITUENTS

Sesquiterpene lactones of the germacranolide type, principally taraxinic acid β-glucopyranosyl ester and its 11,13-dihydro-derivative [2,3]; triterpene esters and free triterpenols such as α- and β-amyrin, lupeol, taraxasterol and cycloartenol [4,5]; the phytosterols β-sitosterol, stigmasterol and campesterol [3,4,6]; *p*-hydroxyphenylacetic acid [2,3]; flavonoids such as apigenin 7-glucoside, luteolin 7-glucoside and two luteolin 7-diglucosides [7,8]; hydroxycinnamic acids such as cichoric, monocaffeoyltartaric and chlorogenic acids [8,9]; the coumarins cichoriin and aesculin [8,9]; furan fatty acids [10]; minerals, particularly potassium (up to 4.5% in dried leaf) [11-13], and carotene [14].

CLINICAL PARTICULARS

Therapeutic indications
As an adjunct to treatments where enhanced urinary output is desirable, for example, rheumatism and the prevention of renal gravel [15].

Posology and method of administration

Dosage
Adults: 4-10 g of the drug or as an infusion, three times daily; 2-5 ml of tincture (1:5, ethanol 25% V/V), three times daily; 5-10 ml of juice from fresh leaf, twice daily [16].

Method of administration
For oral administration.

Duration of administration
No restriction.

Contra-indications
Occlusion of the bile ducts, gall-bladder empyema,

E/S/C/O/P
MONOGRAPHS
Second Edition

obstructive ileus [15].

Special warnings and special precautions for use
None required.

Interaction with other medicaments and other forms of interaction
None reported.

Pregnancy and lactation
No data available. In accordance with general medical practice, the product should not be used during pregnancy and lactation without medical advice.

Effects on ability to drive and use machines
None reported.

Undesirable effects
Dandelion can cause allergic contact dermatitis due to the presence of the sesquiterpene lactone taraxinic acid β-glucopyranosyl ester [17-19].

Overdose
No toxic symptoms reported.

PHARMACOLOGICAL PROPERTIES

Pharmacodynamic properties

In vitro experiments
Aqueous extracts of dandelion leaf restored the inhibition of nitric oxide production by cadmium in mouse peritoneal macrophages in a dose-dependent manner [20] and synergistically activated nitric oxide synthase in these cells treated with recombinant γ-interferon. The results suggested that the effects were due to secretion of tumour necrosis factor-α (TNF-α) induced by the dandelion leaf extracts [21].

A lyophilized dandelion leaf extract showed anti-oxidant activity, reducing secondary lipid peroxidation and enhancing NADPH cytochrome P-450 reductase activity in rat liver microsomes. The IC_{50} for malondi-aldehyde production (within 15 minutes) was 0.55 mg/ml [22]. Lyophilized aqueous leaf extract was found to have greater free radical scavenging activity in the H_2O_2/OH-luminol-microperoxidase system than root extract due to the higher polyphenol and flavonoid contents [23].

Dandelion leaf extracts at concentrations of 100 and 1000 µg/ml inhibited the production of tumour necrosis factor-α and interleukin-1 by rat astrocytes stimulated with lipopolysaccharide and substance P. These findings suggested an anti-inflammatory action in the central nervous system by inhibiting interleukin-1 production [24].

In vivo experiments
In experiments with mice and rats the diuretic and saluretic indices of a fluid extract of dandelion herb, corresponding to approximately 8 g of dried herb per kg body weight, were comparable to those of furosemide at 80 mg/kg body weight [11]. The high potassium content of the leaf ensures replacement of potassium eliminated in the urine [11-13].

A decoction from fresh dandelion leaf (equivalent to 5 g of dried plant), administered intravenously to dogs, doubled the volume of bile secreted from the liver during a 30-minute period [25]. A choleretic effect was also observed in rats following intra-duodenal administration of a dandelion extract; the volume of bile per hour increased by about one third [26]. An alcoholic extract of the whole plant administered intraduodenally to rats increased bile secretion by about 40% over the following 2 hours [27].

Clinical studies
No published clinical data are available.

Pharmacokinetic properties
No pharmacokinetic data are available.

Preclinical safety data
The intraperitoneal LD_{50} in mice of a fluid extract (1:1 from dried dandelion herb) was determined as 28.8 g/kg body weight [11]. Rabbits treated orally with dried dandelion whole plant at 3-6 g/kg body weight showed no visible signs of acute toxicity [28].

REFERENCES

1. Dandelion Leaf. In: British Herbal Pharmacopoeia. Bournemouth: British Herbal Medicine Association.

2. Hänsel R, Kartarahardja M, Huang J-T, Bohlmann F. Sesquiterpenlacton-β-D-glucopyranoside sowie ein neues Eudesmanolid aus *Taraxacum officinale*. Phytochemistry 1980;19;857-61.

3. Kuusi T, Pyysalo H, Autio K. The bitterness properties of dandelion II. Chemical investigations. Lebensm-Wiss Technol 1985;18:347-9.

4. Westerman L, Roddick JG. Annual variation in sterol levels in leaves of *Taraxacum officinale* Weber. Plant Physiol 1981;68:872-5.

5. Akashi T, Furuno T, Takahashi T, Ayabe S. Biosynthesis of triterpenoids in cultured cells and regenerated and wild plant organs of *Taraxacum officinale*. Phytochemistry 1994;36:303-8.

6. Westerman L, Roddick JG. Effects of senescence and gibberellic acid treatment on sterol levels in detached leaves of dandelion (*Taraxacum officinale*). Phytochemistry 1983;22:2318-9

7. Hänsel R, Keller K, Rimpler H, Schneider G, editors.

Taraxacum. In: Hagers Handbuch der Pharmazeutischen Praxis, 5th ed. Volume 6: Drogen P-Z. Berlin: Springer-Verlag, 1994:897-904.

8. Williams CA, Goldstone F, Greenham J. Flavonoids, cinnamic acids and coumarins from the different tissues and medicinal preparations of *Taraxacum officinale*. Phytochemistry 1996;42:121-7.

9. Budzianowski J. Coumarins, caffeoyltartaric acids and their artifactual methyl esters from *Taraxacum officinale* leaves. Planta Med 1997;63:288.

10. Hannemann K, Puchta V, Simon E, Ziegler H, Ziegler G, Spiteller G. The common occurrence of furan fatty acids in plants. Lipids 1989;24:296-8.

11. Rácz-Kotilla E, Rácz G, Solomon A. The action of *Taraxacum officinale* extracts on the body weight and diuresis of laboratory animals. Planta Med 1974;26:212-7.

12. Rácz G, Bodon J, Tölgyesi G. Determination of the mineral content of 41 medicinal plant species by chemotaxonomical and biochemical observations. Herba Hung 1978;17:43-54.

13. Hook I, McGee A, Henman M. Evaluation of dandelion for diuretic activity and variation in potassium content. Int J Pharmacog 1993;31:29-34.

14. Gonzalez A. Lactucae - chemical review. In: Haywood VH, Harborne JB, Turner BL, editors. The biology and chemistry of the Compositae. London: Academic Press, 1977:1081-95.

15. Weiss RF. Lehrbuch der Phytotherapie, 7th ed. Stuttgart: Hippokrates Verlag 1991:162-3.

16. Bradley PR, editor. Dandelion Leaf. In: British Herbal Compendium, Volume 1. Bournemouth: British Herbal Medicine Association, 1992:73-5.

17. Hausen BM. Taraxinsäure-1'-O-β-D-glucopyranosid, das Kontaktallergen des Löwenzahns (*Taraxacum officinale* Wiggers). Dermatosen 1982;30:51-3.

18. Wakelin SH, Marren P, Young E, Shaw S. Compositae sensitivity and chronic hand dermatitis in a 7-year-old boy. Br J Dermatol 1997;137:289-91.

19. Ingber A. Seasonal allergic contact dermatitis from *Taraxacum officinale* (dandelion) in an Israeli florist. Contact Dermatitis 2000;43:49.

20. Kim HM, Lee EH, Shin TY, Lee KN, Lee JS. *Taraxacum officinale* restores inhibition of nitric oxide production by cadmium in mouse peritoneal macrophages. Immunopharmacol Immunotoxicol 1998;20:283-97.

21. Kim H-M, Oh C-H, Chung C-K. Activation of inducible nitric oxide synthase by *Taraxacum officinale* in mouse peritoneal macrophages. General Pharmacol 1999; 32:683-8.

22. Hagymási K, Blázovics A, Fehér J, Lugasi A, Kristó ST, Kéry Á. The *in vitro* effect of dandelion antioxidants on microsomal lipid peroxidation. Phytother Res 2000; 14:43-4.

23. Hagymási K, Blázovics A, Lugasi A, Kristó ST, Fehér J, Kéry Á. In vitro antioxidant evaluation of dandelion (*Taraxacum officinale* Web.) water extracts. Acta Alimentaria 2000;29:1-7.

24. Kim H-M, Shin H-Y, Lim K-H, Ryu S-T, Shin T-Y, Chae H-J et al. *Taraxacum officinale* inhibits tumour necrosis factor-alpha production from rat astrocytes. Immunopharmacol Immunotoxicol 2000;22:519-30.

25. Chabrol E, Charonnat R, Maximin M, Waitz R, Porin J. L'action cholérétique des Composées. CR Soc Biol 1931;108:1100-2.

26. Büssemaker J. Über die choleretische Wirkung des Löwenzahns. Naunyn-Schmied Arch Exp Path Pharmakol 1936;181:512-3.

27. Böhm K. Untersuchungen über choleretische Wirkungen einiger Arzneipflanzen. Arzneim-Forsch/Drug Res 1959;9:376-8.

28. Akhtar MS, Khan QM, Khaliq T. Effects of *Portulaca oleracea* (Kulfa) and *Taraxacum officinale* (Dhudhal) in normoglycaemic and alloxan-treated hyperglycaemic rabbits. J Pak Med Assoc 1985;35:207-10.

TARAXACI RADIX

Dandelion Root

DEFINITION

Dandelion root consists of the dried roots and rhizomes of *Taraxacum officinale* Weber *s.l.*

The material complies with the monograph of the Österreichisches Arzneibuch [1] or the British Herbal Pharmacopoeia [2].

Fresh material may also be used provided that, when dried, it complies with the monograph of one of the above pharmacopoeias.

CONSTITUENTS

Sesquiterpene lactones including eudesmanolides (tetrahydroridentin B and taraxacolide-O-β-gluco-pyranoside) [3], guaianolides (11β,13-dihydrolactucin and ixerin D) [4] and three germacranolide esters, taraxinic acid β-glucopyranosyl ester and its 11,13-dihydro-derivative [4,5] and ainslioside [4]; a lupane-type triterpene (3β-hydroxylup-18(19)-ene-21-one) from fresh roots [6]; benzyl glucoside and the phenylpropanoid glycosides dihydroconiferin, syringin and dihydrosyringin [4]; triterpene alcohols and phytosterols, including taraxasterol [3,7]; the γ-butyrolactone glucoside ester taraxacoside [8]; chlorogenic acids [9], caffeic acid and *p*-hydroxy-phenylacetic acid [10]; potassium [11] and amino acids [12]. In autumn the dried root contains up to 40% of inulin, in spring about 2% [11,13]. The latex was found to contain a serine proteinase (taraxalisin) [14].

CLINICAL PARTICULARS

Therapeutic indications
Restoration of hepatic and biliary function, dyspepsia, loss of appetite [11,15].

Posology and method of administration

Dosage

Adults: 3-5 g of the drug or 5-10 ml of tincture (1:5, ethanol 25% V/V), three times daily [16].

Method of administration
For oral administration.

Duration of administration
No restriction.

E/S/C/O/P
MONOGRAPHS
Second Edition

Contraindications

Occlusion of the bile ducts, gall-bladder empyema, obstructive ileus [15].

Special warnings and special precautions for use

None required.

Interaction with other medicaments and other forms of interaction

None reported.

Pregnancy and lactation

No data available. In accordance with general medical practice, the product should not be used during pregnancy and lactation without medical advice.

Effects on ability to drive and use machines

None known.

Undesirable effects

Dandelion root can produce allergic contact dermatitis due to the presence of the sesquiterpene lactone taraxinic acid β-glucopyranosyl ester [17].

Overdose

No toxic effects reported.

PHARMACOLOGICAL PROPERTIES

Pharmacodynamic properties

In vitro experiments

Lyophilized aqueous extracts of dandelion root were found to have antioxidant properties; they diminished enzymatically-induced lipid peroxidation and reduced cytochrome c with and without NADPH in rat liver microsomes in a concentration-dependent manner. The root extracts were less active than leaf extracts [18].

An ethanolic extract of dandelion root dose-dependently inhibited ADP-induced platelet aggregation with a maximal inhibition of 85% at a concentration equivalent to 0.04 mg of dried root per ml of human platelet-rich plasma. A fraction of the extract containing low molecular weight polysaccharides caused 91% inhibition and a fraction enriched in triterpenes/steroids 80% inhibition of platelet aggregation, both at a concentration equivalent to 0.04 mg of dried root per ml of plasma [19].

A methanolic extract of dandelion root showed strong inhibitory activity towards the formation of leukotriene B_4 from activated human neutrophils (90% inhibition at 3 µg/ml). The butanol-soluble fraction of the extract inhibited leukotriene B_4 formation by 86% at 3 µg/ml, while ethyl acetate- and water-soluble fractions dis-

played only weak activity (32 and 21% inhibition at 3 µg/ml, respectively) [5].

Taraxinic acid β-glucopyranosyl ester from dandelion root inhibited HIV-1 replication in acutely infected H9 cells with an IC_{50} of 1.68 µg/ml. The compound was slightly active against uninfected H9 cell growth with an IC_{50} of 7.94 µg/ml [5].

In vivo experiments

A decoction from fresh dandelion root (equivalent to 5 g of dried plant), administered intravenously to dogs, doubled the volume of bile secreted from the liver during a 30-minute period [20]. A choleretic effect was also observed in rats following intra-duodenal administration of a dandelion extract; the volume of bile per hour increased by about one third [21]. An alcoholic extract of the whole plant administered intraduodenally to rats increased bile secretion by 40% over the following 2 hours [22].

A dry 80%-ethanolic extract of dandelion root, administered orally at 100 mg/kg body weight one hour before oedema elicitation, inhibited carrageenan-induced rat paw oedema by 25%, compared to 45% inhibition of oedema by indometacin at 5 mg/kg [23]. In another experiment, carrageenan-induced rat paw oedema was partially inhibited following intra-peritoneal administration of 100 mg/kg body weight (42% after 3 hours and 29% after 5 hours) [24].

No consistent pattern of diuresis was obtained with extracts (petroleum ether, chloroform or methanol) of dandelion root administered to mice at a dose of 50 mg/kg. Some extracts showed statistically significant natriuretic and kaliuretic effects related to the potassium content of the roots [24,25].

Aqueous and ethanolic extracts of dandelion root, administered orally to mice at the equivalent to 25 g of dried root per kg body weight, showed no hypoglycaemic activity in oral glucose tolerance tests [26].

Clinical studies

No published clinical data are available.

Pharmacokinetic properties

No pharmacokinetic data are available.

Preclinical safety data

The intraperitoneal LD_{50} in mice of a fluid extract (1:1 from dried dandelion root) was determined as 36.6 g/kg [27]. A dry ethanolic extract showed low toxicity in mice and rats when administered in doses up to the equivalent of 10 g (oral) and 4 g (intra-peritoneal) of dried drug per kg body weight [24].

REFERENCES

1. Radix Taraxaci - Löwenzahnwurzel. Österreichisches Arzneibuch.

2. Dandelion Root. In: British Herbal Pharmacopoeia. Bournemouth: British Herbal Medicine Association.

3. Hänsel R, Kartarahardja M, Huang J-T, Bohlmann F. Sesquiterpenlacton-β-D-glucopyranoside sowie ein neues Eudesmanolid aus *Taraxacum officinale*. Phytochemistry 1980;19:857-61.

4. Kisiel W, Barszcz B. Further sesquiterpenoids and phenolics from *Taraxacum officinale*. Fitoterapia 2000; 71:269-73.

5. Kashiwada Y, Takanaka K, Tsukada H, Miwa Y, Taga T, Tanaka S, Ikeshiro Y. Sesquiterpene glucosides from anti-leukotriene B_4 release fraction of *Taraxacum officinale*. J Asian Nat Prod Res 2001;3:191-7.

6. Kisiel W, Barszcz B, Szneler E. A new lupane-type triterpenoid from *Taraxacum officinale*. Polish J Chem 2000;74:281-3.

7. Burrows S, Simpson JCE. The triterpene group. Part IV. The triterpene alcohols of *Taraxacum* root. J Chem Soc 1938;2042-7.

8. Rauwald H-W, Huang J-T. Taraxacoside, a type of acylated γ-butyrolactone glycoside from *Taraxacum officinale*. Phytochemistry 1985;24:1557-9.

9. Clifford MN, Shutler S, Thomas GA, Ohiokpehai O. The chlorogenic acids content of coffee substitutes. Food Chem 1987;24:99-107.

10. Faber K. Der Löwenzahn - *Taraxacum officinale* Weber. Pharmazie 1958;13:423-36.

11. Vogel H-H, Schaette R. Phytotherapeutische Reflexionen. Betrachtungen über *Silybum marianum (Carduus marianus), Taraxacum officinale, Cichorium intybus, Bryonia alba et dioica, Viscum album* und ihre Beziehungen zur Leber. Erfahrungsheilkunde 1977;26: 347-55.

12. Petlevski R, Hadzija M, Slijepcevic M, Juretic D. Amino acids in nettle root, juniper berries and dandelion root (Urticae radix, Juniperi fructus and Taraxaci radix). Farm Glas 2001;57:139-47.

13. Hänsel R, Keller K, Rimpler H, Schneider G, editors. *Taraxacum*. In: Hagers Handbuch der Pharmazeutischen Praxis, 5th ed. Volume 6: Drogen P-Z. Berlin: Springer-Verlag, 1994:897-904.

14. Rudenskaya GN, Bogacheva AM, Preusser A et al. Taraxalisin - a serine proteinase from dandelion, *Taraxacum officinale* Webb. FEBS Lett 1998;43:237-40.

15. Weiss RF. Lehrbuch der Phytotherapie. 7th ed. Stuttgart: Hippokrates Verlag 1991:162-3.

16. Bradley PR, editor. Dandelion Root. In: British Herbal Compendium, Volume 1. Bournemouth: British Herbal Medicine Association, 1992:76-7.

17. Hausen BM. Taraxinsäure-1'-O-β-D-glucopyranosid, das Kontaktallergen des Löwenzahns (*Taraxacum officinale* Wiggers). Dermatosen 1982;30:51-3.

18. Hagymási K, Blázovics A, Lugasi A, Kristó ST, Fehér J, Kéry Á. In vitro antioxidant evaluation of dandelion (*Taraxacum officinale* Web.) water extracts. Acta Alimentaria 2000;29:1-7.

19. Neef H, Cilli F, Declerck PJ, Laekeman G. Platelet anti-aggregating activity of *Taraxacum officinale* Weber. Phytother Res 1996;10:S138-40.

20. Chabrol E, Charonnat R, Maximin M, Waitz R, Porin J. L'action cholérétique des Composées. CR Soc Biol 1931;108:1100-2.

21. Büssemaker J. Über die choleretische Wirkung des Löwenzahns. Naunyn-Schmied Arch Exp Path Pharmakol 1936;181:512-3.

22. Böhm K. Untersuchungen über choleretische Wirkungen einiger Arzneipflanzen. Arzneim-Forsch/Drug Res 1959; 9:376-8.

23. Mascolo N, Autore G, Capasso F, Menghini A, Fasolo MP. Biological screening of Italian medicinal plants for anti-inflammatory activity. Phytother Res 1987;1:28-31.

24. Tita B, Bello U, Faccendini P, Bartolini R, Bolle P. *Taraxacum officinale* W. Pharmacological effect of ethanol extract. Pharmacol Res 1993;27(Suppl.1):23-4.

25. Hook I, McGee A, Henman M. Evaluation of dandelion for diuretic activity and variation in potassium content. Int J Pharmacog 1993;31:29-34.

26. Neef H, Declercq P, Laekeman G. Hypoglycaemic activity of selected European plants. Phytother Res 1995;9:45-8.

27. Rácz-Kotilla E, Rácz G, Solomon A. The action of *Taraxacum officinale* extracts on the body weight and diuresis of laboratory animals. Planta Med 1974;26:212-7.

THYMI HERBA

Thyme

E/S/C/O/P
MONOGRAPHS
Second Edition

DEFINITION

Thyme consists of the whole leaves and flowers separated from the previously dried stems of *Thymus vulgaris* L. or *Thymus zygis* L. or a mixture of both species. It contains not less than 12 ml/kg of essential oil, of which not less than 40% is thymol and carvacrol (both $C_{10}H_{14}O$; M_r 150.2), calculated with reference to the anhydrous drug [1].

The material complies with the monograph of the European Pharmacopoeia [1].

Fresh material may also be used, provided that when dried it complies with the monograph of the European Pharmacopoeia.

CONSTITUENTS

Essential oil containing phenols, predominantly thymol and/or carvacrol, and terpenoids [2-7]; glycosides of phenolic monoterpenoids, eugenol, aliphatic alcohols and acetophenones [8-10]; flavonoids, among which thymonin, cirsilineol and 8-methoxycirsilineol are characteristic [11-13]; biphenyl compounds of mono-terpenoid origin [13,14]; caffeic acid and rosmarinic acid [15-17]; saponins [18,19]; long-chain saturated hydrocarbons and aliphatic aldehydes [20]; and an arabinogalactan [21].

CLINICAL PARTICULARS

Therapeutic indications
Catarrh of the upper respiratory tract, bronchial catarrh and supportive treatment of pertussis [22].
Stomatitis and halitosis [22].

Posology and method of administration

Dosage

Internal use

Herb
Adults and children from 1 year: 1-2 g of dried herb, or the equivalent amount of fresh herb, as an infusion several times a day [22-24].
Children up to 1 year: 0.5-1 g [24].

Fluid extract
Adults and children: Dosage to be calculated in accordance with the dosage for the herb [25].

Tincture (1:10, 70% ethanol): 40 drops up to three times daily [23].

Other equivalent preparations.

Topical use
A 5% infusion as a gargle or mouth-wash [22,23].

Method of administration
For oral administration or topical application.

Duration of administration
No restriction.

Contra-indications
None known.

Special warnings and special precautions for use
None required.

Interaction with other medicaments and other forms of interaction
None reported.

Pregnancy and lactation
No data available. In accordance with general medical practice, the product should not be used during pregnancy and lactation without medical advice.

Effects on ability to drive and use machines
None known.

Undesirable effects
In very rare cases hypersensitivity reactions have been reported [26,27].

Overdose
No toxic effects reported.

PHARMACOLOGICAL PROPERTIES

Pharmacodynamic properties

In vitro experiments

Spasmolytic effects
Bronchospasmolysis is attributed to the flavonoids thymonin, cirsilineol and 8-methoxycirsilineol, shown to be potent spasmolytics by *in vitro* experiments on guinea pig trachea [28,29].

A fluid extract of thyme (67% ethanol; containing 0.072% thymol and 0.005% carvacrol) dose-dependently and reversibly antagonized contractions of isolated guinea pig trachea preparations provoked by barium chloride (49% inhibition), carbachol (42% inhibition), histamine (73% inhibition) and prostaglandin$_{2\alpha}$ (89% inhibition) [30].

Antimicrobial effects
An aqueous extract of thyme (1:1) dose-dependently inhibited *Helicobacter pylori* in a growth inhibition test and two urease activity assays. In a disc zone inhibition test the effect of 1.6 mg of the dried extract was stronger than that of 30 µg of nalidixic acid [31].

Mycobacterium tuberculosis strain H37Rv was inhibited by an acetone extract of thyme with an MIC of 0.5 mg/ml in the agar plate test and in a radiometric assay. In the latter the same activity was confirmed on the growth of the drug-resistant *Mycobacterium tuberculosis* strain CCKO28469V [32].

A fluid extract of thyme (67% ethanol; containing 0.072% of thymol and 0.005% of carvacrol) showed activity towards the pneumotropic bacteria *Moraxella catarrhalis*, *Klebsiella pneumoniae* and *Diplococcus pneumoniae* in disc diffusion tests [33].

Thyme essential oil proved highly antibacterial and antifungal when tested on Gram-positive and Gram-negative bacteria, fungi and yeasts. The activity was mainly attributed to thymol and carvacrol [34-50].

Anti-inflammatory effects
A 96%-ethanolic extract of thyme exhibited significant hyaluronidase-inhibitory activity (p<0.05), reducing the enzyme activity to 35.5% [51].

Hydroperoxide formation from methyl linoleate was inhibited by 97% by a dry extract of thyme (80% methanol; total phenolics 17.1 mg/g, determined as gallic acid) at a concentration of 500 ppm [52].

Formation of the inflammation mediator PGE$_2$ in monocyte-macrophage cell line MM6 was suppressed by a fluid extract of thyme (67% ethanol; containing 0.072% of thymol and 0.005% of carvacrol) with an IC$_{50}$ of about 0.1 µg/ml compared to 100 µg/ml for acetylsalicylic acid and 0.004 µg/ml for indometacin [33].

High antioxidative properties were demonstrated for a dry acetone extract (28.6:1) and a supercritical carbon dioxide extract (18.3:1) of thyme in the carotene bleaching test [53]. Other assays have also confirmed antioxidant activities of thyme extracts of different polarity [33,54,55].

Antioxidative effects of thyme oil have been determined in various test systems and attributed mainly to its phenolic constituents [56-58].

Thyme oil inhibited prostaglandin biosynthesis [59].

Rosmarinic acid has shown anti-inflammatory activity due to inhibition of the classical complement pathway in rats and inhibition of some human PMN functions, when tested at several dosage levels and by several application methods [60,61].

An arabinogalactan isolated from thyme exhibited

significant anti-complementary activity via both classical and alternative pathways in a dose-dependent manner (p<0.01 to p<0.05) [21].

Other effects

The antiviral activity of a fluid extract of thyme (67% ethanol; containing 0.072% of thymol and 0.005% of carvacrol) on influenza A virus and respiratory syncytial virus was determined in a plaque reduction test; the IC_{50} values were 15 µg/ml and 20 µg/ml respectively [33].

In an *in vitro* growth inhibition assay with bloodstream forms of *Trypanosoma brucei* the ED_{50} of thyme essential oil was found to be 0.4 µg/ml [62].

A methanolic extract of thyme significantly promoted Ca^{2+} fluxes into clonal rat pituitary cells (0.001<p<0.01) [63].

A methanolic thyme extract (15:1) inhibited non-enzymatic glycation of bovine serum albumin (82% inhibition at 1 mg/ml) [64].

In vivo experiments

Oral administration of a fluid extract of thyme (ethanol 67% V/V; 0.072% of thymol and 0.005% of carvacrol) at 162 mg/kg body weight significantly reduced carrageenan-induced rat paw oedema for 5 hours (p<0.05). During the first 3 hours the effect was comparable to that of phenylbutazone at 123.4 mg/kg body weight [33].

Intraperitoneal pretreatment of rats with thyme essential oil, thymol or carvacrol at 125 mg/kg body weight protected against hepatotoxicity induced by carbon tetrachloride (administered intraperitoneally at 1 ml/kg body weight). Glutamic pyruvate transaminase levels were significantly lower (p<0.001) than in untreated controls; the levels achieved with the essential oil and carvacrol were comparable to the level after intraperitoneal pretreatment with silymarin at 35 mg/kg body weight. Hepatic concentrations of malondialdehyde, indicating the degree of lipoperoxidation, were significantly reduced (p<0.05) [65].

Daily oral administration of 3.9 mg of thyme essential oil to rats over a period of 17 months resulted in the maintenance of significantly higher levels of polyunsaturated fatty acids (PUFAs) within the retinal phospholipids, particularly of arachidonic (p<0.001) and docosahexaenoic (p<0.05) acids. Based on these findings, a positive influence of thyme on age-related macular degeneration has been discussed [66]. In rats fed with thyme essential oil or thymol at 42.5 mg/kg body weight/day for 21 months the levels of the two PUFAs in phospholipid fractions from liver, brain, kidney and heart tissues were also significantly higher than in age-matched controls (p<0.001 to p<0.05)

[67,68]. Under the same experimental conditions, potential benefits of thyme oil and thymol on age-related changes in antioxidant systems was shown by determination of superoxide dismutase activity (SOD), glutathione peroxidase activity (GSHPx) and total antioxidant status (TAS) in liver, kidney, heart and brain of rats. SOD activity in liver (p<0.05) and heart (p<0.01), and GSHPx activity in liver (p<0.05), kidney (p<0.01) and brain (p<0.05), were significantly higher in thyme oil or thymol treated animals than in age-matched controls. A significantly higher TAS (p<0.001 to p<0.05) was observed in all organs [68,69].

Rosmarinic acid exhibited inhibitory activity in three *in vivo* models in which complement activation plays a role: reduction of oedema induced by cobra venom factor in the rat; inhibition of passive cutaneous anaphylaxis; and impairment of *in vivo* activation by heat-killed *Corynebacterium parvum* of mouse macrophages. However, rosmarinic acid did not inhibit t-butyl hydroperoxide-induced rat paw oedema, indicating selectivity for complement-dependent processes [60].

Clinical studies

In a randomized, double-blind, comparative study, 60 patients with productive cough complaints resulting from uncomplicated respiratory infections were treated with thyme syrup (3 × 10 ml daily, n = 31) or a bromhexine preparation (n = 29) for 5 days. No significant difference was observed between thyme syrup and bromhexine in self-reported alleviation of the complaints on days 2 and 5 of treatment [70].

In an open, multicentre study, 154 children aged 2 months to 14 years (mean 4.4 years) with bronchial catarrh or bronchitis were treated daily with 15-30 ml of thyme syrup, containing 97.6 mg of thyme fluid extract (2-2.5:1) per ml, for a period of 7-14 days (mean 7.9 days); 46 patients did not receive any co-medication. Compared to the start of the treatment an improvement in the intensity of coughing was reported in 93.5% of patients [71].

Pharmacokinetic properties

After oral administration of a tablet or capsule containing thyme extract (70% ethanol, 6-10:1) to healthy volunteers, first traces of thymol were detected in the exhaled air after 30 and 60 minutes respectively; after 140 minutes thymol was no longer detectable in the exhaled air. The increase in concentration of thymol in the exhaled air matched the blood concentration [72,73].

Preclinical safety data

Acute toxicity

A concentrated thyme extract decreased locomotor

activity and caused a slight slowing down of respiration in mice in an acute toxicity test. Doses of 0.5-3.0 g extract/kg body weight corresponding to 4.3-26.0 g of dried plant material, administered orally, produced these effects at all dose levels [74].

The oral LD_{50} of thyme essential oil (*Thymus vulgaris*) has been determined as 2.84 g/kg body weight in rats [75]. The intraperitoneal LD_{50} of *Thymus zygis* oil was found to be 600 mg/kg body weight in female mice [65].

Subchronic toxicity
Increases in weights of liver and testes were observed after oral administration to mice of a concentrated 95%-ethanolic extract from aerial parts of thyme (corresponding to 0.9 g of crude drug) daily for 3 months. 30% of the male animals died, while in the female and control groups only 10% died [74].

Mutagenicity
Thyme oil showed no mutagenic potential in the Ames test with *Salmonella typhimurium* strains TA98, TA100, TA1535 and TA1537, with or without metabolic activation, and no DNA-damaging activity in the *Bacillus subtilis* rec-assay [76].

Clinical safety data
In a study in 21 patients who received thyme fluid extract, neither adverse reactions relating to gastro-intestinal, central and peripheral nervous or respiratory systems, nor adverse skin or psychiatric reactions, were observed [77].

REFERENCES

1. Thyme - Thymi herba. European Pharmacopoeia, Council of Europe.

2. Weiss B, Flück H. Untersuchungen über die Variabilität von Gehalt und Zusammensetzung des ätherischen Öles in Blatt- und Krautdrogen von *Thymus vulgaris* L. Pharm Acta Helv 1970;45:169-83.

3. Stahl-Biskup E. The chemical composition of *Thymus* oils: a review of the literature 1960-1989. J Ess Oil Res 1991;3:61-82.

4. Adzet T, Granger R, Passet J, San Martin R. Le polymorphisme chimique dans le genre *Thymus*: sa signification taxonomique. Biochem Syst Ecol 1977; 5:269-72.

5. Pino JA, Estarrón M, Fuentes V. Essential oil of thyme (*Thymus vulgaris* L.) grown in Cuba. J Essent Oil Res 1997;9:609-10.

6. Panizzi L, Flamini G, Cioni PL, Morelli I. Composition and antimicrobial properties of essential oils of four Mediterranean Lamiaceae. J Ethnopharmacol 1993; 39:167-70.

7. Shatar S, Altantsetseg S. Essential oil composition of some plants cultivated in Mongolian climate. J Essent Oil Res 2000;12:745-50.

8. Skopp K, Hörster H. An Zucker gebundene reguläre Monoterpene, Teil I. Thymol- und Carvacrolglykoside in *Thymus vulgaris*. Planta Med 1976;29:208-15.

9. van den Dries JMA, Baerheim Svendsen A. A simple method for detection of glycosidic bound monoterpenes and other volatile compounds occurring in fresh plant material. Flavour Fragrance J 1989;4:59-61.

10. Wang M, Kikuzaki H, Lin C-C, Kahyaoglu A, Huang M-T, Nakatani N, Ho C-T. Acetophenone glycosides from thyme (*Thymus vulgaris* L.). J Agric Food Chem 1999; 47:1911-4.

11. van den Broucke CO, Dommisse RA, Esmans EL, Lemli JA. Three methylated flavones from *Thymus vulgaris*. Phytochemistry 1982;21:2581-3.

12. Adzet T, Vila R, Cañigueral S. Chromatographic analysis of polyphenols of some Iberian *Thymus*. J Ethnopharmacol 1988;24:147-54.

13. Haraguchi H, Saito T, Ishikawa H, Date H, Kataoka S, Tamura Y, Mizutani K. Antiperoxidative components in *Thymus vulgaris*. Planta Med 1996;62:217-21.

14. Nakatani N, Miura K, Inagaki T. Structure of new deodorant biphenyl compounds from thyme (*Thymus vulgaris* L.) and their activity against methyl mercaptan. Agric Biol Chem 1989;53:1375-81.

15. Litvinenko VI, Popova TP, Simonjan AV, Zoz IG, Sokolov VS. "Gerbstoffe" und Oxyzimtsäureab-kömmlinge in Labiaten. Planta Med 1975;27:372-80.

16. Hegnauer R. Chemotaxonomie der Pflanzen IV. Basel: Birkhäuser Verlag, 1966:328.

17. Lamaison JL, Petitjean-Freytet C, Carnat A. Teneurs en acide rosmarinique, en dérivés hydroxycinnamiques totaux et activité antioxydante chez les Apiacées, les Borraginacées et les Lamiacées médicinales. Ann Pharm Fr 1990;48:103-8.

18. Garcia Marquina JM, Gallardo Villá M. Saponinas del *Thymus vulgaris* L. Farmacognosia (Madrid) 1949; 9:261-76.

19. Hegnauer R. Chemotaxonomie der Pflanzen IV. Basel: Birkhäuser Verlag, 1966:321.

20. Guillén MD, Manzanos MJ. Composition of the extract in dichloromethane of the aerial parts of a Spanish wild growing plant *Thymus vulgaris* L. Flavour Fragrance J 1998;13:259-62.

21. Chun H, Jun WJ, Shin DH, Hong BS, Cho HY, Yang HC. Purification and characterization of anti-complementary polysaccharide from leaves of *Thymus vulgaris* L. Chem Pharm Bull 2001;49:762-4.

22. Czygan F-C, Hiller K. Thymi herba - Thymian. In: Wichtl M, editor. Teedrogen und Phytopharmaka. Ein Handbuch für die Praxis auf wissenschaftlicher

Grundlage, 4th ed. Stuttgart: Wissenschaftliche Verlagsgesellschaft, 2002:607-10.

23. Van Hellemont J. In: Fytotherapeutisch compendium, 2nd ed. Utrecht: Bohn, Scheltema & Holkema, 1988: 599-605.

24. Dorsch W, Loew D, Meyer E, Schilcher H. In: Empfehlungen zu Kinderdosierungen von monographierten Arzneidrogen und ihren Zubereitungen. Kooperation Phytopharmaka: Bonn, 1993:100-1.

25. Hochsinger K. Die Therapie des Krampf- und Reizhustens. Wiener Med Wschr 1931;13:447-8.

26. Spiewak R, Skorska C, Dutkiewicz J. Occupational airborne contact dermatitis cause by thyme dust. Contact Dermatitis 2001;44:235-9.

27. Benito M, Jorro G, Morales C, Peláez A, Fernández A. Labiatae allergy: systemic reactions due to ingestion of oregano and thyme. Ann Allergy Asthma Immunol 1996;76:416-8.

28. van den Broucke C, Lemli J, Lamy J. Action spasmolytique des flavones de différentes espèces de Thymus. Plantes Méd Phytothér 1982;16:310-7.

29. van den Broucke CO, Lemli JA. Spasmolytic activity of the flavonoids from Thymus vulgaris. Pharm Weekbl Sci Ed 1983;5:9-14.

30. Meister A, Bernhardt G, Christoffel V, Buschauer A. Antispasmodic activity of Thymus vulgaris extract on the isolated guinea-pig trachea: discrimination between drug and ethanol effects. Plant Med 1999;65:512-6.

31. Tabak M, Armon R, Potasman I, Neeman I. In vitro inhibition of Helicobacter pylori by extracts of thyme. J Appl Bacteriol 1996;80:667-72.

32. Lall N, Meyer JJM. In vitro inhibition of drug-resistant and drug-sensitive strains of Mycobacterium tuberculosis by ethnobotanically selected South African plants. J Ethnopharmacol 1999;66:347-54.

33. Christoffel V, Schwenk U, Eberhard G, Morgenstern E, Ziska T, Glatthaar B et al. Pharmacological profiling of the Thymus vulgaris preparation BNO 1018. Symposium Phytopharmaka-Forschung 2000. Bonn, 27-28 November 1998.

34. Patáková D, Chládek M. Über die antibakterielle Aktivität von Thymian- und Quendelölen. Pharmazie 1974;29:140-2.

35. Simeon de Bouchberg M, Allegrini J, Bessiere C, Attisso M, Passet J, Granger R. Propriétés microbiologiques des huiles essentielles de chimiotypes de Thymus vulgaris Linnaeus. Riv Ital EPPOS 1976;58:527-36.

36. Janssen AM, Chin NLJ, Scheffer JJC, Baerheim Svendsen A. Screening for antimicrobial activity of some essential oils by the agar overlay technique. Pharm Weekbl Sci Ed 1986;8:289-92.

37. Allegrini J, Simeon de Bouchberg M. Une technique d'étude du pouvoir antibactérien des huiles essentielles. Prod Probl Pharm 1972;27:891-7.

38. Janssen AM. Antimicrobial activities of essential oils - a pharmacognostical study [Dissertation]. Leiden: Rijksuniversiteit te Leiden, 1989:91-108.

39. Farag RS, Salem H, Badei AZMA, Hassanein DE. Biochemical studies on the essential oils of some medicinal plants. Fette Seifen Anstrichmittel 1986; 88:69-72.

40. Lens-Lisbonne C, Cremieux A, Maillard C, Balansard G. Méthodes d'évaluation de l'activité antibacterienne des huiles essentielles: application aux essences de thym et de cannelle. J Pharm Belg 1987;42:297-302.

41. Menghini A, Savino A, Lollini MN, Caprio A. Activité antimicrobienne en contact direct et en microatmosphère de certaines huiles essentielles. Plant Med Phytother 1987;21:36-42.

42. Deans SG, Ritchie G. Antibacterial properties of plant essential oils. Int J Food Microbiol 1987;5:165-80.

43. Vampa G, Albasini A, Provvisionato A, Bianchi A, Melegari M. Étude chimique et microbiologique sur les huiles essentielles de Thymus. Plant Med Phytother 1988;22:195-202.

44. Chalchat JC, Garry RP, Bastide P, Fabre F, Malhuret R. Corrélation composition chimique/activité antimicrobienne: V - Contribution à la comparaison de 2 méthodes de détermination des CMI. Plantes Méd Phytothér 1991;25:184-93.

45. Amvam Zollo PH, Biyiti L, Tchoumbougnang F, Menut C, Lamaty G, Bouchet P. Aromatic plants of tropical Central Africa. Part XXXII. Chemical composition and antifungal activity of thirteen essential oils from aromatic plants of Cameroon. Flavour Fragr J 1998;13:107-14.

46. Hammer KA, Carson CF, Riley TV. Antimicrobial activity of essential oils and other plant extracts. J Appl Microbiol 1999;86:985-90.

47. Dorman HJD, Deans SG. Antimicrobial agents from plants: antibacterial activity of plant volatile oils. J Appl Microbiol 2000;88:308-16.

48. Daferera DJ, Ziogas BN, Polissiou MG. GC-MS analysis of essential oils from some Greek aromatic plants and their fungitoxicity on Penicillium digitatum. J Agric Food Chem 2000;48:2576-81.

49. Inouye S, Takizawa T, Yamaguchi H. Antibacterial activity of essential oils and their major constituents against respiratory tract pathogens by gaseous contact. J Antimicrob Chemother 2001;47:565-73.

50. Viollon C, Chaumont J-P. Antifungal properties of essential oils and their main components upon Cryptococcus neoformans. Mycopathologia 1994;128:151-3.

51. Ippoushi K, Yamaguchi Y, Itou H, Azuma K, Higashio H. Evaluation of inhibitory effects of vegetables and herbs on hyaluronidase and identification of rosmarinic acid as a hyaluronidase inhibitor in lemon balm (Melissa officinalis L.). Food Sci Technol Res 2000;6:74-7.

52. Kähkönen MP, Hopia AI, Vuorela HJ, Rauha J-P, Pihlaja K, Kujala TS, Heinonen M. Antioxidant activity of plant extracts containing phenolic compounds. J Agric Food Chem 1999;47:3954-62.

53. Dapkevicius A, Venskutonis R, van Beek TA, Linssen JPH. Antioxidant activity of extracts obtained by different isolation procedures from some aromatic herbs grown in Lithuania. J Sci Food Agric 1998;77:140-6.

54. Simandi B, Hajdu V, Peredi K, Czukor B, Nobik-Kovacs A, Kery A. Antioxidant activity of pilot-plant alcoholic and supercritical carbon dioxide extracts of thyme. Eur J Lipid Sci Technol 2001;103:355-8.

55. Soares JR, Dinis TCP, Cunha AP, Almeida LM. Antioxidant activities of some extracts of *Thymus zygis*. Free Rad Res 1997;26:469-78.

56. Youdim KA, Dorman HJD, Deans SG. The antioxidant effectiveness of thyme oil, α-tocopherol and ascorbyl palmitate on evening primrose oil oxidation. J Essent Oil Res 1999;11:643-8.

57. Teissedre PL, Waterhouse AL. Inhibition of oxidation of human low-density lipoproteins by phenolic substances in different essential oils varieties. J Agric Food Chem 2000;48:3801-5.

58. Dorman HJD, Surai P, Deans SG. *In vitro* antioxidant activity of a number of plant essential oils and phyto-constituents. J Essent Oil Res 2000;12:241-8.

59. Wagner H, Wierer M, Bauer R. *In vitro* Hemmung der Prostaglandin-Biosynthese durch etherische Öle und phenolische Verbindungen. Planta Med 1986:184-7.

60. Englberger W, Hadding U, Etschenberg E, Graf E, Leyck S, Winkelmann J, Parnham MJ. Rosmarinic acid: a new inhibitor of complement C3-convertase with anti-inflammatory activity. Int J Immunopharm 1988; 10:729-37.

61. Gracza L, Koch H, Löffler E. Isolierung von Rosmarin-säure aus *Symphytum officinale* und ihre anti-inflammatorische Wirksamkeit in einem In-vitro-Modell. Arch Pharm (Weinheim) 1985;318:1090-5.

62. Mikus J, Harkenthal M, Steverding D, Reichling J. *In vitro* effect of essential oils and isolated mono- and sesquiterpenes on *Leishmania major* and *Trypanosoma brucei*. Planta Med 2000;66:366-8.

63. Rauha J-P, Tammela P, Summanen J, Vuorela P, Kähkönen M, Heinonen M et al. Actions of some plant extracts containing flavonoids and other phenolic compounds on calcium fluxes in clonal rat pituitary GH_4C_1 cells. Pharm Pharmacol Lett 1999;9:66-9.

64. Morimitsu Y, Yoshida K, Esaki S, Hirota A. Protein glycation inhibitors from thyme (*Thymus vulgaris*). Biosci Biotech Biochem 1995;59:2018-21.

65. Jiménez J, Navarro MC, Montilla MP, Martin A, Martinez

66. Recsan Z, Pagliuca G, Piretti MV, Penzes LG, Youdim KA, Noble RC, Deans SG. Effect of essential oils on the lipids of the retina in the ageing rat: a possible therapeutic use. J Essent Oil Res 1997;9:53-6.

67. Youdim KA, Deans SG. Beneficial effects of thyme oil on age-related changes in the phospholipid C_{20} and C_{22} polyunsaturated fatty acid composition of various rat tissues. Biochem Biophys Acta 1999;1438:140-6.

68. Youdim KA, Deans SG. Effect of thyme oil and thymol dietary supplementation on the antioxidant status and fatty acid composition of the ageing rat brain. Br J Nutr 2000;83:87-93.

69. Youdim KA, Deans SG. Dietary supplementation of thyme (*Thymus vulgaris* L.) essential oil during the lifetime of the rat: its effects on the antioxidant status in liver, kidney and heart tissues. Mechanisms Aging Dev 1999;109:163-75.

70. Knols G, Stal PC, van Ree JW. Produktieve hoest: tijm of broomhexine? Een dubbelblind gerandomsiseerd ondersoek. Huisarts en Wetenschap 1994;37:392-4.

71. Integrierter Abschlußbericht vom 04.12.1997 für Dentinox Gesellshaft KG, Berlin. Anwendung von Hustagil® Thymian-Hustensaft bei Kindern mit Erkältungskrankheiten der oberen Luftwege oder mit Beschwerden der Bronchitis.

72. Bischoff R, Ismail C, März R, Bischoff G. Exhalations-monitoring mit Online-Analyse Geräten - ppb und sub-ppb Analytik mit neuartigen Sensoren. Biomedizin Technik 1998;43:266-7.

73. Schindler G, Bischoff R, Kohlert C, März R, Ismail C, Veit M et al. Comparison between the concentrations in exhaled air and plasma of an essential oil compound (thymol) after oral administration. In: Abstracts of 3rd International Congress on Phytomedicine. Munich, 11-13 October 2000. *Published as*: Phytomedicine 2000;7(Suppl II):30 (Abstract SL-58).

74. Qureshi S, Shah AH, Al-Yahya MA, Ageel AM. Toxicity of *Achillea fragrantissima* and *Thymus vulgaris* in mice. Fitoterapia 1991;62:319-23.

75. von Skramlik E. Über die Giftigkeit und Verträglichkeit von ätherischen Ölen. Pharmazie 1959;14:435-45.

76. Zani F, Massimo G, Benvenuti S, Bianchi A, Albasini A, Melegari M et al. Studies on the genotoxic properties of essential oils with *Bacillus subtilis* rec-assay and *Salmonella*/microsome reversion assay. Planta Med 1991;57:237-41.

77. Ernst E, März R, Sieder C. A controlled multi-centre study of herbal versus synthetic secretolytic drugs for acute bronchitis. Phytomedicine 1997;4:287-93.

A. *Thymus zygis* oil: its effects on CCl_4-induced hepatotoxicity and free radical scavenger activity. J Essent Oil Res 1993;5:153-8.

TRIGONELLAE FOENUGRAECI SEMEN

Fenugreek

E/S/C/O/P
MONOGRAPHS
Second Edition

DEFINITION

Fenugreek consists of the dried, ripe seeds of *Trigonella foenum-graecum* L.

The material complies with the monograph of the European Pharmacopoeia [1].

CONSTITUENTS

Steroidal saponins, occurring mainly as furostanol 3,26-diglycosides such as trigofoenosides A-G [2-10]. On hydrolysis the saponins yield 0.6-1.7% of spirostanol sapogenins consisting mainly (about 95%) of diosgenin and its 25β-epimer yamogenin in a 3:2 ratio [11-13], together with tigogenin and others [14-16]. Steroidal sapogenin-peptide esters such as fenugreekine are also present [17].

Mucilage polysaccharide, consisting mainly of galactomannan (25-45 %) [2,18,19] with a backbone of β-(1→4)-linked mannose residues, branches of α-(1→6)-galactosyl residues and a small proportion of xylose [2,19].

Other constituents include: trigonelline (= coffearine, the N-methylbetaine of nicotinic acid) [20,21]; protein (rich in tryptophan and lysine); free amino acids, principally 4-hydroxyisoleucine [2,22,23]; saponin-hydrolysing enzymes [24]; proteinase inhibitors which act on human trypsin and chymotrypsin [2,25]; scopoletin and other coumarins [21,26]; flavone glycosides [26,27]; sterols (cholesterol, β-sitosterol) [11]; lecithin and choline [28].

A small amount (< 0.01%) of volatile oil is present, in which alkanes, terpenes, oxygenated and aromatic compounds have been identified [29]. The dominant and characteristic aroma compound in fenugreek is 3-hydroxy-4,5-dimethyl-2(*5H*)-furanone (sotolone), of which 3-25 mg/kg is present in the seeds [22,23].

CLINICAL PARTICULARS

Therapeutic indications

Internal use
Adjuvant therapy in diabetes mellitus [30-37]; anorexia [2,38-40]; as an adjunct to a low fat diet in the treatment of mild to moderate hypercholesterolaemia [29,32,35,39,41-43].

External use
Furunculosis, ulcers, eczema [2,38-40].

Posology and method of administration

Dosage

Internal use
Adults: As adjuvant therapy in diabetes or for hyper-cholesterolaemia, 25 g of powdered seeds or equivalent preparations daily [31,34,37,42,43]; for lack of appetite, 1-6 g of powdered drug up to three times daily with water before meals [2,38,40].

External use
As an emollient, 50 g of powdered seeds boiled in 250 ml of water for 5 minutes then applied as a warm moist poultice [2,38,40].

Method of administration
For oral administration or local application.

Duration of administration
No restriction

Contra-indications
None known.

Special warnings and special precautions for use
Protease inhibitors may still be active in the crude drug; more data are needed to evaluate their lack of toxic effects [2,23].

Interactions with other medicaments and other forms of interaction
The absorption of drugs taken concurrently with fenugreek may be affected by the high mucilaginous fibre content [38,40].

Pregnancy and lactation
Fenugreek should not be used medicinally during pregnancy and lactation [44] since conflicting data have been reported from reproductive toxicity testing in rats [45,46; summarized under Reproductive toxicity].

Low levels of fenugreek are accepted as food flavouring [38,47] and, in this respect, fenugreek has GRAS (Generally Recognized As Safe) status in the USA [48].

Effects on ability to drive and use machines
None known

Undesirable effects
Allergic reactions have been observed in rare cases [2,49].

Overdose
Large doses (e.g. 100 g of fenugreek daily) have been reported to cause minor gastrointestinal symptoms such as diarrhoea and flatulence in 4 out of 10 cases [30,35,41].

PHARMACOLOGICAL PROPERTIES

Fenugreek and its extracts have hypocholesterolaemic, hypoglycaemic, insulin-stimulating and appetite-stimulating effects in animals and humans [2,33,43].

Pharmacodynamic properties

In vitro experiments

Antimicrobial activity
A saponin-rich dry ethanolic extract of fenugreek (drug to extract ratio 9:1) slightly inhibited the growth of fungi (*Candida* sp.) and bacteria (*Escherichia coli*, *Pseudomonas aeruginosa*, *Staphylococcus aureus* and *Streptococcus faecalis*) with a MIC_{50} of 1.25% [50].

A dry ethanolic extract of fenugreek at 100 mg/ml exhibited slight antibacterial activity against *Bordetella bronchiseptica*, *Bacillus cereus*, *B. pumilis*, *B. subtilis*, *Micrococcus flavus*, *Staphylococcus aureus*, *Sarcina lutea*, *E. coli* and *Proteus vulgaris* with inhibition zones of 17-22 mm diameter, compared to 19-32 mm for streptomycin at 1 mg/ml [51].

Furostanol saponins from fenugreek showed no anti-fungal activity but, when transformed by β-glucosidase into spirostanol-type saponins (involving cleavage of glucose at C-26), the latter exhibited strong dose-dependent fungicidal activity against *Rosellinia necatrix*, *Trichoderma viride*, *T. harzianum* (MIC_{50}: 25 µg/ml) and *Candida albicans* (MIC_{50}: 50 µg/ml) [10].

Isolated fenugreekine inhibited replication of *Vaccinia* virus by about 80% when applied at 0.2 mg/ml along with the virus in chorionic allantoic membrane (CAM) cultures [17].

Spasmolytic activity
An aqueous fluid extract (1:1) of fenugreek produced a mild relaxant effect on smooth muscle of isolated rabbit duodenum when applied at 0.5 mg/ml [52].

Mucociliary activity
A decoction from fenugreek showed slight inhibitory activity on mucociliary transport in isolated mucosa from the frog oesophagus [53].

In vivo experiments

Hypocholesterolaemic effects
When fenugreek was added to a hypercholesterol-aemia-inducing diet for rats at levels of 15%, 30% and 60%, faecal excretion of bile acids and cholesterol increased dose-dependently and elevation of serum

cholesterol was strongly inhibited at all levels (p<0.001) [54].

Addition of fenugreek at 30% to the diet of rats fed on a hypercholesterolaemic diet for 4 weeks significantly reduced serum cholesterol, to 210 mg/dl compared to 423 mg/dl in positive control animals (p<0.001). Various fractions (two defatted fractions, a poly-saccharide fraction and crude saponins), in amounts corresponding to 30% of fenugreek, also reduced serum cholesterol to varying extents (p<0.05 for the polysaccharide fraction; p<0.01 for the crude sap-onins), while a lipid fraction and isolated trigonelline had no effect. Serum triglyceride levels were not reduced by fenugreek or the fractions from it. In rats given a hypercholesterolaemic diet for 4 weeks *before* addition of fenugreek at 30%, fenugreek was equally effective in reducing serum cholesterol (p<0.001) [55]. In another study, a dry ethanolic extract from defatted fenugreek added to the diet of hyper-cholesterolaemic rats at 30 g/kg body weight reduced plasma cholesterol levels (p<0.05); the effect was attributed to saponins in the extract [56].

A saponin-rich fraction from fenugreek, given orally to alloxan-diabetic dogs as a dose corresponding to 0.08 g/kg/day of saponins for 21 days, had a significant hypocholesterolaemic effect (p<0.05) similar to that of defatted fenugreek cotyledons. From faecal analysis, about 57% of the saponins had been hydrolysed to sapogenins in the digestive tract of the dogs; smila-genin, diosgenin and gitogenin were detected in the faeces and the sapogenins may have contributed to the hypocholesterolaemic effect [57]. Purified steroid saponins from fenugreek (12.5 mg/day per 300 g body weight for 2-4 weeks) significantly decreased total plasma cholesterol in both normal (p<0.001) and streptozotocin-diabetic (p<0.01) rats without any change in triglycerides [8].

When the soluble gel fraction of fenugreek (consisting mainly of galactomannan) was administered orally to rats, 600 mg was required to reduce starch digestion by 50%, whereas only 80 mg was required to reduce bile salt uptake by 50% [19]. Fenugreek administered orally to rats as a single dose at 50-200 mg/kg also enhanced the total output of bile acids (p<0.05), probably due to increased conversion of cholesterol to bile salts in the liver [58].

Powdered fenugreek added to the diet of normal rats at 2 g/kg and 8 g/kg body weight for 2 weeks signifi-cantly and dose-dependently reduced serum levels of total cholesterol, triglycerides, and LDL- and VLDL-cholesterols (p<0.05 to p<0.01). The same treatment of alloxan-diabetic rats gave similar results and also significantly increased HDL-cholesterol (p<0.05) compared to untreated controls. When roasted seeds were evaluated in these experiments the effects were somewhat less pronounced [9].

Subchronic administration of purified steroid saponins from fenugreek, mixed with food at 12.5 mg/day per 300 g body weight, led to a decrease in total plasma cholesterol in normal (p<0.001) and streptozotocin-diabetic (p<0.01) rats; decreases in VLDL- + LDL-cholesterol (p<0.01) without any change in free cholesterol indicated a reduction in cholesterol esters [10].

Defatted fractions from fenugreek were added to the diet of alloxan-diabetic dogs twice per day for 21 days: a fraction containing 79% of fibre (1.145 g/kg/day) and a fraction containing 22% of saponins (0.365 g/kg/day). The fibre-enriched fraction showed antidiabetic and hypocholesterolaemic activity. The saponin-enriched fraction had a hypolipidaemic effect, reducing elevated cholesterol and triglyceride levels compared to controls [59].

Fenugreek powder as 20%, 30% and 60% of the diet, and three fractions from fenugreek (defatted meal, saponin-free meal or crude saponins; all at levels equivalent to fenugreek seed at 30% of the diet), given for 2 weeks to rabbits pretreated with a high fat diet for 9 weeks, improved plasma lipid profiles. The fenugreek powder and each fraction from it reduced plasma cholesterol and triglyceride levels (p<0.01) with no effect on HDL-cholesterol, and significantly lowered the ratio of plasma total cholesterol to HDL-cholesterol (p<0.01). Compared to fenugreek powder, the crude saponin fraction was the most effective of the 3 extracts and saponin-free meal the least effective [60].

Hypoglycaemic effects
In a glucose tolerance test, a suspension of powdered fenugreek (0.25 g in 5 ml of water) administered once by stomach tube to streptozotocin-induced diabetic rats, reduced postprandial hyperglycaemia [61].

Defatted fenugreek administered orally at 1.86 g/kg body weight daily for 8 days reduced hyperglycaemia in alloxan-diabetic dogs (p<0.05); it also reduced the response to oral glucose in normal dogs (p<0.02) with a decrease in basal levels of plasma glucagon and somatostatin [62]. A fibre-rich fraction from fenu-greek extract (79.4% fibre) induced a reduction in hyperglycaemia (p<0.01) and also exerted hypo-cholesterolaemic effects in alloxan-diabetic dogs [59].

In normal dogs defatted fenugreek (53.9% fibre, 4.8% steroid saponins) added to the diet at 1.86 g/kg daily for 8 days significantly lowered basal levels of blood glucose (p<0.02), plasma glucagon (p<0.01) and plasma cholesterol (p<0.02). Addition of de-fatted seed at this level to the diet of diabetic hypercholesterolaemic dogs similarly decreased cholesterol (p<0.02) and reduced hyperglycaemia (p<0.05) [63].

Isolated trigonelline administered orally to alloxan-diabetic rats at 50 mg/kg body weight had a substantial hypoglycaemic effect, lasting for 24 hours [20]. Coumarin (a minor constituent of fenugreek seeds) at 250 mg/kg and 1 g/kg had a profound hypoglycaemic effect, persisting for at least 24 hours, in alloxan-diabetic and non-diabetic rats but it was toxic at these dose levels [21].

A single 0.5 ml dose of decoctions (1:7.5 or 1:15) from fenugreek, given orally to normal or alloxan-diabetic mice, had dose-dependent hypoglycaemic effects, reaching a maximum after 6 hours (p<0.0005). Hypoglycaemia caused by a dry, ethanolic fenugreek extract (21:1) after oral administration to alloxan-diabetic mice at 200-400 mg/kg was also dose-dependent; the extract at 200 mg/kg had a similar effect to tolbutamide at 200 mg/kg [64].

A decoction of fenugreek (40 g in 300 ml of water) administered intragastrically to fasting rabbits at 4 ml/kg body weight significantly reduced the hyper-glycaemic peak (by17.7%; p<0.01) in a glucose tolerance test [65].

Incorporation of 20% fenugreek into the diet of rats for 2 weeks lowered the peak value of blood glucose by 59% in a starch tolerance test (1 g/kg), whereas no change was observed in a glucose tolerance test [66].

Oral administration of the soluble dietary fibre fraction of fenugreek, composed mainly of galactomannan, to normal and diabetic model (non-insulin-dependent diabetes mellitus, NIDDM) rats at 250 mg/rat had no effect on fasting blood glucose levels, but when fed simultaneously with glucose to the diabetic model rats it had a significant hypoglycaemic effect (p<0.05) [67].

Powdered fenugreek incorporated into their diet for 2 weeks at 2 g/kg or 8 g/kg body weight significantly reduced blood glucose levels in both normal (p<0.05) and alloxan-diabetic (p<0.01) rats compared to untreated controls [68].

Insulin response
A dry hydroethanolic fenugreek extract (12.5% of steroidal saponins, 4.8% of free amino acids), administered orally with food to rats at 10 mg per 300 g body weight daily for 14 days significantly increased plasma insulin levels (p<0.01) compared to controls [69].

Effects on blood lipid peroxidation
Alloxan-diabetic rats were fed on a diet supplemented with fenugreek at 2 g/kg body weight. Biochemical screening after 30 days showed that fenugreek had significantly lowered blood lipid peroxidation (p<0.001), increased plasma glutathione and β-carotene levels and reduced the α-tocopherol level; ascorbic acid was unaltered. The study showed that

disrupted free radical metabolism in diabetic animals may be normalized by fenugreek supplementation [70].

Appetite-stimulating effects
Chronic daily oral administration of a hydroethanolic dry extract of fenugreek seeds (12.5% of saponins, 4.8% free amino acids and 0.002% of the characteristic aromatic compound 3-hydroxy-4,5-dimethyl-2 (5H)-furanone; no protein or lipids) to rats at 10 mg per 300 g body weight for 14 days enhanced food intake by about 20% (p<0.01) and the motivation to eat (p<0.001 on day 14), and was not accompanied by an increase in water intake. The same dose level failed to interact with fenfluramine-induced anorexia, suggesting that serotonergic mechanisms do not play a fundamental role in the observed orexigenic effect. Enhancement of food intake might be related to the aromatic and bitter properties of the seeds. The same extract increased plasma insulin (p<0.01) and reduced total cholesterol (p<0.05) and VLDL-LDL total cholesterol (p<0.05) compared to untreated controls [69].

Purified steroid saponins (12.5 mg/day per 300 g body weight) from fenugreek incorporated into the diet of normal rats significantly increased food intake and the motivation to eat, while modifying the circadian rhythm of feeding behaviour; it also stabilized the food consumption of diabetic rats, resulting in progressive weight gain in these animals in contrast to untreated controls [8,10].

Effect on experimental ulcers
Oral administration of an aqueous fluid extract (1:1) of fenugreek to rats at 1.0 ml/100 g body weight daily for 5 days promoted faster healing of phenylbutazone- and reserpine-induced gastric ulcers compared to controls (p<0.01). The marked demulcent and mild anticholinergic effects of fenugreek may contribute to the rapid healing [52].

Effect on oxalate urolithiasis
Daily oral treatment of rats with fenugreek at 500 mg/kg body weight for 4 weeks significantly decreased the quantity of calcium oxalate deposited in the kidneys (p<0.001) after induction of oxalate urolithiasis by the addition of 3% glycolic acid to the diet [71].

Pharmacological studies in humans
Pharmacological effects of fenugreek studied in humans include effects on blood glucose and/or on blood lipid levels.

In a randomized, crossover study that focused solely on hypolipidaemic effects, 10 apparently healthy, non-obese subjects with asymptomatic hyper-lipidaemia (serum cholesterol > 240 mg/dl) received isocaloric diets for two successive periods of 20 days, the first without and the second with 2 × 50 g daily of debitterized fenugreek powder (free from lipids and saponins). Treatment with fenugreek significantly reduced serum total cholesterol by 24.4%, LDL- and VLDL-cholesterol by 31.7% and triglyceride levels by 37.7% (all p<0.001), while HDL-cholesterol levels were unchanged [41].

In a randomized crossover study, 8 healthy subjects underwent glucose tolerance tests separated by an interval of 1 week, taking 100 g of glucose in 250 ml of water with or without the addition of 25 g of powdered fenugreek. Compared to glucose alone, the addition of fenugreek significantly reduced the rise in plasma glucose after 30 and 60 minutes (p<0.05) and the glucose AUC by 42.4% (p<0.001) [34].

Fenugreek given orally to 30 healthy subjects as 2 × 2.5 g daily for 3 months had no effect on levels of blood lipids or blood sugar (fasting or postprandial) [32].

The germination of fenugreek seeds causes distinct changes with respect to the content of soluble fibre. Germinated fenugreek seed powder was administered to vegetarian volunteers (presumably healthy) with low cholesterol levels in daily amounts of 12.5 g (n = 10) or 18 g (n = 10) for 1 month. Dose-dependent hypocholesterolaemic effects were observed, with significant reductions in plasma total cholesterol and LDL-cholesterol levels in the 18 g group but not in the 12.5 g group. HDL- and VLDL-cholesterol and tri-glyceride levels did not change significantly in either group [72].

Administration of isolated trigonelline, in the amounts present in a therapeutic dose of fenugreek, to diabetic patients did not show any significant hypoglycaemic activity [43] and did not confirm the data in rats [20].

Clinical studies
Hypoglycaemic and hypocholesterolaemic effects of fenugreek have been investigated in both insulin-dependent (type I) and non-insulin-dependent (type II, NIDDM) diabetic subjects and have been reviewed [33,43].

Type I diabetes (insulin-dependent)
Isocaloric diets, with or without the addition of 2 × 50 g daily of debitterized fenugreek powder (free from lipids and saponins), were given to 10 insulin-dependent diabetic patients for periods of 10 days in a randomized, crossover study. An oral glucose tolerance test was performed at the end of each study period. The diet with added fenugreek significantly reduced mean fasting blood glucose levels (p<0.01) and, in the glucose tolerance test, reduced the rise in blood glucose levels at 30, 60 and 90 minutes, thereby significantly reducing the blood glucose AUC (p<0.05). Serum total cholesterol, VLDL- and LDL-cholesterol and triglyceride levels were also significantly reduced, while serum HDL-cholesterol

and insulin levels did not significantly change [30].

Type II diabetes (non-insulin-dependent)
Incorporation of 2 × 12.5 g of debitterized fenugreek powder (free from lipids and saponins) into the meals of 5 non-insulin-dependent diabetic patients daily for 21 days produced a significant improvement in the glucose tolerance test with respect to reduced plasma glucose levels at 0, 30, 60, 120 and 150 minutes (p<0.05) and the glucose AUC (p<0.05); reductions in 24-hour urinary output of glucose (p<0.05) and in serum cholesterol were also observed [34].

In a randomized crossover study, 15 non-insulin-dependent diabetic patients received identical diets with or without the addition of 2 × 50 g of debitterized fenugreek powder (free from lipids and saponins) daily, each for 10 days. Addition of fenugreek to the diet produced a significant fall in fasting blood glucose levels (p<0.01), improved performance in the glucose tolerance test (p<0.01 at 30-120 minutes and for the AUC after glucose load) and 64% reduction in 24-hour urinary glucose excretion (p<0.05). Serum insulin levels were also lower after the fenugreek diet (p<0.05). Significant changes were observed in serum lipids: LDL- and VLDL-cholesterol and triglyceride levels decreased (all p<0.001) without significant change in HDL-cholesterol. In an extension of this study, the same treatment and crossover protocol was followed for 20 days in 5 other non-insulin-dependent (type II) diabetic patients; similar changes, but of higher magnitude, were observed in all parameters [35].

An experimental meal and, separated by an interval of 7 days, the same meal with the addition of 12.5 g of powdered fenugreek was administered to 6 non-insulin-dependent diabetic patients and 6 healthy volunteers. Postprandial blood glucose levels and the glucose AUC showed that fenugreek significantly reduced the glycaemic response (p<0.05) in both groups. A meal containing germinated fenugreek reduced the glycaemic response (p<0.05), but to a lesser extent; boiled fenugreek, with a much lower content of soluble fibre, was largely ineffective [36].

Following a run-in period of 7 days on a prescribed diet, 60 patients with mild, moderate or severe non-insulin-dependent diabetes and a control group of 10 normal subjects included 2 × 12.5 g of powdered fenugreek daily in a similar and isocaloric prescribed diet (at lunch and dinner) for 24 weeks. Inclusion of fenugreek in the diet lowered fasting blood glucose levels, reduced 24-hour urinary sugar excretion (p<0.001) and improved performance in the glucose tolerance test. Insulin levels were also diminished. Glycosylated haemoglobin, measured after 8 weeks of fenugreek treatment, also decreased significantly (p<0.001) [37]. As reported in a separate paper, significant and progressive lipid-lowering effects of fenugreek were also observed in the diabetic patients during this study, with significant reductions in serum total cholesterol, LDL- + VLDL-cholesterol and triglyceride levels (all p<0.001 after 24 months) [42].

Following an overnight fast, 21 non-insulin-dependent diabetic patients consumed a prescribed meal; then 4-7 days later they consumed the same meal to which 15 g of powdered fenugreek had been added. The addition of fenugreek significantly reduced postprandial glucose levels for 2 hours following the meal (p<0.05). No significant effects were observed on cholesterol or triglyceride levels; plasma insulin tended to be lower, but without statistical significance [73].

In a randomized crossover study, 10 non-insulin-dependent diabetic patients consumed isocaloric prescribed diets balanced with respect to carbohydrate, protein and fat content, with or without the daily inclusion of 2 × 12.5 g of powdered fenugreek (and hence more dietary fibre, p<0.001), each for a period of 15 days. Intravenous glucose tolerance tests were performed after each study period; fenugreek treatment significantly reduced mean plasma glucose levels after glucose loading (p<0.05 after 40 minutes; p<0.02 after 60 minutes) and hence the glucose AUC (p<0.05). Furthermore, fenugreek significantly shortened the plasma glucose half-life (p<0.02) due to an increase in its rate of metabolic clearance (p<0.02). There was also a significant increase in erythrocyte insulin receptors (p<0.02). The results suggested that fenugreek can improve peripheral glucose utilization and may exert its hypoglycaemic effect by acting at the insulin receptor as well as at the gastrointestinal level [31].

In a placebo-controlled study, 2 × 2.5 g of fenugreek powder was administered daily for 3 months to 30 non-insulin-dependent diabetics with coronary artery disease (CAD; old, healed myocardial infarction, with or without angina). In comparison with 30 other CAD patients treated with placebo, and with their own baseline values, the patients taking fenugreek had significantly reduced serum total cholesterol and triglyceride levels (both p<0.01 after 3 months vs. baseline) with no significant change in HDL-cholesterol [32]. In the same study, groups of patients with mild (n = 20) or severe (n = 20) type II diabetes but without CAD were given fenugreek powder at the same dose level for 1 month; fasting and postprandial blood sugar levels decreased significantly in the mild NIDDM group (p<0.01) but not in the severe NIDDM group. Remarkably, in the same study, fenugreek given to 30 healthy subjects at 2 × 2.5 g daily for 3 months apparently had no significant effects on blood levels of lipids or glucose (fasting or postprandial) [32].

Diabetes of unspecified type
In an open study, oral administration of 500 mg of

trigonelline produced a transient hypoglycaemic effect for 2 hours in 5 out of 10 fasting diabetic patients; little or no effect was observed in the others. Doubling or quadrupling the dose did not increase the effect and administration of 500-1000 mg of trigonelline three times daily for 5 days did not decrease diurnal blood glucose levels [20].

Pharmacokinetic properties
Trigonelline given orally to cats, dogs and rabbits was excreted unchanged in urine [21].

Preclinical safety data

Acute toxicity
Oral LD_{50} values in rats for constituents of fenugreek have been determined as: 5 g/kg for trigonelline, 3.8 g/kg for scopoletin and 0.72 g/kg for coumarin [21]. The oral LD_{50} of fenugreek absolute (extracted with petroleum ether) in rats was reported as > 5 g/kg [74].

Sub-chronic toxicity
Powdered fenugreek incorporated into the daily diet of rats at levels of 5%, 10% or 20% for 90 days caused no deleterious effects. Weight gain, food intake, haematological parameters and liver enzyme function were comparable to controls and histopathological changes were not significant. Fenugreek appeared to be essentially non-toxic at these dose levels, which equate to at least 1, 2 and 4 times the human therapeutic dose of 25 g/day [43,75].

Daily administration of a saponin-rich ethanolic extract from fenugreek (7.8% saponins) to initially 7-day-old chicks for 21 days, at doses expressed in terms of pure saponins of 10 mg/kg/day intramuscularly, 50 mg/kg/day intraperitoneally or 50 mg/kg/day subcutaneously, caused haemorrhage in the thigh and breast as well as histopathological changes in the liver and kidney [76].

Trigonelline administered orally to rats at 50 mg/kg body weight for 21 days caused no ill-effects. At the same dosage level and duration scopoletin induced minor kidney damage and coumarin inhibited body growth and decreased liver and kidney weight [21].

In spite of the very low toxic potential of fenugreek, proteinase inhibitors occur in the seeds [25] and (in the uncooked state) may still be active and pose a possible toxicological risk. More data are needed to rule this out [2].

Reproductive toxicity
In vitro experiments indicated that aqueous and alcoholic extracts of fenugreek have a stimulating effect on the motility of isolated guinea pig uterus [38,40,77].

Incorporation of fenugreek into the daily diet of pregnant rats at levels of 5% and 20%, corresponding to fenugreek intakes of 890 and 2930 mg/rat/day respectively, for 21 days (commencing on the first day of pregnancy) did not affect pregnancy parameters. The numbers of implantations and resorptions, and placental and fetal weights, were no different from those of control groups [45].

However, in a subsequent study, female rats exhibited high antifertility rates (18% aborted) after daily oral administration of powdered fenugreek at 175 mg/kg body weight, corresponding to about 31.5 mg/rat/day, in days 1-10 of the post-mating period. Teratogenic effects were detected in fetuses in the form of gross, visceral and skeletal anomalies such as everted claw (21% of 44 fetuses examined), inverted claw, shoulder joint defects, kinking of tail (18% of 44 fetuses), neuralpore (18% of 22 fetuses) and non-ossified skull bones (18% of 22 fetuses). The average fetal body weight was 3.15 g compared to 5.36 g in control animals. Remarkably, comparable teratogenic effects were reported from each of the five other traditional herbal drugs investigated in this study: *Asparagus adscendens, Anacyclus pyrethrum, Paeonia officinalis, Mentha arvensis* and *Rosa alba* [46].

The reproductive toxicity data is therefore conflicting. The 1990 study of Sethi et al. [46] reports teratogenic effects, whereas no such effects were observed in the 1986 study of Mital et al. [45], which involved much higher doses of fenugreek (890 or 2930 mg/rat/day as opposed to 31.5 mg/rat/day) and a longer period of administration (21 days versus 10 days). Further studies are needed to clarify these anomalous results.

A dry, crude sapogenin extract from fenugreek (0.6% of steroidal sapogenins; prepared by hydrolysis of defatted seed powder with 2N HCl), administered orally to male rats at 100 mg/day/rat for 60 days, exerted antifertility and antiandrogenic activity. The sperm count and motility of spermatozoa declined significantly (p<0.001) leading to negative fertility tests, and reproductive organ weights and androgen-dependent biochemical parameters in tissues were lower than those of control animals [78].

Clinical safety data
Fenugreek seeds are commonly used as a food flavouring [2,33,38-40,43]. In studies involving the oral administration of fenugreek to a total of 198 subjects at various dosages from 5 g to 100 g per day, only a few subjects experienced minor and reversible adverse effects, mainly in the gastrointestinal tract [30-32,34-35,41,42,73,76,79]; 75 of the subjects received the therapeutic dose of 25 g/day [31,34,42].

No renal or hepatic toxicity and no haematological abnormalities were observed after ingestion of an experimental diet containing 25 g of fenugreek powder daily for 24 weeks by 60 non-insulin-dependent diabetic (NIDDM) patients. Some patients complained of minor gastrointestinal symptoms such as diarrhoea and excess of flatulence, which subsided after 3 to 4 days. A decrease in plasma urea (p<0.05) was interpreted as a protein-sparing effect due to proper utilization of carbohydrate, which then resulted in lower urea levels [43,79].

REFERENCES

1. Fenugreek - Trigonellae foenugraeci semen. European Pharmacopoeia, Council of Europe.

2. Hänsel R, Keller K, Rimpler H, Schneider G, editors. Trigonella. In: Hagers Handbuch der Pharmazeutischen Praxis, 5th ed. Volume 6: Drogen P-Z. Berlin-Heidelberg-New York-London: Springer-Verlag, 1994: 994-1004.

3. Hardman R, Kosugi J, Parfitt RT. Isolation and characterization of a furostanol glycoside from fenugreek. Phytochemistry 1980;19:698-700.

4. Gupta RK, Jain DC, Thakur RS. Furostanol glycosides from *Trigonella foenum-graecum* seeds. Phytochemistry 1984;23:2605-7.

5. Gupta RK, Jain DC, Thakur RS. Furostanol glycosides from *Trigonella foenum-graecum* seeds. Phytochemistry 1985;24:2399-401.

6. Gupta RK, Jain DC, Thakur RS. Two furostanol saponins from *Trigonella foenum-graecum.* Phytochemistry 1986; 25:2205-7.

7. Hardman R. Recent developments in our knowledge of steroids. Planta Med 1987;53:233-8.

8. Petit PR, Sauvaire YD, Hillaire-Buys DM, Leconte OM, Baissac YG, Ponsin GR, Ribes GR. Steroid saponins from fenugreek seeds: Extraction, purification and pharmacological investigation on feeding behavior and plasma cholesterol. Steroids 1995; 60:674-80.

9. Khosla P, Gupta DD, Nagpal RK. Effect of Trigonella foenum graecum (fenugreek) on serum lipids in normal and diabetic rats. Indian J Pharmacol 1995;27:89-93.

10. Sauvaire Y, Baissac Y, Leconte O, Petit P, Ribes G. Steroid saponins from fenugreek and some of their biological properties. Adv Exp Med Biol 1996;405:37-46.

11. Fazli FRY, Hardman R. Isolation and characterization of steroids and other constituents from *Trigonella foenum-graecum.* Phytochemistry 1971;10:2497-503.

12. Hardman R, Brain KR. Variations in the yield of total and individual 25α- and 25β-sapogenins on storage of whole seed of *Trigonella foenum-graecum* L. Planta Med 1972;21:426-30.

13. Bohannon MB, Hagemann JW, Earle FR. Screening

seed of *Trigonella* and three related genera for diosgenin. Phytochemistry 1974;13:1513-4.

14.   Dawidar AM, Saleh AA, Elmotei SL. Steroid sapogenin constituents of fenugreek seeds. Planta Med 1973;24: 367-70.

15.   Knight JC. Analysis of fenugreek sapogenins by gas-liquid chromatography. J Chromatogr 1977;133:222-5.

16.   Gupta RK, Jain DC, Thakur RS. Minor steroidal sapogenins from fenugreek seeds, *Trigonella foenum-graecum*. J Nat Prod 1986;49:1153.

17.   Ghosal S, Srivastava RS, Chatterjee DC, Dutta SK. Fenugreekine, a new steroidal sapogenin-peptide ester of *Trigonella foenum-graecum*. Phytochemistry 1974; 13:2247-51.

18.   Karawya MS, Wassel GM, Baghdadi HH, Ammar NM. Mucilagenous contents of certain Egyptian plants. Planta Med 1980;38:73-8.

19.   Madar Z, Shomer I. Polysaccharide composition of a gel fraction derived from fenugreek and its effect on starch digestion and bile acid absorption in rats. J Agric Food Chem 1990;38:1535-9.

20.   Mishkinsky J, Joseph B, Sulman FG, Goldschmied A. Hypoglycaemic effect of trigonelline. Lancet 1967; 2:1311-2.

21.   Shani (Mishkinsky) J, Goldschmied A, Joseph B, Ahronson Z, Sulman FG. Hypoglycaemic effect of *Trigonella foenum graecum* and *Lupinus termis* (Leguminosae) seeds and their major alkaloids in alloxan-diabetic and normal rats. Arch Int Pharmacodyn 1974;210:27-37.

22.   Girardon P, Sauvaire Y, Baccou J-C, Bessiere J-M. Identification de la 3-hydroxy-4,5-diméthyl-2(5H)-furanone dans l'arôme des graines de fenugrec (*Trigonella foenum graecum* L.). Lebensm-Wiss Technol 1986;19:44-6.

23.   Blank I, Lin J, Devaud S, Fumeaux R, Fay LB. Chapter 3: The principal flavor components of fenugreek (*Trigonella foenum-graecum* L.). In: Risch SJ, Ho CT, editors. Spices - Flavor Chemistry and Antioxidant Properties. ACS Symposium Series 660. Washington DC: American Chemical Society, 1997:12-28.

24.   Elujoba AA, Hardman R. Saponin-hydrolysing enzymes from fenugreek seed. Fitoterapia 1987;58:197-9.

25.   Weder JKP, Haußner K. Inhibitors of human and bovine trypsin and chymotrypsin in fenugreek (*Trigonella foenum-graecum* L.) seeds. Demonstration and purification. Z Lebensm Unters Forsch 1991;192:455-9.

26.   Varshney IP, Sharma SC. Saponins and sapogenins: Part XXXII. Studies on T*rigonella foenum-graecum* Linn. seeds. J Indian Chem Soc 1966:43:564-7.

27.   Wagner H, Iyengar MA, Hörhammer L. Vicenin-1 and -2 in the seeds of *Trigonella foenum-graecum*. Phytochemistry 1973;12:2548.

28.   Yamasaki K, Kikuoka M, Nishi H, Kokusenya Y, Miyamoto T, Matsuo M, Sato T. Contents of lecithin and choline in crude drugs. Chem Pharm Bull 1994; 42:105-7.

29.   Girardon P, Bessiere JM, Baccou JC, Sauvaire Y. Volatile constituents of fenugreek seeds. Planta Med 1985; 51:533-4.

30.   Sharma RD, Raghuram TC, Rao NS. Effect of fenugreek seeds on blood glucose and serum lipids in type I diabetes. Eur J Clin Nutr 1990;44:301-6.

31.   Raghuram TC, Sharma RD, Sivakumar B, Sahay BK. Effect of fenugreek seeds on intravenous glucose disposition in non-insulin dependent diabetic patients. Phytotherapy Res 1994;8:83-6.

32.   Bordia A, Verma SK, Srivastava KC. Effect of ginger (*Zingiber officinale* Rosc.) and fenugreek (*Trigonella foenum-graecum* L.) on blood lipids, blood sugar and platelet aggregation in patients with coronary artery disease. Prostagland Leukotr Essent Fatty Acids 1997; 56:379-84.

33.   Bailey CJ, Day C. Traditional plant medicines as treatments for diabetes. Diabetes Care 1989;12:553-64.

34.   Sharma RD. Effect of fenugreek seeds and leaves on blood glucose and serum insulin responses in human subjects. Nutr Res 1986;6:1353-64.

35.   Sharma RD, Raghuram TC. Hypoglycaemic effect of fenugreek seeds in non-insulin dependent diabetic subjects. Nutr Res 1990;10:731-9.

36.   Neeraja A, Rajyalakshmi P. Hypoglycemic effect of processed fenugreek seeds in humans. J Food Sci Technol 1996;33:427-30.

37.   Sharma RD, Sarkar A, Hazra DK, Mishra B, Singh JB, Sharma SK et al. Use of fenugreek seed powder in the management of non-insulin dependent diabetes mellitus. Nutr Res 1996;16:1331-9.

38.   Barnes J, Anderson LA, Phillipson JD. Fenugreek. In: Herbal Medicines - A guide for healthcare professionals, 2nd ed. London-Chicago: Pharmaceutical Press, 2002: 209-11.

39.   Leung AY, Foster S. Fenugreek. In: Encyclopedia of Common Natural Ingredients used in Food, Drugs, and Cosmetics, 2nd ed. New York: John Wiley, 1996:243-5.

40.   Foenugraeci semen - Bockshornsamen. In: Wichtl M, editor. Teedrogen und Phytopharmaka. Ein Handbuch für die Praxis auf wissenschaftlicher Grundlage, 4th ed. Stuttgart: Wissenschaftliche Verlagsgesellschaft, 2002: 216-9.

41.   Sharma RD, Raghuram TC, Rao VD. Hypolipidaemic effect of fenugreek seeds. A clinical study. Phytotherapy Res 1991;5:145-7.

42.   Sharma RD, Sarkar A, Hazra DK, Misra B, Singh JB, Maheshwari BB, Sharma SK. Hypolipidaemic effect of

fenugreek seeds: a chronic study in non-insulin dependent diabetic patients. Phytotherapy Res 1996; 10:332-4.

43. Al-Habori M, Raman A. Review: Antidiabetic and hypocholesterolaemic effects of fenugreek. Phytotherapy Res 1998;12:233-42.

44. McGuffin M, Hobbs C, Upton R, Goldberg A, editors. *Trigonella foenum-graecum* L. In: American Herbal Products Association's Botanical Safety Handbook. Boca Raton-Boston-London: CRC Press, 1997:117.

45. Mital N, Gopaldas T. Effects of fenugreek (*Trigonella foenum graecum*) seed based diets on the birth outcome in albino rats. Nutr Rep Int 1986;33:363-9.

46. Sethi N, Nath D, Singh RK, Srivastava RK. Antifertility and teratogenic activity of some indigenous medicinal plants in rats. Fitoterapia 1990;61:64-7.

47. Trigonella foenum-graecum L., seeds. In: Flavouring Substances and Natural Sources of Flavourings, 3rd ed. Strasbourg: Council of Europe, 1981:108.

48. Office of the Federal Register. Substances that are generally recognized as safe: Fenugreek. In: Sections 182.10 and 182.20 of the USA Code of Federal Regulations, Title 21, Food and Drugs, Parts 170 to 199. Revised as of April 1, 2000. Washington, DC: National Archives and Records Administration, 2000:445-9.

49. Patil SP, Niphadkar PV, Bapat MM. Allergy to fenugreek (*Trigonella foenum graecum*). Ann Allergy Asthma Immunol 1997;78:297-300.

50. Abbasoglu U, Türköz S. Antimicrobial activities of saponin extracts from some indigenous plants of Turkey. Int J Pharmacogn 1995;33:293-6.

51. Bhatti MA, Khan MTJ, Ahmed B, Jamshaid M, Ahmad W. Antibacterial activity of *Trigonella foenum-graecum* seeds. Fitoterapia 1996;67:372-4.

52. Al-Meshal IA, Parmar NS, Tariq M, Ageel AM. Gastric anti-ulcer activity in rats of *Trigonella foenum-graecum* (Hu-lu-pa). Fitoterapia 1985;56:232-5.

53. Müller-Limmroth W, Fröhlich H-H. Wirkungsnachweis einiger phytotherapeutischer Expektorantien auf den mukoziliaren Transport. Fortschr Med 1980;98:95-101.

54. Sharma RD. Hypocholesterolemic activity of fenugreek (*T. foenum graecum*). An experimental study in rats. Nutr Rep Int 1984;30:221-31.

55. Sharma RD. An evaluation of hypocholesterolemic factor of fenugreek seeds (*T. foenum-graecum*) in rats. Nutr Rep Int 1986;33:669-77.

56. Stark A, Madar Z. The effect of an ethanol extract derived from fenugreek (*Trigonella foenum-graecum*) on bile acid absorption and cholesterol levels in rats. Br J Nutr 1993;69:277-87.

57. Sauvaire Y, Ribes G, Baccou J-C, Loubatières-Mariani M-M. Implication of steroid saponins and sapogenins

in the hypocholesterolemic effect of fenugreek. Lipids 1991;26:191-7.

58. Bhat BG, Sambaiah K, Chandrasekhara N. The effect of feeding fenugreek and ginger on bile composition in the albino rat. Nutr Rep Int 1985;32:1145-51.

59. Ribes G, Da Costa C, Loubatières-Mariani MM, Sauvaire Y, Baccou JC. Hypocholesterolaemic and hypotriglyceridaemic effects of subfractions from fenugreek seeds in alloxan diabetic dogs. Phytotherapy Res 1987; 1:38-43.

60. Al-Habori M, Al-Aghbari AM, Al-Mamary M. Effects of fenugreek seeds and its extracts on plasma lipid profile: a study on rabbits. Phytotherapy Res 1998; 12:572-5.

61. Madar Z. Fenugreek (*Trigonella foenum graecum*) as a means of reducing postprandial glucose level in diabetic rats. Nutr Rep Int 1984;29:1267-73.

62. Ribes G, Sauvaire Y, Baccou J-C, Valette G, Chenon D, Trimble ER, Loubatières-Mariani M-M. Effects of fenugreek seeds on endocrine pancreatic secretions in dogs. Ann Nutr Metab 1984;28:37-43.

63. Valette G, Sauvaire Y, Baccou J-C, Ribes G. Hypocholesterolaemic effect of fenugreek seeds in dogs. Atherosclerosis 1984;50:105-11.

64. Ajabnoor MA, Tilmisany AK. Effect of *Trigonella foenum-graecum* on blood glucose levels in normal and alloxan-diabetic mice. J Ethnopharmacol 1988; 22:45-9.

65. Alarcon-Aguilara FJ, Roman-Ramos R, Perez-Gutierrez S, Aguilar-Contreras A, Contreras-Weber CC, Flores-Saenz JL. Study of the anti-hyperglycemic effect of plants used as antidiabetics. J Ethnopharmacol 1998; 61:101-10.

66. Amin R, Abdul-Ghani A-S, Suleiman MS. Effect of *Trigonella foenum graecum* on intestinal absorption. Diabetes 1987;36:211A (Abstract 798).

67. Ali L, Khan AKA, Hassan Z, Mosihuzzaman M, Nahar N, Nasreen T et al. Characterization of the hypoglycemic effects of *Trigonella foenum graecum* seed. Planta Med 1995;61:358-60.

68. Khosla P, Gupta DD, Nagpal RK. Effect of *Trigonella foenum graecum* (fenugreek) on blood glucose in normal and diabetic rats. Indian J Physiol Pharmacol 1995;39:173-4.

69. Petit P, Sauvaire Y, Ponsin G, Manteghetti M, Fave A, Ribes G. Effects of a fenugreek seed extract on feeding behaviour in the rat: metabolic-endocrine correlates. Pharmacol Biochem Behav 1993;45:369-74.

70. Ravikumar P, Anuradha CV. Effect of fenugreek seeds on blood lipid peroxidation and antioxidants in diabetic rats. Phytotherapy Res 1999;13:197-201.

71. Ahsan SK, Tariq M, Ageel AM, Al-Yahya MA, Shah AH. Effect of *Trigonella foenum-graecum* and *Ammi majus* on calcium oxalate urolithiasis in rats. J Ethnopharmacol 1989;26:249-54.

72. Sowmya P, Rajyalakshmi P. Hypocholesterolemic effect of germinated fenugreek seeds in human subjects. Plant Foods Hum Nutr 1999;53:359-65.

73. Madar Z, Abel R, Samish S, Arad J. Glucose-lowering effect of fenugreek in non-insulin dependent diabetics. Eur J Clin Nutr 1988;42:51-4.

74. Opdyke DLJ. Monographs on fragrance raw materials: Fenugreek absolute. Food Cosmet Toxicol 1978; 16(Suppl):755-6.

75. Udayasekhara Rao P, Sesikeran B, Srinivasa Rao P, Nadamuni Naidu A, Vikas Rao V, Ramachandran EP. Short term nutritional and safety evaluation of fenugreek. Nutr Res 1996;16:1495-505.

76. Nakhla HB, Mohamed OSA, Al Fatuh IMA. The effect of *Trigonella foenum graecum* (fenugreek) crude saponins on Hisex-type chicks. Vet Hum Toxicol 1991; 33:561-4.

77. Abdo MS, Al-Kafawi AA. Experimental studies on the effect of *Trigonella foenum-graecum*. Planta Med 1969;17:14-8.

78. Kamal R, Yadav R, Sharma JD. Efficacy of the steroidal fraction of fenugreek seed extract on fertility of male albino rats. Phytotherapy Res 1993;7:134-8.

79. Sharma RD, Sarkar A, Hazra DK, Misra B, Singh JB, Maheshwari BB. Toxicological evaluation of fenugreek seeds: a long term feeding experiment in diabetic patients. Phytotherapy Res 1996;10:519-20.

URTICAE FOLIUM/HERBA

Nettle Leaf/Herb

DEFINITION

Nettle leaf consists of the dried leaves, and nettle herb of the dried flowering aerial parts, of *Urtica dioica* L., *Urtica urens* L., their hybrids or mixtures of these. The material complies with the Deutsches Arzneibuch (nettle leaf) [1] or the Pharmacopoea Helvetica (nettle herb) [2].

Fresh material may be used provided that when dried it complies with one of the above pharmacopoeias.

A draft monograph intended for the European Pharmacopoeia has been published on nettle leaf [3].

CONSTITUENTS

Caffeic acid esters, principally caffeoylmalic acid in *Urtica dioica* (up to 1.6%) but none in *Urtica urens*; chlorogenic acid (up to 0.5%) and small amounts of neochlorogenic acid and free caffeic acid in both species [4-6].

Flavonoids, principally kaempferol, isorhamnetin, quercetin and their 3-rutinosides and 3-glucosides in the herb [7] and similar flavonol glycosides in the flowers [8].

Minerals (ca. 18% expressed as ash) including potassium (1.8-2.0%) [9,10] and silicon (0.9-1.8%) [11]. The potassium-sodium ratio has been determined as 63:1 in the unprocessed drug [9].

Other constituents include a 13-hydroxyoctadeca-trienoic acid [12], diastereoisomeric 3-hydroxy-α-ionol glucosides [13], scopoletin, sitosterol and its 3-glucoside [14], glycoprotein [15], free amino acids (30 mg/kg) [16] and a relatively high amount of chlorophyll (ca. 2.7%) [14].

Stinging hairs on the leaves contain acetylcholine, histamine, 5-hydroxytryptamine (serotonin) [17,18] and small amounts of leukotrienes [18].

CLINICAL PARTICULARS

Therapeutic indications
Adjuvant in the symptomatic treatment of arthritis, arthroses and/or rheumatic conditions [19-25].

Nettle leaf or herb is also used as a diuretic, for example to enhance renal elimination of water in inflammatory complaints of the lower urinary tract

E/S/C/O/P
MONOGRAPHS
Second Edition

[26-29]. Animal studies have not yet confirmed a diuretic effect after oral administration [30,31] and clinical evidence is limited [32].

Posology and method of administration

Dosage

Internal use
Adults: Hydroalcoholic extracts corresponding to 8-12 g of nettle leaf daily, divided into 2-3 doses [19-23]; 3-5 g of the drug as an infusion up to three times daily [14,26,29,33,34]; tincture 1:5 (25% ethanol) 2-6 ml three times daily [33]; 15 ml of fresh juice up to three times daily [32].

External use
Adults: Fresh nettle leaf applied to the skin in the area of pain for 30 seconds once daily [25].

Method of administration
For oral or topical administration.

Duration of administration
No restriction.

Contra-indications
None known.

Special warnings and special precautions for use
None required.

Interaction with other medicaments and other forms of interaction
None reported.

Pregnancy and lactation
No data available. In accordance with general medical practice, the product should not be used during pregnancy and lactation without medical advice.

Effects on ability to drive and use machines
None known.

Undesirable effects
Gastrointestinal upset or allergic response in a few individuals after oral use [19,20,22-24].

Overdose
No toxic effects reported.

PHARMACOLOGICAL PROPERTIES

Pharmacodynamic properties

In vitro experiments

Anti-inflammatory activity
A nettle leaf hydroethanolic extract (6.4-8:1) and its main phenolic constituent, caffeoylmalic acid, were tested for inhibitory potential on the biosynthesis of arachidonic acid metabolites by rat leukaemic basophilic granulocytes (RBL-1 cells). The extract (0.1 mg/ml) and the isolated acid (1 mg/ml) showed partial inhibitory effects of 20.8% and 68.2% respectively on the 5-lipoxygenase-derived synthesis of leukotriene B_4; caffeoylmalic acid exhibited concentration-dependent activity with an IC_{50} of 85 µg/ml. Both the extract and the acid showed strong concentration-dependent inhibition of the synthesis of cyclooxygenase-derived prostaglandins (IC_{50} of 92 µg/ml for the extract and 38 µg/ml for the acid) [35].

The same extract significantly and dose-dependently reduced lipopolysaccharide (LPS)-stimulated release of two proinflammatory cytokines, tumour necrosis factor-α (TNF-α) and interleukin-1β (IL-1β), in human whole blood from 6 healthy volunteers. After 24 hours, TNF-α concentration was reduced by 50.8 % and IL-1β concentration by 99.7% using the highest tested extract concentration of 5 mg/ml (p<0.001); after 65 hours the inhibition was 38.9% and 99.9% respectively (p<0.001). The extract and LPS stimulated release of interleukin-6 (IL-6) in human blood when used separately, but showed no additive effect when used simultaneously; IL-6 acts antagonistically to IL-1β, decreasing IL-1β-induced PGE_2 synthesis by fibroblasts and synovial cells. Selected constituents of nettle leaf (caffeoylmalic acid, chlorogenic acid, caffeic acid, quercetin and rutin), tested in the same way did not influence the release of TNF-α, IL-1β or IL-6 at concentrations up to 5×10^{-5} mol/litre [36].

Th1 and Th2 cells (T helper cells) have cytokine patterns which regulate cell-mediated and humoral immune responses. Th1 cells produce IL-2 and interferon-γ (IFN-γ), proinflammatory cytokines that induce a cascade of inflammatory responses. Th2 cells produce interleukin-4 (IL-4), IL-5 and IL-10. The cytokine patterns of these Th effector cells are antagonistic and cross-regulated; thus agents that promote Th1 cytokine expression inhibit Th2 cytokine production and vice versa. The water-soluble fraction from a nettle leaf extract (6.4-8.1:1) significantly inhibited phytohaemagglutinin (PHA)-stimulated production of Th1-specific IL-2 (p<0.01) and IFN-γ (p<0.02) in human peripheral blood mononuclear cells (PBMC) in a dose-dependent manner, by 50 ± 32% and 77 ± 14% respectively at the highest concentration tested (equivalent to 400 µg/ml expressed as the total extract). The dose-dependent inhibiting effect on IL-2 and IFN-γ expression was also detected by reverse transcriptase-polymerase chain reaction in PHA-stimulated PBMC. In contrast, the extract fraction enhanced the secretion of Th2-specific IL-4 by PHA-stimulated PBMC, but dose-dependently decreased IL-10 secretion. These results suggest that nettle leaf extract may inhibit the inflammatory cascade in auto-immune diseases such as rheumatoid arthritis [37].

Activation of transcription factor NF-κB is elevated in several chronic inflammatory diseases; in rheumatoid arthritis NF-κB activity is elevated particularly in the synovial lining and endothelial cells. Incubation of HeLa cells with various concentrations of a nettle leaf extract (6.4-8.1:1) before stimulation with tumour necrosis factor (TNF) demonstrated that the extract potently and dose-dependently inhibited the formation of an NF-κB DNA complex and inhibited NF-κB reporter gene activity; in both cases even stronger inhibition was observed with a water-soluble fraction of the extract. Pretreatment with the water-soluble fraction also inhibited NF-κB activation in stimulated Jurkat T, L929 fibrocarcinoma and MonoMac6 cells. Further experiments with stimulated HeLa and Jurkat T cells suggested that the water-soluble fraction of the extract inhibits NF-κB activation not by modification of DNA binding but by preventing the degradation of its inhibitory subunit IκB-α [38].

In an *ex vivo/in vitro* study, 2×670 mg of a nettle leaf extract (6.4-8.1:1) was administered daily for 21 days to 18 healthy volunteers from whom blood samples were taken at 0, 7 and 21 days. Testing of the whole blood samples revealed, in comparison with day 0 values, significant reductions in lipopolysaccharide (LPS)-stimulated release of two cytokines, tumour necrosis factor-α (TNF-α) and interleukin-1β (IL-1β): at day 7 and day 21, release of TNF-α had decreased by 14.6% (p<0.01) and 24.0% (p<0.001), and IL-1β by 19.2% (p<0.01) and 39.3% (p<0.001), respectively. When a water-soluble fraction from the same batch of nettle leaf extract, at various concentrations, was incubated for 24 hours with 0-, 7- and 21-day whole blood samples from the volunteers, concentration-dependent (and time-dependent in the sense of 7- and 21-day samples from the volunteers) inhibition of LPS-induced release of the same cytokines was demonstrated; at the highest concentration of extract fraction (160 μg/ml) incubated with 21-day blood samples, release of TNF-α decreased by 79.5% (p<0.001) and IL-1β by 99.2% (p<0.001) compared to day 0 values of blood untreated with the extract fraction [39].

An extract of nettle herb, prepared as 0.25 mg/ml of a lyophilized aqueous extract in water, produced 93% inhibition of platelet activating factor (PAF)-induced exocytosis of elastase from human neutrophils. The same extract (0.2 mg/ml) showed no activity in a test for inhibition of the biosynthesis of prostaglandins from ^{14}C-arachidonic acid [40].

Articular cartilages contain chondrocytes embedded in a well-developed matrix composed of collagen and proteoglycans. Inflammatory joint diseases are characterized by enhanced extracellular matrix degradation, which is predominantly mediated by cytokine-stimulated upregulation of matrix metalloproteinase (MMP) expression. Besides tumour necrosis factor-α, interleukin-1β produced by articular chondrocytes and synovial macrophages is the most important cytokine stimulating MMP expression under inflammatory conditions. A dry 95%-isopropanolic extract (19-33:1) from nettle leaf and a 13-hydroxyoctadecatrienoic acid (a constituent present in the extract) at 10 μg/ml significantly suppressed interleukin-1β-induced expression of matrix MMP proteins on cultured human chondrocytes: relative expression of MMP-1, MMP-3 and MMP-9 decreased by 63-96% (p = 0.0014 to 0.0057) with the nettle leaf extract and 60-88% (p = 0.0078 to 0.054) with 13-hydroxyoctadecatrienoic acid [12].

Dendritic cells appear to play an important role during the development of rheumatoid arthritis; it has been postulated that dendritic cells present T cells with autoantigens, leading to autoreactivity of T cells in the synovium. In the inflamed joint endothelium is activated. Endothelial cells guide dendritic cells to the inflamed region, where T cells are stimulated; these T cells initiate or enhance the local inflammation, promoting the recruitment of granulocytes and/or macrophages, leading to degradation of the joint. A dry 95%-isopropanolic extract (19-33:1) from nettle leaf exhibited an immunosuppressan effect in preventing the maturation of cultured human myeloid dendritic cells (without affecting their viability), leading to reduced induction of primary T cell responses [41]

Uterine muscle activity
Aqueous extracts of nettle herb produced slight contraction followed by relaxation in isolated uterine smooth muscle from the non-pregnant mouse. Application of the extracts to uterine muscle from the pregnant mouse produced a diametrically opposed effect, increase of muscular tone and contractions of considerable amplitude. The authors concluded that the extracts had adrenolytic activity, similar to the action of dihydroergotamine and inhibiting the effect of adrenaline [42].

In vivo experiments

Diuretic effects
The effects of continuous intravenous perfusion into anaesthetized rats for 1.25 hours of solutions (in isotonic 0.9% saline) of a dry aqueous extract from nettle herb at two dose levels, 4 mg/kg/hour or 24 mg/kg/hour, were compared with the effect of furosemide (as a control diuretic), similarly perfused at 2 mg/kg/hour. Compared to control periods (perfusion of saline only), the nettle herb extracts caused dose-dependent increases in diuresis (urine volume) of 11% and 84% (both p<0.001) and in natriuresis of 28% and 143% (both p<0.001) respectively, while furosemide increased diuresis by 85% and natriuresis by 155% (both p<0.001) [43].

No effect on diuresis or ion excretion could be

demonstrated in rats after oral administration of an aqueous extract of nettle herb at a dose of 1 g/kg body weight [30].

Furthermore, no significant diuretic effect was observed during 2 hours after oral administration to rats of an unspecified ethanolic extract of nettle at 1 g/kg body weight, whereas urinary excretion increased significantly after intraperitoneal administration of 500 mg/kg [31].

Although the potassium-sodium ratio of dried nettle leaf was determined as 63:1, the ratio in a decoction (2 g of dried leaf boiled in 200 ml of deionized water) was found to be much higher at 448:1, the highest ratio in a selection of 8 'official diuretic drugs' investigated [9].

Spontaneous motility

A nettle herb infusion and aqueous extract (3:1) produced dose-dependent reductions in spontaneous motility and body temperature in rats and mice when administered intraperitoneally at doses of 1.739 and 3.748 g/kg body weight for the infusion and 303 and 606 mg/kg for the extract [44]. An aqueous extract of nettle herb at a dose of 750 mg/kg led to a significant reduction in spontaneous activity in mice during the first 16 hours after administration [30].

Hypotensive effects

In the perfusion experiments described above under Diuretic effects [43], the diuretic and natriuretic effects were accompanied by a dose-dependent hypotensive effect. Compared to control periods (perfusion of isotonic 0.9% saline only), perfusion of dry aqueous extract from nettle herb (in isotonic saline) reduced arterial blood pressure by 15% at 4 mg/kg/hour and 38% at 24 mg/kg/hour (both p<0.001), while furosemide at 2 mg/kg/hour reduced arterial blood pressure by 28% (p<0.001). The hypotensive effect was reversible within about 1 hour of recovery after the lower dose of nettle herb extract or furosemide, but was persistent after the higher dose of nettle herb extract, indicating a possible toxic effect at that dose level [43].

Nettle herb produced a rapid but only transient decrease of 31.7% on the blood pressure of anaesthetized rats after intravenous administration of an aqueous extract at a dose of 25 mg/kg body weight [30]. In cats, an aqueous extract (3.3:1) administered by cannula at a dose of 26.6 mg/kg body weight produced a marked hypotensive effect and bradycardia, which was not compensated by subsequent administration of adrenaline [45].

Hyperglycaemic activity

Both an 80%-ethanolic extract and an aqueous decoction of nettle herb, evaporated to dryness, resolubilized and administered to mice at the equivalent of 25 g drug/kg body weight 2 hours prior to glucose load, produced hyperglycaemic effects in an oral glucose tolerance test [46].

Analgesic activity

After administration of nettle herb aqueous extract at a dose of 1200 mg/kg, mice showed much greater resistance to thermal stimulation in the hot plate test at 55°C, taking 190% longer time to react than control animals [30]. On the other hand, no analgesic activity was noted in the hot plate test after oral or intraperitoneal administration to rats of an unspecified ethanolic extract of nettle, although this extract reduced the writhing response to phenylquinone in rats after oral (1 g/kg) and intraperitoneal (500 mg/kg) treatment [31].

Local anaesthetic activity

Local application to the rat tail of 0.05 ml of nettle herb aqueous extract (100 mg lyophilized extract per ml), in the same region as subsequent application of heat in the tail flick test, produced a local anaesthetic effect comparable to that of lignocaine [30].

Clinical studies

Adjuvant treatment of arthritis, arthroses and/or rheumatic conditions

Five open, multicentric, post-marketing surveillance studies have been carried out on patients with arthritic or rheumatic complaints using a preparation containing a dry hydroethanolic extract of nettle leaf (6.4-8:1) at a daily dosage of 2 × 670 mg (corresponding to 9.648 g of dried leaf per day). In each study a proportion of the patients also continued other therapies, primarily non-steroidal anti-inflammatory drugs (NSAIDs), while others received only the nettle leaf extract. Assessments were carried out through patient questionnaires and consultations with physicians. Overall, 80-95% of patients rated the efficacy of the extract, and 93-95% its tolerability, as good or very good [19-23]:

- 152 patients with rheumatic pains, of whom about 60% had degenerative disorders of joints, were treated in a 3-week study. Pain symptoms assessed by a visual analogue scale (VAS) improved in 70% of patients by at least one third: pain at rest by 50%, movement pain by 51%. In patients receiving only nettle leaf extract (n = 12) pain decreased by 43% [19].

- 219 patients, mainly with degenerative or inflammatory joint disorders, were treated in another 3-week study. Pain symptoms (VAS) improved by at least one-third in 70% of patients; in patients with pain of degenerative origin by about 50%. Patients taking only nettle leaf extract found it as effective as the extract + NSAIDs [20].

- 223 patients with arthritis (over 50% gonarthritis, 34% coxarthritis) were treated in a 6-week study. Pain intensity (VAS) decreased by 56% and objective assessment of all findings on joints (reddening, overheating, swelling, pressure pain and joint discharge) improved by 60-65% on average. A reduction in complaint symptomatic of at least 33% from initial values was experienced by 75% of the patients and this was reflected in patients' responses to a Quality of Life questionnaire. Out of the 130 patients initially taking concomitant NSAIDs, 106 (81%) reduced or discontinued their NSAID dosage [21].

- 8955 patients suffering pain and impairment of mobility due to osteoarthritis or rheumatoid arthritis were treated in a 3-week study. The total symptom scores (1-5 point scales for pain at rest, exercise pain and restricted mobility) of 96% of patients decreased by 45% on average and no clinically relevant differences in efficacy were evident between the group taking only the extract compared to those continuing with NSAIDs or other therapy. 64% of those patients who initially continued NSAID treatment reduced (38%) or discontinued (26%) their NSAID dosage later in the study [22]

- 819 patients with gonarthritis were treated in a 12-month study. Symptoms such as pain, joint stiffness and impaired joint function, assessed by a quantitative gonarthritis-specific questionnaire, decreased by 61% on average. The frequency of each of 5 symptoms (swelling, pressure pain, reddening, joint discharge and overheating) decreased significantly (p<0.001) [23].

In an open, randomized 14-day study, patients with acute arthritis received daily either 2 × 100 mg of diclofenac (n = 17) or 50 mg of diclofenac and 50 g of a prepacked stewed nettle leaf purée (water content 95.5%, caffeoylmalic acid content 20 mg) (n = 19). Both groups also received the gastroprotective misoprostol (a prostaglandin analogue). The main criterion of the study was relative improvement in elevated serum levels of C-reactive protein, which decreased by about 70% in both groups. Assessments (verbal rating score 0-4) of physical impairment, subjective pain and pressure pain by patients, and stiffness by physicians, showed improvements in the range 52-77%, with no significant differences between the two groups [24].

An exploratory study was carried out on the alleviation of pain by external application of fresh nettle leaves, which causes urtication. From analysis of recorded, semi-structured interviews between a doctor and 18 people who had tried this self-treatment for joint or muscle pains, 15 out of 18 claimed that nettle treatment worked on every application; 17 out of 18 reported pain relief after the first course of treatment and had found no other treatment as effective as nettle leaf. Onset of pain relief occurred in less than 24 hours in 11 out of 18 patients. The stinging sensation was reported by 14 out of 18 as 'not painful, with a not unpleasant warmth' and, other than 3 cases of localised numbness for 6-24 hours and a few rashes, no side effects were reported [47].

Subsequently a randomized, double-blind, crossover study was carried out involving 27 patients with persistent osteoarthritic pain at the base of the thumb or index finger, none of whom had previously used nettle leaf as a treatment. Existing analgesic or anti-inflammatory treatments were continued during the study. A fresh leaf from pot-grown, non-flowering *Urtica dioica* or *Lamium album* (white deadnettle, as a placebo of similar appearance), handled through plastic, was applied to the affected area once daily for 30 seconds in a standard manner. One week of treatment was followed by a wash-out period of 5 weeks before one week of the alternative treatment. Compared to placebo, significantly greater reductions in scores were observed with nettle leaf on a visual analogue scale for pain (p = 0.026) and the Stanford health assessment questionnaire for disability (p = 0.0027). No serious side affects were reported and the localized rash and itching associated with nettle leaf was acceptable to 23 of the 27 patients [25].

Diuretic effects
In an open 2-week study, 32 patients suffering from myocardial or chronic venous insufficiency were treated daily with 3 × 15 ml of nettle herb pressed juice. A significant increase in the daily volume of urine was observed throughout the treatment, the volume in day 2 being 9.2% higher (p<0.0005) than the baseline amount in patients with myocardial insufficiency and 23.9% higher (p<0.05) in those with chronic venous insufficiency. Minor decreases in body weights (about 1%) and systolic blood pressure were also observed. Serum parameters were unaffected and the treatment was well tolerated apart from a tendency towards diarrhoea [32].

Pharmacokinetic properties
No data available.

Preclinical safety data
The intraperitoneal LD_{50} of an aqueous extract of *Urtica dioica* herb in mice has been determined as 3.625 g/kg body weight [30].

An ethanolic extract of *Urtica dioica* herb showed low toxicity in both rats and mice after oral and intra-peritoneal administration at the equivalent of up to 2 g of dried drug per kg body weight [31].

Clinical safety data

No serious adverse effects were reported from 5 clinical studies in which a total of 10,368 patients took 2 × 670 mg of a dry hydroethanolic extract of nettle leaf (6.4-8:1), corresponding to about 9.7 g of dried leaf, daily for periods varying from 3 weeks to 12 months; the incidence of minor adverse effects (mainly gastrointestinal upsets or allergic reactions) was 1.2-2.7% [19-23]. In a study where 19 patients received 50 g of a stewed nettle leaf purée daily for 14 days, 3 patients reported meteorism [24].

REFERENCES

1. Brennesselblätter - Urticae folium. Deutsches Arzneibuch.

2. Urticae herba - Ortie, Brennesselkraut, Ortica. Pharmacopoea Helvetica.

3. Nettle Leaf - Urticae folium. Pharmaeuropa 2002; 14:142-4.

4. Bauer R, Holz A, Chrubasik S. Kaffeoyläpfelsäure als Leitsubstanz in Brennesselzubereitungen. In: Chrubasik S, Wink M, editors. Rheumatherapie mit Phytopharmaka. Stuttgart: Hippokrates Verlag, 1997:112-20.

5. Schomakers J, Bollbach FD, Hagels H. Brennesselkraut. Phytochemische und anatomische Unterscheidung der Herba-Drogen von Urtica dioica und U. urens. Dtsch Apoth Ztg 1995:135;578-84.

6. Budzianowski J. Caffeic acid esters from Urtica dioica and U. urens. Planta Med 1991;57:507.

7. Ellnain-Wojtaszek M, Bylka W, Kowalewski Z. Zwiazki flawonoidowe w Urtica dioica L. [Flavonoid compounds in Urtica dioica L.]. Herba Pol 1986;32:131-7 and Chem Abstr 1988;109:146304.

8. Chaurasia N, Wichtl M. Flavonolglykoside aus Urtica dioica. Planta Med 1987;53:432-4.

9. Szentmihályi K, Kéry Á, Then M, Lakatos B, Sándor Z, Vinkler P. Potassium-sodium ratio for the characterization of medicinal plant extracts with diuretic activity. Phytotherapy Res 1998;12:163-6.

10. Lutomski J, Speichert H. Die Brennessel in Heilkunde und Ernährung. Pharm unserer Zeit 1983;12:181-6.

11. Piekos R, Paslawska S. Studies on the optimum conditions of extraction of silicon species from plants with water. V. Urtica dioica. Planta Med 1976;30:331-6.

12. Schulze-Tanzil G, de Sousa P, Behnke B, Klingelhoefer S, Scheid A, Shakibaei M. Effects of the antirheumatic remedy Hox alpha - a new stinging nettle leaf extract - on matrix metalloproteinases in human chondrocytes in vitro. Histol Histopathol 2002;17:477-85.

13. Neugebauer W, Winterhalter P, Schreier P. 3-Hydroxy-

14. α-ionyl-β-D-glucopyranosides from stinging nettle (Urtica dioica L.) leaves. Nat Prod Lett 1995;6:177-80.

14. Wichtl M, Grimm U. Brennesselblätter - Urticae folium. In: Hartke K, Hartke H, Mutschler E, Rücker G, Wichtl M, editors. Kommentar zum Deutschen Arzneibuch. Stuttgart: Wissenschaftliche Verlagsgesellschaft, 2000 (13. Lfg):B 53.

15. Andersen S, Wold JK. Water-soluble glycoprotein from Urtica dioica leaves. Phytochemistry 1978;17:1875-7.

16. Lapke C, Nündel M, Wendel G, Schilcher H, Riedel E. Concentrations of free amino acids in herbal drugs. Planta Med 1993;59(Suppl):A627.

17. Collier HOJ, Chesher GB. Identification of 5-hydroxytryptamine in the sting of the nettle (Urtica dioica). Brit J Pharmacol 1956;11:186-9.

18. Czarnetzki BM, Thiele T, Rosenbach T. Immunoreactive leukotrienes in nettle plants (Urtica urens). Int Arch Allergy Appl Immunol 1990;91:43-6.

19. Ramm S, Hansen C. Brennessel-Extrakt bei rheumatischen Beschwerden. Dtsch Apoth Ztg 1995; 135 (39, Suppl.):3-8.

20. Hansen C. Brennesselblätter-Extrakt wirksam bei Arthroseschmerzen. Aktuelle Ergebnisse einer multizentrischen Anwendungsbeobachtung mit Rheuma-Hek. Der Allgemeinarzt 1996:654-7. Also published in different format as: Sommer R-G, Sinner B. IDS 23 in der Rheuma-Therapie. Kennen Sie den neuen Zytokinantagonisten? Therapiewoche 1996;46:44-9.

21. Ramm S, Hansen C. Arthrose: Brennesselblätter-Extrakt IDS 23 spart NSAR ein. Jatros Ortho 1997;12:29-33.

22. Ramm S, Hansen C. Brennesselblätter-Extrakt: Wirksamkeit und Verträglichkeit bei Arthrose und rheumatoider Arthritis. In: Chrubasik S, Wink M, editors. Rheumatherapie mit Phytopharmaka. Stuttgart: Hippokrates Verlag, 1997:97-106. Interim data published as: Ramm S, Hansen C. Brennesselblätter-Extrakt bei Arthrose und rheumatoider Arthritis. Multizentrische Anwendungsbeobachtung mit Rheuma-Hek. Therapiewoche 1996;28:1575-8.

23. Wolf F. Gonarthrose. Brennesselblätter-Extrakt IDS 23 in der Langzeitanwendung. Der Kassenarzt 1998;44:52-4.

24. Enderlein W, Chrubasik S, Conradt C, Grabner W. Untersuchungen zur Wirksamkeit von Brennesselmus bei akuter Arthritis. In: Chrubasik S, Wink M, editors. Rheumatherapie mit Phytopharmaka. Stuttgart: Hippokrates Verlag, 1997:107-11. Also published as: Chrubasik S, Enderlein W, Bauer R and Grabner W. Evidence for antirheumatic effectiveness of Herba Urticae dioicae in acute arthritis: A pilot study. Phytomedicine 1997;4:105-8.

25. Randall C, Randall H, Dobbs F, Hutton C, Sanders H. Randomized controlled trial of nettle sting for treatment

of base-of-thumb pain. J Royal Soc Med 2000;93:305-9.

26. Schilcher H. Brennesselkraut (Urticae herba DAC). In: Phytotherapie in der Urologie. Stuttgart: Hippokrates Verlag, 1992:20-1.

27. Schilcher H. *Urtica*-Arten - Die Brennessel. Z Phytotherapie 1988;9:160-4.

28. Czygan F-C, Hiller K. Urticae folium/herba - Brennesselblätter/-kraut. In: Teedrogen und Phytopharmaka. Ein Handbuch für die Praxis auf wissenschaftlicher Grundlage, 4th ed. Stuttgart: Wissenschaftliche Verlagsgesellschaft, 2002:617-9.

29. Jaspersen-Schib R. Die Brennessel - eine Modedroge - oder mehr? Schweiz Apoth Ztg 1989;127:443-5.
Also published in French as:
Jaspersen-Schib R. L'ortie, drogue à la mode ou mieux que cela? Schweiz Apoth Ztg 1991;129:11-3.

30. Lasheras B, Turillas P, Cenarruzabeitia E. Étude pharmacologique préliminaire de *Prunus spinosa* L., *Amelanchier ovalis* Medikus, *Juniperus communis* L. et *Urtica dioica* L. Plantes Méd Phytothér 1986;20:219-26.

31. Tita B, Faccendini P, Bello U, Martinoli L, Bolle P. *Urtica dioica* L.: Pharmacological effect of ethanol extract. Pharmacol Res 1993;27(Suppl 1):21-2.

32. Kirchhoff HW. Brennesselsaft als Diuretikum. Z Phytotherapie 1983;4:621-6.

33. Urtica. In: British Herbal Pharmacopoeia 1983. Bournemouth: British Herbal Medicine Association, 1983:224-5.

34. Van Hellemont J. Fytotherapeutisch Compendium. 2nd ed. Utrecht: Bohn, Scheltema & Holkema, 1988:625.

35. Obertreis B, Giller K, Teucher T, Behnke B, Schmitz H. Antiphlogistische Effekte von Extraktum Urticae dioicae foliorum im Vergleich zu Kaffeoyläpfelsäure. Arzneim-Forsch/Drug Res 1996;46:52-6.

36. Obertreis B, Ruttkowski T, Teucher T, Behnke B, Schmitz H. Ex-vivo in-vitro inhibition of lipopolysaccharide stimulated tumor necrosis factor-a and interleukin-1β secretion in human whole blood by Extractum Urticae dioicae foliorum. Arzneim-Forsch/Drug Res 1996; 46:389-94. Errata *ibid* 1996;46:936.

37. Klingelhoefer S, Obertreis B, Quast S, Behnke B. Antirheumatic effect of IDS 23, a stinging nettle leaf extract, on *in vitro* expression of T helper cytokines. J Rheumatol 1999;26:2517-22.

38. Riehemann K, Behnke B, Schulze-Osthoff K. Plant extracts from stinging nettle (*Urtica dioica*), an antirheumatic remedy, inhibit the proinflammatory transcription factor NF-κB. FEBS Letters 1999;442:89-94.

39. Teucher T, Obertreis B, Ruttkowski T, Schmitz H. Zytokin-Sekretion im Vollblut gesunder Probanden nach oraler Einnahme eines *Urtica dioica* L.-Blattextraktes. Arzneim-Forsch/Drug Res 1996;46:906-10.

40. Tunón H, Olavsdotter C, Bohlin L. Evaluation of anti-inflammatory activity of some Swedish medicinal plants. Inhibition of prostaglandin biosynthesis and PAF-induced exocytosis. J Ethnopharmacol 1995;48:61-76.

41. Broer J, Behnke B. Immunosuppressant effect of IDS 30, a stinging nettle leaf extract, on myeloid dendritic cells *in vitro*. J Rheumatol 2002;29:659-66.

42. Broncano FJ, Rebuelta M, Lazaro-Carrasco MJ, Vivas JM. Estudio del efecto sobre musculatura lisa uterina de distintos preparados de las hojas de *Urtica dioica* L. An Real Acad Farm 1987;53:69-75.

43. Tahri A, Yamani S, Legssyer A, Aziz M, Mekhfi H, Bnouham M, Ziyyat A. Acute diuretic, natriuretic and hypotensive effects of a continuous perfusion of aqueous extract of *Urtica dioica* in the rat. J Ethnopharmacol 2000;73:95-100.

44. Broncano J, Rebuelta M, Vivas JM, Diaz MP. Estudio de diferentes preparados de *Urtica dioica* L sobre SNC. An Real Acad Farm 1987;53:284-91.

45. Broncano FJ, Rebuelta M, Vivas JM, Gomez-Serranillos M. Étude de l'effet sur le centre cardiovasculaire de quelques préparations de l'*Urtica dioica* L. Plant Méd Phytothér 1983;17:222-9.

46. Neef H, Declercq P, Laekeman G. Hypoglycaemic activity of selected European plants. Phytotherapy Res 1995;9:45-8.

47. Randall C, Meethan K, Randall H, Dobbs F. Nettle sting of *Urtica dioica* for joint pain - an exploratory study of this complementary therapy. Complement Therap Med 1999;7:126-31.

URTICAE RADIX

Nettle Root

E/S/C/O/P
MONOGRAPHS
Second Edition

DEFINITION

Nettle root consists of the whole, cut or powdered, dried roots and rhizomes of *Urtica dioica* L., *Urtica urens* L., their hybrids or mixtures of these.

The material complies with the Deutsches Arzneibuch [1].

CONSTITUENTS

Urtica dioica agglutinin (UDA), approx. 0.1% [2-9], a lectin which can be separated into 6 isolectins [3] and which contains 86 amino acid residues [9]; a mixture of polysaccharides, basically 2 glucans, 2 rhamnogalacturonans and 1 arabinogalactan [7,10,11]; scopoletin [12-14]; β-sitosterol [12-14], β-sitosterol glucoside [13,14] and other sterols and sterol glucosides [14,15]; phenylpropanes (homovanillyl alcohol and its glucoside) [14,16]; lignans such as (+)-neo-olivil and its derivatives [14,16,17], (–)-secoisolariciresinol [18,19], (–)-isolariciresinol and dehydrodiconiferyl alcohol [19], and lignan glucosides [16,20,21]; ceramides [22]; hydroxy fatty acids including (10*E*,12*Z*)-9-hydroxy-10,12-octadecadienoic acid [23] and the isomeric 9,10,13-trihydroxy-11-octadecenoic and 9,12,13-trihydroxy-10-octadecenoic acids [18]; and monoterpene diols and their glucosides [24].

CLINICAL PARTICULARS

Therapeutic indications
Symptomatic treatment of micturition disorders (dysuria, pollakisuria, nocturia, urine retention) in benign prostatic hyperplasia (BPH) [25-50] at stages I and II as defined by Alken [51] or stages II and III as defined by Vahlensieck [50].

Posology and method of administration

Dosage

Daily dose: 4-6 g of the drug as an infusion [48,49]; 300-600 mg of dried native extract (7-14:1, 20% V/V methanol) [25-38] or 378-756 mg of dried native extract (12-16:1, 70% V/V ethanol) [39]; 4.5-7.5 ml of fluid extract (1:1, 45% ethanol) [41] or 15 ml of fluid extract (1:5, 40% ethanol) [42]; comparable extracts at equivalent dosages.

Method of administration
For oral administration.

Stages of Benign Prostatic Hyperplasia as defined by Alken [51]	Stages of Benign Prostatic Hyperplasia as defined by Vahlensieck [50]
Stage I Dysuria, pollakisuria, possibly nocturia, reduction in projection of the urine stream, no residual urine (stage of compensation of the bladder musculature).	**Stage I** No micturition problems More or less marked BPH Urine stream: greater than 15 ml/s maximal flow No residual urine No bladder trabeculation
Stage II Same symptomatic as under I, except with residual urine (incipient decompensation of the bladder musculature).	**Stage II** Intermittent micturition problems (frequency, calibre of urine stream) More or less marked BPH Urine stream: between 10 and 15 ml/s maximal flow No or low (≤50 ml) residual urine No or incipient bladder trabeculation
Stage III Complete stoppage or overflow of the bladder (decompensation of the bladder musculature).	**Stage III** Permanent micturition problems (frequency, calibre of urine stream) More or less marked BPH Urine stream: less than 10 ml/s maximal flow Residual urine more than 50 ml Trabeculated bladder
	Stage IV Permanent micturition problems (frequency, calibre of urine stream) More or less marked BPH Urine stream: less than 10 ml/s maximal flow Residual urine more than 100 ml Overflowing bladder Stoppage of the upper urinary tract

Duration of administration
No restriction.

Contra-indications
None known.

Special warnings and special precautions for use
All cases of difficulty in micturition require clarification by a physician and regular medical checks in order to rule out the need for other treatment, e.g. surgical intervention. Consultation with a physician is particularly necessary in cases of blood in the urine or acute urine retention.

Interaction with other medicaments and other forms of interaction
None reported.

Pregnancy and lactation
Not applicable.

Effects on ability to drive and use machines
None known.

Undesirable effects
Gastrointestinal complaints [29,33,27,39,40]. Rare cases of allergic skin reactions [28].

Overdose
No toxic effects reported.

PHARMACOLOGICAL PROPERTIES

Pharmacodynamic properties

There are four main hypotheses about the pathogenesis of BPH:

Sex hormones
Data relating to dihydrotestosterone (DHT) concentrations in normal and hyperplastic prostates are contradictory. Originally it was assumed that higher levels of sexual hormones in hyperplastic prostate tissue play an etiologic role in the development of BPH. Results from modern methodology show that DHT concentrations in BPH tissue are unchanged or

even lower than in normal tissue [52,53].

Growth factors
The transformation of stroma cells into embryonal cells, known as "embryonal reawake", is a possible cause of BPH. The involvement of transforming growth factors (TGF β) and basic fibroblast growth factors (bFGF) in this process is under discussion [54]. The presence of receptors for epidermal growth factor (EGF) is also associated with the development of BPH [55]. Therapy could consist of reducing the binding of these growth factors to smooth muscle cells of the prostate, thus inhibiting the growth of stroma cells [56].

Sex hormone binding globulin (SHBG)
Increased binding capacity of sex hormone binding globulin (SHBG) to testosterone and dihydro-testosterone results in hyperplasia, as a compensation for the decrease in hormones and an increase in 5α-reductase activity [57,58]. Therapy could consist of a reduction in SHBG binding capacity for androgens. Although this hypothesis seems to be the most probable, the mechanism is still unknown and many biochemical pathways seem to play a role in BPH [43,48,59].

Prostaglandins and leukotrienes
An increased concentration of prostaglandins and leukotrienes is another possible cause of BPH. Therapy could consist of an inhibition of eicosanoid metabolism by inhibiting phospholipase, prostaglandin synthetase and/or lipoxygenase [48,59,60].

In vitro experiments
Significant suppression (average 67%) of SHBG binding capacity by a 10% solution of a 20% metha-nolic extract of nettle root has been demonstrated. It appears that the binding of 5α-dihydrotestosterone to proteins can be influenced by the extract [58]. An aqueous extract of nettle root dose-dependently inhibited the binding of SHBG to solubilized receptors from human prostatic tissue; in the same experiment neither a 70% ethanolic extract of nettle root nor *Urtica dioica* agglutinin were effective [61].

The lignan secoisolariciresinol and a mixture of isomeric (11*E*)-9,10,13-trihydroxy-11-octadecenoic and (10*E*)-9,12,13-trihydroxy-10-octadecenoic acids isolated from nettle root reduced the binding activity of human SHBG; methylation of the mixed hydroxy acids increased their activity by about 10-fold [18].

(10*E*,12*Z*)-9-hydroxy-10,12-octadecadienoic acid isolated from an aqueous-methanolic extract of nettle root inhibited aromatase activity [23,62]. On the other hand, aromatase inhibition by five other compounds isolated from a methanolic extract of nettle root was only weak (less than 1% compared to 4-hydroxy-androst-4-ene-3,17-dione) [63].

A polysaccharide fraction from an aqueous extract of nettle root showed activity in the lymphocyte trans-formation test. Isolated polysaccharides produced significant, concentration-dependent reduction of haemolysis (95% reduction at 1 mg/ml) in classical and alternative complement tests. From these results anti-inflammatory and immunomodulating activities were deduced [7,64,65]. Lectin fractions from *Urtica dioica* agglutinin stimulated the proliferation of human lymphocytes in the lymphocyte transformation test [7,64].

Organic solvent extracts of nettle root inhibited Na+, K+-ATPase activity of human BPH tissue cells by 28-82% at 0.1 mg/ml/ml. Steroidal compounds from nettle root, such as stigmast-4-en-3-one, stigmasterol and campesterol, inhibited the enzyme activity by 23.0-67.0% at concentrations from 10^{-3} to 10^{-6} M. These results suggest that some hydrophobic constituents such as steroids inhibit the membrane Na+, K+-ATPase activity of the prostate, which may subsequently suppress prostate-cell metabolism and growth [66].

A lectin fraction from *Urtica dioica* agglutinin inhibited by 53% the binding of epidermal growth factor (EGF) to EGF receptors in cells cultured from human prostatic tissue [7]. The growth of cells cultured from human BPH tissue was significantly inhibited by 5 different fractions from a 20% methanolic extract of nettle root [67]. *Urtica dioica* agglutinin at 500 ng/ml to 100 μg/ml dose-dependently inhibited the binding of ^{125}I-labelled EGF to its receptor on human A431 epiderm-oid cancer cells [68].

Lignans present in polar extracts of nettle root, (+)-neo-olivil, (–)-secoisolariciresinol, dehydrodiconiferyl alcohol, isolariciresinol and (–)-3,4-divanillyltetra-hydrofuran, as well as the main intestinal metabolites of plant lignans in humans (enterodiol, enterolactone and enterofuran), showed binding affinity to human SHBG. Outstandingly high affinity was exhibited by (–)-3,4-divanillyltetrahydrofuran, which is present only in traces in nettle root [19].

A 20% methanolic extract of nettle root significantly ($p<0.05$), and time- and concentration-dependently, inhibited the proliferation of human prostatic epithelial LNCaP (lymph node carcinoma of the prostate) cells; maximum growth reduction of 30% was obtained on day 5 at a concentration of 10^{-6} mg/ml. In contrast, the extract had no antiproliferative effect on human prostatic stromal cells [69]. Comparable inhibition ($p<0.05$) of proliferation of human epithelial LNCaP cells by a polysaccharide-rich fraction (POLY M) of the same extract was observed over a 7-day period. Again, the inhibition was time- and concentration-dependent, with maximum suppression of 50% on day 6 at concentrations of 10^{-9} and 10^{-11} mg/ml [70]. No cytotoxic effects of the extract [69] or the fraction

POLY-M [70] on cell proliferation were observed.

Nettle root extract inhibited cell proliferation in cultures of prostate tissue taken from BPH patients [71].

It has been shown that *Urtica dioica* agglutinin binds to the cell membrane of prostatic adenoma cells from BPH patients [72] and can inhibit the action of growth factors involved in the regulation of prostate growth [73].

In vivo experiments
10 dogs suffering from BPH, treated daily for 100 days with 90 mg of a nettle root extract (3.5-7:1, 20% V/V methanol) per kg body weight, showed an average decrease of 30% in prostate volume [74]. The same extract did not inhibit testosterone and dihydro-testosterone stimulated growth of the prostate in castrated rats [75].

A crude aqueous fraction from nettle root containing 4 different polysaccharides, administered orally at 40 mg/kg, significantly inhibited carrageenan-induced rat paw oedema by 36.8% after 5 hours (p<0.01) and 63.6% after 22 hours (p<0.005). This anti-inflammatory activity was comparable after 5 hours, and markedly superior after 22 hours, to that exhibited by indo-metacin at 10 mg/kg (42.1% and 27.3% inhibition respectively) [10,11,64].

In a BPH model involving implantation of mouse fetal urogenital sinus tissue into the ventral prostate glands of adult male mice, a 20% methanolic extract of nettle root administered orally for 28 days reduced experimentally-induced prostate growth by 51.3%, compared to 26.5% by an aqueous extract [76]. In the same model, a polysaccharide-rich fraction (POLY-M) from the 20% methanolic extract reduced prostate growth by 33.8% whereas *Urtica dioica* agglutinin increased prostate growth by 20.1% and secoisolarici-resinol by 37.2% [77].

Pharmacological studies in humans
31 men aged between 58 and 82 years with BPH at stages I to II were treated daily for 20 weeks with 1200 mg of a dried nettle root extract preparation (3.5-7:1; 20% V/V methanol). From fine needle aspiration biopsies of the prostate at 4-weekly intervals, morpho-logically significant changes in prostatic adenoma cells were detected that may relate to competitive inhibition of SHBG binding capacity by the extract [78].

Prostatic cells taken by needle biopsy from 33 BPH patients treated with nettle root extract for about 6 months were investigated by fluorescence microscopy. Compared with normal prostatic cells, a decrease in homogenous granules was detected in hyperplastic cells from the BPH patients, indicating that biological

activity in these cells had decreased [79]. The presence of nettle root constituents or their metabolites in prostate tissue obtained (through prostatectomy) from BPH patients treated with nettle root extract was demonstrated by fluorescence microscopy. The granular fluorescence was not observed in prostate tissue from patients not treated with nettle root extract, but could be simulated to some extent by *in vitro* incubation of this tissue with nettle root extract [80].

Morphological examination of prostate tissue obtained by needle biopsy from BPH patients before and 6 months after therapy with nettle root extract confirmed ultrastructural changes in the smooth muscle cells and epithelial cells of the prostate [81].

Clinical studies

*Clinical studies performed with dried native extract of nettle root (7-14:1, 20% V/V methanol) in a preparation containing an equal amount of diluent. As in the published reference papers where mg amounts are stated, **the following dosages relate to the extract preparation, of which only 50% was native extract (7-14:1)***

In a randomized, double-blind, placebo-controlled study with 40 BPH II patients (1200 mg of extract preparation per day, n = 20; placebo, n = 20), statistic-ally significant (p<0.05) decreases in micturition frequency and SHBG levels were observed in the verum group after 6 months [25].

Significant improvements of 14% in average urinary flow rate and 40-53% in residual urine volume were observed in BPH patients (n = 32) who received 600 mg of extract preparation daily for 4-6 weeks in a randomized, placebo-controlled (n = 35), double-blind study [26].

50 BPH I-II patients enrolled in a double-blind, controlled study were treated daily for 9 weeks with 600 mg of extract preparation (n = 25) or placebo (n = 25). A significant increase of 44% in micturition volume (p<0.05) and a highly significant decrease in serum levels of SHBG (p = 0.0005) were observed. The latter effect was probably due to the SHBG binding capacity of the extract [27].

In an open, multicentre study with 5492 patients receiving 600-1200 mg of extract preparation per day for 3-4 months, significant improvements in nycturia and daytime micturition frequency were observed [28]. A 50% decrease in nycturia was reported in an open, multicentre study with 4051 BPH patients who received 1200 mg of extract preparation per day for 10 weeks [29]. In another open, multicentre study, with 4480 BPH patients receiving 600-1200 mg of extract preparation per day for 20 weeks, significant improvements (p<0.01) in urinary flow and residual urine volume were observed [30].

111 BPH patients with nycturia received 1200 mg of extract preparation per day for 10 weeks in an open study. Nocturnal micturition frequency decreased in 55% of cases [31]. 37 out of 39 BPH I-III patients experienced improvements in urinary flow, residual urine, nycturia and pollakisuria after a 6-month treatment with 600-1200 mg of extract preparation per day [32]. In another open study, residual urine decreased in 67 out of 89 BPH patients receiving 600 mg of extract preparation per day for 3-24 months [33].

Significant decreases (p<0.05) in prostate volume and residual urine volume as well as in serum SHBG, oestradiol and oestrone levels were observed in an open study with 253 BPH patients who received 1200 mg of extract preparation per day for 12 weeks [34]. Decreases in prostate volume in 54% of cases and residual urine in 75% of cases were observed in an open study with 26 BPH patients who received 1200 mg of extract preparation per day for 4-24 weeks [35].

Clinical studies performed with other nettle root preparations

In a double-blind, multicentre study, 41 BPH patients were treated daily for 3 months with either 2 × 3 ml of an aqueous extract preparation equivalent to 4.68 g of a fluid extract (1:1, 16% ethanol) (n = 20) or placebo (n = 21). A decrease in residual urinary volume of 19.2 ml in the verum group compared to 10.7 ml in the placebo group, and an increase in maximal urinary flow of 7.1 ml/s in the verum group compared to 4.4 ml/s in the placebo group, were observed. A significantly greater improvement (p = 0.002) in International Prostate Symptom Scores (see Cockett et al. [82]) in the verum group was also reported [40].

Daily treatment for 60 days with 90-150 drops of a fluid extract (1:1, 45% ethanol; Ph. Fr.) led to a 66% decrease in residual urine in an open study with 10 BPH patients [41].

In a open study with 67 BPH patients, a reduction in nocturnal micturition frequency was observed after 6 months of daily treatment with 3 × 5 ml of a fluid extract (1:5, 40% ethanol) [42].

In an open multicentre study involving 1319 patients with BPH and/or prostatitis, daily treatment for 6 months with 378-756 mg of a native extract of nettle root (12-16:1, 70% V/V ethanol) led to substantial improvements in dysuria, nycturia, pollakisuria, urinary flow and residual urine volume. 79.9% of the patients reported an improvement in their quality of life [39].

Pharmacokinetic properties

After oral administration of 20 mg of purified *Urtica dioica* agglutinin (UDA) to patients and healthy volunteers, 30-50% was excreted unchanged in the faeces. The concentration in urine was in the 1-10 ng/ml range and the total amount of UDA in urine was less than 1% of the administered dose. These data confirmed the extreme stability of UDA in the digestive tract and its partial uptake and renal clearance [83].

Preclinical safety data

No data available.

Clinical safety data

Over 16,000 patients have been treated with nettle root extracts in clinical studies [25-35,39-42] and have taken daily doses of up to 756 mg of hydro-alcoholic dry native extract for periods of up to 6 months or, in a few cases, 300 mg of dry native extract for 24 months. The incidence of adverse events was generally under 5%. No serious adverse effects have been reported, the majority of complaints being mild gastrointestinal upsets. In the most recent large open study, involving 1319 patients, the incidence of adverse events probably or possibly related to treatment with nettle root extract was 1.0% [39].

REFERENCES

1. Brennesselwurzel - Urticae radix. Deutsches Arzneibuch.

2. Peumans WJ, De Ley M, Broekaert WF. An unusual lectin from stinging nettle (*Urtica dioica*) rhizomes. FEBS Lett 1984;177:99-103.

3. Van Damme EJM, Broekaert WF, Peumans WJ. The *Urtica dioica* agglutinin is a complex mixture of isolectins. Plant Physiol 1988;86:598-601.

4. Broekaert WF, Van Parijs J, Leyns F, Joos H, Peumans WJ. A chitin-binding lectin from stinging nettle rhizomes with antifungal properties. Science 1989;245:1100-2.

5. Beintema JJ, Peumans WJ. The primary structure of stinging nettle (*Urtica dioica*) agglutinin. A two-domain member of the hevein family. FEBS Lett 1992;299:131-4.

6. Willer F, Wagner H, Schecklies E. Urtica-Wurzel-extrakte. Standardisierung mit Hilfe der ELISA-Technik und der HPLC. Dtsch Apoth Ztg 1991;131:1217-21.

7. Willer F. Chemie und Pharmakologie der Polysaccharide und Lektine von *Urtica dioica* (Lin.) [Dissertation]. Ludwigs-Maximilians-Universität, Munich, 1992.

8. Balzarini J, Neyts J, Schols D, Hosoya M, Van Damme E, Peumans WJ, De Clercq E. The mannose-specific plant lectins from *Cymbidium hybrid* and *Epipactis helleborine* and the (N-acetylglucosamine)$_n$-specific

plant lectin from *Urtica dioica* are potent and selective inhibitors of human immunodeficiency virus and cytomegalovirus replication in vitro. Antiviral Res 1992; 18:191-207.

9. Lerner DR, Raikhel NV. The gene for stinging nettle lectin (*Urtica dioica* agglutinin) encodes both a lectin and a chitinase. J Biol Chem 1992;267:11085-91.

10. Wagner H, Willer F. Zur Chemie und Pharmakologie der Polysaccharide und Lektine von *Urtica dioica*-Wurzeln. In: Rutishauser G, editor. Benigne Prostatahyperplasie III. Klinische und experimentelle Urologie 22. München-Bern-Wien-New York: Zuckschwerdt, 1992:125-32.

11. Wagner H, Willer F, Samtleben R, Boos G. Search for the antiprostatic principle of stinging nettle (*Urtica dioica*) roots. Phytomedicine 1994;1:213-24.

12. Schilcher H, Effenberger S. Scopoletin und β-Sitosterol - zwei geeignete Leitsubstanzen für Urticae radix. Dtsch Apoth Ztg 1986;126:79-81.

13. Chaurasia N, Wichtl M. Scopoletin, 3-β-Sitosterin und Sitosterin-3-β-D-glucosid aus Brennesselwurzel (Urticae radix). Dtsch Apoth Ztg 1986;126:81-3.

14. Chaurasia N. In: Phytochemische Untersuchungen einiger Urtica-Arten unter besonderer Berücksichtigung der Inhaltsstoffe von Radix und Flores Urticae dioicae L. [Dissertation]. Philipps-Universität, Marburg, 1987: 293-7.

15. Chaurasia N, Wichtl M. Sterols and steryl glycosides from *Urtica dioica*. J Nat Prod 1987;50:881-5.

16. Chaurasia N, Wichtl M. Phenylpropane und Lignane aus der Wurzel von *Urtica dioica* L. Dtsch Apoth Ztg 1986;126:1559-63.

17. Schöttner M, Reiner J, Tayman FSK. (+)-Neo-olivil from roots of *Urtica dioica*. Phytochemistry 1997;46:1107-9.

18. Ganßer D, Spiteller G. Plant constituents interfering with human sex hormone-binding globulin. Evaluation of a test method and its application to *Urtica dioica* root extracts. Z Naturforsch 1995;50c:98-104.

19. Schöttner M, Ganßer D, Spiteller G. Lignans from the roots of *Urtica dioica* and their metabolites bind to human sex hormone binding globulin (SHBG). Planta Med 1997;63:529-32.

20. Kraus R, Spiteller G. Lignanglucoside aus Wurzeln von *Urtica dioica*. Liebigs Ann Chem 1990:1205-13.

21. Kraus R, Spiteller G. Phenolic compounds from roots of *Urtica dioica*. Phytochemistry 1990;29:1653-9.

22. Kraus R, Spiteller G. Ceramides from *Urtica dioica* roots. Liebigs Ann Chem 1991:125-8.

23. Kraus R, Spiteller G, Bartsch W. (10*E*,12*Z*)-9-Hydroxy-10,12-octadecadiensäure, ein Aromatase-Hemmstoff aus dem Wurzelextrakt von *Urtica dioica*. Liebigs Ann Chem 1991:335-9.

24. Kraus R, Spiteller G. Terpene diols and terpene diol glucosides from roots of *Urtica dioica*. Phytochemistry 1991;30:1203-6.

25. Fischer M, Wilbert D. Wirkprüfung eines Phyto-pharmakons zur Behandlung der benignen Prostata-hyperplasie (BPH). In: Rutishauser G, editor. Benigne Prostatahyperplasie III. Klinische und experimentelle Urologie 22. München-Bern-Wien-New York: Zuckschwerdt, 1992:79-84.

26. Dathe G, Schmid H. Phytotherapie der benignen Prostatahyperplasie (BPH). Doppelblindstudie mit Extraktum Radicis Urticae (ERU). Urologe [B] 1987; 27:223-6.

27. Vontobel HP, Herzog R, Rutishauser G, Kres H. Ergebnisse einer Doppelblindstudie über die Wirksamkeit von ERU-Kapseln in der konservativen Behandlung der benignen Prostatahyperplasie. Urologe [A] 1985;24:49-51.

28. Tosch U, Müssiggang H. Medikamentöse Behandlung der benignen Prostatahyperplasie. Euromed 1983; (6):334-6.

29. Stahl H-P. Die Therapie prostatischer Nykturie mit standardisierten Extraktum Radix Urticae. Z Allgemeinmed 1984;60:128-32.

30. Friesen A. Statistische Analyse einer Multizenter-Langzeitstudie mit ERU. In: Bauer HW, editor. Benigne Prostatahyperplasie II. Klinische und experimentelle Urologie 19. München-Bern-Wien-San Francisco: Zuckschwerdt, 1988:121-30.

31. Vandierendounck EJ, Burkhardt P. Extractum radicis urticae bei Fibromyoadenom der Prostata mit nächtlicher Pollakisurie. Studie zur Prüfung der Wirkung von ZY 15095 (Simic®). Therapiewoche Schweiz 1986; 2:892-5.

32. Maar K. Rückbildung der Symptomatik von Prostata-adenomen. Ergebnisse einer sechsmonatigen konservativen Behandlung mit ERU-Kapseln. Fortschr Med 1987;105:18-20.

33. Djulepa J. Zweijährige Erfahrung in der Therapie des Prostata-Syndroms. Die Ergebnisse einer konservativen Behandlung mit Bazoton®. Ärztl Praxis 1982;34:2199-202.

34. Bauer HW, Sudhoff F, Dressler S. Endokrine Parameter während der Behandlung der benignen Prostata-hyperplasie mit ERU. In: Bauer HW, editor. Benigne Prostatahyperplasie II. Klinische und experimentelle Urologie 19. München-Bern-Wien-New York: Zuckschwerdt, 1988:44-9.

35. Feiber H. Sonographische Verlaufsbeobachtungen zum Einfluß der medikamentösen Therapie der benignen Prostatahyperplasie (BPH). In: Bauer HW, editor. Benigne Prostatahyperplasie II. Klinische und experimentelle Urologie 19. München-Bern-Wien-New York: Zuckschwerdt, 1988:75-82.

36. Brom S. Benigne Prostatahyperplasie. Rationale Therapie der BPH mit neuen Wirkstoffen. Dtsch Apoth

Ztg 1996;136:607-14.

37. Bracher F. Phytotherapie der benignen Prostata-hyperplasie. Urologe A 1997;36:10-7.

38. Veit M, van Rensen I, Blume H, Ihrig M, Morck H, Dingermann T. Bewertung von Phytopharmaka in der Therapie der BPH. Pharm Ztg 1998;143:1905-27.

39. Kaldewey W. Behandlung der benignen Prostata-hyperplasie und der Prostatitis mit einem standard-isierten Urticae-radix-Extrakt. Ein multizentrische Studie in 279 urologischen Praxen. Urologe B 1995;35:430-3.

40. Engelmann U, Boos G, Kres H. Therapie der benignen Prostatahyperplasie mit Bazoton Liquidum. Ergebnisse einer doppelblinden, placebokontrollierten, klinischen Studie. Urologe B 1996;36:287-91.

41. Goetz P. Die Behandlung der benignen Prostata-hyperplasie mit Brennesselwurzeln. Z Phytotherapie 1989;10:175-8.

42. Belaiche P, Lievoux O. Clinical studies on the palliative treatment of prostatic adenoma with extract of *Urtica* root. Phytotherapy Res 1991;5:267-9.

43. Schilcher H. Pflanzliche Urologika. Dtsch Apoth Ztg 1984;124:2429-36.

44. Vahlensieck W. Konservative Behandlung der benignen Prostatahyperplasie. Therapiewoche Schweiz 1986;2: 619-24.

45. Schilcher H. Möglichkeiten und Grenzen der Phytotherapie am Beispiel pflanzlicher Urologika. Teil 2: Adnexerkrankungen des Mannes und der Frau und Urolithiasis. Urologe B 1988;28:90-5.

46. Schilcher H. Urtica-Arten - Die Brennessel. Z Phyto-therapie 1988;9:160-4.

47. Schilcher H, Boesel R, Effenberger S, Segebrecht S. Neue Untersuchungsergebnisse mit aquaretisch, anti-bakteriell und prostatotrop wirksamen Arzneipflanzen. Pharmakologische und phytochemische Unter-suchungen von Goldrutenkraut, Birkenblättern, Wacholderbeeren, Gewürzsumachwurzelrinde, Lieb-stöckelwurzel, Queckenwurzel und Medizinal-kürbissamen. Z Phytotherapie 1989;10:77-82.

48. Schilcher H. Brennesselwurzel (Urticae radix). In: Phytotherapie in der Urologie. Stuttgart: Hippokrates, 1992:84-8.

49. Jaspersen-Schib R. Die Brennessel - eine Modedroge - oder mehr? Schweiz Apoth Ztg 1989;127:443-5.

50. Vahlensieck W, Fabricius PG. Benigne Prostata-hyperplasie (BPH). Therapeutische Möglichkeiten durch medikamentöse Therapie. Therapiewoche 1996;33: 1796-802.

51. Alken CE. Konservative Behandlung des Prostata-Adenoms und Stadien-Einteilung. Urologe B 1973; 13:95-8.

52. Voigt K-D, Bartsch W. Intratissular androgens in benign prostatic hyperplasia and prostatic cancer. J Steroid Biochem 1986;25:749-57.

53. Walsh PC, Hutchins GM, Ewing LL. Tissue content of dihydrotestosterone in human prostatic hyperplasia is not supranormal. J Clin Invest 1983;72:1772-7.

54. Aumüller G. BPH und Wachstumsfaktoren: Mechan-ismen und Hypothesen. Urologe A 1992;31:159-65.

55. Jinno H, Ueda K, Otaguro K, Kato T, Ito J, Tanaka R. Prostate growth factor in the extracts of benign prostatic hypertrophy. Partial purification and physicochemical characterization. Eur Urol 1986;12:41-8.

56. Schmitt J, Gutschank WM, Heck H, Enderle-Schmitt U, Aumüller G. Cell culture of prostatic stromal tissue. A contribution to pathogenesis and therapy. In: Bauer HW, editor. Benigne Prostatahyperplasie. Klinische und experimentelle Urologie 14. München-Bern-Wien-San Francisco: Zuckschwerdt, 1987:18-22.

57. Streber AS. Künftig mit Pseudo-Testosteron gegen Prostata-Adenom? Ursache für die Vergrößerung der akzessorischen Geschlechtsdrüse ist ein Anstieg des sexualhormonbindenen Globulins. Ärztl Praxis 1981; 33:1045-7.

58. Schmidt K. Die Wirkung eines Radix Urticae-Extrakts und einzelner Nebenextrakte auf das SHBG des Blutplasmas bei der benignen Prostatahyperplasie. Fortschr Med 1983;101:713-6.

59. Nahrstedt A. Pflanzliche Urologika - eine kritische Übersicht. Pharm Ztg 1993;138:1439-50.

60. Miersch W-DE. Benigne Prostatahyperplasie. Konservative und operative Therapien. Dtsch Apoth Ztg 1993;133:2653-60.

61. Hryb DJ, Khan MS, Romas NA, Rosner W. The effect of extracts of the roots of the stinging nettle (*Urtica dioica*) on the interaction of SHBG with its receptor on human prostatic membranes. Planta Med 1995;61:31-2.

62. Bartsch W, Kühne G. Hemmung der Aromatase durch 9-Hydroxy-10-trans-12-cis-octadecadiensäure. In-vitro-Untersuchungen mit einem Inhaltsstoff von Extractum radicis urticae. In: Rutishauser G, editor. Benigne Prostatahyperplasie III. Klinische und experimentelle Urologie 22. München-Bern-Wien-New York: Zuckschwerdt, 1992:108-15.

63. Ganßer D, Spiteller G. Aromatase inhibitors from *Urtica dioica* roots. Planta Med 1995;61:138-40.

64. Wagner H, Willer F, Kreher B. Biologisch aktive Verbindungen aus dem Wasserextrakt von *Urtica dioica*. Planta Med 1989;55:452-4.

65. Willer F, Wagner H. Immunologically active poly-saccharides and lectins from the aqueous extract of *Urtica dioica*. Planta Med 1990;56:669.

66. Hirano T, Homma M, Oka K. Effects of stinging nettle root extracts and their steroidal components on the Na$^+$, K$^+$-ATPase of the benign prostatic hyperplasia. Planta Med 1994;60:30-3.

67. Enderle-Schmitt U, Gutschank W-M, Aumüller G. Wachstumskinetik von Zellkulturen aus BPH unter Einfluß von Extractum radicis urticae (ERU). In: Bauer HW, editor. Benigne Prostatahyperplasie II. Klinische und experimentelle Urologie 19. München-Bern-Wien-San Francisco: Zuckschwerdt, 1988:56-61.

68. Wagner H, Geiger WN, Boos G, Samtleben R. Studies on the binding of Urtica dioica agglutinin (UDA) and other lectins in an in vitro epidermal growth factor receptor test. Phytomedicine 1994;1:287-90.

69. Konrad L, Müller H-H, Lenz C, Laubinger H, Aumüller G, Lichius JJ. Antiproliferative effect on human prostate cancer cells by a stinging nettle root (*Urtica dioica*) extract. Planta Med 2000;66:44-7.

70. Lichius JJ, Lenz C, Lindemann P, Müller H-H, Aumüller G, Konrad L. Antiproliferative effect of a polysaccharide fraction of a 20% methanolic extract of stinging nettle roots upon epithelial cells of the human prostate (LNCaP). Pharmazie 1999;54:768-71.

71. Rausch U, Aumüller G, Eicheler W, Gutschank W, Beyer G, Ulshöfer B. Der Einfluß von Phytopharmaka auf BPH-Gewebe und Explantatkulturen in vitro. In: Rutishauser G, editor. Benigne Prostatahyperplasie III. Klinische und experimentelle Urologie 22. München-Bern-Wien-New York: Zuckschwerdt, 1992:116-24.

72. Sinowatz F, Amselgruber W, Boos G, Einspanier R, Schams D, Neumüller C. Zur parakrinen Regulation des Prostatawachstums: Besteht eine Wechselwirkung zwischen dem basischen Fibroblasten-Wachstumsfaktor und dem Lektin UDA? In: Boos G, editor. Benigne Prostatahyperplasie. Frankfurt: PMI, 1994:79-86.

73. Wagner H, Willer F, Samtleben R. Lektine und Polysaccharide - die Wirkprinzipien der *Urtica-dioica*-Wurzel? In: Boos G, editor. Benigne Prostatahyperplasie. Frankfurt: PMI, 1994:115-22.

74. Daube G. Pilotstudie zur Behandlung der benignen Prostatahyperplasie bei Hunden mit extractum radicis urticae (ERU). In: Bauer HW, editor. Benigne Prostatahyperplasie II. Klinische und experimentelle Urologie 19. München-Bern-Wien-San Francisco: Zuckschwerdt, 1988:63-6.

75. Rhodes L, Primka RL, Berman C, Vergult G, Gabriel M, Pierre-Malice M, Gibelin B. Comparison of finasteride (Proscar®), a 5α reductase inhibitor, and various commercial plant extracts in *in vitro* and *in vivo* 5α reductase inhibition. The Prostate 1993;22:43-51.

76. Lichius JJ, Muth C. The inhibiting effects of *Urtica dioica* root extracts on experimentally induced prostatic hyperplasia in the mouse. Planta Med 1997;63:307-10.

77. Lichius JJ, Renneberg H, Blaschek W, Aumüller G, Muth C. The inhibiting effects of components of stinging nettle roots on experimentally induced prostatic hyperplasia in mice. Planta Med 1999;65:666-8.

78. Ziegler H. Zytomorphologische Untersuchung der benignen Prostatahyperplasie unter Behandlung mit Extract. Radicis Urticae (ERU). Vorläufige Ergebnisse. Fortschr Med 1982;100:1832-4.

79. Ziegler H. Fluoreszenzmikroskopische Untersuchungen von Prostatazellen unter Einwirkung von Extract. Radicis Urticae (ERU). Fortschr Med 1983;101:2112-4.

80. Dunzendorfer U. Der Nachweis von Reaktionseffekten des Extractum Radicis Urticae (ERU) im menschlichen Prostatagewebe durch Fluoreszenzmikroskopie. Z Phytotherapie 1984;5:800-4.

81. Oberholzer M, Schamböck A, Rugendorff EW, Mihatsch M, Rist M, Buser M et al. Elektronenmikroskopische Ergebnisse bei medikamentös behandelter benigner Prostatahyperplasie (BPH). In: Bauer HW, editor. Benigne Prostatahyperplasie. Klinische und experimentelle Urologie 14. München-Bern-Wien-San Francisco: Zuckschwerdt, 1987:13-7.

82. Cockett AT, Aso Y, Denis L, Murphy G, Khoury S, Abrams P et al. 1994 Recommendations of the International Consensus Committee concerning: The International Prostate Symptom Score (I-PSS) and Quality of Life Assessment. In: Cockett ATK, Khoury S, Aso Y, Chatelain C, Denis L, Griffiths K and Murphy G, editors. The 2nd International Consultation on Benign Prostatic Hyperplasia (BPH). Paris, June 27-30, 1993: Proceedings 2. Jersey, Channel Islands: Scientific Communication International, 1993:553-5.

83. Samtleben R, Boos G and Wagner H. Novel enzyme-linked immunoassay for the quantitation of *Urtica dioica* agglutinin (UDA) in stinging nettle extracts and human excretions. In: Abstracts of 2nd International Congress on Phytomedicine. Munich, 11-14 September 1996 (Abstract SL-107). *Published as*: Phytomedicine 1996;3(Suppl 1):134.

UVAE URSI FOLIUM

Bearberry Leaf

DEFINITION

Bearberry leaf consists of the whole or cut dried leaf of *Arctostaphylos uva-ursi* (L.) Spreng. It contains not less than 7.0% of anhydrous arbutin ($C_{12}H_{16}O_7$; M_r 272.3), calculated with reference to the dried drug.

The material complies with the monograph of the European Pharmacopoeia [1].

CONSTITUENTS

The main characteristic constituent of bearberry leaf is arbutin (normally between 5 and 15%) accompanied by variable amounts of methylarbutin (up to 4%) and by small amounts of the free aglycones hydroquinone and methylhydroquinone [2-4]. Other constituents include gallic acid, galloylarbutin and up to 20% of gallotannins [5-10]; flavonoids, especially glycosides of quercetin, kaempferol and myricetin [1,10]; and triterpenes, mainly ursolic acid and uvaol [10].

CLINICAL PARTICULARS

Therapeutic indications
Uncomplicated infections of the lower urinary tract [11-17] such as cystitis, when antibiotic treatment is not considered essential [18-20].

Posology and method of administration

Dosage

Adults: Cold water infusions of the dried leaf corresponding to 400-800 mg of arbutin per day, divided into 2-3 doses; equivalent preparations [12,17]. Not recommended for children.

Method of administration
For oral administration. Patients should be advised to consume plenty of liquid during the treatment [12]. Alkalinization of the urine may be beneficial [12, 16].

Duration of administration
Treatment should be continued until complete disappearance of symptoms (up to a maximum of 2 weeks), but if symptoms worsen during the first week of treatment medical advice should be sought [16].

Contra-indications
Kidney disorders.

E/S/C/O/P
MONOGRAPHS
Second Edition

Special warnings and special precautions for use

The amount of free hydroquinone in bearberry leaf preparations should be controlled. Hydroquinone is a topical irritant and a hepatotoxin [21-23]; oral ingestion of 5-12 g has been fatal [22]. Long term external application of creams containing up to 10% of hydroquinone has caused skin colloid degeneration (ochronosis) [24-26].

Interaction with other medicaments and other forms of interaction

Concomitant acidification of the urine (by other remedies, for instance) may result in a reduction of efficacy [16,17].

Pregnancy and lactation

Bearberry leaf should not be used during pregnancy or lactation [23].

Effects on ability to drive and use machines

None known.

Undesirable effects

Nausea and vomiting may occur due to stomach irritation from the high tannin content of bearberry leaf [17].

Overdose

No reports are available on overdose of bearberry leaf.

PHARMACOLOGICAL PROPERTIES

Pharmacodynamic properties

In vivo experiments

An aqueous extract of bearberry leaves was administered intraperitoneally to 10 male rats as a single dose of 50 mg/kg body weight; a control group of 10 rats received hypotonic saline solution and another group of 10 rats received the diuretic compound hydrochlorothiazide at 10 mg/kg body weight. The urine volume from rats treated with the extract was significantly higher ($p<0.001$ from the 4th to 8th hour after administration; $p<0.05$ over a 24-hour period) than from the controls and was comparable to the volume after hydrochlorothiazide treatment [27].

Pharmacological studies in humans

The active principle of bearberry leaf is believed to originate from transformation of the main constituent arbutin, resulting in an antibacterial effect in the urine (bladder antiseptic). Microbiological investigation in vitro revealed strong antibacterial properties of urine samples obtained from healthy volunteers after consumption of 800 mg of arbutin or bearberry tea containing an equivalent amount of arbutin. This effect was only observed with urine adjusted to pH 8, whilst urine of pH 6 was ineffective [12,13].

In another study, urine samples from healthy volunteers were collected 3 hours after oral administration of 0.1 g or 1.0 g arbutin. In vitro tests for antibacterial activity, involving 74 different strains of bacteria including E. coli, Proteus mirabilis, Pseudomonas aeruginosa and Staphylococcus aureus, were performed in comparison with 20 different synthetic antibacterial substances at their usual urine concentration in therapy. Only gentamicin, nalidixic acid and urine collected after oral administration of 1.0 g of arbutin and adjusted to pH 8 were active against all strains tested [14].

Pharmacokinetic properties

Arbutin, the main constituent of bearberry leaf, is rapidly absorbed after oral administration of the pure substance or bearberry leaf tea or bearberry leaf extract preparations. Urinary excretion of phenolic metabolites occurs within a few hours, with excretion maxima during the first 6 hours and approx. 70-75% of the administered dose being excreted within 24 hours [13,14,28].

Preclinical safety data

Single dose toxicity
No data have been reported for bearberry leaf. The oral LD_{50} of hydroquinone in 2% aqueous solution has been determined as 320 mg/kg in rats, 400 mg/kg in mice, 550 mg/kg in guinea pigs, 300 mg/kg in pigeons, 70 mg/kg in cats and 200 mg/kg in dogs [29].

Repeated dose toxicity
No data have been reported for bearberry leaf.

Reproductive toxicity
No data have been reported for bearberry leaf. However, arbutin is reported to be an experimental teratogen [23].

Genotoxicity
Bearberry leaf has been shown to be non-mutagenic in the Ames test using Salmonella typhimurium strains TA98 and TA100, and in the Bacillus subtilis rec-assay [30]. Hydroquinone was found to be mildly myeloclastogenic in the micronucleus test in SPF mice after oral administration of a toxic dose (200 mg/kg) [31].

Carcinogenicity
No data have been reported for bearberry leaf.

REFERENCES

1. Bearberry Leaf - Uvae ursi folium. European Pharmacopoeia, Council of Europe.

2. Hänsel R, Keller K, Rimpler H, Schneider G, editors.

Arctostaphylos. In: Hagers Handbuch der Pharmazeutischen Praxis, 5th ed. Volume 4: Drogen A-D. Berlin: Springer-Verlag, 1993:328-38.

3. Sticher O, Soldati F, Lehmann D. Hochleistungs-flüssigchromatographische Trennung und quantitative Bestimmung von Arbutin, Methylarbutin, Hydrochinon und Hydrochinonmonomethylaether in Arctostaphylos-, Bergenia-, Calluna- und Vacciniumarten. Planta Med 1979;35:253-61.

4. Linnenbrink N. Vergleichende phytochemische Untersuchung an in vitro-Kulturen. Variabilität der Inhaltsstoffe Arbutin und Methylarbutin bei Arctostaphylos uva-ursi und Arctostaphylos nevadensis. [Dissertation]. University of Hamburg, 1984.

5. Wähner C, Schönert J, Friedrich H. Zur Kenntnis des Gerbstoffs der Bärentraubenblätter (Arctostaphylos uva-ursi L.). Pharmazie 1974;29:616-7.

6. Britton G, Haslam E. Gallotannins. Part XII. Phenolic constituents of Arctostaphylos uva-ursi L. Spreng. J Chem Soc 1965;7312-9.

7. Haslam E, Lilley TH, Cai Y, Martin R, Magnolato D. Traditional herbal medicines - The role of polyphenols. Planta Med 1989;55:1-8.

8. Herrmann K. Über den Gerbstoff der Bärentrauben-blätter. Arch Pharm (Weinheim) 1953;286:515-23.

9. Friedrich H. Beobachtungen über die Hemmung der β-Glukosidase-Aktivität durch Gallotannin und deren mögliche Bedeutung für die Stabilität der Arbutindrogen. Arch Pharm (Weinheim) 1955;288:583-9.

10. Hegnauer R. In: Chemotaxonomie der Pflanzen. Stuttgart: Birkhäuser Verlag, 1962; Volume 4: 65-94, 1989; Volume 8: 418-33.

11. Bradley PR, editor. Uva ursi. In: British Herbal Compendium. Volume 1. Bournemouth: British Herbal Medicine Association, 1992:211-3.

12. Frohne D. Arctostaphylos uva-ursi (L.) Spreng. (Bärentraube). Bonn: Kooperation Phytopharmaka. Unpublished review, 1977.

13. Frohne D. Untersuchungen zur Frage der harndesinfizierenden Wirkungen von Bärentrauben-blatt-Extrakten. Planta Med 1970;18:1-25.

14. Kedzia B, Wrocinski T, Mrugasiewicz K, Gorecki P, Grzewinska H. Antibacterial action of urine containing arbutin metabolic products. Med Dosw Mikrobiol 1975; 27:305-14.

15. Wichtl M, Egerer HP. Bärentraubenblätter - Uvae ursi folium. In: Hartke K, Hartke H, Mutschler E, Rücker G and Wichtl M, editors. Kommentar zum Europäischen Arzneibuch. Stuttgart: Wissenschaftliche Verlags-gesellschaft, Eschborn: Govi-Verlag, 1999 (11. Lfg.):B 5.

16. Weiss RF. In: Lehrbuch der Phytotherapie. 7th ed.

Stuttgart: Hippokrates Verlag, 1991:315-6.

17. Frohne D. Bärentraubenblätter. In: Wichtl M, editor. Teedrogen, 2nd ed. Stuttgart: Wissenschaftliche Verlagsgesellschaft, 1989:72-4.

18. Coe FL, Brenner BM. Abklärung von Erkrankungen der Niere und der ableitenden Harnwege. In: Straub PW, editor. Harrison. Prinzipien der Inneren Medizin. Deutsche Ausgabe. 11th ed. Volume 2. Basel: Schwabe Verlag, 1989:1345-56,1404-12.

19. Furrer HJ, Malinverni R. Harnwegsinfektionen bei Erwachsenen: alte und neue Aspekte. Ther Umsch 1994;51:842-51.

20. Weber R. Die unkomplizierte Harnwegsinfektion. PTA heute 1995;9/2:150-1.

21. Nowak AK, Shilkin AB, Jeffrey GP. Darkroom hepatitis after exposure to hydroquinone. Lancet 1995;345:1187.

22. US Environmental Protection Agency. Extremely Hazardous Substances. Superfund Chemical Profiles. Park Ridge NJ: Noyes Data Corporation, 1988:859-63.

23. Lewis RJ. In: Sax's Dangerous Properties of Industrial Materials, 8th ed. New York: Van Nostrand Reinhold, 1989:1906-7.

24. Champion RH, Burton JL, Ebling FJG, editors. In: Textbook of Dermatology, 5th ed. Oxford: Blackwell Scientific, 1992:1602,2626-8,3029-30,3058-61.

25. Lawrence N, Bligard CA, Reed R, Perret WJ. Exogenous ochronosis in the United States. J Am Acad Dermatol 1988;18:1207-11.

26. Hull PR, Procter PR. The melanocyte: an essential link in hydroquinone-induced ochronosis. J Am Acad Dermatol 1990;22:529-31.

27. Beaux D, Fleurentin J, Mortier F. Effect of extracts of Orthosiphon stamineus Benth., Hieracium pilosella L., Sambucus nigra L. and Arctostaphylos uva-ursi (L.) Spreng. in rats. Phytotherapy Res 1999;13:222-5.

28. Paper DH, Koehler J, Franz G. Bioavailability of drug preparations containing a leaf extract of Arctostaphylos uva-ursi (L.) Spreng. (Uvae ursi folium). Pharm Pharmacol Lett 1993;3:63-6.

29. Woodard G, Hagan CE, Radomski JL. Toxicity of hydroquinone for laboratory animals. Fed Proc 1949; 8:348.

30. Morimoto I, Watanabe F, Osawa T, Okitsu T. Mutagenicity screening of crude drugs with Bacillus subtilis rec-assay and Salmonella/microsome reversion assay. Mutat Res 1982;97;81-102.

31. Gad-El-Karim MM, Sadagopa Ramanujam VM, Ahmed AE, Legator MS. Benzene myeloclastogenicity: a function of its metabolism. Am J Ind Med 1985;7:475-84.

VALERIANAE RADIX

Valerian Root

DEFINITION

Valerian root consists of the dried underground parts of *Valeriana officinalis* L.*s.l.*, including the rhizome surrounded by the roots and stolons. It contains not less than 5 ml/kg of essential oil for the whole drug and not less than 3 ml/kg of essential oil for the cut drug, both calculated with reference to the dried drug, and not less than 0.17 per cent of sesquiterpenic acids expressed as valerenic acid ($C_{15}H_{22}O_2$; M_r 234), calculated with reference to the dried drug.

The material complies with the monograph of the European Pharmacopoeia [1].

CONSTITUENTS

Essential oil containing monoterpenes (such as bornyl esters, camphene and pinenes), sesquiterpenes (including valerenal and valeranone) and less volatile sesquiterpene carboxylic acids (valerenic acid and derivatives) [2-9]; gamma-aminobutyric acid (GABA), glutamine and arginine in relatively high concentrations [10,11]. Valepotriates may be present in the root [12-15], but are unstable and unlikely to be present in finished products [3,4,16,17]. Similarly baldrinals, the decomposition products of valepotriates, are not detected in valerian root preparations [17].

CLINICAL PARTICULARS

Therapeutic indications
Relief of temporary mild nervous tension and/or difficulty in falling asleep [18-35].

Posology and method of administration

Dosage

Adult single dose: 1-3 g of the drug (e.g. as a tea infusion) or equivalent extracts prepared with water or ethanol (max. 70%) [18-22,24,28,29,31,32].
For tenseness, restlessness and irritability, up to 3 times daily. As an aid to sleep, a single dose half to one hour before bedtime [19-21,24], with an earlier dose during the evening if necessary.
Elderly: as for adults.
Children from 3 to 12 years under medical supervision only: proportion of adult dose according to bodyweight, as non-alcoholic preparations.

Method of administration
For oral administration.

E/S/C/O/P
MONOGRAPHS
Second Edition

Duration of administration

No restriction; neither dependence nor withdrawal symptoms are reported.

Contra-indications

Children under 3 years of age.

Special warnings and special precautions for use

If symptoms persist for more than 2 weeks, or the condition worsens, seek medical advice.

Interaction with other medicaments and other forms of interaction

None reported.

Pregnancy and lactation

No data available.

In accordance with general medical practice, the product should not be used during pregnancy and lactation without medical advice.

Effects on ability to drive and use machines

Studies designed to assess the effects of sedatives on vigilance have compared valerian root extract-containing preparations with placebo and benzo-diazepines, using established techniques for testing the capacity to drive vehicles [37-39]. These studies showed that valerian root, administered as 10 ml of syrup corresponding to 4 g of the drug [39], or in combination with other tranquillizing plant drugs [37-39], does not reduce vigilance measured 8 hours after taking the preparation, i.e. there was no morning-after (hangover) effect. A double-blind, randomized, placebo-controlled study showed that neither single nor repeated evening administrations for 14 days of 600 mg of valerian root extract (ethanol 70% V/V; corresponding to 3 g of the drug) have a relevant impact on criteria of driving capability such as reaction time, alertness and concentration the morning after intake [40]. These results do not, therefore, support earlier reports of somnolence the morning after taking a valerian root preparation [21,24].

However, there appeared to be some impairment of vigilance 1-2 hours after administration of valerian syrup [39]. Thus, taking valerian root preparations immediately (up to 2 hours) before driving a car or operating hazardous machinery is not recommended. The effect of valerian preparations may be strength-ened by consumption of alcohol.

Undesirable effects

No adverse effects confirmed.

Withdrawal symptoms have been observed after long term overdosage [41].

Overdose

Valerian root at a dose of approximately 20 g caused benign symptoms (fatigue, abdominal cramp, chest tightness, lightheadedness, hand tremor and mydriasis) which disappeared within 24 hours [42]. If symptoms arise, treatment should be supportive.

PHARMACOLOGICAL PROPERTIES

Since valepotriates, with rather unstable epoxide structures, are generally absent from finished products [16,17] and show poor oral absorption [33,43], their pharmacological properties have been excluded from this section.

Pharmacodynamic properties

In vitro experiments

The interaction of hydroalcoholic and aqueous extracts of valerian root with the GABA-benzodiazepine-chloride channel receptor complex in rat brain has been investigated; they inhibited the uptake and induced the release of radiolabelled GABA in synaptosomes isolated from rat brain cortex [44-46]. Similarly, both extracts displaced [^{3}H] muscimol bound to the $GABA_A$ receptor [47]. The release of GABA was Na^+-dependent and independent of the presence of Ca^{2+} in the external medium, which indicated that valerian extracts release GABA by reversal of the GABA carrier [44,45]. The relatively high GABA concentration in aqueous and hydro-alcoholic extracts might be responsible for the observed activity [11,46,47]. However an ethanolic extract, in which GABA could not be detected, inhibited synaptosomal [^{3}H]GABA uptake and potentiated veratridine- or K^+-stimulated [^{3}H]GABA release from hippocampal slices [48]. Another explanation for the sedative properties of valerian could be the presence of relatively high concentrations of glutamine found in aqueous extracts [11]. An in vitro study demonstrated that hydroxyvalerenic acid and acetoxyvalerenic acid, in physiologically un-realistic amounts, could inhibit the catabolism of gamma-aminobutyric acid at synaptic junctions in the central nervous system [49].

At low concentrations, an ethanol extract enhanced flunitrazepam binding (EC_{50}: 4.1×10^{-10} mg/ml), while at higher concentrations this increase was replaced by an inhibition (IC_{50}: 4.8×10^{-1} mg/ml), suggesting the presence of at least two different biological activities interacting with benzodiazepine sites [48]. The lipophilic fraction of a hydroalcoholic extract also showed affinity for the barbiturate receptor and to a lesser extent for the mitochondrial benzo-diazepine receptors [50]. Another in vitro study demonstrated the interaction of a hydroalcoholic extract of valerian root with adenosine receptors (but not with benzodiazepine receptors) mediating sedation in the rat brain. However, this extract contained 1.38% of valtrate whereas an aqueous extract devoid of valepotriates produced only a weak effect under similar conditions [51].

A hydroethanolic extract showed a dose-dependent inhibitory effect (IC_{50} of near 0.5 mg/litre) on the binding of 2-[^{125}I] iodomelatonin to its binding site. Valerenic acid was not able to influence the binding [52].

Among four 7',9:7',9 diepoxylignans recently found in valerian root, hydroxypinoresinol showed a high affinity for the $5-HT_{1A}$ receptor (IC_{50}: 2.3 μM/litre) [53,54].

In vivo experiments

The essential oil of valerian root and compounds isolated from it (valerenic acid, valerenal, valeranone), injected intraperitoneally, showed central depressive and/or muscle relaxant activity in mice, as assessed from a wide range of pharmacological symptoms [55]. Valeranone also produced a significant, dose-dependent reduction of spontaneous motility in mice during the first 5 hours after intraperitoneal administration [18]. Valerenic acid injected intraperitoneally into mice had a non-specific central nervous depressant effect and prolonged pentobarbital-induced sleeping time [56]. Homobaldrinal (a breakdown product of isovaltrate), administered perorally, showed a high sedative action by inhibition of spontaneous motility in mice [57]. A tincture of valerian root administered intraperitoneally was reported to inhibit spontaneous motility in experiments on mice [58].

The central depressant activity of a dichloromethane extract (50 mg/kg) of valerian root, and a particular fraction from it (10 mg/kg), has been demonstrated *in vivo* [59,60] using what is considered to be the most reliable and elegant method available to date: an autoradiographic tracer method to measure glucose transformations in more than 30 areas of the rat brain after intraperitoneal injection of test substances, as a measure of neuronal activity. Using the same technique, negative results were obtained with the essential oil, valerenic acid and valeranone, as well as with valtrate, didrovaltrate and homobaldrinal, leading to the conclusion that these substances have no central effect [59,60].

Unfettered cats with implanted electrodes showed no changes in their EEGs following oral administration of valerian root extract at 100 or 250 mg/kg body weight; muscle tonus was reduced in 30-40% of the cats [61].

A dry 70%-ethanolic extract (1 g of extract equivalent to 4 g of valerian root), administered intraperitoneally to male mice, was assessed for possible neuro-pharmacological activity [62]. At doses of up to 100 mg/kg bodyweight the extract did not produce overt sedation or tranquillization, since no modifications of spontaneous motility, nociception or body temperature and no palpebral ptosis were observed, whereas diazepam at doses of up to 2 mg/kg clearly reduced spontaneous motility, lowered body temperature and produced a weak ptosis. On the other hand, the extract showed anticonvulsive activity against picrotoxin (3 mg, given intravenously) with an ED_{50} of 6 mg/kg, compared to an ED_{50} of 0.03 mg/kg for diazepam, and also caused a significant prolongation of thiopental-induced anaesthesia ($p<0.05$) with 100 mg/kg of extract. Anticonvulsive activity against picrotoxin was present mainly in a methylene chloride fraction of the extract (ED_{50}: 0.25 mg/kg), although aqueous and n-hexane fractions were not inactive. In similar tests pure valerenic acid (12.5 and 25 mg/kg, but not 6.25 mg/kg) also antagonized picrotoxin but essential oil of valerian (up to 40 mg/kg) and acetoxy-valerenic acid (up to 25 mg/kg) were ineffective. In contrast to diazepam and haloperidol the extract showed no clear-cut, dose-dependent anticonvulsive effect against harman. From the overall results the authors suggested that the observed effects of the extract are caused by an unknown interaction, which may differ from that of diazepam, with the $GABA_A$-benzodiazepine receptor complex [62].

A commercially available dry aqueous alkaline extract of valerian root (drug to extract ratio 5-6:1, standardized on valerenic acid) produced significant sedative effects after oral administration to female mice. In spontaneous motility tests, doses of 20 and 200 mg/kg body weight produced reductions in motility after 120 min of 29% and 36% respectively, the ED_{50} of the extract being calculated as 230 mg/kg. In control animals 5 mg and 25 mg of diazepam resulted in substantial reductions in motility shortly after administration and maximum reductions of 77% and 90% respectively. The extract increased thiopental-induced sleeping time by factors of 1.6 at 2 mg/kg ($p<0.01$) and 7.6 at 200 mg/kg ($p<0.01$) compared to a factor of 4.7 for chlorpromazine at 4.0 mg/kg. Thus the extract exhibited dose-related sedative activity in mice although less pronounced than that of diazepam or chlorpromazine. It showed only weak anticonvulsant properties, increasing the lag time before pentetrazole-induced convulsions by a factor of 1.4 ($p≤0.01$) at a dose level of 500 mg/kg, compared to factors of 3.2 for methaqualone hydrochloride at 100 mg/kg and 2.3 for diazepam at 0.2 mg/kg [63].

In conclusion, despite considerable pharmacological research to confirm the empirically recognized sedative effects [33-35] of valerian root, its active principles and their mode of action remain unclear [36].

Pharmacological studies in humans

Electroencephalographic (EEG) recordings performed in a sleep laboratory on 10 young men who normally slept well showed no changes in objective measures of sleep after administration of 400 mg of valerian root dry aqueous extract (approx. 3:1), taken on three non-consecutive nights [19,20].

Double-blind studies [22] on two groups of healthy young subjects using a similar extract showed that:

a) in a home study, based on subjective assessment and motor activity recordings, doses of 450 mg and 900 mg had a significant, dose-dependent, sleep-promoting effect.

b) in a laboratory study, on the basis of objective assessments, motor activity recordings, polygraphic sleep recordings and all-night spectral analysis of the sleep EEG, a dose of 900 mg produced similar trends but no significant differences from placebo.

In a randomized, placebo-controlled, double-blind study performed in a cross-over design, 12 healthy female volunteers received a single dose of 1.2 g of a valerian root extract (drug to extract ratio 5-7:1) or 10 mg diazepam or placebo. The subjects rated their current state of alertness on a visual analogue scale (VAS) from "wide awake" to "almost asleep". In the VAS results 120 minutes after treatment, valerian extract reached about one third of the diazepam value compared to placebo. 100 mg of caffeine administered 140 minutes after the extract, weakened these effects. Quantitative EEG for 5 minutes under vigilance-controlled reaction time conditions followed by 5 minutes under resting conditions was measured before administration and 120 and 180 minutes after intake; the effects after administration of valerian extract were difficult to distinguish from placebo [23].

Clinical studies
A variety of studies have been carried out to assess the sedative effects of valerian root in humans [19-22,24-32].

In one large scale study with 128 volunteers the effect on their sleep of 400 mg of valerian root dry aqueous extract (approx. 3:1), taken on three non-consecutive nights, was assessed by analysis of subjective sleep ratings. Compared to a placebo, the extract produced significant improvements in sleep latency and in sleep quality, particularly in relatively poor sleepers [19-21].

In a double-blind study on 8 volunteers suffering from mild insomnia, with assessment by subjective ratings and wrist-worn activity meters, 450 mg of a similar extract produced a significant decrease in sleep latency. A higher dose of 900 mg produced no further improvement [24].

Based on subjective evaluation, significant improvements in sleep quality were obtained following oral use of valerian root extract in a double blind study on 27 persons with sleep difficulties. A combination product containing an extract equivalent to 400 mg of root was compared with a control preparation on

randomized successive nights [25].

In a double-blind study with 48 volunteers placed under experimental 'social stress' conditions, valerian root extract at a low dosage (100 mg) showed no apparent sedative effects but reduced subjective feelings of somatic arousal, supporting a hypothetical thymoleptic effect [26].

The effect of treatment with 3×405 mg of valerian root extract daily for 7 days on objective and subjective sleep parameters was investigated in a double-blind study involving 14 elderly female poor sleepers. The dry aqueous alkaline extract had a drug to extract ratio of 5-6:1. Polysomnography was conducted on three nights, at one-week intervals (one week before, one hour before and seven days after commencement of treatment). Six subjects received placebo and eight subjects valerian. Subjects in the valerian group showed an increase in slow-wave sleep (SWS) and a decrease in sleep stage 1. There was no effect on sleep onset time or time awake after sleep onset. Rapid eye movement (REM)-sleep was unaltered. There was also no effect on self-rated sleep quality. It was hypothesized that valerian increases SWS in subjects with low baseline values and thus improves sleep quality only under certain conditions, which still have to be explored [27].

Short-term (single dose) and long-term (14 days) effects of a valerian root extract (drug to extract ratio 5:1; ethanol 70% V/V) on sleep structure and sleep perception were investigated in a randomized, double-blind, placebo-controlled, crossover study involving 16 patients with previously established psycho-physiological insomnia. No effects were observed after a single dose of 600 mg of the extract given 1 hour before bedtime. However, after 14 days of treatment with 600 mg of the extract, slow wave sleep (SWS) latency measured by polysomnographic recordings was significantly reduced in comparison with placebo (13.5 vs 21.3 minutes, p<0.05). The SWS percentage of time in bed was increased after valerian treatment compared to the baseline value (9.8 vs 8.1%, p<0.05). A tendency for shorter subjective sleep latency and a higher correlation coefficient between subjective and objective sleep latencies were observed under valerian treatment [28].

In a randomized, double-blind study, 78 elderly patients with sleep disorders of nervous origin were treated with 270 mg of a valerian root extract (n = 39) or placebo (n = 39) daily for 14 days. Based on psychometric scales and subjective ratings, the verum group showed significant improvements in sleep latency time (p<0.001)and sleep duration (p<0.001) compared to the placebo group [29].

11,168 patients (average age: 51 ± 18 years) participating in an open multicentric study were treated for 10 days with tablets containing 45 mg of a dry extract of valerian root (drug to extract ratio 5-6:1). At the end of the study, the therapy was rated as successful in 72% of the cases with difficulty in falling asleep, in 76% of the cases with discontinuous sleep and in 72% of the patients with restlessness and tension [30].

In a randomized, double-blind, placebo-controlled, multicentric study, 121 patients with insomnia (ICD-10, F 51.0) were treated daily for 28 days with either 600 mg of a valerian root extract (drug to extract ratio 5:1; ethanol 70% V/V; corresponding to 3 g of valerian root) (n = 61) or a placebo (n = 60), taken one hour before retiring to bed. After 28 days the effects were assessed using a standard questionnaire with a self-rating scale. Significant improvements in sleep quality (p = 0.035), rested feeling after sleep (p = 0.032) and general well-being (p = 0.002) were evident in patients in the verum group. The physicians also found significant improvement in patients treated with the valerian root extract, in improvement of insomnia (p = 0.002) and overall therapeutic effect (p = 0.001). The efficacy of the product was rated as very good or good in 66% of cases by the patients and in 61% by the doctors, whereas only 26% of the placebo group received similar ratings from patients and physicians [31].

In a randomized, double-blind, comparative study, 75 non-organic insomniacs were treated 30 minutes before going to sleep with either 600 mg of a valerian root extract (drug to extract ratio 5:1, ethanol 70% V/V) or 10 mg of oxazepam daily for 28 days. Sleep quality improved significantly (p<0.001) in both groups, with no statistical difference between the two groups (p = 0.70) [32].

Pharmacokinetic properties
No data available.

Preclinical safety data
A low order of toxicity was reported for an ethanolic extract of valerian root, the LD_{50} by intraperitoneal injection into mice being 3.3 g/kg. When this extract was administered intraperitoneally to rats daily for 45 days in doses ranging from 400-600 mg/kg no significant changes in weight, blood or urine were observed in comparison with control animals [64].

After administration of an alcoholic extract of valerian root to rats at 300 or 600 mg/kg/day for 30 days, no significant differences in growth, arterial pressure, weight of key organs or haematological and biochemical parameters were found in comparison with control animals [65].

The oral LD_{50} of valerian root essential oil in rats was determined as 15 g/kg body weight, the highest value

of 27 essential oils tested including, for example, peppermint and anise oils. The quantity of essential oil which could be administered to 100 g rats daily over a period of 8 weeks was also determined. With doses of 100 mg or 200 mg all the animals survived and increased in weight, similar to control animals in the first case and differing only slightly in the second case; sedative effects were observed but disappeared during the day and the animals performed normal grooming. With increasing dosage above 200 mg, growth declined and adverse symptoms were reported. At 250 mg daily, 2 out of 5 of the animals perished within 3 weeks [66].

In acute oral toxicity tests the LD_{50} of valeranone was greater than 3 g/kg in both rats and mice [67].

After intraperitoneal administration of valerenic acid to mice of 17-25 g body weight, 50 mg/kg was found to reduce spontaneous motility, 100 mg/kg caused ataxia and 150-200 mg caused muscle spasms, whereas 400 mg/kg caused heavy convulsions leading to the death of 6 out of 7 mice within 24 hours [56].

REFERENCES

1. Valerian Root - Valerianae radix. European Pharmacopoeia, Council of Europe.

2. Hazelhoff B, Smith D, Malingré TM, Hendriks H. The essential oil of *Valeriana officinalis* L.s.l. Pharm Weekbl Sci Ed 1979;1:71-7.

3. Rücker G. Über die "Wirkstoffe" der Valerianaceen. Pharm unserer Zeit 1979;8:78-86.

4. Hänsel R, Schulz J. Valerensäuren und Valerenal als Leitstoffe des offizinellen Baldrians. Bestimmung mittels HPLC-Technik. 2. Mitteilung zur Qualitätssicherung von Baldrianpräparaten. Dtsch Apoth Ztg 1982;122:215-9.

5. Titz W, Jurenitsch J, Gruber J, Schabus I, Titz E, Kubelka W. Valepotriate und ätherisches Öl morphologisch und chromosomal definierter Typen von *Valeriana officinalis* s.l. II. Variation charakteristischer Komponenten des ätherischen Öls. Sci Pharm 1983;51:63-86.

6. Bos R, Hendriks H, Bruins AP, Kloosterman J, Sipma G. Isolation and identification of valerenane sesquiterpenoids from *Valeriana officinalis*. Phytochemistry 1986;25:133-5.

7. Bos R, Woerdenbag HJ, van Putten FMS, Hendriks H, Scheffer JJC. Seasonal variation of the essential oil, valerenic acid and derivatives, and valepotriates in *Valeriana officinalis* roots and rhizomes, and the selection of plants suitable for phytomedicines. Planta Med 1998;64:143-7.

8. Gränicher F, Christen P, Kapetanidis I. Essential oils from normal and hairy roots of *Valeriana officinalis* var. *sambucifolia*. Phytochemistry 1995;40:1421-4.

9. Bos R, Woerdenbag HJ, Hendriks H, Scheffer JJC. Composition of the essential oils from underground parts of *Valeriana officinalis* L.s.l. and several closely related taxa. Flavour Fragr J 1997;12:359-70.

10. Lapke C, Nündel M, Wendel G, Schilcher H, Riedel E. Concentrations of free amino acids in herbal drugs. Planta Med 1993;59(Suppl):A627.

11. Santos MS, Ferreira F, Faro C, Pires E, Carvalho AP, Cunha AP, Macedo T. The amount of GABA present in aqueous extracts of valerian is sufficient to account for [^3H]GABA release in synaptosomes. Planta Med 1994; 60:475-6.

12. Titz W, Jurenitsch J, Fitzbauer-Busch E, Wicho E, Kubelka W. Valepotriate und ätherisches Öl morphologisch und chromosomal definierter Typen von *Valeriana officinalis* s.l. I. Vergleich von Valepotriatgehalt und -zusammensetzung. Sci Pharm 1982;50:309-24.

13. Thies PW, Funke S. Über die Wirkstoffe des Baldrians. I. Mitteilung. Nachweis und Isolierung von sedativ wirksamen Isovaleriansäureestern aus Wurzeln und Rhizomen von verschiedenen Valeriana- und Kentranthus-Arten. Tetrahedron Lett 1966;(11):1155-62.

14. Thies PW. Über die Wirkstoffe des Baldrians. 2. Mitteilung. Zur Konstitution der Isovaleriansäureester Valepotriat, Acetoxyvalepotriat und Dihydrovalepotriat. Tetrahedron Lett 1966;(11):1163-70.

15. Thies PW. Die Konstitution der Valepotriate. Mitteilung über die Wirkstoffe des Baldrians. Tetrahedron 1968; 24:313-47.

16. van Meer JH, van der Sluis WG, Labadie RP. Onderzoek naar de aanwezigheid van valepotriaten in valeriaanpreparaten. Pharm Weekbl 1977;112:20-7.

17. Bos R, Woerdenbag HJ, Hendriks H, Zwaving JH, De Smet PAGM, Tittel G et al. Analytical aspects of phytotherapeutic valerian preparations. Phytochem Analysis 1996;7:143-51

18. Hänsel R, Keller K, Rimpler H, Schneider G, editors. Valeriana. In: Hagers Handbuch der Pharmazeutischen Praxis, 5th ed. Volume 6: Drogen P-Z. Berlin-Heidelberg-New York-London: Springer-Verlag, 1994:1067-95.

19. Leathwood PD, Chauffard F. Quantifying the effects of mild sedatives. J Psychiatr Res 1982/83;17:115-22.

20. Leathwood PD, Chauffard F, Munoz-Box R. Effect of *Valeriana officinalis* L. on subjective and objective sleep parameters. In: Sleep 1982. 6th Eur Congr Sleep Res, Zürich 1982. Basel: Karger, 1983:402-5.

21. Leathwood PD, Chauffard F, Heck E, Munoz-Box R. Aqueous extract of valerian root (*Valeriana officinalis* L.) improves sleep quality in man. Pharmacol Biochem Behav 1982;17:65-71.

22. Balderer G, Borbély AA. Effect of valerian on human sleep. Psychopharmacology 1985;87:406-9.

23. Schulz H, Jobert M, Hübner WD. The quantitative EEG as a screening instrument to identify sedative effects of single doses of plant extracts in comparison with diazepam. Phytomedicine 1998;5:449-58.

24. Leathwood PD, Chauffard F. Aqueous extract of valerian reduces latency to fall asleep in man. Planta Med 1985; 51:144-8.

25. Lindahl O, Lindwall L. Double blind study of a valerian preparation. Pharmacol Biochem Behav 1989;32:1065-6.

26. Kohnen R, Oswald W-D. The effects of valerian, propranolol and their combination on activation, performance and mood of healthy volunteers under social stress conditions. Pharmacopsychiatry 1988; 21:447-8.

27. Schulz H, Stolz C, Müller J. The effect of valerian extract on sleep polygraphy in poor sleepers: a pilot study. Pharmacopsychiatry 1994;27:147-51.

28. Donath F, Quispe S, Diefenbach K, Maurer A, Fietze I, Roots I. Critical evaluation of the effect of valerian extract on sleep structure and sleep quality. Pharmacopsychiatry 2000;33:47-53.

29. Kamm-Kohl AV, Jansen W, Brockmann P. Moderne Baldriantherapie gegen nervöse Störungen im Senium. Med Welt 1984;35:1450-4.

30. Schmidt-Voigt J. Die Behandlung nervöser Schlafstörungen und innerer Unruhe mit einem rein pflanzlichen Sedativum. Therapiewoche 1986;36:663-7.

31. Vorbach EU, Görtelmeyer R, Brüning J. Therapie von Insomnien. Wirksamkeit und Verträglichkeit eines Baldrianpräparates. Psychopharmakotherapie 1996;3: 109-115.

32. Dorn M. Wirksamkeit und Verträglichkeit von Baldrian versus Oxazepam bei nichtorganischen und nichtpsychiatrischen Insomnien: Eine randomisierte, doppelblinde, klinische Vergleichsstudie. Forsch Komplementärmed Klass Naturheilkd 2000;7:79-84.

33. Houghton PJ. The biological activity of valerian and related plants. J Ethnopharmacol 1988;22:121-42.

34. Jaspersen-Schib R. Sédatifs à base de plantes. Schweiz Apoth Ztg 1990;128:248-51.

35. Weiss RF, Fintelmann V. *Valeriana officinalis*, Valerian. In: Herbal Medicine, 2nd ed. (translated from 9th German edition of Lehrbuch der Phytotherapie). Stuttgart-New York: Thieme, 2000:261-4.

36. Hänsel R. Pflanzliche Sedativa. Informierte Vermutung zum Verständnis ihrer Wirkweise. Z Phytotherapie 1990;11:14-9.

37. Gerhard U, Hobi V, Kocher R, König C. Die sedative Akutwirkung eines pflanzlichen Entspannungsdragées im Vergleich zu Bromazepam. Schweiz Rundschau Med (Praxis) 1991;80:1481-6.

38. Herberg K-W. Doppelblinde Crossoverstudie zum Einfluß einer Hopfen-Baldrian-Kombination (Ivel®) und von Placebo allein und in Kombination mit Alkohol auf Verkehrssicherheit und allgemeine Leistungsfähigkeit von Probanden. Köln: TÜV Rheinland (Study No. MI 9218), April 1994.

39. Gerhard U, Linnenbrink N, Georghiadou C, Hobi V. Vigilanzmindernde Effekte zweier pflanzlicher Schlafmittel. Schweiz Rundschau Med (Praxis) 1996; 85:473-81.

40. Kuhlmann J, Berger W, Podzuweit H, Schmidt U. The influence of valerian treatment on "reaction time, alertness and concentration" in volunteers. Pharmaco-psychiatry 1999;32:235-41.

41. Garges HP, Varia I, Doraiswamy PM. Cardiac complications and delirium associated with valerian root withdrawal. JAMA 1998;280:1566-7.

42. Willey LB, Mady SP, Cobaugh DJ, Wax PM. Valerian overdose : a case report. Vet Human Toxicol 1995; 37:364-5.

43. Braun R, Dittmar W, Hübner GE, Maurer HR. In-vivo-Einfluss von Valtrat/Isovaltrat auf Knochenmarkzellen der Maus und auf die metabolische Aktivität der Leber. Planta Med 1984:50:1-4.

44. Santos MS, Ferreira F, Cunha AP, Carvalho AP, Ribeiro CF, Macedo T. Synaptosomal GABA release as influenced by valerian root extract - involvement of the GABA carrier. Arch Int Pharmacodyn 1994;327:220-31.

45. Santos MS, Ferreira F, Cunha AP, Carvalho AP, Macedo T. An aqueous extract of valerian influences the transport of GABA in synaptosomes. Planta Med 1994;60:278-9.

46. Ferreira F, Santos MS, Faro C, Pires E, Carvalho AP, Cunha AP, Macedo T. Effect of extracts of Valeriana officinalis on [³H]GABA. Release in synaptosomes: further evidence for the involvement of free GABA in the valerian-induced release. Rev Port Farm 1996;46:74-7.

47. Cavadas C, Araújo I, Cotrim MD, Amaral T, Cunha AP, Macedo T, Fontes Ribeiro C. In vitro study on the interaction of Valeriana officinalis L. extracts and their amino acids on GABA_A receptor in rat brain. Arzneim-Forsch/Drug Res 1995;45:753-5.

48. Ortiz JG, Nieves-Natal J, Chavez P. Effects of Valeriana officinalis extracts on [³H]flunitrazepam binding, synaptosomal [³H]GABA uptake and hippocampal [³H]GABA release. Neurochem Res 1999;24:1373-8.

49. Riedel E, Hänsel R, Ehrke G. Hemmung des γ-Amino-buttersäureabbaus durch Valerensäurederivate. Planta Med 1982;46:219-20.

50. Mennini T, Bernasconi P, Bombardelli E, Morazzoni P. In vitro study on the interaction of extracts and pure compounds from Valeriana officinalis roots with GABA, benzodiazepine and barbiturate receptors in rat brain. Fitoterapia 1993;64:291-300.

51. Balduini W, Cattabeni F. Displacement of [³H]-N⁶-cyclohexyladenosine binding to rat cortical membranes by a hydroalcoholic extract of Valeriana officinalis. Med Sci Res 1989;17:639-40.

52. Fauteck J-D, Pietz B, Winterhoff H, Wittkowski W. Interaction of Valeriana officinalis with melatonin receptors: a possible explanation of its biological action. In: Abstracts of 2nd International Congress on Phyto-therapy. Munich, 11-14 September 1996. Published as: Phytomedicine 1996;3(Suppl 1):76 (Abstract SL-56).

53. Hölzl J. Baldrian - Ein Mittel gegen Schlafstörungen und Nervosität. Dtsch Apoth Ztg 1996;136:751-9.

54. Bodesheim U, Hölzl J. Isolierung, Strukturaufklärung und Radiorezeptorassays von Alkaloiden und Lignanen aus Valeriana officinalis L. Pharmazie 1997;52:386-91.

55. Hendriks H, Bos R, Allersma DP, Malingré TM, Koster AS. Pharmacological screening of valerenal and some other components of essential oil of Valeriana officinalis. Planta Med 1981;42:62-8.

56. Hendriks H, Bos R, Woerdenbag HJ, Koster AS. Central nervous depressant activity of valerenic acid in the mouse. Planta Med 1985;51:28-31.

57. Wagner H, Jurcic K, Schaette R. Vergleichende Untersuchungen über die sedierende Wirkung von Baldrianextrakten, Valepotriaten und ihren Abbau-produkten. Planta Med 1980;38:358-65.

58. Torrent MT, Iglesias J, Adzet T. Valoración experimental de la actividad sedante de la tintura de Valeriana officinalis L. Circular Farmacéutica 1972;30:107-12.

59. Krieglstein J, Grusla D. Zentral dämpfende Inhaltsstoffe im Baldrian. Valepotriate, Valerensäure, Valeranon und ätherisches Öl sind jedoch unwirksam. Dtsch Apoth Ztg 1988;128:2041-6.

60. Grusla D, Hölzl J, Krieglstein J. Baldrianwirkungen im Gehirn der Ratte. Dtsch Apoth Ztg 1986;126:2249-53.

61. Holm E, Kowollik H, Reinecke A, von Henning GE, Behne F, Scherer H-D. Vergleichende neurophysio-logische Untersuchungen mit Valtratum/Isovaltratum und Extractum Valerianae an Katzen. Med Welt 1980; 31:982-90.

62. Hiller K-O, Zetler G. Neuropharmacological studies on ethanol extracts of Valeriana officinalis L.: behavioural and anticonvulsant properties. Phyto-therapy Res 1996;10:145-51.

63. Leuschner J, Müller J, Rudmann M. Characterisation of the central nervous depressant activity of a commercially available valerian root extract. Arzneim-Forsch/Drug Res 1993;43:638-41.

64. Rosecrans JA, Defeo JJ, Youngken HW. Pharmacological investigation of certain Valeriana officinalis L. extracts. J Pharm Sci 1961;50:240-4.

65. Fehri B, Aiache JM, Boukef K, Memmi A, Hizaoui B. Valeriana officinalis et Crataegus oxyacantha: Toxicité

par administrations réitérées et investigations pharmacologiques. J Pharm Belg 1991;46:165-76.

66. von Skramlik E. Über die Giftigkeit und Verträglichkeit von ätherischen Ölen. Pharmazie 1959;14:435-45.

67. Rücker G, Tautges J, Sieck A, Wenzl H, Graf E. Untersuchungen zur Isolierung und pharmako-dynamischen Aktivität des Sesquiterpens Valeranon aus *Nardostachys jatamansi* DC. Arzneim-Forsch/Drug Res 1978;28:7-13.

ZINGIBERIS RHIZOMA

Ginger

E/S/C/O/P
MONOGRAPHS
Second Edition

DEFINITION

Ginger consists of the dried, whole or cut rhizome of *Zingiber officinale* Roscoe, with the cork removed, either completely or from the wide flat surfaces only. Whole or cut, it contains not less than 15 ml/kg of essential oil, calculated with reference to the anhydrous drug.

The material complies with the monograph of the European Pharmacopoeia [1].

CONSTITUENTS

Essential oil (0.25-3.3% V/m) [2-4] containing monoterpenes, mainly geranial (citral a) and neral (citral b), and sesquiterpenes (30-70%), mainly β-sesquiphellandrene, β-bisabolene, *ar*-curcumene and α-zingiberene [3-5]; pungent principles (4-7.5% w/w) [6] consisting of the gingerols, shogaols and related phenolic ketone derivatives [7-10]; other constituents include diarylheptenones [11]; diterpenes [12,13]; 6-gingesulphonic acid [14] and monoacyldigalactosyl glycerols [14].

CLINICAL PARTICULARS

Therapeutic indications
Prophylaxis of the nausea and vomiting of motion sickness [15-19], and as a postoperative antiemetic for minor day-case surgical procedures [20,21].

Posology and method of administration

Dosage

Adults and children over 6 years: 0.5-2 g of the powdered drug daily in single or divided doses [22]; for the prophylaxis of motion sickness, 30 minutes before travel.

Method of administration
For oral administration.

Duration of administration
No restriction.

Contraindications
None known.

Special warnings and special precautions for use
None reported.

Interaction with other medicaments and other forms of interaction

May enhance absorption of sulphaguanidine [23].

Pregnancy and lactation

No data available. In accordance with general medical practice, the product should not be used during pregnancy and lactation without medical advice.

Effects on ability to drive and use machines

None known [24].

Undesirable effects

Heartburn has been reported in a few cases [25,26].

Overdose

No toxic effects reported.

PHARMACOLOGICAL PROPERTIES

Pharmacodynamic properties

In vivo experiments

Acetone extracts of ginger (150 mg/kg) and metoclopramide (25 mg/kg) provided significant (p<0.01) complete protection from emesis in *Suncus murinus* when administered orally 1 hour before the administration of cyclophosphamide (300 mg/kg subcutaneously). 6-Gingerol (25 mg, 50 mg/kg orally) also provided complete anti-emetic protection [27].

Methanolic extracts of ginger inhibited the emetic action of copper sulphate pentahydrate in leopard and ranid frogs when administered orally. Emetic latency was prolonged by 157% by a chloroform extract at a dose of 1 g/kg body weight. The shogaols and gingerols showed anti-emetic activity at 20 and 50 mg/kg [28].

Extracts of ginger prepared with acetone (drug to extract ratio 28.5:1) or 50% ethanol (drug to extract ratio 21:1) were administered intragastrically to dogs at 25-200 mg/kg body weight 30 minutes after intravenous cisplatin emetic challenge at 3 mg/kg. The acetone extract significantly reduced the mean number of emetic episodes (p<0.05) to 1.3 at 200 mg/kg compared to 13.7 for the cisplatin control. Furthermore, the emetic latency increased to 137 minutes at 100 mg/kg compared to 103 minutes for the cisplatin control (p<0.05). Similar protection was exhibited by the ethanolic extract. The reduction in the number of emetic episodes by acetone or ethanolic extracts was less than that observed (0.8) after intravenous administration of the 5-HT$_3$ receptor antagonist granisetron at 0.5 mg/kg. Aqueous extract of ginger was ineffective. The acetone and ethanolic extracts were ineffective against apomorphine emetic challenge at 25 µg/kg body weight [29].

Intragastric pretreatment of rats with the same extracts, or with ginger juice (2.2:1 from fresh rhizomes), partially reversed the inhibitory effect of cisplatin on gastric emptying. Compared to controls, this reversal was significant with the acetone extract at 200 mg and 500 mg/kg body weight (p<0.01), the ethanolic extract at 500 mg/kg only (p<0.01), and ginger juice at 4 ml/kg (p<0.001). The reversal of gastric emptying produced by the acetone extract at 500 mg/kg and ginger juice at 4 ml/kg was more than that produced by odansetron (a 5-HT$_3$ receptor antagonist) at 3 mg/kg given orally 30 minutes before cisplatin (61%, 76% and 58% respectively) [30].

The hydrophilic free radical initiator 2,2'-azobis(2-amidinopropane) dihydrochloride was used to induce emesis and retching in young male chickens. 10-Shogaol administered orally at 10 mg/kg body weight inhibited emesis by 80.6% compared to controls (p<0.01); doses of 20 and 50 mg/kg had lower inhibitory values. A dose of 50 mg/kg of 10-gingerol produced 84.9% inhibition of emesis (p<0.001) with lower doses resulting in lesser inhibition [31].

Pharmacological studies in humans

In a double-blind, placebo-controlled, cross-over comparative study with hyoscine (0.6 mg) and cinnarizine (15 mg) in 16 healthy male volunteers, ginger (1 g, taken orally) did not reduce the symptoms of motion sickness induced by cross-coupled stimulation [32]. Ginger (0.5 g or 1 g, taken orally) did not reduce the incidence of motion sickness compared to placebo in a double-blind comparative trial with, *inter alia*, hyoscine (0.6 mg) and dimenhydrinate (100 mg) in groups of healthy volunteers (n = 8) using standardized NASA techniques to create motion sickness [33]. In a placebo-controlled, cross-over comparative study of ginger and hyoscine (0.6 mg) in groups of healthy volunteers (n = 8), ginger (0.5-1 g, taken orally) provided no protection against motion sickness [25].

A placebo-controlled, single-blind, single dose comparison of ginger (940 mg taken orally), dimenhydrinate (100 mg) and placebo showed that ginger was superior to dimenhydrinate. This study involved three randomly allocated groups (n = 6) of students with self-rated high susceptibility to motion sickness, who were asked to spend a maximum of 360 seconds in a revolving chair. The mean length of time each group spent in the chair before nausea or vomiting occurred were as follows; placebo group 90.0 seconds, dimenhydrinate group 216.2 seconds and for the ginger group 335.8 seconds [15].

In a double-blind, placebo-controlled, crossover study, vertigo induced by caloric stimulation of the vestibular system in healthy volunteers (n = 8) was significantly reduced (p<0.05) by ginger (1 g taken orally) [16].

The effect of a ginger extract on fasting and post-prandial gastroduodenal motility was studied in a randomized, double-blind, placebo-controlled, two-period crossover study in 12 healthy volunteers. After fasting since 10.00 pm the previous day, each volunteer took 200 mg of extract (equivalent to 2 g of ginger) or placebo at 8.00 am, followed by a second dose at 12.00 noon and then a standardized meal at 12.30 pm. The results showed that the interdigestive antral motility, measured using stationary manometry, was significantly increased by ginger (p = 0.021) during phase III of the migrating motor complex. There was also a significantly increased motor response (p = 0.025) to the test meal in the gastric corpus [34].

Clinical studies

No significant differences in physician-observed effectiveness for motion sickness were noted in a double-blind comparison of ginger (2 × 250 mg every 4 hours, n = 30) and dimenhydrinate (2 × 50 mg every 4 hours, n = 30), carried out on a group of passengers on a cruise liner in rough seas. It was concluded that the two treatments had equivalent activity although fewer side effects were reported with the ginger capsules [17].

A double-blind, placebo-controlled study in naval cadets on board a sailing vessel in heavy seas showed that, compared to placebo (n = 39), ginger (1 g taken orally, n = 40) significantly reduced the tendency to vomiting and cold sweating (p<0.05) [18].

In a study of 1741 tourist volunteers on whale safaris, 203 were given ginger (250 mg) two hours prior to departure; the remainder were assigned to other treatments. 78.3% of those taking ginger reported no seasickness. Ginger was found to be as effective as cinnarizine, cyclizine, dimenhydrinate, meclozine and hyoscine [19].

Children aged 6-13 years suffering from hyper-ketonaemia were given ginger (n = 12) at a dose of 500 mg every 4 hours (mean daily dose 1.25 g) or metoclopramide (n = 12) at a dose of 0.5-1 mg/kg body weight, divided into 3 daily doses (mean daily dose 25.17 mg), in a double-blind comparative study. In the opinion of the physicians ginger was significantly more effective than metoclopramide (p<0.0005). Ginger was significantly better at preventing vomiting (p<0.05) than the metoclopramide [35].

In a double-blind placebo-controlled randomized study in 60 women who had major gynaecological surgery, ginger (1 g administered orally) was compared to metoclopramide (10 mg intravenously). Pre-operatively administered ginger significantly reduced the recorded incidence of postoperative nausea compared to placebo (p<0.05). The numbers of incidences of nausea were similar in the ginger and metoclopramide groups (n = 20). Administration of a postoperative antiemetic was significantly less in the ginger and metoclopramide groups than in the placebo group (p<0.05) [20].

Powdered ginger (4 × 250 mg daily) given orally for 4 days in a randomized, double-blind crossover study involving 27 pregnant women, gave significantly greater relief of the symptoms of hyperemesis gravidarum than placebo (p = 0.035) [36].

In a randomized, double-blind study in 120 women who presented for elective laparoscopic gynaeco-logical surgery on a day-stay basis, ginger (1 g, taken orally) significantly reduced postoperative nausea (p = 0.006) compared to placebo. Three groups (n = 40) received metoclopramide (10 mg) or ginger (1 g) or placebo (1 g) preoperatively. The incidence of nausea was similar in the metoclopramide (27%) and ginger (21%) groups and less than in the placebo group (41%). Postoperative antiemetics were required more often in the placebo group (38%) than in the metoclopramide (32%) or ginger (15%) groups, only the difference between placebo and ginger being statistically significant (p = 0.02) [21].

Three groups of 36 female patients were enrolled in a randomized, double-blind, controlled trial and received placebo or 0.5 g or 1 g of ginger, each in combination with oral diazepam, as pre-medication 1 hour prior to gynaecological laparoscopic surgery under general anaesthesia. The incidence of moderate or severe postoperative nausea was 22, 33 and 36%, while the incidence of vomiting was 17, 14 and 31%, in groups receiving 0, 0.5 or 1 g of ginger respectively. In this study, therefore, ginger was ineffective in reducing the incidence of postoperative nausea and vomiting; in fact, the incidence tended to increase as the dose of ginger increased [37].

In a double-blind, placebo-controlled comparative study, 120 patients scheduled for gynaecological laparoscopy were randomly allocated to receive either placebo (n = 28), 1.25 mg of droperidol (n = 29), 2 g of ginger (n = 27) or 1.25 mg of droperidol combined with 2 g of ginger (n = 27). There were no statistical differences in postoperative nausea scores or vomit-ing frequency between the four groups [38].

Systematic review of clinical studies

A systematic review has been published [39] of six randomized, double-blind, placebo-controlled clinic-al trials of ginger for nausea and vomiting. Pooled data from three trials on postoperative nausea and vomiting [20,21,37] indicated a non-significant difference between ginger (1 g taken before the operation) and placebo based on pooled absolute risk reduction for the incidence of post-operative nausea. The other three trials, one each on sea-sickness [18], morning sickness during pregnancy [36] and chemotherapy-induced nausea, collectively favoured ginger over placebo [39].

Pharmacokinetic properties

Following a bolus intravenous dose of 6-gingerol (3 mg/kg) in cannulated rats, the gingerol cleared very rapidly from plasma. A two-compartment open model was found to best describe the data. The terminal half-life was 7.23 minutes and total body clearance was 16.8 ml/min/kg. Serum protein binding was 92.4% [40].

Preclinical safety data

Acute toxicity
A dry 80%-ethanolic extract was well tolerated by mice after oral administration (by gavage) at 2.5 g/kg body weight, with no mortality or side effects except mild diarrhoea in 2 out of 10 animals; doses of 3.0 and 3.5 g/kg caused 20 and 30% mortality respectively within 72 hours of administration due to involuntary contractions of skeletal muscle [41].

The acute oral LD_{50} in rats and the acute dermal LD_{50} in rabbits of ginger oil exceeded 5 g/kg body weight [42].

Mutagenicity and carcinogenicity
Ginger was found to contain an antimutagenic factor which reduced the number of His+ revertants induced by tryptophan pyrolysate (a known mutagen) incubated with *Salmonella typhimurium* strain TA98 using S9 liver homogenate as activator [43]. Ginger was also effective against mutagenic pyrolysis products from a number of other amino-acids as well as from tryptophan [44].

The addition of ginger juice to solutions of 2(2-furyl)-3-(5-nitro-2-furyl)acryl amide (AF2) and N-methyl-N'-nitro-N-nitrosoguanidine (NTG) markedly increased mutagenesis by these two chemicals in the Hs30 strain of *E. coli* B/r. After fractionation of the plant juice 6-gingerol was found to be a potent mutagen. However, ginger juice significantly suppressed mutagenesis by 6-gingerol and also suppressed spontaneous mutations. Gingerol may be activated by the presence of certain kinds of mutagen and thus would not be suppressed by the antimutagenic components of the juice [45].

Comparison of the mutagenicity of 6-shogaol, zingerone, curcumin and 6-gingerol in the Hs30 strain of *E. coli* B/r showed that zingerone had only 4% of the mutagenicity of shogaol, which in turn was 10^4 times less mutagenic than 6-gingerol [46]. Ginger rhizome was negative in the *Bacillus subtilis* spore rec-assay but gave positive results in the Ames test using *Salmonella typhimurium* strain TA100 in the presence and absence of S9 activation mixture; results with strain TA98 were negative [47]. Similar results were reported with Zingiberis siccatum rhizoma [48].

Other researchers also found that ginger extract did not induce revertants in *Salmonella typhimurium* strain TA98 or in TA1538, with or without S9 activation. They did, however, confirm that it was mutagenic in strains TA 100 and TA 1535 in the presence of S9 mixture. Zingerone was again non-mutagenic in all four strains, whereas gingerol and shogaol were mutagenic after activation in strains TA 100 and TA 1535, with gingerol the most potent and the effect being dose-dependent. The extract and the pure compounds were non-toxic to the bacteria. These workers also found that zingerenone suppressed the mutagenicity of co-administered shogaol and gingerol in a dose-dependent fashion. Yet again there was no reduction in bacterial survival. It was concluded that the weak mutagenic effect of the plant extract was the result of the combined action of pro- and antimutagenic fractions present in the rhizome [49].

An aqueous extract of ginger reduced the mutagenicity of benzo[a]-pyrene in *Salmonella typhimurium* strains TA98 and TA100 [50]. From another study ginger was reported to be strongly mutagenic (200-500 revertants per plate) when tested against strain TA102 but of intermediate mutagenicity in strain TA98 [51].

Oil of ginger was recorded as a positive in a rec-assay using the *Bacillus* DNA repair test for genotoxicity [52]. Unpublished observations that ginger showed no toxic effect in the SOS Chromotest for genotoxicity have been reported [53].

A ginger tincture showed no genotoxic effects in a somatic segregation assay using *Aspergillus nidulans*, which detects chromosomal damage caused by aneuploidy and some clastogenic effects as well as mitotic crossover [54].

The clastogenic effects of an aqueous extract of ginger administered orally by gavage at 0.5, 1, 2, 5 and 10 g/kg body weight, and of ginger oil administered intraperitoneally at 0.625, 1.25 and 2.5 ml/kg body weight, were investigated in groups of male mice (n = 5). Chromosome damage was studied in preparations made from bone marrow cells following injection of colchicine into all mice. The genotoxicity of the ginger extract was significantly greater (p<0.05) than that of the vehicle control, but was low in comparison with the positive control (cyclophosphamide, 10 mg/kg body weight). The degree of clastogenicity of ginger oil was higher than that of the extract. It was concluded that the observed marginal genotoxicity of ginger extract resulted from a combination of pro- and anticlastogenic fractions present in ginger [55].

Neither ginger nor its purified constituents have been subjected to systematic investigations in mammalian cell cultures. Antitumour effects of ginger in human and mouse cancer cells have been reported [8]. High doses (1 mg/ml) of various ginger components, e.g. gingerols, gingerdione and dehydrogingerdione, showed cytotoxic effects in primary cultured rat hepatocytes [56]. Ginger extracted into synthetic plasma did not alter prothrombin time in an *in vitro* model using pooled human plasma [57].

Clinical safety data

In patients with coronary artery disease, ginger (4 g daily for 3 months) did not affect platelet aggregation induced by either adrenaline (epinephrine) or ADP, and no changes in fibrinolytic activity or fibrinogen levels were observed. However, a single dose of 10 g of ginger did produce a significant reduction (p<0.05) in agonist-induced platelet aggregation [58].

No adverse reactions to ginger, in comparison with placebo, were noted in the studies included in the systematic review [39]. Other studies report low levels of mild gastric disturbances (eructation, pressure on stomach), headache and somnolence [17,24,37].

No side effects were observed in the study involving 27 patients suffering from hyperemesis gravidarum, who ingested 4 × 250 mg of ginger daily for 4 days. One spontaneous abortion and one legal abortion (for personal reasons) were recorded. None of the 25 infants subsequently delivered had deformities and all had Apgar scores of 9-10 after 5 minutes [36].

REFERENCES

1. Ginger - Zingiberis rhizoma. European Pharmacopoeia, Council of Europe.

2. Govindarajan VS. Ginger - chemistry, technology and quality evaluation: Parts 1 and 2. CRC Crit Rev Food Sci Nutr 1982;17:1-96 and 189-258.

3. Connell DW. The chemistry of the essential oil and oleoresin of ginger (*Zingiber officinale* Roscoe). Flavour Industry (London) 1970;1(Oct):677-93.

4. Lawrence BM. Major tropical spices - ginger (*Zingiber officinale* Rosc.). Perfumer Flavorist 1984;9(Oct/Nov):1-40.

5. MacLeod AJ, Pieris NM. Volatile aroma constituents of Sri Lankan ginger. Phytochemistry 1984;23:353-9.

6. Steinegger E, Stucki K. Trennung und quantitative Bestimmung der Hauptscharfstoffe von Zingiberis rhizoma mittels kombinierter DC/HPLC. Pharm Acta Helv 1982;57:66-71.

7. Connell DW, Sutherland MD. A re-examination of gingerol, shogaol and zingerone, the pungent principles of ginger (*Zingiber officinale* Roscoe). Aust J Chem 1969;22:1033-43.

8. Hikino H. Recent research on oriental medicinal plants. In: Wagner H, Hikino H, Farnsworth NR, editors. Economic and Medicinal Plant Research, Volume 1. London: Academic Press, 1985:53-85.

9. Connell DW, McLachlan R. Natural pungent compounds. IV. Examination of the gingerols, shogaols, paradols and related compounds by thin-layer and gas chromatography. J Chromatogr 1972;67:29-35.

10. Yoshikawa M, Hatakeyama S, Chatani N, Nishino Y, Yamahara J. Qualitative and quantitative analysis of bioactive principles in Zingiberis rhizoma by means of high performance liquid chromatography and gas liquid chromatography. On the evaluation of Zingiberis rhizoma and chemical change of constituents during Zingiberis rhizoma processing. Yakugaku Zasshi 1993; 113:307-15.

11. Endo K, Kanno E, Oshima Y. Structures of antifungal diarylheptenones, gingerenones A, B, C and iso-gingerenone B, isolated from the rhizomes of *Zingiber officinale*. Phytochemistry 1990;29:797-9.

12. Huang Q, Iwamoto M, Aoki S, Tanaka N, Tajima K, Yamahara J et al. Anti-5-hydroxytryptamine$_3$ effect of galanolactone, diterpenoid isolated from ginger. Chem Pharm Bull 1991;39:397-9.

13. Tanabe M, Chen Y-D, Saito K, Kano Y. Cholesterol biosynthesis inhibitory component from *Zingiber officinale* Roscoe. Chem Pharm Bull 1993;41:710-3.

14. Yoshikawa M, Hatakeyama S, Taniguchi K, Matuda H, Yamahara J. 6-Gingesulfonic acid, a new anti-ulcer principle, and gingerglycolipids A, B and C, three new monoacyl-digalactosylglycerols, from Zingiberis rhizoma originating in Taiwan. Chem Pharm Bull 1992;40:2239-41.

15. Mowrey DB, Clayson DE. Motion sickness, ginger and psychophysics. Lancet 1982;i:655-7.

16. Grontved A, Hentzer E. Vertigo-reducing effect of ginger root. A controlled clinical study. ORL 1986; 48:282-6.

17. Riebenfeld D, Borzone L. Randomised double-blind study to compare the activities and tolerability of Zintona® and dimenhydrinate in 60 subjects with motion sickness. Unpublished Pharmaton report, 1986.

18. Grontved A, Brask T, Kambskard J, Hentzer E. Ginger root against seasickness. A controlled trial on the open sea. Acta Otolaryngol (Stockh) 1988;105:45-9.

19. Schmid R, Schick T, Steffen R, Tschopp A, Wilk T. Comparison of seven commonly used agents for prophylaxis of seasickness. J Travel Med 1994;1:203-6.

20. Bone ME, Wilkinson DJ, Young JR, McNeil J, Charlton S. Ginger root - a new antiemetic. The effect of ginger root on postoperative nausea and vomiting after major gynaecological surgery. Anaesthesia 1990;45:669-71.

21. Phillips S, Ruggier R, Hutchinson SE. *Zingiber officinale* (ginger) - an antiemetic for day case surgery. Anaesthesia 1993;48:715-7.

22. Wichtl M. Zingiberis rhizoma - Ingwer. In: Wichtl M, editor. Teedrogen und Phytopharmaka, 4th ed. Stuttgart: Wissenschaftliche Verlagsgesellschaft, 2002:653-6.

23. Sakai K, Oshima N, Kutsuna T, Miyazaki Y, Nakajima H, Muraoka T et al. Pharmaceutical studies on crude drugs 1. Effect of the Zingiberaceae crude drug extracts on sulfaguanidine absorption from rat small intestine. Yakugaku Zasshi 1986;106:947-50.

24. Kirchdorfer AM, Heister R. Report on a field study with Zintona® in the prophylaxis and treatment of motion sickness. Unpublished Pharmaton report 1983.

25. Stewart JJ, Wood MJ, Wood CD, Mims ME. Effects of ginger on motion sickness susceptibility and gastric function. Pharmacology 1991;42:111-20.

26. Desai HG, Kalro RH, Choksi AP. Effect of ginger and garlic on DNA content of gastric aspirate. Ind J Med Res 1990;92:139-41.

27. Yamahara J, Rong HQ, Naitoh Y, Kitani T, Fujimura H. Inhibition of cytotoxic drug induced vomiting in suncus by a ginger constituent. J Ethnopharmacol 1989;27:353-5.

28. Kawai, T, Kinoshita K, Koyama K, Takahashi K. Anti-emetic principles of *Magnolia obovata* bark and *Zingiber officinale* rhizome. Planta Med 1994;60:17-20.

29. Sharma SS, Kochupillai V, Gupta SK, Seth SD, Gupta YK. Antiemetic efficacy of ginger (*Zingiber officinale*) against cisplatin-induced emesis in dogs. J Ethnopharmacol 1997;57:93-6.

30. Sharma SS, Gupta YK, Reversal of cisplatin-induced delay in gastric emptying in rats by ginger (*Zingiber officinale*). J Ethnopharmacol 1998;62:49-55.

31. Yang Y, Kinoshita K, Koyama K, Takahashi K, Tai T, Nunoura Y, Watanabe K. Novel experimental model using free radical-induced emesis for surveying anti-emetic compounds from natural sources. Planta Med 1999;65:574-6.

32. Stott, JRR, Hubble MP, Spencer MB. A double blind comparative trial of powdered ginger root, hyoscine hydrobromide and cinnarizine in the prophylaxis of motion sickness induced by cross coupled stimulation. Advisory Group for Aerospace Research and Development, Conference Proceedings 1985;372,39:1-6

33. Wood CD, Manno JE, Wood MJ, Manno BR, Mims ME. Comparison of efficacy of ginger with various antimotion sickness drugs. Clin Res Pract Drug Reg Aff 1988;6:129-36.

34. Micklefield GH, Redeker Y, Meister V, Jung O, Greving J, May B. Effects of ginger on gastroduodenal motility. Int J Clin Pharmacol Ther 1999;37:341-6.

35. Careddu P. Treatment of periodic acetonemic vomiting:

36. Fischer-Rasmussen W, Kjaer SK, Dahl C, Asping U. Ginger treatment of hyperemesis gravidarum. Eur J Obstet Gynecol Reprod Biol 1990;38:19-24.

37. Arfeen Z, Owen H, Plummer JL, Ilsley AH, Sorby-Adams RAC, Doecke CJ. A double-blind randomized controlled trial of ginger for the prevention of post-operative nausea and vomiting. Anaesth Intens Care 1995;23:449-52.

38. Visalyaputra S, Petchpaisit N, Somcharoen K, Choavar-atana R. The efficacy of ginger root in the prevention of postoperative nausea and vomiting after outpatient gynaecological laparoscopy. Anaesthesia 1998;53:506-10.

39. Ernst E, Pittler MH. Efficacy of ginger for nausea and vomiting: a systematic review of randomized clinical trials. Brit J Anaesth 2000;84:367-71.

40. Ding G, Naora K, Hayashibara M, Katagiri Y, Kano Y, Iwamoto K. Pharmacokinetics of [6]-gingerol after intravenous administration in rats. Chem Pharm Bull 1991;39:1612-4.

41. Mascolo N, Jain R, Jain SC, Capasso F. Ethno-pharmacologic investigation of ginger (*Zingiber officinale*). J Ethnopharmacol 1989;27:129-40.

42. Opdyke DLJ. Monographs on fragrance raw materials: ginger oil. Food Cosmet Toxicol 1979;12:901-2.

43. Kada T, Morita K, Inoue T. Anti-mutagenic action of vegetable factor(s) on the mutagenic principle of tryptophan pyrolysate. Mutat Res 1978;53:351-3.

44. Morita K, Hara M, Kada T. Studies on natural desmutagens: screening for vegetable and fruit factors active in inactivation of mutagenic pyrolysis products from amino acids. Agric Biol Chem 1978;42:1235-8.

45. Nakamura H, Yamamoto T. Mutagen and anti-mutagen in ginger, *Zingiber officinale*. Mutat Res 1982;103:119-26.

46. Nakamura H, Yamamoto T. The active part of the [6]-gingerol molecule in mutagenesis. Mutat Res 1983;122:87-94.

47. Morimoto J, Watanabe F, Osawa T, Okibsu T. Mutagenicity screening of crude drugs with *Bacillus subtilis* rec-assay and *Salmonella*/microsome reversion assay. Mutat Res 1982;97:81-102.

48. Yamamoto H, Muzutani T, Nomura H. Studies on the mutagenicity of crude drug extracts I. Yakugaku Zasshi 1982;102:596-601.

49. Nagabhushan M, Amonkar AJ, Bhide SV. Mutagenicity of gingerol and shogaol and antimutagenicity of zingerone in *Salmonella*/microsome assay. Cancer Lett 1987;36:221-33.

50. Sakai Y, Nagase H, Ose Y, Sato T, Kawai M, Mizuno M. Effects of medicinal plant extracts from Chinese herbal medicines on the mutagenic activity of benzo[a]pyrene.

comparison of drugs. Unpublished Pharmaton report 1986.

Mutat Res 1988;206:327-34.

51. Mahmoud I, Alkofahi A, Abdelaziz A. Mutagenic and toxic activities of several spices and some Jordanian medicinal plants. Int J Pharmacognosy 1992;30:81-5.

52. Kuroda K, Yoo YS, Ishibashi T. Rec-assay of natural food additives, Part 2. Seikatsu Eisei 1989;33:15-23, through Chem Abstr 111:38126.

53. Backon J. Ginger as an antiemetic: possible side effects due to its thromboxane synthetase activity. Anaesthesia 1991;46:705-6.

54. Ramos Ruiz A, De la Torre RA, Alonso N, Villaescusa A, Betancourt J, Vizoso A. Screening of medicinal plants for induction of somatic segregation activity in *Aspergillus nidulans*. J Ethnopharmacol 1996;52:123-7.

55. Mukhopadhyay MJ, Mukherjee A. Clastogenic effect of ginger rhizome in mice. Phytother Res 2000;14:555-7.

56. Hikino H, Kiso Y, Kato N, Hamada Y, Shioiri T, Aiyama R et al. Antihepatotoxic actions of gingerols and diarylheptanoids. J Ethnopharmacol 1985;14:31-9.

57. Jones SC, Miederhoff P, Karnes HT. The development of a human tissue model to determine the effect of plant-derived dietary supplements on prothrombin time. J Herbal Pharmacotherapy 2001;1:21-34.

58. Bordia A, Verma SK, Srivastava KC. Effect of ginger (*Zingiber officinale* Rosc.) and fenugreek (*Trigonella foenumgraecum* L.) on blood lipids, blood sugar and platelet aggregation in patients with coronary artery disease. Prostagland Leukotr Essent Fatty Acids 1997; 56:379-84.

INDEX

556